HOLISTIC MIDWIFERY

A Comprehensive Textbook
for Midwives in Homebirth Practice

VOLUME I:
Care During Pregnancy

Revised

ANNE FRYE, CPM
B.A. Holistic Midwifery

Illustrated by Rhonda Wheeler

with a Foreword by
Veronika Kolder, MD

and an Introduction by
Robbie Davis-Floyd, PhD

Labrys Press
Portland, Oregon

December 2013, reprint of August 2006 printing, 1500 copies
  Labrys Press, all rights reserved.

ISBN-13: 978-1-891145-55-1
ISBN-10: 1-891145-55-X

Library of Congress Control no. 98-104092

Previous printings:
  3136 copies, First ed. paperback, September, 1995
  4322 copies, revised ed. paperback, February, 1998, with typographical corrections and a
    number of minor revisions
  762 copies, August 2006, reprint of 1998 printing, with minor corrections (pp. 353-355,
    1003)
  1507 copies, March 2008, reprint of August 2006 printing
  1956 copies, September, 2010, reprint of August 2006 printing (correction on p. 262)

Other publications by Anne Frye and Labrys Press:
  UNDERSTANDING DIAGNOSTIC TESTS IN THE CHILDBEARING YEAR
  HOLISTIC MIDWIFERY, A COMPREHENSIVE TEXTBOOK FOR MIDWIVES IN HOMEBIRTH
    PRACTICE: Vol. II: Care during Labor and Birth
  HEALING PASSAGE: A MIDWIFE'S GUIDE TO THE CARE AND REPAIR OF THE TISSUES INVOLVED
    IN BIRTH
  UNDERSTANDING FEMALE PELVIC ANATOMY IN 3D, Windows-based interactive program and
    vignettes formatted for DVD players that introduce selected soft-tissue regions of the female
    pelvis

For more information or customer service, please contact:
  Labrys Press, 7528 NE Oregon St., Portland, OR 97213 USA
  (503) 255-3378, FAX (503) 255-1474,
  I have three domain names, all of which take you to the same homepage:
  http://www.midwiferybooks.com
  http://www.annefrye.com
  http://www.LabrysPress.com   E-mail me at: midwiferybooks@gmail.com

  Call or visit the web site regarding current editions and pricing. Please report any defects in
materials or workmanship as soon as they are noted. A mechanism for posting errors you may
discover in the text can be found on the web site. Noted errors along with corrections can be found
there as well.

  Each of us is responsible for our own health and well-being. The information in this book
is based on the knowledge, research and experiences of the author and other competent sources.
However, since each woman and baby are unique, the author and publisher can assume no liability
for the use of information contained herein. Since theories and clinical recommendations both are
constantly being refined, research should be done to determine current practice trends, if there is any
question regarding recommendations. Readers are encouraged to seek appropriate medical
consultation and care whenever indicated.

To my sister Healers
Witches
Wise Women

Midwives

Who for hundreds of years
Were burned
and tortured
and died
by the millions
as your children looked on.

To those who locked arms and walked into the sea
Rather than submit to the inquisitor's torments.

For the wisdom that went with you
Mostly unwritten, but never forgotten.

For all you knew and shared
The care you gave
And the courage it took
To continue in the face of truly
Overwhelming odds,

For your strength; a source of continuing inspiration,

To you, dear Sisters,

I dedicate this book.

<u>Acknowledgements</u>

After several logistical mishaps, this book got underway and finally finished. Thanks to Hilary Schlinger for her careful content editing of the entire text. Rhonda Wheeler saved the day with her beautiful and rapidly produced drawings as time was getting short. Elsa Del Toro and Holly Scholles posed for the cover photo, which I took. Kathy Pollock did a thorough job of proofreading the original manuscript so that I could prepare the revised edition. Thanks for content editing must also go to Jennifer Braun, Susan Claypool, Laura Davis, Robbie Davis-Floyd, Carla Hartley, Veronika Kolder, Clarebeth Loprinzi-Kassel, Polly Malby, Kirsten Meagher, Mark Nichols, MARI Patkelly, Holly Scholles, Karyn Stardancer, Clove Tsindle and Nancy Wainer-Cohen as well as all the midwives who sent in tricks of the trade. Your expertise and suggestions enriched this book and are greatly appreciated.

Thank you, one and all, for your invaluable help and support!!

Foreword

Ten years ago in August, I had the good fortune to meet Anne Frye under a shady tree in Michigan. We were both attending the Michigan Women's Music Festival and had sought out a gathering of midwives. A physician in the early years of my training in obstetrics and gynecology, I definitely felt like the outsider at that gathering. But, a shared concern for birthing women and my genuine respect for Anne's knowledge and academic bent lead us to stay in touch and become friends.

Today, again a warm summer day, I am writing this foreword with my newborn daughter on my lap. Although I am an obstetrician and have practiced in hospital settings, my daughter was born at home. We were attended by the independent midwives in our community.

Why would I, or any woman, choose to give birth at home with midwives? This textbook has answered that question.

Over the past 25 years, the courageous North American midwives that have practiced outside medical institutions have been creating a new standard of maternity care. Anne's book is a milestone in this historic process and the culmination of the modern North American homebirth movement to date.

This textbook should dispel some of the mistaken beliefs held by my colleagues; that midwives are unskilled and uneducated; that they irrationally resist the application of modern obstetrical practices; that they do not know how to identify or deal with complications when these arise.

In fact, quite the contrary is true. This book clearly demonstrates that independent midwifery care is well thought out, and, if anything, provides a broader and more holistic model of health care than institutionalized medicine has. A look at Anne's section on working with women who are survivors of abuse will prove just how important this subtle and yet profoundly healing shift in focus can be.

When considered together with her previous publications, Anne has truly given us a gold mine of information that is not readily available elsewhere. She offers thought provoking reservations regarding the application of tests, technology and drugs. And yet, Anne is at her strongest when it comes to prevention and the herbal and homeopathic treatment of common pregnancy problems. Here the traditional midwife shines through and the reader reaps the benefits of Anne's many years of experience and keen observation. There is much to be learned in these pages for anyone who attends pregnant and birthing women today.

In closing, I would like to thank the many practitioners who will be studying this textbook. There will always be those mothers who, like me, know intuitively that they can best birth their children at home. In takes deep dedication and courage to attend homebirth despite the medical and legal antagonism midwives face today. Know that the work you do is vitally important to women, their infants and their families. And let this outstanding textbook inspire you to a lifetime of learning in the service of those for whom you labor.

Veronika E. B. Kolder, M.D.
July 24, 1995

Preface

What a job!! Even contemplating writing this book was overwhelming. Finally, after having entered 80 pages into the computer, I managed to format my hard drive and erased it all. Fortunately, the most valuable data was in hard copy so I could reenter it into the computer. Writing the rest has sometimes been easy, and sometimes it has been like pulling teeth.

Why do it? First off, I felt destined to do it. From the moment I stepped out of clinical training, I have felt guided and compelled to share what I know. For decades midwives have had no comprehensive texts of our own. We have relied on obstetrical texts based on a male medical model of birth. Midwifery textbooks, first from England and then the only United States nurse-midwifery text, have been all that was available for midwifery based book learning. While all of these texts have useful information to share, none of them are written from the point of view of homebirth practice, apprenticeship training, or out-of-hospital midwifery model care.

Raven Lang put homebirth and midwifery care back into the mainstream consciousness with the publication of The Birth Book in 1972. Ina May Gaskin has given us a real feel for what it is like when women create a subculture where birth is not feared and is woman-centered in her landmark book Spiritual Midwifery. Elizabeth Davis has given us a wonderful, detailed overview of independent home-based midwifery in her beautifully written book Heart and Hands: A Guide to Midwifery. These books offer lots of information without being overwhelming in their scope, and are useful for both beginning midwives and parents. Carolyn Steiger has made a monumental contribution to validating apprenticeship training in her thorough book Becoming a Midwife. Carla Hartley has also given us a detailed introduction to midwifery study and apprenticeship training from her perspective in Helping Hands: The Apprentice Workshop. My own book Understanding Diagnostic Tests in the Childbearing Year has been used extensively throughout North America to help establish a more truly midwifery-based standard of care, relating maternal physiology and nutrition to the interpretation of laboratory tests. My other book, Healing Passage, is now a standard textbook in many nursing and independent midwifery programs in the United States, and both of these books are beginning to be known abroad. Nan Koehler's book Artemis Speaks and several others have also contributed to the growing library of texts which seek to articulate our unique standard of care and body of knowledge. However, none of these books are comprehensive textbooks in the way I envision this series will be. This book, therefore, does not seek to replace any of these valuable contributions; it will hopefully inspire a new category of texts to which other midwives will contribute as well.

Repeatedly, the medical world has said if we want to make something "true" we must document it. While efforts are underway to gather statistics from North

American independent midwives, it is equally important to have a range of textbooks that discuss in detail the hows and whys of the way we practice without apology to the medical model of care. If we want to validate a different standard of care, then we must document, explain and support that standard in a way that is accessible to others who wish to examine it. We must begin to write down what our ancient midwifery foremothers passed down from mother to daughter by oral tradition so that the priceless gems of knowledge we are re-membering will not be lost again. Medical model practitioners reading this text may be put off by the number of "folk remedies" recommended and wonder how safe or effective they may actually be. I would remind them that there were no randomized controlled trials to test the safety or efficacy of ultrasound, fetal heart monitoring, epidurals, oxytocin, numerous drugs, separation of mothers and babies, or even hospital birth prior to their routine use! Indeed, few such trials have been done to date on any of these interventions. With that in perspective, I have included remedies which I personally know to be effective or which other midwives have recommended as effective from their experience and have been used, in many cases, for centuries without harmful effects.

During my career, I have often wished that I knew what other midwives have learned. At a difficult birth, I would think "Wouldn't it be great to be able to turn to a reference text which contained many different ways other midwives have successfully dealt with the problem I'm confronting?" There is no textbook that offers a wide range of knowledge in this way. This series of texts should change all that.

These three volumes, when finished, will be midwifery from soup to nuts. No one textbook can contain everything and mine is colored by my own experience and practice style. I hope, however, that it inspires other midwives to write down what they know from their own experiences, so that in the future we have many more resources to assist us as we creatively care for women giving birth.

Anne Frye
B.A. Holistic Midwifery
July 27, 1995

Notes on the revised edition: This revision does not represent a fully new edition. However, with the help of Kathy Pollock's professional proofreading skills, many of the technical errors and typos missed in going over the first printing have been corrected. The number of pages I could replace for a reprint was limited, so I balanced fixing typos with incorporating some exciting new information that I learned since the book was first put into print. I trust it will continue to serve you well in your studies while I get back to writing volume II!

Anne Frye
January 30, 1998

Table of Contents: Volume I, Care During Pregnancy

xiv

Introduction

I am honored to be asked to write an introduction for what is truly an historic work—the most comprehensive textbook ever written by an independent midwife, for independent midwives who specialize in homebirth. In this massive three-volume series, midwife/author Anne Frye covers all aspects of midwifery care for pregnancy, birth, and the postpartum period; she is contemplating a fourth volume on well-woman care. These works offer a thorough description of the midwifery standard of care which has been evolving over the past 25 years throughout North America. Midwives have dared to step outside the boundaries of biomedicine to serve the increasing numbers of women who want to reclaim women's trust in childbirth as a natural process, and in themselves as birth-givers; in so doing, midwives have reconstructed ways of being *with woman* that were almost lost.

This reclaiming and reconstruction of the ancient tradition of women attending women in childbirth was made possible by independent midwives' willingness to practice outside of the hospital, in settings in which women could rediscover their own ways of birthing, and midwives could rediscover how best to support them. While respecting medical understandings and techniques, this work goes far beyond the limitations of the technomedical "management" of birth to articulate the broader and more responsive holistic approach to the care of mothers and babies. In presenting a midwifery standard of care that is valid in its own right, Holistic Midwifery makes an invaluable contribution to the world, to birthing women, and to the health care community.

The approach to the care of the parturient woman presented in these pages is, in many ways, ineffable. The essence of the holistic approach cannot be expressed in print, but only felt, lived and experienced in the one-on-one interaction that you, the midwife, engage in with the women for whom you care. There is an intimacy to that interaction rarely found in medicalized settings. Your attentiveness when she reports her dreams of pregnancy and birth, the space you create to receive her when she needs to talk about her uncertainties, her terrors, her wishes for this baby, this birth, your intuitive understanding when she can't find the words—these constitute the ineffable and inexpressible essence of holistic midwifery.

To be sure, all these things can happen in the hospital when the caregivers there are attentive and loving; the difference is that in the hospital, these ineffable aspects are generally considered "fluff," secondary in importance to the overall goal of producing a healthy baby. In my book, Birth as an American Rite of Passage, I argue that the cultural management of hospital birth in the West is undergirded by a paradigm that I have called *the technocratic model of birth*. (A *technocracy* is a society organized around an ideology of technological progress.) This paradigm holds that the body is a machine, and metaphorizes the male body as the prototype of the properly functioning body-machine. Female bodies, insofar as they deviate from the male standard, are by definition inherently defective machines, and female reproductive processes are therefore in constant danger of malfunction, and in need of constant monitoring by other, more perfect machines.

I have come to understand that this technocratic model of birth is but part of a larger, and culturally dominant, technocratic model of health care. This powerful paradigm underpins both the creation and the ongoing cultural construction of Western techno-scientific medicine. I identify its primary characteristics as follows:

Characteristics of the Technocratic Model of Care: *Basic principle* = **separation**
1. Mechanization of the body.
2. Isolation and objectification of the patient.
3. A focus on curing disease, repairing dysfunction.
4. Aggressive, interventionist approach to diagnosis and treatment.
5. Alienation of practitioner from patient.
6. Reliance on external diagnosis.
7. Supervaluation of technology.
8. Hierarchical organization, the patient as subordinate to practitioner and institution.
9. Authority and responsibility inherent in the practitioner.

In any North American hospital, there are to be found a number of practitioners who work exclusively within this technocratic model. They define its central core, and thereby set the standards by which insurance companies will abide and around which lawsuits will revolve. At the same time, in the same hospitals, there will be many who work to soften the hard edges of techno-scientific medicine, who practice under a modified paradigm—the humanistic model of health care.

Precepts of the Humanistic Model of Care: *Basic underlying principle* = **respect**.
1. The individual is to be valued as unique and worthy.
2. The body is an organism, not a machine.
3. The whole person should always be considered.
4. The needs of the individual and the institution should be balanced.
5. Information, decision-making, and responsibility should be shared between patient and practitioner.
6. Empathetic communication—including eye contact, touch—is essential to healing.

This paradigm (also known as the "bio-psycho-social model") calls for a conversation-centered approach to illness and health care, and offers rich opportunities to patients and practitioners for teamwork in the treatment and healing process. An excellent description of this model and its benefits can be found in Arthur Kleinman's The Illness Narratives. Nevertheless, many health care practitioners, including homebirth midwives, feel that this humanistic paradigm, while a step in the right direction, simply does not go far enough outside the technocratic model to make an essential difference in health care. It is possible to be humanistic in style while being entirely biomedical in treatment—in birth terms, you can hold a laboring woman's hand and whisper loving words of encouragement even as she is hooked up to the IV and the monitor. Those practitioners who would prefer to encourage the woman to eat, drink, and walk, or to avoid the hospital altogether, adhere to a holistic paradigm which is radically—and even subversively—challenging to the dominant technocratic model of health care.

Characteristics of the Holistic Model of Care: *Basic principle=connection*
1. Views the body as an energy system interlinked with other energy systems.
2. Insistence that total healing requires attention to the body-mind-spirit-emotions-family-community-environment.
3. A focus on creating and maintaining health and well-being.
4. Nurturant, relational approach to diagnosis and treatment.
5. Essential unity of practitioner and client.
6. Respect for the value of inner knowing.
7. Technology at the service of the individual.
8. Lateral, webbed organization--networking.
9. Authority and responsibility inherent in the individual.

It is this holistic paradigm that provides the foundation for this book, as well as for exponential growth in recent years of the field of holistic medicine. Each tenet of this paradigm has profound implications for the treatment of the individual as a whole person. Let us examine them as they apply to midwifery care.

(1.) To say that *the body is an energy system interlinked with other energy systems* is to move far beyond the narrow view of the body-as-machine and a mechanistic, cause-and-effect approach to the treatment of the body-machine's dysfunctions. Another common term for holistic medicine is "energy medicine." Defining the body as an energy system provides a powerful charter for the development and use of forms of medicine and treatment that work energetically—acupuncture, homeopathy, intuitive diagnosis, Reiki, hands-on healing, therapeutic touch. This view acknowledges the possibilities that a pregnant woman's health can be influenced by such subtleties as the "bad vibes" generated by anger or hostility or the electro-magnetic fields created by power plants and microwaves, that an unborn baby can be negatively imprinted by a mother's long-term resentment of the pregnancy or her abandonment by her mate. It is the reason why midwives pay attention to their body wisdom as they sense the energetic rhythms of a woman's pregnancy and birth, and why, like other holistic practitioners, midwives work with the invisible subtleties of energy flow, blockage, and release.

(2.) To say that *total healing requires attention to the body-mind-spirit-emotions-family-community-environment* is to acknowledge that no one explanation of a diagnosis, no one drug or therapeutic approach, will sufficiently address an

4

individual's health problems; rather, such problems must be addressed in terms of the whole person and the whole environment in which she lives. The most commonly asked question in holistic health is "What is going on in your life?" This question, which has become almost a cliche, expresses the holistic view that illness and accidents are more than the mere result of happenstance. An obstetrician whom I recently interviewed had injured his right arm twice in one year, and was finally willing to accept the injuries as a message from his body to slow down and re-evaluate his Type A approach to life. The holistic paradigm does not stop at the simplistic explanation that the sore throat you just developed, the cough you can't shake, are the straightforward result of bacteria invading your body. Bacteria permeate us constantly; most of the time, our immune system protects us. If it is too weak to do so, we must ask, what has weakened it? And there we confront the findings of increasing numbers of scientists that the immune system is depleted by exhaustion, emotional stress, a negative attitude, anxiety and fear, the cruelty of a colleague, the alcoholism of a family member, the loss of a loved one, toxins in the air and the water, the stresses of technocratic life.

(3.) It is easy to see why the practitioners of technomedicine are so resistant to the holistic approach—it is simpler to prescribe a tranquilizer or set a bone than to pay attention to the interconnections of the patient's emotional, mental, and spiritual states, the possibility of dysfunctions in her family life, her socioeconomic condition, the poisoning of her environment. The *focus on creating health and well-being* of the holistic model means that holistic practitioners must do all they can to help with all of the above—one reason why many midwives and other holistic practitioners are also environmental activists and/or advocates for the poor and underprivileged. While no one person can do it all, a truly holistic approach to health care does not ignore a host of other problems in favor of focusing on a small range of symptoms that can be treated with drugs and techniques.

(4.) If the patient is pregnant and overdue, it is far easier to order an induction or schedule a Cesarean than to spend time talking with her about, say, her anxiety about the pain of labor, her fear that the child will be deformed, her worry that she will not be able to return to work or keep her husband after the baby comes. Midwives who understand that the uterus is not a mechanism but a responsive part of the whole will see such common medical diagnoses of dysfunction as "incompetent cervix," "post-dates pregnancy," "failure to progress," "uterine atony" as completely missing the point. They will hug and cry with the mother whose labor stops at eight centimeters, and offer her a pillow to pound and permission to scream as loudly as she wants to, for they know the baby's descent into her vagina may be triggering bodily memories of sexual abuse. They will ask the woman who loses her urge to push if she is afraid to let this baby be born. If they sense that the mother-in-law who has come to watch is terrified of birth, they will ask her to leave the room, for they know that the woman's labor might be affected by this fear. Holistic midwives understand that this *relational and nurturing approach* will provide the mother with the safe space she needs to move through psychological blockages and go on to give birth. And they will attend that birth in the environment the mother chooses, because they know that women give birth most easily wherever they feel the safest and most nurtured. It is worth repeating that, in the holistic view, *total healing requires attention to the body, mind, spirit, family, community, and environment.*

(5.) *Connection* is the fundamental value underlying the holistic paradigm of health care and the primary marker of its relational approach, as is strongly evidenced in the *essential unity of practitioner and client.* Even the term "client" implies a mutually cooperative, egalitarian relationship, in contrast to the relationship of subordination, of waiting on the practitioner's convenience, implied by the technocratic term "patient." Deepak Chopra, a physician, author, and primary spokesperson for the holistic health movement, insists that the best way to diagnose is to "become one" with the client—a far cry from the clinical detachment taught in medical schools. Midwives' high value on relationship and connection makes them especially adept at achieving this unity.

(6.) Like other holistic practitioners, midwives have high *respect for the value of inner knowing.* Their deep trust in the body and in their ability to connect psychically and spiritually with the women they attend makes them willing to consciously rely on intuition for decision-making during childbirth. This is not to say that midwives devalue logical, linear thought. As this book will attest, midwives are comfortable with their inductive and deductive abilities, and keenly aware that these are culturally supervalued. The voice of reason is loud and aggressive; the harder task is to identify and heed the truths spoken by the still, small, and culturally devalued inner voice—a voice that can only be heard if the midwife remains connected, not only to the mother and child, but also, and most importantly, to herself. The midwives I interviewed for a recent study on intuition as authoritative knowledge in homebirth (Davis-Floyd and Davis 1996) insisted that the degree of connection they are able to maintain with mother and child depends on the degree of connection they maintain to the flow of their own thoughts and feelings. So basic is the importance of this internal connectedness that many of them actively seek it during and even before birth. As Elizabeth Davis, author of Heart and Hands: A Guide to Midwifery, explained:

> Sometimes, especially when I've been doing a lot, it's hard for me to clear myself and arrive at the birth open. So before I leave, I lie down and just try to unwind and unfold my concerns of the day and open to myself, so that I can also be open to the woman and her birth.

The worth of this enterprise of "staying open to the woman and her birth" is affirmed by the outstanding safety record that contemporary home birth midwives like Elizabeth Davis and Anne Frye are achieving—a record that compares most favorably with the interventionist, expensive, and often iatrogenic "active

6

management" of labor and birth in many hospitals.[1] "Staying open" frees midwives from the narrow restraints imposed by technomedical protocols, allowing them to expand their definitions of normal to encompass the range of behaviors and signs actually exhibited by pregnant women as they labor and birth. Independent midwives are often willing to expand protocol parameters to reflect their intuitions, their body knowing, about the actual circumstances of individual labors, rather than reshaping labor to fit protocol parameters. They see a labor that is unlike other labors, not as a dysfunction to be fixed, but as a meaningful expression of the birthing woman's uniqueness, to be understood and dealt with on its own terms.

(7.) Many hospital-based practitioners place such high value on technology that women who do not have repeated ultrasound scans, and laboring women who are not hooked up to intravenous lines and electronic fetal monitors, appear to be inadequately cared for. In the realm of technobirth, the machines seem to carry more potency than human touch. In the face of such technological tyranny, the laboring woman's own bodily knowing and experience are often ignored.

Such profound subordination of the mother to the machine is not part of holistic midwifery practice. This is not to say that midwives are anti-technology. On the contrary, holistic midwives, as this book will demonstrate, develop extensive familiarity with a myriad of technologies that can be applied to facilitate birth, from stethoscopes to IV lines and oxygen machines. The difference is that these technologies are not allowed to dominate the birth, but rather are kept in their proper place, *at the service of the individual* and the unfolding process of her birth.

(8) Whereas the technocratic system of health care is unabashedly stratified and hierarchical, a diagram of the relationships among holistic practitioners and their clients would show a *lateral, webbed organizational structure*. Attendees at the 1993 conference of the Midwives' Alliance of North America in San Francisco physically created such a web during the closing ceremonies. Four hundred and fifty midwives formed a giant circle around the edges of an otherwise-empty ballroom. They passed around balls of yarn in many colors. Each participant looped the yarn that came to her around her wrist, until all were physically linked with yarn forming a giant rainbow-hued web which filled the ballroom, linking everyone through myriad connections. Spontaneously lifting the giant web into the air by lifting their arms, the midwives quickly discovered that, if one person moved

---

1. It is essential that this statistical record be as thorough and comprehensive as possible; I urge all midwives to keep careful statistics on the births they attend, using the MANA data collection form described in the statistics chapter of this volume, and to send these in for tabulation. As Michel Odent often says, "science will save us." The excellent outcomes of 11,814 midwife—attended births in freestanding birth centers have already been documented (Rooks et.al. 1989). When statistics are available on many thousands of midwife-attended home births in the U.S., it will become increasingly difficult for the American obstetrical community to continue to insist on the superiority of birth in the hospital.

her arm, the whole web moved in response. And, if a ball of yarn got stuck in the middle, at least thirty people had to move in synchrony for one person to retrieve it. This was a perfect ritual and symbolic demonstration of the kinds of relationships these midwives share, and of the high value they place on human interconnectedness—a value you will see expressed throughout this book.

(9) *Authority and responsibility inhere in the individual.* This is a real sticking point in the technocracy, which insists on keeping everyone hooked into the system, and reacts, often with vengeance, when any one person or group tries to detach. The routine use of IV lines in the hospital is the perfect symbolic expression of this phenomenon: the IV is the umbilical cord to the hospital, graphically demonstrating that the pregnant woman is dependent on the institution for her life and that of her baby. In the technocracy, we are all dependent on institutions for our lives. Through that dependence, we can to some extent be controlled. Society's need for control over its citizens is the reason why the system is set up to place responsibility for life and death in the institution and its authority figures, for along with that kind of responsibility goes a great deal of power. Taking individual responsibility for illness and health, for death and for life, then, is equivalent to religious heresy: it is to re-claim the power that "properly" belongs to society for oneself. Yet that is precisely what many in the holistic health movement are doing, and this is especially true for those who give birth at home.

Here midwives depart dramatically from technocratic norms. Because the system is set up to give obstetricians and the hospital ultimate responsibility for birth outcome, these agents feel justified in taking control of the birth process. Midwives see their proper role as a nurturant and supportive one; they seek to empower birthing women with all the information they can provide, leaving ultimate decision-making authority in the woman's hands, as is evidenced in the "Informed Choice Agreements" used extensively by midwives across North America (see the Statement of Informed Disclosure chapter in the Initiating Contact and Establishing Care section).

It is a basic tenet of holistic healing that individuals must take responsibility for their own health and well-being. I am currently conducting research on holistic physicians (Davis-Floyd and St. John, in press); I often hear them express frustration when their clients come to them expecting a "quick fix," as these holistic MDs want very much to work with people who will realize their responsibility for what they eat and the kind of lives they choose to lead. The lawsuits that proliferate in the technocracy are the direct result of the displacement of responsibility onto institutions and technomedical authority figures. If each citizen of the technocracy would reclaim that responsibility, the system would transform. In their willingness to serve, rather than to control, women and babies, midwives as primary health care practitioners are paving the way for that transformation.

* * *

8

The comprehensive scope of Holistic Midwifery underscores the wide range of expertise necessary to practice as a competent midwife, from palpation skills to fostering the emotional and spiritual connection between the pregnant woman, her growing baby, and her family. It documents that midwives, educated through a variety of routes, can and do offer excellent, skilled, and knowledgeable care—a quality of care so high, in fact, that it constitutes a challenge to technomedical practitioners to see if they can match the standards set by independent midwives.

As you begin Holistic Midwifery's Volume I, Care During Pregnancy, keep in mind that while all modern obstetrical textbooks cover prenatal care, no textbook has ever provided coverage as thorough as this one does. Medical texts emphasize the actual birth and the management of problems as they arise—an outcome-oriented approach. The mere fact that this series starts out addressing the prenatal period at such length points out one of the most fundamental differences in care philosophy: midwives focus on process, not outcome. As should be evident from our discussion above, midwives know that *the quality of the pregnancy and birth process directly influences the quality of its outcome.* Like mother and unborn child, the two are inseparable. Just how important their connection is will become ever more clear as you travel through these pages. Sisters, enjoy your journey!

Robbie E. Davis-Floyd, Ph. D.
Research Fellow, Dept. of Anthropology, University of Texas
Author, Birth as an American Rite of Passage
Editor (with Carolyn Sargent) Childbirth and Authoritative Knowledge: Cross-Cultural Perspectives

References:

Davis-Floyd, Robbie, Birth as an American Rite of Passage. U. of Calif. Press, Berkeley, 1992.
Davis-Floyd, Robbie E., Davis, E., "Intuition as Authoritative Knowledge in Midwifery and Home Birth." In Childbirth and Authoritative Knowledge: Cross-Cultural Perspectives, eds. Robbie Davis-Floyd and Carolyn Sargent. University of California Press, Berkeley CA. In press, forthcoming Fall 1996.
Davis-Floyd, Robbie E. & St. John, G., From Doctor to Healer: Physicians in Transition. Rutgers University Press, in press.
Kleinman, Arthur, The Illness Narratives. New York: Basic Books, 1988.
Rooks, Judith P., et.al. "Outcomes of Care in Birth Centers: The National Birth Center Study," New England Journal of Medicine Vol. 321, 1989 pp. 1804-11.

An Overview of the Text

First, I'll review what is included, then we'll talk a bit about how to study the book. The book is divided into sections covering general topics; each section is then divided into chapters. Because of the scope of this three volume series, detailed information is covered in a logical order from prenatal to postpartum and interconceptional concerns. This volume assumes that the woman has already decided to proceed with her pregnancy and will cover the prenatal period up to the threshold of labor. Issues regarding unwanted pregnancy will be covered in Volume III. Even though it is important to discuss such topics as vaccinations and infant circumcision with clients during prenatal care, those topics will be addressed in separate chapters in the postpartum volume.

Practice Makes Perfect: This section is an overview of setting up practice. It briefly introduces many of the issues and concerns which the fledgling primary attendant will face. I have offered many tidbits of knowledge based upon my own experience. I do not address these topics in depth, however. Valuable information may also be found in Carolyn Steiger's book Becoming a Midwife and Carla Hartley's workbook Helping Hands, The Apprentice Workbook, and there are many books on the market which discuss operating a small business.

General Anatomy and Physiology: While most midwifery textbooks do not attempt to cover general anatomy and physiology, I thought it would be useful to include a section emphasizing those aspects most relevant to midwifery practice. Certainly an understanding of basic anatomy and physiology is helpful in clinical practice. A ten pound textbook is not required to gain such an understanding. At the risk of being insulting to some, I have assumed no background knowledge in this chapter. While all of us presumably know that we see with our eyes and hear with our ears, there may be much anatomical information that is obvious to some of us but certainly not all. Some may not want the level of detail I provide, while others undoubtedly will want more. For more detailed information, a full-scale anatomy and physiology textbook is recommended.

The rest of the text is devoted to prenatal care proper. Each section is written with the student midwife in mind; therefore the fundamental basics of each topic are discussed, as well as advanced techniques.

Sustaining Health and Well-being During Pregnancy: Prenatal care begins and ends with how the mother can best take care of herself during pregnancy. Nutrition is covered thoroughly, as are exercise and the effects of various harmful substances. Emotional and physical abuse issues are addressed, as well as environmental hazards.

10

Basic Skills: The book moves from the principles of anatomy and physiology and the basic underpinnings of how to keep things in balance to an explanation of the skills you need to perform prenatal care. Each skill is explained in its entirety, as it will be used throughout pregnancy. Additional skills that are most commonly applied for labor, birth and the postpartum period are explained in Volumes II and III.

Initiating Contact and Establishing Care: This section begins to synthesize knowledge gained from the previous chapters. The midwife meets clients for the first time and establishes her relationships with them. I present the ways to address each woman's unique situation as well as potential problems you may encounter.

An Overview of Prenatal Care: This section introduces the concept of prenatal care visits (their purpose), what you are doing in prenatal visits, what is generally included in each visit throughout pregnancy and some of the issues which will be dealt with on an ongoing basis such as childbirth education, the handouts you will use and examples of some of the forms you will need to record your findings.

Prenatal Care: First, Second and Third Trimesters: These sections cover the respective weeks of pregnancy; addressing normal changes, fetal development, highlights of each prenatal visit, basic lab work and a section on problems which are typically, nbut not necessarily exclusively, associated with that period of pregnancy.

Problems That Can Occur at Any Time: This section deals with all those problems that are not distinctly associated with a particular trimester. It is also referred to as the general problems section in some places for the sake of brevity.

Preexisting Medical Conditions: This section begins with a discussion of how to screen for medical conditions. Guidelines are included to help you decide if you are qualified to work with a woman who has a particular medical condition. A range of medical conditions is included so that this book can serve as a first reference when women call you with unusual histories.

How this book relates to my other books: My books are designed to complement each other. While I have repeated some of the most basic and important information from the other books, most of the time I have made reference to pertinent topics for you to cross reference. You will find it valuable to acquire all of my books in order to make these references meaningful. If something comes up that is not addressed in this text, look in one of the other texts to see if it is addressed. For example, the multitude of infections which are mentioned in Diagnostic Tests are not reproduced here, but I expect you to know where to look for them.

The Index: I have done my best to be sure the entries in this index are consistent with those in my other books. Always look in the index of any of my books first if you are not sure where to find a bit of information. I have tried to reference each topic in at least two ways to better ensure you can find what you are looking for.

Studying this text: As you may have gathered from the above categories, information builds on itself as you move through the text. For example, basic anatomy and physiology is presented first so that you will have some orientation as you learn to do a general physical exam. The basics of keeping a pregnancy healthy and what a healthy pregnancy looks like at different stages are covered before discussion centers on problems which may arise. Basic skills are offered before prenatal care is discussed. This way, the student midwife can study sections one after another, while more experienced midwives can easily find the information they need to review.

References: References to specific information are noted by naming the author and the year of publication in parentheses just after the pertinent text. If the notation appears inside the period of a sentence: (sample). it means that the sentence itself contains the references. If a reference is found at the end of several sentences or a paragraph, it means all the preceding information was, at least partially, derived from that source. If my knowledge was enhanced significantly by a specific author, a reference is noted at the end of that section to that effect: *i.e.*, (section based on Jones, 1990) If my knowledge or most references overlapped, no source is mentioned. The sources of all the remedies and products mentioned are found in the Appendix.

Vocabulary changes: There are a few major changes which I have made in the vocabulary used in this book. Changing terminology is not something I take lightly, since I feel it can often generate confusion. However, some terms are so clearly reflective of the (male) medical model or so negate women's experiences that I have chosen to risk confusion, with the hope that these new terms can become commonplace:

Abortion/miscarriage: Most texts refer to the loss of a pregnancy, regardless of the reason, as an abortion. This text will use the term **miscarriage** when referring to the spontaneous loss of a pregnancy and the term **abortion** when referring to the induced termination of a pregnancy.

Braxton-Hicks contractions: The normal uterine activity which takes place throughout pregnancy is referred to by mainstream medicine as Braxton-Hicks contractions. Because Dr. Braxton-Hicks—a male—never had a uterine contraction and because this name communicates nothing to the woman about the purpose of the contractions, this text will refer to these as **toning contractions**. Other midwives like to use the term "practice" or "preparatory" contractions. Toning contractions will be discussed more thoroughly later in the text.

Cesarean: To emphasize the fact that a Cesarean is major surgery, I shall refer to Cesarean section as a surgical delivery or birth.

Episiotomy: When the female perineum is cut, clitoral circulatory tissues and nerves are cut as well. To help dispel the cavalier attitude regarding this form of routine genital mutilation which takes place in the United States and other Western countries, this text will refer to this procedure by the name clitorotomy: to cut the clitoris.

Vagina: Most midwives I have talked to have been appalled to learn that the word vagina means "sheath for a sword." When I asked Sheila Kitzinger (who has done extensive research into word origins used in obstetrics) if there wasn't a friendlier word in some other language, she said that most words from other languages meant something even worse! I guess the patriarchy doesn't think much of women's genitals other than how they can serve men. In fact, the term vagina was first applied to women by Roman soldiers who collected vaginas for their swords. They began to joke about the "vagina" collection they had back home; thus the term was associated with women's genitals. The obvious lack of respect, sadomasochism and overt misogyny implied in this word have lead me to conclude that midwives should launch a campaign for the adoption of a more enlightened term.

After discussing this with other midwives and brainstorming for possible words to use instead of vagina, we decided that **yoni** was probably the most suitable, although it technically refers to the female genitals in general. Yoni is an East Indian word and was the primary object of Tantric worship, representing the Great Mother, the source of all life; it seems much more appropriate. Therefore, this book will replace the word vagina with either the term birth passage or yoni. For the sake of continuity with other texts, Latin words which incorporate the word vagina (such as pubovaginalis) will remain unchanged. When the word vagina appears in the documents of an organization, it will also remain unchanged.

VBAC: Now that I've decided to change the term vagina to yoni, what about the phrase vaginal birth after Cesarean? I have decided to call it yoni birth after Cesarean: YBAC.

BECOMING A MIDWIFE

The Philosophy of Midwifery

In modern times, philosophy regarding maternity care has been divided into two systems of belief referred to as the "medical model of care" and the "midwifery model of care." The midwifery model teaches women to trust pregnancy and birth as physiological processes, becoming attuned to what is normal in such a way that deviations from normal are easily recognized. The female body is seen as uniquely and inherently normal in its own right. It finds the medical model misplaced in assuming that a normal, healthy process is inherently dangerous. Midwives focus on preventive care by emphasizing the importance of good nutrition and exercise, and the elimination of substance abuse. They foster healthy family relationships to prevent complications which result from high levels of fear and stress. The midwifery model's trust and confidence in the natural processes of pregnancy and birth and focus on birth as primarily a social (not a medical) event create a haven of normalcy which counteracts the hysteria surrounding birth in our culture today.

The medical model teaches practitioners to be skeptical of the natural process of pregnancy and birth. This skepticism arises from the underlying notion (which permeates all medical teaching) that maleness is inherently normal and femaleness is inherently deviant; therefore the most non-male thing the female body does, which is to reproduce, is highly suspect—a problem waiting to happen. The expectation of, detection of, and management of problems is paramount in the medical model. The ultimate goal of bio-technical medicine is to avoid death.

In short, while the medical model seeks to avoid death at all costs, the midwifery model seeks to support the life-giving processes of pregnancy and birth. It leaves no stone unturned in its quest to achieve optimal health and well-being for those mothers and babies seeking care. Robbie Davis-Floyd, an anthropologist who has done extensive work in exploring birthing practices in the west from a cultural perspective, has created a wonderful list of contrasts between what she terms the technocratic model versus the holistic model of birth. (Birth as an American Rite of Passage, U. of Calif. Press, Los Angeles, 1992)

THE TECHNOCRATIC MODEL OF BIRTH	THE HOLISTIC MODEL OF BIRTH
Male-centered	Female-centered
Women = objects	Women = subjects
Male body = norm	Female body = norm
Female = defective male	Female is normal on her own terms
Classifying, separating approach	Holistic, integrating approach
Mind is above & separate from body	Mind and body are one
Body = machine	Body = organism
Female body = defective machine	Female body = healthy organism
Female reproductive processes dysfunctional	Female reproductive processes healthy
Pregnancy & birth inherently pathological	Pregnancy & birth inherently healthy

THE TECHNOCRATIC MODEL OF BIRTH	THE HOLISTIC MODEL OF BIRTH
Doctor = technician	Midwife = nurturer
Hospital = factory	Home = nurturing environment
Baby = product	Mother/baby inseparable unit
Baby grows itself through mechanical process	Connection between growth of baby & state of mother
Fetus is separate from mother	Baby & mother are one
Safety of fetus pitted against emotional needs of mother	Safety of baby & emotional needs of mother are the same
Best interests of mother & fetus antagonistic	Good for mother = good for baby
Supremacy of technology	Sufficiency of nature
Importance of science, things	Importance of people
Institution = significant social unit	Family = essential social unit
Action based on facts, measurements	Action based on body knowledge & intuition
Only technical knowledge is valued	Experiential & emotional knowledge valued as highly as or more than technical knowledge
Best prenatal care is objective, scientific	Best prenatal care stresses subjective empathy, caring
Health of baby during pregnancy ensured through drugs, tests, techniques	Health of baby ensured through physical & emotional health of mother & her attunement to the baby
Labor = a mechanical process	Labor = a flow of experience
Time is important; adherence to time charts during labor is essential for safety	Time is irrelevant, the flow of the woman's experience is important
Birth must occur within 24 hours	Labors can be short or take several days
Once labor begins, is should progress steadily; if it doesn't, pitocin necessary	Labor can start & stop, following its own rhythms
Some intervention necessary in all births	Facilitation (proper food, effective positioning, support) is appropriate, interventions are usually inappropriate
Pain is unacceptable	Pain is acceptable
Analgesia & anesthesia for pain during labor	Mind/body integration, labor support for pain
Environment is not relevant	Environment is the key to safe birth
Uterus = an involuntary muscle	Uterus = responsive part of whole woman
Woman is hooked up to machine with frequent exams by staff	Woman does what she feels is appropriate
Once a surgical birth always a surgical birth for many women	VBAC normal
VBAC is high risk	VBAC = low risk
Cesarean for breech presentation or twins	Squatting or hands and knees for breech, twins often born via the birth canal
Birth = a service medicine owns & supplies to society	Birth = an activity a woman does that brings new life
Obstetrician = supervisor, manager, skilled technician	Midwife = skillful guide
Doctor is in control	The midwife supports, assists
Responsibility belongs to the doctor & the system	Responsibility is the mother's

What It Means to Be a Midwife

Midwifery practice means something different to each one of us. The midwife is a guide and assistant in directing the life force which comes through during pregnancy to grow the baby and nourish the mother, and which manifests as birthing energy during labor so that the baby can be born. While midwifery has a profoundly spiritual aspect, you need not consider yourself "spiritually oriented" to have a feeling for the power of birth or to have an intuitive understanding that birthing energy can be blocked by non-physical issues.

In fact, the feeling that midwifery is a spiritual calling and that we are handmaidens to the process of life entering the planet can cause starry-eyed wanna-bes to have an overly romantic notion of midwifery practice. The reality of long hours, enormous responsibilities, split second, sometimes life and death decision-making and often low pay bring reality home to many who drop out early on. For those who persevere, a unique, ever challenging and wondrous career lies ahead.

Midwifery as a Calling:

Many midwives feel that they were selected and given the work of attending births. Many, myself included, can describe a specific series of events which support this feeling, and most describe a continually evolving spiritual connection with birth, birthing energy and the intimate work of attending women through this life passage.

My own story goes like this: As a child, midwifery was my favorite game. I was always putting dolls up someone's shirt and catching babies. The entire experience of birth held continual fascination for me. At about eight years of age, I discovered that a friend of my mother was pregnant, and she was about five months along. I fantasized that no one would be in the neighborhood the day she went into labor. Right around that age I also had a very significant dream. In this dream I was near the water, in a fog. On a dock, surrounded by people, a woman was laboring to birth. Into the midst of this crowd I went to assist her, although there were no anatomical details in the dream.

Years later, after having become disenchanted with the education I was receiving to become an art therapist for emotionally disturbed children, I moved to San Francisco. After getting a job at a local Co-op, a sister employee turned to me and told me she was going to a school in town called the Holistic Childbirth Institute and was planning to become a midwife. Bells went off, heaven opened up, I remembered my dream of long ago and I knew in the deepest sense of the word that THAT was my destiny: to become a midwife. Without any doubts, I began to pursue that end as only a single-minded Aries can.

Two months later I was enrolled at the Holistic Childbirth Institute (HCI), which promised to make their first two years of childbirth educator training a prerequisite to a midwifery program (which never happened). Two and a half years later upon graduation from HCI, I was accepted at the Maternity Center in El Paso, Texas where I obtained my clinical training. After six months of training, three other classmates and I opened The Rising Moon Birth Place in El Paso, where I practiced for an additional nine months. From there, I practiced as a primary attendant for births for short periods of time in Atlanta, Detroit, and Syracuse and for 9 years in New Haven CT, totaling 17 years in and out of practice and attending over 500 births, plus teaching across the country.

The path to midwifery is full of surprises, growth producing experiences and painful lessons. One is called at once to be a constant student, a channel of energy, a guardian of a natural and sacred process and an advocate for the rights of women and newborns when they are most vulnerable. Not crossing the line which divides humble self confident assurance and arrogant knowitallism takes a certain amount of spiritual equilibrium. Midwifery is not a responsibility to be taken lightly. It calls upon you to be the best you can be: the best advocate, guide, healer, counselor, mother, comrade and confidant of the women seeking your care. Western culture has split up the extended family and left women with small children isolated and alone while their middle class spouses work, or in a position where they must find work themselves while their tiny babies stay in day care. As midwives, we deal with problems, decisions and responsibilities which our foremothers did not have to face. Overseeing the safe passage of both mother and baby is an awesome task. Additionally, being on constant call is a unique burden carried by many who choose to offer non-institutionally based care.

If you are new to the idea of midwifery, I suggest that you examine your reasons for choosing it carefully. Put aside the strokes you think you will get and the visions of candle-lit births, and imagine yourself taking charge in a crisis and being strong with women so that they can find their own strength. Imagine yourself cleaning up body fluids and coming home exhausted, only to have the phone ring again with another woman in labor; making love, only to have the beeper go off; at the movies, only to have to leave. Such is the "romantic" life of the midwife. It helps immensely to see your relationship to birth as a primary relationship, one which will often supersede everything else in your life in order to commit yourself to the life that is non-institutional midwifery care.

While there are some who intellectually select midwifery as a career, feeling called into the service of birth adds a special, spiritual dimension which enlarges and gives meaning to the experience as nothing else can. It provides a context for your work to be purposeful and directed. It opens the way for developing intuitive and insightful skills. For me, the calling of midwifery has provided endless challenges, rewards and spiritually enlightening experiences. While each midwife and potential midwife must search out for herself what this work means to her, reaching for the deeper side of practice will inevitably result in an understanding of how midwifery, in the truest sense, can be a personal spiritual path.

18

A Very Brief History of Midwifery and Birthing Care in the United States

The history of midwifery is the history of women healers, revered from time immemorial for their knowledge and skills. That status began to change in the Western world with the advent of Christianity and the takeover of Europe by the Roman Catholic church. From the 1300s until the 1600s, the Roman Catholic Church ravaged Europe and Great Britain with the Inquisition. This brutal attempt to "abolish paganism from the civilized world" (as defined by the Church) brought a holocaust that murdered, by some estimates, nine million "witches," many of whom were midwives or other healers and 85% of whom were women. The "Age of Reason" slowly saw an end to this terror, as medical science replaced the Church as the repository of "truth." Midwifery slowly reemerged throughout Europe, gradually defining the parameters of the profession.

Midwifery was practiced widely among native North American peoples. The white colonial invaders also imported their own midwives. In colonial America it was common for adult women to have witnessed many births. In communities where the women were generally healthy, birth was seen as a straightforward social affair to be supported by female relatives and friends. New midwives were self-selected or appointed from the ranks of community women who attended many of the local births in groups as friends of the laboring mother. Near the turn of the 20th century many more midwives trained in various European nations emigrated to the larger cities. Beginning in 1619, black slaves brought from Africa included midwives among their number. These women evolved into the Grand midwife in rural and poor urban areas during the early 1900s, particularly in the South.

In colonial America, birth was at first considered beneath the dignity of the male medical doctor. After 1750, however, more and more men were returning from medical education abroad to practice in colonial towns and cities. The medical community began to see that attending women during birth was a way to make an entrance into the medical care of families. At first women were reluctant to have male attendants, and many doctors who did attend births had little or no practical experience. In response to this lack of training, maternity hospitals were established for the very poor, allowing medical students access to birthing women.

As men became more involved with birth, theories regarding how pregnancy and labor occur became less magical and moved to more scientific and mechanical explanations. The dissection and fragmentation of the process was well underway, removing the spiritual aspects of birth from its physical components. This made birth seem more manageable and less overwhelming to the men now overseeing it, who had no personal reference for what birth was like.

The prevalence of maternal postpartum infection, then known as childbed fever, increased dramatically during the decades when more women were under the routine care of doctors. Doctors, unlike midwives, tended to have broader based practices. They would often go from the activity of examining cadavers to the bedside of laboring women without washing their hands. Thus, women attended by physicians had more postpartum infections. Various things were used to deal with this problem; after it became apparent that contagion could be transmitted from woman to woman via care providers, hospitals reacted with extreme efforts at antisepsis in order to prevent infection. Many of these invasive treatments (enemas, shaves, douches with bichloride of mercury, etc.) only made matters worse. This added fuel to the argument that birth was indeed dangerous and needed to be in expert hands in a setting where emergencies could be handled immediately: the hospital. The combination of inappropriately applied methods of hygiene, the use of dangerous drugs, inadequate nutrition in the women receiving care, and crude surgical techniques caused many women to die from childbirth-related infections, drug overdoses and injuries.

In the early 1900s childbirth was still seen as an essential function of womanhood. As women became more outspoken, means were sought to relieve the mother from the physical burdens of labor. Pain relief for childbirth was first available in the form of chloroform and ether in the 1840s, but was not widely used. During the 1910s, feminists of the day campaigned to import from Germany a new method of anesthesia for labor popularly referred to as "Twilight Sleep." This was a combination of the psychedelic amnesic drug scopolamine and the sedative morphine. These drugs could only be administered in a hospital setting, causing many more middle and upper class women to seek institutionalized care for the first time. This greatly assisted the transfer of birth from the relative safety of the home environment into the hospital. Hospitals catering to the middle and upper classes of the day were well appointed and well staffed and much quieter than today's institutions. This is where the notion that the hospital is a safe haven of rest for birthing mothers originated. Desire for these modern conveniences quickly accelerated as more and more women sought out "safe, sanitary and scientific" hospital care.

Throughout the 1900s the issue of the "midwife problem" was increasingly discussed in medical journals and by public health officials. Midwives were stereotyped as dirty, ignorant immigrant women out to make a buck off of other poor women. The most vehement opponents of midwives were physicians in private practice and obstetrical specialists who saw midwives as a direct economic and turf threat. They also saw midwives as taking valuable cases away from medical students, thereby impeding educational pursuits. At the same time it was recognized that there were not enough well-trained doctors to eliminate midwifery entirely. Therefore the midwife was seen as a necessary evil to be gradually phased out as more doctors who were willing to treat the poor became available.

Public health officials took a more moderate view, seeing that midwives were not going to disappear, especially in those communities where no other services were available to replace them. Health departments throughout the South offered simple manuals and training for midwives which included information on basic hygiene and the warnings signs of problems. Midwives were admonished to use no drugs other than silver nitrate for the baby's eyes, and to register the birth. A few Northern areas had a more ambitious approach. Bellevue Hospital in New York began a school for midwives in 1911, with other hospitals in New Jersey and Philadelphia quickly following suit. Public health authorities found that these graduates had better outcomes than did doctors, borne out by statistics reflecting lower maternal and infant mortality rates.

However, as the onslaught of derogatory literature continued in the professional and popular press, the midwife was seen as "other than American." With the restriction of immigration in 1919, no new midwives were being incorporated into ethnic communities. Immigrant women, eager to be full-fledged citizens, modern and up-to-date, flocked to clinics to have their babies with doctors.

The first vision of a more medically acceptable type of midwife came from Mary Breckinridge, a British-trained midwife, who founded the Frontier Nursing Service in 1925. She was not seen as dirty or backward the way a non-English speaking woman may have been since she was English and medically trained. She and her associates offered home-based care to remote rural women in Appalachia; but her vision of a network of such services for the rural poor was never realized, as roads were built and even rural women had more access to hospitalized care.

In the 1930s a uniquely U.S. American practitioner, the professional nurse-midwife, began to evolve. The Maternity Center Association (MCA) of New York (founded in 1918 to provide maternity services) began to train public health nurses as midwives in 1932. These few early nurse-midwives supervised the remaining immigrant midwives and also attended births for the urban poor in an MCA rural project. The medical profession viewed nurse-midwifery practice as an appropriate source of care for poor women. Nurse-midwives themselves never intended to infringe upon the physician's role as birth attendant for the middle class. Their number remained small until public demand for more hospital options, as well as homebirth and independent midwifery, increased public awareness of alternatives. Women birthing both in and out of hospital began to demand different kinds of care on a wider scale.

Throughout the early 1900s, independent midwifery, although marginalized almost out of existence, still persisted. In ethnic communities and rural areas elder midwives practiced up until the 1960's, with excellent results. Many of these Grand midwives carried with them the last of the pure apprenticeship training tradition where their work was passed on to them by a relative or the neighborhood midwife. Health departments continued to give short courses of study to Grand midwives and grant them licenses. In some places they were forbidden to keep records or statistics; thus their historically excellent care is largely invisible today except to the communities they have served. As laws were removed from the books and not updated, the Grand midwives were gradually phased out of existence by the obstetric community. It seemed that non-institutionally based midwifery might indeed die a quiet death in North America.

In the late 1960's evidence of a new generation of grass roots midwives began to emerge. In Santa Cruz, California, Raven Lang, along with a group of other women, formed a birthing center, offering prenatal care and homebirth to women in their community. The first book out of the "new" midwifery movement was Raven's The Birth Book published in 1972, which described a midwifery model of care in a modern context. Its publication heralded the rebirth of home-centered, apprentice trained midwifery in North America. Shortly after that, in 1975, Ina May Gaskin published the first edition of Spiritual Midwifery, describing the evolution of her midwifery experience and health care system in a rural, self-sufficient alternative community in Tennessee.

Shari Daniels opened The Maternity Center in the mid-1970s, providing one of the only institutional settings for clinical training of independent midwives in the United States at the time. Other proprietary schools sprang up along the Texas/Mexico border. Prompted by community demand, a groundswell of midwives, either apprenticeship-trained, self-taught, or schooled in Texas, started to practice across the United States and Canada regardless of their legal status in their local jurisdiction. In March of 1981 Carla Hartley began to offer the first formal academic training for at-a-distance apprentice-based learning, Apprentice Academics Midwifery Home Study Course, which evolved from the program she devised for her own apprentices.

The presence of non-nurse midwives with out-of-hospital experience began to influence the way birth was viewed in North America. As more women began to demand options and some to choose homebirth, the medical profession loosened up on such things as the number of support persons permitted to accompany a woman in labor, and the use of delivery rooms. Postpartum hospital stays shortened and childbirth classes became ever more popular. Paralleling these changes, nurse-midwives worked within the institutional system, risking ridicule and often their employment itself to stand up for women rights regarding such things as the elimination of routine shaves and enemas and the right to be accompanied in labor by a significant other of the woman's choice.

Today, nurse-midwives are legally practicing in every state and independent midwives exist in all states and provinces of Canada regardless of legality of practice. There is a wide spectrum in the legal status of independent midwives, ranging from licensure, certification or legal acceptance to complete censure. It is estimated that there are approximately 6,000 independent midwives and about 5,000 nurse-midwives practicing in North America today, with more being trained all the time.

For reference and further reading:

Ulrich, Laurel, A Midwife's Tale, Knopf Pub., New York, NY 1990.
Wertz, Richard & Wertz, D., Lying-In, A History of Childbirth in America, Schocken Books, New York, NY 1979.

The Kind of Midwifery Preparation You Want

The educational route that you choose along your path to primary practice will depend upon your need for academic structure, credentials, the legal restrictions in the area you choose to practice, your financial situation, the flexibility of your lifestyle and the accessibility of the training programs themselves. If you intend to practice legally in your state, you should inquire about the minimum education required in order to do so. The route you choose will influence your ability to practice midwifery in a hospital setting. If you want to establish a homebirth practice, your training needs to emphasize creative thought and the development of judgement skills independent of immediate access to other health care providers. If you're at home, there is no neonatal team outside the door waiting for the word from you! Finally, you must make a decision about which educational route best serves your individual learning style.

We do not learn midwifery in an emotional vacuum. Your personal experiences will impact how you receive the information, what parts of it are hard to learn, and what you tend to block out. For example, when you read about miscarriage you may find yourself immersed in feelings of sadness and loss if you, your mother or another significant person in your life has experienced pregnancy loss. Part of being a midwife is learning to midwife yourself. At each point in your learning experience, do your best to stay connected to your emotional reality and take time to reflect upon each experience as you are more involved on a clinical level. Don't hesitate to seek support from other midwife students or a therapist if need be. Talk about what is coming up; cry about it, celebrate it. Being present with your total experience will greatly enhance your own learning and healing and will make you a clear emotional, mental and spiritual channel for helping others.

Options for midwifery training:

In general, midwifery training consists of theoretical (book-learning) and clinical experience. Books offer a way of comparing the opinions of experienced practitioners as well as supplying more perspective for you to bring to your clinical training. Clinical training involves learning hands-on skills. The magic "minimum number" of births considered necessary to become a competent midwife varies widely. Many CNMs become credentialed after having attended only 15 to 20 births, while some direct entry programs require 100. Most schools fall somewhere in between, with similar minimum requirements for prenatal and postpartum visits.

No one can tell you how many births *you* need to feel ready to assume the multi-level responsibilities involved in competent midwifery practice. Ina May Gaskin says it is not numbers *per se* that indicate someone is ready, but whether one can competently deal with an emergency. More hands-on experience is needed if you plan to work out-of-hospital, since you will lack immediately available back-up support in a fully independent practice.

Formal education: One option to consider is that of formal schooling. Established programs offer the following advantages: structured curriculum, teachers and advisors who can serve as resources, easy access to libraries and other learning aides, some assurance that what you are learning is accepted up-to-date bio-technical medical practice, supervised clinical learning experiences (in most cases), and a formal acknowledgement at the completion of the course (such as a title like CNM, a diploma or a certificate).

On the down side, institutionally-linked training can carry with it impersonal interaction and a lack of creativity in teaching in favor of supporting the status quo educational and medical opinions of the day. Learning can become a rote process of trying to get through each course with enough knowledge to pass tests rather than an internal and transformative experience. Other disadvantages of formal schooling include the likelihood that non-bio-technical means of treatment or a variety of alternatives to standard medical practice will not be covered in your education. (This may not be true of some programs; ask!) Structured learning is geared to move students through material at a set pace and in a certain order which may not suit your personal learning style. The clinical portion of your training may not encourage independent action and in some cases may be very limited. Some direct-entry programs require you to find your own clinical learning site. Be sure to discuss how continuity of care is prioritized in the program as well.

Another pitfall is that it is easy to walk away from a structured learning environment feeling like you have "arrived" and now are armed with all necessary information. While you will probably have all the basic information you need to start a practice, you never know it all. Whatever your training, it will have been biased by the opinions of the instructors. Regardless of the route you choose, no program will cover all there is to learn. Once you're out that door you are just beginning!

Last but not least, a credential is often seen as a guarantee of competence by the public as well as your peers. As such it fosters an aura of expertise and a false sense of security for your clients. For nurse-midwives, malpractice insurance and formal relationships with the medical community are required in many areas in order to practice. This, too, influences your relationship with your clients, and, practically speaking, where you can actually practice (because insurance companies may not cover out-of-hospital practices).

Certified Nurse-Midwifery is the most widely recognized and best paid type of midwifery practiced in the United States. As a CNM, you are able to work for a good salary in a structured environment with hospital privileges if you so desire. CNMs practice legally in all states, although practice is regulated and in some states homebirth practice by CNMs is not allowed. Most places require CNMs to have a formal arrangement with a physician for collaboration, including direct supervision in some places. In practical terms this prevents many CNMs from having homebirth practices since they may not be able to find a doctor willing to do this. Or, the doctor might be willing to provide back-up, but is unable to do so because of restrictions from his own malpractice insurance. The relationship between physicians and CNMs varies widely from area to area; some CNMs face very hostile situations while others enjoy a great deal of freedom of practice. CNM training could take as long as six to eight years if you not already a registered nurse (RN). There are a few three year programs which include a crash RN course the first year, and which require a BA or BS as a prerequisite.

Generally, training as a registered nurse (a two to four year program) is followed by an additional one to two years of specialized training in nurse-midwifery. Some states, such as Oregon, require CNMs to have a Master's degree to practice. Most CNMs have spent a year or two in obstetrical nursing before they apply to nurse-midwifery school; it is here that CNM educational programs generally expect that students will obtain the "watch and wait" skills of a good midwife. As a CNM you are trained to work with essentially normal women and function as part of a "health care team" in a hospital or clinic setting, and to rely upon the immediate availability of other specialists for assistance in the event of a problem. Programs vary from conventional classroom format to modular and at-a-distance learning. Most of these include clinical training at a hospital which has a neonatal intensive care unit (level 3) during the experiential portion of the program. How much hands-on learning you will receive and in what setting varies greatly from program to program; this should be thoroughly researched when choosing a school.

Formally schooled direct-entry midwifery is the European model of midwifery education. It does not require a registered nursing degree as a prerequisite, but most programs require a high school diploma and some may require a number of basic college level prerequisites such as chemistry, anatomy and physiology, microbiology, nutrition, etc.. Be sure to check with the programs you are considering about prerequisites. Attendance at a 3-year program such as the Seattle Midwifery School or the Traditional School of Midwifery in Florida fulfills the necessary educational requirements to take a state recognized direct-entry licensure test which may be recognized in other states (ask).

A number of other schools, such as the *Maternidad La Luz* in El Paso, Texas, offer classes but focus on hands-on experience. Birthingway Midwifery School and Sage Femme in Portland, Oregon offer classes and varying degrees of access to clinical training as well. Miami-Dade Community College in Florida is the first place in the United States to offer direct entry schooling within an accredited college environment. The National College of Midwifery in Taos, New Mexico grants both undergraduate and graduate degrees in midwifery, but is currently unaccredited. Schools may offer hands-on clinical training in a birthing center, clinic, or homebirth practice setting, while others offer classroom study only. A few offer only clinical training with no structured classroom learning.

Your choice of program will depend upon your background, your need for an accredited program, etc.. Florida and other states are beginning to offer state-run midwifery programs. Be sure to discuss whether they are approved by the North American Registry of Midwives as an evaluation agency (see next chapter). You should contact different schools and discuss their programs to get a feel for which one might be right for you.

Because midwifery programs are being developed so rapidly, it would be impossible to include an up-to-date list in a textbook. For a current listing of midwifery programs of all types, write to MANA, P.O. Box 175, Newton, KA 48103.

Apprenticeship: Another option is independent, self-directed study and apprenticeship. This requires the most self-discipline but also allows the most flexibility. You must be highly motivated and able to manage your time and resources to work out a program of individualized study and experience. This route fosters the kind of responsibility-taking and inner motivation that will be required of you as you start to practice, especially if you intend to do homebirths. Many students begin by taking a course in childbirth education (the International Cesarean Awareness Network, Association of Labor Assistants and Childbirth Educators [ALACE] and ACHI are among several offering programs), then teaching classes for pregnant parents. You can start a study group with other interested women in your area. As you gain basic knowledge and skills you would seek a local midwife with whom you can apprentice. She will become your mentor, and attending births with her will offer you the clinical experience you need.

If you feel the need for some structure in your educational process, The Ancient Arts Midwifery Institute offers the Apprentice Academics Home Study Course, an in-depth correspondence course which guides you through learning all the textbook essentials which you can take before or concurrent with clinical training.

One advantage of the apprentice route is that you learn what you feel you need to when you feel it is necessary. An apprenticeship can take as long as necessary for you to feel competent. Along with this, no one declares you competent; this is an inner knowing which you arrive at when you are ready, with the support and input of your midwife/mentor. Your clinical experience will be one on one, you will usually have more time between births to reflect on your experiences, and you will have a more personal relationship with the women you see.

Disadvantages to this route include the lack of a structured learning environment. Finding a midwife to apprentice with is difficult for some, and the midwife you choose may have no aptitude for teaching. If you and the midwife do not get along, there may be no other options in your local area. It can be difficult to obtain clinical experience in areas in which your midwife/teacher lacks expertise, or which she does not include in practice (for example, many independent midwives do not do well-woman gynecological care). In most states you will have no credential to acknowledge your educational route, although the midwife you work with could certainly write you a letter of recommendation or verify your skills. A few states, such as New Mexico, South Carolina and New Hampshire accept apprenticeship as a route of entry to licensure or certification. The North American Registry of Midwives (NARM) certification (see next chapter) also offers a way to both validate skills and gain certification after completion of an apprenticeship. Your records of workshops, study groups and births attended (and in what capacity) can help document your learning. In fact, careful documentation of each and every thing you do during your apprenticeship is essential, as well as a file of documents showing completion of any course work. Two books are available to help with the necessary documentation: Practical Skills Record for Midwives and Practical Skills Guide for Midwifery, both are written by Pam Weaver and Sharon Evans and may be ordered directly from Morningstar Publishing Co., 18195 Plainview, Bend, OR 97701.

Talk to midwives in your community who have arrived at their practice via different educational routes. You should write to a variety of programs for further information. With this in hand, you should be able to make an informed decision about the kind of midwifery education that best suits your needs now and in the future. Good Luck!

Formal Validation Processes for Midwives in the United States

Independent (direct-entry) midwives: For a number of years after independent midwifery was "reborn" in force in North America, there was great division among midwives about the wisdom of credentialing of any kind. Some midwives believed that credentials serve only as a formal entry into a patriarchal, hierarchal structure; over the last 150 years, only institutions have issued credentials, and most independent midwives were not training in any kind of institution. There was concern that those midwives who had credentials would inevitably be seen as "better-than" those that did not. Midwives have felt credentialing had the potential to co-opt and undermine our attempts to re-member our lost midwifery heritage which is being regained by working outside of institutions and increasingly outside the modern, western medical paradigm. Thus, many independent midwives resisted formal schooling and credentialing.

However, the pressing need to create some form of validation process in the face of increasing numbers of midwives being prosecuted and even occasionally jailed became ever more obvious during the 1980s. For some time it was felt that local jurisdictions were best equipped to do this, since each area had different competence requirements due to the fact that some were much more rural than others. Throughout the 1970s and 80s midwives worked within their immediate communities, and a number of local professional organizations came up with creative validation mechanisms for apprenticeship models of education. The question of whether national certification was desirable or even possible remained a subject of huge debate.

At the national Midwives's Alliance of North America (MANA) conference of 1986, the MANA membership voted to establish a Registry Board which would develop a test of academic knowledge which would be open to midwives of all educational backgrounds. Those that passed the test would be listed in a Registry of Midwives. Once established, the testing process was requested for use by various state governments as they formulated criteria for regulating independent midwifery.

In 1991, the North American Registry of Midwives (NARM) began work on a national certification process which requires the passage of the registry exam and includes additional validation of clinical skills. Midwives from all over the country were involved in its development.

Not everyone is pleased with these developments and not all midwives will seek formal validation. However, it was felt that if independent midwives didn't develop their own certification process someone else would, and probably to the dissatisfaction of most. The NARM process recognizes midwives from all educational backgrounds and focuses on competency-based assessment. In doing so, it challenges the current paradigm which requires formal institutionally-based learning in order to "arrive" at a profession and, by recognizing all educational routes, it helps ensure that midwives will not all become "cookie-cutter" mimics of each other. In these respects, it represents a major shift from standard certification processes and seems a promising solution to the "problem" of formal validation.

NARM administers the national certification process. You may write to them and get details regarding how your educational process can be validated and what the testing mechanism entails. NARM certification standards are based upon the Midwives's Alliance of North America Core Competencies for Basic Midwifery Practice, which are included in the following chapter.

In addition, independent midwifery programs of education are being accredited by the Midwifery Educators Accreditation Counsel (MEAC). This body recognizes all routes of entry into the profession as valid (apprenticeship as well as formal schooling). As of publication, it is in the process of gaining recognition as the only body authorized to accredit midwifery programs by the United States government; nurse-midwifery programs are accredited through a nursing accrediting body.

Nurse-midwives: Nurse-midwives must first complete a nursing program and take their state Nursing Boards. Nurse-midwives receive a credential at the end of the successful completion of an American College of Nurse-Midwifery (ACNM) approved educational program which provides training in the nursing specialty of midwifery. The credential received depends upon the program; it may be anything from a certificate all the way up to a PhD. Graduates must then pass the ACNM certification exam, thereby becoming Certified Nurse-Midwives, in order to practice in most states.

MANA: The Midwives Alliance of North America

MANA was founded in 1982 to provide a meeting ground for all type of midwives. Because the American College of Nurse-Midwives (ACNM) was not open to expanding their membership to include independent midwives, the majority of the MANA membership has been composed of non-nurse-midwives, although many nurse-midwives are MANA members and have played important roles in the organization's evolution. MANA has gone through many changes; membership has grown, and MANA has developed a comprehensive set of documents for use by the midwifery community. While their intent has remained essentially the same over the years, language refinement and a constant effort to demedicalize terminology has been the thrust of many revisions.

The MANA Statement of Values and Ethics: This document is intended as a consciousness-raising tool for individual midwives and groups to explore their own values and moral responses in a variety of situations. The values expressed, while not held universally by all midwives, reflect essential precepts for a great many. The statement does not focus on a list of do's and don'ts, but offers many specific statements regarding issues relevant to midwifery practice and then offers a way to evaluate how to make the most ethical decision in individual situations.

MANA Core Competencies for Midwifery Practice: This document is intended to outline the basic areas of competency which a midwife needs in order to responsibly enter primary practice. It focuses on repeatable skills which can be observed and evaluated. The equally important but less tangible skills of intuition, rapport with people, sensitivity, ability to make judgement calls and to integrate many levels of knowledge are included in the Guiding Principles of Practice. Without all these skills a midwife is nothing more than a birth technician, and a dangerous one at that, because it is those intangible skills which are so often the most important. This document places the core competencies appropriate to well-woman care outside of pregnancy in a separate section. This was done for two reasons: first, competent midwifery need not include the provision of well-woman care and secondly, some midwives do not wish to offer care which has to do with contraception due to their religious convictions.

Core competency documents are used by educational programs as a blueprint for the development of a more detailed curriculum which includes learning objectives. The self-taught midwife can also use them as a guide for her academic and clinical study.

MANA Standards for the Art and Practice of Midwifery: These standards outline responsible parameters of practice for midwives. Standards are intended to outline generalities only; they do not recommend specific protocols. Those are left to the individual midwife, based on her training and expertise. (See the chapter on

30

Protocols of Practice in the Practice Makes Perfect section for more information).

References and further reading:

Schlinger, Hilary, Circle of Midwives: Organized Midwifery in North America, MANA, 1992.

The MANA Statement of Values and Ethics

We, as midwives, have a responsibility to educate ourselves and others regarding our values and ethics and to reflect them in our practices. Our exploration of ethical midwifery is a critical reflection of moral issues as they pertain to maternal/child health on every level. This statement is intended to provide guidance for professional conduct in the practice of midwifery, as well as for MANA's policy making, thereby promoting quality care for childbearing families. MANA recognizes this document as an open, ongoing articulation of our evolution regarding values and ethics.

First, we recognize that values often go unstated and yet our ethics (how we act), proceed directly from a foundation of values. Since what we hold precious, that is, what we value, infuses and informs our ethical decisions and actions, the Midwives Alliance of North America wishes to explicitly affirm our values [1] as follows:

I. Woman as an Individual with Unique Value and Worth

A. We value women and their creative, life-affirming and life-giving powers which find expression in a diversity of ways.
B. We value a woman's right to make choices regarding all aspects of her life.

II. Mother and Baby as Whole

A. We value the oneness of the pregnant mother and her unborn child; an inseparable and interdependent whole.
B. We value the birth experience as a rite of passage; the sentient and sensitive nature of the newborn; and the right of each baby to be born in a caring and loving manner, without separation from mother and family.
C. We value the integrity of a woman's body and the right of each woman and baby to be totally supported in their efforts to achieve a natural, spontaneous vaginal birth.
D. We value the breastfeeding relationship as the ideal way of nourishing and nurturing the newborn.

---

1. The membership largely agrees with the values that follow. However, some may word them differently or may leave out a few. This document is intended to prompt personal reflection and clarification, not to represent absolute opinions.

III. **The Nature of Birth**

A. We value the essential mystery of birth.[2]

B. We value pregnancy and birth as natural processes that technology will never supplant.[3]

C. We value the integrity of life's experiences; the physical, emotional, mental, psychological and spiritual components of a process are inseparable.

D. We value pregnancy and birth as personal, intimate, internal, sexual, and social events to be shared in the environment and with the attendants a woman chooses.[4]

E. We value the learning experiences of life and birth.

F. We value pregnancy and birth as processes which have lifelong impact on a woman's self esteem, her health, her ability to nurture, and her personal growth.

IV. **The Art of Midwifery**:

A. We value our right to practice the art of midwifery. We value our work as an ancient vocation of women which has existed as long as humans have lived on earth.

B. We value expertise which incorporates academic knowledge, clinical skill, intuitive judgement and spiritual awareness.[5]

C. We value all forms of midwifery education and acknowledge the ongoing wisdom of apprenticeship as the original model for training midwives.

D. We value the art of nurturing the intrinsic normalcy of birth and recognize that each woman and baby have parameters of well-being unique unto themselves.

E. We value the empowerment of women in all aspects of life and particularly as that strength is realized during pregnancy, birth and thereafter. We value the art of encouraging the open expression of that strength so women can birth unhindered and confident in their abilities and in our support.

---

2. Mystery is defined as something that has not or cannot be explained or understood; the quality or state of being incomprehensible or inexplicable; a tenet which cannot be understood in terms of human reason.

3. Supplant means to supersede by force or cunning; to take the place of.

4. In this context internal refers to the fact that birth happens within the body and psyche of the woman: ultimately she and only she can give birth.

5. An expert is one whose knowledge and skill is specialized and profound, especially as the result of practical experience.

F. We value skills which support a complicated pregnancy or birth to move toward a state of greater well-being or to be brought to the most healing conclusion possible. We value the art of letting go.[6]

G. We value the acceptance of death as a possible outcome of birth. We value our focus as supporting life rather than avoiding death.[7]

H. We value standing for what we believe in in the face of social and political oppression.

V. **Woman as mother:**

A. We value a mother's intuitive knowledge of herself and her baby before, during and after birth.[8]

B. We value a woman's innate ability to nurture her pregnancy and birth her baby; the power and beauty of her body as it grows and the awesome strength summoned in labor.

C. We value the mother as the only direct care provider for her unborn child.[9]

D. We value supporting women in a non-judgmental way, whatever their state of physical, emotional, social or spiritual health. We value the broadening of available resources whenever possible so that the desired goals of health, happiness and personal growth are realized according to their needs and perceptions.

E. We value the right of each woman to choose a care giver appropriate to her needs and compatible with her belief systems.

---

6. This addresses our desire for an uncomplicated birth whenever possible and recognizes that there are times when it is impossible. That is to say, a woman may be least traumatized to have a Cesarean and a live baby, but a spontaneous vaginal birth, in this case, is not possible. We let go of that goal to achieve the possibility of a healthy baby. Likewise, the situation where parents choose to allow a very ill, premature or deformed infant to die in their arms rather than being subjected to multiple surgeries, separations and ICU stays. This too, is a letting go of the normal for the most healing choice possible within the framework of the parent's ethics given the circumstances. What is most healing will, of course, vary from individual to individual.

7. We place the emphasis of our care on supporting life (preventive measures, good nutrition, emotional health, etc.) and not pathology, diagnosis, treatment of problems, or heroic solutions in an attempt to preserve life at any cost of quality.

8. This addresses the medical model's tendency to ignore a woman's sense of well-being or danger in many aspects of health care, but particularly in regard to her pregnancy.

9. This acknowledges that the thrust of our care centers on the mother, her health, her well-being, her nutrition, her habits, her emotional balance and, in turn, the baby benefits. This view is diametrically opposed to the medical model which often attempts to care for the fetus/baby while dismissing or even excluding the mother.

34

F. We value pregnancy and birth as rites of passage integral to a woman's evolution into mothering.
G. We value the potential of partners, family and community to support women in all aspects of birth and mothering.[10]

VI. The nature of relationship:

A. We value relationship. The quality, integrity, equality and uniqueness of our interactions inform and critique our choices and decisions.
B. We value honesty in relationship.
C. We value caring for women to the best of our ability without prejudice against their age, race, religion, culture, sexual orientation, physical abilities, or socioeconomic background.
D. We value the concept of personal responsibility and the right of individuals to make choices regarding what they deem best for themselves. We value the right to true informed choice, not merely informed consent to what we think is best.
E. We value our relationship to a process larger than ourselves, recognizing that birth is something we can seek to learn from and know, but never control.
F. We value humility in our work.
G. We value the recognition of our own limits and limitations.
H. We value direct access to information readily understood by all.
I. We value sharing information and our understanding about birth experiences, skills, and knowledge.
J. We value the midwifery community as a support system and an essential place of learning and sisterhood.
K. We value diversity among midwives; recognizing that it broadens our collective resources and challenges us to work for greater understanding of birth and each other.
L. We value mutual trust and respect, which grows from a realization of all of the above.

Making decisions and acting ethically:

These values reflect our feelings regarding how we frame midwifery in our hearts and minds. However, due to the broad range of geographic, religious, cultural, political, educational and personal backgrounds among our membership, how we act based on these values will be very individual. Acting ethically is a

---

10. While partners, other family members and a woman's larger community can and often do provide her with vital support, in using the word potential we wish to acknowledge that many women find themselves pregnant and mothering in abusive and unsafe environments.

complex merging of our values and these background influences combined with the relationship we have to others who may be involved in the process taking place. We call upon all these resources when deciding how to respond in the moment to each situation.

We acknowledge the limitations of ethical codes which present a list of rules which must be followed, recognizing that such a code may interfere with, rather than enhance, our ability to make choices. To apply such rules we must have moral integrity, an ability to make judgments, and we must have adequate information; with all of these an appeal to a code becomes superfluous. Furthermore, when we set up rigid ethical codes we may begin to cease considering the transformations we go through as a result of our choices as well as negate our wish to foster truly diversified practice. Rules are not something we can appeal to when all else fails. However, this is the illusion fostered by traditional codes of ethics.[11]   MANA's support of the individual's moral integrity grows out of an understanding that there cannot possibly be one right answer for all situations.

We acknowledge the following basic concepts and believe that ethical judgements can be made with these thoughts in mind:

> *Moral agency and integrity are born within the heart of each individual.
> *Judgments are fundamentally based on awareness and understanding of ourselves and others and are primarily derived from ones own sense of moral integrity with reference to clearly articulated values. Becoming aware and increasing our understanding are on-going processes facilitated by our efforts at personal growth on every level. The wisdom gained by this process cannot be taught or dictated but one can learn to realize, experience and evaluate it.
> *The choices we can or will actually make may be limited by the oppressive nature of the medical, legal or cultural framework in which we live. The more our values conflict with those of the dominant culture, the more risky it becomes to act truly in accord with our values.
> *The pregnant woman and midwife are both individual moral agents unique unto themselves, having independent value and worth.
> *We support ourselves and the women and families we serve to follow and make known the dictates of our own conscience as our relationship begins, evolves and especially when decisions must be made which impact us or the care being provided. It is up to all of us to work out a mutually satisfactory relationship when and if that is possible.

---

11. Hoagland, Sarah, paraphrased from her book Lesbian Ethics.

It is useful to understand the two basic theories upon which moral judgments and decision making processes are based. These processes become particularly important when one considers that in our profession, a given woman's rights may not be absolute in all cases, or in certain situations the woman may not be considered autonomous or competent to make her own decisions.

One of the main theories of ethics states that one should look to the consequences of the act (i.e. the outcome) and not the act itself to determine if it is appropriate care. This point of view looks for the greatest good for the greatest number. The other primary ethical theory states that one should look to the act itself (i.e. type of care provided) and if it is right, then this could override the net outcome. This is a more process oriented, feminist perspective. As midwives we weave these two perspectives in the process of making decisions in our practices. Since the outcome of pregnancy is ultimately an unknown and is always unknowable, it is inevitable that in certain circumstances our best decisions in the moment will lead to consequences we could not foresee.

In summary, acting ethically is facilitated by:

*Carefully defining our values.
*Weighing our values in consideration with those of the community
    of midwives, families and culture in which we find ourselves.
*Acting in accord with our values to the best of our ability as the
    situation demands.
*Engaging in on-going self-examination and evaluation.

There are both individual and social implications to any decision making process. The actual rules and oppressive aspects of a society are never exact, and therefore conflicts may arise and we must weigh which choices or obligations take precedence over others. There are inevitably times when resolution does not occur and we will be unable to make peace with any course of action or may feel conflicted about a choice already made. The community of women, both midwives and those we serve, will provide a fruitful resource for continued moral support and guidance.

Bibliography:

Cross, Star, MANA Ethics Chair, 1989, unpublished draft of MANA Ethics code.
Daly, Mary, GynEcology: The Metaethics of Radical Feminism, Beacon Press, Boston, 1978.
Hoagland, Sarah Lucia, Lesbian Ethics: Toward New Value, Institute of Lesbian Studies, Palo Alto, CA, 1988.
Johnson, Sonia, Going Out of Our Minds: The Metaphysics of Liberation, Crossing Press, Freedom, CA 1987.

MANA Core-Competencies for Midwifery Practice

GUIDING PRINCIPLES OF PRACTICE:

The midwife provides care according to the following principles:

A. Midwives work in partnership with women and their chosen support community throughout the care-giving relationship.
B. Midwives respect the dignity, rights and the ability of the women they serve to act responsibly throughout the care-giving relationship.
C. Midwives work as autonomous practitioners, collaborating with other health and social service providers when necessary.
D. Midwives understand that physical, emotional, psycho-social and spiritual factors synergistically comprise the health of individuals and affect the childbearing process.
E. Midwives understand that female physiology and childbearing are normal processes, and work to optimize the well-being of mothers and their developing babies as the foundation of care-giving.
F. Midwives understand that the childbearing experience is primarily a personal, social and community event.
G. Midwives recognize that a woman is the only direct care provider for herself and her unborn baby; thus the most important determinant of a healthy pregnancy is the mother herself.
H. Midwives recognize the empowerment inherent in the childbearing experience and strive to support women to make informed decisions and take responsibility for their own well-being.
I. Midwives strive to ensure vaginal birth and provide guidance and support when appropriate to facilitate the spontaneous processes of pregnancy, labor and birth, utilizing medical intervention only as necessary.
J. Midwives synthesize clinical observations, theoretical knowledge, intuitive assessment and spiritual awareness as components of a competent decision making process.
K. Midwives value continuity of care throughout the childbearing cycle and strive to maintain continuous care within realistic limits.
L. Midwives understand that the parameters of "normal" vary widely and recognize that each pregnancy and birth are unique.

GENERAL KNOWLEDGE AND SKILLS:

I. The midwife provides care incorporating certain concepts, skills and knowledge from a variety of health and social sciences, including but not limited to:

38

A. Communication, counseling and teaching skills.
B. Human anatomy and physiology relevant to childbearing.
C. Community standards of care for women and their developing infants during the childbearing cycle, including midwifery and bio-technical medical standards and the rationale for and limitations of such standards.
D. Health and social resources in her community.
E. Significance of and methods for documentation of care throughout the childbearing cycle.
F. Informed decision making.
G. The principles and appropriate application of clean and aseptic technique and universal precautions.
H. The selection, use and care of the tools and other equipment employed in the provision of midwifery care.
H. Human sexuality, including indications of common problems and indications for counseling.
I. Ethical considerations relevant to reproductive health.
J. The grieving process.
K. Knowledge of cultural variations.
L. Knowledge of common medical terms.
M. The ability to develop, implement and evaluate an individualized plan for midwifery care.
N. Woman-centered care, including the relationship between the mother, infant and their larger support community.
O. Knowledge of various health care modalities[1] as they apply to the childbearing cycle.

CARE DURING PREGNANCY
II. The midwife provides health care, support and information to women throughout pregnancy. She determines the need for consultation or referral as appropriate. The midwife uses a foundation of knowledge and/or skill which includes the following:

A. Identification, evaluation and support of maternal and fetal well-being throughout the process of pregnancy.
B. Education and counseling for the childbearing cycle.
C. Preexisting conditions in a woman's health history which are likely to influence her well-being when she becomes pregnant.
D. Nutritional requirements of pregnant women and methods of nutritional assessment and counseling.

---

1. Health care modalities may include but are not limited to such practices as bio-technical medicine, homeopathy, naturopathy, herbology, Chinese medicine, chiropractic, etc.

E. Changes in emotional, psycho-social and sexual variations that may occur during pregnancy.
F. Environmental and occupational hazards for pregnant women.
G. Methods of diagnosing pregnancy.
H. Basic understanding of genetic factors which may indicate the need for counseling, testing or referral.
I. Basic understanding of the growth and development of the unborn baby.
J. Indications for, and the risks and benefits of bio-technical screening methods and diagnostic tests used during pregnancy.
K. Anatomy, physiology and evaluation of the soft and bony structures of the pelvis.
L. Palpation skills for evaluation of the fetus and uterus.
M. The causes, assessment and treatment of the common discomforts of pregnancy.
N. Identification of, implications of and appropriate treatment for various infections, disease conditions and other problems which may affect pregnancy.
O. Special needs of the Rh- woman.

CARE DURING LABOR, BIRTH AND IMMEDIATELY THEREAFTER:

III. The midwife provides health care, support and information to women throughout labor, birth and the hours immediately thereafter. She determines the need for consultation or referral as appropriate. The midwife uses a foundation of knowledge and/or skill which includes the following:

A. The normal processes of labor and birth.
B. Parameters and methods for evaluating maternal and fetal well-being during labor, birth and immediately thereafter, including relevant historical data.
C. Assessment of the birthing environment, assuring that it is clean, safe and supportive, and that appropriate equipment and supplies are on hand.
D. Emotional responses and their impact during labor, birth and immediately thereafter.
E. Comfort and support measures during labor, birth and immediately thereafter.
F. Fetal and maternal anatomy and their interactions as relevant to assessing fetal position and the progress of labor.
G. Techniques to assist and support the spontaneous vaginal birth of the baby and placenta.
H. Fluid and nutritional requirements during labor, birth and immediately thereafter.
I. Assessment of and support for maternal rest and sleep as appropriate during the process of labor, birth and immediately thereafter.
J. Causes of, evaluation of and appropriate treatment for variations which occur during the course of labor, birth and immediately thereafter.

40

K. Emergency measures and transport procedures for critical problems arising during labor, birth or immediately thereafter.
L. Understanding of and appropriate support for the newborn's transition during the first minutes and hours following birth.
M. Familiarity with current bio-technical interventions and technologies which may be commonly used in a medical setting.
N. Evaluation and care of the perineum and surrounding tissues.

POSTPARTUM CARE:

IV. The midwife provides health care, support and information to women throughout the postpartum period. She determines the need for consultation or referral as appropriate. The midwife uses a foundation of knowledge and/or skill which includes but is not limited to the following:

A. Anatomy and physiology of the mother during the postpartum period.
B. Lactation support and appropriate breast care including evaluation of, identification of and treatments for problems with nursing.
C. Parameters of and methods for evaluating and promoting maternal well-being during the postpartum period.
D. Causes of, evaluation of and treatment for maternal discomforts during the postpartum period.
E. Emotional, psycho-social and sexual variations during the postpartum period.
F. Maternal nutritional requirements during the postpartum period including methods of nutritional evaluation and counseling.
G. Causes of, evaluation of and treatments for problems arising during the postpartum period.
H. Support, information and referral for family planning methods as the individual woman desires.

NEWBORN CARE

V. The entry-level midwife provides health care to the newborn during the postpartum period and support and information to parents regarding newborn care. She determines the need for consultation or referral as appropriate. The midwife uses a foundation of knowledge and/or skill which includes the following:

A. Anatomy, physiology and support of the newborn's adjustment during the first days and weeks of life.
B. Parameters and methods for evaluating newborn wellness including relevant historical data and gestational age.

C. Nutritional needs of the newborn.

D. Community standards and state laws regarding indications for, administration of and the risks and benefits of prophylactic bio-technical treatments and screening tests commonly used during the neonatal period.

E. Causes of, assessment of, appropriate treatment and emergency measures for newborn problems and abnormalities.

PROFESSIONAL, LEGAL AND OTHER ASPECTS

VI. The entry-level midwife assumes responsibility for practicing in accord with the principles outlined in this document. The midwife uses a foundation of knowledge and/or skill which includes the following:

A. MANA's documents concerning the art and practice of midwifery.

B. The purpose and goal of MANA and local (state or provincial) midwifery associations.

C. The principles and practice of data collection as relevant to midwifery practice.

D. Laws governing the practice of midwifery in her local jurisdiction.

E. Various sites, styles and modes of practice within the larger midwifery community.

F. A basic understanding of maternal/child health care delivery systems in her local jurisdiction.

G. Awareness of the need for midwives to share their knowledge and experience.

WELL-WOMAN CARE AND FAMILY PLANNING

VII. Depending upon education and training, the entry-level midwife may provide family planning and well-woman care. The practicing midwife may also choose to meet the following core competencies with additional training. In either case, the midwife provides care, support and information to women regarding their overall reproductive health, using a foundation of knowledge and/or skill which includes the following:

A. Understanding of the normal life cycle of women.

B. Evaluation of the woman's well-being including relevant historical data.

C. Causes of, evaluation of and treatments for problems associated with the female reproductive system and breasts.

D. Information on, provision of or referral for various methods of contraception.

E. Issues involved in decision-making regarding unwanted pregnancies and resources for counseling and referral.

MANA Standards and Qualifications
for the Art and Practice of Midwifery

The midwife recognizes that childbearing is a woman's experience and encourages the active involvement of family members in care.

1. Skills: Necessary skills of a practicing midwife include the ability to:

> *Provide continuity of care to the woman and her family during the maternity cycle
> *Assess and provide care for the woman and her family during the maternity cycle
> *Identify and assess deviations from normal
> *Maintain proficiency in lifesaving measures by regular review and practice; and
> *Deal with emergency situations appropriately.

> *In addition, a midwife may choose to provide well-woman care.

It is affirmed that judgement and intuition play a role in competent assessment and response.

2. Appropriate equipment: Midwives are equipped to assess maternal, fetal and newborn well-being; to maintain a clean and/or aseptic technique; to treat maternal hemorrhage; and to resuscitate mother or infant.

3. Records: Midwives keep accurate records of care provided for each woman such as are acceptable in current midwifery practice. Records shall be held confidential and provided to the woman on request.

4. Data collection: Midwives collect data for their practice on a regular basis. It is highly recommended that this be done prospectively, following the guidelines and using the data form developed by the MANA Statistics and Research Committee.

4. Compliance: Midwives will inform and assist parents regarding the Public Health requirements of the jurisdiction in which the midwifery practice will occur.

5. Medical consultation and referral: All midwives recognize that there are certain conditions when medical consultations are advisable. The midwife shall make a reasonable attempt to assure that her client has access to consultation and/or referral to a medical care system when indicated.

6. Screening: Midwives respect the woman's right to self-determination within the boundaries of responsible care. Midwives continually assess each woman regarding her health and well-being relevant to the appropriateness of midwifery services. Women will be informed of the assessment. It is the right and responsibility of the midwife to refuse or discontinue services in certain circumstances. Appropriate referrals are made in the interest of the mother or baby's well-being or when the required or requested care is outside the midwife's legal or personal scope of practice as described in her protocols.

7. Informed choice: Each midwife will present accurate information about herself and her services, including but not limited to:

> *Her education in midwifery
> *Her experience level in midwifery
> *Her protocols and standards
> *Her fees for services
> *The services she does and does not provide
> *The responsibilities of the pregnant woman and her family

8. Continuing education: Midwives will update their knowledge and skills on a regular basis.

9. Peer review: Midwifery practice includes an on-going process of review with peers.

10. Protocols: Each midwife will develop protocols for her services that are in agreement with the basic philosophy of MANA and in keeping with her level of understanding. Each midwife is encouraged to put her protocols in writing.

(revised January, 1997)

References

American College of Nurse-Midwives' documents
ICM membership and joint study on maternity, FIGO, WHO, etc., revised 1972.
New Mexico regulations for the practice of lay midwifery, revised 1982.
North West Coalition of Midwives Standards for Safety and Competency in Midwifery.
Varney, Helen, Nurse-Midwifery, Blackwell Scientific Pub., Boston, MA, 1980.

ACNM: The American College of Nurse-Midwives

In their first years of growth, nurse-midwives had no formal professional association. During the mid-1940's the National Organization of Public Health Nurses (NOPHN), a professional organization, established a section for nurse-midwives. A few years later, reorganization of the professional nursing organizations in the United States led to nurse-midwifery being assigned to the Maternal and Child Health National League for Nursing Interdivisional Council, but it was felt that the concerns of this group were too broad to be a forum for nurse-midwives. Therefore the ACNM was founded in 1955 to serve as the professional organization for nurse-midwives.

The formation of the ACNM provided a base from which CNMs have been able to work for recognition of nurse-midwifery within the context of the medical system, and to formulate educational standards and core competencies for nurse-midwifery schools. The ACNM also has a set of documents which include Core-Competencies, Standards and Practice, and a Code of Ethics for nurse-midwifery practice. Copies of these documents can be obtained from The American College of Nurse-Midwives, 1522 K Street NW, Washington, DC 20005, (202) 289-0171.

Today, the ACNM has some 5,000+ members and is working to expand the scope of nurse-midwifery practice to be more autonomous and embrace multiple practice sites while still remaining acceptable to the mainstream medical community. A more detailed history of the development of nurse-midwifery in the United States may be found in the text Nurse-Midwifery, by Helen Varney, CNM.

References and further reading:

Varney, Helen, Nurse-Midwifery, Blackwell Scientific Pub., Boston, MA 1980.

PRACTICE MAKES PERFECT

Setting Up a Practice

Establishing your first primary practice necessitates some degree of competence in a variety of areas: organizing, accounting, decorating, advertising, negotiation and diplomacy, not to mention midwifery! If you have come to your practice by way of apprenticeship you have probably had a chance to sort out what will and won't work in your own practice. If you have just completed a more formal midwifery program, the task may appear more daunting.

Setting up your office: The details of beginning a practice can seem overwhelming to those who have never done anything like this before. Here are some ideas from my own experience:

The office environment: You'll need some kind of office space. This can be a separate room in your own or your midwifery partner's home, your living room, your clients' home (if you plan to do home visits for all of your care), or an office space which you have rented or borrowed in a location outside your home. One option is to convert a garage or similar building into a separate office on your own property. This space should be pleasant, clean, easy to heat and cool, child-proof and private. A near-by bathroom is a big plus too. Typical office furnishings are a sturdy futon-type couch, large sturdy comfortable chairs, a thick rug, file cabinets, a book shelf, a desk (against the wall, not between you and your clients) a toy box and chairs. A living-room type atmosphere works well to create a relaxed environment and a feeling that you are all in this together; it will do much to help women open up to you and feel at ease.

Women have been so put off by the "typical" medical environment of the doctors's office that you can go a long way toward making women feel at ease by the way your office is set up. Depending upon the kind of care you provide you may feel the need for such things as an examination table with stirrups; however, these tables can be very intimidating. Whenever possible, place frankly medical-looking furniture and large equipment in a separate room or behind a modesty screen. Most examinations can also be done with women lying on a firm day bed or even the carpet/floor space in the center of the room.

How you arrange your office will depend upon where you practice, how many women you see each day and other variables. Wherever it may be, make it cozy, inviting, and have it look more like a home than a typical office. (See the chapter on Caring for Women Who Have Disabilities in the Special Circumstances section for details regarding making your office space accessible.)

Filing system: There are all kinds of fancy filing systems available at office supply stores, but your system need not be expensive or elaborate. For prenatal files, get 12 stiff cardboard file divider/organizer tabbed inserts and label them for each month of the year. File your clients first by the month they are due, then by last name, in each monthly slot. For postpartum records, transfer files to a separate set of twelve labeled dividers under the heading "postpartum" and again organize them by both month of birth and last name. When you finish a woman's care, store her file in another location, arranged by either the date she gave birth or by last name.

At first, manila folders can be used to keep each individual file organized. Once a bit more money is coming in you may want to punch holes in your charts and use a three ring binder to neatly organize active files, removing those charts to manila folders for storage after the care cycle is over.

Your chart forms can be color coded for ease of use, with initial history forms in one color, prenatal and intrapartum in others and postpartum yet another so you can pull what you want at a glance.

Computer, anyone? Deciding whether to use a computer in your practice will depend, to a certain extent, upon how comfortable you feel with technology and how big your practice is. You can, of course, keep almost everything on computer; your appointments, bookkeeping, your resumes and informed disclosures, statistics, etc. A computer will allow you to update your books, create handouts and perform other office chores almost painlessly. However, it will still be necessary for you to have a paper chart on each client, primarily for the ease of taking it with you.

Talk to a local computer wizard about what type of equipment is most suited to your specific needs. Since technology is changing daily, most of my suggestions about specific hardware will be long out of date by the time you read this, so I will refrain. Some things you might want to consider are: a hard drive of at least 500 megabyte capacity, a 486 chip or higher, a "green" machine (energy efficient), a low radiation emission monitor and a laser printer (now quite affordable). Be sure your hardware and software (programs you'll use) are compatible before you invest. Wordperfect, the most popular word processor (fancy typewriter) works with virtually any printer, but not all programs do. If you're going to use a computer, I highly recommend a back-up device, such as a tape back-up system (you should at least back up your hard drive to removable floppy disks), as well as a utility program (like Norton utilities) and an anti-virus program.

Money issues in your practice: Money is one of the most difficult issues for many women starting out as midwives. As women, our work in the world is devalued, often invisible. Work to clear up your "stuff" around money. Ambivalent feelings about charging people will only cause confusion when clients don't pay, beg off or short change you. It can also create confusion around the issue with the other midwives with whom you work. (More discussion regarding money can be found in the chapter on Money Matters in the section on Initiating Contact and Establishing Care).

Bookkeeping: Since most midwives are less than expert financiers, this is probably their most dreaded aspect of setting up practice. One simple way to keep your books is to open a separate checking account for your practice. Deposit all money and checks into that account and write as many business-related expenses as possible on checks from that account. All you need are your receipts, cancelled checks and a filled in check register showing whose money was deposited and where it went. Personal money should be withdrawn from this account and deposited into another account that you use for personal expenses only. In a partnership practice, you could open a business account, write all business related expenses from that account and pay yourselves each a salary based upon what you earn from each client.

Every month or two go through your receipts, staple your receipts to each check and file them according to expense category (business, postage, car, etc.). Use ledger sheets to itemize expenses in various categories; you will need a total for each area of expense. This way all is in order when tax time rolls around.

Keep a separate record of maintenance and mileage use for your car, as well as any driving you do to homevisits, midwifery meetings or births; this is deductible as business use of the vehicle.

Collecting money from clients: This, too, can be as simple or as complicated as you want it to be. For years I worked with a simple system: each client had a signed Responsibility Agreement in her chart. When a payment was made, in cash or by check, it was recorded on her form and then the payment was placed in an envelope. The person making the payment, the amount and who the check was made out to were written on the outside of the envelope. A glance at the envelope would tell how the money was splitting up so far.

After a week or so when money had accumulated in the envelope, all those to be paid would be present for tallying up the total amount and dividing it appropriately. If the writing of checks had left an uneven amount to be divided, this could be taken care of by writing an IOU to the midwife owed and putting it in the envelope. That IOU would be paid from the next batch of checks or the midwife with the extra money would write a check from her business account to the one needing more to make up the difference. In this way each one of us had her own income recorded and no one was responsible for any books other than those for her own income. Business expenses were shared as necessary purchases arose.

Get an accountant: Unless you feel adept at understanding tax laws, get an accountant. Ask around and get several recommendations; do not pick someone out of the phone book. An unscrupulous accountant or tax preparer can cause the IRS to red flag your return; you may get audited merely because they are after him! Together with a good accountant, you can work out a system which will be the easiest for you. Here are some questions to ask prospective accountants:

*What services do you offer?
*How much do you charge?
*Do you have a preference for how I set up my books?
*Can I provide a summary sheet of expenses for tax purposes?
*If I get audited, will you represent me? Must I be present as well?
*How often do those for whom you do taxes get audited?
*Do you charge an additional fee to represent me for an audit if you
   have done my taxes for that year?

In addition, discuss with them how they view such things as home offices, and any other areas of potential high risk. You might want to explore whether or not incorporating your business is in your best interest. The conversation will also give you a good idea of how willing the person is to work with you and how easy it will be for you to communicate.

Paying assistants and partners: It is least cumbersome to have your clients make a check out directly to other people with whom you work. That way, you do not have to deal with filing taxes for them as your employees. If you do need to hire others as employees, be sure to check out state and federal guidelines about what you need to do in the way of taxes, benefits and unemployment insurance to avoid problems with an audit later on.

<u>Working with other midwives and health professionals:</u> As a responsible midwife, you must have some plan in the event that a woman or newborn needs care which you cannot provide. Finding other practitioners who will consult with you may be very easy or almost impossible, depending upon where you live. Fortunate is the midwife who lives in a state where naturopaths or chiropractors attend births, for they are more likely to be open to working with midwives. Family practice doctors are next in line, along with nurse-midwives and finally obstetricians. Your choice of who you can work with may be limited by legal constraints in your state as well as by their own malpractice concerns. The ideal situation involves a practitioner who has hospital privileges who knows that a woman is planning a homebirth with you. In the event of a problem, you would call the backup practitioner for consultation, referral or transport to the hospital, depending on the circumstances. Back-up may vary depending on a woman's particular circumstances, for example, one practitioner may provide care for women having YBACs while another might not. Presenting yourself in a reasonable, professional manner, being familiar with enough medical terminology to sound educated and not waiting until a serious situation has developed before seeking consultation are important components of developing a good reputation in your local community. A local professional group of alternative practitioners may already exist or you could consider starting such a group; this will provide network opportunities as well as peer support.

Knowing exactly who to approach can be tricky. Certainly talking to other midwives is a good way to find out who is friendly in your area, but be sure they understand that you are looking for avenues for consultation yourself. You won't win friends by going in and disrupting a carefully developed relationship that another midwife has worked hard to create.

One of the best ways to track down other friendly practitioners is to follow up on those who are known to the women who seek your care. Occasionally a woman will happen to tell a doctor she is planning a homebirth and the doctor will surprise you by being fairly supportive. These are the ones to pursue, carefully. This can be done by sending another woman to them and having her request back-up as well. She does so by asking the practitioner if they will meet her in the hospital if a problem should arise prenatally or during birth which necessitates a transport. That way the doctor is engaging with her, not you. If ongoing simultaneous prenatal care is taking place, your recommendations may differ significantly from those of a bio-technical provider. The practitioner should be clear that the woman is making her own decisions, not merely doing what she was told by you. Many medical model practitioners seem to think that women are blank slates to be written upon, rather than individuals capable of making informed, self-directed choices: encourage women to clarify this for other care providers.

It is much more difficult to get another practitioner to offer you *carte-blanche* back-up directly, although informal alliances and the possibility of telephone consultation often develop as other practitioners grow more comfortable with the women you send them and the care you provide.

Working with local hospitals: Again, what is possible will vary greatly from place to place depending upon whether you are in a rural or urban area, your legal status and the general climate of support (or lack thereof) in the medical community. Naturally, transport will be easier if you have a supportive care provider with privileges at the hospital you plan to use. When no specific support is available, be aware of which providers are supportive and the hospitals where they work. You will then be able to call, ask who is on call and then select the best of the bunch in an emergency.

In a large city, you can always take a woman to a federal or state funded general hospital that deals with obstetrics and not risk being turned away. They must accept anyone for care. Not so with private hospitals. There are plenty of stories of midwives bringing critical emergencies to private hospitals only to be rejected due to the parents' lack of insurance, the hospital's reluctance to deal with the situation or the absence of an obstetrics department.

Back-up may also need to be geared to a mother's insurance or medical card limitations. For example, a woman who participates in a prepaid health plan such as Kaiser will have to go there unless she is willing to pay out-of-pocket for care elsewhere.

Depending upon your community, you may have to deal with several different hospitals in larger urban areas. Hospital attitudes, policies and services can differ greatly from one to the next, even those within the same city. For example, while teaching hospitals are often *not* a good choice for a planned hospital birth (too willing to experiment), they may be more open-minded when dealing with crises or unusual situations (such as a breech or twin birth) because of the opportunity this affords their students. Don't wait to be surprised that one hospital will not allow extra support persons while another lets you and everybody else into the birthing room. Investigate the hospitals in the communities you serve so you don't waste time taking a woman in for care that is unavailable or into an environment that is unduly hostile. Your choice of where to take a woman will also be influenced by how emergent the problem that has arisen seems to be. If time is not of the essence, you and the parents have more leeway in selecting which hospital will offer the best overall experience. In a crisis, you'll usually need to go for the closest possible reasonable care. Before you leave for the hospital, you will often be able to give the parents a good idea of what is likely to occur, depending upon what the problem may be.

Generally, in most settings, once you transport you are in the role of support person only. The medical personnel will do all the hands-on care and be in charge of management. Your role, in this case, is as an advocate, encouraging the parents to carefully consider their options.

Arranging back-up care for special circumstances: While your willingness to assist women who have breeches, twins or a history of previous surgical births is all well and good, you will then faced with the issue of what to do should a problem arise. The surrounding medical community may welcome you with open arms regardless of the circumstances. For the majority of midwives however, this will not be the case. Because of the prevailing fear of unusual births as well as fear of litigation, back-up with a specific care provider knowledgeable about the woman's situation will simply be unavailable in many areas. If so, you will have to resort to transport to the hospital emergency room in the event of a problem. The parents should understand this aspect of the choice they are making; not having a specific practitioner to call upon does increase the overall risk to a certain extent. In an emergency, if the hospital staff refuses to believe the woman or listen to you, you could have a real crisis on your hands. To complicate the situation further, you may put yourself on the line legally if you declare that you are her midwife, although in an emergency you may have no choice due to the need to communicate directly about the woman's condition. Finally, you must weigh the cost of supporting one woman to have a birth at home which you know will cause an uproar among bio-medical providers, thus putting you in the political hot seat and possibility jeopardizing your ability to care for the rest of the women in your community who would choose to birth at home.

For example, when women wanting YBACs came to me in the mid-1980s for homebirths, the local medical community was quite reluctant to do such births in the hospital, much less sanction them at home. I was practicing in New York, where independent midwifery was a felony. I let it be known to the birthing community that if women started having YBACs unattended, the medical community would have little to say if the midwives began to help. The month that one mother had her 4th child YBAC at home (after three Cesareans) and two women died in the hospital from complications of elective repeat Cesareans was when the tables turned. After that, we began to attend YBACs and the medical community did not protest. The bottom line for change is that the choice and the responsibility must ultimately rest with the women we care for; when they are clearly ready to take the responsibility for their decisions, we as midwives have an ethical obligation to assist. I have, on occasion, suggested that a woman screen her calls with her answering machine and not respond to clinic practitioners hassling her about something when it was obvious to both of us that it wasn't a problem.

In the meantime, you will have to do your best to make clear to women the precarious nature of proceeding with prenatal care and a homebirth without prearranged back-up. As a midwife you are taking on a more complex situation on many levels when you agree to help a woman carrying breech, with twins or another unusual pregnancy; you will need a solid relationship with the parents in order to do so.

Working with apprentices: You will probably be approached, sooner or later, by women who want to apprentice with you in your practice. Carolyn Steiger has already done a fine job of outlining creative ways to work within the midwife/apprentice relationship in her book Becoming A Midwife and Carla Hartley has addressed this vital area in Helping Hands as well. I certainly feel no need to repeat their words here. Here are just a few things to consider from the primary midwife's point of view:

*Do you feel you are a good teacher? If not, let potential apprentices know the limitations of working with you from the beginning.
*How long have you been in primary practice? You probably want to get on your feet, feel established, and have a sense of yourself as a primary attendant before you take on the added complexity of teaching someone else.
*What do you know and feel intuitively about this person? *Choose apprentices that you feel good about and can trust.* Do not make the mistake of taking on a questionable person because it is your "duty" as a trained midwife, or because she has nowhere else to turn for training. It is not your responsibility to train everyone who requests an apprenticeship. It also isn't necessary for every apprentice you have to be your best friend, but you should get a

good, clear feeling from anyone you are going to be taking to births.

*Be clear about what you expect from an apprentice from the start. For example, while she cannot be expected to take on the clinical/skills aspect of the practice immediately, she can be expected to take on the time commitment for appointments for each birth she plans to attend.

*Establish check points at specified intervals to evaluate your work together and to determine if it should continue. This way, if things aren't working out, you have a planned way to evaluate the relationship before tension builds up and a real problem exists.

*If you originally felt good about someone and have second thoughts later, pay attention to these feelings and follow through with a talk or even a dismissal from training, if this seems appropriate. Remember, it is *your* practice.

*The mother's needs come first. Be sure and check with her about her feelings regarding your apprentices. If she feels uncomfortable with someone, try to find out why while affirming her right to make the choice not to have the apprentice there. Find someone else to help you for that birth.

*Discuss what costs are involved for the apprentice (Does she need her own car? a beeper?, etc.) What she can be expected to be paid and at what point? Some midwives pay apprentices a stipend to cover basic expenses, while others charge apprentices for their training. Be clear from the onset what the arrangement will be, and whether there is a point in the future when you will be paying her for her newly acquired skills.

*Encourage the apprentice to enroll in local study groups or classes, or find other means of getting more input than just what she learns from you. This way she gets a broader educational base and the responsibility is not solely on you to make sure everything is covered.

*Encourage her to read Becoming a Midwife and Helping Hands, The Apprentice Workbook. You should review them as well. Even if you don't follow the recommendations exactly, they can help give you ideas of how to evaluate her progress and deal with various situations as they arise. She may also want to purchase Practical Skills Guide for Midwifery, a manual which outlines basic midwifery skills in a step-by-step fashion. (Order from Morningstar Pub. Co., 18195 Plainview, Bend, OR 97701.)

*Once an apprentice is selected, be clear about what her responsibilities are at each stage of her learning; especially in the event of an emergency.

As for yourself, check with NARM about how you can assist in validating the training experiences of your apprentices.

Making your practice known in the world: Advertising your practice can be tricky, especially if you are not practicing legally. While you want the women in your community to know their options, you don't want to wave a red flag in the face of the medical community.

You can get the word out into the community that you are beginning your practice via word-of-mouth, advertising, or both. For those who have been trained via apprenticeship, women are probably already aware that your training is over and you are beginning to practice on your own. When, where and how you advertise will also depend upon how well known the midwifery option is in your community.

Many midwives do not advertise at all. Information about their practice is spread by word-of-mouth from one woman to another. Midwives also give talks or slide shows at various childbirth-related functions and this gives women a chance to meet and talk with them.

Discreet classified ads can be published in the local paper. Some avoid using the inflammatory word "midwife" in favor of advertising their childbirth classes for homebirth or sibling participation, or a homebirth support group. This way, women know you are hooked into the homebirth community and will call you. You could simply say something like: "Interested in having a homebirth?" and give a phone number.

Display ads can be used if you are clearly legal. Look for local newspapers that focus on women's and community issues. Be sure your ad includes your name, the name of your practice and a phone number. You may want to avoid giving out your address if you are in a volatile community in which your ad could be misconstrued as a place someone may want to vandalize (especially if you use phrases such as "choices in childbirth"). Also, try to make your ad matter-of-fact rather than enticing, since we don't want to be guilty of luring women into our care, as hospital ads so often do.

If you go to the expense of having a separate telephone line for your business, you can take out an ad in the yellow pages. This will be expensive (depending upon the size of the ad) but many use the yellow pages as a resource.

Business cards and flyers are other good ways of letting the world know about your practice. One or both can sometimes be posted in health food stores, groceries, community centers, libraries, maternity stores, and book stores.

Health Care Modalities

A number of different philosophies regarding healing and wellness have become more well known over the past 20 years. Western bio-technical medicine is the dominant modality in North America, suggesting that it is "the best," which is simply not true; it is one of many valid approaches. Being aware of a wide range of options allows us to recommend the least interventive modalities as a first line of treatment for many conditions. Of course, experts in various modalities will not always be available in every community, and your clients will have to decide what course of action they feel most comfortable with as well.

There are many different healing modalities and this list is not exhaustive of all the options out there. Here is a basic overview of some of the main therapies:

Aromatheraphy: This involves the use of natural fragrances to influence the health and emotional well-being, often in conjunction with other healing modalities as well. The Complete Book of Essential Oils and Aromatheraphy, by Valerie Ann Worwood provides an thorough explanation of its uses.

Ayurvedic medicine: Ayurveda is a holistic system of medicine that is widely used in India. It teaches that humanity is a microcosm, a universe within; therefore, our existence is indivisible from the totality of cosmic manifestation. Ayurvedic teaching says that every human being has four biological and spiritual instincts: religious, financial, procreative and the instinct toward freedom. Balanced good health is the foundation for the fulfillment of these instincts. Ayurvedic philosophy includes consideration of the influences of heredity, time (the interplay between one's age and the seasons), and methods which allow our bodies to obtain their own good health. There is much focus on building a strong immune system. Ayurveda teaches that all creation, including the human constitution, is composed from the five elements of nature: ether, air, fire, water and earth. Which elements are present and to what degree in each individual are unique to each person but basically fall into three general groupings or doshas: *pitta* (fire and water), *vata* (air and ether), and *kapha* (water and earth). Each is the combination of two of the five elements. Usually a person is a combination of all three doshas. In order to live in a way that promotes health and longevity: we must discover our distinctive makeup or *prakriti;* balance is the goal. Imbalance or *vikruti* is the basis of disease. Diet, herbs, level of physical activity, the weather, and even menstruation and pregnancy are a few of the factors that can aggravate and increase the doshas. Adjusting these factors can bring the body back into balance. More detail regarding Ayruvedic medicine can be found in the books Ayurveda: The Science of Self-Healing, by Dr. Vasant Lad and After the Baby's Birth . . . A Woman's Way to Wellness, by Robin Lim.

Bio-technical medicine: This is standard Western mainstream allopathic medicine as we know it: drugs (especially antibiotics) and surgery being two of its most widely used treatments. This philosophy views "normal" as what is true for the majority and implicitly considers white males the most normal population of all. Allopathic means opposite and this modality is based upon the principle that opposites cure. Therefore if you have a bacterial infection you take an antibiotic, designed to kill the bacteria. In many cases, this modality uses large doses of medicines over a length of time to effect a change or suppression of symptoms. Surgery is also widely used to grossly affect the condition of the body. When the body is very ill, bio-technical medicine tends to pile on drugs to try to manage the symptoms. Although this modality recognizes that the body can heal and rejuvenate itself, it has little or no understanding of the body's vital force or how to work with it to allow the body to effect its own healing. There is also a focus on biochemical processes without much regard for nonphysical influences on one's health status. Bio-technical medicine is at its best in crisis situations and injuries which require physical repair. Bio-technical physicians use diagnostic techniques which rely on laboratory tests to a great extent.

Chinese medicine: Like Ayruvedic medicine, the Chinese have a completely different philosophy of how the body functions and of health than Western medicine. Chinese medicine strives to enhance recuperative power, immunity and the capacity for pleasure, work and creativity. All creation is seen as the result of the union of two polar opposites *Yin* and *Yang*: earth and heaven, winter and summer, night and day, cold and hot, wet and dry, inner and outer, body and mind. Harmony of *yin* and *yang* means health while disharmony leads to disease. The goal of Chinese medicine is to restore harmony.

Each human being is seen as a world in miniature. The body is comprised of the basic constituents *Qi* (chee), **moisture**, **blood**, *Shen* (spirit) and *Jing* (essence). *Qi* is the animating force that gives us our capacity to move, think, feel and work. Moisture is the liquid medium which protects, nurtures and lubricates tissues. Blood is the material foundation out of which we create bones, nerves, skins, muscles and organs. *Shen* is the immaterial expression of the person, and *Jing* represents the body's reproductive and regenerative substance. Thoughts and feelings, the fourth constituents, are acknowledged as being inextricably linked to physiology.

Chinese medicine also recognizes five functional systems known as organ networks: Liver, Heart, Spleen, Lung and Kidney. Networks govern particular tissues, mental faculties and physical activities by regulating and preserving *Qi*, moisture, blood *Shen* and *Jing*. However, these organ networks do not correlate with the function of the physical organs as they would in Western medical thought. For example, in addition to fluid metabolism, the kidney stores the essence responsible for reproduction, growth and regeneration. It controls the teeth, bones, marrow, brain, inner ear, pupil of the eye, and lumbar region, and is associated with fear, the will, and the capacity for sharp thinking and perception. Problems such as retarded growth, ringing in the ears, low back pain, paranoia, fuzzy thinking, weak vision, apathy, or despair are viewed as dysfunctions of the kidney network. The heart not only propels blood through the vessels, but houses the spirit and governs the mind. Symptoms such as anxiety, restless sleep, angina, and palpitations occur when the heart is agitated. The spleen is in charge of the assimilation of foods and fluids, and well as ideas. When this network is disturbed indigestion, bloating, fatigue, scattered thinking and poor concentration occur. The liver is responsible for the storage of blood, flow of *Qi*, and evenness of temper. When the liver is imbalanced, tension in the neck and shoulders, high blood pressure, headaches, cramping, moodiness, and impulsive behavior may follow. The lung sets the body's rhythm, defends it boundaries, and affords inspiration. Lung network problems may cause tightness in the chest, skin rashes, vulnerability to colds and flus, rigid thinking, or melancholy.

Five body climates are also recognized: wind, dampness, dryness, heat and cold. These forces can cause imbalance within the body, weakening or obstructing the movement of *Qi* in the organs. Internal wind manifests as vertigo, unsteady movement, and trembling. Dampness becomes phlegm and edema in the body. Dryness causes chapping or cracking of mucus membranes. Cold retards circulation and depresses metabolism. Finally heat causes tissue inflammation.

Qi, moisture and blood circulate within a web of pathways that link the organ networks with the organism as a whole. Health exists when everything flows smoothly. All illness is understood as a result of either the depletion or congestion of *Qi*, moisture or blood. Depletion leads to weakness, lethargy, frequent illness, poor digestion, and inadequate blood flow. Congestion results in aches, tension, tenderness, pain, a distended abdomen, irritability and swelling.

Diagnosis is accomplished by first establishing what the symptoms are via a thorough interview. The practitioner then feels for nine pulse points in each wrist, and examines the color and form of the face, tongue and body. This information is interpreted in the context of the person's present and past complaints, work and living habits, physical environment, family health history, and emotional life.

Balance is achieved by regulating the *Qi*, moisture and blood in the organ networks: weak organs are tonified, congested channels are opened, excess is dispersed, tightness is softened, agitation is calmed, heat is cooled, cold is warmed, dryness is moistened and dampness is drained. Treatment may incorporate acupuncture, herbal remedies, diet, exercise and massage.

Acupuncture is based on the idea that *Qi* courses through channels in the body like streams in a landscape. Acupuncture points are located in small depressions in the skin called "men" or "gates." These gates are opened and closed to adjust circulation in the channels and to expel noxious influences from them. Thin needles are inserted into the points to communicate from the outside to the inside. Acupuncture mobilizes *Qi*, moisture and blood, invigorating proper function of muscles, nerves vessels glands and organs. Herbal remedies are often used as well; these are aimed at the underlying causes of the symptoms based on traditional Chinese diagnosis. They rarely cause unwanted side effects. (Beinfield & Krongold, 1991)

Chiropractic adjustment: Chiropractic medicine involves the use of physical manipulations to align the spinal bones properly. It originated with the concept that a straight spine would enhance one's spiritual experience of life. It soon became apparent that the by-products of spinal manipulation included many physical benefits which had not been intended or anticipated. Over time, chiropractic adjustments began to be focused on total physical well-being. The theory is that the nervous system affects every function in the body; therefore a well functioning nervous system enhances health and can significantly alter or alleviate physical symptoms.

There are several varieties of chiropractic care. Standard chiropractic finds spinal vertebrae which are out of alignment (subluxations) and, using hand manipulations, adjusts the bones so that they are in alignment. Classical chiropractic care only attends to the alignment of the spinal bones. Additional techniques have come into favor in recent years, including various pelvic manipulations. "Toftness" is a technique which uses a non-electronic energy focusing device to help the doctor locate energy blocks in the spine. An activator (spring-loaded device) is used to gently jar the bones back into place. In Network Chiropractic, the practitioner senses energy blocks with her hands and then uses a very light touch to redirect the energy of the spine; after these subtle adjustments begin to make changes, the practitioner may feel it appropriate to use more standard structural adjustments from time to time.

Hands-on energy healing: There are a wide variety of hands-on healing methods such as Reike, therapeutic touch, ortho-bionomy and polarity. Crystals are sometimes used to channel energy as well. All of these techniques work with the body's energy to balance the system and achieve greater well-being. They can be used in conjunction with other modalities.

Homeopathy: Homeopathy is based on the principle of "like cures like" and the law of similars. In homeopathic prescribing, minute doses of every conceivable substance are carefully prepared in various dilutions for use as remedies. Homeopathy views the body as constantly trying to achieve a perfect state of balance. Sometimes the best it can do is manifest a physical state that produces illness. When this occurs, a homeopathic remedy that in large (material) doses would produce similar symptoms is given in a highly potent, but physically dilute, therapeutic dose. The homeopathic remedy selected would be the mineral, plant, or animal substance that would most closely produce those symptoms in a healthy individual (which is known as "proving" the remedy).

To find the right remedy, questions are asked of the person regarding every aspect of their acute or chronic condition. In addition, personal preferences, habits, moods, etc. are inquired about so that a "symptom picture" emerges. For example, if a person is jittery, hyper, can't sleep well at night, and has loose stools, these would be noted down. In addition, any information such as what may make the symptoms better or worse, times of day the symptoms were most apparent, food preferences, and a host of other details would be obtained.

The homeopathic practitioner then goes to a resource known as a repertory and starts to look up the symptoms described, noting down what remedies are associated with each. As research proceeds, some remedies may be repeated from symptom to symptom. Repeated remedies are noted, and the choice narrows down. Finally, a symptom picture emerges, and the remedy is chosen. (The more acute the condition, the less precise this symptom picture must be.) In classic homeopathy, one remedy is taken at a time to decide if it is effective, and it is changed as necessary. While most prepared remedies recommend taking 3 to 5 pellets in a dose, a person need only take one for it to be just as effective, regardless of the size of the pellet.

Because of this individualization of prescription, several remedies often apply to what we think of as the same condition (the flu, for example); different people will have different reactions to an illness considered the "same" by bio-technical standards. When the remedy matches the symptoms precisely enough, it fits the energy pattern of the body at that moment like a key in a lock, adding a burst of energy and creating an avenue for the body to manifest balance in a more harmonious way. When a remedy is chosen perfectly, this can be a truly miraculous transformation. If the remedy does not match, usually nothing changes.

Remedies are commonly prepared by using one of two dilution methods; the decimal or centesimal. In decimal (X potency) dilutions, one part of the remedial substance is combined with 9 parts of inert solution. It is then percussed, or shaken, by being lightly pounded (as in the hand) for a time and then diluted again. One part of that solution is then added to 9 parts of inert solution, and so it goes, each dilution being one X of potency. When 26X is reached, a chemist cannot find any of the original remedy in the preparation. Even so, the more dilute the remedy, the more potent it is considered to be. This is because the dilution and percussion process releases and raises the vibrational quality of the remedial substance on a molecular level. The centesimal (C potency) scale is prepared the same way except dilutions are 1 to 99. Sometimes the C scale is referred to as D potency; they are the same.

The higher the potency of any remedy, the more precisely it must be prescribed to be effective. Higher potencies are used for constitutional (deep acting) prescribing, acute symptoms when you think the prescription is precise and symptoms are severe, and in cases where the chosen remedy seems to be working but has not been entirely effective.

Dry grafting: I am now going to tell you a well kept homeopathic secret. It will be hard to believe, but it is absolutely true; I have tested it myself with a number of remedies. In order to make duplicate remedies all you need to do is:

* *Start with medicated pellets that were obtained from a homeopathic pharmacy.
* *Obtain new glass bottles and lids (small tube-shaped bottles are great, you can label the top and stand them up in a tin or other small box)
* *Write out labels for each new remedy you want to make (check stationary stores for small round labels that fit the tops of the bottles)
* *Place two or three medicated pellets of the desired remedy in the bottom of the new bottle
* *Fill the same bottle with new, blank, unmedicated pellets (be sure to do this over a plate, not over the big bottle of blank pellets. Dispose of any that drop on the plate. These precautions ensure that you do not accidently potentize your entire supply of blank pellets.) If you like, you can add a drop of grain alcohol, but I have not found this to be essential.
* *You now have a duplicate remedy of your original that is as potent as the first!! Amazing but true.
* *Be sure to cap and label this remedy before you go on to make the next, all remedies look alike!
* *Never reuse old bottles to make new remedies unless they are to be the same remedy and potency.
* *You can also fill up your partially used medicated remedies with blank pellets and achieve the same result.
* *You can make dry grafts from dry grafts as well; these are also just as good as new!

For further information regarding homeopathic medicine, refer to the following books and suppliers for equipment:

Everybody's Guide to Homeopathic Medicines, by Stephen Cummings and Dana Ullman (a basic primer, you don't need to know anything about homeopathy to read this)

The Science of Homeopathy, by George Vithoulkas (in depth philosophy and methodology of classical homeopathy)

Homeopathic Medicine for Women, by Dr. Trevor Smith (a variety of women's health issues are addressed)

Homeopathy for Pregnancy, Birth, and Your Baby's First Year, by Miranda Castro, St Martin's Press, New York, 1993.

Sources of homeopathic remedies, books and education:

Homeopathic Educational Services, 2124 Kitteredge, Berkeley, CA 94704.
(415) 649-0294, 9 am to 6 pm. Monday through Friday, Pacific time; (800)
359-9051 toll free ordering; books, tapes, computer programs, and remedies.
InterNatural, P.O. Box 580, South Sutton, NH 03273. (603) 927-4237
National Center for Homeopathy, 1500 Massachusetts Ave., NW—Suite 42,
Washington, D.C. 20005 (203) 223-6182; newsletter, conferences, books,
summer courses.
International Foundation for Homeopathy, 2366 Eastlake Ave., E., Suite 301,
Seattle, WA 98102, (206) 324-8230; professional and lay courses and a
listing of classical homeopathic practitioners.
Foundation for Homeopathic Education and Research, 2124 Kitteredge St,
Berkeley, CA 94704; sponsors research.
Pacific Academy of Homeopathic Medicine, 105 El Cerrito Plaza Professional
Building, El Cerrito, CA 94530; videos and seminars for beginning to
advanced students.
Rocky Mountain Homeopathic Press, P.O. Box 10265, Sedona, AZ 86336; send
SASE for information on books, family care and midwifery workshops.

Homeopathic pharmacies:

Boiron-Bornemann, Inc. Homeopathic manufacturing pharmacists, 1208
Amosland Rd., Norwood, PA 19074. (800) 258-8823. Large selection of
single homeopathic remedies, but very stuffy about dealing with midwives.
Boericke & Tafel, 1011 Arch St., Philadelphia, PA 19107, (800) 276-2820.
Dolisos, 3014 Rigel Ave., Las Vegas, NV 89102, (800) 365-4767. They are quite
happy to provide you with a credit account as a midwife and can supply you
with a full range of remedies and blank pellets as well.
Hahnemann Medical Pharmacy, 828 San Pablo Ave, Albany, CA 94706, (510)
527-3003.
Luyties Pharmaceutical Co., 4200 Laclede Ave., St. Louis, MO 63108, (314)
533-4600.
Standard Homeopathic Co., 154 W. 131st, Los Angeles, CA 90061. In
(800) 624-9659; also very stuffy about dealing with midwives.
Apothecary Products, Inc., 11531 Rupp Dr., Burnsville, MN 55337. (800) 328-
2742; order screw cap vials for remedies, the 1 dram size is easy to carry.

Herbology: Herbs offer a powerful alternative to bio-technical drug therapy, one
which has been time-tested for hundreds of thousands of years by indigenous
healers world wide (more research trials than the few decades drugs can boast).

They are nourishing, healing, and help to restore the body and its organs so that it can, in turn, balance the system and overcome dis-ease. Herbs are very different than drugs in many respects. Instead of isolating one active agent, they offer a whole complex of supportive, nutritive agents to facilitate the action of the most potent ingredients. Here is a summary of how to prepare herbs for medicinal use. For more detailed information, Susun Weed and Billie Potts have written books that are both accurate and specific in the preparation and use of herbs for health and healing. (See references at end of chapter for books on herbal healing.)

To prepare herbs for medicinal purposes:

Gathering plant materials: Fresh plant materials should be gathered when the energy of the plant is in the part to be used; leaves before the plant flowers; flowers when the plant is flowering with the blooms fully open and perfect; in the spring or fall for roots when the energy has returned to the root; barks in early spring when the sap is rising; seeds in the late fall.

Tinctures made with dry herbs: Use 1 ounce herb by weight to 5 liquid ounces 100 proof vodka. Place both in a jar with a well fitting lid. Let sit in a dark space for 6 weeks or more. This method is suitable for tincturing dried roots, barks, and seeds, but not dried leaves or flowers.

Tinctures of fresh herbs: You may wash herbs if necessary and dry with a towel. Pack a jar full with cleaned herbs. Cover with 100 proof vodka. Cap and let sit for at least 6 weeks. Flowers, leaves, and stems as well as all other plant parts may be tinctured in this way.

Tinctures may be drawn off for use and the plant materials left in the remaining solution if you like. A glass turkey baster is ideal for this purpose; they can be purchased in kitchen specialty stores.

Medicinal strength water-based infusions: Use only dried herbs—the rehydration process ruptures the dried cell membranes and releases the medicinal properties into the water. Always boil the water, then turn off the heat for 2 minutes so the temperature drops below boiling. This will help preserve the enzymes in the herbs. Pour the water over the herb and let it steep covered for the designated amount of time. Refrigerate what is not taken immediately.

> **Roots & Barks:** use 1 pint water to 1 oz. herb; steep 10 hours.
> **Light textured leaves (Nettles):** use 1 qt. water to 1 oz. herb; steep for 6 hours or more.
> **Leathery leaves (Uva Ursi or Rosemary):** 1 qt. water to 1 oz. herb, allow to steep 10 hours.
> **Flowers & oily leaves (Peppermint):** 1 qt. water to 1 oz. herb, steep

½ to 1 hour, depending upon the potency of the herb being prepared.

Seeds: 1 pt. water to 1 oz. seeds, allow to steep ½ hour.

Medicinal oils: Use only fresh plant materials gathered after the dew has been burned off by the sun. Carefully brush or scrub off dirt, but do not wash plant materials. Chop the plant material. Pack firmly into an absolutely dry jar, leaving a little space at the top. Cover plant material with olive oil, leaving no air space at the top. Use a dry chopstick to work the oil down into the plant material, leaving no air pockets. Place in a cool, dry, dark place with something absorbent beneath the jar, as oil frequently overflows the top as the plant's gases are released. These are tricky to make. Some materials, especially Comfrey, will mold during this process and should be watched closely and shaken gently every few days. If an air space forms between the oil and the lid, be sure to add more oil so no air space is left. Stain carefully and decant after 6 weeks. Do not leave plant material in oil past six weeks as it may go rancid. (Olive oil is preferred because it will not go rancid at room temperature and is good for the skin.)

Dried herbs in capsules: Capsules are often the least effective way to take herbs. A powdered herb has been maximally exposed to air, and loses potency rapidly. On the other hand, a capsuled herb will have a milder effect on the body. There are just a few exceptions mentioned in the text, capsuled ginger for nausea and Collinsonia root tablets for varicose veins being among them. Otherwise, infuse the herb, tincture it, eat it or buy commercially freeze-dried herbs in capsules for maximum potency.

Use of herbs in pregnancy: Remember that, while herbs are basically safe and natural they can also have powerful effects, as well as some side effects. Use herbs wisely. The herbs mentioned in my texts are safe to use as directed during pregnancy; others are not. Research those you are unsure of, especially in oil form. Pennyroyal, in particular, is not safe in any form, yet it can be found is some uterine tonic combinations. Be careful!

Sources of herbal products: It is very important to obtain high quality herbs and herbal preparations. Here are some sources you can count on:

Earth's Harvest, 2557 NW Division, Gresham, OR 97030, (800) 428-3308; offers a variety of prepared yoni remedies as well as other remedies.
Eclectic Institute, 11231 S. E. Market St., Portland, OR 97216. (800) 332-4372; source of freeze dried herbs in capsules and tinctures.
Equinox Botanicals, Rt. 1, Box 71, Rutland, OH 75775; source for Labor Enhancement formula, Echinacea tincture, Spring Dandelion root tincture, and Prenatal Uterine Tonic tincture.

Herb Pharm, Box 116, Williams, OR 97554; high quality single herb tinctures and loose dry herbs.
Nature's Herb Company, 281 Ellis St., San Francisco, CA 94102; premixed vaginal bolus by the pound and many other mixes and hard-to-locate items.
Frontier Cooperative Herbs, Box 69, Norway, Iowa 52318. (319) 227-7991; excellent high quality bulk herbs.
NF formulas, 9775 SW Commerce Circle, Suite C-5, Wilsonville, OR 97070, in Oregon dial (800) 325-9326, all others call (800) 547-4891; many fine herbal preparations and natural vitamin supplements for pregnancy.
Wish Garden Herbs, Box 1304, Boulder, CO 80306.

<u>Naturopathic medicine</u>: Naturopaths use a variety of healing modalities such as herbs, hydrotherapy, homeopathy, physical manipulations, dietary adjustments, special diagnostic tests and a holistic philosophy of care to deal with disease and ill health. Sometimes a naturopath will specialize in one modality—for example, primarily working with homeopathy or body work.

<u>Medical astrology</u>: The natal or birth chart is calculated based on the time, date and place of birth. It shows the essential characteristics of a person and can also be symbolically progressed or advanced according to a person's age to obtain information as the life unfolds. The daily positions of the planets (transits) also impact the expression and experiences represented in the birth chart. All these techniques can be used by a skilled astrologer to assist in understanding the health trends in a person's life. Astrology could, for example, help distinguish whether a suspected problem will have a severe consequence. There may be astrological counselors in your area who have experience with medical astrology. If you are interested, you might want to take classes and become proficient yourself. Basic character analysis can also help you understand how to deal with clients on a psychological and emotional level.

References and further reading
Beinfield, Harriet, and Korngold, Efren, <u>Chinese Medicine: How it Works</u>, published by the authors, to obtain copies call 1-800-873-3946.
Lust, John, <u>The Herb Book</u>, Bantam Pub. through Benedict Lust Pub., Simi Valley, CA, 1974.
<u>Peterson's Field Guide to Wild Flowers</u> & <u>Peterson's Field Guide to Medicinal Plants</u>. Can be found in local book stores.
Potts, Billie, <u>Witches Heal</u>, 2nd ed., DuReve Pub., 1988.
Shiloh, Jana, "Homeopathic Remedies for Labor and Birth," <u>Mothering</u>, No. 56, Jul/Aug/Sept. 1990, pp. 61-65.
Weed, Susun, <u>Wise Woman Herbal for the Childbearing Year</u>, Ash Tree Pub., Box 64, Woodstock, NY 12498. This is the best, most complete book on herbs in pregnancy. Most of the preparations in this text have been derived from my personal experience, that of other midwives or Susun's book; excellent sections on how to prepare herbs, theory, and exact details of usage.

How to Gather and Tabulate Statistics

NOTE: It will help to read the Statistics in Perspective section of the Informed Disclosure example before reading this chapter.

I would like to give you some idea of how to go about tabulating your statistics. If you have a computer or someone you know is willing to help you on theirs, that's wonderful. If not, you can still do a good job with hand tabulation.

Your statistics form:

Statistics provide a means of communicating about birth outcomes which are accepted worldwide. Therefore, gathering statistics on the births you attend is very important to furthering midwifery in general and for letting your local community know how you practice.

The Midwives' Alliance of North America (MANA) has developed a form which specifically addresses homebirth practice. It is designed to gather data which will reflect the different ways midwifery is practiced and thus demonstrate that diverse practice styles can lead to healthy births for mothers and babies. Developed by an epidemiologist and the MANA statistics committee, it gathers a lot of information in its four page format. I strongly encourage you to use the MANA form (see copy at the end of this chapter) and to encourage your state association or licensure board to adopt it as well. Results can be entered into Epi 5, a medical statistics program, and tabulated right from your computer. (For a sample of this form, write the MANA statistics committee, 36 Glen Ave. Ottawa, ONT, K1S 2Z7, [613] 730-0282.)

Always attempt to fill out the statistical form at or shortly after each birth. This way details are fresh in your mind and it gets done. This is infinitely easier than trying to go back through all your charts, months or years later, and gather up the information. Try to tabulate your statistics every four to six months or at least once a year, depending upon how active your practice is. That way you will have a reasonable number of forms to work with at one time.

Tabulating data:

Using the MANA form and sending in your forms to be tabulated will allow you to pull your statistics from the big pool; you can tabulate your personal statistics on your own computer. If you must tabulate data by hand, to avoid confusion, try to keep the number of statistics forms which you are totalling up small. I have tried many methods of coming up with totals, and have found the following to be the least confusing: Let's say you are trying to total all the first-time mothers. Simply go through your sheets, separate out those for first-time mothers in a stack and count them up. Then go through the remaining stack and withdraw all mothers who had their second through fourth child and count them up. Finally add up all those who had their fifth child or greater and add them up. You now have three subtotals, all of which should add up to your grand total. You can do this with every data parameter you are tabulating.

Which information you include in the statistical data you share with clients will depend upon how much detail you want. At the very least, total births, total surgical and forceps deliveries, total deaths and total transports and their outcomes are good places to start. See the chapter on the Statement of Informed Disclosure to see how statistics can be presented in some detail in your disclosure document.

Calculating percentages and mortality rates:

Percentages: A percentage reflects the number of times something happens in relationship to 100. Therefore 1 is 1% of 100 and 20 is 20% of 100. You can calculate percentages for numbers other than 100 either by hand or by using a calculator. Let's say you had a total of 56 births last year. Two of these ended in surgical deliveries. What percentage is 2 out of a total of 56? Divide 2 by 56; this equals 0.035714285. Multiplying that result by 100 equals 3.5714285. Round that off to the nearest hundredth of the total figure; this gives you 3.57% (round up for a figure 5 or above, round down or leave it as is for amounts below five). If the result had been 3.8350301 you could round this off to 3.84%. Therefore 2 is 3.57% of 56. If you have a percent button on your calculator enter it like this: 2 ÷ 56 %. In general: # of events ÷ total of all births X 100 = %.

Maternal mortality: Maternal mortality is based upon the number of deaths per 100,000 total births. This is because few women die in childbirth today in industrialized countries. Let's say you have the unfortunate experience of having a mother die from a bad reaction to anesthesia after being transported for a manual removal of the placenta after birth. This constitutes 1 maternal death out of a grand total of the 452 births you have attended in your midwifery career. To calculate maternal mortality, divide 1 by 452 and multiply the result by 100,000. This gives a result of 221.2 deaths per 100,000 births. Of course this assumes that the death rate will remain steady until a total of 100,000 births is reached, and thus gives a very unfair gauge of what may occur in actual practice.

Infant mortality: Infant mortalities include deaths from birth through the first year of life, thus including factors such as accidents, malnutrition, disease and abuse. Mortality is calculated based on the number of events per 1000 total births (not a percentage). Let's say you had 1 fetal death at term due to birth defects out of the 56 total births above. The fetal mortality rate projects how many babies would die if they continued to die at the same rate for your next 944 births. To get this answer you figure as follows:

1 ÷ 56 = 0.017857142. Multiply 0.017857142 by 1000 = 17.857142 per 1000. Round this off to 17.9 per 1000. That is: # of deaths ÷ total of all births X 1000 = infant/fetal mortality rate per 1000 births.

Fetal, neonatal and perinatal mortality: These rates are estimated by calculating all fetal and infant deaths per 1000 total births from a certain point in gestation through a specified amount of time (days or weeks) after birth. There are several definitions in use:

Late fetal mortality: deaths after 28 weeks gestation up through birth.

Neonatal mortality: infant deaths from birth to less than 29 days old.

Perinatal mortality: Def. 1 Infant deaths of less than 7 days and fetal deaths with stated or presumed gestation of 28 weeks or more.

Perinatal mortality: Def. 2 Infant deaths of less than 28 days and fetal deaths with stated or presumed gestation of 20 weeks or more.

Perinatal mortality: Def. 3 Infant deaths of less than 7 days and fetal deaths with stated or presumed gestation of 20 weeks or more.

To obtain the number of deaths for each definition, you use the same basic formula: # of deaths ÷ total births (including those ending in death) X 1000 = death rate per 1000 total births

References and further reading:

Jordan, B., Birth in Four Cultures, 4th ed., Waveland Press, Inc., Prospect Hts, Il, 1993.
Stewart, David, The Five Standard of Safe Childbearing, NAPSAC Pub., Marble Hill, MO 1981.

Please note: in general code: 1=yes, 0=no, ?=don't know; blank=does not apply

DEMOGRAPHIC

Midwife Code   1**

Midwife's Code for
   Identifying This Birth   1

Client's Municipality _____

Population (1=city >1,000,000, 2=city >250,000,   2
   3=town >10,000, 4=small town (<10,000), 5=rural)

Postal (ZIP) Code

Mother's: Age

   Last grade of high school completed

   Post secondary education (years)

   Occupation _____   *3

   Ethnic Origin (1=Caucasian, 2=African
     or Caribbean, 3=Native American, 4=Asian,
     5=Other_____)

   Special group (1=Hispanic, 2=Amish,
     3=Francophone, 4=other_____)

   Natural hair colour (1=brown, 2=black, 3=red,
     4=blond)

Partner status at time of birth (1=married couple,
   2=unmarried couple, 3=female partner,
   4=separated/divorced, 5=single, 6=couple,
   marital status not known, 7=other_____)

Partner's: Age

   Last grade of high school completed

   Post Secondary education (years)

   Occupation _____

Family socio/economic level (midwife's evaluation)
   (1=low, 2=medium, 3=upper)

PREVIOUS PREGNANCY AND DELIVERY HISTORY

Number of previous :   pregnancies

                miscarriages   4

                induced abortions

                stillbirths   4

                live births

Number of previous :   home births

                caesarean sections

                VBAC's

                episiotomies

                postpartum hemorrhages

Other previous pregnancy or delivery concern(s)
   (1=gest <37 wks, 2=gest>42 wks, 3=hypertension,
   4=breech, 5=pre/eclampsia, 6=IUGR, 7=birth defect,
   8=shoulder dys, 9=other_____)

PRESENT PREGNANCY CONCERNS

Maternal problems: (1=pregnancy-induced
   hypertension,2=chronic hypertension,3=pre-eclampsia,   5
   4=eclampsia, 5=gestational diabetes, 6=diabetes
   mellitus, 7=persistent anemia (Hct<30 or Hb<10 g/dl),
   8=Rh sensitized,9=other_____)

Infection (1=genital herpes,
   2=chlamydia, 3=urinary tract infection, 4=yeast,
   5=gonorrhea, 6=other_____)

                           1st 2nd 3rd

Bleeding in trimester: (1=light, 2=heavy)

Fetal problems: (1=suspected IUGR, 2= birth
   defect diagnosed in utero(_____),
   3=intrauterine death, 4=other_____)

Midwife perceives emotional/social problems   6
   <---- (specify and describe in margin of form)

BREECH AFTER 28 WEEKS GESTATION

1st time breech noticed (week of gest. from LMP)

Last time breech (week of gest. from LMP)

Breech turning exercises (# of times)

External cephalic version   by midwife   :

(attempts: sucesses)   by physician   :

Other procedures (1=_____)

** 1,2,3 etc. are footnotes: see page 4 for clarifications

PRENATAL CARE

Week (from LMP) any prenatal care began

Week (from LMP) midwife prenatal care began

Prenatal classes (1=this preg, 2=other preg, 3=both)

Two most important reasons for choosing intended   7
   place of birth (as stated by mother)
   (1=desire for natural birth, 2=effect on baby, 3=control,
   4=social pressure, 5=cost, 6=safety, 7=family unity,
   8=atmosphere, P=partner preference, H= "high risk",
   9=other_____)

Number of prenatal visits: with a midwife
                  estimated with G.P.
                  estimated with obstetrician

Payment (1=client paid, 2=Blue Cross/Shield,
   3=commercial insurance, 4=HMO (other prepay),
   5=Champus,6=Medicaid,7=universal government health
   insurance, 8=other_____)

PRENATAL DETAILS

Mother's height (or estimate)   feet   inches

Mother's prepregnancy weight (pounds)

Weight gain during pregnancy (pounds)

Method of conception (1=coitus, 2=artificial
   insemination, 3=in vitro, 4=other)   1st 2nd3rd

Ultrasound (# of times each trimester)

Other prenatal testing (1=triple screen,
   2= chorionic villus sampling, 3=AFP, 4=amniocentisis,
   5=biophysical profile, 6=non stress test, 7=GTT,
   8=random glucose, 9=other_____)

Tobacco, Alcohol or Recreational Drugs

Mother smoked cigarettes during pregnancy

   Number of months

   Average # of cigarettes per day

Alcohol during pregnancy

   Average number of drinks per month

Marijuana/THC/hashish   (1=occasional, 2=regular)

Other illegal drugs   (1=occasional, 2=regular)

Drug type (1=cocaine, 2=other_____)

Prescription drugs in pregnancy (1=antibiotics,
   2=antifungals, 3=antiemetics, 4=antihypertensives,
   5=other (specify)_____)

Mother's overall nutrition in pregnancy (midwife's
   assessment)(1=excellent, 2=good, 3=fair, 4=poor)

Diet during pregnancy (1='meat & potatoes', Primary
   2=whole foods and meat, 3=junkfood, Secondary
   4=ovo-lacto vegetarian, 5=vegan vegetarian,
   6=macrobiotic, 7=other_____)

Mother restricted calorie intake to limit weight gain

Herbs to ease labour(last 6 wks)(1=daily, 2=less often)

Activity level during majority of pregnancy (1=very
   active, 2=active, 3=sometimes active, 4=sedentary)

Perineal Massage or Stretching

   Estimated # of times during 3rd trimester

Mother reports a history of sexual abuse
   (1=yes before puberty, 2=yes after puberty,
   3=before and after puberty, 4=mother prefers
   not to answer, 5=midwife did not ask)

Risk Factors Why a Home Birth Was Not or Could Not Have Been Initiated, Or Was Outside of Home Birth Protocol (Answer for All clients)   8

Reasons: (1=preterm/post-term,
   2=breech or malpresentation, 3=multiple birth,
   4=hypertension, 5=anemia, 6=diabetes,
   7=pre-eclampsia/eclampsia, 8=placenta previa/
   abruptio, 9=other(specify)_____)

Woman Stopped Using This Midwife For Primary Care Before Labour Began

Reasons:(1=miscarriage, 2=referral for   4
   complications, 3=client moved, 4=client chose birth
   centre, 5=client chose hospital, 6=changed midwives,
   7=cost, 8=stillbirth, 9=other_____)

Gestation when midwife primary care stopped   9

* Code will be added later

Midwives' Alliance of North America

Please note: in general code: 1=yes, 0=no, ?=don't know; blank=does not apply

INTENDED BIRTH PLACE, GESTATION, ATTENDANTS

Midwife Code

Birth Number

Planned during pregnancy to have: (1=home birth, 2=birth centre birth, 3=hospital birth)   10

Began labour intending to deliver: (1=at home, 2=in birthing centre, 3=in hospital)

Referral after first assessment in labour

Gestation – midwife's best estimate before   Weeks   Days
birth based on all available information

Mother certain about dates (1=yes ,2=fairly, 3=not)

Attendants at labour and birth

Attendants during labour

Attendants at birth
(1=mother's partner, 2=midwife, 3=2nd midwife,
4=midwife apprentice, 5=friends, 6=children age 1–4,
7=children 5+, 8=other family members, 9=FP or GP,
N=nurse, B=obstetrician, S=other   )

LABOUR SUMMARY

	Day	Month	Year
Date of birth			

Place of birth (1=home, 2=freestanding birth centre,
3=hosp birth room, centre or "LDR", 4=hosp separate
lab/del/rec, 5=hosp OR, 6=other   )

Midwife's role in hospital (if applicable) (1=primary
care giver, 2=doctor's assistant, 3=labour coach,
4=midwife's assistant, 6=not present, 7=   )

Length of Labour:

Total time:	Days	Hours	Minutes
Early Labour		:		11
1st stage		:		12
2nd stage (full dilation)		:	
3rd stage		:	

Approximate total time the woman in labour had a:

	Hours	Minutes
midwife present before birth	:	
apprentice only before birth	:	
midwife present after birth	:	

Amount of time before birth

membranes ruptured	Hour	Minute	AM/PM
Actual time of birth		:	

Plateaus, Reversals, Anterior Lip or Pushing Before Full Dilation

	Dilation		Hours	Minutes
1st stage plateaus	cm	:		
(stayed at same centimetre	cm	:		
assessment for > 2 hours)	cm	:		
	cm	:		

			to	
Cervical reversal (from what cm to what cm)				

	Hours	Minutes
Anterior lip longer than 1 1/2 hours	:		13
Pushing before full dilation	:	
2nd stage plateau(full dilation & no pushing)	:		14

Positions and Mobility

Positions of potential concern   Stage 1
occurring during active labour   Stage 2
(1=posterior, 2=breech, 3=head deep transverse,
4=tranverse lie, 5=acynclitism, 6=face & brow)

Baby's position at delivery (1=anterior, 2=posterior,
3=frank breech, 4=footling breech,5=complete breech,
6=head deep trans, 7=transverse lie, 8=face, 9=brow)

Mother's mobility during labour   Stage 1
(1=mother changed positions frequently,   Stage 2
2=mother didn't choose to take many positions
3= movement restricted by anaesthetic or attachments,
4=movement restricted by staff)

Mother's final delivery position (1=semi-sitting,
2=hands & knees, 3=squatting, 4=standing,5=on side,
6=on back, 7=stirrups, 8=birthing stool, 9=deBy birth
stool, M=McRoberts(thigh hyperflexion),
0=other   )

Underwater birth

LABOUR AND BIRTH PROCEDURES

Induction, Augmentation or IV

Induction (1=pitocin, 2=prostag, 3=nipple stimulation,
4=castor oil, 5=art rupture of memb < 5 cm,
6=art rupture of mem >= 5cm, 7=stripping of membranes,
8=intercourse,   By midwife
9=other   )   By physician
Time until labour started (hours)

Augmentation   By midwife
(use induction codes)   By physician

I.V. initiated (stage)

Other Procedures During Labour

Number of vaginal examinations

Doppler use (1=1st stage, 2=2nd stage, 3=1st and 2nd)

Use of water (0=none,1=bath, 2=shower,   Stage 1
3=jacuzzi, 4=other   )   Stage 2

Drugs (1=analgesics, 2=tranquillizers, 3=sedatives,
4=alcohol, 5=other   )

Medicinal herbs (specify) (1=   )

Other procedures (1=body massage, 2=enema,
3=catheterization,4=other   )

Nourishment during active labour (0=nothing, 2=only
clear fluids or jello, 3=other fluids, 4=solid food)

Perineal Care

Active perineal guidance in 2nd stage
(0=midwife remained passive,1=manual support,
2=massage,3=compresses,4=oils/lubricants,
5=verbal guidance,6=other   )

Episiotomy (1=medio lateral by physician,2=median,
physician,3=medio lateral,midwife, 4=median,midwife)

Perineal tear & degree (0=no tear,1=1st, 2=2nd,
3=3rd(into anal sphincter), 4=4th (into rectal mucosa))

Episiotomy or tear repair (0=no repair)

Local anaesthetic for repair

Labial tear(1=slight, 2=required suture)

Clitoral/urethral tear (1=slight, 2=required suture)

Cervical laceration (2=required suture, 3=extensive)

Hospital or Birth Centre Procedures

Electronic fetal monitoring:(1=internal,2=ext,3=both)

Fetal scalp sample

Cord blood gases

Anaesthesia (1=epidural,2=general,3=pudendal,
block,4=entonox,5=other   )

Forceps (1=outlet,2=low,3=mid,4=rotation,5=other)

Vacuum extraction

Caesarean section

Reason(s) for C-section (1=failure to progress,
2=fetal distress, 3=meconium, 4=not vertex lie,
5=maternal exhaustion, 6=other   )

Midwife considers C-Section necessary
(0=no, 1=yes, 2=possibly, 3=probably)

Apgars (hospital staff assessment)   1 minute
5 minute

TRANSPORT FROM PLANNED HOME BIRTH OR PLANNED BIRTH CENTRE BIRTH

Did the midwife consider transport an emergency?

Transport by– (1=car, 2=ambulance, 3=other)

Labour stage at transport (1=first, 2= second,
3=third, 4=postpartum)

Length of time before or after birth that decision to
transport was made (hrs/mins)

Minutes from decision to arrival at hospital

Reason(s) for transport   Primary reason
(1=failure to progress,   Secondary reason
2=sustained fetal distress, 3=malpresentation,
4=thick meconium, 5=abruptio/praevia, 6=hemorrhage,
7=retained placenta, 8=maternal exhaustion, B=baby's
condition, 9=other   )

Midwife and clients reception at hospital
(1=supportive,2=indifferent,3=unsupportive,4=hostile)

Please note: in general code: 1=yes, 0=no, ?=don't know; blank=does not apply

LABOUR AND DELIVERY FACTORS

Midwife

Birth Number

Delivery Factors

Preterm labour (< 37 weeks)	
Compound presentation	
Shoulder dystocia (1=minor, 2=moderate, 3=severe)	
# of resolution techniques tried	
Most effective tech(_____)	
Fetal bradycardia (prolonged FHT < 110)	
Fetal tachycardia (prolonged FHT > 160)	
Late or deep decels (1=1st stage,2=2nd,3=1 & 2)	
Midwife thinks emotional or social factors may have affected course of labour(<—write details in margin)	
Cord problems (1=only 1 or 2 vessels, 2=very short, 3=around neck tightly, 4=around neck 2+ times, 5=cord prolapse, 6=other_____)	
Other complications (1=shock, 2=uterine prolapse, 3=placenta previa, 4=abruptio placenta, 5=hematoma, 6=embolism, 7=ruptured uterus, 8=anaesthesia complications, 9=other_____)	

Meconium

Stage when meconium noticed	
Density (1=thin, 2=moderate, 3=thick)	
Consistency (1=particulate, 2=well dissolved)	
Colour (1=yellow,2=light green,3=dark green, 4=brown, 5=colour darkened during labour)	

Blood Loss

Prophylatic to avoid hemorrhage (1=oxytocin, 2=sheperd's purse, 3=other_____)	
Estimated blood loss milliliters	
or cups (use 2 decimals – e.g. 1.00, 2.25)	
Postpartum hemorrhage(> 500 ml or 2 1/4 cups)	
Action(s) taken for blood loss (1=fundal massage, 2=nipple stimulation, 3=external bimanual compression, 4=internal bimanual comp, 5=IV fluids, 6=blood transfusion, 7=other_____)	
Drugs (1=pitocin,2=methergine(ergotrate),3=_____	
Herbs:(1=_____)	
D & C	

NEWBORN DATA (first 4 hours)

Number of babies (complete this page for each baby)	
Sex (1=girl, 2=boy)	
Birthweight grams	
OR lbs. ozs	
Apgar (midwife's assessment) 1 minute	
5 minute	
Any clinical evidence that baby is preterm	
Any clinical evidence that baby is postterm	
Stillbirth(1=death before labour, 2=during labour)	
Birth defects(1=minor,2=serious,3=life threatening)	
Specify_____	

Procedures

Resuscitation: (1=suction on the perineum, 2=DeLee, 3=bulb suctioning, 4=tactile stim, 5=oxygen, 6=ambubag, 7=mouth to mouth, 8=chest compressions, 9=intubation, R=respirator, W=wall)	
Eye prophylaxis (1=silver nitrate, 2=erythromycin (ilotycin), 3=sterile water, 4=other_____)	
Vitamin K given (1=oral, 2=IM)	

Immediate neonatal complications

Complications: (1=respiratory distress, 2=meconium aspiration, 3=IUGR, 4=metabolic (hypoglycemia,hypocalcemia), 5=prematurity, 6=seizures, 7=birth injuries_____, 8=other_____)	
Transfer to neonatal intensive care unit	

DELIVERY OF PLACENTA AND MEMBRANES

Cord clamped (1=immediately (before pulsing stopped), 2=after pulsing stopped, 3=after placenta delivered, 4=other_____)	
Cord clamped –# of minutes after birth	
Mother's postion waiting to deliver placenta (1=lying down, 2=standing, 3=squatting, 4=sitting, 5=hands & knees, 6=several positions)	
Method: (1=maternal effort, 2=controlled cord traction,3= manual removal, 4=D&C)	
Membranes appear: (1=complete, 2=incomplete)	
Placenta appears: (1=complete, 2=incomplete)	
Anatomical variations of placenta (1=infarcts, 2=calcium deposits, 3=succenturiate, 4=accreta, 5=other_____)	

POSTPARTUM CARE AND BREASTFEEDING

Number of postpartum visits with midwives	
Estimated postpartum visits: other caregivers	
Final midwife postnatal visit or contact (week)	
Number of weeks breastfed in first 6 weeks	
Number of weeks before any supplement (7=>6 weeks)	
Circumcision in first 6 weeks	

INFANT'S HEALTH IN FIRST 6 WEEKS

Newborn health problems in first 6 weeks (1=jaundice beyond normal physiologic level, 2=sepsis/infection, 3=respiratory distress, 4=failure to thrive,5=premature/immature,6=seizures,7=birth trauma, 8=other (specify)_____)	
Jaundice level if measured (mmol/litre)	

Newborn hospitalized in first 6 weeks

Number of days in neonatal intensive care unit	
Number of days newborn hospitalized in first 6 weeks	
Reason(1=born there,2=baby's cond,3=mother's cond)	
Baby's problem(s) (use newborn health problems)	

Newborn died in first 6 weeks of life

No. of days after birth that death occurred	
Underlying cause of death (1=birth defects, 2=prematurity, 3=other(specify)_____) (Provide details about death in margin ——>)	

MOTHER'S HEALTH IN FIRST 6 WEEKS

Postpartum infections (1=yeast, 2=delayed perineal healing/infection, 3=breast, 4=urinary tract, 5=uterine, 6=febrile episode(>100.4 after first 24 hours))	
Other Postpartum Complications (1= late hemorrhage(after 24 hrs), 2=hypertension, 3=cervical/uterine prolapse, 4=hematoma, 5=pulmonary embolism, 6= thrombophlebitis, 7=eclampsia, 8=anemia (<10 mg), 9=other (Specify)_____)	
Postpartum depression (1=moderate, 2=severe)	
# of days mother hospitalized in first 6 weeks	
Maternal Death	
Underlying cause _____	
(Please provide details about death in margin ——>)	

INFANT'S & MOTHER'S HEALTH at 6 WEEKS

Infant (1=good,no problems, 2=residual problems)	
Mother (1=good,no problems, 2=residual problems)	

FORM COMPLETION

Form filled out by: (initials)

	Day	Month	Year
Date majority of form filled out			

MANA thanks you for spending the time to contribute to its data collection by carefully filling out this form.

Form developed by Kenneth C. Johnson, PhD and Betty~Anne Daviss-Putt. Many thanks to 26 midwives, 5 epidemiologists, 2 psychologists and 1 graphic artist who provided invaluable feedback.
Contact: Betty~Anne Daviss-Putt
36 Glen Avenue, Ottawa, Ontario, CANADA K1S 2Z7
Phone (613) 730 0282 or 432 5701, Pager 593-4917

Protocols of Practice

In order to understand the concept of protocols, it is helpful to first establish some definitions. A **standard** is a specific statement that generally outlines how to carry out an ethical belief. For example, if a midwifery organization sets forth the well-being of mothers and babies as a value, the membership's ethic might be to practice responsibly. One of the standards related to responsibility might be the ability to control a hemorrhage at a birth. **Protocols** outline in detail the specific steps an individual midwife will take to actually carry out the standards set forth. Protocols are generally not set up by the midwifery organization; instead they reflect individual practice. Following our example, one midwife may choose to carry certain herbs and to know bi-manual compression, while another may feel she is not practicing responsibly unless she also carries oxytocin and knows how to set up IVs. Both are fulfilling the stated standard to the extent that they personally feel is necessary to practice responsibly. Protocols arise out of a complex interaction between a midwife's values, ethics, skills and individual concepts of moral integrity/responsibility as well as the education and training she has had and the practice setting in which she works.

Formulating a protocol document: Writing a set of practice protocols can benefit you in a couple of ways. It helps remind you of all the steps you want to take in exploring a situation with a client; have some copies duplicated and make them available to clients and other collaborating health care professionals. Protocols can also provide a certain amount of legal protection in case your practice is questioned. Demonstrating that you followed your protocols will be of great assistance to you if the care you provided is reviewed. Ideally, you can write your protocols on a computer so they can easily be modified as your experience grows.

When formulating your protocols, you can start by making a list of topics which need to be addressed. You might use the table of contents in these and other textbooks to help you formulate such a list. While most protocols focus only on how problems might be handled, I encourage you to include your guidelines regarding how you support maternal and fetal well-being as well as emotional and psychological factors. You should also gather the latest regulations on practice from any midwifery organizations or licensing boards to which you must answer. Next, you can outline what you would do in each circumstance. Introduce the document by explaining its purpose. The following offers an example of how a protocol document might be introduced:

> Protocols outline the most likely course of action in given circumstances which may arise during your midwifery care. In mainstream medicine, protocols focus on actions taken when problems occur, and are usually written in a difficult-to-decipher shorthand. Since the primary focus of our care is on prevention, our protocols for

normal situations are included in addition to those pertinent to complications.

In non-critical situations various options and recommendations will be discussed prior to any action being taken. In cases of critical emergency (which most often takes place at the actual time of birth) time may not be available for discussion before action must be taken. The most probable steps for these cases are outlined herein. Please feel free to ask questions about any of these situations at any time.

Our protocols are presented with the understanding that it is impossible to unequivocally state what will be done in individual situations. To simply follow rules by rote precludes the possibility of considering each woman and circumstance with all their unique variables. We have formulated this statement as to our process after careful evaluation of our usual procedures; it accurately reflects our most likely course of action. Please review the following information with these thoughts in mind.

This could be followed by a table of contents and then a logical progression of information from the establishment of care through the last postpartum visit. Here is one example of a typical entry for a protocol regarding a therapeutic agent:

The Use of Evening Primrose Oil:

Any woman who fits into any of the following categories and who is not a DES daughter will be advised to take 1 to 3 500 mg. capsules daily of Evening Primrose Oil (or Black Currant oil or Borage oil), usually starting at the 36th week of gestation:

*First time mothers
*Women who have had anovulatory cycles
*Women who have taken oral contraceptives or had a progesterone-
    releasing IUD
*Women with cervical surgery, tearing or injury
*First-time YBAC candidates
*Women with severe surgical adhesion problems (one capsule every
    other day throughout pregnancy to increase at 36 weeks as above
    if indicated)

Doses may be adjusted according to parity and the reason for treatment (e.g. less daily for multiparas). DES primigravidas will be assessed for supplementation on an individual basis.

Some of your options for care may be limited by state or local standards for midwives practicing under rules of certification and licensure in your area. When this is so, you can plainly state the case in your protocols, for example:

> <u>Breech presentation</u>: If a breech presentation persists past the 36th week of pregnancy, the guidelines of the Oregon Midwifery Association require that a consult be arranged with a collaborating physician in preparation for a possible hospital birth. State guidelines do not permit certified midwives to attend planned breech births at home at this time. Should the baby's position convert to vertex prior to the onset of labor, we will proceed with homebirth as planned.

Whose protocols are "correct"? Disagreements may arise within the midwifery community as to what constitutes an appropriate protocol. For example, the midwife who carries IVs may accuse the one who does not of practicing unsafely; this is an example of how ethical decisions are challenged, but also reflects how rules evolve out of a thought process which assumes that there is one right answer for every situation. Coming together as a community to review and discuss various approaches to practice can be educational as well as supportive, as each midwife shares her unique knowledge with others. Such sharing will help in minimizing such conflicts.

Legal Issues

Your legal status will greatly impact your practice as a midwife. If you are practicing totally illegally, you will have to be careful about how you make yourself known in the community and how you approach other care providers for back-up. Do your best to make no apologies for your existence. The more paranoid you are, the more likely you will manifest problems for yourself. You do need to talk with your clients about both the legal status of midwifery in your area and the particulars of what this means in the event of a transport.

Transports in an illegal climate can mean that you cannot tell the hospital staff you are a midwife; in order to stay with the woman once she is hospitalized you must pass yourself off as a labor support person. In some cases the medical community will be so hostile that you cannot accompany women into the hospital at all. If you are practicing illegally, exactly what your parameters of care are, your restrictions about getting lab work done, and your rapport or lack thereof with local doctors and nurse-midwives all need to be carefully spelled out with clients. You also need to carefully weigh your choices regarding who you take on as a client and when and if you will transport in certain situations. If you are so afraid of your legal status that you would hesitate to transport a woman who needs medical care, you have no business practicing at all.

Your income is another area of concern if you practice illegally. Some midwives only accept cash, some claim insurance some of the time, some file taxes under a related professional title (childbirth educator and counselor is commonly used). You must talk with accountants and find one willing to work with your illegal status (ask around).

If you practice legally without regulation you are in the best situation possible for developing a truly midwifery-based standard of care. Of course legal practice does not necessarily mean the medical community will offer you open-handed support, but at least it means you can transport without fear that you will be arrested on the hospital doorstep.

If you are state licensed or certified, you are practicing with rules imposed by the government; these frequently do not reflect a truly midwifery model of care. In Wyoming, for example, midwives are allowed to attend homebirths but are not allowed to do prenatal care!! Ridiculously narrow protocols are another problem which accompanies legal practice in many areas. Such rules are largely due to practitioners from a medical model of care who have little understanding of midwifery care or philosophy and are trying to apply hospital-based standards to the homebirth environment. This often sets up a frustrating and, in many respects, unworkable situation in which midwives are not allowed to do their best for women.

Working With Other Midwives

As a midwife you must decide how you will manage your practice and with whom you will work. There are several options:

Solo practice: This means that you are the only primary midwife in your practice. This is, at best, a hard row to hoe. You must be on call constantly, and there is no one to relieve the burden of responsibility no matter how tired, sick or needed you may be by others in your life. It means you will be solely responsible for caring for both mother and baby in an emergency; this is sometimes simply humanly impossible if both need emergency care simultaneously. While you will most likely want to take apprentices with you to births, they cannot be expected to share the responsibility the way a full-fledged partner could. Sometimes midwives in solo practice in adjoining or overlapping geographic areas make arrangements to "take call" for each other or offer mutual support, should the need arise.

Partnership practice: This affords the individual midwife more flexibility in terms of personal time as well as providing the woman seeking care with more perspectives in the event of a question about her condition. Two experienced midwives are on hand at the birth if both mother and baby need attention. Two midwives allow for more rest at births and this makes for a generally saner existence. Of course, this means you must share the wealth and have a practice load which allows both of you to make a living. In some partnership practices, midwives alternate call, taking an apprentice with them to births and only having both primary midwives at the birth in exceptional circumstances (breech or twin births for example). It is nice to find a partnership that balances the weaknesses and strengths of each midwife.

Group practice: Several midwives may decide to start a practice together. The more midwives you have working together, the better it is for them in terms of call time, time off and multiple opinions readily at hand if a problem comes up. On the down side, the women you care for may feel the brunt of this by not being able to pick who they will see for care or have at their birth. If you choose group practice, try to work out an equitable arrangement which balances your needs with women's needs for continuous care. (See chapter on Maintaining Continuity of Care in the section on An Overview of Prenatal Care for some ideas.)

The Midwifery Community

Ah, the midwifery community, that haven of sisterly refuge to which we can always turn when things are difficult, when we have questions, when we need unconditional, undying and unending support. In the best of all possible worlds this may be our vision of midwifery community, but it is far from reality. While there certainly are groups of midwives who function together well, work side by side, and shoulder burdens as well as joys equally, there are many communities where turf battles over clientele exist, where one midwife is seen as better or worse than the rest, or where judgments and condemnations are on the tip of everyone's tongue when a problem occurs at a birth.

This is inevitable because, for all the high calling that we feel for midwifery as a practice, we are still only human. Furthermore, we are women who have generations of oppression behind us. We have learned well to turn on each other when the patriarchy does not support us. The horizontal oppression and emotional violence that can occur in any women's community are frightening. When one midwife has a problem or when we question her skill, it is easy to turn to judgements and recriminations rather than objectively examining the situation or case and deciding upon the best course of action. Often we tend to point the finger lest we be targeted as a problem as well.

To ward off these admittedly regrettable responses to stress within our individual communities, it helps for midwives to strategize together about what means will be used to deal with difficult issues, before those issues arise. As these policies are formulated, each midwife must search her heart as to whether she would feel these procedures fair if she had to undergo them herself.

An individual midwife can also take steps to be sure that she keeps her relationship with the other midwives in her community as clear as possible. Here are some ideas of how you might go about doing this:

* *When moving to a new community, visit the area and contact and connect with as many midwives as possible. Talk to them about their work and practice style, who may need a partner and whatever other aspects of moving to the area seem pertinent. Find out about the receptivity of the local medical community to midwifery and what the legal status of midwifery is in that jurisdiction.
* *Discover what, if any, midwifery associations exist in the area. If there is more than one, find out as much as you can about why this is so.
* *Try to be objective about gossip you hear regarding one midwife or a group of midwives. Get both sides of the story whenever possible. Each time the situation is brought up, try to get as much data as you can from each individual you talk to so that a more

total picture of the situation emerges. Don't offer your opinion, instead tell others you need to talk to the midwife herself and encourage others to do the same.

*If you have a problem birth and there is no structure for addressing this in the birthing community, call a midwifery community meeting *yourself* to have a peer review of the case. Some areas are now calling the process "peer support"; try to bring this attitude to your meetings. Go over your chart with those who attend, asking them to keep the proceedings of the meeting confidential. This way, you will defuse much of the gossip and exaggeration that inevitably crop up around sticky situations such as these. You let your community know that *you* recognize that you are not perfect and welcome their input.

*Try not to let insecurity or minimal experience make you afraid to call upon the expertise of other midwives if the need arises. Likewise, avoid a cock-sure attitude that, because you are quite experienced, the other midwives in your community have nothing to offer you in the way of growth-producing input. Remember, even if the other midwives have been to far fewer births than you, those were different births than any you have attended. It is quite possible they could have gleaned valuable information even though they have a more limited experience base.

*If you have special expertise or experience to offer, make yourself available to your community as a resource. This does not mean that you should endlessly do things for other midwives or their clients free of charge, but it does mean that it helps if you are generous with your knowledge. At the same time do not use it as an ego trip to put other midwives "in their place."

What if your community seems to have a "problem" midwife? It seems that many communities of midwives have one midwife or a small group of midwives that the rest of the community views as a thorn in its side. Although the issue is surely charged, try to distinguish what is really a problem from what others would prefer to be different. Is the midwife's practice dangerous? If so, how? Does she do things that you would not choose to do? If so, what have her outcomes been? (For example, just because you are afraid of breech births and refuse to do them does not mean that if she feels fine about them and does them successfully, *she* is the one with the problem.) Is her knowledge base dangerously lacking or merely different from your own? For example, when I first moved to Detroit, no midwives there used or carried oxytocin, but I had to admit that they dealt with hemorrhage quite adequately when it came up. Just because a midwife works differently than you do does not mean she is incompetent. Is a "spiritual" midwife refusing to intervene in the case of a problem? A very important question to ask is "What are her outcomes?" If her clients clearly understand that this is the way she practices, what her outcomes have been, and that other birth attendants with different ideas are available, they are free to make that choice. Is it not so much something specific, but everything in general? Does this midwife lie to you or her clients? Does she misrepresent things at meetings or to others about the midwifery community in general? Do you suspect that she has less experience than she claims to have? Is she not dealing with problems simply because she isn't detecting them? These are bigger and more real problems that are, unfortunately, harder to deal with. The best you can do is to encourage the midwifery community to deal with her as directly as possible. If letters, groups discussions, etc. do not produce satisfactory results, the group's only recourse may be to take whatever steps are already in place to deal with someone who is not willing or able to work with the rest of the birthing community. This is a painful and inadequate solution, but may be the limit of your ability to influence the situation.

What if you seem to be the problem? If your midwifery community as a whole has problems, try to evaluate your role in these problems. If many of your colleagues are urging you to change your practice or get psychological help, or if you seem to be the constant focus of strife in your community, consider that perhaps they see something that you are unaware of. Midwifery is a demanding profession and puts us in a position to be seen as a heroine by birthing women. As such, it offers powerful psychological reinforcement for those of us who are extremely co-dependent and need to be needed, or have other emotional issues which have not been brought to consciousness. Be humble enough to at least admit that there may be a kernel of truth to what is being said. Most of all, get an objective opinion from a counselor or therapist so that you are not bringing dangerous psychological imbalances to the women seeking your care. This is a set-up for making poor judgements or compounding an already volatile situation. In therapy, you can not only get a grip on your personal situation, but can find new ways to communicate with others in your community and, hopefully, come to a more balanced relationship all around.

BASIC ANATOMY AND PHYSIOLOGY FOR MIDWIVES

An Introduction to Anatomy and Physiology for Midwives

No other comprehensive midwifery textbook attempts to cover general anatomy and physiology. You may be wondering why it is included here. Midwives need a basic knowledge of how the body works. While this understanding varies given the healing modalities you choose to use, having an understanding from the Western medical viewpoint is helpful in reading other medical texts and conversing with bio-technical medical care providers. This section can also help you when you do general physical exams on mothers or babies, in the study of embryology, when interpreting lab tests, when trying to understand the impact of a particular disease condition or infection on the body, and in understanding what might be going on when a woman explains her symptoms. Only by understanding what is normal can you then confidently assess what is abnormal. A knowledge of basic A&P facilitates this understanding.

Each chapter will be introduced with a brief explanation highlighting just a few of the ways the information can help you in practice. If you are in primary practice, it is my hope that this section will provide you with pertinent information on each topic without belaboring unnecessary details. Throughout, I have attempted to include slightly more information than you will typically need to ensure that this text can serve as a primary reference for this type of information. This section explains what is normal in a nonpregnant woman first. The last chapter then goes through each organ system and describes the changes that occur during pregnancy. I have chosen to place this information together in a separate chapter because you may find it necessary to reference these changes specifically and I thought this the best way to make the information accessible.

The A&P section covers the functioning of the physical body from the most basic biochemical level to the interrelationship of the organ systems within it. Much of the information that is most distant from what you will need to know in clinical practice is given as brief definitions and included primarily for reference.

For years, the human body has been described in bio-technical as a complex machine. Actually the body is an expression of the spirit within, an energy filed in constant interaction with all other energy fields. As such, it is infinitely more complicated and integrated than any machine we know. However, as I attempt to simplify this information as much as possible, some of my writing may also tend to reflect this mechanistic language. While, the male body is often put forth in textbooks as the "norm," this book, in its drawings and explanations, will assume discussion of the female body as the "norm" unless otherwise noted. After all, all fetuses start out female and midwives are primarily dealing with the female body. Keeping these things in mind, this section is a crash course in A & P for midwives. Please note that all references are placed at the end of this entire section, rather than at the end of each chapter.

<u>Anatomy and Physiology: An Overview</u>

Let's start with some basic definitions. **Anatomy (ah-NAT-oe-me)** refers to the study of bodily parts and the relationships between them. **Physiology (fiz-e-OL-oh-gee)** deals with the functions of the body parts, i.e. how they work. The human body is organized into interacting networks as follows:

Chemical—the most basic level includes all atomic and molecular substances essential for maintaining life.

Cellular—chemicals are organized into cells, the smallest body part capable of self-sufficient life.

Tissues—groups of similar cells and the substances between them that perform special functions.

Organs—different kinds of tissues joined together in a definite form as a functional unit; for example, the brain, the liver, and the placenta are all organs.

Systems—consist of a group of organs which all have a common function such as the digestive system or the skeletal system.

Organism—all parts considered together; an individual animal or plant.

Life processes: Organisms are differentiated from non-living things by certain processes they undergo which support physical life, such as **metabolism (me-TAB-oh-lizem)** which is the sum total of all the chemical processes that occur in the body. The **catabolism (cah-TAB-oh-lizem) phase** of this process provides the organism with the energy needed to sustain life by breaking down chemical compounds into usable parts. The **anabolism (ah-NAB-oh-lizem) phase** uses that energy to combine or synthesize various chemical substances that form the cells. Many bodily functions contribute to metabolism, such as:

*Ingestion**—the taking in of foods

*Absorption**—the uptake of substances by cells

*Assimilation**—the formation of absorbed elements into substances required by the cells

*Respiration**—the exchange of gases with the environment

*Secretion**—the production or release of a useful substance by the cells

*Excretion**—the elimination of wastes produced by the metabolic process

These processes help the body to maintain a state of **homeostasis** or balance. As part of this balancing act, the body also has two other activities which further its existence:

Growth: an increase in the size and/or number of existing cells.

Reproduction: the formation of new cells for growth, repair or replacement, or the creation of an entirely new individual.

Very Basic Chemistry

The understanding of basic chemistry may not seem very relevant to daily clinical midwifery practice. However, when you are struggling to understand such technical procedures as the pH level of fetal scalp blood samples, fetal acid status in relationship to fetal distress in labor, and why it is important for women to eat enough salt in pregnancy, some basic chemistry will help you to grasp those concepts more clearly. This chapter is intended to provide you with background and reference information.

All things which exist are made up of **energy**. On the physical plane, energy takes the form of **matter**, which is anything which occupies space and has mass (i.e., substance or weight). Matter may exist in a solid, liquid or gaseous state. All forms of matter are made up of a limited number of building units called **chemical elements**. These are substances which cannot be broken down into simpler substances by ordinary chemical reactions. There are currently 89 recognized naturally occurring chemical elements. There are 20 additional artificial elements and that number is gradually increasing. Elements are designated by letter abbreviations, usually derived from the first or second letter of the Latin or English name. These are called **chemical symbols**. Examples of such symbols are: **H** for hydrogen, **C** for carbon and **O** for oxygen.

About 26 elements are normally found in the human body, with oxygen, carbon, hydrogen and nitrogen making up 96% of the body's weight. In practical terms, about 45 to 75% of adult body weight is made up of water. Together with carbon, nitrogen, calcium and phosphorus, these chemicals constitute about 99% of the total body weight. Twenty other elements in trace amounts compose the remaining 1%. Here is a list of the main chemical elements in the human body:

Chemical element	How the element functions in the body:
Oxygen (O)	Found in water and organic molecules, functions in cellular respiration
Carbon (C)	Found in all organic molecules
Hydrogen (H)	Found in water, all foods, and most organic molecules
Nitrogen (N)	Found in all protein molecules and nucleic acid molecules
Calcium (Ca)	Found in bones and teeth; required for blood clotting, intake and output of substances through cell membranes, motility of cells, movement of chromosomes before cell division, glycogen metabolism, neurotransmission and muscle contraction
Phosphorus (P)	Part of many proteins and nucleic acids; required for normal bones and teeth, found in nerve tissue
Chloride (Cl)	Combined with sodium, it helps move water between cells
Sulfur (S)	Part of many proteins, especially contractile proteins of muscles

Chemical element	How the element functions in the body:
Potassium (K)	Required for growth and important in conduction of nerve impulses and muscle contraction
Sodium (Na)	Combined with chloride it is a component of bone, essential in maintaining blood fluid balance and is needed for conduction of nerve impulses
Magnesium (Mg)	Component of many enzymes
Iodine (I)	Vital to functioning of thyroid gland
Iron (Fe)	Essential part of hemoglobin and respiratory enzymes

<u>**Atoms and molecules**</u>: Elements are pure substances that cannot be decomposed into simpler substances. Atoms are the smallest units of elements that enter into chemical reactions. An element is therefore a quantity of atoms which are all alike. Atoms consist of two basic parts, the **nucleus** and the **electrons**.

The centrally located nucleus contributes most of an atom's weight and contains positively charged particles called **protons (p^+)** and may contain uncharged or neutral particles called **neutrons (n^0)**. Together they are referred to as the **nucleus**. Because of the presence of the protons, the nucleus itself has a positive charge. It is the number of protons that distinguishes one type of atom from another. **Electrons (e^-)** are negatively charged particles that orbit the nucleus in unfixed three-dimensional variously shaped clouds called **orbitals**. This path is irregular and may occur anywhere in the

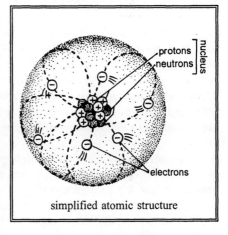

simplified atomic structure

cloud. This is called its **path of probability**, because there is no guarantee it will be found in this area, but there is a good chance it will be. In nature, most atoms exist in a charged state. If there are more protons than electrons, that atom has a net positive charge and is called a **cation**. Other atoms have a net negative charge; that is, they have more electrons than protons, and are called **anions**.

Molecules are groups of atoms bonded together. Molecules are made of the same type of atom (oxygen—O_2). A compound contains two or more different types of atoms. An example is water—H_2O, consisting of two atoms of hydrogen and one atom of oxygen. Molecules and compounds can have a positive or negative charge. For example, phosphate molecules have a negative charge (PO_4^-).

Chemical processes: When atoms combine with or break apart from other atoms, a **chemical reaction** occurs, which produces new products with different properties. These reactions are the foundation of all life processes on the physical plane.

The atoms in molecules and compounds are held together by forces of attraction called **chemical bonds**, which can be either ionic or covalent. Chemical reactions are the making or breaking of bonds between molecules.

Molecules and compounds are formed when atoms are able to take on or give up additional electrons and therefore combine to balance their electrons. Atoms which give up electrons are called **electron donors**. Those which tend to pick up electrons are called **electron acceptors**. Ionic bonding results from the electrostatic interaction between ions. When a positively charged atom and a negatively charged atom are attracted to each other, an **ionic bond** is formed.

A **covalent bond** occurs when neither of the combining atoms loses or gains an electron; instead they share one, two or three electron pairs. Two atoms of the same type may form a covalent bond. Covalent bonds are far more common in organisms than ionic bonds and are far more strong and stable.

A **hydrogen bond** consists of a hydrogen atom covalently bonded to one oxygen atom or one nitrogen atom, but attracted to another oxygen or nitrogen atom. This weak bond can serve as a bridge between or within molecules, but does not form a molecule by itself because of the weakness of the bond. A few elements already have the maximum number of electrons in their outermost energy level and therefore do not naturally seek to combine with other elements. These are called **inert elements** or **noble gases**; an example is helium.

Elemental atoms of the same type may have differing numbers of neutrons in their nucleus giving them different nuclear masses. Due to this variation, the atomic weight for a given element is only an average. Atoms of a given element with differing numbers of neutrons are called **isotopes**.

Radioisotopes are isotopes that are unstable because they continuously undergo alteration of their nuclear structure as they try to form a more stable configuration. This nuclear "decay" process causes the atoms to emit radiation. Radioisotopes are used in several medical tests, where their path is followed through the body by detecting their radiation emission.

Most of the chemicals in the body exist in the form of compounds. **Inorganic compounds** are small, ionically bonded molecules that lack carbon. Some are vital to bodily function; they include water, many of the salts, as well as acids and bases. **Organic compounds** are molecules which contain carbon.

Energy: Chemical reactions produce **energy**, which is the capacity to do work. **Potential energy** is inactive or stored, and **kinetic energy** is the energy of motion. Energy exists in several different forms:

> **Chemical energy** is released or absorbed in the breakdown or formation of chemical bonds. This energy is utilized when we metabolize food.
>
> **Mechanical energy** is that which is directly involved in movement.
>
> **Radiant energy,** such as heat and light, travels in waves. Some heat is released during breakdown processes in the body; this helps maintain body temperature.
>
> **Electrical energy** is the result of the flow of charges, electrons or charged atoms called ions. It is essential for the conduction of nerve impulses. Our muscles will not work without the electrical impulses from the attached nerves.

Energy can be transformed from one form into another.

Acids, bases and salts: Bodily fluids are mostly water and must maintain a fairly constant balance of acids and bases to sustain life. A solution is acidic when it contains a large amount of the hydronium (H^+) ion, a proton. An acid compound, such as hydrochloric acid (HCl), will tend to give up H^+ ions. A solution is defined as basic or alkaline if it contains high concentrations of the hydroxyl (OH^-) ion. A basic compound, sodium hydroxide (NaOH) will tend to give up OH^- ions. A salt is a compound that contains a cation other than H^+ and an anion other than OH^-. Acids and bases combine with one another to form salts.

When molecules of inorganic compounds such as acids, bases, or salts are dissolved in water, they undergo **ionization (i-on-i-ZA-shun)**; that is, they break apart into ions. Such atoms are called **electrolytes (e-LECK-trow-lites)** because they will conduct an electric current. Electrolytes in the body consist of essential minerals which help maintain normal fluid balance, conduct electrical impulses in the nerves and muscles, and make up the skeletal system among many other functions. Serum electrolytes consist of ions dissolved in the blood that are responsible for maintaining pH in the body.

What is pH? The term **pH (potential of hydrogen)** is used to describe the degree of acidity or alkalinity (basicity) of a solution. pH is discussed by using a scale of 1 to 14, with 1 being the most acidic and 14 being most alkaline; 7.0, the midpoint of the scale, is neutral; that is, it is neither acid nor alkaline. A solution becomes more acidic as its hydrogen ion concentration rises. A pH of 5.0 is more acid (i.e., less alkaline) than one of 6.0. The difference between the two figures is negative and logarithmic; each number is a multiple of -10. Each value represents an enormous difference in hydrogen concentration. A pH of 7.20 is a 40% increase

86

of hydrogen compared to 7.35. Each whole pH number represents a tenfold change from the previous value. The range of blood pH compatible with life is 6.8 to 7.8. When an organism's delicate acid/base ratio is altered, an excessively acid or alkaline state results.

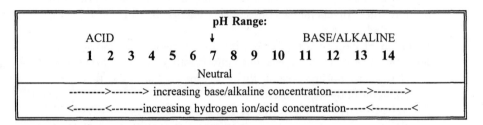

Biochemical reactions (reactions that occur in living systems) are very sensitive to small changes in the pH balance. A **buffer system** is a reserve of molecules which are utilized as needed to help resist large swings in pH; its essential function is to react with strong acids or bases in the body and replace them with weak acids or bases that will change the pH values only slightly. Carbonic acid and bicarbonate are both produced by the body and are important buffers involved in the maintenance of normal blood pH.

Organic compounds: Organic compounds always contain carbon and hydrogen. Carbon is a unique life-supporting element. Because it has four electrons in its outer shell, it can combine with a variety of other atoms, including other carbon atoms, to form straight chains, or branched chains and ring-shaped molecules. Organic compounds, held together almost entirely by covalent bonds, include carbohydrates, fats, proteins, nucleic acids (DNA and RNA) and adenosine triphosphate (ATP).

Carbohydrates are a large group of organic compounds known as **sugars** and **starches**. Their principal function is to provide the most readily available source of energy to sustain life. They are mainly composed of carbon, hydrogen and oxygen. There are three basic types of carbohydrates:

Monosaccharides (mon-oh-SACK-ah-rides) are simple sugars containing three to seven carbon atoms. Glucose and fructose are in this category. Although they have the same types of atoms, they are arranged differently, resulting in two different sugars.

Disaccharides (die-SACK-ah-rides) consist of two monosaccharides which are chemically joined. This combining process results in the loss of a water molecule and is called **dehydration synthesis**. Sucrose, or white table sugar, is an example of this carbohydrate; it is a combination of fructose and glucose. Disaccharides can be broken down into small molecules by adding water; this is called **digestion**.

Polysaccharides (pol-e-SACK-ah-rides) are long chains of monosaccharides joined together through dehydration synthesis; they lack the sweetness of sugars. One of the main polysaccharides is glycogen.

Lipids, or fats, are composed of carbon, hydrogen and oxygen. Among these are fats, phospholipids (lipids that contain phosphorus), steroids, carotenes, vitamins E and K and prostaglandins. A fat molecule (triglyceride) consists of one molecule of glycerol and three of fatty acids. Lipids form via a dehydration process as water is lost. Fats represent the body's most highly concentrated source of energy, but are 10 to 12% less efficient as body fuels than are carbohydrates. There are several varieties of fats:

A **saturated fat** contains no double bonds between any of its carbon atoms, and all the carbon atoms are bonded to the maximum number of hydrogen atoms; thus this fat is saturated with hydrogen atoms. Most of these are animal fats which remain solid at room temperature.

Unsaturated fat contains one or more double covalent bonds between its carbon atoms and is not completely saturated with hydrogen atoms. Examples are olive and peanut oil which remain liquid at room temperature.

Polyunsaturated fats contain two or more double covalent bonds between their carbon atoms. Corn, safflower and sunflower oils are examples of polyunsaturated fats.

Prostaglandins (pros-tah-GLAN-dens) are a large group of membrane-associated fats composed of 20 carbon fatty acids containing five carbon atoms joined to form a ring. They are called local hormones because they are produced by cells in certain localized areas of the body (such as the uterine musculature) and influence the functioning of their neighbor cells. Although synthesized in minute amounts, they simulate hormones and are involved in the regulation of many hormonal responses.

Proteins are complex structures responsible for many bodily activities. Proteins in the form of enzymes speed up many essential biochemical reactions. Antibodies are proteins that provide defenses against disease conditions. Chemically, proteins always contain carbon, hydrogen, nitrogen and oxygen. Many also contain sulfur and phosphorus. **Amino acids** are the building blocks of proteins. The bonds between amino acids are called peptide bonds. Amnio acids combine to form more complex molecules, called polypeptides, while water molecules are lost through dehydration synthesis. At least 20 different amino acids are found in proteins. Specific combinations of some of these amino acids produce different types of proteins.

Nucleic (new-CLAY-ick) acids are large organic molecules containing carbon, hydrogen, oxygen, nitrogen and phosphorus. The basic units of nucleic acids are **nucleotides**. Each of these contains three basic parts:

1. A nitrogen base; these are ring-shaped structures containing carbon, hydrogen, oxygen and nitrogen. They can be one of five possible nitrogen bases: the double-ringed structures of adenine and thymine (called purines) or the single ringed structures of cytosine, guanine and uracil (called pyrimidines).
2. A pentose sugar (either deoxyribose or ribose)
3. A phosphate group

Deoxyribonucleic (dee-ox-see-rye-bow-new-KLAY-ick) acid (DNA) is a molecule consisting of two strands of chemicals with crossbars (a ladder), which twist about each other to form a spiral staircase shape. The uprights of the ladder consist of alternating phosphate groups and deoxyribose portions of the nucleotides. The rungs of the ladder have two halves which consist of paired nitrogen bases. Adenine always pairs with thymine, and cytosine always pairs with guanine. **Genes** are segments of DNA molecules. They determine our inherited traits and control bodily activities throughout our lifetime. When a cell divides, its hereditary information is passed on to the next generation of cells via the genes.

Ribonucleic acid (RNA) is single stranded and its sugar is ribose. It does not contain thymine, but does contain the nitrogen base uracil. RNA has a specific role to perform with DNA in protein synthesis reactions.

Adenosine (a-DEN-oh-sin) triphosphate (try-FOSS-fate) (ATP) is essential to the life of the cell, because it stores energy for various cellular activities. It consists of the phosphate groups adenine and the ribose sugar. When its energy is released, another type of molecule, **adenosine diphosphate (ADP)**, is formed. ADP can be converted back to ATP using the energy supplied by various breakdown reactions, especially that of glucose.

Cyclic adenosine-3',5'-monophosphate (cyclic AMP) is a molecule of adenosine monophosphate with the phosphate attached to the ribose sugar at two places. It functions in certain hormonal reactions.

The Structure of Cells

A knowledge of cellular structure is useful in midwifery in understanding how certain microbes get into the system, in the study of embryology, in understanding how gamete (ova and sperm) production occurs, and in learning how the body heals tissues.

A **cell** is the basic living, structural and functional unit of an organism. **Cytology** is the study of cells. In discussing the structure of cells, it is easiest to look at a generalized cell model, since there are many different types of cells in the body. There are three basic parts of a cell:

   *Plasma (cell) membrane** is the outer, limiting membrane separating the cell's internal parts from the extracellular fluid and external environment.
   *Cytoplasm** is the substance between the nucleus (center) of the cell and the plasma membrane that surrounds it. It contains **organelles** which are tiny permanent structures within the cells. Each one has a characteristic make up which is highly specialized for specific cellular activities. **Inclusions**, the secretions and storage products of cells, are also found within the cytoplasm
   *Nucleus**, an organelle, is the "control center" of the cell where cellular function is mediated.

Cellular chemistry:

The plasma membrane consists of phospholipids and proteins, as well as smaller amounts of cholesterol, glycolipids (combined lipids and carbohydrates) water, carbohydrates and ions.

A double layer of phospholipids forms the basic fabric of the plasma membrane. Various proteins within this layer assist in transferring substances in and out of the cell; they also help recognize other live cells, various hormones, nutrients and other chemicals. These proteins serve as enzymes that stimulate cellular reactions such as respiration. They may also assist in changing the shape of the cell membrane during cell division, movement and digestion.

Cellular functions: A membrane is **permeable** to a substance if it allows the free passage of that substance. The cell's **plasma membrane** has the ability to permit certain substances to enter and exit while restricting the passage of others. This is called **selective permeability**. The movement of substances across cell membranes is essential to life. Transport processes can be divided into active and passive transfer. **Passive processes** occur without assistance from the cells when the concentration of a substance is high outside the cell and low inside of it; thus the force of the external pressure pushes the molecules into the cell. There are several varieties:

Diffusion depends on the tendency of molecules to scatter themselves evenly throughout their environment; it occurs when there is a greater movement of molecules from a region of higher concentration to a region of lower concentration. This movement continues until the molecules are evenly distributed, when they begin to flow back and forth at an equal rate.

Facilitated transport occurs when molecules combine with protein carrier molecules in the plasma membranes and are released into the cytoplasm.

Osmosis is the movement of pure water molecules through a selectively permeable membrane, such as a blood vessel, from an area of higher particle concentration to an area of lower particle concentration. (Particles include salt and serum albumins.) The more dissolved solids the solution contains, the greater the movement of water into the solution from an area containing fewer solids. Osmosis is an important force in the movement of water between various parts of the body and is key to understanding why sufficient salt and protein maintain a pregnant woman's circulating blood volume.

Filtration moves solvents such as water and dissolved substances such as sugar across a selectively permeable membrane by gravity or by mechanical pressure, usually created by water. This always occurs from an area of higher pressure to one of lower pressure.

Dialysis is the diffusion of solid particles across a selectively permeable membrane by separating the smaller molecules from the larger molecules. This probably does not take place in the body and is mainly employed through the use of artificial kidney machines.

Active processes occur when energy from outside or inside the cell contributes to movement of a substance across the membrane. In this case the concentration of the molecules on the outside of the cell is lower than it is within it.

Endocytosis occurs when the cell membranes surrounds a substance, encloses it and brings it into the cell.

Exocytosis occurs when the cell exports substances by reverse endocytosis.

Cellular structure: The main body of the cell inside the membrane and external to the nucleus is called the **cytoplasm**. It is a jelly-like, semitransparent, elastic fluid containing suspended particles such as proteins, carbohydrates, lipids and inorganic substances. A series of minute tubules and filaments form a cytoskeleton, which provides the cell with support and shape. Cytoplasm is the site of some chemical reactions whereby new substances are synthesized for cellular use. It also readies chemicals for transport to other parts of the cell or to other cells and helps excrete waste.

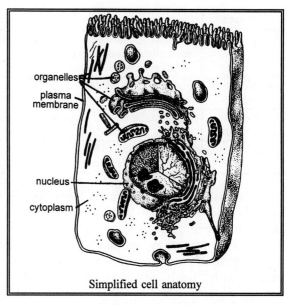

Simplified cell anatomy

Organelles are structures which provide a system of compartmentalization so that cellular processes do not interfere with each other. These structures assume specific roles in growth, maintenance, repair and control within the cell.

Organelle	Function
Nucleus	The largest structure within the cell. Contains genes and controls cellular activities
Ribosomes	Sites of protein synthesis
Endoplasmic Reticulum (ER)	Contributes to mechanical support; conducts intracellular nerve impulses in muscle cells; assists intracellular exchange of materials with cytoplasm; provides a surface for chemical reactions; provides a pathway for transporting chemicals; serves as a storage area; together with Golgi Apparatus synthesizes and packages molecules for export
Golgi Apparatus	Works with ER to export substances; forms lysosomes (to break down molecules); secretes lipids; synthesizes carbohydrates; combines carbohydrates with proteins to form glycoproteins for secretion
Mitochondria	Site of production of adenosine triphosphate (ATP)
Lysosomes	Digest substances & foreign microbes, may be involved with bone removal
Peroxisomes	Contains several enzymes related to hydrogen peroxide metabolism
Microfilaments	Form part of cytoskeleton; involved in muscle cell contraction; provide support & shape; assist in cellular & intracellular movement

Organelle	Function
Microtubules	Form part of cytoskeleton; provide support & shape; act as intracellular conducting channels; assist in cellular movement; form the structure of some specialized cell parts
Intermediate filaments	Form part of cytoskeleton; may provide structural reinforcement for some cells
Centrioles & centrosome	Help organize cellular components during division
Flagella & cilia	Allow movement of the entire cell (flagella) or movement of particles along the cell's surface (cilia)

Inclusion bodies are stored substances in the cytoplasm. They include **melanin,** the pigment in skin, hair and eyes that screens out ultraviolet rays; **glycogen** (stored glucose) and **lipids** (stored in fat cells) both of which can be broken down for energy, and **mucus** which provides lubrication and protection.

Extracellular materials are substances outside of the cell membrane. These include body fluids which provide a medium for dissolving, mixing and transporting substances.

Within the cell, complex activities take place to produce and reproduce proteins of various kinds for use by other cells and organs. Incompletely understood processes serve to maintain and repair DNA molecules, which carry the genetic code for the organism.

Cellular reproduction: The above structures contribute to cell maintenance on a daily basis. However, cells may become damaged, diseased or worn out and then die; but most cells have a programmed lifespan. **Cell division** is the process by which cells reproduce themselves. It consists of the division of the nucleus and the cytoplasm, a process known as **mytosis.**

When any cell reproduces it must duplicate its chromosomes so that the genetic information can be passed to the new cell. A **chromosome** is a tightly coiled DNA molecule that is partly covered by a protein which causes changes in the length and thickness of the chromosome. The hereditary information of the genes is contained in the DNA portion of the chromosome. During the metabolic phase of division the cell prepares to double all of its components so that it may reproduce itself. Remember that DNA is a molecule consisting of two strands of chemicals with crossbars (a ladder) which twist about each other to form a spiral staircase shape. When DNA replicates, it partially uncoils and splits in half down the middle of each "stair rung" at the point where the nitrogen bases are connected. It now looks like a ladder cut lengthwise down the middle. Each exposed nitrogen base then searches out its complimentary nitrogen base from the cytoplasm in the cell. This pairing continues until each of the two strands of split DNA have formed two new DNA strands. Thus one chromosome becomes two. Most somatic cells in humans have two sets of 23 chromosomes each, a total of 46 chromosomes, making them **diploid** cells. The second set is a duplicate. Two chromosomes that are alike (a pair) are called **homologous (ho-MOL-oh-gus)**.

Two types of division occur:

Somatic cell division occurs when a single parent cell duplicates itself. This process consists of a nuclear division which occurs through **mitosis** and cytokinesis. It ensures that each new daughter cell has the same number and kind of chromosomes as the original parent cell. Each cell is identical in genetic makeup after this process is complete. This is the type of division which increases the number of body cells. During a 24 hour period the average adult must replace billions of cells from different parts of the body.

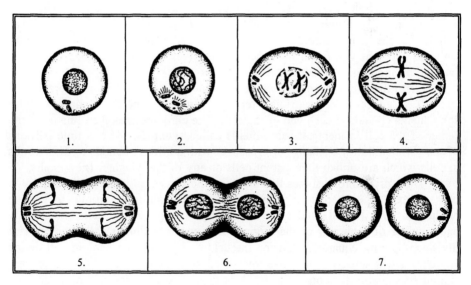

1. Before division, the nucleus contains chromatin (chiefly consisting of DNA). The contrioles are close together.
2. The chromatin condenses into 46 chromosomes and the centrioles start to move to opposite sides of the cell. Spindle fibers develop around them.
3. Each chromosomes doubles itself. The nucleus' membrane begins to break and disappear and it's contents mix with the cytoplasm. Centrioles reach opposite sides of the cell.
4. Spindle fibers stretch across the cell. Chromosome pairs line up in the center (only two pairs are shown).
5. Two halves of each chromosome pair separate and move to opposite sides of the

cell.

6. Two new nuclear membranes develop. The chromosomes turn back into chromatin. Two new cellular membranes develop, cytokinesis. The cell division is almost complete.

7. The two new cells are born—identical in all respects to the parent cell and each other.

Reproductive cell division is the unique process by which sperm and ova are reproduced in preparation for conception. **Gametes**, or sex cells, have only half the chromosomes of somatic cells. Their special division process causes them to give up one set of duplicate chromosomes so that the mature gamete has only 23. These are called **haploid (HAP-loyd) cells**, meaning "one-half."

This process begins with a parent cell containing a full compliment of 46 chromosomes. Cell reproduction consists of a nuclear division called **meiosis** plus cytokinesis. A diploid parent cell divides into two daughter cells each with half the original number of chromosomes. Unlike other cells, reproductive cells must leave only half of the genetic information in each new cell. That half can then match up with the half that will be in the other **gamete** (sex cell) it combines with, thus creating a unique genetic pattern.

First, the chromosomes shorten and thicken, the nuclear membrane and nucleoli disappear, the centrioles replicate and a spindle of these cellular components appears at each end of the cell. The chromosomes then line up in the center of the cell in identical pairs; this is called **synapsis**. At this time portions of one chromatid may exchange or **crossover** with portions of another. This results in cells which are unlike their parent cells or any of the daughter (new) cells.

The paired chromosomes line up along the equatorial plane of the cell, with one member of each pair on either side. (This pairing is unique to gamete production.) As the cell divides into two, each resulting daughter cell contains only one member of each pair of the original chromosomes; this is called **equatorial division**. During equatorial division the centromeres of each haploid cell divide and chromatids separate and move toward opposite poles of the cell in a process similar to somatic division. The DNA is then replicated and a further division occurs, resulting in four haploid cells. All four of these develop into sperm in men, but only one of the four will develop into an ovum in women.

Anatomical Terminology

There are a number of special terms used to describe the location of the various parts of the body. These terms provide a universal and consistent reference for discussions. While they may be a bit technical to use with the average client, it is a good idea to familiarize yourself with them so you sound knowledgeable when talking to other health care providers. To start, you should know that there is a universally accepted stance which is referred to as the **anatomical position**. This positioning is the starting point for defining the references in the chart which follows. In the anatomical position, the body is standing erect and facing forward, the feet are together, and the arms are hanging at the sides with the palms facing forward. The following pages contain tables describing directional references commonly used in anatomy and physiology textbooks.

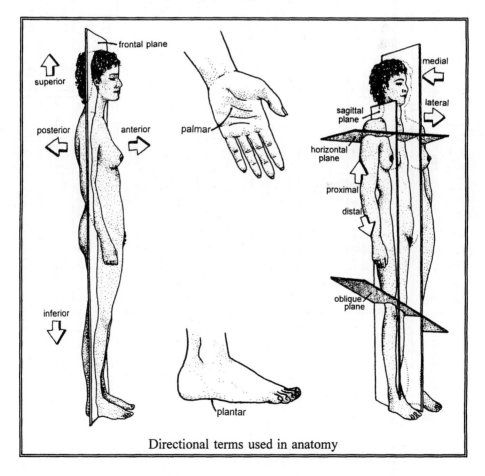

Directional terms used in anatomy

Directional terms describing the location of structures within the body as a whole:

Term	Definition	Example
Superior (cephalad)	Toward the head or the topmost part	The heart is superior to the stomach
Inferior (caudal)	Away from the head or toward the lower part (toward the feet)	The stomach is inferior to the heart
Anterior (ventral)	Toward the front of the body	The rib cage is anterior to the heart
Posterior (dorsal)	Toward the back or spine	The esophagus is posterior to the trachea
Medial	Nearer the middle or midline of the body	The ulna bone is on the medial side of the forearm
Lateral	Farther from the midline of the body	The ascending colon is lateral to the bladder
Intermediate	Between two structures	The heart is located intermediate to the lungs
Ipsilateral	On the same side	The left leg and left arm are ipsilateral
Contralateral	On the opposite side	The left leg and right arm are contralateral
Proximal	Toward (nearer) the trunk of the body; toward the attached end of a limb	The wrist is proximal to the fingers, the shoulder is proximal to the wrist
Distal	Farther from the attachment of an extremity to the trunk, a structure, or from the point of origin	The fingers are distal to the wrist, the wrist is distal to the forearm
Superficial	Toward the surface	The skin is superficial to the internal organs
Deep	Away from the surface	The muscles of the arm are deep to the skin surface
Parietal	Pertaining to or forming the outer wall of a body cavity, or the membrane lining the walls of a body cavity	The pleural membrane is a parietal structure
Visceral	An internal organ or body cavity or a membrane covering an internal organ	The abdominal cavity
Plantar	Special term referring to the sole of the foot	The sole of the foot is the plantar surface, the upper surface is dorsal
Palmar	Special term referring to the palm of the hand	The palmar surface of the hand and the outer or dorsal surface
Upper extremities	Upper limbs	Shoulders, upper arms, forearms, wrists & hands
Lower extremities	Lower limbs	Thighs, legs, ankles & feet

Term	Definition	Example

Body cavities	Spaces containing internal organs:
	The **Dorsal cavity** contains the cranial & spinal cavities:
	   Cranial—The skull
	   Spinal cavity—bony spinal canal
	The **Ventral cavity** includes the following:
	   Thoracic—chest area above the diaphragm, subdivided into:
	     Pleural cavity
	     Pericardial cavity
	     Mediastinum, containing the mass of tissues and organs separating the two lungs
	
	   Abdominal (peritoneal)—From below the diaphragm to a line running from the sacral promontory to the pubic bone
	   Pelvic—the area contained by the pelvic girdle
		Contains the brain
		Contains the spinal cord
		
		Contains the lungs
		Contains the heart
		Contains the esophagus, heart, attached blood vessels, trachea, thymus gland, some nerves & pericardial cavity (everything but the lungs)
		
		Contains the liver, gallbladder, stomach, pancreas, spleen, kidneys & intestines
		Contains the bladder, sigmoid colon, rectum & internal reproductive organs

Plane	Imaginary flat surfaces obtained by "cutting" through the body along specific lines, as follows:
	   Sagittal (SAJ-i-tal)—vertical plane dividing the body into right and left halves (also called cross-section)
	   Frontal (coronal [koh-ROW-nall]—divides the body along the side into front and back halves
	
	   Horizontal (transverse)—divides parallel to the ground (cuts the body in half)
	   Oblique (intermediate)—between horizontal & longitudinal
		A midsagittal section of the pelvic bones shows them cut down the middle, from front to back (the left or right half)
		A frontal section of the head would divide it from the top of the head, down through the ears to the neck. The face half would be the frontal section.
		A transverse section of the torso would cut the body through the waist
		An oblique section of the body would be cut at a 45° angle between the horizontal & vertical planes

98

Term	Definition	Example
Quadrants upper right, upper left, lower right, lower left	**Upper right quadrant**	Liver, pancreas, upper right small intestines, upper right ascending & transverse colon, right kidney
	Upper left quadrant	Stomach, spleen, upper left small intestine, upper left descending & transverse colon, left kidney
	Lower right quadrant	Lower right small intestine & ascending colon, appendix, right uterine tube & ovary
	Lower left quadrant	Lower left small intestine & descending colon, left uterine tube & ovary
Body Regions right hypochondriac region, epigastric region, left hypochondriac region, lumbar region, umbilical region, lumbar region, iliac (inguinal) region, hypo-gastric (pubic) region, iliac (inguinal) region	General areas of the body: **Axial** **Appendicular** **Abdominal**—subdivided into 9 regions by drawing 2 vertical lines downward from the centers of the collarbones; 1 horizontal line at the lower edge of the rib cage, & another horizontal line placed at the upper edges of the hipbones.	Head, neck, thorax (chest), abdomen & pelvis Upper & lower extremities
	Upper abdominal regions: (roughly upper third of abdomen) *Right hypochondriac region* *Epigastric region* *Left hypochondriac region*	Behind lower right rib cage From lower sternum to lower border of rib cage (stomach area) Area behind lower left rib cage
	Middle abdominal regions: (roughly mid-third of abdomen) *Right lumbar region* *Umbilical region* *Left lumbar region*	From lowest border of right rib cage to hipbone Area in center of the abdomen From lowest border of left rib cage to hipbone
	Lower abdominal regions: (roughly lower third of abdomen) *Right iliac (inguinal)* *Hypogastric (pubic)* *Left iliac (inguinal)*	From top of right hipbone to level of crotch Area from lower mid-abdomen to crotch Area from top of left hipbone to level of crotch

The Tissues

Understanding different tissues will help when you are trying to understand about embryology, yoni and cervical examinations, how healing occurs, how the uterus works, and how disease affects the body.

A **tissue** is a group of similar cells and their intercellular substance functioning together to perform a specialized activity. The branch of science dealing with the study of tissues is called **histology**. There are four basic types of tissues which are classified according to their structure and function:

> **Epithelial (ep-i-THEE-lee-all) tissue** which covers body surfaces, lines body cavities and forms glands.
> **Connective tissue** protects and supports the body and its organs and binds organs together.
> **Muscular tissue** is responsible for movement.
> **Nervous tissue** initiates and transmits nerve impulses that coordinate body activities.

Epithelial tissue: **Epithelium** is divided into two types. One type covers and lines body areas; it forms the skin and the outer covering of some organs and lines body cavities and the inside of the respiratory and digestive tracts, blood vessels and ducts. It is, along with nerve tissue, found in the organs that are sensitive to smell and hearing. The second variety constitutes the secreting portion of glands. Both types of epithelium consist largely or entirely of closely packed cells with little or no intercellular materials between them. They are arranged in continuous sheets that may be either single or multilayered. Nerves may pass through this sheet, but blood vessels do not. Epithelial tissues are firmly adhered to connective tissues which hold them in place and prevent tearing. There are subcategories of epithelial tissue:

> **Simple epithelium** is specialized for absorption or filtration, and is located in areas that have minimal wear and tear. Its cells are arranged in a single layer. It lines all blood and lymphatic vessels, including the heart, air cells in the lungs, and certain tubules of the kidney.

> **Stratified (layered) epithelium** is not specialized as above; it is relatively thick, and is found in areas with a high degree of wear and tear. It's cells are stacked in several layers. It lines the skin, mouth, pharynx, esophagus, yoni and anal passage.

Pseudostratified epithelium has only one layer of cells; however, since not all cells reach the surface, it gives the appearance of a multilayered structure. It lines the respiratory tract.

Epithelial cells also have different shapes. These basic categories include:

Squamous (SKWAY-mus) epithelial cells which are flattened and scale-like. They are attached to each other like a mosaic. Squamous epithelium lines all blood and lymphatic vessels, including the heart, air cells of the lungs, and certain tubules of the kidney.

Cuboidal cells are cube-shaped in cross section, sometimes appearing as hexagons. They line the glands and digestive tract.

Transitional cells often have a combination of shapes and are found where there is a high degree of distention or expansion in the body. They range in shape from cube-like, columnar, to polyhedral and squamous, depending upon their location and function. These cells line the urinary tract and kidneys.

Glandular epithelial cells secrete hormones. These cells lie in clusters deep within the covering and lining epithelium, usually within columnar or cuboidal epithelium. A **gland** consists of one (unicellular) or more (multicellular) highly specialized epithelial cells which produce and discharge substances. **Exocrine (X-oh-krin) glands** secrete their products into ducts (tubes) that empty at the surface covering or lining epithelium or directly onto a free surface, such as the skin. These secretions include oil, wax, perspiration, and digestive enzymes. **Endocrine (EN-do-krin) glands** are ductless and secrete products into the blood stream. These secretions are always hormones, chemicals that regulate various physical activities.

Connective tissue: Connective tissue is the most abundant tissue in the body. This internal tissue binds and supports other structures, is highly vascular and thus has a rich blood supply. Its cells are widely scattered with considerable intercellular material. The intercellular substance largely determines the tissue's qualities and may consist of fluid, semifluid, mucoid (mucus-like) or fibrous material. In cartilage this material is firm but pliable. In bone it is much harder and not pliable. The cells may store fat, ingest bacteria and cell debris, form anticoagulants, or give rise to antibodies that protect against disease. There are several kinds of connective tissues:

Connective tissue proper is called **loose** or **areolar (a-RE-oh-lar)** and is one of the most widely distributed connective tissues in the body. It consists of loosely woven fibers and several kinds of cells embedded in a semifluid intercellular substance. There are also a number of cells found in loose connective tissue such as those for tissue repair and protection as well as pigmentation and fats. Several different varieties of this type of tissue are continuous throughout the body. It is present in the mucus membranes and around blood vessels, body organs and nerves. Combined with fat (adipose) tissue it forms the subcutaneous layer of the skin. Three types of fibers are found between the cells of loose connective tissue. They are:

>   **Collagenous (KOHL-ah-gin-us) (white) fibers** which are very tough and resistant to pulling force. They are somewhat flexible because they are wavy. Collagen fibers often occur in bundles and are made of the protein **collagen**.

>   **Elastic (yellow) fibers** are smaller and freely branch and rejoin one another; they are made of a protein called **elastin**.

>   **Reticular fibers** are also made of collagen plus a glycoprotein. They are long and thin and branch extensively. They provide support and strength and form the framework of many soft organs.

Adipose tissue is specialized for fat storage. It is found wherever loose connective tissue is located, such as in the subcutaneous layer of the skin, around the kidneys and heart, in the marrow of long bones, as padding around joints, and behind the eyeball. It is a major energy reserve and supports and protects various organs.

Dense (collagenous) connective tissue is characterized by more closely packed fibers and less intercellular material. The fibers may be regularly or irregularly arranged. In areas where tension is exerted in various directions, the fibers are interwoven in sheets that are irregular in orientation. It forms most fasciae, part of the skin layer, bone and cartilage coverings or linings, and capsules around some organs. Regularly arranged fibers are found in areas which receive tension in one direction only. The most common type is found in **tendons** (which attach muscles to bones), many **ligaments** (which hold bones together at joints) and **aponeuroses, (ap-oh-new-ROW-sees)** which are flat bands that join one muscle to another or to bone.

>   **Elastic connective tissue** is primarily made up of freely-branching elastic fibers. It will stretch and then snap back into shape. It forms part of the cartilage in the walls of elastic arteries and in the larynx, the trachea, the bronchial tubes and the lungs.

Reticular connective tissue consists of interlacing fibers. It forms a support for many organs and helps bind together the cells of smooth muscle tissue.

Cartilage is capable of enduring considerably more stress than the tissues discussed above. It has no blood vessels or nerves of its own. It consists of a dense network of collagenous (tough and resistant to pulling) and elastic fibers firmly embedded in chondroitin sulfate, a jellylike substance.

Osseous (OS-e-us) tissue (bone), together with cartilage, forms the skeletal system. Bone is classified as either compact (dense) or spongy (cancellous) depending on how the intercellular substance and cells are organized. The bony skeleton supports the soft tissue, works with muscles to provide for movement, stores minerals and produces several kinds of blood cells.

Vascular tissue (blood) is a liquid connective tissue that consists of an intercellular substance called plasma and the blood cells and cell-like structures that float and are transported within it.

<u>Muscle tissue:</u> Muscles consist of highly specialized cells that are modified for contraction. They are capable of providing motion, maintenance of posture and heat. There are three varieties:

Skeletal muscle tissue is attached to bones. It is voluntary; i.e., its activity is consciously controlled. It is also striated; that is, the cells contain alternating bands that are perpendicular to the long axis of the cells.

Cardiac muscle forms most of the walls of the heart. It is involuntary; that is, it functions automatically. It is striated as well.

Smooth muscle tissue is in the wall of hollow internal structures such as blood vessels, the stomach, intestines, uterus and urinary bladder. It is nonstriated (therefore smooth), and functions as involuntary muscle.

<u>Nervous tissue:</u> The nervous system consists of two basic kinds of cells: **neurons** and **neuroglia**. Neurons or nerve cells are highly specialized cells that are capable of picking up stimuli, converting it to impulses and conducting the impulses to other neurons, muscle fibers or glands. Neuroglia are cells that protect and support neurons.

Membranes: The combination of an epithelial layer and an underlying connective tissue layer constitutes an epithelial membrane. There are three types:

> **Mucus membrane** lines body cavities that open directly to the exterior. It secretes mucus that prevents the tissues from drying out.
>
> **Serous membrane** or **serosa** are thin layers of loose connective tissue which line a body cavity that does not directly open to the exterior. It also covers the organs that lie within the cavity. The part attached to the cavity wall is called the **parietal portion,** the part that covers the organs themselves is called the **visceral portion.**
>
> **Cutaneous membrane** is also called the skin layer.
>
> **Synovial membranes** do not contain epithelium. They line the cavities of joints and are composed of loose connective tissue with elastic fibers and varying amounts of fat. These membranes secrete synovial fluid into the joints which lubricates the ends of bones as they move in the joints and nourishes the cartilage covering the bones.

Tissue repair: Tissue repair is the process by which new tissue replaces or repairs damaged cells. The repair will either result in a near-perfect reconstruction of the damaged area or be accomplished by producing scar tissue (a new connective tissue), depending upon the type of cells involved. (See Healing Passage for more details regarding the process of tissue healing.)

The Organ Systems of the Body: An Overview

The different parts of the human body are grouped into **systems**, sets of organs which function together. There are 11 organ systems:

1. **Integumentary**—the skin and structures derived from the skin such as hair, fingernails, and sweat and oil glands. All of these structures protect internal body parts and provide sensory information through touch.
2. **Skeletal**—includes all the bones and joints in the body and their associated connective tissues (such as cartilage); provides mobility as well as soft tissue protection and support.
3. **Muscular**—all the muscles in the body; allows for movement, maintains posture and produces heat.
4. **Nervous**—includes the brain, spinal cord, nerves and sense organs, such as the eye and ear, all of which process and react to sensory input.
5. **Endocrine**—all the glands that produce hormones which regulate bodily functions.
6. **Cardiovascular**—the blood, heart and blood vessels. These organs distribute oxygen and nutrients to cells, carry away waste products and carbon dioxide, maintain the acid-base balance of the body (pH), protect against disease, prevent hemorrhage by forming blood clots and help regulate body temperature.
7. **Lymphatic**—includes the lymph fluid, lymph vessels and organs containing lymphatic tissue and storing white blood cells (called lymphocytes) such as the spleen, thymus gland, lymph nodes and tonsils. This system returns proteins and plasma to the cardiovascular system, filters body fluid, produces white blood cells, and protects against disease.
8. **Respiratory**—includes the lungs and passageways leading into and out of them. The lungs supply oxygen, eliminate carbon dioxide (a waste gas) and help regulate the acid-base (pH) balance of the body.
9. **Digestive**—a long tube extending from the mouth to the anus and the associated organs such as the salivary glands, liver, gallbladder, and pancreas. It performs the physical and chemical breakdown of food for use by the cells and eliminates indigestible food stuffs as waste.
10. **Urinary**—the organs which produce, collect and eliminate urine. This system regulates the chemical composition of blood, eliminates wastes, regulates fluid and chemical (or electrolyte) balance and volume, and helps maintain the acid-base balance of the body.
11. **Reproductive**—the organs that produce, transport and store reproductive cells, serve as sites for fertilization and the development of the fetus. This system includes the mammary glands.

The Integumentary System

A basic overview of the structure of the skin will assist you in your midwifery by enhancing your understanding of how the body protects itself. The skin helps to protect the body by:

1. **Regulating body temperature** in response to changes in environmental temperature or exercise. The sweat glands produce perspiration which helps lower the body's temperature back to normal.
2. **Protecting the internal organs by covering the body,** thereby providing a physical barrier for underlying tissues against injury and contamination.
3. **Eliminating wastes via perspiration** which releases small amounts of salts, water and other organic compounds.
4. **Synthesizing vitamin D** when exposed to ultraviolet radiation from the sun.
5. **Receiving certain stimuli** via nerve endings and receptors that detect temperature, touch, pressure and pain.
6. **Certain skin cells help to increase immunity.**

The skin is made up of two layers. The **epidermis** is the outer, thinner portion of the skin which is composed of epithelium (cells which cover a surface). The epidermis is attached to the inner, thicker, connective tissue portion of the skin layer called the **dermis**. Beneath the dermis is the **subcutaneous layer**, which is also called the **superficial facia** or **hypodermis**. This layer consists of areolar (tiny spaces) and fat tissues. Fibers from the dermis extend down into the superficial facia and attach the skin to the subcutaneous layer. The facia is attached to underlying tissues and organs.

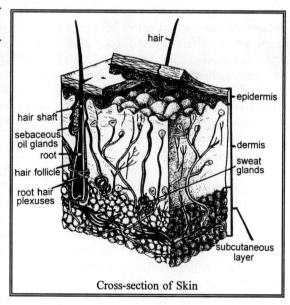

Cross-section of Skin

In addition, the skin has some specialized structures, as follows:

Hair, an outgrowth of the epidermis, is distributed over the body surface. Its primary function is protection. Each hair consists of a **shaft** and a **root**. Surrounding each root is the **hair follicle**, which sheaths the root and provides it with nourishment and an anchor in the skin surface. Around each follicle are nerve endings called **root hair plexuses (PLEK-us-is) (networks)** which are sensitive to touch. Hair growth is controlled by both general metabolism and androgenic hormones. Hair grows in three cycles. The anagen or growth phase lasts 2 to 6 years for individual hairs, during which the hair follicle is steadily forming new hair shaft keratin. The catagen or transition phase then begins lasting 2 weeks, when the growing bulb involutes. Then the telogen, or resting phase starts, lasting 2 to 4 months when the hair is no longer growing, but remains loose in the follicle until it falls out. (Gleicher, 1985, p. 1148)

Nails are hardened epidermal cells which form a clear, solid covering over the dorsal surface of the ends of the fingers and toes. Each consists of a nail body (the visible part), the free edge, (the tip which continues to grow out from the digit), and the root, which is hidden in the skin at the base. The nails help protect the surfaces they cover as well as assisting with grasping and manipulation of small objects.

Glands: There are three types of glands within the skin layer:

Sebaceous (se-BAY-shus) or oil glands are typically connected to hair follicles; those not in follicles open directly onto the skin surface. These are found in the lips, labia minora, glans penis and eyelids. The sebaceous glands secrete an oily substance called **sebum** (SEE-bum), a mixture of fats, cholesterol, proteins and inorganic salts. Sebum helps keep hair and skin moist and pliable, prevents excessive evaporation of water and inhibits the growth of certain bacteria.

    Sudoriferous (soo-door-IF-err-us) or **sweat glands** can be divided into two types. **Apocrine sweat glands** are found under the arms, in the pubic region and the areolae (pigmented portion) of the nipples. The mammary glands are a type of apocrine gland and will be discussed separately. Most apocrine glands open into hair follicles and begin functioning at puberty, secreting sweat of a characteristic odor.

    Eccrine (ESEE-rean) sweat glands are found throughout the skin layer except for the edges of the lips, nail beds, glans penis, clitoral glans, labia minora and eardrums. They are most numerous in the palms of the hands and soles of the feet. They empty into skin pores, openings which allow the elimination of perspiration and other wastes.

    Ceruminous (see-ROO-me-nus) glands are found in the external ear canal and produce **cerumen**, or earwax, which protects the ear from the entry of foreign objects.

The Skeletal System

Understanding the skeletal framework of the body will assist midwives in knowing more about how joints move in order to protect babies from injury during birth due to mishandling; in visualizing the skull bones of the infant when assessing the babies position during internal exams; in understanding how the baby moves down and out of the mother's pelvis; and in knowing how blood cells are made. The skeleton performs several basic functions:

1. **Supports the body** by providing a framework which cradles soft tissues and provides a point of attachment for many muscles.
2. **Protects many internal organs from injury** by providing a strong, resilient casing.
3. **Bones assist movement** because they serve as levers to which muscles are attached. Muscle contraction causes the bones to move and allows us to walk or grasp.
4. **Some mineral elements (primarily calcium and phosphorus) are stored in the bones** and can be distributed to other parts of the body as needed.
5. **Blood cell production**. The center of many bones is composed of a soft, spongy substance called **red marrow**. Red marrow produces red blood cells, some white blood cells, and platelets.

The skeleton is made up of two types of connective tissue: cartilage and bone. Like other connective tissues, bone or **osseous (OS-ee-us)** tissue contains a great deal of intercellular substance surrounding widely separated cells. These spaces provide channels for blood vessels and make the bones lighter. A delicate hormonal balance allows for the utilization and replacement of calcium to maintain the strength of the bones. Various vitamin deficiencies or imbalances in the body's ability to maintain optimum calcium levels can cause the bones to be either too weak or too heavy. Bones grow rapidly in the newborn but this growth slows in adulthood, and skeletal injuries can take months to heal in certain parts of the body. There are four basic types of bones:

Long bones have greater length than width, they consist of two ends **(epiphyses)** and a middle **(diaphysis)**. They are slightly curved for strength. The thighs, legs, toes, arms, and forearms all contain long bones.

Short bones are somewhat cube-shaped and nearly equal in length and width; examples are the wrist and ankle bones.

Flat bones are thin and composed of two or more parallel plates

108

enclosing a spongy layer. Examples include the skull bones, sternum, ribs and scapulas.

Irregular bones have complex shapes and cannot be grouped with the others. They include the bones of the spinal column and some facial bones.

In addition to these basic bone types, the **sutural (SOO-chur-all) bones** are small bones between the joints of certain skull bones. **Sesamoid (SEZ-ah-moid) bones** are small bones in areas where considerable pressure develops, such as the wrist, and the patella, or kneecaps.

The adult skeleton consists of a total of 206 bones which are divided into two groups. The **axial (up and down) skeleton** consists of the ribs, breastbone, skull bones and backbone. The **appendicular skeleton** contains the bones of the free appendages (that is the arms and legs) plus the girdles of the shoulder and pelvis.

The Axial skeleton: The **skull** contains 8 cranial bones (which form the dome of the head and encase the brain) and 14 facial bones which create the contours of the face and support the eyes, nose and mouth. The **nasal sinuses** are delicate bony cavities surrounded by the facial bones to either side of and above the nose. The skull rests on the superior end of the spinal column.

Certain bones and landmarks of the skull are important to know when discussing fetal positioning in relationship to the mother and on the newborn physical exam. Each of the cranial bones is mobile in the fetus and newborn. There is a gap that is bridged by a small amount of connective tissue where the edges of the skull bones meet. These gaps are referred to as **sutures**.

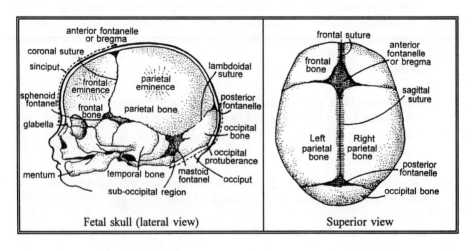

Fetal skull (lateral view)   Superior view

Larger membrane-filled spaces are also present in the fetal and newborn skull; these are called **fontanelles (fon-tah-NELLS)**. The two which are significant in midwifery are the **anterior (frontal) fontanelle** and the **posterior (occipital [ok-SIP-it-all]) fontanelle**. Together, the location of the skull bones, fontanelles and suture lines can assist you in determining the position of the head during prenatal care and in labor.

Articulations of the skeleton: The skeleton is articulated (joined) in various locations to assist in movement, since the bones are too rigid to bend without being damaged. The points of contact between bones or between cartilage and bones are commonly known as **joints**. Joints are classified by function, taking into account the degree of movement they permit:

Synarthroses (sin-are-THROW-sees) are immovable joints
Amphiarthroses (am-fee-are-THROW-sees) are slightly moveable
Diarthroses (die-are-THROW-sees) are freely moveable

They are also classified by structure:

Fibrous joints have no joint cavity; The bones are held together by fibrous connective tissue. Examples are the sutures in the skull, the meeting place of tibia and fibula, and the roots of the teeth.

Cartilaginous joints have no joint cavity; the bones are held together by cartilage. An example is the symphysis pubis.

Synovial joints form a space between articulating bones. The bones are united by a surrounding articular capsule that encloses the synovial cavity and often by accessory ligaments as well. A small amount of synovial fluid is secreted within the joint which helps lubricate the bones and ease motion. The knee is a synovial joint.

The various movements of the body create friction between moving parts. To reduce this friction, saclike structures called **bursae** are located within the body tissues. Bursae resemble joints in that their walls consist of connective tissue lined with a synovial membrane. Bursae are filled with fluid similar to synovial fluid and are located between the skin and bone in places where skin rubs over bone as well as between tendons and bones, muscles and bones, and ligaments and bones.

Movements of various joints: Having a basic understanding of the way joints move will assist you when doing a physical exam on either the mother or the newborn.

MOVEMENT	DEFINITION	EXAMPLE
Gliding	One surface moves back & forth & from side to side over another without angular or rotary motion	The joints between the wrist bones
Flexion	Usually involves a decrease in the angle between the anterior surfaces of articulating joints (includes the knee & toes)	Bending the head forward, bending the knee or the elbow
Extension	Usually involves an increase in the angle between the anterior surfaces of articulating bones (includes the knee & toes)	Straightening the head, arm or knee
Hyper-extension	Continuation of extension beyond the anatomical position	Bending the head backward, extending the entire arm backward
Abduction	Movement of a bone away from the midline	Moving the arm straight out in front of you; spreading fingers
Adduction	Movement of a bone toward the midline	Returning the arm to your side; moving fingers together
Rotation	Movement of a bone around its longitudinal axis; may be medial or lateral	Shaking the head "no," holding arm straight & turning palm up, then down
Circumduction	Movement in which the distal end of a bone moves in a circle while the proximal end remains stable to make a 360° rotation	Moving the outstretched arm in a circle

Below are listed some specialized movements of the body:

MOVEMENT	DEFINITION
Inversion	Movement of the sole of the foot inward at the ankle joint
Eversion	Movement of the sole of the foot outward at the ankle joint
Dorsiflexion	Flexion of the foot at the ankle joint
Plantar flexion	Extension of the foot at the ankle joint
Protraction	Movement of the mandible (jaw) or clavicle forward on a plane parallel to the ground
Retraction	Movement of a protracted part backward on a plane parallel to the ground (nipple shrinkage in response to cold air)
Supination	Movement of the forearm in which the palm is turned anterior to the ground
Pronation	Movement of the flexed forearm inward towards the body so that the palm is facing posterior or inferior
Elevation	Movement of a part of the body upward (lifting the hand)
Depression	Movement of a part of the body downward (lowering the hand)

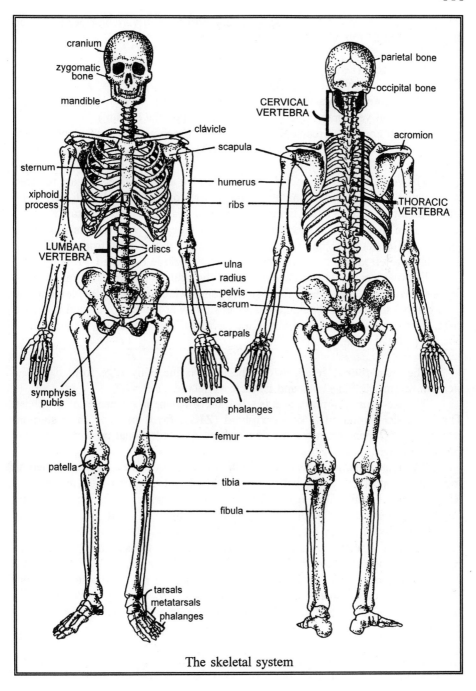

The skeletal system

The **vertebral column** or **spine** is composed of 26 vertebral bones, which are distributed as follows:

*7 **cervical** (neck) vertebrae
*12 **thoracic** vertebrae (behind the thoracic cavity)
*5 **lumbar** vertebrae (supporting the lower back)
*5 **sacral** vertebrae (fused into one bone called the sacrum)
*4 to 6 **coccygeal (cock-SIGH-GEE-all)** vertebrae, fused into one or two bones called the **coccyx (COCK-six)**

The vertebrae of the cervical, thoracic, lumbar and sacral regions are referred to by using a system which numbers the bones from superior to inferior. The letters C (for cervical), T (for thoracic), L (for lumbar) and S (for sacral) are used to designate those regions respectively. Each group of vertebrae is numbered separately; for example, the first lumbar vertebrae counting down from the level of the skull is referred to as L1. The first thoracic vertebrae is labeled T1, and so on.

Between each adjacent vertebrae from the skull to S1 are **discs** made up of fibrous cartilage. These discs form strong joints which allow for movement and absorb shocks. The spinal column curves in slightly at the neck, out behind the rib cage, in at the lower back and out at the sacrum. This curvature helps maintain posture and distribute weight evenly.

The term **thorax** refers to the chest. It is the bony cage formed by the sternum, costal cartilage, ribs and thoracic vertebrae.

The **sternum**, or breastbone, is a flat, narrow bone in the center of the chest. The lower tip is referred to as the **xiphoid (ZIGH-foyd) process**. The sternum forms an attachment point for the ribs and provides additional protection for the heart and lungs.

The **ribs** make up the sides of the thoracic cavity. They increase in length from the topmost (first) through the seventh. The lower ribs then decrease in length to the twelfth rib. Each rib articulates (connects) to its corresponding thoracic vertebrae along either side of the spinal column. The rib articulations are flexible to allow for easy breathing and motion.

The first through the seventh ribs are attached to the sternum by a strip of cartilage called **costal cartilage**. These are called the **true ribs**. The remaining five pairs are referred to as **false ribs** because they do not have a direct frontal attachment point. Rather, the cartilage of ribs 8, 9, and 10 merge into one attachment and ribs 11 and 12 have no frontal attachment and are therefore said to be **floating**.

Appendicular skeleton: consists of several groups of bones as well:

The **pectoral (PECK-tore-all)** or shoulder girdles are bones which attach the bones of the arms to the axial skeleton. They consist of two clavicles and two scapulae. The **clavicles (KLAV-i-culls)**, or collarbones, are long and slender with a double curvature. They are found just above the first rib and below the neck. The clavicles transmit force from the upper body to the trunk.

The **scapulae (SCAP-you-la)** or shoulder blades are large, triangular, flat bones situated in the dorsal part of the thorax between the levels of the second and seventh ribs. The part of the scapula which connects with the clavicle is called the **acromion (ah-CROW-me-on)** and is often referred to in discussing fetal position when the baby is lying transverse (sideways).

The **upper extremities (arms)** consist of 60 bones. The bones of each arm include a **humerus (HYOO-mer-us)** or upper arm bone, the **ulna** (inner) and **radius** (outer) bones in the forearm, 8 **carpals** or wrist bones, 5 **metacarpals** (palm bones, and 14 **phalanges** (fa-LAN-gees) in the fingers of the hand.

The **lower extremities (legs)** consist of a total of 60 bones. The **femur** or thighbone is the longest and heaviest bone in the body. The **patella**, or kneecap, is a small, triangular bone in front of the knee joint. The lower leg is made up of one larger bone called the **tibia** (inner side) and the **fibula** (a long, small bone of the outer side of the leg). The seven ankle bones are referred to as **tarsals**. The bones of the foot are similar to those in the hand, with 5 **metatarsal** bones and 14 **phalanges**. They are arranged in two arches, which enable the foot to support weight and provide leverage while walking.

The **pelvic girdle**, or simply the **pelvis**, is an important anatomical feature for midwives to learn in detail, for it is the bony passage through which the baby must pass in order to be born. It also cradles and protects the reproductive organs. It will be helpful to refer to the illustrations on the following page as you review the material below. This section discusses the bony features of the pelvis. Later, in the Pelvimetry chapter (Skills section), the significance of the pelvic structures in relationship to birth will be discussed in detail.

The pelvis is made up of four bones: the 2 hip bones on each side are the **innominate (eh-NOME-e-nate) bones**. Each joins one side of the sacrum in back (the **sacroiliac joint**) and the **symphysis pubis** in front. The fourth bone is the **coccyx** at the tip of the sacrum.

The two **innominate bones** are each formed by the fusion of three bones (the ilium, the ischium and the pubis) around the **acetabulum (as-e-TAB-you-lum)** (the socket joint for the femur).

The **ilium** is the uppermost pelvic bone which flares to form what we commonly think of as the hips. It has a main body, which is fused with the ischial body, and an **ala** (or wing). The anterior superior iliac spine forms an attachment for the inguinal ligament. The posterior superior iliac spine marks the level of the second sacral vertebra, indicated by dimples in the overlying skin. The iliac crest

114

extends from the anterior superior iliac spine to the posterior superior iliac spine.

The **ischium** consists of a body in which the superior and inferior rami (branches) of the pubis merge. The main part of the ischium forms part of the acetabulum. The superior ramus is behind and below this part. The inferior ramus is fused with the inferior ramus of the pubis. Each ischium has an ischial spine (a pointed landmark), which is used extensively when discussing the location of the baby in the pelvis. The ischium forms an attachment for the levator ani muscle, the main muscle of the pelvic floor. The curved lowermost portions of each ischium are the bones on which we sit, called the tuberosities.

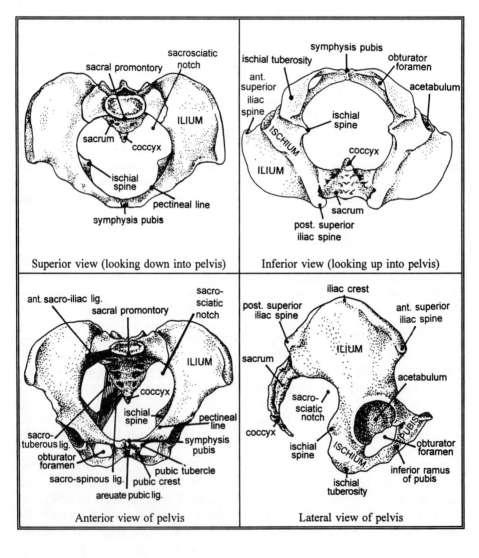

Superior view (looking down into pelvis)

Inferior view (looking up into pelvis)

Anterior view of pelvis

Lateral view of pelvis

The **pubis** consists of a body and two rami or bony branches. The body on each side is joined in the front center to form the symphysis pubis. This joint becomes softened with the hormones of pregnancy and allows some pelvic mobility to facilitate birth. The levator ani muscles attach to the inner side of the pubic bone. The pubic crest is the superior border of the pubic body. The pubic spines form the ends of the crest where the superior ramus meets the body of the pubis in front. The two front ends of the superior ramus are joined to the body of the pubis as the pubic spine and the other end joins the body of the ilium, where it merges to help shape the acetabulum. The inferior pubic ramus merges with the inferior ramus of the ischium.

The **sacrum** is shaped like an inverted triangle; its base at the top supports the spinal column, the apex (end) is below. It usually consists of 5 vertebrae fused together; rarely there are 4 or 6. The sacrum flares on each side where it joins the innominate bones at the sacroiliac joints. These joints allow for sacral mobility during birth. Very rarely, one of these wings is missing (Naegele's pelvis), creating an obliquely contracted pelvic cavity. If both wings are missing (Robert's pelvis), a narrow pelvis opening is the result. The upper surface of the first sacral vertebra is joined to the lower surface of the fifth lumbar vertebra. The sacrum curves backward, causing its inner surface to contribute to the bowl shape of the pelvic cavity. The anterior superior edge of the first sacral vertebra protrudes into the inner pelvic space and is referred to as the **sacral promontory**.

The **coccyx** (tail bone) is composed of four small vertebrae. The top edge of the first coccygeal vertebra articulates with the lower edge of the fifth sacral vertebra to form the sacrococcygeal joint. Rarely this joint is fused. The pelvic floor muscles and anal sphincter are attached to the coccyx.

The pelvic shape of each sex has unique characteristics. The male pelvis is heaver and more suited for the heaver male frame, and has no cartilage in the symphysis pubis. The female pelvis is lighter, more rounded, and ideally suited for childbearing. There are two other intermediate shapes as well. Together, these four conformations make up the basic pelvic types. Of course, an individual often has a pelvis which includes features which are a mixture of these shapes. These details will be thoroughly discussed in the chapter on Pelvimetry in the Skills section (the art of examining the pelvis to determine its size and shape).

The Muscular System

The uterus of a woman at the end of her pregnancy is the strongest muscle in her body. Although the uterus and the perineal muscles are the ones of primary concern in midwifery, this chapter will give you an overview of the entire muscular system. Since the uterus' primary work is so connected to labor, we will discuss it in detail in the second volume of this textbook. The perineal muscles are discussed later in this section.

The contraction and relaxation of muscles provides for the motion of various body parts. Muscle tissue constitutes 40 to 50% of the total body weight and is composed of highly specialized cells. The study of muscles is called **myology**. Muscle tissue has four principal characteristics that assume key roles in maintaining the body's balance:

Excitability is the ability of muscle tissue to receive and respond to stimuli. A stimulus is a change in the internal or external environment strong enough to initiate a nerve impulse (action potential).

Contractility is the ability to shorten and thicken, or contract, when a sufficient stimulus is received.

Extensibility is the ability of muscle tissue to be stretched (extended). Many skeletal muscles are arranged in opposing pairs. While one is contracting, the other is relaxed and is undergoing extension.

Elasticity is the ability of muscle tissue to return to its original shape after contraction or extension.

Through these various processes, muscle performs three important functions: motion, maintenance of posture, and heat production.

Muscles are typed according to their location, microscopic structure and nervous control.

Skeletal muscle is attached to bones and moves parts of the skeleton and is the only type under voluntary control.

Cardiac muscle tissue forms the bulk of the wall of the heart.

Smooth muscle is involved in maintaining our internal environment. It is located in the walls of hollow internal structures, such as blood vessels, the stomach and the intestines.

Muscles are surrounded by a sheet of fibrous connective tissue called **fascia (FASH-ee-ah)** and are attached to bones by tendons. Nerve impulses from the brain causes various chemical reactions which lead to contraction of the muscle fibers. A contraction temporarily shortens the fibers and thereby moves the bone or other structures to which the muscle is connected. Once the nerve impulse is terminated, the muscle fibers relax or lengthen once again and are at rest. A sustained partial contraction of a group of muscle fibers produces **muscle tone**. The muscles require adequate oxygen, and other nutrients and chemical substances to work at their best.

The skeletal muscles: The term "muscle tissue" refers to all the muscles in the body. Generally, however, when we refer to the muscular system we are thinking solely of the skeletal muscles and the connective tissue that make up individual muscle organs, such as the biceps in the upper arm. (Muscles which are located within the structure of an organ, such as the cardiac muscle, will be discussed separately as part of that organ.) There are nearly 700 skeletal muscles. You should be familiar with some of the terms which are used to name these muscles.

*   ***Muscle names may indicate the direction of muscle fibers.** **Rectus** fibers run up and down in relationship to the midline. **Oblique** muscles are diagonal to the midline. **Transverse** fibers run at a 90° angle to the midline.
*   ***A muscle is often given a Latin name according to location**; e.g. the temporalis is near the temporal bone.
*   ***Muscular size is another distinguishing feature.** The term maximus means largest, minimus means smallest, longus, is long and brevis, short. For example, the gluteus maximus and gluteus minimus are, respectively, the largest and smallest gluteus muscles.
*   ***Some muscles are named for their number of origins.** The **origin** is the site of attachment to a stationary bone. The biceps brachia has two origins, the quadriceps femoris has four. The attachment of muscle tendon to a movable bone is called the **insertion**.
*   ***Other muscles are named for their shape.** Examples are the deltoid (triangular) and trapezius (meaning trapezoid).
*   ***Muscles may be named for both their origin and insertion**, for instance the sternocleidomastoid originates on the sternum and clavicle and inserts at the mastoid process of the temporal bone.
*   ***Muscles may be named according to their action.** For example, the levator (productive of upward movement) ani muscles of the pelvis contract upwards, lifting the pelvic contents slightly.

Muscles associated with birth: Midwifery is mainly concerned with the skelet muscles of the pelvis. This group of muscles surrounds, supports and contr openings of the anus, yoni and urethra, and contract and relax during doing so they stimulate the nerves in the clitoral structures and pleasure. Since they are an integral part of the sexual organ in the chapter on The Female Sexual and Reproductive Syste

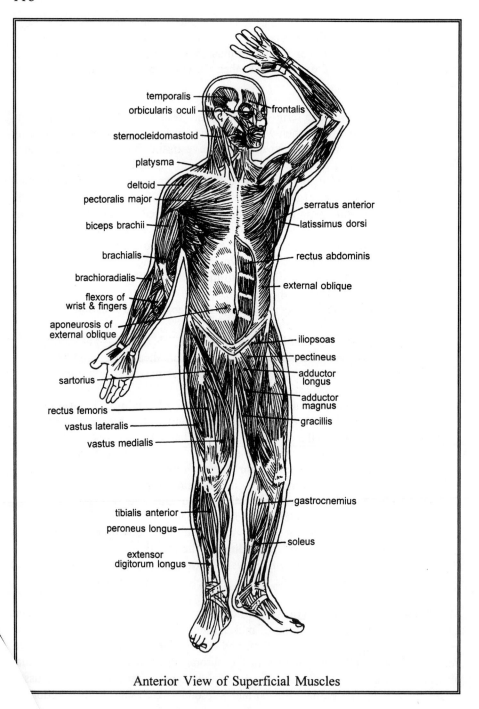

temporalis

orbicularis oculi

frontalis

sternocleidomastoid

platysma

deltoid

pectoralis major

biceps brachii

brachialis

brachioradialis

flexors of wrist & fingers

aponeurosis of external oblique

sartorius

rectus femoris

vastus lateralis

vastus medialis

serratus anterior

latissimus dorsi

rectus abdominis

external oblique

iliopsoas

pectineus

adductor longus

adductor magnus

gracillis

tibialis anterior

peroneus longus

extensor digitorum longus

gastrocnemius

soleus

Anterior View of Superficial Muscles

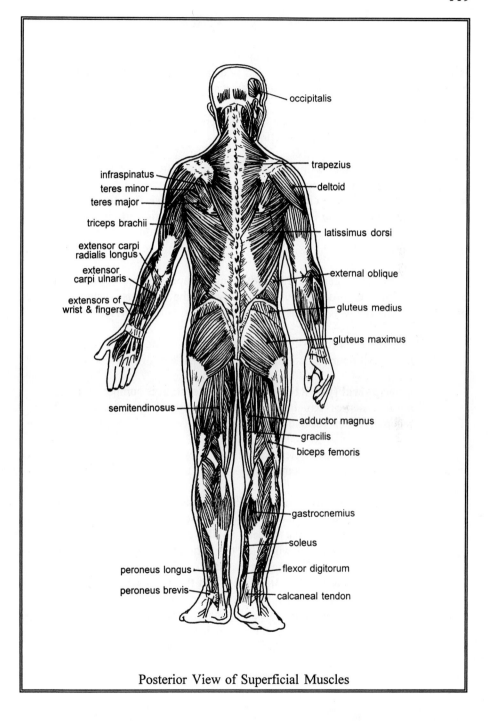

Posterior View of Superficial Muscles

The Nervous System

Knowledge of the nervous system will assist you in understanding how pain is felt, how pain medications work, and will give you a basis for understanding normal neurological responses in the mother and newborn.

The **nervous system** is the body's control center and communications network. It serves three basic functions:

1. It senses changes within the body and in the outer environment; this is the **sensory function**.
2. It interprets these changes; this is the **integrative function**.
3. It responds to the interpretation by initiating action in the form of muscular contraction or glandular secretions; this is the **motor function**.

The nervous system is the body's most rapid means of maintaining a balanced internal environment. The study of the nervous system is called **neurology**. The nervous system is organized into two main divisions:

*The **central nervous system (CNS)** consists of the brain and spinal cord. All neurological impulses are either sent or received by the CNS.
*The **peripheral (per-RIF-er-al) nervous system** is composed of the various nerves which connect the brain and spinal cord with receptors, muscles and glands.

Further, the nervous system functions in two other ways which produce voluntary and involuntary movement.

*The **somatic nervous system (SNS)** conducts impulses to and from skeletal muscles and is under our conscious control.
*The **autonomic nervous system (ANS)** conveys impulses to and from smooth muscles which are not normally under our conscious control, such as the heart and glands. It is divided into the **parasympathetic nervous system** and the **sympathetic nervous system**. Each uses a different chemical transmitter where the nerve fibers reach their target organ; each is built differently and has a different effect on the organ it serves. For example, the parasympathetic system inhibits the heartbeat and the sympathetic system accelerates it.

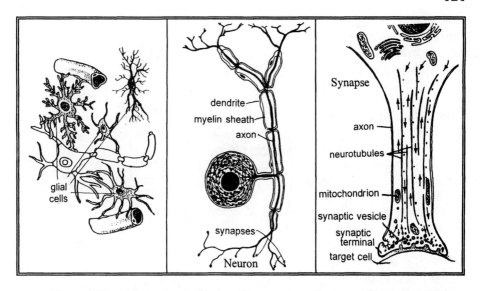

dendrite
myelin sheath
axon

synapses

Neuron

Synapse

axon

neurotubules

mitochondrion

synaptic vesicle

synaptic terminal

target cell

glial cells

The nervous system is made up of two types of nerve cells. A nerve is a bundle of motor and sensory fibers, together with connective tissue and blood vessels. **Neurons** are the nerve cells which are responsible for conducting energy (impulses) from one part of the body to another. The typical motor neuron looks like a ball (the cell body) with a number of fine, rootlike fibers projecting from it. These **dendrites** carry impulses toward the cell. Also projecting from the cell body is a single long fiber called an **axon**. It is the main conducting fiber of the cell. At its far end the axon divides into several small branches, each ending in a number of tiny knobs. The axon carries messages away from the cell. Although all neurons have these basic components, they vary in structure as far as size and shape. Four types of **neuroglia** or **glial cells** perform functions of support and protection. They are the smaller of the two and outnumber the neurons by 5 to 10 times. They twine around nerve cells or line certain structures in the brain and spinal cord. Neuroglia also bind nervous tissues to other structures and produce a protective nerve covering called the **myelin (MY-lynn) sheath** which increases the speed of impulse transmission and insulates and maintains the axon.

Sensory nerves carry messages from the sense organs to the CNS. **Motor nerves** carry directions from the CNS to the peripheral nervous system. The major nerves, of which there are 43, actually arise in the central nervous system.

Nerve impulses are conducted from one neuron to another across tiny gaps called **synapses** between the axon knobs and the dendrites of an adjacent cell. A complex interaction of chemicals called **nerve transmitter substances** transmit the information from one nerve to the next. Cold slows these impulses and heat speeds them up.

The spinal cord and the brain: The **spinal cord** is a roughly cylindrical column of nerve tissues about 16 to 18 inches (42 to 45 cm.) long, which is enclosed within a channel formed by the spinal vertebrae from the lower brain to the lower back (L2). Below this point it extends as a non-nervous fibrous tissue to the coccyx. The spinal cord is made up of collections of neurons and bundles of nerve fibers. The **gray matter** (the nerve collections) is shaped roughly like a sideways H in cross section, with a posterior and anterior

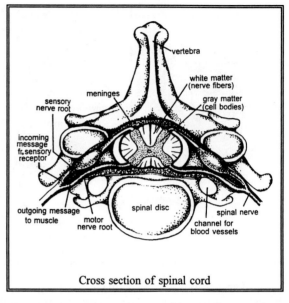

Cross section of spinal cord

horn (protruding area) in front and in back. The anterior horn is composed of motor neurons while the posterior horn contains cellular bodies of connector neurons and sensory neurons. The gray matter is surrounded by **white matter** which is divided into three columns. It contains ascending and descending nerves which connect the brain and the spinal cord in both directions. The descending nerves send motor impulses from the brain to the peripheral nervous system while the ascending nerves channel sensory impulses to the brain.

The spinal cord is encased and protected by the vertebral column which forms a canal for it to pass through as well as providing openings so that nerves can exit the canal and make contact with the peripheral nervous system. The **meninges (me-NIN-gees)** surrounding the spinal cord is a three layer membrane which covers the brain and the entire spinal cord up to each point of its exit from the spinal column through the openings in between the vertebral bones (the intervertebral foramina). The spinal cord is supported and suspended within this sheath by membranous extensions which protect the spinal cord from shocks and sudden displacement.

Each spinal nerve is attached to the spinal cord by two roots, one of which carries motor fibers and the other, sensory fibers. These roots carry messages to and from the spinal cord-like wires on an electrical lead. At a short distance from the spinal cord each nerve splits into branches which further divide into smaller branches, forming a network of nerves which radiate all over the body.

The spinal cord has two main functions. It acts as a two-way conduction system between the brain and the peripheral nervous system. Secondly, it controls simple reflex actions. **Reflexes** are rapid, involuntary responses to changes in the internal and external environment which attempt to keep the body in balance. Those significant to midwifery practice are discussed in the chapter on the Physical Exam (Skills section) and in a later volume in a chapter on the Newborn Exam.

The 12 pairs of **cranial nerves** emerge from the underside of the brain. They supply the sense organs and muscles in the head. Some cranial nerves, such as the optic nerve, contain only sensory fibers. The **vagus nerve** supplies the digestive organs, heart and air passages in the lungs.

The nerves in the spinal cord can analyze some relatively simple input, but the more complex work of impulse interpretation is done in the brain.

The 31 pairs of spinal nerves are named and numbered according to the region and level of the spinal cord from which they emerge. The first cervical pair emerges between the atlas and the occipital bone. All others leave the spinal cord through channels between adjoining vertebrae. There are eight pairs of cervical nerves, 12 pairs of thoracic nerves, five pairs of lumbar nerves, five pairs of sacral nerves and one pair of coccygeal nerves. Each pair of nerves controls certain parts of the body. When there is a neurological disturbance or damage, the areas of influence can be examined to determine what part of the spinal cord is injured. A simplified look at these relationships follows:

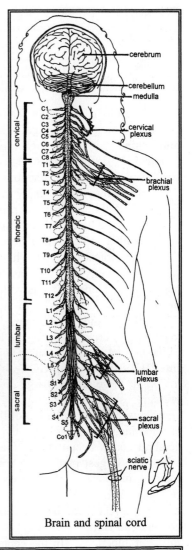

Brain and spinal cord

ORIGIN	AREA OF INFLUENCE:
Cervical C1-C5	Skin & muscles of the head, neck, and upper part of the shoulders
Brachial C5-C8 & T1	Upper extremities and shoulder region
Thoracic T2	Under the arms and the back of the arm
T3 & T6	Intercostal muscles and skin of the anterior & lateral chest
T7-T11	Intercostal muscles; abdominal muscles & overlying skin, deep back muscles & skin of the dorsal thorax

ORIGIN	AREA OF INFLUENCE:
Lumbar L1-L4	Anterolateral abdominal wall, external genitals, and part of the upper legs
Sacral L4-L5 & S1-S4	Buttocks, perineum and lower extremities, including the legs and feet

The **brain** is roughly shaped like a mushroom and is the largest organ in the body, weighing an average of 3 pounds (1300 grams). It has 3 regions: the **hindbrain**, the **midbrain (mesencephalon [mess-in-SEF-ah-lon])** and the **forebrain**. Each of these regions is also divided into separate areas which are responsible for distinct functions and are all connected to other parts of the brain.

Brain functions usually involve the participation of thousands of different neurons. Although many sensory neurons terminate and many motor neurons originate in the brain, the majority of the brain's neurons are **interneurons**, whose job is to filter, analyze and store information.

The largest part of the hindbrain is the **cerebellum**. This area is concerned with motor activities such as unconscious muscular movements that maintain posture and balance. It acts with other areas to coordinate body movements. The **brain stem** links the brain to the spinal cord and includes parts of the hindbrain, the midbrain and the forebrain. Here incoming and outgoing messages come together and cross over, for the left side of the body is governed by the right side of the brain and vice-versa. The brain stem is made up of the **medulla oblongata (me-DULL-la ob-long-GOT-ah)**, the **pons** and the **reticular formation** of the midbrain; these are in charge of life sustaining functions such as heart rate, blood pressure, swallowing, coughing, breathing and unconsciousness. Control of consciousness is also the job of the reticular formation, which decides which input is important enough to alert the brain. If its action is slowed or prevented, the cerebral cortex becomes inactive and unconsciousness results.

The largest part of the brain is known as the **cerebrum**. It is essential to thought, memory, consciousness and the higher mental processes such as abstract reasoning and decision making. It is equally divided down the middle into two halves, the **cerebral hemispheres**, which are joined by nerve fibers known as **corpus callosum**. Each side is a mirror image of the other, yet has completely different functions. In the center of the cerebral hemispheres is a collection of nerve cells known as the **basal ganglia**. This control system coordinates muscle activity allowing the body to perform specific types of unconscious movement.

The **thalamus (THAL-ah-muss)** is an oval structure above the midbrain. It lies in two masses on either side of the third ventricle in the center of the brain. It is the principal relay station for sensory impulses that reach the cerebral cortex from the spinal cord, brain stem, cerebellum, and parts of the cerebrum.

The **hypothalamus** lies at the base of the brain beneath the two cerebral hemispheres. It is a collection of specialized nerve centers which connect with other areas of the brain as well as the pituitary gland. It controls eating, sleeping and body temperature along with other vital functions. It also forms links with other areas involved with the senses, behavior and memory. Together the thalamus and hypothalamus are known as the **diencephalon (die-in-SEF-ah-lon)**.

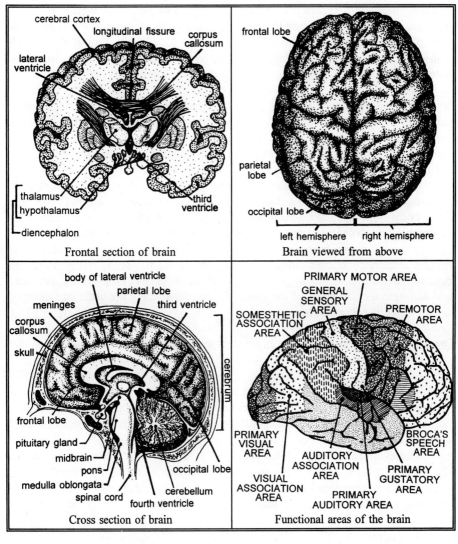

Frontal section of brain

Brain viewed from above

Cross section of brain

Functional areas of the brain

The **cerebral cortex** is the 1/8 inch (3 mm.) thick, wrinkled layer of gray matter covering the outside of the cerebrum. This part of the brain is so highly developed that it forms folds in order to fit into the skull. Within the folds are deep groves which divide each hemisphere into four areas called **lobes**. Each lobe has two or more specific functions. The temporal lobes are involved with hearing and smell, the parietal lobes with touch and taste, the occipital lobes with movement, speech and complicated thinking. Each of these lobes is subdivided into specific areas which connect with other parts of the body.

The brain and spinal cord are hydrated, nourished, and protected by the **cerebrospinal fluid**. There is 80 to 150 ml. (3 to 5 oz.) of clear, watery fluid that flows around the meninges and through the **ventricles** (cavities) of the brain. The fluid is made continuously from blood by specialized cells within the brain's ventricles. These ventricles are all connected and are numbered from the top to the bottom. The first and second are the largest of the four.

Peripheral nervous system: The peripheral nervous system acts to relay sensory and motor messages between the central nervous system and the body's muscles, glands, and sense organs. It plays virtually no part in the analysis of sensory signals or the initiation of motor signals. Both of these activities and many other processes occur in the central nervous system.

One of the main functions of the nervous system is to monitor and respond to **sensations**. A sensation is a state of awareness of external or internal conditions of the body. In order for a sensation to register, first a **stimulus**, or change in the environment capable of initiating a response from the nervous system, must occur. Next a receptor or sense organ must convert the stimulus to a nerve impulse. This impulse is then conducted along a neural pathway to the brain. The brain then translates the impulse into a specific type of sensation. Pain, pleasure, pressure, cold and heat are just a few of the types of sensations which the brain can interpret and to which it can initiate response.

The senses: The senses of sight, hearing, taste, touch and smell are all specialized extensions of the nervous system. We will review each of them individually.

The **eyes** are the organs of **sight** and work like very sophisticated cameras. As light bounces off of objects, images are transmitted to the brain. The rays of light are then bent by the structures of the eye to form tiny, perfect images of much larger objects.

The eyes are surrounded and protected by a number of accessory structures. The **eyebrows** form a transverse arch at the junction of the upper eyelid and the forehead. They resemble hairy scalp, with coarse hairs that are directed to the side. They help protect the eyes from foreign objects, perspiration and the direct rays of the sun.

The upper and lower **eyelids** or **palpebrae (PAL-pee-brea)** shade the eyes during sleep, protect them from excessive light and foreign objects, and spread lubricating secretions over the eyeballs. They are made up of epidermis, connective tissues, muscles and a tarsal plate. The **tarsal plate** is a thick fold of connective tissue that forms the inner surface of the eyelids. The **conjunctiva (con-JUNK-**

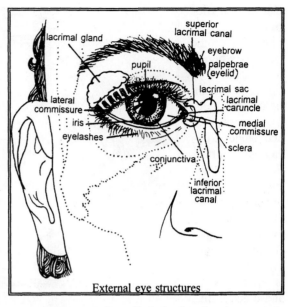

External eye structures

tea-va) is a thin mucus membrane which lines the inner surface of the eyelids and the very edges of the eyeball. Projecting from the outer border of each eyelid is a row of short hairs called the **eyelashes** which also protect the eyes from sun and foreign objects. The space between them that exposes the eyeball is called the **palpebral fissure**. Its angles are known as the **lateral commissure (KOM-eh-sure)**, which is narrow and on the outer side of the face, and the **medial commissure**, which is broader and near the nose. The reddish elevation in the corner of the eye is called the **lacrimal caruncle (CAR-uncle)**; it contains oil and sweat glands.

The **lacrimal apparatus** is the term used for a group of structures that makes and drains away tears. These consist of glands, ducts and canals. Each **lacrimal gland** is above the outer side of the eye and is about the size of an almond. Six to twelve excretory ducts empty tears onto the conjunctiva of the upper eyelid. Tears wash over the eye when blinking occurs and then drain into the tiny ducts found in the corner of the eye. They then flow into the **lacrimal sac** which transports the tears into the nasal passages. Tears contain mucus, salts and a bactericidal enzyme called lysozyme. They clean, lubricate and moisten the eyeballs.

The **eyeball** in an adult is about 2.5 cm. (1 inch) in diameter. It is surrounded by four main muscles which allow it to move. The eyeballs are covered by a white protective layer called the **sclera**. Beneath this layer is the **uveal tract** which consists of three layers of connective tissue containing blood vessels, tiny muscles which change the thickness of the lens and produce fluids, and the iris.

Light enters the eye through the **cornea**, the first lens of the eye. The cornea forms a centrally located five-layered transparent covering over the inner eye structures. It is attached to the sclera all around its edges. After passing through the cornea, light then passes through a fluid-filled chamber between the cornea and the iris.

The **iris** is what gives the eye its color. Its center (the **pupil**) is open. Like a camera shutter it dilates and contracts to allow the appropriate amount of light to enter the interior of the eye. In dim light the pupil gets bigger to let in more light; in bright light it contracts. Excitement, fear and some drugs can also affect the size of the pupil independent of the amount of available light. Behind the iris is the **lens**, which is soft, elastic and transparent.

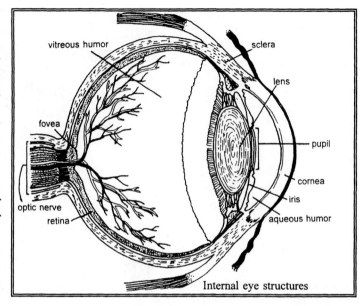

Internal eye structures

Behind the lens is the main interior chamber of the eye. It is filled with a substance called the **vitreous humor**, which has a jelly-like texture and makes the eyeball feel firm and rubbery. Running through its center is the **hyaloid canal**, the remains of a channel which carried an artery during fetal development. The back of this chamber is lined with a light-sensitive layer called the **retina**. It is made up of two different types of light sensitive cells called **rods** and **cones**, these pick up light and color respectively. The cones are also responsible for clear images, and are most plentiful in the area known as the **fovea** or **macula**, the focus of the sharpest image in the back of the eye. The retina surrounding the macula registers the edges of our visual field, known as peripheral vision.

All light-sensitive cells are connected into one main nerve cable to the brain called the **optic nerve**. The optic nerves from each eye meet just beneath the brain, cross over at the **optic chiasma (ki-AZ-mah)** and combine information as it is delivered to the visual cortex of the brain, where image information is interpreted. A large artery runs the length of the nerve and emerges at the back of the eye, where its smaller vessels spread over the surface of the retina. A corresponding vein removes blood along the same route.

The **ears** provide the sense of **hearing** and **balance**. The **outer ear** is the shell-shaped external ear structure which gathers sound waves. The **middle ear** has an assembly of bones which amplifies sounds; the **inner ear** converts sound vibrations into electrical impulses and assists with balance.

Sound waves are produced by the vibrations of air molecules, their size and energy of the waves determines loudness, which is measured in decibels (dB). The number of vibrations or cycles per second make up frequency; the more vibrations, the higher the pitch of the sound. This is expressed as hertz (Hz). The audible range is approximately 20 to 20,000 Hz per second, although humans are most sensitive to sounds in the 500 to 4000 Hz range. Hearing loss usually takes place in the higher frequency range first.

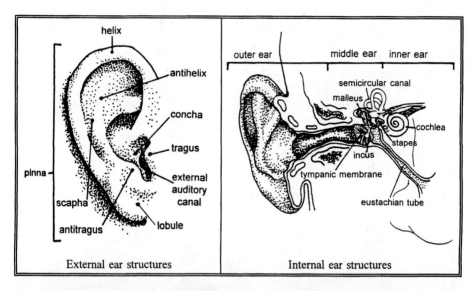

External ear structures   Internal ear structures

The fleshy outer ear or **pinna** functions as a sound receptacle. In its center is a bony canal leading to the eardrum (**tympanic membrane**). Sound causes this membrane to vibrate, which triggers three gear-like bones, the **ossicles** behind the tympanic membrane, to begin to vibrate. The **malleus** attaches to the eardrum; the **stapes** attaches to the inner ear, and the **incus** connects the two. These bones work together to amplify the eardrum movement 20-fold. The ossicles reside in a chamber where the **eustachian (you-STAY-shee-un) tube** also begins; it forms a narrow channel which opens behind the tonsils in the throat. It equalizes air pressure on each side of the eardrum.

The inner ear transmits sound waves to the brain for interpretation. Hearing and balance mechanisms occupy a chamber filled with fluid called **endolymph**. Sound waves travel from the stapes and permeate this fluid. This causes tiny hairs attached to nerve fibers lining the **cochlea (KOK-le-ah)** to vibrate and send nerve impulses via the **cochlear nerve** to the auditory center in the brain.

The inner ear also contains the organs of balance, which are attuned to the position of the head. Here a maze of fluid-filled tubes called **semicircular canals** are situated at various angles and levels. Fine particles of chalk are suspended in a thick jelly-like substance within these tubes. The particles move according to the head's position, thereby stimulating sensitive hairs. The resulting nerve impulses are interpreted by the brain, which then directs balance accordingly. The eyes play a vital role in balance as well, since they offer important information about how the body is situated in its environment.

The sense of **smell** is probably the oldest and least understood of the five senses. It is closely linked with the sense of taste. The sensory receptors for smell are located in two separate passages in the roof of the nasal cavity, beneath the frontal lobes of the brain. This is called the **olfactory** area; it is tightly packed with millions of odor sensing cells. Each cell has about a dozen fine hairs called **cilia** which project into a layer of mucus. The mucus keeps the cilia moist and acts to trap odorous substances. It is thought that tiny particles dissolve in the mucus and stick to the cilia, which causes the cells to send off electrical signals to the brain via the olfactory nerves. Thus a substance must release particles of the chemical from which it is made into the air in gaseous form in order to stimulate the sense of smell. The olfactory center in the brain is closely connected to the **limbic system** where emotions, moods and memories are located; therefore smells often evoke vivid memories.

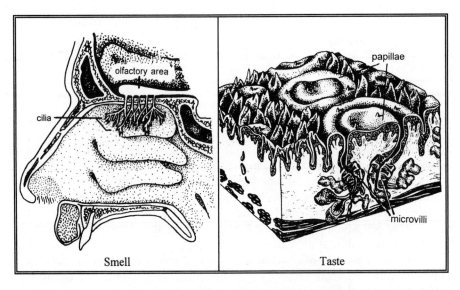

Smell   Taste

The sense of **taste** is limited in range and versatility and presents less information than any other sense. It is considerably aided by the sense of smell; without smelling, the ability to taste is greatly impaired. Tasting is also triggered by the chemical content of foods. Particles stimulate nerve impulses that are transmitted to the brain and interpreted. The **taste buds** are central to this process. About 9,000 taste buds stud the surface of the tongue. They are contained within many small projections called **papillae**. These are mainly located on the upper surface of the tongue, but some can be found on the palate and even in the throat.

Each taste bud consists of groups of receptor cells. These have fine hair-like projections called **microvilli** that stick out into the surface of the tongue through fine pores in the papilla. These projections are linked to nerve fibers which lead to the brain. The taste buds respond to only four basic tastes. Sweet buds are at the tip of the tongue, while sour, salt and bitter buds are progressively further back. Chemicals must be in liquid form in order to be tasted. This is accomplished by the production of **saliva**, a digestive fluid that starts to secrete and break down food as soon as it enters the mouth. The brain simultaneously interprets such things as the texture and temperature of foods.

The sense of **touch** is a specialized activity in the skin surface. Root hair plexuses are wrapped around the base of fine hairs in the skin, and respond to any stimulation of the hair. Free nerve endings are the most widely distributed touch receptors in the body and respond to pain, thermal stimuli and light touch. Various other receptors, grouped into discs called corpuscles, are modified cells which respond to different stimuli. Tactile Merkel's and Meissner's corpuscles respond to light touch (skin is not indented). Lamellated (Pacinian) corpuscles, corpuscles of Ruffini and bulbous corpuscles (of Krause) respond to touch-pressure. The external temperature greatly affects touch reception, with cold dulling the sense of touch considerably. Each variety of touch receptor transmits its impulses to the brain, where the sensory information is sorted out and a response initiated.

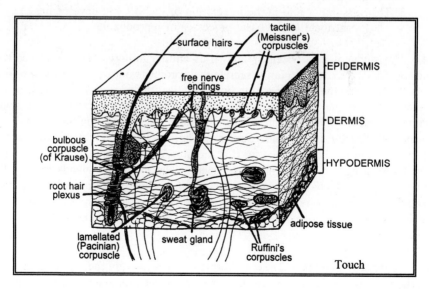

132

The Endocrine System

Pregnancy and birth have much to do with how hormones work in the body; therefore an overall understanding of the endocrine system will be directly useful to your practice.

Two regulatory systems help send and receive sensory messages and correlate body signals: the nervous system and the endocrine system. These two systems work together to keep the body going, each stimulating and inhibiting the other as appropriate. The **endocrine system** affects bodily activity by releasing chemical messengers, called **hormones**, into the bloodstream. Hormones carry messages to virtually all parts of the body. The response of the area most sensitive to the influence of a particular hormone may take from less than a minute to several hours to occur. Although hormonal effects are extremely varied, they can be categorized into four broad areas:

1. They help control the internal environment by regulating its chemical composition and volume.
2. They respond to marked changes in environmental conditions to help the body cope with emergency demands such as infection, trauma, stress, etc.
3. They assume a role in the integration of growth and development.
4. They contribute to the basic processes of reproduction.

The study of this system is known as **endocrinology**. The body has two kinds of glands. **Exocrine glands** secrete their products onto a free surface or into ducts which carry the hormones into body cavities, the center of an organ, or the surface. **Endocrine glands** secrete their hormones into the extracellular space around the secretory cells; the hormones then pass into capillaries and are transported directly in the bloodstream. The amount of hormone released is dependent upon the body's need for it at the time. Most hormones are released in short bursts triggered by the nervous system. The endocrine glands include the **pituitary (hypophysis), thyroid, adrenals (suprarenals), pineal (epiphysis cerebri)**, and the **thymus gland**. In addition several organs such as the **pancreas, ovaries, testes, kidneys, stomach, small intestines,** and **placenta** contain endocrine tissue.

There are three main classes of hormones. **Amines** are the simplest; they are modified forms of the amino acid tyrosine. Examples include some adrenal and thyroid hormones. Hormones derived from **proteins** and **peptides** consist of chains of amino acids varying from simple to complex. Examples are oxytocin and insulin. **Steroids** are derived from cholesterol. They include some adrenal hormones and are fat-soluble. Steroids and thyroid hormones alter cell function by entering the cell membranes and interacting within the cell itself. Once released by a cell, hormones are carried to a **target cell** that responds in a specific way. Almost all body cells are target cells of some sort, but each has specific receptors which make its surface sensitive only to certain hormones.

Prostaglandins (pros-tah-GLAN-dens) or **PGs** are potent membrane-associated, biologically active lipids that are secreted into the blood in small quantities. They are called local or tissue hormones because their site of action is the immediate area in which they are produced. They are synthesized by nearly every mammalian cell and tissue and are released as a result of chemical and mechanical stimuli. Prostaglandins are classified into several groups designated by letters A through I (i.e. PGA through PGI). Each group is further divided based on the number of double chemical bonds in the fatty acids. Thus PGE_2 has two double bonds, PGE_1 has one. Prostaglandins are believed to regulate and modify cell metabolism, and may help modulate the response of cells to stimuli. They can also be rapidly deactivated, especially in the lungs, liver and kidneys. Their broad range of biological activity indicates their importance in normal physiology.

The **pituitary gland** or **hypophysis (hi-POF-i-sis)** is found at the base of the brain (the hypothalamus). It can be divided into two halves that function separately. The pituitary works in coordination with the hypothalamus and higher brain centers to produce and control hormones essential to normal fertility and lactation. The pituitary is considered the master gland of the body. It not only produces its own hormones, it influences the hormone production of other glands as well.

The **posterior pituitary** works in concert with the hypothalamus, the body's link between the nervous system and the glands, which is connected to the pituitary stalk. It produces oxytocin and **antidiuretic hormone (ADH)**, also known as vasopressin. **Oxytocin** controls uterine activity during labor and breastfeeding. ADH governs the body's water-balancing mechanism. The hypothalamus feeds these hormones to the posterior pituitary and orders their release based on signals from the body. The hypothalamus and posterior pituitary gland function as a self-contained unit.

The **anterior pituitary** produces 7 hormones: **melanocyte-stimulating hormone** (increases skin pigmentation), **thyroid stimulating hormone** (TSH), **adrenocorticotropic hormone** (ACTH; stimulates the adrenal glands to produce cortisone), **prolactin** (regulates milk production), **growth hormone** (controls body growth), **follicle stimulating hormone** (FSH, stimulates ovum production), and **luteinizing hormone** (LH, induces ovulation and helps maintain early pregnancy).

The **thyroid** (found in the front center of the neck) is an endocrine gland responsible for regulating oxygen use, stimulating the burning of calories for energy, enhancing the function of epinephrine, and controlling the rate at which various organs function. It also controls the metabolism of food, and the growth and development of bone, nerve tissue and muscle.

The thyroid gland produces three hormones: **calcitonin (kal-si-TOE-nin (CT), thyroxine (thigh-ROCKS-en)** (T_4) and **triiodothyronine (tri-ee-oh-doe-THIGH-row-nen)** (T_3). Calcitonin is one of the hormones which regulate calcium metabolism. T_3 and T_4 are chemically similar; both are frequently referred to as "thyroid hormone," with T_3 being more potent and T_4 being much more plentiful.

Thyroid hormones are produced under the influence of a negative feedback system. The principle organs involved in this process are the hypothalamus, anterior pituitary and thyroid gland. The hypothalamus sends directions via its messenger hormone, thyroid releasing factor (TRF), to the anterior pituitary gland and regulates the release of thyroid stimulating hormone (TSH). TSH directs the thyroid gland to produce and release more thyroid hormone. This chain of events is cycled on and off by the hypothalamus. Fluctuations in serum thyroid hormone levels trigger the release of TRF by the hypothalamus. (Smith, 1990)

The thyroid takes iodine from the blood, combines it with tyrosine (an amino acid), and converts it into T_3 and T_4, which it then stores and releases when necessary. More than 99% of T_3 and T_4 is transported to cells by three carrier proteins in the bloodstream: thyroxine binding globulin (TBG), thyroxine binding prealbumin and albumin. TBG binds most of the thyroid hormone released by the thyroid gland. Less than 1% of T_3 and T_4 remains in the free, unbound state, which is the only metabolically active form. The small portion of thyroid hormone not bound to protein (free hormone) is the true determinant of function, since it is the only form available to the tissues. If function is extremely abnormal, all body systems may feel the effects.

The small **parathyroid glands** are located on the back of or inside each thyroid lobe and are responsible for the regulation of calcium in the body. Parathyroid hormone (PTH), also called parahormone, increases as calcium levels fall, prompting release of calcium from the bones to raise blood levels. Three forms exist: intact glandular hormone, multiple **N-terminal (mid-molecular) fragments**, and **C-terminal fragments** (both types of terminal fragments are byproducts of hormone breakdown).

The **adrenal glands** or **suprarenals** sit like little caps on top of each kidney. Each is divided into two regions that produce different hormones. The outer layer, or cortex, produces three classes of hormones: **mineralocorticoids** help control water and mineral balance, **glucocorticoids** help regulate normal metabolism and resistance to stress, and **gonadocorticoids** (sex hormones) supplement hormones produced by the gonads. All in all, the cortex produces at least 40 steroid hormones which are collectively referred to as corticosteroids.

Aldosterone accounts for 95% of the mineralocorticoid activity. It regulates salt excretion by the kidneys and is involved in carbohydrate usage. The glucocorticoids consist of **cortisol** (or hydrocortisone), **corticosterone**, and **cortisone**. All help to stimulate the production and storage of glucose, reduce fat inflammation after trauma, and are vital to immune function. Of the three, cortisol accounts for 95% of their activity.

The **inner layer, or medulla** of the adrenals, produces **adrenalin** (or epinephrine), which prepares the body for physical action (the "fight or flight" response), and **noradrenalin** (or norepinephrine), which regulates blood pressure.

The **pancreas** is classified as both an endocrine and exocrine gland. It is a flat organ located behind and slightly below the stomach. It has three kinds of cells: **alpha cells** which secrete **glucagon** (which increases blood glucose levels), **beta cells** that secrete **insulin** (which decreases blood sugar levels) and **delta cells** which secrete **growth hormone-inhibiting factor** (GHIF) and **somatostatin** (which inhibits the secretion of insulin).

The **ovaries** and **testes** are paired oval bodies referred to as gonads. The **ovaries** are the female organs located in the pelvis that secrete **estrogens** and **progesterone**, which are responsible for the development and maintenance of the female sexual characteristics. They regulate the female reproductive system along with gonadotropic hormones from the pituitary gland. They also produce **relaxin**, which softens connective tissues in preparation for birth.

The **testes** are the male gonads, and are found in the scrotum. They produce **testosterone**, the main male sex hormone which maintains male sexual character-istics. They also produce **inhibin**; this inhibits the secretion of follicle stimulating hormone thereby controlling sperm production.

The **pineal gland (epiphysis cerebri)** is attached to the roof of the third ventricle in the brain. It is a covered pine cone-shaped gland measuring 3 to 9 mm in length, 3 to 6 mm in width, and 3 to 5 mm in thickness. It is encased in a capsule and consists of masses of cells called **pinealocytes**. Although calcification of the gland begins at puberty, this may actually increase its activity. Its function remains somewhat obscure. It secretes the hormone **melatonin** which appears to inhibit reproductive activities by acting on other hormones. Another hormone, **adrenoglomerulotropin** may help stimulate the adrenal cortex to secrete aldosterone.

The **thymus gland** consists of two flat, symmetrical encapsulated lobes found just above and in front of the heart. Each lobe is divided into many lobules, each consisting of a dense cortex of lymphoid tissue containing thymocyte cells and a medulla which contains less densely packed thymocytes. It is quite large in infants and grows rapidly for the first 2 years of life. It reaches a weight of 30 grams at puberty, then slowly begins to reduce in size and is replaced by fat and connective tissues. It plays a major role in the function of the immune system. Its hormones include **thymosin, thymic humoral factor (THF), thymic factor (TF)** and **thymopoietin**. These hormones promote the maturation of special white blood cells called T cells.

Other endocrine tissues include those found in the **stomach** which produce gastric hormones and the **placenta** which produces pregnancy-related hormones. When deprived of oxygen the **kidneys** trigger the production of a hormone that stimulates red cell production. The **skin** produces vitamin D when exposed to sunlight. And the **cardiac muscle** produces a hormone that regulates the blood pressure.

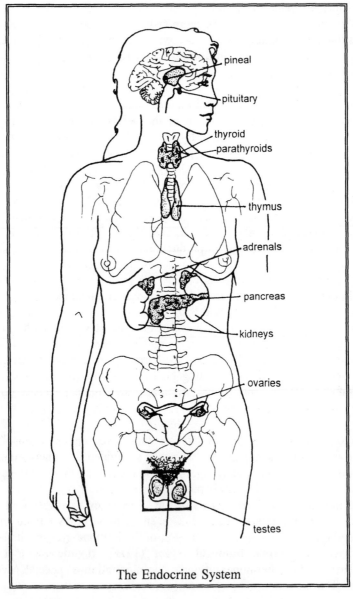

The Endocrine System

The Cardiovascular System

The cardiovascular system is comprised of the blood, heart and blood vessels. Study of the heart and blood vessels will help you understand how nutrients are exchanged for waste products between the mother's system and that of the fetus, how blood clotting occurs, the differences between fetal and adult circulation, and how to interpret certain lab results.

The **blood** is a fluid which carries mobile cells, providing a means of nourishment and waste disposal for specialized cells that are in fixed locations and cannot carry out an independent existence. The study of the blood and blood-forming tissues is called **hematology**. Blood is normally contained within a network of closed vessels. Substances within the blood interact with **interstitial fluid** (also called **intercellular** or **tissue fluid**), which surrounds the cells and exchanges substances with the bloodstream. Blood transports oxygen, nutrients, hormones and enzymes. These substances diffuse from tiny blood vessels called capillaries into the interstitial fluid, where they are exchanged for wastes from the cells. The blood can also transport disease-related substances.

Blood is a thick, adhesive fluid made up of formed elements (cells and cell-like structures [45% of total volume]) and a fluid which transports them and other substances called **plasma** (55% total volume). The thickness (or viscosity) of water is 1.0; the thickness of blood ranges from 4.5 to 5.5 due to the presence of many blood cells. The average woman has 4 to 5 liters of blood when she is not pregnant. Blood is a complex liquid which performs these critical functions: **transportation of vital substances, regulation of pH, and protection from blood loss** via the clotting mechanism.

Blood cell formation takes place in the ends of the humerus and femur, sternum, ribs, vertebrae and pelvis as well as in lymphoid tissue. Red blood cells, platelets and some white cells (**leukocytes**) are produced in red bone marrow (myeloid tissue). Undifferentiated cells in the red bone marrow are transformed into immature cells called **hemocytoblasts (he-mow-SIGH-toe-blasts)** that eventually develop into a variety of mature red and white blood cells. Other types of white cells arise from the spleen, tonsils and lymph nodes. (For more details about the different types of blood cells see the chapter on The Complete Blood Count in <u>Diagnostic Tests</u>). Red cells are mainly responsible for the transport of oxygen. White cells of various types help protect the body against disease conditions.

Platelets are also carried by the plasma. They are the smallest cells in the body, with about 250 million to every milliliter of blood. Their basic function is to form a plug at the site of injury when bleeding must be stopped.

Plasma transports many of the body's important substances. Each liter of plasma contains about 2½ ounces (75 grams) of protein composed of two types; albumin and globulin. Albumin is the most abundant type of protein found in the blood. It is made by the liver and serves as a food source for the tissues. Albumin works with sodium to hold fluid in the circulating blood volume, preventing its leaking into surrounding tissues through a process called **osmosis**. **Globulins** comprise about 38% of plasma proteins and function as antibodies against specific foreign substances.

Hemostasis is the process that stops bleeding. It is regulated within the system so that the blood will circulate freely. The smooth lining of the blood vessels and adequate blood flow inhibit coagulation. In addition, the intrinsic fibrinolytic system breaks up clots that form due to abnormal processes, thus minimizing life-threatening blockages.

Clotting can be triggered in three ways: vascular spasm, platelet plug formation and blood coagulation (clotting). Normal hemostasis (stabilization of bleeding) can be divided into two basic reactions. Primary hemostasis occurs with the immediate response of platelet adhesion to exposed, torn skin fibers at the site of vessel injury. As the platelets aggregate (stick together) and vessels contract, the lesion is sealed off. During secondary hemostasis or coagulation, fibrin reinforces the initial platelet plug; this is a necessary step to stop bleeding in larger injuries.

There are two mechanisms that trigger blood to coagulate:

*The **extrinsic pathway** is activated when a blood vessel is cut or damaged. Tissue trauma releases agents that stimulate the clotting response.

*The **intrinsic pathway** is activated under certain abnormal conditions during which blood clots within a vessel, even though there has been no external trauma and blood loss is not a factor. It may be triggered by an irritation of the blood vessel lining, which may occur with infection, degeneration, a concentrated blood volume, or foreign material in the blood stream.

*Although different coagulation factors are involved with each pathway, the basic steps in the clotting process are similar when an injury or insult occurs. The common final pathway of either of these mechanisms is the formation of a fibrin clot.

There are twelve clotting factors, including calcium (which is necessary for all clotting to take place). Eight of these are proteins synthesized by the liver. All factors are normally found inactive in the plasma. Platelets, though not considered factors, play an essential role in the clotting mechanism.

Not all blood is the same. There are almost 400 red cell factors currently identified. Typing is determined by the presence or absence of certain sugars on the red blood cell. Human blood can be divided into four major groups or factors:

A, B, AB, and O. Each major factor has a specific antigen (a protein causing the formation of antibodies) called an agglutinogen or isoantigen (the prefix "iso" refers to agents which the body produces with no outside stimulation). The antigens of the ABO group are unique in that they are not limited to the surface of the red blood cells; they are found in many other tissues as well. It is thought that 80% of the white western population are "secretors" of A and B antigens in their saliva and gastric juice. Sensitization may occur in the absence of blood mixing through contact with their own body fluids (i.e. within an individual's own system). It is by virtue of this unique blood antigen production that Anti-A and Anti-B antibodies are said to occur naturally. Major blood group isoantibodies are maintained at a fixed level. AB blood recognizes A, B and O as compatible. Type O has a "functionally silent" antigen and therefore recognizes both A and B blood as foreign. (Lloyd, 1987) Here is how it breaks down:

Blood Group	Isoantigen on RBC	Isoantibodies in serum
O	silent	Anti-A & Anti-B (universal donor)
A	A	Anti-B
B	B	Anti-A
AB	A & B	Neither Anti-A nor Anti-B (universal recipient)

The percentage of people with the various blood types varies from race to race. The following proportions are based on United States populations:

Blood Group	Caucasians	African-Americans
O	45%	46%
A	41%	27%
B	10%	20%
AB	4%	7%

The rest of the blood antigens are referred to as **minor factors**, since isoantibodies are not present with these blood factors. When a foreign minor blood factor is introduced into the bloodstream and identified within the body, inherent antigens on the host RBCs are stimulated to form antibodies. The antibodies remain in the system and will destroy the same factor during future exposures. (More details can be found in the chapter on Blood Types and Incompatibilities in Diagnostic Tests).

The study of the heart is referred to as **cardiology**. The **heart** is a large muscular organ that weighs about 12 ounces and is about as large as the person's fist. It straddles the midline of the chest, with its larger end to the left. The right end of the heart lies behind the right border of the sternum. The heart projects out as a rounded triangle to the left of the sternum with its point below the left nipple. This pulsating point is called the **apex beat**. The heart is contained within a stabilizing yet flexible pouch called the **pericardium**.

The interior of the heart has four muscular chambers which pump the blood. Each chamber is a three-layer muscular bag with walls which contract and push blood onward. The chambers are arranged in pairs. The two upper ones are called the right and left **atria**. The atria are separated by a partition called the **interatrial septum**. It has an oval depression called the **fossa ovalis**, which is the closed-over location of the foramen ovale, an opening present during fetal development. The two lower chambers are the right and

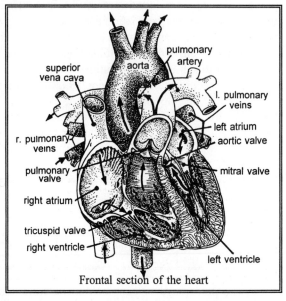

Frontal section of the heart

left **ventricles**, which are separated by an **interventricular septum**. Blood flows from one chamber to another through a series of one-way valves. The **tricuspid valve** connects the right atrium to the right ventricle; blood exits the right side of the heart through the **pulmonary valve**. The **mitral valve** connects the left atrium to the left ventricle; blood exits the left side of the heart through the **aortic valve**.

The heart pumps blood throughout two separate circulatory systems. First, it pumps clean blood from the lungs out to the arteries via the **aorta**, which is the main artery of the body. Arterial blood is circulated throughout the body, delivering food and oxygen to the tissues. Waste products are deposited in the blood in exchange and the blood flows through the veins to return to the heart.

The right atrium receives blood from the veins. The **superior vena cava** brings blood from locations above the heart. The **inferior vena cava** brings most of its blood from locations below the heart. The right atrium empties blood into the right ventricle. It pumps the blood into the lungs via the right and left pulmonary arteries. In the lungs carbon dioxide is exchanged for oxygen. Oxygenated blood then returns to the heart via the pulmonary vein which empties into the left atrium. The blood then passes into the left ventricle; and the whole circuit begins again—the left ventricle pumps blood into the ascending aorta, which branches into several channels from which blood is delivered to the rest of the body. The blood is channeled from one chamber to another by way of one-way valves which open and shut in sequence as the blood moves through the heart.

The autonomic nervous system supplies the heart and can affect how fast or slow it beats, but it does not initiate contraction. The heart has a special self-regulating system called the **conduction system**. This system generates its own electrical impulses which stimulate the heart to beat. Each portion of the cardiac cycle (heart beat) produces a different electrical impulse. Therefore, much can be learned about the function of the heart by applying electrodes to the chest and recording the impulses on a graph. This test is called an **electrocardiogram**.

When the heart beats, the two atria contract while the two ventricles relax, and vice versa. The term **systole (SIS-toe-lee)** refers to the phase of contraction. The term **diastole (die-AS-toe-lee)** refers to the phase of relaxation. A cardiac cycle refers to the systole and diastole of all the chambers. The activity of the heart is regulated by the rest of the body's needs. When cells are very active, more nutritive substances are needed and the heart rate increases. The sound of the heartbeat comes from the blood flow created by the closure of valves. The first sound can be described as a long booming sound which occurs soon after ventricular systole begins. The second sound is shorter and sharper and occurs at the end of ventricular systole. A brief pause occurs before the next cycle begins.

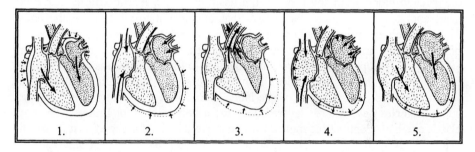

1. Blood filling the atria from the lungs and rest of the body flows into the ventricles from the contraction of the atria.
2. As the atria begins to relax, the ventricles begin to contract, the tricuspid and mitral valves close to keep blood from back-flowing to the atria. Pressure builds in the ventricles.
3. The ventricles contract. With build-up of internal pressure in the ventricles, the aortic and pulmonary valves are pushed open to allow blood to flow to the lungs and rest of the body.
4. The ventricles begin to relax. The decrease in internal pressure causes the aortic and pulmonary valves to close, preventing blood from flowing back into the ventricles. Blood starts to flow into the atria.
5. The atria fill with blood from the lungs and the rest of the body. Rising internal pressure pushes open the tricuspid and mitral valves, allowing blood to flow into the ventricles.

The amount of blood ejected from the left ventricle into the aorta per minute is called the **cardiac output (CO)**. It is determined by the amount of blood pumped by the left ventricle during each beat and the number of heartbeats per minute. The amount of blood ejected by a ventricle during each systole is called the **stroke volume (SV)**. Stroke volume depends on the amount of blood that enters the ventricle during diastole and the amount left in the ventricle following its systole. In a resting adult, stroke volume averages 70 ml. with the average heart rate ranging between 60 to 75 beats a minute. Factors such as stress or exercise tend to increase stroke volume, heart rate and cardiac output. During rest or relaxation stroke volume, heart rate and cardiac output tend to decrease. Under certain conditions stroke volume may fall dangerously low; in the case of hemorrhage for example, stroke volume falls because the blood volume has dropped and the heart muscles are not being adequately stretched. The body will attempt to maintain a safe cardiac output by increasing the rate and strength of the contractions of the heart muscles.

Blood vessels are tubes which form a network carrying blood throughout the body. They are the third part of the cardiovascular system. **Arteries** carry oxygenated blood from the heart to the tissues. Large, elastic arteries leave the heart and divide into muscular vessels that branch out to all parts of the body. These branch again into smaller vessels called **arterioles**, which enter tissues and branch into the smallest vessels called **capillaries**, where nutrients and wastes are exchanged. Groups of capillaries come together to form small veins called **venules** before leaving the tissues. These form progressively larger tubes called **veins** which carry the deoxygenated, waste-laden blood back to the lungs for cleaning.

Arteries have a three layered wall and a hollow core, or **lumen**. They are elastic and have contractible muscles which move the blood along after it leaves the heart. They can also constrict in an attempt to stop bleeding, but since arterial blood is under a great deal of pressure, this does not always work.

Capillaries connect veins and arteries by forming a one cell layer tube within tissues through which nutrients and wastes are exchanged.

Veins are composed of essentially the same three coats as arteries, but they have considerably less elastic tissue and smooth muscle and contain more white fibrous tissue. The pressure in veins is much less than in the arteries; therefore venous walls are not as strong. There are also valves in the veins to prevent back flow because the force of gravity tends to pull upwardly flowing blood downwards. Contractions of the skeletal muscles surrounding veins milk the blood upward. Breathing helps move venous blood—during inspiration the diaphragm moves downward, causing a decrease in pressure in the chest cavity, which causes blood to move up from the abdomen to the chest. During expiration, back flow is prevented by the valves.

The alternating expansion and elastic recoil of an artery with each heartbeat is called the **pulse**. The **blood pressure** is the pressure in the arteries exerted by

143

the left ventricle when it undergoes systole (contraction) and the pressure remaining in the arteries when the ventricle is in diastole (relaxation).

The major blood vessels are illustrated on the following pages:

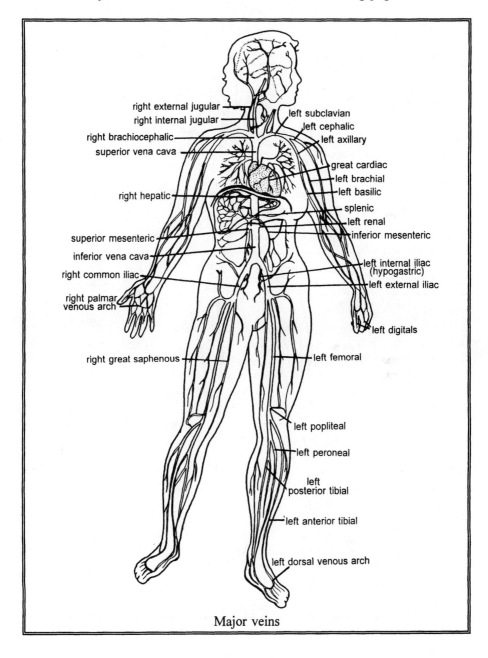

Major veins

144

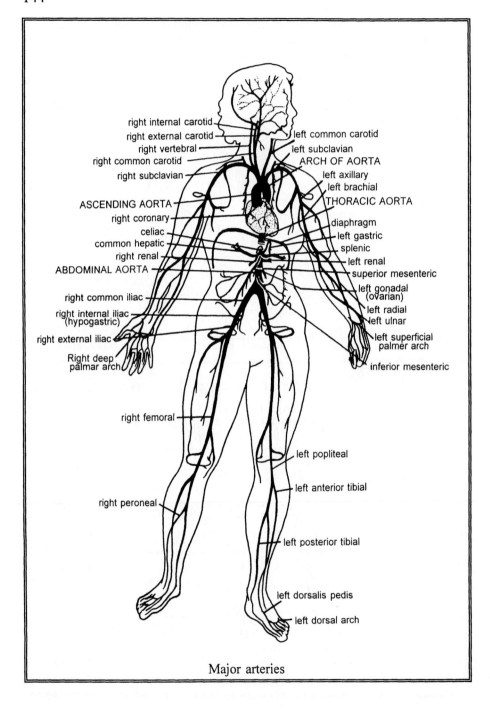

right internal carotid
right external carotid
right vertebral
right common carotid
right subclavian

left common carotid
left subclavian
ARCH OF AORTA
left axillary
left brachial

ASCENDING AORTA
right coronary
celiac
common hepatic
right renal
ABDOMINAL AORTA

THORACIC AORTA
diaphragm
left gastric
splenic
left renal
superior mesenteric

right common iliac
right internal iliac
(hypogastric)
right external iliac
Right deep
palmar arch

left gonadal
(ovarian)
left radial
left ulnar
left superficial
palmer arch
inferior mesenteric

right femoral

left popliteal

left anterior tibial

right peroneal

left posterior tibial

left dorsalis pedis
left dorsal arch

Major arteries

The Lymphatic System

Understanding the lymphatic system will help you when learning about the immune system, various diseases and how to prevent illness.

The **lymphatic (lim-FAT-ick)** system consists of a fluid called lymph, a network of vessels called lymphatics which transport lymph, the lymph nodes, spleen, and thymus gland as well as the bone marrow, where leukocytes are made.

Tiny lymph vessels (capillaries) are found throughout the body except in avascular tissue, the central nervous system, splenic pulp and bone marrow. Unlike blood capillaries they do not connect to other structures, but end in a blind pouch. Lymph capillaries unite to form larger vessels called lymphatic vessels. These resemble veins in structure, but have thinner walls and more one-way valves and contain lymph nodes at various intervals. Lymphatics of the skin travel in loose subcutaneous tissue and generally follow veins. Internal lymphatic vessels usually follow arterial pathways and form networks around them.

Lymph is a clear fluid which seeps through capillary walls and bathes the cells, bringing them oxygen and nutrients and cleansing away toxins. Some returns to the capillaries, but a significant amount is passively transported through the thin lymphatic vessels, since there is no active pump. Muscle action, close contact with arterial pulses, postural changes, passive compression and respiration all help lymph fluid to move through the system. Lymph flow is much more easily obstructed by pressure from clothing, such as a bra, than is the case with the circulatory system.

Lymph nodes are small oval structures located along the length of the lymphatics. They are found throughout the body, usually in groups and range from 1 to 25 mm. (.04 to 1 inch) in length. White blood cells called lymphocytes are produced and stored within the nodes. The **tonsils** are groups of large lymphatic nodules embedded in a mucus membrane. They are arranged in a ring at the junction of the oral cavity and the pharynx. There are three forms: the **pharyngeal** tonsil or **adenoid** is in the posterior wall of the throat. A pair of **palatine tonsils** are situated on either side of the back of the throat, and the **lingual tonsils** are at the base of the tongue. The tonsils protect against the entry of foreign substances, and produce lymphocytes and antibodies.

The **spleen** is an oval mass about 12 cm. (5 inches) in length. It is the largest mass of lymphatic tissue in the body. It is located on the left side of the body between the top of the stomach and the diaphragm. It is molded around adjacent organs and the diaphragmatic muscle, and is contained within a capsule of connective tissue. It contains lymphatic tissue, lymphocyte cells, venous sinuses filled with blood and bands of splenic tissue called **cords**. These splenic cords are filled with erythrocytes (red blood cells) and various kinds of white blood cells. The spleen does not filter lymph fluid since it contains no lymphatic vessels. It produces **B lymphocyte cells**, which develop into antibody-producing plasma cells. The spleen also consumes bacteria and unusable red blood cells and platelets. The spleen stores blood and releases it according to the body's needs, such as during a hemorrhage.

The **thymus gland** is a double lobed organ located in the upper chest behind the sternum and between the lungs. It is composed of an outer layer called the cortex and a central medulla. The cortex is made up of tightly packed lymphocytes held together by fibrous tissue. The medulla consists of thymus cells and scattered lymphocytes in a cellular mass. The thymus gland is large and quite active in the first few years of life. It reaches its maximum size during puberty (up to 1½ oz. or 45 gm.). The thymus gland of an infant is very large compared to the rest of the body; by old age it has atrophied so that little or no tissue remains. It is thought that the thymus helps lay the foundation for the way the body will respond to infection, in particular making sure the body does not turn its activities against itself in the process. **T** or **thymus cell lymphocytes** are under the control of the thymus. There are two types of T-lymphocytes: T-helper cells assist B cells in producing antibodies; T-suppressor cells prevent B cells from producing antibodies. The thymus may regulate and destroy those lymphocytes which could cause harm to the body; this appears to be the case because it destroys about 95% of the new lymphocytes it produces.

The immune response: The immune response is the body's reaction to the entry of foreign substances which occurs through the activation of white blood cells known as lymphocytes. It appears that foreign organisms that enter the body are taken to nearby lymph nodes or to the spleen by lymph vessels. Here, monocytes (white blood cells) differentiate into macrophages which surround and engulf the organism and present it to T and B cells. These recognize the organism's protein or antigen and set up an antibody (gamma globulin) mechanism to destroy future organisms of the same type. There are a number of other antimicrobial substances that the body produces as well. **Interferon** protects uninfected host cells from viral infection. **Complement** becomes attached to microbes by antigen-antibody complexes and causes their break-up. **Properdin** works in a similar fashion.

The immune response is also responsible for allergies. Normally harmless substances such as pollen may induce the production of antibodies causing the body to release certain substances such as histamines (inflammatory agents) into the tissues which have a disruptive effect on blood vessels and muscle tissues. In a similar manner, organ transplants and tissue grafts from other people cause the body to try and reject the foreign tissues, thus complicating transplant procedures.

Women are best endowed immunologically: antibody levels are higher, delayed hypersensitivity reactions are more intense, and response to vaccines is more brisk than in men. This may be why there is more autoimmune disease in young women than in men. The difference in male/female immune response may in part be accounted for by an immune-enhancing role of estrogens and the immunosuppression which is associated with androgens.

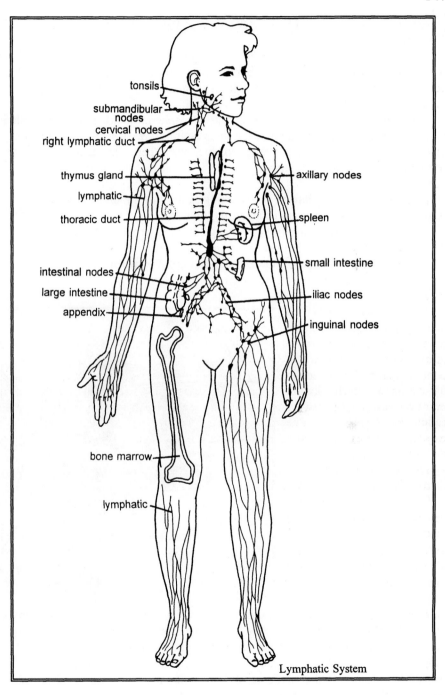

tonsils

submandibular
nodes

cervical nodes

right lymphatic duct

thymus gland

lymphatic

thoracic duct

intestinal nodes

large intestine

appendix

bone marrow

lymphatic

axillary nodes

spleen

small intestine

iliac nodes

inguinal nodes

Lymphatic System

The Respiratory System

A knowledge of respiration will help you understand how oxygen works in the body and (when you have a newborn that must be hospitalized) to interpret tests concerning pH and oxygen saturation in newborns.

The exchange of gasses between the atmosphere, the blood and the cells is called **respiration**. The cardiovascular and respiratory systems participate equally in this process: if one system fails, so does the other. There are three basic processes involved in respiration:

> ***Pulmonary ventilation** or breathing is the inspiration (inflow) and
> expiration (outflow) of air in the lungs.
> ***External respiration** is the exchange of gases between the lungs and
> the blood.
> ***Internal respiration** is the exchange of gases between the blood and
> the cells.

The **nose** forms the pathway by which air enters the body in the normal course of breathing. It consists of a bony bridge with a projection of cartilage which divides into two narrow passageways called **nasal fossae**. The external openings of the nose are called **nostrils**.

The **throat** is the area that leads into the respiratory and digestive tracts. It extends from the oral and nasal cavities to the esophagus and trachea. The **pharynx** channels food and liquids into the digestive tract and air into the lungs. It

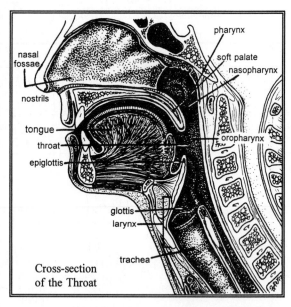

Cross-section
of the Throat

extends from the back of the mouth to a little way down inside the neck, and is lined with muscles. It is shaped like an inverted cone, extending for 5 inches (12 cm.) behind the arch at the back of the mouth to where it joins the gullet or esophagus. Its upper end is rigid because it is surrounded by skull bones. The lower end is joined to the elastic cartilages of the larynx. It is divided into three sections. The **nasopharynx** lies above the level of the soft palate and forms the back of the nose. It contains the adenoids and the openings for the eustachian tubes on either side. The **soft palate** is below this area in the back of the throat; upward movement of this palate closes off the nasopharynx during swallowing to prevent food from going up the nose. The **oropharynx** is at the back of the mouth and forms part of the airway between the mouth and the lungs. Its squeezing action helps shape sounds of speech as they come from the larynx. The lowermost or laryngeal section is involved entirely with swallowing. The movements of the pharynx must be coordinated so that food and air are directed into the appropriate tubes. This is achieved by a plexus (network) of nerves which supply the area.

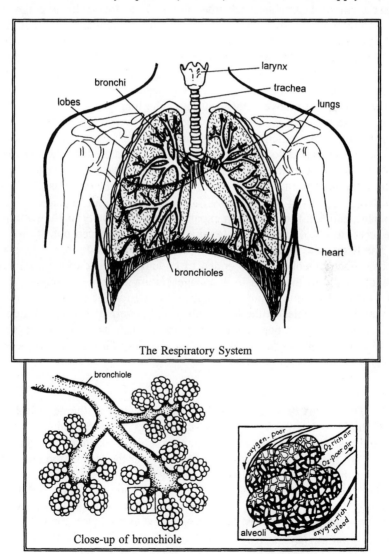

The Respiratory System

Close-up of bronchiole

The **trachea** or windpipe is made up of hoops of cartilage and looks like a vacuum cleaner hose. It takes air from the pharynx to the bronchi. The respiratory tract from the mouth and nose to the bronchi is lined with mucous membrane.

The **lungs** fill most of the thorax. The right lung is the largest, since the heart takes up more room on the left side of the thorax. Each lung is divided into sections called **lobes**: the right lung has three lobes (upper, middle and lower) and the left has two. The lobes are separate from each other and are demarcated by fissures or groves on their surface. The lungs are formed by a dense network of tiny tubes. The largest of these are the **bronchi**, which divide off into two main tubes at the end of the trachea, each entering one lung. Inside the lung, the bronchi continue to branch off into increasingly smaller tubes, eventually terminating in air sacs called **alveoli**.

The lungs are held open by surface tension created by a fluid produced by the **pleural membrane**. This membrane is the thin lining surrounding the lungs within the chest wall and is composed of two layers which slide over each other and allow the lungs to move with breathing. The lung's wet surface sticks to the lining the same way two panes of glass stick together when wet. When the chest expands the lungs are pulled out and the air is taken in. Most of the work is done by the muscular sheet called the diaphragm, which separates the chest cavity from the abdominal cavity at the lower border of the rib cage. In chest breathing, on inhalation the diaphragm contracts as it rises to expand the chest cavity, it relaxes on exhalation, the chest wall partially collapses, and the air is forced out. With abdominal breathing, the diaphragm expands toward the belly to allow more air to fill the lower lobes of the lungs, in expiration the air is forced out.

The lungs take in oxygen and get rid of carbon dioxide, or waste gas, from the body. Each alveolus is surrounded by a dense network of capillaries which bring blood cells to the lungs to exchange carbon dioxide for oxygen. Adults breathe about 12 times a minute when at rest. The rate of breathing is regulated by the respiratory center in the brain and by the levels of carbon dioxide in the blood. When more carbon dioxide is present, such as when under stress or exercising, the brain speeds up the breathing rate until the gas balance is returned to normal or until the stress ceases.

Speech: The **larynx** or voice box is found in the center of the neck at the top of the trachea. The larynx closes off the trachea, as when coughing, and plays a specialized and complex role as the organ of speech. Positioned over it is the **epiglottis**, the flap-valve which comes down to cover the **glottis** (the opening from the back of the throat into the larynx). The **vocal cords** consist of two delicate ligaments, shaped like lips which open and close as air passes through them. They vibrate during speech or vocalization, moving together for high pitched sounds and apart for low pitched ones. The mouth assists with speech by helping to shape sounds with the tongue and palate.

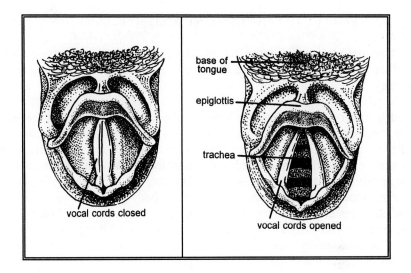

base of tongue

epiglottis

trachea

vocal cords closed

vocal cords opened

The Digestive System

Understanding the digestive process will help you understand how nutrients are utilized in the body and the changes which take place in digestion during pregnancy.

Digestion is the process that breaks down food into substances that can be absorbed and used by the body for energy, growth and repair. Organs which are attached to the digestive tract produce **enzymes,** chemicals that assist this process. The organs of digestion are divided into two main groups. The first is comprised of the gastrointestinal (GI) tract or alimentary canal, a continuous tube about 28 feet (9 m.) long running through the front of the body cavity and extending from the mouth to the anus. The second group of organs are accessory structures such as the teeth, tongue, salivary glands, liver, gallbladder and pancreas. These assist with the breakdown of food substances in various ways. There are five main functions of the digestive system:

1. **Ingestion** of food into the body (eating)
2. **Movement** of food along the digestive tract
3. **Digestion** or the breakdown of food by both chemical and mechanical processes
4. **Absorption** of chemical substances for use by the cells
5. **Defecation** or the elimination of indigestible substances from the body

Digestion begins in the **mouth** or **oral cavity** where food is broken into smaller particles via chewing. The **teeth** are hard, bone-like structures implanted in sockets around the jaws. There are two sets of teeth. Twenty deciduous (baby) teeth begin to appear at about 6 months of age. This process is usually complete by age 3. After age 6 lower, then upper, baby teeth are replaced by permanent teeth. By the time a person is in her early twenties she usually has all 32 adult teeth.

Each tooth has two parts: the **crown** is the part visible above the gum line; the **root** is imbedded within the jawbone and held in place by ligaments. Front teeth have one root, those further back have two or three. Most of the tooth is made from a hard substance called **dentine** which contains living cells. The dentine in the crown is covered by a protective layer of **enamel,** an extremely hard and cell-free insensitive tissue. The root is covered

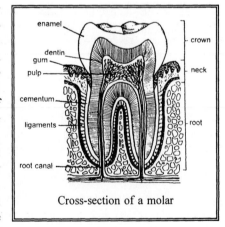

Cross-section of a molar

with **cementum**, a substance that is similar to dentine and helps anchor the tooth in its socket. In the center of each tooth is a hollow cavity known as a pulp chamber filled with a sensitive connective tissue known as **dental pulp**. This extends from inside the crown to the end of the root, which is open to allow blood vessels and nerves into the pulp chamber.

There are several types of teeth which perform different functions. **Incisors** have a narrow blade-like edge which cut food like scissors. **Canines** are pointed and adapted for tearing, while **molars** and **premolars** are used for grinding. The teeth form an even, semi-oval arch with the incisors at the front and canine, premolars and molars placed progressively further back in the mouth.

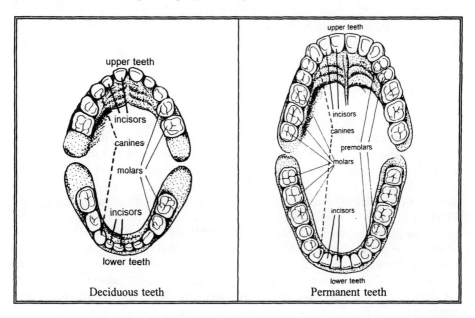

| Deciduous teeth | Permanent teeth |

The **salivary glands** secrete salivary amylase (AM-i-lass), an enzyme which begins to break down carbohydrates into maltose and glucose; and lysozyme, an enzyme which acts as a mild antiseptic. They also keep the mouth moist and pliable and aid in swallowing and tasting. There are 3 pairs of salivary glands in the face and neck; the **parotids**, the **submandibulars** and the **sub-linguals**, with many smaller glands scattered throughout the mouth. Each is composed of branching tubes that are packed together and lined with secretory cells. The parotids are the largest of these glands and are the main producers of salivary amylase. Saliva empties from the parotid ducts into the cheeks.

The submandibular glands lie under the jaw below the back teeth, and the sublingual glands are centrally located below the tongue. Both discharge fluid from ducts which open on either side of the frenulum (the small strip of tissue that joins the base of the tongue to the floor of the mouth). These glands secrete a mixture of mucus and **ptyalin (TIE-ah-lynn)**, an enzyme which breaks down starch and sugars.

Once food is chewed and mixed with saliva the tongue pushes the food up against the roof of the mouth (the hard palate) and into the muscle-lined cavity at the back of the throat (the pharynx) so that it can go down the esophagus. Normally the soft palate and the epiglottis (a flap which closes off the trachea during swallowing) prevent food from entering the trachea.

The **esophagus (e-SOF-a-gus)** lies behind the trachea just

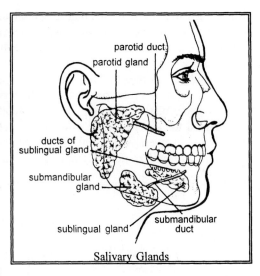

Salivary Glands

below the level of the notch found at the top of the sternum between the clavicles. It is an elastic tube about 10 inches (25 cm.) long and about 1 inch (2.5 cm.) in diameter. The esophagus is made up of four layers as is the rest of the GI tract: a lining of mucus membrane, a submucous layer, a thick layer of muscle, and a protective outer covering. The esophagus actively pushes the food along into the stomach by a series of involuntary wave-like contractions called **peristalsis (per-i-STAL-sis)**. There is no real constricting muscle, or sphincter, that separates the esophagus from the stomach. Stomach juices are normally kept in place because of the muscular lining of the esophageal walls and the fact that the tubular esophagus gets pinched off as it passes through the diaphragm. When this mechanism is inadequate, reflux or back washing of stomach juices occurs. Since stomach juice is acidic, this burns the esophagus and causes indigestion and heartburn.

The **stomach** is located in the upper left abdomen and is shaped like an elongated C. It forms a muscular enlargement of the gastrointestinal tract; its wall is a thick layer of muscle lined with epithelial membrane. The primary job of the stomach is to serve as a reservoir for food where a special juice called pepsin can begin the digestion of proteins. Gastric lipase (digests milk fats, especially in children) and rennin (digests milk in infants) are also secreted to break down food for further digestion. Food is mixed with gastric juices to form a pulp, which is then forced past the pyloric sphincter (which closes the stomach off) into the duodenum. The stomach empties all its contents, called **chyme**, into the duodenum within two to six hours after ingestion.

The **duodenum (do-oh-DEE-num)** is a 10 inch (25 cm.) horseshoe-shaped tube curved around the fat end of the pancreas, attached to the lower end of the stomach and forming the first part of the small intestines. The mucosa of the duodenum secretes mucus and digestive enzymes, helping to neutralize hydrochloric acid from the stomach and protecting the lining of the duodenum from acidic damage. Bile from the gallbladder and enzymes from the pancreas also enter the duodenum via a common duct. These fluids assist the process of digesting carbohydrates, proteins and fats.

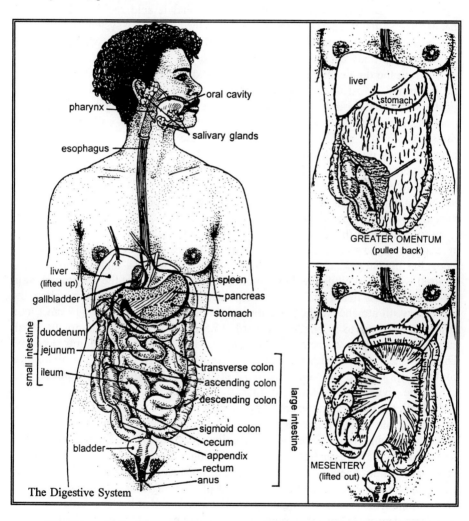

The Digestive System

Bile is a thick, bitter, yellow or greenish fluid made in the liver. It is essential in the breakdown of fats as well as serving as a means of eliminating the remains of old blood cells. It is stored, concentrated (up to 10 times) and released from the **gallbladder**, a pear-shaped muscular sac about 3 to 4 inches (7 to 10 cm.) long. The gallbladder is located in a depression on the underside of the liver.

The **pancreas** is a soft gland about 6 inches (12.5 cm.) long and 1 inch (2.5 cm.) thick. It is shaped roughly like a carrot with the fat end curved back on itself. It is made up of small clusters of glandular epithelial cells, about 1% of which form the endocrine portion of the gland. The remaining 99% forms the exocrine portion of the organ; this produces a mixture of digestive enzymes called pancreatic juices which breakdown carbohydrates, protein, nucleic acid and fat. (Remember that endocrine glands secrete their products into the circulatory system and exocrine glands secrete their products onto a free surface or into ducts which carry the hormones into body cavities, the center of an organ, or the surface.)

From the duodenum, chyme enters the next portion of small intestines called the **jejunum**. Most of the nourishment from the food is absorbed here, leaving mostly water and food waste behind. The inner lining of the jejunum consists of a series of circular folds lined with tiny hair-like projections called villi. Each villus contains a capillary and a tiny branch of the lymphatic system known as a lacteal. When digested food contacts the villi, glycerol, fatty acids and dissolved vitamins enter the lacteals. From there they are carried throughout the lymphatic system and enter the bloodstream. The capillaries in the villi absorb amino acids, sugars, vitamins and minerals directly into the hepatic portal vein which takes the substances directly to the liver.

The **ileum** is the last 12 feet (3.5 meters) of the small intestines. It is similar in structure to the rest of the small intestines. It consists of muscular layers which move the digested food along as well as layers of mucosa and an inner lining covered with villi. While the duodenum is fixed to the back of the abdominal wall, the jejunum and ileum are loosely stabilized by a fan-like structure called the **mesentery**. It attaches to the posterior abdominal wall with a 6 inch (15 cm.) long base and fans out to a length of 6 yards (5.5 meters) and attaches to the small intestines. This allows them to float, more or less, within the abdominal cavity. The mesentery, along with the rest of the protective covering for the abdominal contents, are collectively called the **peritoneum**, the lining of the abdomen.

The **liver** weighs three to four pounds (1.4 to 1.8 kg.). It is found underneath the diaphragm, where it is protected by the lower ribs. It is divided into two lobes; the right is the largest, occupying the entire upper portion of the abdomen's right side. The left lobe is smaller, reaching the midpoint of the upper left abdomen. The liver has about 500 functions; these can basically be divided into making new chemicals and neutralizing poisons and wastes. All the blood which leaves the digestive system must first pass through the liver. The lining of veins on the liver is made of highly specialized cells called Kupffer cells (after the man who identified them) that remove bacteria and excess red cells. The liver then takes out nutrients for its own use and for storage, and passes the remainder into the body's general circulation. The liver breaks down and recreates protein molecules into useable forms, a process referred to as synthesis. Protein is used to build new cells, blood elements, and hormones. Fats are broken down into forms which are used to renew or build fatty tissues. During the digestive process toxic byproducts are produced. These are further processed, converted or neutralized by the liver into substances the body can safely dispose of.

The liver also breaks down all forms of sugar into glucose, the body's primary energy food. When glucose is in the bloodstream, the hormone called insulin acts as the chemical doorway which allows glucose to enter the cells to be utilized. The level of glucose in the body is balanced by the presence of insulin and other hormones. The liver releases glucose for immediate use and converts and stores extra glucose as glycogen (a loose-knit mesh of glucose molecules). When glycogen stores become depleted as the result of excess energy use or lack of food intake, the body must break down either protein or fat for energy. Fat breakdown produces ketones. There are three types of ketones: aceto-acetic acid and betahydroxy-butyric acid and acetone. Acetone is a waste product of fat breakdown and is not useful; the other two ketones can be readily converted to energy.

The liver also produces about 1 3/4 pints (1 liter) of bile daily. Bile contains water (95%) and a wide range of chemicals such as bile salts, mineral salts, cholesterol and bile pigments called bilirubin. Bile is continuously made in small quantities by every cell in the liver. Bile mineral salts help neutralize stomach acids and break down fats so digestive chemicals can work on them. They may also assist in the absorption of fats and fat soluble vitamins through the intestinal wall. Bile salts are not destroyed after use; 80% to 90% of them are carried back to the liver for further use.

From the end of the ileum, digested food passes into the **large intestine**. Here the absorption of nutrients is completed, certain vitamins are manufactured, and feces (solid wastes) are formed and expelled. The large intestine is about five feet (1.5 meters) long and averages 2.5 inches (6.5 cm.) in diameter. It extends from the ileum to the anus and is attached to the posterior abdominal wall by its **mesocolon**, another membranous attachment of peritoneum. The large intestine is divided into four parts or regions: the cecum, colon, rectum and anal canal.

The opening from the ileum into the large intestine is covered by a fold of mucus membrane called the **ileocecal sphincter** or **valve**, which allows materials to pass slowly into the large intestine. Hanging below the ileocecal valve is the **cecum**, a blind pouch about 2.5 inches (6 cm.) long. Following a meal the **gastroileac reflex** causes any chyme in the ileum to be forced into the cecum. Attached to the inner side of the cecum is a small tube-shaped projection about 3 inches (8 cm.) in length called the **appendix**. It may serve as a means of combating infection since it contains a large collection of lymph glands, however its exact purpose in humans remains obscure.

The open end of the cecum merges with a long tube called the **colon**, which is divided into three sections: the **ascending colon** (coming up the right side of the body) the **transverse colon** (passing horizontally across the upper abdomen) and the **descending colon** (which comes down the left side of the body). The **sigmoid colon** begins at the left iliac crest, projects inward to the midline and ends as the rectum at about the level of the third sacral vertebra. Unlike the small intestine, the lining of the large intestine has no villi or circular folds. It contains columnar epithelium which absorb water, and goblet cells which secrete lubricating mucus into the colon. The colon walls are made up of muscle, mucosal tissue and glands.

Colonic movements begin when chyme passes through the ileocecal valve. Movement of material through the colon is stimulated as each section of the colon is filled. When distention reaches a certain point, the walls contract and squeeze the contents further along. Finally mass peristalsis occurs as a wave of muscular contractions begin moving food from the transverse colon into the rectum.

The last stage of digestion takes place in the large intestine and occurs through bacterial, not enzymatic, action. Bacteria ferment any remaining carbohydrates and release hydrogen, carbon dioxide and methane gas, which contribute to gas in the colon. They also convert any remaining proteins into amino acids and break them down into simpler substances. Several vitamins, including some of the B vitamins and vitamin K, are synthesized by bacterial action and absorbed. After 3 to 10 hours the chyme becomes solid or semisolid as a result of water absorption and is now known as **feces**. Feces are made up of water, inorganic salts, sloughed off epithelial cells from the mucosa of the alimentary canal, bacteria, products of bacterial decomposition and undigested parts of food.

The **rectum** forms the last eight inches (20 cm.) of the GI tract and lies anterior to the sacrum and coccyx. The last inch (2 to 3 cm.) of the rectum is called the **anal canal**, the opening of which is called the **anus**. It is kept closed by a set of sphincter muscles which open to allow the passage of stool or feces. As the rectum fills with fecal material, pressure-sensitive nerves tell us the lower bowel is full and needs to be emptied.

Protective coverings: The abdominal cavity is lined with a serous membrane known as the **peritoneum (per-uh-tuh-NEE-uhm)**. The **parietal peritoneum** lines the abdominal cavity and the **visceral peritoneum** forms a closely applied covering over most of the organs in the abdomen. Between these membranes is a space called the **peritoneal cavity** or **coelom**, a sac containing a small amount of serous fluid which allows the organs to move. Retroperitoneal organs lie behind this cavity and are more or less fixed in place. They are covered, but not surrounded, by peritoneum and include the pancreas, most of the duodenum, the abdominal aorta, inferior vena cava, ascending and descending colons and the kidneys. Superficially, the organs in the abdomen are draped by a protective covering called the **greater omentum**, which extends from underneath the liver, over the stomach and other organs as an extensive folded membrane containing a large amount of fat, plasma cells and white blood cells. It stops at the pelvic cavity. Numerous lymph nodes and vessels within the peritoneum guard against infection, but if inflammation should occur, the greater omentum wraps around the site and walls off the area. The lesser omentum extends from the liver to the top of the stomach and a small portion extends from the duodenum to the liver.

The Urinary System

Understanding the urinary tract helps you to understand blood volume expansion that takes place during a well-nourished pregnancy, how the mother's body maintains an adequate blood volume in the event of blood loss, and the impact of urinary tract infection on the pregnancy in general.

The primary function of the urinary system is to help keep the body in balance by controlling the composition and volume of blood. It does so by removing and restoring selected amounts of water and solids. The metabolism of nutrients results in the production of waste products which must be eliminated; the urinary tract helps with this process. The urinary system consists of two kidneys, two ureters, one urinary bladder and a single urethra. The branch of medicine that deals with the function of the urinary tract is call **urology (you-ROL-oh-gee)**.

The **kidneys** are reddish organs shaped like kidney beans. They are located just above the waist between the levels of the last thoracic and third lumbar vertebrae, and are partially protected by the 11th and 12th pairs of ribs. The right kidney is slightly lower than the left because it is slightly displaced by the liver. Both are surrounded by fibrous tissue and fat which encases and protects them.

The body of each kidney can be divided into an outer cortex layer and an inner medulla. The medulla contains 5 to 14 striated triangular structures called renal pyramids which fan out from the inner curve of the kidney. The renal pyramids contain thousands of tiny filtering units or **nephrons (NEF-rons)**. Each nephron can be divided into two parts: the filter, or **glomerulus (glow-MER-yoo-lus)** and the **tubules**, where water and essential nutrients are extracted from the blood. The nephrons control blood concentration and volume by removing selected amounts of water and solids, regulating blood pH, and removing toxic wastes.

The glomerulus consists of a knot of tiny blood capillaries which have very thin walls. Water containing dissolved waste products can pass freely across these walls into the collecting system of tubules on the other side. The holes in the capillaries form a biological sieve and are so small that certain large molecules, such as proteins, cannot normally pass through. This network is so extensive that it often contains almost 25% of the blood volume, and filters about 4½ fluid ounces (130 ml.) from the blood every minute. The amount of filtered blood produced in the capsular space each minute is called the **glomerular filtration rate (GFR)**.

Each glomerulus is surrounded by a **Bowman's capsule**, which is the beginning of its tubule. Here almost all the filtered water and salt is reabsorbed, thereby concentrating the urine. To reabsorb all this water, the pituitary gland secretes antidiuretic hormone (ADH) which changes the permeability of the tubule walls and regulates the amount of water that is reabsorbed. The adrenal hormone aldosterone regulates the exchange of sodium and potassium salts, which helps to regulate blood pressure. The parathyroid gland secretes parathyroid hormone which regulates calcium reabsorption. The kidneys themselves produce a hormone called renin, the level of which depends upon the amount of salt in the blood stream and which helps to control blood pressure. The tubules connect the glomeruli to a collecting system made up of minor and major **calyces** or drainage ducts (singular calyx) which ultimately drain urine into a reservoir known as the **renal pelvis**. From there urine flows into the bladder via the ureters.

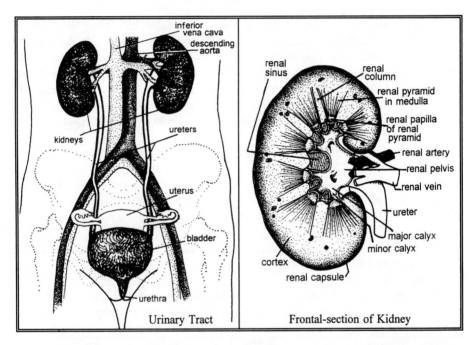

| Urinary Tract | Frontal-section of Kidney |

Urine is the by-product of kidney activity. It is a sterile, deionized fluid containing uric acid, minerals, vitamins, antibodies and waste products. Normally 1 to 2 quarts (1,000 to 2,000 ml.) are produced daily. As urine is formed it flows into the renal pelvis where it drips down either of two tubes beginning in the kidneys and opening into the bladder. These **ureters (YOU-re-ters)** are extensions of the renal pelvis; they extend 10 to 12 inches (25 to 30 cm.) to the urinary bladder and are about ½ inch (1.7 cm.) thick. They are muscular tubes which move the urine along by contracting, with the help of gravity and pressure. The ureters enter the bladder along its top, lateral edge on either side. Since the ureters pass beneath the bladder for a few centimeters before opening into it, the pressure from the full bladder helps to prevent reflux (urine washing back up the ureters).

The urinary bladder is a 4-layered, hollow muscular bag found in the pelvic cavity behind the symphysis pubis. It is in front of the yoni and below the uterine fundus; it is attached to the lower part of the anterior uterine surface. When full it becomes pear-shaped and rises into the abdominal cavity. It is held in place by folds of peritoneum. If you draw an upside-down, broad based triangle the urethral opening is found at its lower-most apex. The two upper points of the triangle are where the ureters open into the bladder. The bladder walls consist of a lining of mucus membrane (which is folded to facilitate stretching), mucosa, muscle and peritoneum (which lies over the top of the bladder). The bladder forms a holding area for urine, which is expelled by a process known as **micturition (mick-too-RISH-un)** or urination. This is brought about by a combination of nerve impulses.

The **urethra** is a small tube leading from the floor of the bladder to the exterior of the body. It runs parallel with the anterior wall of the yoni and is approximately ¼ inch (6 mm.) wide when not dilated. Its walls have three layers: mucus membrane, spongy tissue called the urethral sponge and an outer muscle layer. The spongy layer also contains the **female prostate glands**, multiple tubular structures which open into the urethral lumen and secrete a thin, clear fluid in some women during orgasm (Sevely, 1987).

The Female Sexual and Reproductive System

Reproduction is the means by which we create new life. It occurs within our bodies on a cellular level as cells are constantly aging, dying and being replaced. Reproduction is also the process by which a new human being starts out as a single cell and develops into a whole individual. The organs of the male and female reproductive systems produce the specialized cells which join to grow into a new organism. These organs may be grouped by function. Both sexes have **gonads**, special glands which produce gametes or reproductive cells and the hormones which support these processes. Special **ducts** or tubes then transport, receive and store gametes and provide a place for fertilization to occur. The female reproductive organs house and nourish the developing fetus. Accessory glands produce other materials which support gametes.

The female organs of reproduction include the ovaries which produce ova (eggs) and the hormones progesterone, estrogen and relaxin; the uterine or egg (fallopian) tubes which transport the ova to the uterus; the uterus (womb); the yoni; the clitoris; and other features of the genitals. The mammary glands or breasts are specialized sweat glands which produce milk to nourish babies; they are therefore considered part of the female reproductive system. Because the muscles of the pelvis are so directly involved in sexual response and childbirth, they are discussed in this chapter.

The external genitals and related internal structures: (Refer to the illustration on the page following these descriptions and keep in mind that the normal female genitalia may vary considerably from woman to woman.)

Mons veneris/mons pubis (mons vee-NEAR-us/PEW-biss): The pad of fatty tissue covering the pubic bone, visible as a hair-covered triangular area on the lower abdomen when a woman is standing with her legs together. After puberty (when the hair appears) this area is sometimes referred to as the **escutcheon (es-CUT-chin).**

Vulva (VUHL-va)/pudenda (pew-DEN-da): This term refers collectively to the labia (majora and minora), the shaft and glans of the clitoris, and the openings of the urethra and yoni. The vulva extends from the pubic bone to the point in front of the anal opening.

Labia Majora (LAY-bee-ah ma-JOR-ah): These large, fleshy, fatty, hair-covered lips originate from the mons veneris and extend between the legs on either side from front to back, ending at the lower border of the introitus of the yoni. They are 7 to 8 cm. in length, 2 to 3 cm. in width, and 1 to 1.5 cm. thick, forming a protective pad above and beside the clitoris. The round ligaments of the uterus terminate at the level of their upper borders.

Labia minora (LAY-bee-ah meh-NOR-ah): These are the soft inner lips of the vulva found inside and parallel to the labia majora. Their structure is similar to mucous membrane. The hood of the clitoris is a tent of this tissue. The labia minora proper begin just below the clitoral glans. They extend as two ruffled lips whose width decreases as they descend to merge with and encircle the lower border of the mouth of the yoni, thus forming the fourchette. This tissue is less stretchable than that of the yoni.

Fourchette (foor-SHET): The delicate, semicircular, membranous tissue formed by the labia minora as they merge at the lower border of the mouth of the yoni (This is also the lower border of the vestibule of the vulva).

Vestibule (VES-tah-bule) of the vulva: The space extending from below the clitoral hood and the inside of the labia minora down to the fourchette of the yoni. The clitoris, urethra and opening of the yoni are situated within the vestibule.

Clitoris (KLIH-tore-iss): Research done by male anatomists has left the impression that the clitoris is a tiny knob of nerves beneath the junction of the labia minora and that the yoni is the central feature of the female genitalia. (Since men have been doing the research, and the yoni is a major interest of theirs, no wonder!) Although texts go on at length about male anatomy, only one textbook, written by feminist researchers, explores clitoral anatomy in similar depth (A New View of A Woman's Body by the Federation of Feminist Women's Health Centers). Feminist research has revealed the clitoris as an elaborate organ. In fact, almost every structure of the female genitalia is either an extension of clitoral tissue or involved in its support, protection, or function. The clitoris itself consists of:

> **Shaft/corpus (CORE-pus)/body:** A 2 cm tubular body that contains two parallel columns of erectile tissue. It extends along the lower center surface of the symphysis pubis, projects forward slightly from beneath the clitoral hood, and terminates with the glans.

> **Glans:** The glans is the nerve-filled, exposed tip immediately beneath the lip of the hood at the end of the shaft.

> **Crura (CREW-rah):** The crura form an inverted V-shape of erectile tissue about 1 cm above the glans beginning where the shaft divides with two long, pointed arms. The two 7.5 cm-long arms extend beneath the rami of the pelvis to the ischial spines of erectile tissue. They are covered by the ischiocavernosus muscles. (The singular form is crus [krus]).

Hood/prepuce/foreskin: The uppermost portion of the labia minora forms a tent over the shaft. The hood covers and protects the shaft from direct stimulation.

Frenulum (FREN-you-lum) of the clitoris: The junction of the labia minora just below the glans.

Clitoral sponge/Bulb of the vestibule (VEST-tah-bule): Dense circulatory tissue lying just beneath the inner edge of the labia majora to either side of the yoni. The clitoral sponge is shaped roughly like an inflated (i.e. fat) wishbone. The narrow, joined end extends from beneath the shaft of the clitoris. Its two arms are 3 to 4 cm. long, 1 to 2 cm wide, and 0.5 to 1 cm. thick and curve around either side of the yoni. The arms are joined across the bottom by the perineal sponge. This erectile tissue becomes engorged with blood during sexual excitement and, to a lesser extent, with the blood volume expansion of pregnancy. The front and sides of the sponge are covered by the bulbocavernosus muscle.

The perineum (PEAR-ih-KNEE-um): The skin-covered tissue between the anus and the mouth of the yoni. It is usually about 4 cm. long or more.

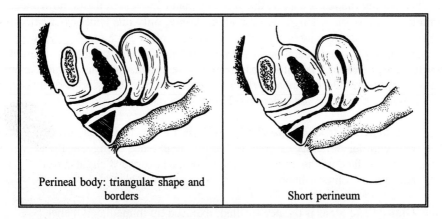

| Perineal body: triangular shape and borders | Short perineum |

Perineal (PEAR-ih-KNEE-all) body: A 4 cm. 3-dimensional equilateral triangle of soft tissue which rests on top of the anal sphincter behind the perineum. The triangle's back point meets the center edge of the pubovaginalis portion of the levator ani muscle. The top side borders the lower third of the yoni floor, and the front side is the perineal skin surface, with the triangle pointing toward the anus. The center of the perineal skin surface is about 1.5 to 2.5 cm. from the central point of the superficial transverse muscle (the first layer of the central point of the perineum). The top edge of this muscle lies about 1.25 cm. below the surface of the mucosa of the yoni. In a short perineum the perineal body may be almost nonexistent, bringing the openings of the yoni and anus closer together.

Perineal sponge: the vascular tissue within the perineal body that becomes engorged with blood during sexual excitement. It is an extension of the clitoral sponge and is severed when an episiotomy is performed.

Since the yoni and urethra are surrounded by clitoral tissue, this makes them clitoral orifices, and places a routine clitorotomy (episiotomy) in the category of not only genital, but clitoral mutilation.

Internal structures which are also found in the genital area include:

Urethral meatus (you-REE-thrall mee-A-tuss): The mouth of the urethra just below the clitoral glans, about 0.5 to 1.4 cm. below the junction of the labia minora. Like the opening of the yoni, it is surrounded by clitoral circulatory tissue.

Urethra (you-REE-thrah): The 4 cm. long tube through which urine passes. It is centrally located above the upper wall of the yoni. (See the previous chapter for a more detailed description).

Urethral sponge: A spongy encasement of clitoral circulatory tissue that sheathes the length of the urethra.

Paraurethral (Skene's) ducts and glands: Two tiny ducts may lie either just inside or outside the urethral meatus at about 4 and 8 o'clock. They drain the glands positioned to the side of and behind the meatus.

Yoni or birth passage (vagina): The yoni is the passageway for the menstrual flow and the passageway through which a baby passes in order to be born. The yoni allows indirect access to sensitive vascular and nerve tissues of the clitoris and the female prostate glands during sexual activity. The yoni allows sperm to enter the cervix via sexual

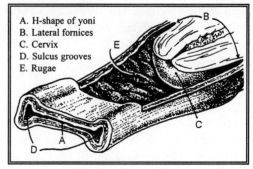

A. H-shape of yoni
B. Lateral fornices
C. Cervix
D. Sulcus grooves
E. Rugae

intercourse (the insertion of the penis into the yoni) or by introduction of semen in or near the opening of the yoni. It is a circular, muscular, normally collapsed, H-shaped passage; the H-shape is most obvious after a woman has just given birth. The tissue of the yoni is constructed of squamous epithelium (mucosa), beneath

166

which is a layer of connective tissue and a thin, two-layer muscular coat. The side walls have longitudinal ridges, and the top and bottom walls have transverse ridges called *rugae* (**RUE-gay**).

The upper (top) wall is beneath the pubic bone and is usually 5 to 7.5 cm. long. The urethra parallels the upper wall of the yoni from above. The deeper portion of the upper yoni wall is in contact with the bladder. The ureters run on either side of the yoni outside the upper lateral fornices. The uterine arteries are also in this area, one on either side as well. The bottom wall is above the rectum. It is 7.5 to 10 cm long; its lower third contacts the perineal body. The upper third contacts the pouch of Douglas (lowermost area of the abdominal cavity).

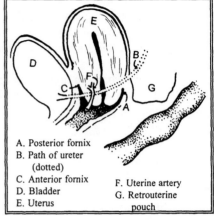

A. Posterior fornix
B. Path of ureter
   (dotted)
C. Anterior fornix
D. Bladder
E. Uterus
F. Uterine artery
G. Retrouterine
   pouch

The middle third of the birth passage is bounded on either side and from below by the pubovaginalis portion of the levator ani muscle.

Within the yoni the following structures and landmarks are identified:

Sulcus (SULL-kuss) grooves: The grooves present on either side of the birth passage where the wall and the floor meet; there are two upper and two lower grooves. They may not be obvious until after the birth of a first baby.

Fornices (FORE-nih-sees): The lower portion of the cervix protrudes into the upper end of the yoni. The space created between the body of the cervix and the wall of the yoni is referred to as the fornix (FORE-nex). The lateral fornices are adjacent to the ureters and uterine arteries. The posterior fornix is deepest, bordering the pouch of Douglas. The anterior fornix borders the bladder's base.

Vault: The upper third of the yoni into which the cervix protrudes; the fornices.

Cervix (SER-viks): The mouth of the uterus which protrudes into the upper end of the yoni. It dilates during birth to allow passage of the baby. The cervix is constructed so that the sides are less fibrous and less muscular than the front and back lips. The cervical orifice is called the **os** (oss).

The mucosa of the yoni: The 1 cm-deep soft, vascular lining of the yoni. It is loosely attached to underlying structures and contains secretory tissue; there are no glands that produce yoni discharge. The pH of secretions vary with ovarian activity and average 4.0 in adults; pH is lowest midcycle and highest premenstrually.

The External Genitals:

Key:

A. Mons veneris
B. Labia majora
C. Labia minora
D. Clitoral hood
E. Clitoral glans
F. Frenulum
G. Paraurethral glands
    and ducts*
H. Urethral meatus
I. Yoni opening
J. Hymenal ring*
K. Greater vestibular glands
    and ducts*
L. Vestibule of the vulva
M. Fourchette
N. Perineum
O. Anus

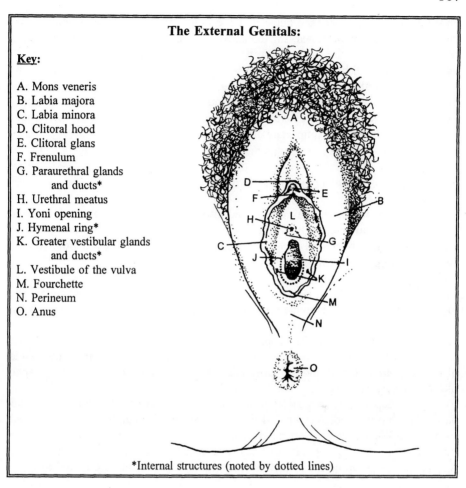

*Internal structures (noted by dotted lines)

Introitus (in-TRO-ih-tus): The mouth of the yoni. Because it is surrounded by clitoral circulatory tissue, it may be thought of as a clitoral orifice.

Vestibule (VEST-tah-bule) of the yoni: The space that extends from the external opening of the yoni to the depth of the hymenal ring.

Greater vestibular (VEST-TIB-you-lar) (Bartholin's) glands: Two pea-sized glands located at a depth of 2 cm on either side of the yoni, just beneath and behind the lower edge of the clitoral sponge. Their 2 cm-long ducts open at 4 and 8 o'clock between the introitus and the hymenal ring.

Hymenal (HI-men-all) ring: The hymen is a circular band of ruffled connective tissue approximately .5 to 2 cm inside the opening of the yoni. It is made of elastic and collagenous tissue but contains no muscle fibers. The virginal hymen presents as a membrane of varying thicknesses. The size of the opening also varies widely. Sometimes the hymen is imperforate, if so this is discovered at puberty when the menstrual blood begins to back up and create pressure. Other variations include a perforated membrane, and a membranous septum which may partially block the introitus. In multiparas and some nulliparas, the hymen appears on either side as tags of skin, known as *caruncules myrtiformes* (KAR-ung-kulls MUR-tee-form). The hymen is an important landmark during suturing.

An overview of perineal/clitoral musculature:

The pelvic muscles may be divided into two basic groups: the **pelvic floor** and the **urogenital triangle** with the **deep transverse muscle**. The mid-point of the perineal body is central to all of these muscles and the central point of the perineum is where they all meet.

The most shallow layer of muscles (closest to the skin) is called the **urogenital triangle**. It is made up of the superficial transverse, bulbocavernosus, and ischiocavernosus muscles. The ischiocavernosus forms the top point and two lateral sides of the triangle. The superficial transverse muscle completes the bottom edge of an open triangular framework. The bulbocavernosus runs from the inside of the top point down behind the superficial transverse (bottom edge) and is shaped like a pair of parentheses.

The deep transverse muscle (or urogenital diaphragm) forms a solid triangular base of muscle immediately behind the open urogenital triangle. It is perforated by the urethra and yoni. Together, these two layers of muscles fit inside the inverted V shape of the pubic arch and are in the same plane. Each muscle is distinct but made up of fibers that are difficult to discern with the naked eye.

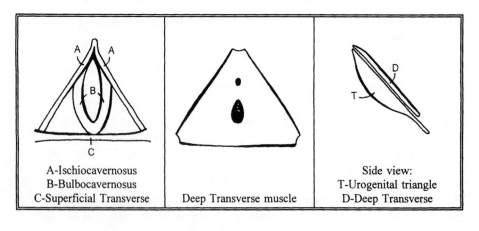

| A-Ischiocavernosus
B-Bulbocavernosus
C-Superficial Transverse | Deep Transverse muscle | Side view:
T-Urogenital triangle
D-Deep Transverse |

Behind the urogenital triangle is the **pelvic floor**. It is made up of several muscles which function collectively and are referred to as the levator ani (Kegel) muscle. To understand their general shape, imagine an inverted teardrop-shaped bowl. Now imagine removing a V-shaped area from the central edge of the rounded end and removing a narrow U-shaped area from the pointed tip down toward the central base of the bowl. The lower sacrum and coccyx project into the V-shaped area. The U-shaped area fits up behind the yoni, and the midpoint of the U attaches to the central point of the perineum. The tips of the pointed ends attach to the pubic bone.

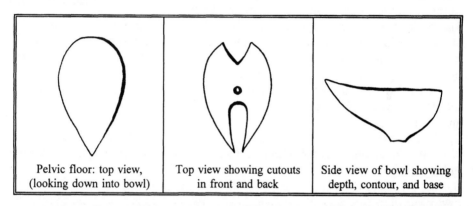

| Pelvic floor: top view, (looking down into bowl) | Top view showing cutouts in front and back | Side view of bowl showing depth, contour, and base |

The sides of the bowl attach to the muscular lining of the pelvic side walls (the obturator internus muscles) at the level of the ischial spines. The bowl has a small round base, which is formed by the anal sphincter.

The relationship between the pelvis, the angles of the urogenital triangle and deep transverse muscle, and the pelvic floor (levator ani) are shown in a simplified form below without any other details:

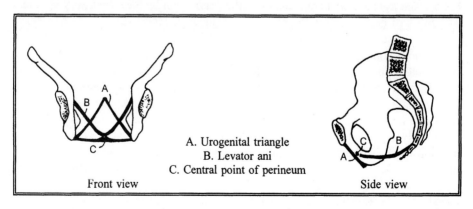

A. Urogenital triangle
B. Levator ani
C. Central point of perineum

Front view   Side view

Anal sphincter (A-null SFINCK-ter): The external muscle that closes the

170

rectum—a strong, circular band about 1.9 cm wide. It is shaped like an oval cone with one-third of the tip end removed. Its fibers form the bottom part of a figure-eight, which merges at the 12 o'clock point with the bulbocavernosus muscle. This is the most superficial (shallow) muscle in the genital area, with only a thin covering of skin and mucous membrane. It forms a tapered muscular shelf upon which the perineal body rests. The topmost posterior edge of the sphincter forms the base of the central point of the perineum.

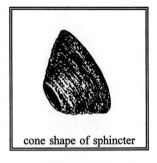

cone shape of sphincter

The other muscle attachments are usually slightly above and behind the top edge at the 12 o'clock point. It merges into a strip of tissue, the **anococcygeal body (A-no-cock-SIGH-gee-ahl)**, which connects it to the coccyx. The sphincter is the most distinctly visual muscle in the perineal body.

If the perineum is short, the perineal body forms a thin pad of tissue above the sphincter, and the central point of the perineum lies behind (not slightly above and behind) the back edge.

A more detailed description of these muscles can be found in Healing Passage.

Internal reproductive organs:

Ovaries: The ovaries, or female gonads, are a pair of glands about the size of unshelled almonds. They are positioned in the upper pelvic cavity, one on each side of the uterus. The ovaries are held in position by a series of ligaments and are attached to the broad ligament of the uterus. They are anchored to the uterus by the ovarian ligament and are attached to the pelvic wall by the suspensory ligament. The **hilus** of each ovary is the point of entrance for blood vessels and nerves.

A loose layer of epithelium covers the outer ovary. Inside, a layer of collagenous connective tissue covers a deeper layer, or stroma, which is composed of an outer dense cortex and a loose inner layer known as the medulla. The cortex contains ovarian follicles, which are immature ova and their surrounding tissue in various stages of development. Unlike males, who constantly produce new sperm, females have all their eggs in immature form at birth, and hormonal influences cause only one to develop each month. (In those rare instances when two eggs develop at once, there is a potential for conceiving fraternal twins.) During the menstrual years, the ovary also contains a **vesicular ovarian (Graafian) follicle**—a larger fluid-filled swelling containing an immature ovum and the surrounding tissues. This follicle secretes hormones called estrogens. Finally, during a woman's menstrual years, the ovaries always have a **corpus luteum**, a glandular body that develops from a ruptured ovarian follicle after the ovum is released (ovulation). It produces the hormones progesterone, estrogen and relaxin.

Uterine or egg tubes: The **uterine** or **egg (Fallopian) tubes** or **oviducts** are a pair of passageways. The funnel-shaped, open distal end of each tube is called the **infundibulum (in-fun-DEE-bue-lum)**. Each has a fringed end; these finger-like projections are referred to as **fimbriae (FIM-brie-ah)**. The tube's widest and longest portion is called the **ampulla** (about two-thirds of its length) which leads to the **isthmus** on either side and comprise the last third of its length. Each uterine tube enters the uterine horn where it forms a narrow, thick walled opening into the cornu (or horn) of the uterus, which enlarges to form the uterine cavity. The uterine tubes are about 10 to 12 cm. long and about 1 cm. in diameter.

Each tube has three layers. The internal mucosa has two types of cells lining its lumen—ciliated and nonciliated, or secretory cells. Ciliated cells propel the ovum toward the uterine cavity. Nonciliated cells provide nourishment to the developing ovum as it travels down the tube on its way to the uterus. The middle layer of smooth muscle and the outer layer of longitudinal muscle produce peristaltic contractions which also assist this process. During ovulation, the fimbriae gather around the ovary and sweep the ovum into the ampulla, which is where fertilization usually occurs. If no fertilization occurs, the ovum degenerates.

The epithelial lining of the uterine tubes undergoes cyclic changes similar to those in the uterus but without shedding. These changes consist of a resting phase, a premenstrual phase, a menstrual stage and a post-menstrual phase.

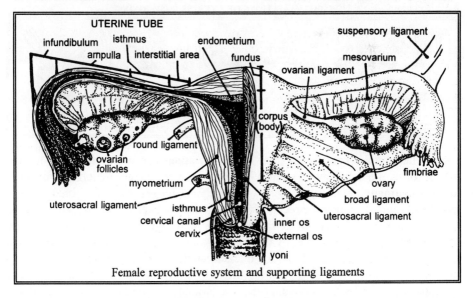

Female reproductive system and supporting ligaments

Uterus: The uterus is situated between the urinary bladder and the rectum. It is about 3 inches (7.5 cm.) long, 2 inches (5 cm.) wide and 1 inch (2.5 cm.) thick and is shaped like an inverted pear. It is divided into three regions: the dome-shaped portion above the uterine tubes called the **fundus**, the largest tapering central portion called the **body**, and the inferior narrow portion which opens into the yoni called the **cervix**. Between the body and the external cervix is a ½ inch (1 cm) region called the **isthmus**. The junction of the isthmus and the upper end of the cervical passage is called the **inner os**. The **external os** or mouth of the cervix opens into the yoni. The interior of the uterus is called the uterine cavity and the interior of the cervix is called the cervical passage.

In the majority of women the uterus is flexed forward over the bladder. This **anteflexion** causes the cervix to enter the yoni at nearly a right angle, with the os pointing toward the woman's lower sacrum. The position of the uterus is maintained by a pair of **broad ligaments** which attach the uterus to either side of the pelvic cavity. Uterine blood vessels and nerves pass through these ligaments. Posteriorly, the **uterosacral ligaments** attach the uterus to the sacrum on either side of the rectum. The **cardinal (lateral cervical) ligaments** extend below the bases of the broad ligaments between the wall of the pelvis and the cervix and yoni. The **round ligaments** are bands of fibrous connective tissue between the layers of the broad ligaments. They extend from just below the uterine tubes to the external genitalia. These ligaments usually maintain the uterus in an anteflexed position, however some women may have a posteriorly tilted or **retroflexed** uterus. The uterine body and fundus may also be positioned in a variety of other ways.

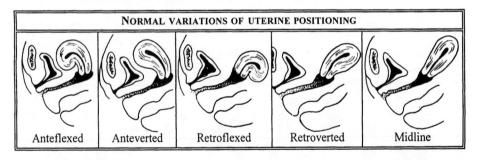

NORMAL VARIATIONS OF UTERINE POSITIONING				
Anteflexed	Anteverted	Retroflexed	Retroverted	Midline

The uterus is made up of three layers of tissue. The **perimetrium** or **serosa** which forms the outer layer is part of the visceral peritoneum, which becomes the **broad ligament** on either side. Anteriorly it drapes over the bladder and posteriorly it drapes over the rectum forming a deep pocket called the **retrouterine pouch** (also known as the **cul de sac** or **pouch of Douglas**). The middle layer, the **myometrium**, forms the bulk of the uterine wall. It is composed of three layers of smooth muscle fibers which are thickest at the fundus and thinnest near the cervix. The inner layer of the uterus, the **endometrium**, is a mucous membrane composed of two layers containing numerous glands. The innermost layer is the **stratum functionalis** which is shed during menstruation. The **stratum basalis** is a permanent second layer which generates a new functionalis following menstruation.

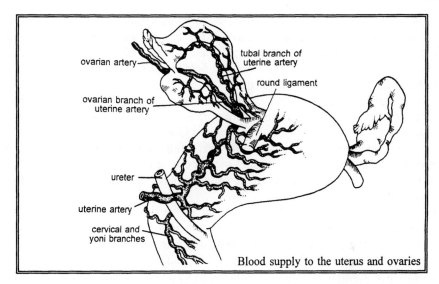

ovarian artery

tubal branch of
uterine artery

round ligament

ovarian branch of
uterine artery

ureter

uterine artery

cervical and
yoni branches

Blood supply to the uterus and ovaries

Blood is supplied to the uterus by branches of the internal iliac artery called the **uterine arteries**. These main vessels branch into smaller arteries arranged in a circular pattern in the myometrium and further divide in the endometrium into straight arterioles which transport the materials for creating the functionalis. There are also spiral arterioles which penetrate the functionalis and change markedly during the menstrual cycle. The uterus is drained by the uterine veins.

A chief purpose of the ovaries and uterus is to prepare the body for a possible pregnancy and to support, house and nourish a developing baby during pregnancy. This is accomplished via the **menstrual cycle**, which consists of a series of changes in the endometrium of a nonpregnant woman. These changes prepare the uterine lining to accept a fertilized ovum. If no fertilization occurs, the endometrial lining is shed. The **ovarian cycle** is a corresponding monthly series of events which leads to the maturation and release of an ovum.

Female hormones: The menstrual and ovarian cycles and the changes of puberty are controlled by a hormone from the hypothalamus called **gonadotropin releasing factor (GnRF)** which stimulates the release of **follicle stimulating hormone (FSH)** from the anterior pituitary. FSH stimulates the development of the ovarian follicles and the secretion of estrogens by the follicles. GnRF also causes the release of **luteinizing hormone (LH)** from the anterior pituitary. LH stimulates the further development of the ovarian follicles, brings about ovulation, and stimulates the production of estrogens, progesterone and relaxin by ovarian cells.

Estrogens, the growth hormones, have three main functions: the development and maintenance of the female reproductive structures, especially the endometrial lining of the uterus and secondary sex characteristics (body hair, fat distribution to breasts, abdomen, mons pubis and hips, voice pitch, broad pelvis); control of fluid and electrolyte balance; and the increase of protein anabolism. At least six different estrogens have been found in female plasma. Only three, however, are present in significant quantities. They are *beta*-estradiol, estrone, and estriol. Of these, ß-estradiol exerts the major effect.

Progesterone is the hormone of maturation and works with estrogens to prepare the endometrium for implantation of a fertilized ovum and the mammary glands for milk secretion. High levels inhibit GnRF and prolactin.

Relaxin goes to work near the end of pregnancy when it relaxes the ligaments and other connective tissues in the body to help with opening the cervix and allowing maximal flexibility in the pelvic joints to facilitate birth. It also helps to increase sperm motility.

The menstrual cycle lasts from 24 to 35 days, and averages 28 days in the majority of women. This cycle may be understood as a three phase process: menstruation, the preovulatory phase and the postovulatory phase.

Menstruation, or the menses, is the periodic shedding of the endometrial lining, which consists of tissue fluid, blood, mucus and epithelial cells. It is caused by a sudden reduction in estrogens and progesterone when fertilization has not occurred. If pregnancy does occur, changes take place which maintain the levels of these hormones. The menses lasts about five days during which an average total of 25 to 65 ml. (2/3 to 2 oz.) of fluid is discharged, although some women lose considerably more fluid than this. As the functionalis lining of the uterus is released, patchy areas of bleeding develop from small areas of tissue detaching one at a time. The uterine glands also discharge their contents and collapse, releasing tissue fluid. These secretions flow through the cervix and out of the yoni. When the flow is complete the entire functionalis has been shed and only the basalis layer remains, leaving the endometrium very thin.

Even as bleeding is taking place, the **ovarian cycle** is also beginning. **Ovarian follicles**, called primary follicles, begin to develop due to the release of FSH from the anterior pituitary. A follicle is a spherical area in the cortex of the ovary containing an oocyte (immature ovum) and is surrounded by a layer of cells. Each ovary contains about 200,000 follicles.

During the early part of the menstrual phase 20 to 25 primary follicles start to produce very low levels of estrogen. A clear membrane called the **zona pellucida** develops around the potential ovum. About 20 primary follicles develop into secondary follicles on day four to five of the menses due to an increase in the number of cells in the protective layer. These cells differentiate and begin to secrete **follicular (fo-LICK-you-lar) fluid**. This fluid moves an immature ovum to the edge of the secondary follicle and then fills the follicular cavity.

The **preovulatory phase** is the second part of the menstrual cycle and covers the time between menstruation and ovulation. It varies in length more than the other phases, but usually lasts from days 6 to 13 in a 28 day cycle.

175

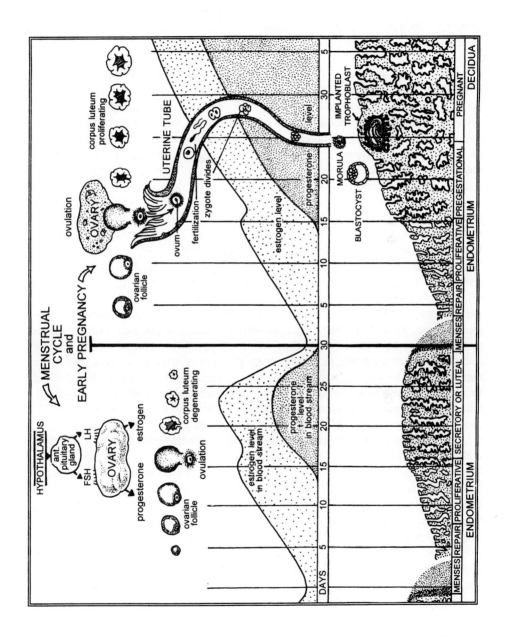

During this phase FSH and LH stimulate the ovarian follicles to produce more estrogens which, in turn, stimulate the endometrium to thicken to a depth of 4 to 6 mm.. Because of this proliferation of tissue, and the increase in estrogen production by the follicles, this is referred to as either the proliferative phase or the follicular phase.

At this point one of the secondary follicles in the ovary matures into a **vesicular ovarian (Graafian) follicle** which is ready for ovulation. Estrogen and LH levels steadily increase as maturation approaches. Small amounts of progesterone may be released by the vesicular ovarian follicle a day or two before ovulation. Just before ovulation takes place estrogen levels inhibit GnRF which in turn suppresses FSH levels. At the same time, the high estrogen level causes the anterior pituitary to release a surge of LH, leading to the rupture of the vesicular follicle, thus releasing the immature ovum.

Immediately after rupture the vesicular ovarian follicle collapses. Its cells enlarge, change character and form the **corpus luteum** or yellow body. The blood within the ruptured follicle clots, forming the **corpus hemorrhagicum**. This clot is eventually absorbed by the remaining follicular cells.

The **postovulatory phase** is the most consistent in duration. It lasts from days 15 to 28 in a 28-day cycle, typically covering the 14 to 15 days prior to the onset of bleeding, regardless of the length of the preovulatory phase. This is the period between ovulation and the first day of the next menses. After ovulation, LH stimulates the development of the corpus luteum, which secretes increasing amounts of estrogens and progesterone. Progesterone prepares the endometrium to receive a fertilized ovum by stimulating the secretory endometrial glands, vascularizing the superficial endometrium, thickening the endometrial glycogen storage and increasing tissue fluid. This preparation peaks about one week after ovulation, which corresponds to the anticipated arrival of a fertilized ovum. The level of FSH gradually increases and LH slowly drops during this phase.

If fertilization and implantation do not occur, the rising levels of progesterone and estrogens from the corpus luteum inhibit GnRF and LH secretion. As a result the corpus luteum degenerates and becomes the **corpus albicans**, which simply means white body. This results in a drop in progesterone and estrogen levels produced by the degenerating corpus luteum, which initiates endometrial shedding. The decreased levels of progesterone and estrogens cause the pituitary to release FSH in response to increased levels of GnRF from the hypothalamus. Thus a new ovarian cycle is initiated.

If fertilization and implantation do occur, the corpus luteum is maintained for the first 3 to 4 months of pregnancy by a placental hormone known as human Chorionic Gonadotropin (hCG). During this time the corpus luteum secretes estrogens and progesterone. The placenta also secretes estrogen and progesterone to support the pregnancy and breast development for lactation. Once placental hormone production begins, the role of the corpus luteum gradually diminishes and its work is finally replaced by hormones produced by the placenta.

Mammary glands: The breasts are modified sudoriferous (sweat) glands that lie over the upper chest and are attached to the underlying muscles by connective tissue. Children have similar breast structures. At puberty, estrogens cause the female breasts to develop which prepares them for lactation. Each breast consists of 15 to 20 **lobes** or compartments separated by fatty tissue. The amount of fat or adipose tissue surrounding and protecting these lobes determines the size of the breasts. The lobules are held in place by connective tissue (Cooper's ligaments) which surrounds them much like the membrane of an orange wedge holds its contents in place and runs between the skin and deep fascia to support the breast. Each lobe has several smaller compartments or **lobules** composed of connective tissue in which grape-like clusters of milk secreting cells called **alveoli (al-VEE-oh-lie)** are embedded. Each alveolus is surrounded by a set of tiny myoepithelial cells which contract to eject the milk into ductules, or secondary tubules, which enlarge into collecting **lactiferous** or **mammary ducts**. As they near the nipple, the ducts widen into reservoirs called **ampullae (am-POO-lah)** or **lactiferous (lack-TIFF-er-us) sinuses** where milk is stored.

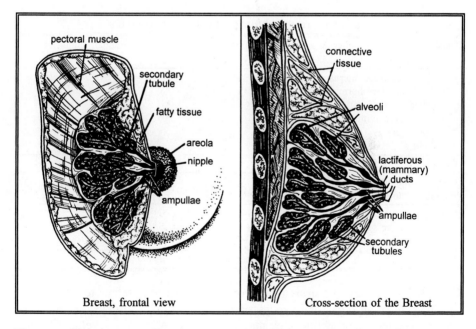

Breast, frontal view   Cross-section of the Breast

The ampullae narrow as they approach the nipple. Each lactiferous duct conveys milk from a lobe to the exterior. Glandular tissue extends towards the underarm area partly beneath the lateral border of the pectoralis majora muscle; this tissue is known as the **axillary tail**. The circular pigmented area of skin surrounding the nipple is called the **areola (a-RE-oh-la)**. Small prominences in the areola contain modified sebaceous **(Montgomery's)** glands.

Variations and Abnormalities of the Female Reproductive System

The overall incidence of female reproductive anomalies is unknown but thought to occur in 1 in every 700 women. Septate uteri make up 80% of all such abnormalities. It appears that only Class I anomalies are related to infertility, although increased rates of miscarriage as well as abnormal presentation of the fetus, and placental complications have been associated with most other types. However, most women with uterine abnormalities have normal fertility and can carry a pregnancy to term. The structures which become the mature uterus and yoni are referred to as Muellerian ducts during embryologic development.

In some cases uterine abnormalities are found in conjunction with deformities of the skeletal (especially the lumbosacral spine) and renal systems (Rokitansky-Küster-Hauser complex). Therefore, whenever reproductive abnormalities are found, women should be checked for urinary tract anomalies as well (and vis versa). There may be renal agenesis, ectopia (misplacement) of the kidney or pelvic kidneys on one side.

CLASSIFICATION OF MUELLERIAN DUCT ANOMALIES
Class I Segmental Muellerian agenesis or hypoplasia: Yoni; Cervical; Fundal; Tubal; or combination of these defects
Class II Unicornuate uterus 　With rudimentary horn: 　　With a communicating endometrial cavity 　　With a noncommunicating cavity 　　With no cavity 　Without any rudimentary horn
Class III Uterus didelphys
Class IV Bicornuate uterus 　Complete to the internal os; Partial; Arcuate
Class V Septate uterus 　With complete septum 　With incomplete septum
Class VI Uterus with internal luminal changes (T-shaped cavity)

Class I: Muellerian Agenesis or hypoplasia: Agenesis refers to the lack of development of an organ and hypoplasia refers to incomplete development. The yoni, cervix, uterus, or uterine tubes may be affected. Abnormal development may also occur as a combination of defects in more than one of these structures. On bimanual exam, the absence of the yoni or uterus will be detectable. Absence of the uterine tubes is more rare and may not be as easily distinguished. Hypoplasia of the birth passage may be surgically corrected. However, it is associated with an absence of the uterus in 80 to 90% of cases. Surgical correction will leave the yoni heavily scarred and may necessitate surgical delivery of babies. The following drawings depict the main varieties of these defects:

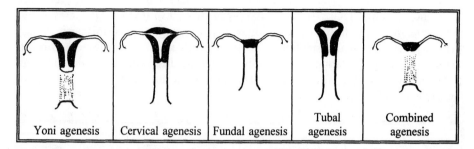

| Yoni agenesis | Cervical agenesis | Fundal agenesis | Tubal agenesis | Combined agenesis |

Class II: Unicornuate uterus: Usually one normal horn exists alone or together with a partially developed horn. On bimanual exam, the uterus may be felt to one side of the midline. The smaller horn may or may not communicate externally; 90% do not open into the yoni. Those with a unicornate uterus generally do not have problems conceiving but are more prone to first or second trimester miscarriage as well as breech presentation. If implantation occurs in a communicating rudimentary horn the uterus may rupture by the end of the second trimester; alternatively, the placenta may implant in the smaller horn and the baby may grow in the larger one, resulting in a trapped placenta and a serious problem at the time of birth. If a small horn with an open cavity does not communicate with the yoni, menstrual fluids become backed up during adolescence and surgical removal of the horn will be necessary.

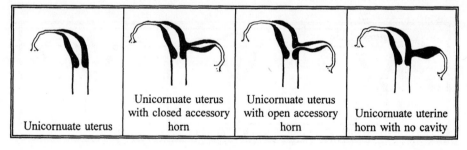

| Unicornuate uterus | Unicornuate uterus with closed accessory horn | Unicornuate uterus with open accessory horn | Unicornuate uterine horn with no cavity |

Class III: Uterus didelphys: This is a double uterus consisting of two separate structures which may be hard to differentiate from a bicornuate defect on bimanual exam. It is frequently found with a double or septate yoni as well. When the yoni is normal, one of the uterine structures may be obstructed and retention of menstrual flow on that side may result. There is no notably increased risk of pregnancy complications with uterus didelphys.

180

Class IV: Bicornuate uterus: This defect results in two separate uterine horns (cavities) of equal size and is associated with an increased incidence of premature labor and abnormal fetal position. Thirty-five percent of these pregnancies end in late second trimester miscarriage. Women experiencing repeated miscarriage may wish to pursue surgical correction. On palpation, these uteri feel large and heart-shaped, with an indentation in the midline of the fundus. The most minimal form of this defect is called an arcuate uterus which has a thickening in the midline of the fundus.

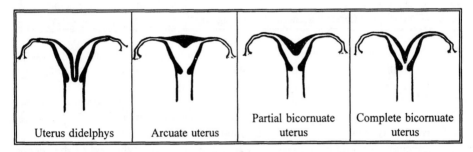

| Uterus didelphys | Arcuate uterus | Partial bicornuate uterus | Complete bicornuate uterus |

Class V: Septate uterus: The single uterine cavity is divided either partially or completely by a thin longitudinal septum. The septum is made up of fibromuscular tissue similar to myometrium but poorly supplied with blood vessels. The septum may be partial, limited to the fundus, or may span the entire length of the uterus. Fertility is not impaired but miscarriage is as high as 67%, almost twice as high as for those with bicornuate uteri.

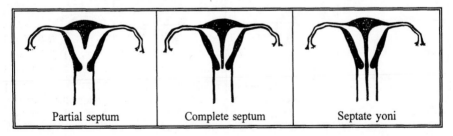

| Partial septum | Complete septum | Septate yoni |

Thirty-three percent of women with septate uteri experience preterm labor and 28% have an abnormal fetal position; inadequate septal blood flow and decreased intrauterine volume are suspected reasons. The risk of postpartum hemorrhage is increased and intrauterine adhesions sometimes form as the placental site heals. If the placenta attaches to the relatively avascular septum, this can result in placenta accreta. Surgical removal of the septum is indicated for women desiring to concieve. The improvement in pregnancy outcome is dramatic after surgery, with 88% of women carrying a normal pregnancy and only 5% miscarrying.

Septate yoni: Septa in the yoni are among the most common of genital tract abnormalities, occurring in .2 to 5. per 1,000 live births. They are usually found with bicornate or septate uteri and do not usually cause infertility. The septum may need to be divided to allow penetration of the yoni or normal birth.

DES-related anomalies:

From 1948 to 1971, a potent synthetic nonsteroidal estrogen called diethylstilbestrol (DES) was widely prescribed for 4 to 6 million women in the United States. The daughters of these women are at increased risk for a number of reproductive problems; more than 50% will have some kind of DES-related reproductive abnormality. The most common anomaly involves adenosis in the yoni. Columnar or glandular epithelium (similar to that which normally lines the cervical passage, uterine endometrium or uterine tubes) is found in the yoni or on the exposed surface of the cervix. This is most often noted in the fornices of the yoni. The rate of adenosis is around 35% in exposed women and is most frequently seen when DES was given to their mothers for long periods of time in high doses during early pregnancy. Adenosis results from the arrest of the normal upward growth of squamous epithelium which lines the yoni during the 10th through the 18th weeks of embryonic development. On internal exam you may note a strawberry appearance varying from 1 mm. spots to extensive areas, especially in the upper yoni. This tissue may transform into normal mucosa over time in some women.

Structural abnormalities of the yoni, cervix, uterus and perhaps the uterine tubes may be present in up to 48% of DES-exposed daughters. Women who have cervical or intrayoni structural abnormalities or epithelial changes in the yoni all to be at increased risk for uterine abnormalities as well. The uterus and yoni begin formation during the first week of gestation, with major development beginning at 4 to 5 weeks. The uterus and yoni are first divided by a septum which disappears to create a single channel by 7 weeks. This timing makes reproductive structures a prime target for teratogenic effects of agents administered to the mother in early pregnancy.

Class VI: Internal luminal changes: DES exposure may result in a T-shaped endometrial cavity, an abnormally small uterine cavity, uterine constriction, constriction rings near the insertion points of the uterine tubes, other irregularities in the shape of the endometrial cavity, adhesions within the uterine cavity and bulbous dilation of the lower cervical segment. The uterine tubes may be shortened and convoluted with withered fimbria and a pinpoint os. The yoni may have an incomplete, transverse or longitudinal ridge or septum as well.

182

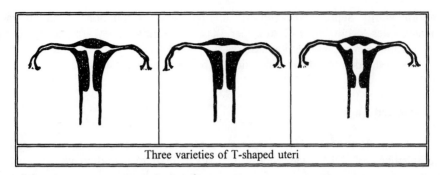

Three varieties of T-shaped uteri

A number of cervical anomalies have been noted in DES-exposed daughters, which may be referred to by different terms depending upon the source. Sometimes all such abnormalities are lumped under the term cockscomb. Structural changes of the cervix and yoni have also been noted to regress with age; this is not true, however, for abnormalities of the uterus.

CERVICAL ABNORMALITY	ALSO KNOWN AS:	DESCRIPTION
Cockscomb	Hood, transverse ridge	Raised ridge, usually on anterior cervix
Collar	Rim, hood, transverse ridge	Flat rim partially or completely encircling the cervix
Peudopolyp		A circular, constricting groove around the cervix, anterior or posterior cervical passage may be thicker than usual.
Hypoplastic cervix	Immature cervix	Cervix is less than 1.5 cm. in diameter
Altered fornix of yoni		May have no fornix or only a partial fornix, cervix & yoni may be fused

(Jefferies, et.al., 1984)

The reproductive potential of the woman will depend upon the extent of the defects found. A higher rate of ectopic pregnancy, preterm birth, intrauterine fetal death and miscarriage has been noted in DES daughters when compared with unexposed women. (Buttram & Gibbons, 1979; Herbst, et.al., 1972; Lichtman & Papera, 1990)

Anatomic variations and disorders of the breast:

Fibrocystic changes (lumpy breast tissue) are normal during the reproductive years. This condition is not usually aggravated by pregnancy.

Polymastia: Extra (supernumerary) nipples refers to the presence of glandular breast tissue along the milk line, which includes the underarm area. This may cause problems of engorgement or leaking of milk if there is enough tissue present.

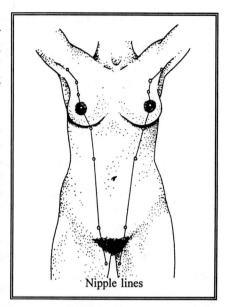

Nipple lines

Depression or inversion of one or both nipples may be normal if the nipple has always been that way. Nipple inversion which has gradually or suddenly developed in a previously erect nipple is a likely sign of an underlying tumor which is pulling the nipple inward. In these cases, a consultation with a breast specialist should be obtained without delay. Another normal nipple variation includes a fissured or cracked nipple. Other nipple and areola variations are illustrated below:

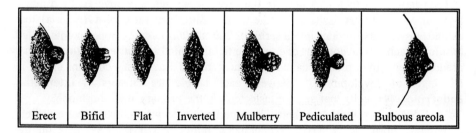

| Erect | Bifid | Flat | Inverted | Mulberry | Pediculated | Bulbous areola |

No nipples: In this condition, the lactiferous ducts open directly into a depression in the center of the areola.

Poorly developed breast tissue: This rare condition may occur in one or both breasts and may be indicated by one breast being significantly smaller than the other or by the lack of normal breast changes that occur with pregnancy.

The Male Sexual and Reproductive System

While the male reproductive system is not a focus of your attention in midwifery, it will be helpful to familiarize yourself with its basic anatomy and physiology. The male reproductive organs consist of the testes or male gonads which produce sperm, a number of ducts which transport the sperm, and accessory glands that add secretions to the sperm that together constitute the semen. There are several supporting structures, including the penis.

The scrotum: The **scrotum** is the external pouch which holds the testes. It consists of loose skin and superficial fascia which form a supporting container. Externally, it appears as a single pouch separated into two lateral portions by a ridge called the **raphe (RA-fee)**. Inside, it is divided into two sacs, each containing one testis. The external location of the scrotum and the contraction of its muscle fibers help to bring it closer or further away from the body, thus regulating temperature within the scrotum. The production and survival of sperm requires a temperature that is 5.4°F (3°C) lower than that inside the body.

Testes: The **testes** or **testicles** are a pair of oval glands measuring about 2 inches (5 cm.) long by 1 inch (2.5 cm.) in diameter. Each testis is covered by a dense layer of white fibrous tissue called the **tunica albuginea (al-byoo-GIN-ee-a)** that extends inward and divides into a series of 200 to 300 internal compartments called **lobules**. Each lobule contains one to three tightly coiled **seminiferous tubules** that produce sperm by a process called spermatogenesis. Each testis contains sperm in all stages of development. Between each tubule are clusters of **interstitial endocrinocytes**, cells that secrete testosterone, the primary male hormone.

When a boy reaches puberty the anterior pituitary begins to secrete follicle stimulating hormone (FSH) and luteinizing hormone (LH). FSH acts on the seminiferous tubules to initiate spermatogenesis. LH contributes to this process and also stimulates the secretion of **testosterone (tes-TOSS-ta-rone)**. This primary male hormone controls the functioning of the male sex organs and stimulates other maturation processes such as widening the shoulders, narrowing the hips, growth of body hair and deepening of the voice. Another anterior pituitary hormone called **inhibin** regulates the secretion of FSH, thus controlling sperm production.

In humans, **spermatogenesis (sper-ma-ta-GIN-ah-sis)**, or the production of sperm, takes two to three weeks. Spermatozoa are created and matured at the rate of about 300 million per day. It is composed of a head, a midpiece and a tail. Within the **head** are the nuclear (genetic) material as well as enzymes that help the sperm penetrate into the ovum. The **midpiece** carries the mechanism which helps the sperm swim. The **tail** propels the sperm along its way. Each spermatozoa is highly adapted for reaching and being received by a female ovum.

Immature sperm move through the seminiferous tubules to straight tubules which lead to a network of ducts in the testis called the **rete testis**. The sperm then move through a series of passageways called **efferent ducts**, located in the **epididymis (ep-I-did-ah-mass)**. This comma-shaped organ lies along the posterior border of each testis and consists primarily of a tightly coiled tube, the **ductus epididymis**. This is the site of sperm maturation. Sperm require ten days plus 18 hours to complete their maturation to the point where they can fertilize an ovum. The ductus epididymis also stores sperm for up to four weeks and propels them toward the urethra during ejaculation by peristaltic action of its smooth muscle. After four weeks, sperm that have not been ejaculated are reabsorbed.

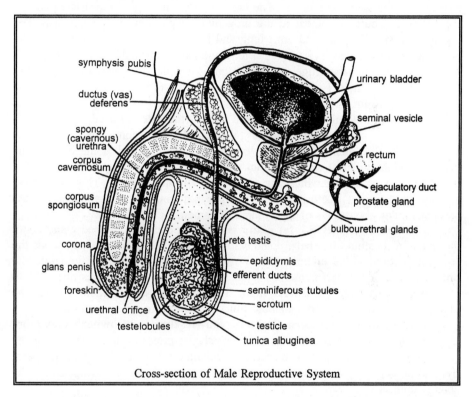

Cross-section of Male Reproductive System

The **ductus deferens** begins where the ductus epididymis becomes less convoluted. It is about 18 inches (45 cm.) long and ascends along the posterior border of the testes, penetrates the inguinal canal and enters the pelvic cavity where it loops over the side and down the posterior surface of the urinary bladder. The widened end of the ductus deferens is known as the **ampulla (am-POOL-la)**. The ductus deferens has a three-layer muscular wall which carries sperm along to be stored in the ampulla. Since the vas deferens is accessible via the scrotum, it is the tube severed during vasectomy or male sterilization.

The testicular artery, autonomic nerves, veins, cremaster muscle (which raises and lowers the testicles) and lymphatics follow the path of the vas deferens. These structures are collectively referred to as the **spermatic cord**. This cord passes through the inguinal canal, an oblique passageway in the anterior abdominal wall just above and parallel to the medial half of the inguinal ligament. This canal is about 1.6 to 2 inches (4 to 5 cm.) in length.

Behind the urinary bladder are the **ejaculatory (e-JACK-you-lah-tore-e) ducts**. Each one is about 1 inch (2 cm.) long and is formed by the union of the ducts from the seminal vesicle and vas deferens. These ducts eject sperm into the prostatic urethra. The **urethra** is the last duct in the system, serving as a common passageway for sperm and urine. The urethra passes through the prostate gland, a supportive muscular layer called the urogenital diaphragm, and the penis. The urethra is about 8 inches (20 cm.) long and is divided into three portions. The prostatic urethra is 1 inch (2 to 3 cm.) long and passes through the prostate gland. As it passes through the urogenital diaphragm it is called the membranous urethra which is about ½ inch (1 cm.) long. The last 6 inches (15 cm.) passes through the corpus spongiosum of the penis known as the **spongy (cavernous) urethra**. Finally it enters the bulb of the penis and ends at the external urethral orifice.

The pair of **seminal vesicles (VES-i-kuls)** are convoluted pouch-like structures about 2 inches (5 cm.) in length, lying behind and at the base of the urinary bladder in front of the rectum. These accessory sex glands secrete the liquid portion of semen which serves to transport the sperm. This is a thick, alkaline fluid rich in fructose (a sugar) which they pour into the ejaculatory duct and constitutes about 60% of the volume of semen.

The **prostate (PROS-tate) gland** is a single, doughnut-shaped gland about the size of a chestnut. It is behind and below the urinary bladder and surrounds the superior portion of the urethra. The prostate secretes an alkaline fluid into the prostatic urethra through numerous ducts. Prostate fluid constitutes about 13 to 33% of the total volume of seminal fluid. Since an acidic environment (such as the yoni) is hostile to sperm, this alkaline fluid contributes to sperm mobility.

The pair of **bulbourethral (bul-bow-you-RE-thral)** or **Cowper's glands** are about the size of peas and are located beneath the prostate on either side of the membranous urethra. They also secrete an alkaline substance that protects sperm by neutralizing the acid environment of the urethra. Their ducts open into the spongy urethra.

Seminal fluid is a mixture of sperm and the secretions of the various glands just described. The average volume of semen for each ejaculation is 2.5 to 5 ml. and the average number of sperm ejaculated is 50 to 100 million/ml. This large number is required because only a small percentage of sperm make it to the ovum; only one actually achieves fertilization. Once ejaculated, sperm have a life expectancy of about 48 to 72 hours within the female reproductive tract. Semen contains an antibiotic known as seminalplasmin which has the ability to destroy a number of bacteria and it may help to ensure fertilization.

Once ejaculated into the yoni, some of the liquid semen coagulates rapidly to form a plug in the cervix and prevent the back flow of semen into the yoni.

This occurs due to the presence of **vesiculase**, a clotting enzyme produced by the seminal vesicles. This clot liquifies after 5 to 20 minutes due to the action of a prostatic enzyme.

The **penis** is the male organ used to introduce sperm into the yoni, and eliminate urine from the bladder. It is cylindrical in shape and consists of a body, root, and a glans penis. The **body** is composed of three cylindrical masses of tissue, each one bound by fibrous tissue. The two masses on the top and the sides are called the **corpora cavernosa**. The smaller midventral mass is called the **corpus spongiosum penis**. All three consist of erectile tissue permeated by blood sinuses. During sexual excitement the

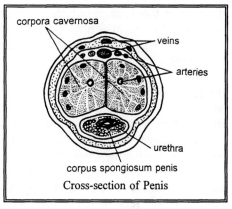

Cross-section of Penis

arteries supplying the penis dilate and large quantities of blood enter the blood sinuses. Expansion of these spaces compresses the veins draining the penis so most of the blood is retained. This results in an erection; the penis becomes longer, stiffer and rises to a 110° or 120° angle from the body when the man is standing. The penis relaxes when the arteries constrict and pressure on the veins is relieved. During male orgasm or ejaculation when the majority of semen is released, the smooth muscle sphincter at the base of the bladder is closed by expansion of the corpus spongiosum. Thus semen and urine do not mix and semen does not enter the bladder. Small amounts of semen may be released prior to ejaculation as well; therefore, if the penis is near the yoni, ejaculation does not have to occur for fertilization to take place.

The penis is attached to the body at the **root**. This area consists of the **bulb of the penis** and the expanded portion of the base of the corpus spongiosum and the crura of the penis, which is the separated and tapered upper end of the corpora cavernosa. The bulb of the penis is attached to the inferior surface of the urogenital diaphragm and enclosed by the bulbocavernosus muscle.

The tip of the penis consists of a slightly enlarged region called the **glans penis** which is shaped like an acorn. The edge of the glans is called the **corona**. The glans is protected by a loosely fitting retractable covering of skin known as the **prepuce (PRE-pyoos)** or **foreskin**. Some cultures practice circumcision, the removal of the foreskin for religious, cultural or supposed hygienic reasons. This is usually done in infancy among Western peoples, but some African tribes include it in rites of puberty. Removal of the foreskin leaves the glans unprotected. In most instances, anesthesia is not used. Circumcision amounts to genital mutilation; sometimes ritually performed as a religious rite. There is no medical basis for its removal in the normal male.

How Pregnancy Impacts Maternal Anatomy and Physiology

Now that we have reviewed basic, nonpregnant female anatomy, we can look at some of the changes which occur in each organ system during pregnancy. Understanding normal physiologic responses to pregnancy is a key to your confident provision of prenatal care. Only by knowing what is normal can you understand whether a problem exists.

Integumentary system: The skin is influenced by the increased hormones of pregnancy. It is normal for pregnant women to perspire more than usual, and the odor of their perspiration may be altered. Oiliness of the skin increases due to increased activity of the sebaceous glands. The hair appears to grow faster during pregnancy, beginning about the third month of gestation. This is due to the prolongation of the anagen, or growth phase, of the hair growth cycle with a decreased number of hairs in resting and hair loss phases. By two to four months after birth, this process is basically reversed resulting in the appearance of rapid hair loss; a return to the normal cycle occurs by 6 to 12 months postpartum.

The skin stretches due to weight gain. *Striae gravidarum* or stretch marks may appear on the enlarging breasts, abdomen and thighs. These occur when the deeper layer of the dermis ruptures and the epidermis is thinned out, producing little scars of bluish pink appearance in the current pregnancy. Stretch marks from past pregnancies appear more silvery. Stretch marks can also be caused outside of pregnancy by weight gain and subsequent loss.

In some women increased pigmentation of the skin occurs which may, in part, be due to the action of estrogen and adrenal hormones, although the physiologic causes remain obscure. The *linea alba*, the white line between the recti muscles of the abdomen, may become a dark line (the *lina negra*); in some women this extends from above the navel down to the border of the pubic hair. The *lina negra* is most commonly seen in darker skinned Caucasians and women-of-color. The breasts, especially the areola, and the vulva may darken as well.

Facial discoloration may appear as tanned, bronzed, or freckled blotches called the mask of pregnancy or chloasma. Exposure to sunlight will darken these splotches even more. Chloasma is a symptom of folic acid deficiency.

Skeletal system: Absorption of calcium increases in the small intestines, starting early in pregnancy. Calcium absorption has doubled by the beginning of the third trimester and remains elevated during postpartum when the woman is lactating. Calcium is progressively retained throughout pregnancy, and maternal bones utilize what the fetus does not. There is therefore no great change in the mineral content of maternal bones during pregnancy. However, bone content can diminish during breastfeeding if calcium and phosphorus intake is inadequate. Bone mass lost during lactation is recovered after weaning. At least three studies correlate breastfeeding with ultimately higher maternal bone mass (Mothering, 1995).

A change in a woman's gait is often noticeable as pregnancy advances. The enlarged uterus causes the balance of the body to be altered; the shoulders are thrown back and the lumbar curve is increased almost to lordosis, which, along with relaxation of the pelvic joints and ligaments during the later weeks of pregnancy, may lead to backaches.

Muscular system: Throughout pregnancy the muscles, tendons and ligaments are increasingly influenced to relax by the action of progesterone and relaxin. This allows maximal opening of the pelvic bones during birth. The byproduct of this process is generalized muscle relaxation which causes the joints to be looser in their attachments. Activities which a woman may ordinarily do with ease outside of pregnancy can cause pulled muscles or even more severe damage. Women should be conscious of this tendency when planning exercise routines or when engaging is any strenuous activity, even those they are accustomed to doing. These hormonal effects are generalized and relaxation of all smooth muscles throughout the body are affected; the ureters, veins, arteries, intestines and sphincter of the stomach relax as well. The result of these effects are discussed under each appropriate organ system.

The senses: Visual alterations during pregnancy vary widely from woman to woman due to hormonal and fluid balance changes. Tear production decreases during pregnancy, particularly during the third trimester. The cornea is about 70% water, and is affected by the generalized changes in extracellular fluid. Central corneal thickness increases by levels as high as 16 microns. This can cause an alteration in visual acuity with a tendency to myopia (nearsightedness). Corneal sensitivity is reduced, which can lead to a woman being unaware of eye irritants. These changes reverse themselves after the birth. (Imafidon & Imafidon, 1992)

Taste is generally dulled during pregnancy while the sense of smell is often heightened. Touch can be heightened as well and some parts of the body may become extremely sensitive. (See chapter on Ear Problems and Hearing Impairment in the section on Problems That Can Occur at Any Time).

Endocrine system: The elevated estrogen of pregnancy causes Thyroid Binding Globulin levels to double at about 12 weeks gestation in relation to nonpregnant values and return to normal by 6 weeks postpartum. A higher TBG level presents more binding sites for the thyroid hormone. As more thyroid hormone becomes protein bound, the thyroid gland produces and releases more hormone as a compensatory measure, resulting in an elevated serum T_4 level. While the amount of protein-bound hormone is higher, unbound, free active hormone remains unchanged, leaving the normal woman basically euthyroid (i.e., with normal hormone levels). It is unclear whether the thyroid gland enlargement frequently noted in normal pregnancy is due to elevated T_4 levels or to the thyroid's efforts to trap iodine more efficiently to compensate for the increased renal clearance of iodine during pregnancy. The fetal thyroid system develops independently of the mother's endocrine system. The placenta effectively blocks maternal thyroid hormones from reaching the fetus except when the maternal hormone levels are extremely elevated. (based on Smith, 1990)

The concentration of hormones secreted by the parathyroid and the size of the glands themselves increase in order to meet fetal calcium requirements. Hormone concentration reaches its highest level between 15 and 35 weeks of pregnancy, returning to normal or even below normal levels before labor begins.

The pituitary gland enlarges during pregnancy and returns to normal size after birth. After birth, there is no significant change in the size of the pituitary's posterior lobe, however the anterior lobe increases in weight with each pregnancy. In rare cases, pituitary enlargement puts pressure on the optic nerves, resulting in restriction of the visual field; vision will spontaneously return to normal after the birth as the glandular size recedes.

Estrogen (primarily estriol E_3) is secreted by the ovaries and adrenal cortex; levels increase 1000-fold in pregnancy. It influences the growth and function of the uterus and breast, is responsible for external genital changes, and increases the pliability of connective tissue. Estrogen decreases gastric secretions, increases skin pigmentations as well as sodium and water retention and increases the clotting ability of fibrinogen. The elevated estriol levels in the third trimester, which may stimulate prostaglandin production, are also due to estrogen. Estrogen may influence the emotional mood swings of pregnancy.

Progesterone production increases ten-fold during pregnancy. It is produced by the corpus luteum of the ovary for the first seven weeks after which the placenta takes over production. Progesterone is responsible for the development of the decidual cells in the endometrium and may play a role in the suppression of the maternal immunologic response to the fetus. It decreases the contractibility of the pregnant uterus and helps develop the lobes of the alveolar system of the breasts. It influences the hypothalamus to cause extensive fat storage in the mother, stimulates the respiratory center, increases the basal body temperature, increases the amount of sodium excreted by the kidneys, relaxes smooth muscle, and decreases gastrointestinal motility as well as the muscle tone of the bladder and ureters.

Prostaglandins are produced by the mother's body as well as by the fetus and the placenta. They help to soften the cervix and prime the body for labor.

Prolactin is produced by the fetal and maternal pituitary glands and by the uterus. Blood levels become elevated by 8 weeks gestation and reach a peak of 200 ng/ml. at term. Prolactin works to sustain milk production and regulate milk composition during lactation, and enhances the mother's ability to attach emotionally to her newborn.

Oxytocin is produced by the hypothalamus and sent to the pituitary for release. It stimulates uterine contractions as well as milk let down and ejection. Distention of the cervix and yoni stimulates the release of oxytocin and prostaglandins during labor.

Circulatory and cardiovascular system: During pregnancy the blood volume and cardiac output both increase. The number of endometrial blood vessels is greatly increased as the uterus enlarges and the placenta becomes a highly vascular structure. There is generalized dilation of the arteries (which is probably controlled by estrogen and prostaglandin). These factors combine to lower vascular resistance, which influences the amount of force it takes to pump the blood.

Cardiac output (how much blood the heart pumps) rises during the first few weeks and is 30 to 45% above nonpregnant levels by the 20th week, where it remains until term. The heart's stroke volume is increased by 10% (to 75 ml.) and cardiac output is further augmented by the 10 to 15% increase in the cardiac rate during pregnancy. The enlarging uterus causes the diaphragm to rise. This displaces the heart to the left and upward. Blood viscosity (thickness) is lower in pregnancy and slight twisting (torsion) of the large abdominal blood vessels occurs because of the enlarged uterus. In late pregnancy the uterus partially impairs venous return from the inferior vena cava, accounting for the lower cardiac output that can be measured when the woman lies on her back. Cardiac demands increase significantly during labor and delivery. Pain increases sympathetic muscle tone, and uterine contractions induce wide swings in systemic venous return. Blood vessel walls are more permeable as well. Evidence of these changes include full and bounding pulses or, in some women, an overall rise in blood pressure.

Mild anemia, increased stroke volume and more rapid ejection of blood from the heart explain the frequent occurrence of benign ejection systolic heart murmurs in pregnant women. A venous hum of pregnancy may be heard at the root of the neck, which is loudest above the clavicle and when the woman is sitting up with her head turned to one side. The physiologic third heart sound is often accentuated during pregnancy. It is also common for the mother's pulse rate to rise 10 to 15 points as pregnancy advances. A mammary souffle (soft swooshing sound) may also be detected due to the increased vascularity of the breasts. Some shortness of breath and edema may also occur. Pericardial effusion is defined as an escape of fluid into the membrane which encases the heart. A small silent pericardial effusion is quite common in normal pregnancy and is not a problem.

Immune system: A subdued immunological reaction to the foreignness of the blastocyst appears to aid implantation and favors a large placenta and healthy fetal growth. The reason for this privileged immunological reaction to the conceptus is not fully understood. Some theories include:

*That the uterus is an immunologically privileged site.
*The conceptus is nonimmunogenic.
*The maternal immune system is altered during pregnancy.
*The placenta is an immunologic barrier.
*Animal studies have found that certain proteins can mask the conceptus; a similar mechanism may be present in women.

Once the pregnancy is established, placental and hormonal factors combine to prevent the maternal system from rejecting the fetus. Although there may be changes in the maternal immune system, women have no predisposition to infectious disease during pregnancy, with the exception of a few viral illnesses (of which poliomyelitis is most problematic).

Respiratory system: During pregnancy, oxygen consumption rises 15 to 20% (to about 45 ml/min.). Roughly one-third of this increase is necessary for the metabolism of the fetus and placenta. The remainder is used to support the increased maternal metabolism. Carbon dioxide excretion likewise increases. Pco_2 (partial pressure of carbon dioxide dissolved in plasma) levels do not change very much during pregnancy. There is a 40% increase in tidal volume (the amount of air inhaled and exhaled) in pregnancy, from 500 to 700 ml., but not any increase in respiratory rate. Residual volume is reduced by 20% (the volume of air in the lungs that remains at the end of expiration and with which the incoming air is diluted). These changes are prompted by progesterone.

Breathlessness is a normal finding in most pregnant women. This may be due to the combination of the lungs' slight displacement upwards as the growing uterus encroaches on the thorax and restricts free movement of the diaphragm, and the deeper respirations necessary to ensure increased oxygen consumption.

In comparison to the heart, pregnancy puts little stress on the respiratory system; respiratory failure is rare. When it occurs it is usually associated with severe asthma, overwhelming infection, or connective tissue disorders.

Digestive system: An increase in dental caries has been traced to elevated levels of acidophilic organisms in the mouth due to the hormones of pregnancy. Gum tissue may become softer and bleed more easily which is partially mediated by hormonal changes but also indicates the need for more vitamin C and bioflavinoids. Some women experience hypersalivation (technically known as ptyalism).

Many women experience nausea and vomiting in early pregnancy due to the sudden increase in hormones in conjunction with hypoglycemia. Food cravings and sensitivities to smell are also common and may aggravate gastrointestinal discomfort. Gastric secretions of hydrochloric acid and pepsin are reduced.

As pregnancy advances, the intestines are displaced to either side of and behind the uterus. The stomach is displaced upwards into the diaphragm. Heartburn may occur because the sphincter between the stomach and esophagus is relaxed by the hormones of pregnancy, causing stomach acids to more easily backwash into the lower esophagus. Gastric emptying time and intestinal motility are decreased, which may cause increased bloating and constipation in some women. The gallbladder takes longer to empty due to smooth muscle relaxation; this may result in gallstone formation in susceptible women. The transit time of food through the gastrointestinal tract (usually spanning approximately 14 to 48 hours) is normally prolonged during late pregnancy by as much as 40%, which enhances the absorption of nutrients.

The anatomical position of the liver is not altered until the second trimester. In the third trimester it may occupy a more posterior-superior position with displacement to the right. Therefore, if you can feel the liver during palpation suspect underlying disease or liver stress.

Urinary system: The ureters are liable to be compressed by the uterus as it rises out of the pelvis. This, in combination with the increased hormones which cause laxity of all muscles, reduces peristalsis in the ureters. Stasis of urine can occur as it gets caught in bends or dilated areas which may develop in the ureters causing pregnant women to be more susceptible to the growth of urinary tract bacteria.

Frequency of urination is common during pregnancy, beginning as early as the sixth week. The uterus is still within the pelvic cavity and becomes slightly more antiflexed with the weight of the pregnancy. This produces pressure on the bladder, simultaneously stretching the bladder base, thus stimulating the urge to urinate. As the uterus rises out of the pelvis (usually around the 12th week) many women are relieved of the increased urgency. In late pregnancy the uterus again presses on the bladder. This, in combination with the general relaxation of the muscles gives rise to greater frequency of urination. Slight urinary incontinence also occurs in some women near term.

The kidneys work harder during pregnancy. The kidneys increase by about 1 cm. in length and the calyces, renal pelvis and ureters dilate markedly. The glomerular filtration rate (GFR) and effective renal plasma flow (ERPF) increase by about 50% in normal pregnancy, beginning shortly after conception, and all increments in the size of the kidneys are present by the second trimester. The GFR reduces by about 15% during the third trimester (measured as 24 hour creatinine clearance). These changes in flow and filtration rates must be taken into account when assessing kidney function during the course of pregnancy, especially in a woman with known renal disease.

Adaptations of pregnancy: the liver, nutrition, and blood volume expansion: (Note: I will use the term metabolic toxemia to discuss liver malfunction resulting from protein/calorie deficiencies. Pre-eclamptic syndrome is a bio-technical term encompassing all conditions which produce the same secondary symptoms).

Pregnancy is a normal physiological condition, and the processes associated with it have a normal function, not a pathological one. The physical changes in the body of a pregnant woman are extensive. Quite simply, everything changes! Although many of these changes are recognized in current medical practice, some of them are poorly understood. Probably the least understood is the relationship between maternal nutrition, blood volume expansion and the increased demand on the liver. Understanding this process is critical to understanding healthy pregnancy. Over the decades, a number of physicians (Pinard, Dodge, Frost, Mitchell, Thompkins, Wiehl, Ross, Hamlin, and others) have proven this nutritional link in their clinical practices. Unfortunately, their work has been largely ignored. The most recent of these researchers is Tom Brewer, a general practitioner who worked extensively with poor pregnant women. He has articulated this process and its link to metabolic toxemia in modern, scientific terms. For a summary of the relevant research, see <u>Maternal Nutrition and Child Health</u>, by Douglas Shanklin.

First, we will get an overview of how some of the adaptations of pregnancy interrelate to maintain the mother and baby in a healthy state. The following changes are of major significance:

I. The formation, implantation, and growth of the placenta. The placenta begins to form during the early weeks of pregnancy, with normal growth dependent upon the nutrients available from the uterine lining and the maternal bloodstream. The placenta implants into the uterine wall by eating its way into the capillary bed of the endometrium (uterine lining). Protein fibers anchor the placenta in place. Open maternal arteries deliver maternal blood into pools that form beneath the placenta. These pools are referred to as the lake of maternal blood. With each maternal heartbeat tiny jets of maternal blood shoot up and bathe the cotyledons which are thin membranes that encase fetal capillaries. This allows exchange between the fetal and maternal blood streams permitting the transfer of maternal nutrients and oxygen to the baby and of waste products from the baby to the mother. Once waste products are exchanged for nutrients, blood repools beneath the placenta and drains into open maternal veins so it can be recirculated and replenished. This special circulatory mechanism is called an Arterial-Venous (A-V) shunt; there is no direct capillary connection. It allows maternal and fetal exchanges between blood streams with no mixing of the two in normal situations.

II. The expansion of the maternal blood volume by 50% to 60% The amount of blood in a pregnant woman's circulation increases as pregnancy advances, with peak volume occurring at 28 to 30 weeks. For a woman whose pre-pregnant weight was 130 lbs., blood volume increases about 2.1 quarts (from 3.5 to a total of 5.6 quarts). This occurs because the mother's body must provide support for an increasingly larger and more complex organ: the placenta. Adequate blood volume expansion provides good profusion of the placental surface. It is the amount of blood and the pressure of the blood which bathes the placental surface that stimulates placental growth. Gradual blood volume expansion results in continued adequate exchange of nutrients and wastes as the baby grows. Additional fluid is also a protection against shock, should the mother lose excess blood after birth.

Maintaining this dramatically expanded blood volume is made possible by the increased activity of the body's salt and water retention mechanisms, by an adequate intake of dietary salt, and by an increase in the synthesis of albumin (a protein which attracts water into the circulation) by the liver. With plasma volume expanding 50% to 60%, the red blood cells, which only increase by 30%, are correspondingly diluted. Plasma volume expansion begins as early as eight weeks and plateaus at 28-30 weeks of pregnancy (Davidson 1974; Christensen, 1958). Red cell volume begins to rise at 18 weeks of pregnancy and continues to rise until term (Norton & Kass, 1968). This is the mechanism of the physiologic "anemia" of pregnancy. It is therefore normal for the hemoglobin to drop about two grams by 28 weeks (and sometimes more, especially with multiple gestations). Some women will then experience a slight rise as term approaches; others will not. The only normal exception to this basic rule is when women live at higher altitudes, where hemoglobin changes are less dramatic. The higher the altitude, the more you must rely on liver enzyme, albumin and total protein levels in lab results to monitor for any problems (see the chapter on Toxemia both in the section on Problems Associated With the Third Trimester and Diagnostic Tests for more information).

III. The growth of the uterus. Before pregnancy, a well-nourished uterus will produce an endometrial lining that supports firm placental implantation. During pregnancy, the uterus changes from an organ weighing a few ounces to one that weighs about two pounds. Maternal nutrition influences how well this cellular hypertrophy takes place and the quality of the new tissues that develop.

IV. The increased demand on liver function. The liver performs over 500 metabolic functions. Three of these are of particular importance during pregnancy:

> **Albumin synthesis:** The liver selectively combines amino acids into protein molecules. Albumin, which is similar to egg white, is the primary blood protein. It has an osmotic pressure which attracts an appropriate amount of fluid into the bloodstream.

> **Hormone metabolism:** The liver clears the bloodstream of hormones. In pregnancy, hormone levels rise to the equivalent of 100 birth control pills a day! The liver converts these hormones into products that are returned to the circulation and excreted by the kidneys.

> **Detoxification:** The liver metabolizes toxic by-products of digestion which enter the bloodstream from the lower bowel, as well as toxins from environmental sources. Digestion slows down in normal pregnancy to enhance absorption of nutrients; therefore toxic by-products have a more favorable environment in which to develop, thus increasing the demand on the liver.

Liver-related demands increase as pregnancy advances. Maintaining liver function at peak efficiency requires a well-balanced diet with enough protein, calories, vitamins, salt, other minerals, and fluids to meet the demands of increased metabolic activity. The liver can only make albumin from dietary protein. If the diet is inadequate in any essential nutrient, the pregnancy suffers. If calories are inadequately supplied in the mother's diet, she will burn protein for her energy needs. Malnutrition due to a lack of either calories or high quality proteins can result in many complications of pregnancy, labor, birth and postpartum.

Adequate blood volume expansion by 28 weeks serves as a foundation for adequate transport of nutrients to the baby during the last trimester, when she begins to put on more weight and store nutrients for after the birth as well as rapidly develop her brain. If the blood volume has not expanded adequately during the first 28 weeks, the mother's body is inadequately prepared to cope with the increased fetal demand and secondary symptoms of metabolic toxemia of late pregnancy become manifest during the last trimester. Increased fetal and placental demands place more stress on the liver to increase blood volume, which it cannot do without proper nourishment. As a result, metabolism becomes increasingly deranged. The kidneys respond to an inadequate blood volume by reabsorbing larger amounts of water and salt as they filter the blood. This reabsorbed fluid and salt is returned to the circulation. If there isn't enough albumin or sodium to hold this reabsorbed fluid within the circulatory system, much of it leaks out into the tissues through the blood vessel walls. The kidneys continue to reabsorb fluid at one end and the fluid keeps leaking out of the capillaries at the other. Pathological weight gain and edema are the result, with eventual reduction in urinary output as the body desperately tries to maintain the blood volume. (Jones, 1993)

Secondary symptoms of toxemia may present before 28 weeks in a severely compromised woman. A symptom is secondary when it may be associated with a variety of underlying causes. Some secondary symptoms are more likely to be related to inadequate blood volume expansion than others. Inadequate blood volume expansion eventually affects other metabolic processes. The symptoms of a contracted blood volume and liver compromise include:

*Intrauterine growth retardation: poor placental function produces a poorly nourished baby.

*Hypovolemia (low blood volume) threatens placental function and brings the mother into labor in a state bordering on dehydration. This is reflected in a high or rising hemoglobin and hematocrit during pregnancy.

*Nausea, tiredness, insomnia and general malaise develop due to chronic hypoglycemia and liver damage.

*Pathological swelling (see above)

*High blood pressure: the mother's body tries to compensate for a contracted blood volume by attempting to adequately supply the placenta, although it doesn't have a large enough blood volume to do so properly. In response to a low or falling blood volume, the kidneys produce renin which constricts blood vessels. This is the same mechanism which raises the blood pressure in order to preserve vital organs after blood loss (such as hemorrhage) occurs.

Hypertension is a late sign of toxemia. A woman's blood pressure may not rise until she is on the verge of convulsions, may not rise until after convulsions occur, or may not rise at all. (See chapter on Hypertension in Pregnancy in the section on Problems That Can Occur At Any Time.)

*Headaches and visual disturbances due to nerve irritation resulting from excessive swelling, vasoconstriction and high blood pressure.

*Epigastric pain from liver damage (under the ribs on the right side).

*Lab results reveal an elevated hemoglobin and, eventually, high liver enzymes as the liver experiences more stress. As the situation becomes more critical, low total protein and albumin levels will be noted since the liver is unable to manufacture blood proteins because it is not receiving the amino-acids necessary to do so.

*Hyperreflexes due to extreme stress and nervous system irritability.

*Proteinuria (protein in the urine), a very late sign of true toxemia caused by kidney damage due to excessive filtering of thick blood and reabsorption of fluids.

*Oliguria: urine production falls off as the body desperately tries to preserve minimal blood volume. When this begins, kidney shutdown is not far behind.

*Maternal convulsions due to neurological irritation in the brain leading to coma and possibly death.

*Liver damage and rupture characteristic of toxemia

Other complications often related to malnutrition include:

*Abruption of the placenta: poor implantation and underlying clots cause separation before birth. Clots form easily when the blood volume is contracted because the blood is thicker.

*Prematurity: if blood volume reaches a critical low, the mother's body rejects the pregnancy in an effort to maintain a balance.

*Stillbirth: a weak fetus/inadequate placenta cannot maintain life either before or in conjunction with the stress of labor.

*Poor healing of the perineum or uterus.

*Infections in the mother or baby before, during, or after the birth.

*Maternal nutritional anemias.

*Weak contractions, long labors, maternal exhaustion in labor.

*Postpartum hemorrhage and coagulation deficiencies.

The primary disease entity in otherwise normal pregnancy is Metabolic Toxemia of Late Pregnancy (called eclamptic toxemia after the onset of convulsions). According to modern medicine, the mechanism is unknown. Treatments vary, but all have centered around treating secondary symptoms via weight and salt restriction, rest, diuretics, antihypertensive drugs, and sedatives. These therapies increase the problem to critical proportions, since they attempt to treat only secondary symptoms and do not deal with the underlying cause.

But what about current toxemia research which says diet is not a factor and which doesn't even mention the liver? Today research is focusing on the possibility that toxemia is a recessive genetic condition (keep in mind that pellagra and beriberi were both thought to be genetic conditions before researchers figured out that they are due to vitamin deficiencies; the "pellagra belt" of the 1930's was also the toxemia belt!). Much of the research regarding the minutia of biochemical changes ignores what is going on in the mother's external environment. The majority of studies make no attempt *at all* to ascertain the quality of the diets of the women they are researching. Often women from low socio-economic clinic populations are used for research, and many enter the study in an already compromised state, even though the study assumes them to be healthy based on a lack of recognized symptoms. While these studies may be discovering valid biochemical processes which take a pathological turn in the presence of a low blood volume, none of them are asking the right questions regarding why the blood volume is low in the first place.

There is much research to show that poor nutrition causes unhealthy pregnancies. Numerous studies, reports, and articles over the years have whole-heartedly supported this view. In an otherwise normal pregnancy, malnutrition leading to a breakdown of liver function with all its concomitant problems is the main thing that goes wrong. In pregnancies complicated by other medical conditions such as diabetes this lack of understanding only compounds the risks for both mother and baby. Enabling the liver to do its job by giving it good food is where all reasonable prenatal therapy needs to begin.

A political issue: The fact that the cause of toxemia in human pregnancy is "not known" is an enormous political issue. It is a feminist issue. While Tom Brewer's work is among the most recent in proving the value of nutrition, it has been largely ignored because he has not performed controlled studies, where one group of women would be intentionally deprived of an adequate diet, because he considers it unethical. It appears that the medical community does not want to recognize the simple truths of the nutrition/toxemia connection.

As long as the scientific community continues to focus on the results of disease (i.e., the detection and management of complications *after* they arise), they will be running on the same old treadmill. Where would all the specialists and producers of medical technology and drugs be if it were suddenly "discovered" that when women eat well in pregnancy, eliminate drugs and stop substance abuse, almost all complications disappear?! It is a discovery they can't afford to make. It is one we can't afford not to make! Pretending not to know is just another way of denying women power over their bodies, their births, and their lives.

References and Further Reading in Anatomy and Physiology:

Brewer, Tom, Metabolic Toxemia of Late Pregnancy, Keats Pub. Co., New Canaan, CT, 1982.

Buttram V. & Gibbons, W., "Muellerian anomalies: A Proposed classification (an analysis of 144 cases)," Fertility and Sterility, Vol. 32, No. 1, July 1979.

Carola, Robert, Harley, J., & Noback, C., Human Anatomy and Physiology, McGraw-Hill Pub. Co., New York, 1990.

Christsensen, P., "Tubular reabsorption of glucose during pregnancy," Scand. J. Clin. Lab. Invest., Vol. 10, No. 364, 1958.

Davidson J., "Changes in renal function and other aspects of homeostasis in early pregnancy," J. Ob/Gyn Br. Commonwealth, Vol. 81, No. 1003, 1974.

Gleicher, Norbert, ed. Principles of Medical Therapy in Pregnancy, Plenum Pub., New York, 1985.

Greenhill, J., Principles and Practice of Obstetrics, W. B. Saunders, Co., Philadelphia, PA, 1951.

Herbst, A, et.al., "Vaginal and cervical abnormalities after exposure to stilbestrol in utero," Ob & Gyn, Vol. 40, No. 2, Sept. 1972, pp. 287-298.

Imafidon, Chris, & Imafidon, J., "Commentaries: Contact Lenses in Pregnancy," Brit. J. of Ob/Gyn, Nov. 1992, Vol. 99, pp. 865-868.

Jefferies, et.al., "Structural anomalies of the cervix and vagina in women enrolled in the Diethylstilbestrol Adenosis (DESAD) Project," Amer. J. or Ob & Gyn, Vol 148, No. 1, Jan. 1, 1984, p. 60.

Jones, Joy, "Brewer Pregnancy Diet," in Rothman, B, ed., Encyclopedia of Childbearing, Oryx Press, Phoenix, AZ, 1993.

Lichtman, Ronnie, & Papera, Susan, Gynecology: Well-woman Care, Appleton & Lance, Norwalk, CT, 1990.

Lloyd, Thomas, CNM, "Rh-factor incompatibility: A primer in prevention," J. of Nurse-Midwifery, Vol. 32, No. 5, Sept/Oct 1987, pp. 297-306.

Mittendorf, Robert, "Managing the DES-exposed woman: an update," Contemp. OB/GYN, Sept. 1994, p. 62.

Mashburn, Jane, et.al., "Hematocrit Values during pregnancy in a nurse-midwifery population," J. of Nurse Midwifery, Vol. 37, No. 6, Nov/Dec 1992, pp. 404-410.

McGovern, Cheryl, "Recognizing a Tubal Pregnancy," MCN, Vol. 3, Sept./Oct. 1978, p. 303-5.

Mothering, Good News: Lucid Breastfeeding, Vol. 74, Spring 1995, p. 31, cited from New Beginnings, July/Aug. 1994, pp. 110-111.

Myles, Margaret, Textbook for Midwives, 6th ed., E. & S. Livingstone, Ltd., London, Eng., 1968.

Neeson, Jean, Clinical Manual of Maternity Nursing, J. B. Lippincott Co., Phil., PA, 1987.

Norten C., & Kass, E., "Bacteriuria of pregnancy-a critical reappraisal," Annu Rev. Med., Vol. 19, No. 431, 1968.

Olds, Sally, et.al., Obstetric Nursing, Addison-Wesley Pub., Co., Menlo Park, CA, 1980, p. 219.

Sevely, Josephine L., Eve's Secrets: A New Theory of Female Sexuality, Random House, New York, NY, 1987.

Shanklin, Douglas & Hodin, Jay, Maternal Nutrition and Child Health, Charles C. Thomas, Pub., Springfield, IL, 1979.

Singer & Grismaijer, Dressed to Kill: the Link Between Breast Cancer & Bras, Avery, NY, 1995

Smith, Judy, "Pregnancy Complicated by Thyroid Disease," J. of Nurse-Midwifery, Vol. 35, No. 3, May/June, 1990, p. 143-149.

Tortora, Gerard & Anagnostakos, N., Principles of Anatomy and Physiology, 5th ed., Harper & Row Publishers, New York, NY 1987.

200

NOTES:

SUSTAINING HEALTH AND WELL-BEING DURING PREGNANCY

Individualizing Your Care

One of the biggest differences between the medical model of care and the midwifery model is the individualization of the care that midwives provide. While some practitioners take this to mean knowing a woman's name and making sure she has time to have her questions answered, most midwives have a broader and deeper understanding of this concept. To truly individualize care means to strive for an in-depth understanding of a particular woman: her unique physical, emotional and mental circumstances with regard to her physical well-being and living environment as well as her hopes and fears about birth. Individualization of care enters into every aspect of our interaction with women.

While "normal values" are given throughout this book, I have tried to give you some sense of what it means to apply normal values to each woman and her baby. Normal results of lab tests, for example, are distributed on a bell curve, with most people falling somewhere in the center. However, a person can be perfectly normal and have lab results that fall outside the considered normal range. Taking into account parameters such as a woman's sense of well-being, her physical size and shape and her emotional milieu can help you detect a variation which for her is truly a normal variation and not a problem. For example, at the same time that you are encouraging a woman to "follow these nutritional guidelines as closely as possible," you will be getting a feel for how much is really enough by evaluating how her baby is growing and how the woman is feeling more than by the number of portions she is eating per day. As you become more experienced, you will be able to detect what is truly normal, developing a "psychic radar system" which goes off when a problem is in front of you. The only way you will really learn this is during your actual, hands-on training, but its importance cannot be overemphasized. How to apply the "normal range" to a particular woman will grow as you become more experienced.

As you read through this section, and indeed, through the whole book, please keep the concept of individualized care in mind. Let your first question always be "what is reflective of health and well-being for this woman before me?", not "what does the book say is normal?" This does not mean you should ignore normal parameters entirely, but it does mean that you have to look at the woman first. All too often in medical circles, the statistics are referred to without regard for the woman's condition at all. This not only means unnecessary interventions are used; downright harm is done more often than not.

An important element of this learning process includes continuity of care. Continuity of care refers to continuous, uninterrupted care from one or more consistent care providers. Being able to individualize care involves connecting with each woman, baby and family well enough to make an accurate judgement about what particular variations are truly normal for *that woman*. If you do not have the opportunity to study within a practice where women are seen by the same midwife each time she comes, some continuity can be achieved by conversing with other midwives involved in a woman's care, from chart review before each appointment and from talking to the woman herself to follow-up on chart notes. Be aware, however, that it is easy to leave a training program feeling confident when, in reality, you never had the opportunity to be truly responsible for helping a woman work through her problems visit by visit, be they emotional or physical. If you see a woman once or twice, notice that she is small-for-dates in her uterine growth, and never see her again, how can you know if her size/date discrepancy was due to a normal variation or a problem? You can review the chart, you can talk to your supervisors and you can ask other students who were involved in her care. But, only by following a woman consistently will you learn the subtle nuances that separate midwifery care from the 5-minute prenatals offered in medical model clinics.

Basic Nutrition

NOTE: Read the chapter on How Pregnancy Impacts Maternal
Anatomy and Physiology in the A & P section before studying
nutrition.

The importance of nutrition during pregnancy: Adequate nutrition is the single most important physical factor in determining the outcome of pregnancy. Good nutrition can make up for a multitude of problems and deficiencies in other areas of a pregnant woman's life. When a woman's work environment is stressful, when she has closely spaced pregnancies or when she has health-compromising medical conditions, good nutrition with adequate amounts of a variety of foods will provide the necessary cushion of protection both mother and developing baby need to make it through birth with a minimum of problems. What constitutes an adequate diet during pregnancy includes increased amounts of protein, salt and calories and other nutrients over and above what a nonpregnant woman needs due to the physiological changes that take place to support the pregnancy. Proper nourishment is protective because it allows the blood volume to expand adequately, preventing toxemia and bringing mother and baby to labor with the maximum reserves for withstanding the stress of birth.

The relationship between maternal and fetal well-being and maternal nutrition has been well documented, although why this relationship exists is not well understood among mainstream practitioners and has not been given high priority in the medical model of care. Although some understanding of maternal blood volume expansion is now more commonly acknowledged by medical practitioners, how and why this process occurs and the critical relationship between adequate blood volume and adequate diet is still a mystery in their minds. Common sense would tell you that you can't grow a healthy baby with poor nutrition and an insufficient quantity of food. Ask any contractor, "If you use inferior materials and have less than you need can you construct a quality home?" The answer, no doubt, will be "of course not." Yet the average obstetrician's view concerning what constitutes adequate dietary intake during pregnancy is, "there needs to be more research." Veterinarians are not waiting for more research. They clearly see the cause and effect relationship between adequate maternal nutrition and healthy baby animals, and act accordingly.

Nutrition is the relationship of food to the health of the human body. Good nutrition implies that all the essential nutrients are supplied in adequate amounts and are being properly utilized to maintain optimal health and well-being. Deficiencies result whenever inadequate amounts of essential nutrients are provided to tissues that must function normally over a long period of time.

In this chapter we will review basic nutrition. In the next chapter we will explore how to apply nutrition in the clinical setting to maximize the prospect of a healthy pregnancy and the birth of a perfectly formed, vibrant, intelligent and immunologically resilient newborn.

The study of the nutritional content of foods is a relatively new science. More is being discovered about nutrition all the time, including the discovery of previously unrecognized nutritive substances. Nutritional supplements touted as complete may actually be lacking substances that have not yet been identified. Therefore it is important to emphasize the need for a whole foods diet rather than dependence upon nutritional supplements, although supplements can be helpful in certain situations when currently recognized nutrients are known to be lacking or deficient in the diet.

A whole foods diet consists of as much unprocessed food in its natural form as possible. This means whole grain flour and bread products (no white enriched flour); natural cheeses rather than cheese foods or other processed products; real eggs and not egg substitutes. The typical American diet is the most processed and denatured diet in the world. It can be a simple matter to direct women to whatever traditional or ethnic diets they may also be familiar with. If American foods are all they know, a transition from processed to whole food equivalents of those foods they like is appropriate.

With this in mind and the fact the people eat foods, not vitamins and minerals, we need to know what foods to recommend and in what amounts. However, it is also important to understand what nutrients are found in different foods and how these nutrients support health and well-being.

There are basically five kinds of nutritive substances found in foods: proteins, fats, carbohydrates, vitamins and minerals. Protein, fats and carbohydrates are discussed in the chapter on Very Basic Chemistry in the Anatomy and Physiology section. Vitamins and minerals are defined as follows: **Vitamins** are organic nutrients required in tiny amounts to maintain growth and normal metabolism. **Minerals** are inorganic substances which may appear in combination with each other or with organic compounds which are required for physiological processes.

Vitamins function with chemicals called **enzymes** which have numerous essential functions within the body. Enzymes have two parts: a protein molecule and a coenzyme which is often a vitamin or something made from a vitamin. Enzymes are responsible for the delivery of nutrients to the cells and elimination of wastes from the cells. They also play a major role in growth, metabolism, cellular reproduction and digestion.

Minerals exist in the body in organic and inorganic combinations. They act as catalysts for many biological reactions such as muscle response, neurological transmissions, digestion and the utilization of nutrients from foods. They are important in the production of hormones. They also help to maintain fluid balance and normal pH within the body. Minerals and vitamins coexist and work together.

On the following pages, you will find an overview of the major, currently recognized nutrients and why they are important.

NUTRIENT	IMPORTANCE	DEFICIENCY SYMPTOMS/RESULTS	TOXICITY LEVEL/EFFECTS
Carbohydrate	Provides energy for bodily functions; assists digestion & assimilation of foods.	Loss of energy; fatigue; excessive protein breakdown; disturbed balance of water, sodium, potassium & chloride	Intake should not exceed that needed to maintain desirable body weight (or, in pregnancy, maternal/fetal well-being)
Fat	Provides energy; serves as a carrier for fat soluble vitamins A, D, E & K; supplies essential fatty acids needed for growth, health, & smooth skin	Eczema or skin disorders; retarded growth	Same as above
Protein	Necessary for growth & development; formation of hormones, enzymes & antibodies; maintains acid-alkali balance; source of heat & energy	Fatigue; loss of appetite; diarrhea & vomiting; stunted growth; edema	Same as above
Vitamin A (fat soluble)	Necessary for growth & repair of body tissues, & for health of eyes; promotes germ killing enzymes; maintains healthy skin, aids in bone & tooth formation; destroys carcinogens	Night blindness; rough, dry, scaly skin; increased susceptibility to infections; fatigue; insomnia; depression; loss of smell & appetite; lusterless hair; brittle nails; inflamed eyelids; birth defect in animals	May cause nausea, vomiting, diarrhea, skin problems, hair loss, headaches, appetite loss; fat soluble. Vit. C helps reduce toxicity
Beta-Carotene	Water soluble vitamin converted to Vit. A by liver; same benefits as fat soluble A	Same	Essentially nontoxic, may turn skin slightly orange-yellow in high enough dosages
B Vitamins (water soluble)	Necessary for carbohydrate, fat & protein metabolism; aids nervous system function; helps maintain muscle tone in gastrointestinal tract; maintains health of hair, eyes, mouth & liver	Dry, rough, cracked skin; acne; dull, dry or gray hair; fatigue; poor appetite; gastrointestinal tract disorders	Relatively nontoxic, (see individual components)
Vitamin B₁ (Thiamine)	Necessary for carbohydrate metabolism; helps maintain healthy nervous system; stabilizes appetite; stimulates growth & good muscle tone	Gastrointestinal disorders; fatigue; loss of appetite; nerve & heart disorders; if severe, can cause beriberi in newborns	No known oral toxicity
Vitamin B₂ (Riboflavin)	Necessary for carbohydrate, fat & protein metabolism; aids in formation of red blood cells & antibodies; maintains cell respiration	Eye problems; cracks & sores in mouth; dermatitis; retarded growth; digestive disturbances; if severe in late pregnancy, may be associated with prematurity or stillbirth	No known oral toxicity
Niacin (B₃) Nicotinic acid, Niacinamide	Necessary for carbohydrate, fat & protein metabolism; helps maintain health of skin, tongue & digestive system	Dermatitis & nervous disorders (pellagra); hot flashes, nausea, vomiting; sweating; palpitations; headaches; insomnia; bad breath; digestive disturbances; sore mouth & gums	No real toxic effects; niacin or nicotinic acid doses over 100 mg. may cause tingling & itching sensation, flushing & head throbbing due to dilation of blood vessels lasting about 15 min., then subsiding. Niacinamide avoids side effects but can cause depression; liver damage may occur w/doses over 2 gms daily
Pantothenic acid (B₅)	Aids in formation of some fats; helps release energy from carbohydrates, fats & proteins; aids in utilization of some vitamins; improves resistance to stress	Vomiting; restlessness; increased susceptibility to infection; gastrointestinal disturbances; depression; fatigue	No known toxicity level

NUTRIENT	IMPORTANCE	DEFICIENCY SYMPTOMS/RESULTS	TOXICITY LEVEL/EFFECTS
Vitamin B_6 (Pyridoxine)	Necessary for carbohydrate, fat & protein metabolism; aids in formation of antibodies; helps maintain sodium/phosphorus balance	Anemia; mouth disorders; nervousness; muscular weakness; dermatitis; dandruff; water retention	Megadoses (2,000 to 6,000 mg/day) have been associated with neuropathy with sensory ataxia, profound distal limb impairment & vibratory sensations.
Vitamin B_{12}	Essential for normal cell formation; necessary for carbohydrate, fat & protein metabolism; maintains healthy nervous system	Pernicious anemia; brain damage; nervousness; neuritis	No known oral toxicity with intakes as high as 600-1,200 mcg.
Biotin	Necessary for carbohydrate, fat & protein metabolism; aids in utilizing other B vitamins	Dermatitis; grayish skin color; depression; muscle pain; impairment of fat metabolism; poor appetite	No known oral toxicity
Choline	Normal nerve transmission; aids metabolism & transport of fats; helps regulate liver & gallbladder	Fatty liver; hemorrhaging kidneys; high blood pressure	No known oral toxicity even with intake as high as 50,000 mg. daily for 1 week
Folic acid (Folacin)	Used in red blood cell formation; aids metabolism of proteins; necessary for growth & division of body cells	Poor growth; gastrointestinal disorders; anemia; poor memory; neural tube defects in the fetus; possibly small babies	No known toxicity
Inositol	Necessary for formation of lecithin; may be directly connected with metabolism for fats; including cholesterol; vital for hair growth	Constipation; eczema; hair loss; high blood cholesterol	No known toxicity
PABA (Paraamino- benzoic Acid)	Stimulates GI bacteria to produce folic acid; acts as a coenzyme in breakdown & utilization of proteins; aids in red blood cell formation.	Fatigue; irritability; depression; nervousness; constipation; headaches; digestive disorders; graying hair	Continued high ingestion may be toxic to the liver, kidney & heart; symptoms are nausea & vomiting
Pangamic acid (B_{15})	Helps eliminate hypoxia; promotes protein metabolism; stimulates nervous & glandular system	Diminished oxygenation of cells; nervous disorders	500 mg. tolerated daily with no toxic effects
Vitamin C (water soluble)	Maintains collagen; helps heal wounds and fractures; strengthens blood vessels; helps resist infections; aids iron absorption; stimulates T-effector cell activity; reduces lipid production in the brain	Bleeding gums; swollen or painful joints; slow-healing wounds & fractures; bruising; nosebleeds; impaired digestion	Essentially nontoxic; extremely high doses near term may result in the birth of a baby who develops neonatal scurvy (Vit. C def.)
Vitamin D (fat soluble)	Improves absorption & utilization of calcium & phosphorus required for bone formation; maintains stable nervous system & normal heart action	Poor bone & tooth formation; softening of bones & teeth; inadequate absorption of calcium; retention of phosphorus in kidneys; possibly fetal malformations of face, heart & skull	High serum calcium levels (enhanced by antacids); kidney stones; nausea & vomiting; calcification of soft tissues (including the placenta)
Vitamin E Tocopherol (fat soluble)	Protects fat soluble vitamins; protects red blood cells; essential in cellular respiration & protection; inhibits coagulation of blood by preventing clots	Rupture of red blood cells; muscular wasting; abnormal fat deposits in muscles	Essentially nontoxic
Vitamin K (fat soluble)	Necessary for formation of prothrombin; needed for blood coagulation	Low prothrombin levels; tendency to bleed & bruise easily	Synthetic vitamin K may be toxic; injection in newborns has been linked to childhood cancers

NUTRIENT	IMPORTANCE	DEFICIENCY SYMPTOMS/RESULTS	TOXICITY LEVEL/EFFECTS
Bioflavonoids (Vitamin P) citrin, rutin, hesperidin, flavone, flavonals (water soluble)	Helps increase strength of capillaries & membranes; not true vitamins (although sometimes called Vitamin P, but help enhance the absorption of vitamin C & they should be taken together	Tendency to bleed & bruise easily	No known toxicity, but extremely high doses may cause diarrhea
Unsaturated fatty acids	Respiration of vital organs; helps maintain resilience & lubrication of cells; helps regulate blood clotting; essential for normal glandular activity	Brittle, lusterless hair; brittle nails; dandruff; diarrhea; varicose veins	No known toxicity; may cause metabolic disturbances & weight gain if taken in excess
MINERALS: Boron	Assists calcium uptake & promote bone health	Loss of calcium through the urine; bone weakness	Do not take more than 3 mg. daily.
Calcium	Sustains development & maintenance of strong bones & teeth; assists normal blood clotting, muscle activity, nerve & heart function	Tetany; softening bones; back & leg pains; brittle bones; insomnia; irritability; depression; lowered pain threshold	No know oral toxicity; excessive intake may cause side effects such as leg cramps
Chlorine	Regulates acid/base balance; maintains osmotic pressure; stimulates production of hydrochloric acid; helps maintain joints & tendons	Loss of hair & teeth; poor muscle contractility; impaired digestion	Excessive intake of sodium chloride (salt) may have adverse effects
Chromium	Stimulates enzymes in metabolism of energy & synthesis of fatty acids cholesterol & protein; increased effectiveness of insulin	Depressed growth rate; glucose intolerance; atherosclerosis	No known toxicity
Cobalt	Functions as part of B_{12}; maintains red blood cells; activates many enzymes in body	Pernicious anemia; impaired respiration; skin sores	Excessive intake may have side effects
Copper	Aids formation of red blood cells; part of many enzymes; works with vitamin C to form elastin	General weakness; impaired respiration; skin sores	Excessive intake may have side effects
Fluorine (Fluorides)	May reduce tooth decay by discouraging growth of acid-forming bacteria	(See chapter on Fluoride in this section)	Intake has side effects (see Chapter on Fluoride in this section)
Germanium (Ge-132)	Improves cellular oxygenation	Not described but many illnesses respond well to this mineral (infections, arthritis, cancer, allergies)	No side effect have been noted
Iodine (iodide)	Essential part of thyroxine; necessary for preventing goiter; regulates production of energy & rate of metabolism; promotes growth	Enlarged thyroid gland; dry skin & hair; loss of physical & mental vigor; cretinism; goiter; suppression of thyroid hormone synthesis & congenital hypothyroidism in children born to iodine-deficient mothers	Up to 1000 mcg. daily produced no toxic effects in persons with a normal thyroid
Iron	Necessary for hemoglobin & myoglobin formation; helps in protein metabolism; promotes growth	Weakness; paleness of skin; constipation; anemia	Excessive intake may be toxic

NUTRIENT	IMPORTANCE	DEFICIENCY SYMPTOMS/RESULTS	TOXICITY LEVEL/EFFECTS
Magnesium	Acts as catalyst in the utilization of carbohydrates, fats, proteins, calcium, phosphorus and possibly potassium	Nervousness; muscular excitability; tremors; depression	3,000 mg. daily may be toxic in some people with kidney malfunctions
Manganese	Enzyme activator; helps carbohydrate & fat production & normal skeletal development; maintains sex-hormone production	Paralysis; convulsions; dizziness; ataxia; blindness & deafness in infants; diabetes; loss of hearing	Excessive intake may have side effects in some people
Molybdenum	Acts in oxidation of fats & aldehydes; aids mobilization of iron from liver reserves	Premature aging; impotence	Excessive intake may be toxic
Nickel	Helps hormone, lipid, membrane & glucose metabolism	Aggravates iron-deficiency anemia	Excessive intake may be toxic
Phosphorus	Works with calcium to build bones & teeth; utilizes carbohydrates, fats & proteins; stimulates muscular contractions	Loss of weight & appetite; irregular breathing; pyorrhea; fatigue; nervous disorders	No known toxicity
Potassium	Works to control activity of heart muscles, nervous system & kidneys	Poor reflexes; respiratory failure; cardiac arrest; nervous disorders; constipation; irregular pulse; insomnia	No known toxicity
Selenium	Works with vitamin E; preserves tissue elasticity; essential in production of glutathione peroxidase which stimulates increased antibody response to germs	Premature aging; SIDS (sudden infant death syndrome)	Excessive intake may be toxic
Sodium	Maintains normal fluid levels in cells & health of nervous, muscular, blood & lymph systems	Muscle weakness; muscle shrinkage; nausea; loss of appetite; intestinal gas	Very high sodium intake (14-28 grams daily) may cause potassium to be lost in the urine, abnormal fluid retention, dizziness & swelling
Sulfur	Part of amino acids; essential for formation of body tissues; part of B vitamins; helps tissue respiration; necessary for collagen synthesis	Sluggishness & fatigue	Excessive intake may be toxic
Vanadium	Inhibits cholesterol formation; helps bone, teeth, and cartilage development	Decreased reproductive ability; increased infant mortality.	Excessive intake may be toxic
Zinc	Component of insulin & male reproductive seminal fluid; aids digestion and metabolism of phosphorus; aids wound healing	Retarded growth; delayed sexual maturity; prolonged wound healing; stretch marks; irregular menses; diabetes; loss of taste & appetite; central nervous system damage in the fetus	Relatively nontoxic; excessive intake may have side effects

(Abrams, 1990; Balch & Balch, 1990; Dunne, 1990)

210

Free radicals and antioxidants:

There is a group of vitamins, minerals and enzymes called antioxidants that help protect our body from the formation of free radicals. Free radicals are atoms or groups of atoms that can cause damage to cells, impair immune function and lead to infectious and degenerative diseases. There are three known free radicals: superoxide, hydroxyl and peroxide. They may be formed by exposure to radiation and toxic chemicals, overexposure to the sun, or through the action of various metabolic processes such as the use of stored fat molecules for energy. Free radicals are normally kept in check by the neutralizing action of free radical scavengers. Some of these are produced in the body, such as the four enzymes superoxide dismutase (SOD), methione reductase, catalase, and glutathione peroxidase. Vitamins A, E, C, *Beta*-carotene and hesperidin, as well as the mineral selenium, are also antioxidants. (Balch, 1990) The vitamins and minerals are discussed in the previous table. Other important antioxidants are as follows:

ANTIOXIDANT	COMMENTS	SOURCES
Gamma-Linoleic acid (GLA)	Regulator of T-lymphocytes; made from linoleic acid; if vitamins B_6, niacin, C or A are lacking, conversion may be blocked. Hydrogenated oil and a high-fat diet also inhibit conversion.	Vegetable oil, Evening Primrose oil, black currant seed oil, borage oil
L-Cysteine (amino acid)	Contains sulfur; needed to produce glutathione; used by the liver & lymphocytes to detoxify chemicals and germ poisons & tobacco smoke, environmental pollutants & alcohol, which all suppress the immune system	Protein rich foods
L-Glutathione (amino acid)	Protects from harmful effects of metals, drugs, cigarette smoke & alcohol	Protein rich foods
Superoxide Dismutase (SOD)	A healthy body produces about 5 million units of SOD and catalase daily. SOD revitalizes the cells & reduces the rate of cell destruction, removes superoxide, and aids in using zinc, copper & manganese. Free radical production increases with age while SOD production is reduced. Supplements must be enterically coated to allow tablet to pass into the small intestines before it dissolves.	Barley grass, broccoli, Brussels sprouts, cabbage, wheatgrass & most green plants
Coenzyme Q_{10}	Vitamin-like substance similar to vitamin E found in human tissue, powerful antioxidant which supports the immune system	Mackerel, salmon & sardines

Getting nutrients from food sources:

Nature intends for us to get the nutrients we need from foods. While it may benefit pharmaceutical companies to market supplements, it does not benefit people to depend upon them for nutrition. A supplement will contain only those nutrients which are recognized as important, often with a focus on the "active" substances, the chemicals that seem to effect changes within the body. In addition, a supplement which is not derived from natural sources will be a petrochemical substance which has the same molecular composition as the natural nutrient but is not the same. Petrochemical substances do not break down in the body the same way that natural ones do (McKenna, 1993).

A whole food is a carefully balanced nutritive complex which provides everything the food has to offer, whether we are aware of its value or not. This includes "passive" ingredients which may help to balance or support the more active ingredients. Since science does not focus on passive ingredients, their value is not well understood; since nature put them there, they are, no doubt, equally important. Foods also offer us the vital force of the plant. This energy is renewing and sustaining to our whole being, not just the physical body. In order to know what foods are high in which nutrients, the following table is offered as a guide. While it does not cover every food item that exists, you can figure out what a food might offer by comparing it with the color and variety of foods that are listed. Many herbs offer concentrated sources of nutrients, and qualify as whole foods.

Nutrient	Food sources
Carbohydrates	Whole grains, sweeteners, fruits, vegetables (esp. starchy & root)
Fats	Butter, vegetable oils, meat fats, milk products, nuts & seeds
Protein	Meats, fish, poultry, soy, eggs, milk products, whole grains, beans
Water	Beverages, fruits & vegetables
Vitamin A	Liver, eggs, yellow fruits & vegetables, dark-green fruits & vegetables, dairy products
B VIT: B_1 (Thiamine)	Nutr. yeast, whole grains, brown rice, blackstrap molasses, organ meats, meats, fish & poultry, egg yolks, legumes, nuts
B_2 (Riboflavin)	Nutritional yeast, whole grains, blackstrap molasses, organ meats, egg yolks, legumes, nuts
B_6 (Pyridoxine)	Meats, whole grains, organ meats, blackstrap molasses, wheat germ, legumes, green leafy vegetables
B_{12}	Organ meats, fish & pork, eggs, cheese, milk & milk products, fermented soy products produced by Ohsawa America, South River & Yamazaki
Biotin	Egg yolks, liver, unpolished rice, nutritional yeast, whole grains, sardines, legumes
Choline	Egg yolks, organ meats, nutritional yeast, wheat germ, soybeans, fish, legumes, lecithin

Nutrient	Food sources
Folic acid	Dark-green leafy vegetables, organ meats, nutritional yeast, root vegetables, whole grains, oysters, salmon, milk
Inositol	Whole grains, citrus fruits, nutritional yeast, molasses, meat, milk, nuts, vegetables, lecithin
Niacin (B$_3$)	Lean meats, poultry & fish, nutritional yeast, peanuts, milk & milk products, rice bran
PABA	Organ meats, wheat germ, yogurt, molasses, green leafy vegetables
Pangamic acid (B$_{15}$)	Nutri. yeast, rare steak, brown rice, sunflower, pumpkin & sesame seeds
Pantothenic acid (B$_5$)	Organ meats, nutritional yeast, egg yolks, legumes, whole grains, wheat germ, salmon
Vitamin C	Citrus fruits, acerola cherries, alfalfa sprouts, cantaloupe, strawberries, broccoli, tomatoes, green peppers
Bioflavonoids (Vitamin P)	Citrus fruits (white inner peel) fruits, black currents, buckwheat
Vitamin D	Salmon, sardines, herring, vit. D-fortified dairy products, egg yolks, organ meats
Vitamin E	Cold-pressed oils, eggs, wheat germ, organ meats, molasses, sweet potatoes, leafy vegetables
Vitamin K	Green leafy vegetables, egg yolks, safflower oil, blackstrap molasses, cauliflower, soybeans, alfalfa sprouts
Unsaturated fatty acids	Vegetable oils, sunflower seeds
MINERALS: Boron	Leafy vegetables, fruits, nuts and grains
Calcium	Green leafy vegetables, shellfish, molasses, sesame seeds, sea weeds
Chlorine	Table & sea salt, seafood, meats, ripe olives, rye flour, sea vegetables
Chromium	Honey, grapes, raisins, corn oil, whole grain cereals, nutritional yeast
Cobalt	Organ meats, oysters, clams, poultry, milk, green leafy vegetables, fruits
Copper	Organ meats, seafood, nuts, legumes, molasses, raisins
Germanium (Ge-132)	Aloe vera, comfrey, garlic, ginseng, skiitake mushrooms, onions
Fluoride	Tea, seafood
Iodine	Seafood, kelp, iodized salt
Iron	Organ meats & meats, eggs, fish & poultry, blackstrap molasses, cherry juice, green leafy vegetables, dried fruits
Magnesium	Seafood, whole grains, dark green vegetables, molasses, nuts
Manganese	Whole grains, green leafy vegetables, legumes, nuts, pineapple, egg yolks
Molybdenum	Legumes, whole grain cereals, milk, kidney, liver, dark green vegetables
Phosphorus	Fish, meat, poultry, eggs, legumes, dairy, nuts, whole grain cereals
Potassium	Lean meat, whole grain, vegetables, dried fruit, legumes, sunflower seeds
Selenium	Tuna, herring, nutri. yeast, wheat germ, bran, whole grains, sesame seeds
Sodium	Seafood, table salt, celery, processed foods, dairy products, sea weeds
Sulfur	Fish, red hot pepper, garlic, onions, eggs, meat, cabbage, brussels sprouts, horseradish
Vanadium	Fish
Zinc	Pumpkin seeds, sunflower seeds, seafood, organ meats, mushrooms, nutritional yeast, soybeans, oysters, herring, eggs, wheat germ, meats

Nutrients that function together when taken in supplemental form: When women you work with resort to taking a supplement for one reason or another, if they try to mimic nature as much as possible they will derive the maximum benefit from the supplement. To do this they must have some idea of which nutrients work together in their bodies. Remember that the understanding of vitamin and mineral relationships is extremely basic and cannot possibly duplicate the delicate and complex balance found when nutrients are taken in their natural forms.

213

NUTRIENT	MORE EFFECTIVE COMBINED WITH:	ANTAGONISTS TO ASSIMILATION
Vitamin A	Vitamin B complex (helps preserve stored A) Choline (protects from toxic effects of A) Vitamin C (helps prevent oxidation) Vitamin D (1 part D to 10 parts A) Vitamin E (acts as an antioxidant) Unsaturated fatty acids, calcium, phosphorus Zinc (helps absorption of A)	Air pollution, alcohol, arsenicals, aspirin, corticosteroid drugs, Dicumarol, mineral oil, nitrates, phenobarbital, thyroid hormone
Vitamin B complex	Vitamin C, E Calcium & Phosphorus	Alcohol, antibiotics, aspirin, corticosteroid drugs, diuretics
B_1 (Thiamine)	Vitamin B complex, Vitamin B_2 (riboflavin), folic acid, niacin, Vitamin E Sulfur & Manganese Vitamin C (helps prevent oxidation)	Alcohol, antibiotics, excess sugar
B_2 (Riboflavin)	Vitamin B complex, niacin, B_6 (B_2 & B_6 doses should be about the same), Vitamin C	Alcohol, antibiotics, oral contraceptives
Niacin (B_3)	Vitamin B complex, B_1, B_2 Vitamin C (helps prevent oxidation)	Alcohol, antibiotics, excess sugar
Pantothenic acid (B_5)	Vitamin B complex, B_6, B_{12} Biotin & Folic acid (aids absorption) Vitamin C (protects against oxidation) Calcium, Sulfur	Aspirin, methylbromide (insecticide fumigant for some foods)
Vitamin B_6 (pyridoxine)	B complex, Pantothenic acid, Vitamin C Magnesium, Potassium, Linoleic acid, Sodium B_1, & B_2 (dosages of these & B_6 should be about the same)	Cortisone, estrogen, oral contraceptives

NUTRIENT	MORE EFFECTIVE COMBINED WITH:	ANTAGONISTS TO ASSIMILATION
Vitamin B_{12}	B complex, Choline, Folic acid, Inositol, Calcium, Potassium, Sodium B_6, Vitamin C & Iron (enhances absorption)	Dilantin, oral contraceptives
Pangamic acid (B_{15})	B complex, Vitamins C & E	
Biotin	B complex, B_{12}, Folic acid, Pantothenic acid, Vitamin C, Sulfur	Antibiotics, Avidin (from raw egg whites) sulfa drugs
Choline	Vitamin A, B complex, Inositol, Linoleic acid B_{12} & Folic acid (help synthesis)	Alcohol, excess sugar
Folic Acid	B complex, B_{12}, Biotin, Pantothenic acid Vitamin C (helps protect against oxidation)	Alcohol, anticonvulsants, oral contraceptives, phenobarbital
Inositol	B complex, B_{12}, Choline, Vitamins C & E, Linoleic acid	Antibiotics
PABA (Para-aminobenzoic) acid	B complex, Folic acid, Vitamin C	Sulfa drugs
Vitamin C	All vitamins & minerals, Bioflavonoids Calcium & Magnesium (help body use C)	Alcohol, antibiotics, antihistamines, aspirin, baking soda, barbiturates, cortisone, DDT, estrogen, oral contraceptives, petroleum, smoking, sulfonamides
Bioflavonoids (Vitamin P)	Vitamin C	
Vitamin D	Vitamin A (10 parts A to 1 part D) Choline & Vitamin C (help prevent toxicity) Unsaturated fatty acids, Calcium, Phosphorus	Alcohol, corticosteroid, oral contraceptives, Dilantin
Vitamin E	Vitamins A, B complex, B_1 Inositol & Manganese (helps utilize E) Vitamin C (protects against oxidation) Unsaturated fatty acids, Selenium	Air pollution, antibiotics, chlorine, hypolipidemic drugs, inorganic iron, mineral oil, oral contraceptives, rancid fats & oils

215

NUTRIENT	MORE EFFECTIVE COMBINED WITH:	ANTAGONISTS TO ASSIMILATION
Unsaturated fatty acids	Vitamins A, C, D & Phosphorus Vitamin E (helps prevent oxidation & depletion)	
Vitamin K	no information available	Air pollution, antibiotics, anticoagulants, mineral oil, radiation, rancid fats & oils
Calcium	Vitamins A, C, & iron (aid in absorption) Vitamin D (helps reabsorb calcium in kidney tubules & helps retain & utilize calcium) Unsaturated fatty acids (helps make calcium available to tissues) Magnesium (2 parts calcium to 1 part magnesium) Boron, Manganese, Phosphorus, hydrochloric acid	Aspirin, corticosteroid drugs, thyroid hormone
Chlorine	No information available	
Chromium	No information available	
Cobalt	Copper, iron, zinc	
Copper	Cobalt, iron, zinc	
Fluorine	No information available	No information available
Iodine	No information available	
Iron	Folic acid, Calcium, Cobalt, Copper, Phosphorus B_{12} (helps Iron function in the body) Vitamin C (aids absorption) Hydrochloric acid (needed for assimilation of Iron)	Antacids, aspirin, EDTA (food preservative) Vitamin E
Magnesium	Vitamin B_6, C & D Calcium (1 part Magnesium to 2 parts Calcium) Phosphorus, Protein	Alcohol, Corticosteroid, diuretics
Manganese	B_1, Vitamin E, Calcium, Phosphorus	Antibiotics
Molybdenum	No information available	
Nickel	No information available	
Phosphorus	Vitamins A, D, unsaturated fatty acids, Iron, Manganese, Protein Calcium (1 part phosphorus to 2.5 parts calcium)	Alcohol, antacids, aspirin, corticosteroid drugs, diuretics, thyroid hormone

NUTRIENT	MORE EFFECTIVE COMBINED WITH:	ANTAGONISTS TO ASSIMILATION
Potassium	B_6, Sodium	Aspirin, corticosteroids, diuretics, sodium
Selenium	Vitamin E	
Silicon	No information available	
Sodium	Vitamin D	
Strontium	No information available	
Sulfur	B complex, B_1, Biotin, Pantothenic acid	
Tin	No information available	
Vanadium	No information available	
Zinc	Vitamins A, B_6, E, Calcium, Copper, Phosphorus	Alcohol, chelating compounds (remove excess copper), corticosteroid drugs, diuretics, oral contraceptives

References and further reading:

Abrams, Richard, Will It Hurt the Baby?, Addison, Wesley Pub. Co., Inc., New York, 1990.

Balch, J., & P. Balch, Prescription for Nutritional Healing, Avery Pub., Garden City, NY 1990.

Dunne, Lavon, Nutrition Almanac, McGraw-Hill Pub., New York, 1990.

McKenna, Joan, "Syphilis and AIDS," workshop, MANA conf., San Francisco, CA, Fall, 1993.

Nutrient Needs During Pregnancy

The table which follows this chapter covers the needs of both nonpregnant and pregnant women for most of the recognized nutrients. Before studying this table it is important to understand what these requirements are based upon. The National Research Council has come up with recommended daily allowances (RDA) of nutrients which are supposedly required to maintain "good" health. While an individual may need more or less nutrients than the amounts stated, the idea is that most will be adequately supplied by following the RDA. These allowances have replaced the old MDR (minimum daily requirement) standards, the minimum amount needed to avoid clinical disease. However, the RDA standard has many drawbacks as well. They are based on women between the ages of 18 and 35 who weigh 128 pounds, are 5' 4" tall, live in a temperate climate, and are moderately active and healthy. Many women do not fit into these categories. In addition, we are not interested in maintaining a minimal level of health as much as optimizing the health of both mother and baby. Therefore, these recommendations are to be considered as *baseline values only*, recognizing that almost all women will need more nutrients than this chart indicates. An increase in food intake will naturally increase the intake of all nutrients.

Also included is a column for nutrient amounts from a chart published in Prescription for Nutritional Healing, called the Optimum Daily Allowance (ODA) for nonpregnant people (no recommended quantities were given for pregnant women). These quantities need to be adjusted somewhat for height and weight, but will give you an idea of what natural health authorities consider closer to optimal intake. As you can see, some are considerably more than the RDA recommends, even during pregnancy.

Minerals and water soluble vitamins are usually measured in milligrams. Trace elements are given in micrograms (1000 micrograms = 1 milligram). Fat soluble vitamins are most often given in International Units (IU) or United States Pharmacopoeia (USP).

While every nutrient is important in maintaining a healthy pregnancy, some nutrients have been studied more thoroughly than others regarding their effect upon pregnancy. This attention to individual nutrients tends to be a "can't see the forest for the trees" approach, since a diet adequate in all nutrients would also not be deficient in any given nutrient. Not surprisingly, every nutrient thus far studied has been found to offer essential benefits to the health of pregnancy.

Protein: Proteins are made up of amino acids, of which there are approximately 29 commonly found varieties. Of these, eight are known as essential amino acids, which means they are not synthesized by our bodies but must come from outside food sources. These are: tryptophan, leucine, lysine, methionine, phenylalanine, isoleucine, valine, and threonine. At least 12 of the non-essential amino acids are produced within the body using available chemical substances.

Food products derived from animals such as meat, dairy and eggs contain these essential amino acids in the proper balance. Therefore ovo-lacto vegetarians, who eat eggs and dairy products, will generally obtain adequate supplies of all the amino acids from some of their food choices, and do not need to be concerned about how much of what amino acid they may be ingesting.

Vegetable foods also contain all the amino acids. However, few of them supply the essential amino acids in the exact proportions the human body needs and some do not contain one or more essential amino acids. One of the first books addressing the vegetarian diet, Diet for a Small Planet, (Francis Lappé, 1991) emphasized the importance of combining foods to ensure that the amino acids in vegetable protein sources complimented each other, making a balanced protein. For example, rice and beans are each high in the amino acids the other is low in or lacks; combining them in the same meal offers a complete protein complement like that found in animal products. You will note that this idea is supported in the food charts in this text which suggest combining various high protein vegetable foods to make a complete protein.

Protein quality is not such an issue if one is getting sufficient calories from a varied diet. It is estimated that when caloric intake is adequate, only 20% of the RDA needs to be complete protein; that is about 9 grams for an adult nonpregnant woman. For safety's sake, of the 80 to 100 grams of protein needed daily during pregnancy, we can assume that about 30% of that needs to be total protein, or about 30 grams a day (and maybe 60% with twins). The rest of the daily intake can come from incomplete protein sources.

In addition, the body has mechanisms for ensuring that its protein needs are met. As the caloric value of food goes up, so does the efficiency with which protein is utilized. If you are getting enough calories, the effective quality (biological value) of the protein you eat actually rises. Secondly, short term dietary deficiencies in the quality of proteins can be made up by drawing from a pool of amino acids within the small intestines, where about 80 to 90 grams of complete protein are supplied daily from the breakdown of cells in the normal course of metabolism. (Robertson, et al., 1986)

In pregnancy, calorie and protein requirements become greater, and the lack of sufficient quantities of either one has more serious immediate consequences. It therefore becomes more important to pay some attention to combining protein sources during pregnancy to be sure one is getting adequate proteins and calories. Increased calorie intake makes protein more available because protein is not being burned for energy needs. This is of critical importance, particularly in those who limit their food choices.

A healthy balance can be reached by the pregnant vegetarian, keeping in mind this understanding of how protein is used. The more varied her diet and the more animal products (such as dairy and eggs) she is willing to eat, the less she must worry about combining foods to achieve a complete protein balance. When the diet is limited, calorie needs become harder to meet and protein combining becomes more important, not only to meet protein needs but to ensure that the overall calorie intake is high enough to meet her energy needs as well. There are many vegan suggestions for balancing proteins in the food charts; here is an additional table showing which foods compliment each other:

Food	Deficient Essential Amino acids	Complimentary protein combinations	
Grains	Lsoleucine & Lysine	Rice + Legumes Corn + Legumes Wheat + Legumes Wheat + peanut + milk Wheat + sesame + soybean Rice + nutritional yeast	
Legumes	Tryptophan & Methionine	Legumes + rice Beans + wheat Beans + corn Soybeans + rice + wheat Soybeans + corn + milk Soybeans + wheat + sesame Soybeans + peanuts + sesame Soybeans + peanuts + wheat + rice Soybeans + sesame + wheat	
Nuts & seeds	Lsoleucine & Lysine	Peanuts + sesame + soybeans Sesame + beans Sesame + soybeans + wheat Peanuts + sunflower seeds	
Vegetables	Lsoleucine & methionine	Lima beans or Green beans or Brussels sprouts or Cauliflower or Broccoli	+ Sesame seeds or Brazil nuts or mushrooms
		Greens + millet or rice	

(Worthington, et. al., 1977)

How much protein is really needed? How much protein is needed by the pregnant woman? While focusing on good food choices, I know that many midwives do not emphasize protein and calories as this text suggests. There has been much talk in recent years about the fact that North Americans eat far too much protein. Many midwives wonder if this goes for pregnant women as well. While I would agree that many people eat more protein that they need, the nutrient needs of the pregnant woman are entirely unique. Because many of the special demands of tissue building can only be met with adequate protein, pregnant women are an exception to this rule. Midwives may also worry that women will have *huge* babies if they eat lots of protein. However, many midwives have only a vague idea of the connection between blood volume expansion, the development of toxemia and the physiological demands on the liver. Once you understand how all the related factors work together, you should feel comfortable with women eating good foods to appetite from the diet suggestions without rigidly adhering to a one-size-fits-all attitude regarding diet during pregnancy. (I practiced on that premise very successfully for years, and most of the babies I saw were between 7.5 and 9.5 pounds.) At the same time, you will be able to intelligently troubleshoot problems as they arise *because you know why they are occurring.* This is the crucial factor, one that isn't articulated in most other texts.

I agree that some women can have very healthy pregnancies and babies eating less than the 80 to 100 grams recommended. When the digestive system is functioning optimally and the protein intake is from high quality vegetable sources, a greater percentage will be biologically available than when a woman eats a predominately meat or processed foods diet. An organic diet will also provide more nutrients than one that is not organic, regardless of the protein sources. However, as the midwife, you must be constantly comparing fetal growth and well-being and the mother's sense of well-being as well as signs of blood volume expansion (detected by a dropping hemoglobin) with the dietary choices being made. If there is any doubt about the adequacy of the diet, protein and calories from whole foods are the first places to investigate, regardless of the type of diet being chosen.

For vegetarians who eat a very limited diet, getting all the necessary nutrients will be more difficult. Spirolina and Blue-green algae are both excellent sources of high quality protein which have many accompanying vitamins and minerals. Powdered forms should be used, since the woman will need to be taking a tablespoonful or more daily to supplement her dietary intake of protein.

Amino acid supplements: Although supplemental amino acids are available, taking an isolated amino acid in high doses is generally not advisable, with a few exceptions. Supplements containing L-Arginine, L-phenylalanine, DL-phenyla-lanine, or L-tryptophan should be avoided during pregnancy (Balch, 1990). L-lysine is frequently recommended in 500 mg. doses to minimize herpes outbreaks; there are no reported problems with this dosage whether or not pregnancy is a factor.

Calories: Adequate calorie intake is vital to a healthy pregnancy. Since calories are utilized solely for energy needs, their intake must be adequate to meet the extra metabolic demands of pregnancy. If calories are insufficient, the body will burn available protein for energy instead. When protein is burned due to a lack of sufficient calories, less amino acids will be available for fetal growth and development, for albumin production to expand the blood volume, and to help with uterine muscle growth. This relationship cannot be reversed—that is, if extra calories are ingested but protein needs are not met, the body cannot convert calories to protein in the same way. The pregnancy will suffer in this situation. Calorie needs must be adequate to meet a woman's activity and stress levels, to compensate for special situations such as multiple gestation, and to meet a woman's particular metabolic needs. If a woman is not obese and her ingested calories are just one-third less than she requires, half of her protein intake will be burned for energy. (Brewer, 1983) In addition, the increased need for other essential nutrients will go unmet if an insufficient quantity of food is eaten.

Doctors and midwives will often suggest a diet which provides plenty of protein (90 to 100 grams) but only 1,500 to 2,000 calories. Reasoning that the woman is eating a high protein diet, midwives may dismiss a woman's diet as a causative factor when she develops toxemia or premature labor. Quite often midwives will state that a woman was eating well but she became toxemic anyway. A woman can be making good food choices and still not be getting what she needs; women must eat enough calories *and* protein from nutrient-rich sources to meet their particular requirements.

Sodium: Sodium is a necessary component of a healthy diet and is essential to the proper maintenance of fluid balance within the body. In 1974 the American College of Obstetricians and Gynecologists stated that low sodium diets are not useful during pregnancy. This was after decades of obstetrical recommendation for severe salt restriction to limit weight gain and edema, in a misguided attempt to prevent toxemia. The facts are that the secondary symptoms of sodium deficiency are similar in many respects to the secondary symptoms of true toxemia.

Sodium works together with albumin to maintain normal circulating blood volume. Too little sodium can cause the body's fluid balance to be upset and lead to a decrease in blood volume after just two weeks of sodium restriction. This occurs because the imbalance allows fluid to seep into the spaces between the cells which surround the blood vessels, causing swelling.

In addition, a low sodium diet can lead to elevated blood pressure. The kidneys will begin to release the hormone renin as the blood volume becomes more and more reduced, which causes arterioles to constrict and thus raises the blood pressure. This is a protective mechanism normally activated when blood volume drops due to hemorrhage. When blood volume is reduced due to a lack of available amino acids from which the liver can make more albumin, or because fluid which should be in the circulation has leaked into the surrounding tissues, the body acts as though a hemorrhage has occurred. Sodium deficiency can also cause impaired kidney function, decreased urine volume and increased excretion of serum uric acid; all signs of more severe metabolic toxemia. Mothers and infants who have died due to toxemia show abnormal cellular changes in kidney tissue similar to the changes noted in cases of severe sodium depletion.

The pregnant woman requires additional sodium for a variety of uses: some goes to the baby, some to the amniotic fluid and some to expand the plasma volume. The increase in breast and uterine tissue requires additional sodium and some sodium is lost due to vomiting and increased sweating.

If a woman has a high sodium diet before pregnancy, her body will simply excrete less than usual in order to meet the increased demands of gestation. If she has been restricting her salt intake, however, she may not get enough to meet her needs. The rule of thumb is to salt foods to taste. If she is experiencing swelling or increased perspiration (for example she is working in her garden or it is a hot summer) she should *increase* her salt intake somewhat to make up for the additional loss of sodium but not so much that her food becomes unpalatable. If more table salt is unacceptable, she can take sodium tablets instead.

Be sure to discuss the role of sodium in the diet, because many women may have already been informed by misguided doctors, friends or relatives that they should restrict their salt intake. If a woman has been doing so for some time, her appetite for salt may be altered to the point that she does not recognize when she is craving salt. It is important to point this out and explain the physiology of why salt is so essential during pregnancy.

There is much confusion over the relationship between sodium and elevated blood pressure. The original studies which "proved" this connection noted a higher incidence of elevated blood pressure in regions where there was high salt consumption. Although such a study is not specific enough to prove that a relationship exists, it nevertheless was presented as such. Furthermore, table salt intake is not the same as sodium intake. Table salt is actually 40% chlorine. Naturally occurring sodium, which is found in foods and combined with other elements, does not seem to have any affect on the blood pressure. Only sodium combined with chlorine seems to affect blood pressure and then only in salt-sensitive persons. About half of those who have essential hypertension have been discovered to be salt sensitive. Risk factors include chronic renal disease, age over 50, family history of hypertension and being of African American descent. Studies "proving" a correlation between salt restriction and lowered blood pressure may actually be linking high blood pressure to junk foods in general. This is because a low salt diet often eliminates high fat foods such as chips, processed meats and bacon. (Seaver, 1992)

Fluids: If the blood volume is to expand, the body must have sufficient fluids on board to assist in this process. Encourage women to drink clear, uncarbonated liquids to thirst. It is important to ask about how much they typically drink during the day. Many North Americans are chronically dehydrated, especially women, who may have trained themselves to drink very little, often because of embarrassing childhood experiences regarding having to ask to go to the bathroom in school or similar circumstances. Encourage women to drink freely. To help with this, she could fill a 2 quart container and see how much is left by the end of the day. Adequate fluid intake supports the maintenance of amniotic fluid volume and helps the kidneys and liver will work more efficiently as well. However, overhydration is equally problematic. Too much fluid can cause an undesirable diuretic effect and excessively dilute blood components. Additionally, overhydration can cause lab values to be skewed, confusing the clinical picture when a problem is suspected.

B$_{12}$: B$_{12}$ deficiency is associated with megaloblastic anemia (see <u>Diagnostic Tests</u> for a full discussion). Women who restrict their intake of meat or dairy products are at high risk for being B$_{12}$ deficient. Any woman choosing such a diet should strongly consider taking a supplement containing B$_{12}$. Single doses of 5 micrograms result in a 70% absorption rate. The amount actually absorbed is lowered as the intestinal content of B$_{12}$ increases; therefore recommend that women take 3 to 5 micrograms not more than two or three times weekly. (Dunne, 1990)

B$_6$: B$_6$ is essential for the utilization of carbohydrates. When it is lacking, an amino acid is converted into a harmful substance with binds to insulin, rendering the insulin useless and impairing the body's use of glucose. B$_6$ also helps the body release glycogen, which is stored glucose.

B$_6$ deficiencies interfere with protein use in a number of ways: hydrochloric acid production is decreased, which in turn decreases protein absorption. Protein is burned for energy needs and causes that which is absorbed to be used improperly. Lack of B$_6$ can therefore contribute to the development of toxemia. Deficiencies can also lead to some of the symptoms of toxemia such as edema, headaches, abnormal brain wave patterns and convulsions. Since B$_6$ is required for the conversion of amino acids into neurotransmitters which regulate moods and brain chemistry, a deficiency can affect a woman's emotional outlook. B$_6$ deficiency interferes with the sodium/potassium balance in the body, which helps regulate how fluids are used in the system. B$_6$ supplementation of edemic women can bring swelling down, probably due to the two-fold effect of helping them utilize protein better as well as regulating tissue fluids.

Women who supplement any B vitamins must be aware that taking an isolated B vitamin can create deficiencies in the rest: therefore a balanced B-complex supplement should be chosen, with an additional tablet of the isolated vitamin to be taken for a limited period of time (no more than 2 to 3 weeks). During that time, she can increase her intake of foods rich in the vitamin she needs, and begin to taper off the extra supplement. Foods high in B$_6$ include:

Rice bran	Tuna	Prune juice
Beef liver	Salmon	Dark turkey meat
Sesame seeds	Coconut	Acorn squash
Chickpeas	Dry sunflower seeds	Raisins
Wheat bran	All-bran cereal	Spinach
Baked potato w/skin	Wheat germ	Amaranth
Banana	Avocado	Brewer's yeast
Rye flour (dark)	Filberts	Plantain
Mussels (raw)	Chicken livers	Refried beans
Mackerel	Beef round steak (lean)	Corn flour

Folic acid: Folic acid acts as a coenzyme in DNA synthesis, making it important for healthy cell division and replication. It also plays a vital role in protein metabolism and neurological development. Folic acid significantly reduces the risk of neural tube defects. (Summers & Price, 1993)

Calcium: Calcium is the most abundant mineral in the body and has many important functions. It strengthens bones and teeth, helps transmit nerve impulses, is essential to normal blood clotting, maintains parathyroid function, balances the blood pH, and protects against the effects of lead and carcinogens. Normally, 99% of the calcium is stored in the bones and teeth with the rest in the blood stream and the cells. If blood levels of ionized calcium fall below normal, symptoms such as tetany, convulsions, cardiac and respiratory failure and coma can result. Calcium is moved from the blood to the bones and back again under a complex hormonal system which responds to calcium levels in the body.

During pregnancy, parathyroid hormone levels tend to rise, causing more calcium to be removed from the bones, decreasing the loss of calcium from the kidneys and increasing its absorption from the gastrointestinal tract. Absorption of calcium increases in the small intestines, starting early in pregnancy. Calcium absorption has doubled by the beginning of the third trimester and remains elevated postpartum when the woman is lactating. Calcium is progressively retained throughout pregnancy, and maternal bones utilize what the fetus does not. There is therefore no great change in the mineral content of maternal bones during pregnancy. However, bone content can diminish during breastfeeding if calcium and phosphorus intake is inadequate. Bone mass lost during lactation is recovered after weaning. At least three studies correlate breastfeeding with ultimately higher maternal bone mass (Mothering, 1995). Over the last 3 months of pregnancy, the mother supplies about 25 g of calcium to be laid down in the fetal bones; this is about 20 mml of calcium daily. The diet must provide 1.2 to 1.5 grams of calcium daily to meet this demand. (Gleicher, 1985) The most assimilable form is calcium citrate maleate, although the citrate and carbonate forms work well for some women. It can be taken together with magnesium in a citrate, tartrate, aspartate or glycinate form (which is the only one that doesn't cause loose stools).

Iron: Much has been made about the need for iron in pregnancy. While adequate iron intake is certainly important, some of this concern arose out of the misinterpretation of the hemoglobin drop which normally accompanies blood volume expansion. Iron deficiency is discussed in depth in <u>Diagnostic Tests</u>. Be sure to review that information. Any iron supplement which you recommend should be easily utilized, which means never prescribe ferrous sulfate. In this form it causes constipation and is hard on the liver. Other forms such as ferrous citrate or ferrous gluconate are much better choices.

References and further reading:

Abrams, Richard, Will It Hurt the Baby?, Addison, Wesley Pub. Co., Inc., New York, 1990.

Balch, J., & P. Balch, Prescription for Nutritional Healing, Avery Pub., Garden City, NY 1990.

Dunne, Lavon, Nutrition Almanac, McGraw-Hill Pub., New York, 1990.

Gleicher, N. Principles of Medical Therapy in Pregnancy, Plenum Pub., NY, 1985, p. 1028.

Mothering, Good News: Lucid Breastfeeding, Vol. 74, Spring 1995, p. 31, cited from New Beginnings, July/Aug. 1994, pp. 110-111.

Robertson, L., et. al., The New Laurel's Kitchen, Ten Speed Press, Berkeley CA, 1986, pp. 335-460.

Seaver, Althea, "Feeling Fine" Avoiding Some Common Discomforts of Pregnancy," Midwifery Today, No. 21, Spring, 1992, pp.22-4.

op. cit., "Nutrition for Two: Sodium in Pregnancy," Midwifery Today, Winter 1991-2, No. 20, pp. 22-4.

op. cit., handout, Nutrition in Pregnancy workshop, Midwifery Today conf., Eugene, OR, 1992.

Summers, Lisa, Price, R., "Preconception Care: An Opportunity to Maximize Health in Pregnancy," J. of Nurse-Midwifery, Vol. 38, No. 4, July/Aug. 1993, pp. 188-198.

Worthington, Bonnie, et. al., Nutrition in Pregnancy and Lactation, C.V. Mosby Co., St. Louis, MO, 1977.

NUTRIENT	ODA	AMOUNT (RDA)		REASONS FOR INCREASED NEED
		NONPREGNANT	PREGNANT	
Protein	25-30 gm. (170 lb. ♂)	44 gm.	80-100 gm.^	Rapid fetal & placental growth; amniotic fluid, uterine & breast growth; increased maternal blood volume; storage for labor & birth
Calories	--	1800	2600-3000^^	Increased maternal metabolism & energy needs; protein sparing
Carbohydrates	--	300 grams	*	Vitamins and energy needs
Fats	--	66 grams	*	Fat soluble vitamins and energy needs
Vitamin A	10,000 IU	4000 IU	5000 IU	Cell development & tissue growth; tooth formation; bone growth
Vitamin D	400 IU	200 IU	400 IU	Helps absorb calcium & phosphorus; mineralization of fetal bone & tooth buds
Vitamin E	600 IU	8 IU	10 IU	Tissue growth; cell wall integrity; red blood cell integrity
Vitamin C	3,000 mg.	60 mg.	80 mg.	Tissue formation; health of connective & vascular tissue; increases iron absorption
Bioflavonoids	500 mg.	--	--	Work with Vitamin C to promote blood vessel & tissue health; build strong amniotic membranes; have an antibacterial effect
Folic acid	400 mcg.	400 mcg.	1 - 2 mg.	Increased metabolic demand in pregnancy, prevention of megaloblastic anemia, increased heme production & cell nucleus material
Niacin	100 mg.	13 mg.	15 mg.	Coenzyme in energy & protein metabolism
Riboflavin	50 mg.	1.2 mg.	1.5 mg.	Coenzyme in energy & protein metabolism
Thiamine	50 mg.	1.0 mg.	1.4 mg.	Coenzyme for energy metabolism
B₆	50 mg.	2.0 mg.	2.6 mg.	Coenzyme in protein metabolism, increased fetal growth requirement
B₁₂	300 mcg.	3.0 mcg.	4.0 mcg.	Coenzyme in protein metabolism, especially vital cells proteins & formation of red cells
Biotin	300 mcg.	100-200 mcg.***	same	
Choline	100 mg.	500-900 mg.**	same	
Inositol	100 mg.	1 gram**	same	
PABA	25 mg.	no RDA	no RDA	
Pantothenic acid	100 mg.	4-7 mg.***	4-7 mg.	
Vitamin K	100 mcg.	70-140 mcg.***	same	
Calcium	1,500 mg.	800 mg.	1200 mg.	Fetal bone formation; increased maternal calcium metabolism

NUTRIENT	ODA	AMOUNT (RDA)		REASONS FOR INCREASED NEED
		NONPREGNANT	PREGNANT	
Phosphorus	--	800 mg.	1200 mg.	Fetal bone and tooth formation; increased maternal phosphorus metabolism
Iron	10 mg.	10 mg.	18+ mg.	Increased maternal red cell volume; fetal iron storage; blood loss postpartum
Iodine	225 mcg.	150 mcg.	175 mcg.	Increased metabolism; increased thyroxine production
Magnesium	750 mg.	300 mg.	450 mg.	Coenzyme in energy & protein metabolism, enzyme activator, tissue growth, cell metabolism, muscle action
Potassium	99 mg.	1875-5675 mg.***	same	
Sodium	--	1100-3300 mg.***	to taste	Increases water retention, which is needed to promote expanded blood volume
Chromium	150 mcg.	.05-.2 mcg.***	same	
Copper	3 mg.	2-3 mg.***	same	
Fluoride	--	1.5-4 mg.♦	same	
Manganese	2 mg.	2.5-5 mg.***	same	
Molybdenum	30 mcg.	.15-.5 mg.***	same	
Selenium	200 mcg.	.05-.2 mg.***	same	
Zinc	30 mg.	15 mg.	25 mg.	Increased tissue growth

^The RDA requirements are +30 grams above nonpregnant levels, which is not enough for most women

^^The RDA requirements are +300 over nonpregnant levels, which is not enough for most women

*No increased requirement set, but it is necessary to increase intake of fats and carbohydrates to meet the extra calorie needs of pregnancy

**No requirement set, this is the average daily intake

***Adequate daily intake, no standards have been set

♦There is controversy over the need for fluoride in the diet at all (see chapter on Fluoride, this section)

-- No recommendations were given

228

Dietary Counseling for Pregnancy:
Helping Women Get the Foods They Need

NOTE: Read the chapter on the How Pregnancy Impacts Maternal Anatomy and Physiology in the Anatomy and Physiology Section before studying this chapter.

With the background just reviewed regarding nutrients and their sources, we are still left with real women who want to know what they need to eat during pregnancy. Food choices are influenced by many things; a woman's dietary history (i.e., what she grew up eating), her personal food preferences, her ability and desire to cook and prepare foods, the preparation time she has available, the kitchen equipment available to her, what the rest of her family prefers to eat, and how much money she has to spend on foods. Cultural influences play a role in what and how much women eat as well. With our cultural hatred of fat, many women have trained themselves to not eat very much and to ignore their hunger. This must be kept in mind when talking to women about adequate dietary intake. Food choices are also influenced by emotional factors such as what a person grew up eating, and familiarity of tastes and preparation methods. Especially during pregnancy, "comfort foods" from childhood can play a big role in what a woman will choose to eat, and dietary counseling should steer her to the more nutritious varieties of foods she likes.

Finances can play a role in dietary choices. Fortunately the foods that are more packaged, processed and stripped of nutrients are usually more expensive as well. Therefore with some coaching and the willingness to eat an optimally healthy diet, most women can afford to get what they need regardless of their economic status.

Remember that many people will tell you they have a good diet as long as they have food on the table three times a day. You must therefore probe further for the specifics of their diet. A review of the different variations of three basic kinds of diets; omnivorous, ovo-lacto vegetarian and vegan, will lead us into the nuts and bolts of dietary counseling.

Omnivorous diet: This is the broadest type of diet, meaning that a person eats some of a wide variety of foods: meats, poultry, fish, dairy products, eggs, vegetables, legumes, nuts, seeds, fruits and grains. It provides the widest choice of foods to meet the increased protein and calorie needs of pregnancy. Meat and dairy products provide concentrated sources of protein, and therefore omnivores need to eat less food to meet their protein and calorie needs than those on a more restricted diet.

Unfortunately, many people who "eat everything" will literally eat just about anything, and they often have not thought about the nutritional aspects of their food choices. This does not apply to everyone, of course, and an omnivorous diet can be an extremely good one. Commercially processed meats and dairy products contain many chemicals, concentrated pesticides and antibiotics given the animals because they are kept in unhealthy conditions; therefore, eating organic meats can reduce the intake of these substances and will be less stressful for the body to process. Again, make sure food choices are as unprocessed as possible and prepared to retain the maximum amounts of nutrients.

Ovo-lacto Vegetarian: This diet includes eggs (ovo) and dairy (lacto) products as well as all fruits, vegetables, legumes, nuts, seeds and grains. It technically eliminates fish, red meats and poultry from the diet, although some people call themselves vegetarian and still eat fish or poultry on occasion. Always ask women to define exactly what they mean when they describe their dietary choices. While this diet limits a woman's choices for protein rich foods to a certain extent, it is quite possible for an ovo-lacto vegetarian to have a perfectly healthy pregnancy.

Vegan: This diet includes all vegetables, nuts, seeds, grains and fruits but eliminates meats, eggs, and dairy products. Although it is possible to have a healthy pregnancy as a vegan, a mother's choices for protein and calorie rich foods are even more limited. In addition, this diet is high in fiber, which tends to fill the woman up quickly. This means she must be willing to eat those foods which contain the protein she needs (such as nuts, seeds and soy products). Women on a vegan diet may find themselves suddenly craving meats or dairy foods which they have not eaten for years. This indicates a need for more protein. A woman is often willing to expand her diet to include some dairy products or fish during her pregnancy. The more a woman is willing to expand her dietary choices the easier it will be for her to get what she needs without getting bored with those things she can eat. Encourage women to drink fortified soy milk (such as Westsoy Plus) which brings the levels of calcium, Vitamins A and D and riboflavin up to the equivalent of whole milk.

Fruitarian: This variation of the vegan diet includes fruits, nuts, seeds and, in some cases, raw vegetables with very few, if any, cooked foods or grains. It is extremely difficult to support a healthy pregnancy on a fruitarian diet, primarily because it lacks many food sources of complex carbohydrates and a variety of foods high in calories and protein. Encourage such women to expand their diets as much as they are willing. They must be scrupulously careful about getting enough protein and calories every day, because fruitarian women will have little or no reserve body fat to carry them through a period of inadequate dietary intake. Spirolina and Blue green algae are particularly helpful sources of protein and minerals for these women, if they will eat them!

Macrobiotic: Macrobiotics is based on the oriental concept of yin (passive, female) and yang (active, male). Foods such as fruits, sugar and liquids are very yin while meats, dense foods such as root vegetables and salts are more yang. Brown rice and other grains fall between these two extremes and are considered very balanced. This Japanese diet is a variation on the vegan approach, but it allows eating fish in small quantities.

There is an emphasis on eating foods grown within a 200 mile radius of the home to ensure that foods are appropriate to the climate in which one lives. Tropical fruits are not desirable outside of a tropical environment. The diet ideally varies with the seasons, with macrobiotics eating young plants in the spring, salads, fruits, and desserts in the summer, squash, kale and winter root vegetables in the fall and winter. Pressure cooking, baking, steaming, boiling, and pickling are preferred food preparation styles, with a minimum of raw or chilled foods. Miso and certain soy products are used extensively.

In keeping with these considerations, the ideal macrobiotic diet consists of 50 to 60% grains (with brown rice being the main grain), 5% soup, 25 to 30% vegetables, 5 to 10% beans and sea vegetables plus other foods. Generally speaking, red meat, pork, many fruits, dairy products, strong spices, plants from the Nightshade family (potatoes, tomatoes and eggplant), and eggs are avoided altogether. Acceptable fruits (for the climate), fats, sweets and liquids are taken in strict moderation. However, even with these restrictions, macrobiotic diets can consist of a wide variety of foods.

People who are themselves well-balanced in their choice to eat macrobiotically are usually quite willing to expand the variety in their diet, listening to their bodies about what they need rather than to a book. Encourage women to eat widely (i.e. from a variety of foods) and to eat what they feel they need during pregnancy, even if this means including some foods they would ordinarily not choose to eat.

Some macrobiotic communities feel that small babies are "better." This is largely due to a misinterpretation of macrobiotic philosophy with the underlying assumption that "yang is better," and yang is more compact than yin, which is expansive. The son of Michio Kushi—the founder of macrobiotic principles in the United States had never heard of this notion when I had the opportunity to work with his family! It was his understanding that, while huge babies (11 pounders and up) are considered large by macrobiotic standards, 7, 8 and even 9 pound babies are not considered too big. Also, many macrobiotics drink minimal amounts of water, so it is important to discuss fluid intake in detail.

Outlining a basic diet for pregnancy:

The basic diet for pregnancy should include the foods presented in the following tables or their equivalents daily. Simply put, this diet requires the daily intake of:

1 quart of milk per fetus (or the equivalent)
2 eggs a day (or the equivalent)
2 other servings of protein-rich foods
2 servings of green vegetables
5 servings of grain products
3 pats of butter
1 iron rich food weekly (for omnivores, others may need more)
5 Yellow or orange vegetables weekly
3 Baked potatoes weekly

It is important to tell a woman out loud that she should eat good foods from the suggested lists to appetite, drink to thirst and salt to taste. Well meaning friends or relatives may have given her inaccurate advice (such as to restrict her salt intake); therefore, it is imperative that you make sure she understands exactly how she needs to eat and why. In addition, you cannot assume that just because a woman has seen another care provider she has been given any advice on appropriate dietary choices for pregnancy. This is particularly true if she has seen a mainstream obstetrician.

The basic diet outlined above must be varied to meet the needs of different types of diets. Gail Brewer refined this concept considerably in her book The Brewer Medical Diet for Normal and High Risk Pregnancy. The following tables have been consolidated and somewhat modified, but are based on those found in her excellent book (now out of print).

Personalizing the diet plan: What each woman actually needs to eat to have a healthy pregnancy and baby varies considerably. To individualize a diet plan, you must take the following things into account: dietary type (omnivore, etc.), number of fetuses, activity level, stress level, pre-pregnancy weight, metabolic rate and complications in previous pregnancies. The following guide can be used as a rough indication of how a woman should adjust her diet to meet her specific needs throughout her pregnancy:

PHYSICAL FACTOR	DAILY CALORIES	DAILY PROTEIN
Baseline nonpregnant requirement	2000	46 g.
Preconception	Increase to 2250	Increase to 56-70 g.
>20 weeks pregnancy	Increase to 2600-2750	Increase to 80-100 g.
Poor nutrition/low wt. beginning of preg.	+500 calories to basic diet	+20 g. to basic diet
Less than 16 years of age	+200 to basic diet	+20 g. to basic diet
Activity/Stress factors	+220 per factor	+20 g. per factor
Multiple gestation	+500 per extra fetus	+30 g. per extra fetus

In addition, how accustomed a woman is to eating a whole foods diet, how well her body absorbs nutrients, and how well her digestive system works overall will influence how much food she needs to eat in order to maintain her well-being. When confronted with the food tables given in this chapter, most women are shocked at the amount of food they are expected to consume. Many women who are still early in their pregnancy declare that they are not this hungry. A gradual increase in appetite will coincide with the gradual increase in maternal blood volume and fetal growth.

Activity level: The following chart can help you figure out how to gauge a woman's activity level and the corresponding nutrient requirements.

HOW OFTEN DOES SHE:	DAILY	WEEKLY	SELDOM
Walk 3 miles in 1 hour or less			
Do 1 hour of yoga			
Swim laps for ½ hour			
Ride a bike at 10 mph for 45 minutes			
Aerobic dance or calisthenics for 1 hour			
Garden work for 1 hour			
Vigorous sex for 40 minutes			
Run 2 miles in 20 min. or less			
Iron clothes for 1 hour			
Ski downhill or X-country 20 minutes (minus lift time)			
Wash and polish car for 1 hour			
Play ½ hour of tennis singles or 45 minutes of doubles			
Wash windows for 1 hour			
Work on a factory assembly line for 1 hour			
Wait tables 1 hour			
Play handball for 20 minutes			
Chop wood for 30 minutes			
Type for 2 hours			
Skip rope for 20 minutes			
Stand for 1½ hours (shopping or at work)			
Walk 1 mile in 30 min. or less with a 20-pd. child in a backpack			

Each of the activities listed burns about 200 calories. If there are five or more checks in the daily column, the woman is very active and may need extra calories in order to meet the demands of her life-style. If she engages in one or more activities for longer than the time period given, she should mark a check for each time period. For example, an employee who stands for 6 hours daily at work would have four checks in the daily column, accounting for 800 calories right there. It is easy to see how an active woman can easily fall behind on her calorie requirements. To the basic diet, add 220 calories and 20 grams of protein for each regular activity. (Brewer, 1983)

Stress level: Stressful situations add to a woman's overall calorie and nutrient requirements. For each relevant factor, add 220 calories and 20 grams of protein to the basic diet. Stress factors that can be identified include:

Divorce in process	Worry about parenting
Moving	Lack of a personal support community
Working two jobs (or one very demanding	(no friends or family nearby)
job)	Substance abuse or recovery
Relationship problems	Feeling unsafe (living in a dangerous
Difficulties with children	neighborhood, etc.)
Ill parent or close relative	Abusive relationships
Financial difficulties	Worries about other aspects of life
Lack of sufficient sleep	Loss of a relationship during pregnancy
Skipping meals	Facing other difficult situations
Worries and fear about pregnancy/birth	Closely spaced pregnancies
Breastfeeding	

Pre-pregnancy weight considerations: For nutritional considerations, a woman's pre-pregnancy weight is most significant if she was underweight when she conceived. Underweight women have no fat reserves to carry them through bouts of nausea or illness when their calorie intake may fall off. Women with extra pounds are not placing themselves at greater risk for problems, as long as they eat a good diet during pregnancy. In fact some women-of-size will gain little weight and a few may actually lose a few pounds. Weight loss should never be a goal during pregnancy, although increasing the activity level is a fine idea. (Brewer, 1983) (See the next chapter as well as the chapter on Working with Women-of-Size in the Special Circumstances section.)

Metabolic rate: Finally you must consider a woman's metabolic rate and how that impacts her nutritional needs. Metabolism may be simply defined as how fast a woman burns the food she eats. Talk to the woman about how she eats and look at her body type to get an idea how her metabolism works outside of pregnancy. If she has a tendency to gain weight regardless of how moderate her dietary intake, and has trouble losing weight even if she increases her activity level, her metabolism is slow. If she burns up her food quickly and is slim whether she is very active or not, then she has a faster metabolism. It is often the case that women with faster metabolisms are naturally more active. The faster the metabolism outside of pregnancy, the more difficult it will be to meet her needs for calories during pregnancy, because her metabolism rate will rise even more. In some cases it may be necessary for her to curtail some of her activities in order to spare calories (for example walking one mile daily rather than her usual five).

Past pregnancy complications: During your initial history interview, you will uncover the details of any past pregnancy complications. While not all complications are nutritionally related, many of them are; these are listed in the chapter on How Pregnancy Impacts Maternal Anatomy and Physiology. Most women will be unable to reconstruct what they ate in a previous pregnancy but will recall whether they were told to restrict weight gain or dietary intake or even if they were given appetite suppressants to curtail weight gain. They will remember nausea, feeling hungry, and being scolded for gaining too much. Remember too, that often women are treated for toxemia when, in fact, their secondary symptoms are benign and their blood volume is adequately expanded (demonstrated by a full term baby of good weight).

Correcting the damage done by low salt diets: If a woman comes to you for care who has been placed on a salt restricted diet by her previous care provider it is important that she make up for this serious nutritional lack as soon as possible. In Europe, many doctors still prescribe low salt diets. Therefore, the Pre-Eclamptic Toxemia Society (PETS) in Germany has devised a remedial regime for such women: Mix ½ Tbsp. of salt into 1 liter of mineral water. Drink this within two hours and eat well, including plenty of protein, green vegetables, and whole grains. Incorporate another ½ tablespoon of salt into this dietary intake. Diuresis will increase considerably and headaches should start to subside within a few hours of beginning this program. After this initial dose of salt, the woman should continue to add salt to her drinking water and liberally to her foods and follow the dietary recommendations in this chapter. If she finds eating salt in this quantity distasteful, salt tablets can be obtained at a drug store and will accomplish the same thing. Once edema and other symptoms have resolved, she can continue to eat well and salt her food to taste. (James, 1989)

Determining if a woman is hypertensive due to chloride-sensitivity: If you or a client is concerned that her hypertensive tendencies may be related to sensitivity to the chloride in table salt, the test described above can also be used to detect whether this is so. Have the woman mix ½ to 1 Tbsp. of table salt in one liter of mineral water and drink it within a short time. Any rise in blood pressure three to four hours afterwards is probably due to chloride sensitivity. If so, the blood pressure should fall again following six hours of no additional intake of table salt. While I do not recommend going in a low salt diet per se, the woman can try avoiding adding salt to her foods at the table and get the extra sodium she needs from natural sources. Sea weeds, seafoods, celery and dairy products are all good sources of natural sodium. (Kuse, Midwifery Today Conf workshop, 1997)

Working with the food lists

Taking all this into account, the food lists on the following pages may be presented and discussed with each woman. These lists simplify the task of making sure calorie and protein intake is adequate; the portions take into account all the other nutrients as well. Women should be encouraged to choose different foods in each group from day to day to vary their nutrient intake; the wider the dietary food choices, the better. While most women will not eat exactly the recommended amounts of food every day, the goal is to strive to follow the diet plan as closely as possible and to choose foods of high nutritional value. This means eliminating empty calories and junk foods which tend to cause undesirable difficult-to-lose weight and provide nothing in the way of nourishment but calories. It is far better to get calories from nutrient-rich foods.

You will note that the foods in different groups often overlap, which means that many of the foods given as sources of a particular nutrient are also quite high in other nutrients. Therefore you will note some repetition from table to table. However, in order for the diet to be adequate, women must eat the portions as stated in the following tables. They cannot use one portion of food which appears in two tables to count for portions from two different categories. For example, count ¼ cup of cottage cheese as either a meat substitute or a dairy choice, not both. The more narrowly a woman eats (that is, the less variety she has in the choices she makes), the more important this becomes, because getting adequate calories and protein becomes increasingly more difficult when the dietary choices are limited.

Specific questions may arise concerning cholesterol, extra protein, more calories, and sodium from women concerned about the possible health risks. The protein, calorie and sodium questions are answered in the chapter on Nutrition in Pregnancy in this section. The cholesterol question is addressed in a special chapter in Diagnostic Tests.

Each woman is an individual; with an idea of what you mean by "eat a lot," and a reminder list of the wide variety of foods available, each woman will usually find a dietary balance that is right for her, as long as she is not restricting intake or weight gain. With your firm understanding of the relationship between her intake and the physiological demands of pregnancy, you will be able to troubleshoot any problems as they arise by ordering laboratory tests when indicated and by offering appropriate dietary advice.

Food choices to be made from each of the food lists which follow:	Daily portions for different diets		
	Omnivore	Ovo-Lacto	Vegan
Milk products & milk substitutes	4	4	4
Calcium replacements	as needed	same	same
Eggs	2	2	omit
Meats, seafood or vegetarian protein sources	6	6	8
Dark green vegetables	2	2	2
Grains, starchy vegetables & fruits	5	5	5
Vitamin C foods	2	3	4
Fats & oils	3	5	9
Vitamin A foods	1	2½	4
Liver or other iron rich foods	4 oz. 1 X wkly	5 daily*	5 daily*
Vitamin & mineral supplements	as needed	as needed	as needed
Salt and other sodium sources	to taste	to taste	to taste
Water	to thirst	to thirst	to thirst
Multiple gestations require 30 grams of protein & 500 calories per extra fetus in addition to the basic daily diet above	+4 Milk or milk substitute choices or +2 Meat, seafood or vegetarian protein sources per extra baby		

*See box for iron sources for those who don't eat liver

Milk products & substitutes (8 grams protein each)
For each low-fat choice, add 1 or 2 extra fat & oil portions
For each unfortified soy choice, select 2 from calcium sources
Every 3 unfortified soy choices, +1 portion from Vit. A foods

Food	Portion
Cow's milk:	
Buttermilk from whole milk	1 cup (8 oz.)
Evaporated, whole reconstituted	1 cup
Evaporated whole, from can	½ cup
Nonfat, dry, powdered	1/3 cup
Nonfat, reconstituted	1 cup
Skim	1 cup
2% fat	1 cup
Whole	1 cup
Yogurt	1 cup
Ice milk	1 cup
Ice cream (all natural)	1 cup
Goat's milk	1 1/8 cup
Cheese:	
Cheddar, Swiss, Muenster, Jack, feta, etc. (not cream)	1¼ oz.
Cottage or ricotta	¼ cup
Parmesan or Romano, grated	3 tbsp.
Trios Cheese Tortellini (12 g.)	2½ oz.
Soy Products:	
Soy milk, whole, fluid (check brand)	9 oz.
Soybean curd (tofu)	4 oz.
Soy cheese (except cream cheese)	1 1/3 oz.

Ovo-Lacto Vegetarian Food Sources of Protein (7 grams each or as noted) Vegans may add ½ cup fortified soy milk to each item to make 10.5 grams of complete protein (meets 1½ portions of protein choices)			
Food (grams protein if > 7 g.)	**Portion**	**Food**	**Portion**
Legumes, cooked:		**Shelled Nuts & seeds:**	
Black beans	½ cup	Almonds	2 oz.
Chick peas (garbanzos)	½ cup	Brazil nuts	2 oz.
Red, white, pinto beans	½ cup	Cashews	1½ oz.
Cowpeas (black-eyed peas)	½ cup	Chestnuts	4 oz.
Fava beans (broad beans)	½ cup	Filberts	2 oz.
Kidney beans (red, white)	½ cup	Hickory nuts	2 oz.
Lima beans, mature	½ cup	Peanuts, roasted	¼ cup
Split peas	½ cup	Peanut butter	2 tbsp.
Mung beans	½ cup	Pecans	3 oz.
Turtle beans	½ cup	Pignolias	2 Tbsp.
Lentils	1/3 cup	Pistachios	1½ oz.
Soybeans	1/3 cup	Pumpkin seeds	1 oz.
Soybean curd/tofu (firm 10 g.)	3½ oz.	Sesame seeds	¼ cup
Grains:		Sunflower seeds	3 Tbsp.
Amaranth flour (8 g.)	2 oz.	Walnuts, Black	1 oz.
Barley	1/3 cup, dry	Walnuts, English	2 oz.
Bread, whole wheat or rye	3 slices	**Vegetables:**	
Buckwheat flour, dark	2/3 cup	Artichoke, cleaned	7 oz.
Bulgur	1/3 cup, dry	Asparagus, cleaned	7 oz.
Couscous	1/3 cup, dry	Brussel sprouts	5 oz.
Cornmeal	3/4 cup	Broccoli	2 cups
Egg noodles, cooked	1 cup	Cauliflower	7 oz.
Gluten flour	¼ cup	Collard greens, cooked	6 oz.
Millet	1/3 cup, dry	Corn, fresh or frozen	2 ears
Oatmeal	2/3 cup, dry	Kale, cooked	6 oz.
Pasta, durum wheat, cooked	1¼ cup	Lima beans, baby	3 oz.
Pasta, high protein, cooked	2/3 cup	Mung bean sprouts	6 oz.
Rice, all types	½ cup, dry	Mushrooms, cleaned	7 oz.
Rye flour	½ cup	Mustard greens, cooked	7 oz.
Seitan (prepared wheat gluten meat)	2 oz.	Peas, green	4 oz.
Spelt flour	5 oz.	Potatoes, whole	2 large
Triticale flour	½ cup	Soy bean sprouts	4 oz.
Wheat bran	3/4 cup	Spinach, cleaned	7 oz.
Wheat germ	¼ cup	Turnip greens, cooked	7 oz.
Whole wheat flour	½ cup	Yams, whole	2
Tempeh:			
Lightlife Corn/Jalapena Tempeh (17 g.)	4 oz.		
3 Grain Tempeh (12 g.)	4 oz.		

238

Prepared Meat Alternatives (This is a representative sample of these foods; for those not listed read labels)

Brand name & product	Protein (grams)	Portion
Breakfast meat alternatives:		
Lightlife Fakin Baken	13 g.	3 strips
Loma Linda Little Links (cnd)	8 g.	2 links
Morningstar Farms Strips	3.2 g.	3 strips
Morningstar Farms Links	14.5 g.	3 links
Morningstar Farms Patties	18.2 g.	2 patties
sausage, simulated meat product	4.6 g.	1 link
sausage simulated meat product	7 g.	1 patty
Soy Boy Soysage	7 g.	2 oz.
Worthington Stripples	4.2 g.	4 strips
Hotdog alternatives:		
Tofu Pups hotdogs	9.3 g.	1 link
Lean Links	5 g.	1 link
Loma Linda Big Franks (canned)	10 g.	1 link
Loma Linda Corn Dogs (frzn)	7 g.	1 corn dog
Loma Linda Sizzle Franks (cnd)	10 g.	2 franks
SmartDogs	20 g.	1 link
Soy Boy Not Dogs	6 g.	1 link
White Wave Healthy Franks	7 g.	1 link
Worthington Veja-links	8.2 g.	2 links
Yves Veggie Chili Dogs	11 g.	1 link
Fish & seafood alternatives:		
Loma Linda Ocean Fillet (frzn)	11 g.	1 fillet
Loma Linda Ocean Platter (dry)	8 g.	¼ cup
Loma Linda Vege-Scallops	14 g.	6 pieces
Worthington Veg Scallops	16.9 g.	½ cup
Mixes:		
Arrowhead Mills Seitan	22 g.	¼ dry/2.5 oz. mixed

Brand name & product	Protein (Grams)	Portion
Stew alternatives:		
Lightlife Sloppy Joe (tempeh)	8.7 g.	4 ⅓ oz.
Lightlife Chia's Chilie	8.7 g.	4 ⅓ oz.
Loma Linda Stew Pac (cnd)	10 g.	2 oz.
Burgers, steaks & patties:		
Lightlife Lemon Grill Tempeh	9.7 g.	1 patty
Lightlife American Grill Tempeh	12.5 g.	1 patty
Loma Linda Chik-Patties (frzn)	14 g.	1 patty
Loma Linda Sizzle Burger (frzn)	15 g.	1 burger
Loma Linda Swiss Steak w/Gravy	9 g.	1 steak
Loma Linda Patty Mix	9 g.	¼ cup
Loma Linda Redi-Burger (cnd)	14 g.	½" slice
Loma Linda Vita-Burger granules, dry	10 g.	3 Tbsp.
Loma Linda Veggie Burger	22 g.	½ cup
Millstone burger-like	13 g.	4 oz.
Millstone burger mix	10 g.	1 oz.
Millstone Veggie Burger	20 g.	½ cup
Mud pie Veggie Burgers	8 g.	1 patty
Worthington Stakelets	14.4 g.	1 piece
Worthington Vegetarian Burger	21.8	½ cup
Luncheon meat alternatives:		
Loma Linda Bologna (frzn)	14 g.	2 slices
Loma Linda Roast Beef (frzn)	11 g.	2 slices
Loma Linda Salami (frzn)	13 g.	2 slices
Loma Linda Sandwich Spread (cnd)	4 g.	3 Tbsp.
Loma Linda Turkey (frzn)	10 g.	2 slices
Loma Linda Vegelona (cnd)	18 g.	½" slice
Yves Deli Slices (frzn)	8 g.	2 slices

KEY: frzn–frozen cnd–canned dry–nonperishable; must add water

Vegetarian Protein Combinations (soy food portions may be combined with any of the complementary foods to create complete protein--7 grams per combination)			
Soy foods	**Amount**	**Complementary foods**	**Amount**
Soy milk, unfortified	1 cup	Almonds, filberts or walnuts	1 oz.
Soybeans, cooked	¼ cup	Brazil nuts or cashews	3 oz.
Tempeh	1 patty/3 oz.	Pumpkin, sesame or	
Tofu	½ oz.	sunflower seeds	2 oz.
Soy nuts	1 oz.	Cowpeas (black-eyed peas)	3½ oz.
Okara	7 oz.	Mushrooms	dry
Miso	4 tbsp.	Millet	3½ oz.
Yuba, dried	½ oz.	Whole wheat flour	3½ oz.
Soy yogurt	1 cup	Gluten flour	dry
		Wheat germ	1 cup
		Brewer's yeast	3 ½ oz.

Fresh Dark Green Vegetables	
Food	**Portion**
Broccoli, cooked	1 cup
Brussels sprouts, cooked	1 cup
Spinach, raw	2/3 cup
Greens: collards, turnip, beet, mustard, dandelion, kale, cooked	2/3 cup
Lettuce, raw (Romaine)	½ cup
Endive, raw	½ cup
Watercress, raw	½ cup
Bok Choy, raw	1 cup
Swiss chard, raw	1 cup
Sprouts, bean or alfalfa, raw	½ cup
Asparagus, cooked	½ cup

Vitamin C rich foods	
Food	**Portion**
Cabbage, raw	1 cup
Cauliflower, cooked	1 cup
Cantaloupe	½ medium
Grapefruit, preferably pink	½
Grapefruit juice	2/3 cup
Lemon	1
Lime	1
Orange	1
Orange juice	½ cup
Papaya	½ cup
Pepper, green or red, raw	1
Potatoes, cooked in skins	2
Strawberries, fresh	½ cup
Tangerines	2
Tomato	1 large
Tomato juice	1 cup
Tomato puree	2/3 cup

Whole Grains (provide carbohydrates & B vitamins)	
Food	**Portion**
Bread, whole wheat or rye	1 slice
Bagel	½
English muffin	½
Dinner roll or biscuit	1
Hotdog or hamburger bun	½
Corn tortilla (6" diameter)	1
Corn bread 2" x 2" X 1"	1 piece
Corn or bran muffin	1
Pancake, 5" diameter	1
Waffle, 5" diameter	1
Crackers:	
Buttery snack type	5
Graham, full oblong	1
Matzo 6" X 4"	½
Saltines	6
Rice cakes, puffed	2
Cereals:	
Shredded wheat	1 biscuit
Bran flakes	½ cup
Granola	½ cup
Unsweetened boxed	3/4 cup
Puffed type, boxed	1 cup
Cooked (oatmeal etc.)	½ cup
Wheat germ	¼ cup
Grits, cooked	½ cup
Popcorn, popped	3 cups
Pasta, cooked	½ cup
Rice, cooked	½ cup
Flour	2½ tbsp.

Calcium Sources (about 100 mg. calcium each) Eat 1 to 2 portions for every unfortified soy choice	
Food	**Portion**
Almonds	2 oz. or 36 nuts
Anchovies	2½ oz.
Beef tripe	3 oz.
Bok choy, cooked	1/3 cup
Brazil nuts	2 oz. or 12 nuts
Bread crumbs, wheat	3½ oz.
Brewer's yeast	5 tbsp.
Broccoli, cooked	1 cup
Buckwheat flour	3/4 cup
Carob powder	¼ cup
Caviar, sturgeon	1½ oz.
Collard greens, cooked	1/3 cup
Dandelion green, cooked	3/4 cup
Dulse (seaweed)	1 oz.
Eggs, whole	4
Fennel	1 large stalk
Filberts	2 oz. (½ cup chopped)
Floradex + calcium	½ capful
Herring	3 oz.
Kale, cooked	½ cup
Kelp (seaweed)	½ oz.
Molasses, blackstrap	2 tsp.
Muffins, wheat or corn	2
Mussels	5 oz.
Mustard green, cooked	½ cup
Okra, cooked	3/4 cup
Olives, black	4 oz.
Oysters	4 oz.
Pancakes, wheat	4 (5" diameter)
Peanuts, roasted	5 oz.
Pistachios	3½ oz./2/3 cup
Sardines	1 oz.
Scallops	3½ oz.
Sesame seed meal	2 tbsp.
Shrimp, cleaned	3½ oz.
Smelt	1 oz.
Soybeans, cooked	1 cup
Soybean curd (tofu)	3½ oz.
Soy flour, full fat	2 oz.
Soy flour, defatted	1 oz.
Soy protein, textured	3½ oz.
Sunflower seeds	3½ oz./2/3 cup
Tortillas made w/lime	2
Waffles, wheat	3
Walnuts, English	2 oz.
Wheat germ	4½ oz.

Fats & Oils (8 grams of fat each)	
Food	**Portion**
Butter	1 Tbsp.
Margarine	1 Tbsp.
Mayonnaise	1 Tbsp.
Soy mayonnaise	1 Tbsp.
Vegetable oil	1 Tbsp.
Avocado	¼
Coconut, grated	3 Tbsp.
Peanut butter	2 Tbsp.
Sausage	1 link
Cream, light	¼ cup
Cream, heavy or whipping	2 Tbsp.
Cream cheese	2 Tbsp.
Sour cream	1½ Tbsp.
French fries	10
Potato chips	10
Lard	1 Tbsp.
Bacon, crisp	2 strips
Salad dressing	2 Tbsp.
Olives	10
Almonds, whole	10
Brazil nuts, whole	5
Cashew nuts	10
Pecans, chopped	2 Tbsp.
Pecans, whole	4
Peanuts, chopped	2 Tbsp.
Peanuts, whole	30
Walnuts, chopped	2 Tbsp.
Walnuts, whole	12

Vitamin A Foods (7,000 IU each)	
Food	**Portion**
Apricots, fresh	7 (1000 IU each)
Cantaloupe, 5" diameter	½
Carrots, cooked	½ cup
Nectarines, whole	3
Papaya	2 cups pieces
Peaches, dried	4 halves
Pumpkin, canned	½ cup
Sweet potato or yam	1
Sour cherries, canned	½ cup
Watermelon	3 slices
Winter squash, cooked	½ cup

Meats, Poultry, Dairy & Seafood (7 grams protein per portion)	
Food	**Portion**
Beef, any cut, cooked	1 oz.
Lamb, any cut, cooked	1 oz.
Pork, any cut, cooked	1 oz.
Organ meats (liver, heart kidney, sweetbreads), cooked	1 oz.
Poultry: chicken, cornish hen, duck, pheasant, turkey, goose, cooked	1 oz.
Veal, any cut, cooked	1 oz.
Deli meat (4" X 1/8")	1 slice
Frankfurter	1
Fish, fresh or frozen, cooked	1 oz.
Shellfish: clams, oysters, scallops shrimp, cleaned	5
Canned seafood: crab, lobster, salmon, tuna	¼ cup
Sardines, canned	3
Anchovies	1 oz.
Cheese: hard or semihard	1 oz.
cottage or ricotta	¼ cup
Parmesan or Romano, grated	3 Tbsp.

Starchy Vegetables & Fruits (provide carbohydrates)			
Food	**Portion**	**Food**	**Portion**
Corn kernels	1/3 cup	Blackberries	½ cup
Corn on the cob	1 ear	Blueberries	½ cup
Lima beans	½ cup	Cantaloupe	½
Parsnips	2/3 cup	Cherries	½ cup
Peas, green	½ cup	Cranberry juice	½ cup
Potato, white	1 small	Cranberry sauce	2 Tbsp.
Potato, mashed	½ cup	Dates	2
Potato chips	15	Figs, fresh or dried	2
Baked beans, canned	¼ cup	Grapefruit	½
Cooked beans, peas, lentils	½ cup	Grapefruit juice	½ cup
Beets, cooked	1 cup	Grapes, purple	1 cup
Carrots, cooked	1 cup	Grapes, green or white	½ cup
Carrots, raw	2	Lemonade	1/3 cup
Cucumber	1 large	Orange	½
Onion, raw	1 2½" diameter	Orange juice	½ cup
onion, cooked	3/4 cup	Papaya	½ cup pieces
Pumpkin, cooked	½ cup	Peach	1
Sauerkraut, prepared	1 cup	Pear	½
Winter squash, cooked	1/3 cup	Persimmon	½
Summer squash, cooked	1½ cup	Pineapple	½ cup pieces
Sweet potato	½	Pineapple juice	1/3 cup
Tomato, raw	1½	Plum	2
Turnips, cooked	1¼	Prunes, cooked	3
Apple	½	Prune juice	¼ cup
Apple juice	1/3 cup	Raisins	2 Tbsp.
Applesauce	¼ cup	Raspberries	½ cup
Apricots, fresh	3	Strawberries	1 cup
Apricot nectar	1/3 cup	Tangerine	1
Avocado	1 cup pieces	Cornstarch	1 Tbsp.
Banana	½	Tapioca, dry	1 Tbsp.

Iron sources for those who don't eat liver			
Food	**Portion**	**Food**	**Portion**
Brewers or nutritional yeast (1.4 mg.)	1 Tbsp.	Pumpkin seeds (17 mg.)	½ cup
Blackstrap molasses (3.2 mg.)	1 Tbsp.	Rice bran (7.8 mg.)	½ cup
Prune juice (10.5 mg.)	1 cup	Wheat germ (.5 mg.)	1 Tbsp.
Dulse seaweed (42.8 mg.)	1 oz.	Tofu (raw, 13.2 mg.)	½ cup
Kelp, seaweed, dried (28.4 mg.)	1 oz.	Amaranth grain (7.4 mg.)	½ cup
Clams, canned, drained (22.3 mg.)	½ cup	Kidneys, braised (13.1 mg.)	3½ oz.
Oysters, eastern (13.4 mg.)	3½ oz.	Sesame seeds (5.2 mg.)	½ cup

PROTEIN SUPPLEMENT POWDERS				
Producer/Brand name	**Protein source**	**Portion**	**Calories**	**Protein**
Amino Fuel	dairy	2 heaping scoops	280	20 g.
Bahama Diet/Dick Gregory's	soy	22.4 g.	90	15 g.
Diet Pep	milk	3 scoops	210	15 g.
Soy Protein Isolaste/Fearn	soy	1 scoop	50	13 g.
Original Vegetable Protein/Naturaide	soy	2 rounded Tbsp.	105	25 g.
Vanilla Vegetable Protein/Naturaide	soy	2 rounded Tbsp.	100	24 g.
Milk & Egg Protein +/Naturaide	dairy	2 heaping Tbsp.	115	26 g.
Natural Beginning	soy	1 scoop	70	10 g.
Perfection/USA Sports Labs	?	1 heaping scoop	98	20.5 g.
Protesoy/Nutritional Factors	soy	2 Tbsp.	70	16 g.
Source of Life Energy Shake	soy	2 rounded Tbsp.	116	15 g.
Spiru-tein	soy	1 heaping scoop	94	14 g.
Spirolina	micro-algae	1 heaping Tbsp.	36	6 g.
Staminex	meat	3 heaping Tbsp.	120	16.2 g.

Commercial Milks from Vegetable Sources (1 qt. cow's milk offers 30 g. protein/500 calories)				
Brand/flavor*	**Serving**	**Calories**	**Protein**	**Calcium (% daily allowance)**
Ah Soy carob	6 oz.	160	4 g.	2%
Edensoy original	8.45 oz.	140	10 g.	10%
Edensoy carob	8.45 oz.	160	8 g.	8%
Edensoy vanilla	8.45 oz.	150	8 g.	8%
Grainissance Amazake Almond shake	8 oz.	272	7 g.	4%
Miller Farms Foods Solait Soy milk	1 oz. powder	135	6 g.	5%
Soy Moo	8 oz.	130	7 g.	15%
Vitasoy Creamy Original	8.45 oz.	160	10 g.	8%
Vitasoy Vanilla Delite	8.45 oz.	190	7 g.	8%
Westbrae unsweetened soy milk	8 oz.	100	7 g.	8%
Westbrae w/oil (yellow box)	8 oz.	150	7 g.	6%
Westbrae Westsoy Plus plain (+A,D, calcium, B₂)	8 oz.	130	6 g.	30%
Westbrae + carob	8 oz.	160	6 g.	30%
Westbrae flavored soy shakes (vanilla malt, etc.)	6 oz.	250-270	6-7 g.	10%

*There are many brands of milk alternatives which do not contain enough protein for pregnancy. Some of these are Grainissance Amazake Original (4 g. per 8 oz.), Rice Dream (2 g. per 8 oz.) Naturally Tofu by Souvex Natural Foods (2 g. per Tbsp.), and White Almond Beverage by Whole & Healthy (1 g. per 6 oz.). Any brand not mentioned must be checked for nutrient content before being used as a milk substitute. (Brewer, 1983) Unfortified soy milk may be fortified by adding 2 Tbsp. safflower oil (to boost calories if needed), 1 Tbsp. powdered calcium supplement (lactate is good), 25 mcg. B_{12} tablet, ½ tsp. salt, ¼ tsp. liquid lecithin (holds oil in suspension), 1 Methionine/C-complex tablet finely crushed and 4 Tbsp. honey or maple syrup per liter.

Here is a sample dietary history which has been analyzed using the preceding lists. The checklist is composed of the various food categories. The number in parentheses is the number of daily portions required and the number to the right represents the portions actually eaten. As you get more familiar with the lists, you will be able to make a quick visual assessment. While learning, find each food item on one of the lists striking out each food as you go (remembering to count each portion only once). Put a tick mark by its category, then add up the ticks.

1 Day Diet History	Checklist
2 whole wheat muffins w/butter & **jam** **Orange juice** Mo's 24 herb tea w/ 1 tsp. **honey** 1 hot dog on roll w/sauerkraut & **relish** Fresh corn on cob w/butter **Apple juice** ½ **apple, ½ mandarin orange, banana** Lentil soup ½ cup macaroni & cheese Fresh asparagus w/butter **Slice custard pie w/scoop ice cream** Dish of plan yogurt w/nuts & **raisins**	Milk (4) 3 Eggs (2) 1 Protein (6) 2½ Dark Greens (2) 1 Grains, starchy veg./fruits (5) 8¼ Vitamin C foods (2) 1½ Vitamin A foods (1) none Fats & oils (3) 4 Iron rich food (4 oz. weekly) none

Note that this woman is eating a lot of sweet foods (bold items) and is low in most categories.

References and further reading:

Brewer, Gail, The Brewer Medical Diet for Normal and High Risk Pregnancies, Simon & Schuster, New York, 1983.

James, Dawn, "New Thoughts About Pre-eclampsia," presentation 9/15/89, Royal College of Medicine, London Eng. President, Pre-eclamptic Toxemia Society, Ty Iago, Carmel, Caernarvon, Gwynedd, LL54 7AB, Wales, U.K. Telephone 028-688-0057.

Nutrition, Healthy Babies and Maternal Weight Gain

No matter how well a woman eats, her efforts can be undermined by inappropriate advice regarding weight gain during pregnancy. Because of the lack of recognition of the connection between maternal nutrition, weight gain and healthy babies, much confusion still prevails about the appropriate amount to gain during pregnancy. A discussion of maternal nutrition is not complete without putting mainstream medical advice regarding weight gain into perspective with what makes sense.

For decades the medical profession has focused intensively on the amount of weight a woman gains and how rapidly she gains it. This is partly because rapid weight gain is a secondary symptom of toxemia (brought on by pathological fluid retention). Fear of toxemia led doctors to severely restrict weight gain during pregnancy to as little as 15 to 20 pounds for many years. The latest recommendations from the American College of Obstetrics and Gynecology on maternal nutrition in pregnancy offers a much more elaborate formula for calculating how much an individual woman should gain which takes into account the mother's pre-pregnancy weight. However, the primary focus on the amount of weight gained has not changed. (ACOG Technical Bulletin, 1993)

The facts are that a woman who eats well will gain what she needs to gain to have a healthy pregnancy, period. While one may be able to point to some general trends in healthy weight gain there is no magic number of pounds which represents what all women need to gain. Neither is there a magic pattern of gain that will apply to every woman. Both will vary according to each woman's physiologic make-up. To hold a woman to a pattern of gain or to set a limit on how much she can gain for the entire pregnancy, no matter how "reasonable" or individualized that limit is considered to be, sets a woman up for trouble.

In one of the most comprehensive studies of maternal weight gain (Hytten & Thompson, 1970), one of the few that took maternal nutrition into account with no weight gain restrictions placed on the women, it was found that the distribution of weight gain over the last 20 weeks of pregnancy looked like this:

WEEKLY LOSS/GAIN IN LAST 20 WEEKS	% OF TOTAL WOMEN STUDIED
Lost ¼ pound	2%
Gained 1 pound	25%
Gained 2 pounds	2%

The other 71% of the women studied gained somewhere in between these ranges. (I cite this study to underscore the fact that a broad range is possible and nothing, by itself, should be considered abnormal.) A more recent study showed that weighing mothers is of little use in predicting small-for-dates infants and that it generates anxiety in women. It concluded that routine weighing of women with a normal weight at their initial physical should be abandoned. (Dawes &

Grudzinskas, 1991)

Very often I hear from midwives or read childbirth books that encourage women to eat well early in pregnancy and then have a fit when women begin to gain "too much" or have gaining spurts. By placing the primary focus on the number of pounds gains the point of good nutrition is lost, and the midwife or doctor unwittingly sabotages the woman's health. Our Western culture is highly focused on fatness; women are especially prone to feeling guilty about getting large and eating too much. Even suggesting an upper limit of weight to gain or focusing on how much weight is gained from visit to visit without reference to nutrition supports a woman in feeling that the weight, not her diet, is the most important issue. This will inevitably lead to many women reducing their intake in the last months of pregnancy, precisely when fetal growth needs are most critical.

What to tell women about weight gain: Tell women to focus on what they eat, not what they gain; that there is no normal amount of weight to gain during pregnancy. In fact, most healthy women gain 35 to 45 pounds during pregnancy. Since each woman is an individual, it is impossible to say what any one will gain. Therefore it is best not to give women any number which they can become attached to as "enough." The thin, underweight woman may gain more, the woman-of-size may gain much less. As long as the dietary choices are good ones, any weight gained will be different than that gained by eating junk food and empty calories, because empty calories create more fat than nutrient-rich foods.

You should instead praise women for gaining weight. They need to hear that gaining is desirable, that their baby is growing nicely, that getting bigger is what *you* want to see! If a woman is concerned about how much she might gain, I make a deal: if she will eat, I won't ask her to weigh herself at each visit (in Norway, weight is not usually checked at prenatals). Instead of focusing on weight gain you should be asking a woman how she is doing with her diet and if any changes have occurred which increase her stress and activity levels so you can counsel her concerning necessary dietary changes. When women see that your primary concern is what they are eating, not what they are gaining, their focus will shift as well.

While you may be less concerned about what a woman is gaining, you still need to be aware when she is gaining little or nothing. If the woman is overweight whose baby is growing and diet is good, there is *usually* no cause for alarm as long as she has not been ill, under unusual stress or the like; even so, this mother may have a weight gain spurt as her blood volume peaks around 28 weeks. However, if the woman is thin and not gaining, there is probably cause for concern (but this must also be correlated with fetal growth). Review the diet; make sure her calorie intake is adequate and that she is not exercising excessively to burn fat. Discuss how she is feeling as her abdomen gets larger; she could easily be obsessing over "getting fat." This needs to be addressed as soon as a problem is noted.

It is perfectly normal for women to have weight gain spurts and lags during pregnancy. You may note that a woman has gained little or nothing but the baby feels larger than last visit. Likewise you may note that a woman has gained several pounds but the baby feels about the same size. These variations are perfectly normal. Often, women have a weight gain spurt of 5 to 10 pounds between the 24th to the 28th week of pregnancy, reflecting an increase in blood volume. Conversely, if women have no such spurt followed by a sudden gain in the third trimester, this could be caused by retained fluid from true toxemia. However, any time a woman improves her nutrition you are likely to see a corresponding weight increase as the body stores fat and the blood volume catches up. By following a number of women throughout their pregnancies and taking the emphasis off of weight and putting it on nutrition you will get a feel for the wide range of normal variation that exists in maternal weight gain during healthy pregnancy.

Weight gain and eating disorders: For those who have had serious eating disorders, their changing body image will be even harder for them to integrate. You need to speak honestly about her history and if any behaviors are still going on (binging and purging, etc.). If the woman was very thin at the onset of her pregnancy, it becomes more important to be sure she is gaining. Getting on a scale may be very difficult for such women. If you feel it is necessary, weigh the mother yourself and do not tell her the result. If a problem develops, discuss needed dietary changes, without reference to the number of pounds. Offer these women frequent opportunities to discuss their changing shapes and ask how they are doing with not falling back into old patterns related to their eating disorder. There may be support groups in your area for such women; check it out.

Research in maternal weight gain and newborn health: Studies which examine the correlation between neonatal problems, maternal weight gain during pregnancy, and newborn weight have discovered that as a mother gains more the newborn's birth weight goes up and the rate at which certain newborn problems occur goes down. However, this focus on maternal weight gain sidesteps the important question of *what* a woman has been eating to gain the weight and produce the healthy infant! The only way to optimize the baby's growth is through excellent maternal nutrition. The weight of both the mother and the baby are statistics which can be easily gathered, but using these as the focus of study still leaves many women and their care providers in the dark about some of the most important physiological processes of pregnancy, and about how to prevent nutrition-related complications such as metabolic toxemia.

With good dietary advice most women will have larger babies than they would otherwise. They may then be confronted by the medical model view that some babies are "too large." Today there is much focus being placed on the "large for gestational age" infant whose mother may be labeled a gestational diabetic. The baby of a truly diabetic woman whose diabetes is undiagnosed or poorly controlled can have serious problems, as it is often born prematurely and has characteristic signs of being truly large for gestational age. Unfortunately medical statistics do not differentiate the large, fragile baby of the uncontrolled diabetic from the large, robust and very healthy baby of a well nourished, healthy mother. If women eat well, they will often have babies that exceed the 8 lb. 14 oz. weight (listed as an upper limit on the scale below) that are every bit as healthy and sound as the babies in category 4 in the table below. If a baby does not grow adequately, it is subject to many problems which a larger baby is less likely to have. Some of these are:

*Perinatal mortality (stillbirth or early infant death)
*Small head circumference (indicating poor brain development)
*Mental retardation
*Cerebral palsy
*Learning problems
*Visual and hearing defects
*Poor growth and development

The following table demonstrates how much more at risk for problems smaller babies can be. Well-nourished women will usually have babies that weigh 6 lb. 8 oz. or more, although factors such as genetics must be taken into account.

| Category | Newborn birth weight | | Comments |
	Grams	Pounds	
1	≤2500	5 lb. 8 oz.	Many problems as listed above
2	2500-2999	5 lb. 8 oz. to 6 lb. 10 oz.	3X higher incidence of the same problems than #3
3	3000-3500	6 lb. 10 oz. to 7 lb. 12 oz.	Improved health over #2
4	3500-4000	7 lb. 12 oz. to 8 lb. 14 oz.	Higher intelligence & less disability

(Varney, 1980)

As little as 120 grams (4 oz.) in birth weight can make a difference in the overall health of a newborn. The need for adequate maternal nutrition cuts across all economic and class lines. Good maternal nutrition means that every baby will have the chance to fully realize its genetic potential and the optimal chance of having a healthy body and a productive life.

Research and further reading

Dawes, MG & Grudzinskas, J., "Repeated measurement of maternal weight during pregnancy. Is this a useful practice?," p. 189 & "Patterns of maternal weight gain in pregnancy," p. 195, Br J. of OB Gyn, Vol. 98, No. 2, Feb. 1991.
Hytten, F. & Thomas A, "Maternal Physiological Adjustments," Maternal Nutrition and the Course of Pregnancy, Washington D.C.: Committee on Maternal Nutrition Food and Nutrition Board, National Research Council, National Academy of Sciences, 1970.
ACOG Technical Bulletin, "Nutrition during Pregnancy," No. 179, April 1993.
Varney, Helen, Nurse-Midwifery, "Chapter 8, Nutritional Management Throughout Pregnancy," Blackwell Scientific Pub., Boston, MA, 1980.

248

Helping Women Cope with Food Cravings

Food cravings often signal the need for particular nutrients in the diet. One way to broach this subject is to ask, "Do you crave anything in particular?," since women can crave both foods and non-nutritive substances when pregnant.

Sweets: Note how often a woman is eating something sweet. For this evaluation any sweet counts: candy, cakes, cookies, ice cream and sodas, as well as fruit and fruit juices. The better the overall diet, the more likely it is that a woman will choose fruit instead of junk. However, a large amount of sweets of any kind almost always signals the need for more protein and calories to meet the needs of pregnancy. The body knows sweets will bring the blood sugar up quickly (and sweets are often potent comfort foods, since they were often the treats of childhood). The first order of business is to increase protein intake and be sure green vegetable intake is adequate. Every time she craves a sweet she should eat protein instead.

Often the notion of eliminating unhealthy foods and empty calories is interpreted as the "treat-less" diet plan for pregnancy. This doesn't have to be the case. If a woman wants a cookie or some ice cream, encourage her to have a high protein snack and some vegetables first and then choose "treat" foods that meet her nutritional needs. For example cookies made of honey, whole wheat flour, eggs, nuts, raisins, oatmeal, etc. are not junk food!! As you can see, they provide a variety of nutritious ingredients rolled into one good-tasting form. Suggest making a huge batch of something and freezing it in small packets to keep a few treats around without unrealistically expecting a busy woman to be sitting home making cookies for herself all the time. Just about any food craving can be met with a nutritious substitute in this manner. Even the desire for soda can be offset by mixing sparkling water with pure fruit juice or buying a similar commercially prepared product. These foods should be taken in moderation, with primary attention given to eating foods from the lists in the previous chapter.

Carbonated drinks: Sometimes the desire for carbonated drinks has to do with a dependency on caffeine. However, many women just enjoy carbonated drinks. While one here and there is not going to hurt, a steady diet of any carbonated beverage is not good. Their is discussion in the natural health care community that the carbonic and phosphoric acids in some carbonated drinks may pull calcium out of the bones and a lot of carbonation can lead to diuresis. Once women understand this, hopefully curtailing their intake won't seem so hard.

Salt: Salt cravings may mean a woman simply needs more salt, but they can also signal the need for additional protein, since sodium is often found in protein foods. Olives, pickles, chips, and highly processed foods are all very salty. She can go ahead and eat these foods if they are nutritious. Encourage her to avoid foods such as processed meats, lots of chips or other empty calorie salt sources.

Non-nutritive substances (Pica):   Sometimes women crave non-nutritive substances such as clay, coffee grounds, ice, flour, baking soda, dry milk of magnesia, paraffin and corn starch. These cravings indicate severe dietary deficiencies such as a lack of minerals or calories.   Ice, clay, sand or soil cravings has been associated with iron deficiency.   Ingestion of starch may interfere with iron absorption in some women. Women who are extremely poor and hungry will tend to crave such things because they will, at least, allay the hunger. For example, cornstarch or laundry starch provide empty calories.

A variety of symptoms have been associated with pica such as intestinal and pyloric obstruction, prematurity, toxemia and perinatal mortality; in the majority of cases these are all directly due to nutritional imbalances. Parotid gland enlargement may occur in women who eat starch.

It is important to realize that pica is common in some cultural traditions and is not necessarily limited to pregnancy. Women may have a variety of beliefs concerning pica: that it will relieve nausea (some clays have a magnesium content similar to antacid preparations), prevent vomiting, "help babies," relieve dizziness, cure swollen legs, relieve headaches or ensure beautiful children. Note that many of these symptoms are often associated with inadequate nutrition. Denial of a craving is felt by some to cause a birthmark to appear on the baby.

In some rural Southern areas beliefs regarding dietary restriction during pregnancy may still prevail such as avoiding milk, eggs, fish, vegetables, grapefruit, tomatoes, butter, liver and beans, bacon, ham or onions as well as green foods after the birth. Ironically, these are the kinds of foods the mother needs in abundance.

If you discover that a woman is experiencing pica, ask what she is craving and how much she is actually ingesting. Does she crave the substance only now, or when she is not pregnant as well? How much of it does she eat outside of pregnancy? Carefully review the diet diaries of any woman who has such cravings and help her figure out what is missing. (Luke, 1977) Often, women who ate a substance as a child will again crave it during pregnancy. This is probably a combination of psychological comfort coupled with the particularly acute nutritional needs of the moment. In order to effectively assist a woman in replacing the substance she is craving with foods, explore the reasons why the pica is present.

Comfort foods: Some women find themselves craving foods they haven't eaten for years. These are often foods they were given as children during illness or as a reward for good behavior. Comforting memories are rekindled, even if the woman is not conscious of this link. Try to help women gravitate toward nutritious choices of the types of foods she is craving. An occasional indulgence in a special less-than-nourishing food is not going to do any harm, but allowing them to take the place of better dietary choices on a regular basis is not a good idea.

References and further reading:

Luke, Barbara, "Understanding Pica in Pregnant Women," Maternal Child Nursing, Vol. 2, No. 2, March/April 1977, p. 97-100.

Vitamin and Mineral Supplements During Pregnancy

No supplement, however balanced and complete, can take the place of a whole foods diet which is adequate in protein, calories and associated nutrients. When the diet is adequate, supplementation is often not necessary. This is more true when the diet is made up of organic foods, spring water and fresh farm raised meats, cheeses and hearty grains. For the working woman, one living in a more polluted city environment, a teenager, a woman carrying a multiple pregnancy, or the busy mother who cannot afford to buy organic vegetables or doesn't have the space in her yard to grow them, nutritional supplementation can help bridge the gap between her dietary reality and the needs of her pregnancy. Supplements will also benefit those who come to you with little nutritional reserve, such as those with signs and symptoms of nutritional deficiencies, very thin women, those with a history of extreme weight swings or those who have followed a number of imbalanced dietary fads, those whose previous pregnancies have been complicated or closely spaced (less than 2 years apart), women who have a history of poor eating habits, eating disorders or recent illness, and those who have digestive disorders or liver damage. Supplementation also benefits women who insist on limiting their dietary choices regardless of the health consequences, those who have not learned to balance the diet they have chosen, women whose allergies limit their dietary choices, those who have a history of substance abuse or regular prescription drug use (birth control pills?), and, finally, very poor women. (Seaver, 1992)

Any recommendation of supplements must come with a discussion of striving for the best quality food intake possible. Vitamins are an assistance, nothing more. A woman who brings a dietary history to their pregnancy which includes many processed and refined foods needs to know that she cannot eat junk and think that her vitamins make up for it!!

With these concepts firmly in mind, supplementation can be considered, with an eye to the woman's individual circumstances. Many of the common problems of pregnancy can be corrected with the addition of a particular supplement; these problems will be discussed throughout this book. Generally, if a woman is healthy without undue stresses in her life and her hemoglobin is within acceptable limits in early pregnancy, she may not need to take any supplements.

Special consideration must be given to women who have limited dietary patterns. The following table summarizes potential deficiencies which can result from dietary choices which limit the types of foods a woman will eat:

TYPE OF DIET	THOSE WHO EAT:	MAY BE DEFICIENT IN:
Omnivore (meat)	No dairy products	Calcium, Vit. D
Ovo-lacto	Mainly dairy for protein	B_6, iron & copper
Vegan	No animal products	Calcium, riboflavin, B_{12}, Vit. D, calories, zinc & protein
Raw foods	No animal products	Same as for vegan plus thiamin, niacin, & B_6

Excessive stress from any of a hundred sources (other kids, job, home life etc.) may prompt you to recommend a multi-vitamin and mineral supplement. Most natural supplements such as those produced by Optinatal, Rainbow Light, and NF Formulas require that a woman take up to six tablets per day to achieve the dosages outlined on the bottle. Depending upon her diet, life circumstances and how her body tolerates supplements, she can choose to take 1 to 6 tablets daily.

Iron has been routinely prescribed to the pregnant woman for years, primarily due to a misunderstanding about the meaning of the hemoglobin reduction that normally occurs during pregnancy. For a thorough review of this process, consult the Anemia in Pregnancy chapter in Diagnostic Tests. Many pregnant women do not need additional iron. For those that need only minimal support, using cast iron skillets and combining foods rich in iron and vitamin C in the same meal can help in getting the additional iron needed for pregnancy.

Vitamin C is used up by living in a polluted environment and by stress; therefore supplementing vitamin C can be important for many women during pregnancy. Vitamin C, along with its associated nutrients, the bioflavinoids, helps to strengthen all bodily membranes. It will make the amniotic sac strong, elastic and resilient, thus greatly minimizing the possibility of early rupture of membranes. The mineral zinc is also important for tissue integrity and adequate amounts assist in maintaining intact membranes as well (Sikorski, et.al., 1990). Since our soil is very zinc depleted, supplementation is often needed.

VITAMIN & MINERAL SUPPLEMENTS	
SUPPLEMENT	DOSAGE
B_{12}	3 to 5 micrograms 2 or 3 times weekly
Folic acid	1 to 2 mg. daily w/no Hx of spinal defects
	4 mg. daily w/Hx of child w/spinal defects
Prenatal Multi vitamin & mineral	
(Optinatal/NF Formula/Rainbow Light)	As indicated for an individual woman
Vitamin C with bioflavinoids	500 to 1000 mg. daily
Vitamin E (for varicose veins)	200 to 800 IU daily (as indicated)
Iron supplement	1 to 3 tablets daily (only if indicated)
Zinc	25 to 40 mg. after a meal

If a woman comes to you for pre-conception counseling, she may begin to take prenatal vitamins three to six months prior to conception, especially if she is a smoker, has a history of drug or alcohol abuse, has had a very poor diet or has a poor birthing history. Many studies indicate that folic acid plays an important role in reducing the incidence of neural tube defects in the baby. The addition of folic acid to the supplement program may be particularly important if the woman or the biological father have a familial history of neural tube defects, if she lives in a highly polluted area or an area with high radon levels, many nuclear power plants or other nuclear industries, or if she cannot get fresh vegetables. Additional folic acid is most necessary during the first three months of pregnancy, and

252

supplementation is ideally begun at least a month prior to conception, especially if one of her children already has a neural tube defect. (Niebyl, 1995)

In women carrying multiple gestations, additional supplementation is desirable. Recommend two to three times the normal daily dosage of Prenatal multi-vitamins (how much should depend on the individual woman's overall diet, stress and activity levels as well as how many fetuses she is carrying).

Megadoses of vitamins: Some practitioners recommend megadoses of certain vitamins for women during pregnancy. A megadose is an amount many hundreds and sometimes many thousands of times in excess of the recommended daily allowance. These recommendations stem from the idea that certain nutrients will significantly boost the mother's health and eliminate common complaints and problems.

While there are certain instances where large doses of vitamins may be required for a period of time (for example, you might advise a woman with the flu to take 500 mg. of vitamin C every few hours for the duration of the illness), megadoses of vitamins are not usually necessary on a routine basis. An exception to this general rule might be a woman who has a preexisting medical condition that is greatly benefitted by megadoses of certain nutrients. In such cases, the woman still needs to be aware that very high doses of some nutrients may be harmful to her unborn baby.

High doses of any water soluble vitamin may, in some cases, produce marked symptoms of deficiency in the newborn because of the rapid drop in blood levels once the baby is not being supplied with nutrients via the umbilical cord. For example, a baby whose mother takes more than 5 grams of vitamin C daily throughout pregnancy may develop scurvy (vitamin C deficiency disease) shortly after birth. The fat soluble vitamins A and D can be stored in the body and rise to toxic levels. Pregnant women should not take more than 25,000 IUs of fat soluble vitamin A or more than 4,000 IUs of vitamin D daily. While complete information regarding which nutrients may cause problems in high doses during pregnancy is not available, the table in the chapter on Basic Nutrition describes some of the best known pregnancy-related risks associated with certain nutritional supplements.

References and further reading:
Balch, J., & Balch, P., Prescription for Nutritional Healing, Avery Pub., Garden City, NY 1990.
Kutsky, Roman, Handbook of Vitamins, Minerals and Hormones, 2nd ed., New York, Van Nostrand Reinhold, 1981.
Seaver, Althea, handout from workshop on Nutrition in Pregnancy given at Midwifery Today Conf. Eugene, OR, 1992.
Sikorski, R., et.al., "Zinc status in women with premature rupture of membranes at term," OB/GYN, Vol. 76, No. 4, October, 1990, pp. 675-677.
Niebyl, J., "Folic acid supplementation," Contemp. Ob Gyn, Vol. 40, No. 6, June 1995, p. 43.

Food Additives

Food additives are a potential health hazard. A diet which emphasizes whole, unprocessed foods will contain a minimal amount of food additives. However, even with such a diet, pesticides are still a concern. Washing vegetables well before preparing them will help to minimize but will not eliminate the intake of pesticides. Certain pesticides have been acknowledged as causing higher cancer rates in children as well as a variety of birth defects. Families living or working on or near farms which use chemical sprays are most at risk (Food Safe News, Fall, 1993). Remember that luncheon meats, sausages, and other processed meats are high in nitrites, a highly toxic additive which is carcinogenic. Encourage women to read the labels on any packaged foods they purchase and to avoid those items which list words not familiar as common foods. A good rule of thumb is: if it isn't on your kitchen shelf or you can't pronounce it, avoid it!

Dairy animals are being given bovine growth hormones to increase milk production, in addition to numerous other drugs. Women should ask their grocers which, if any, brands of milk are not using growth hormone; local health food stores should have such information. While such drugs are not strictly additives, they serve to indirectly contaminate the product and should be avoided whenever possible. How they will affect the body after long-term use is not known.

Irradiation of foods is also being promoted to enhance longevity, kill microorganisms and thus reduce the use of pesticides. The public has been reluctant to accept irradiation as a suitable preservative method, therefore few irradiated foods are actually being sold. Irradiation causes the production of unique radiolytic substances (URI) the ultimate effect of which is unknown. Irradiation destroys vitamins as well. At this time, fresh foods must be labeled with a stylized flower emblem to show they have been irradiated. However, processed foods, such as canned soups, may contain irradiated ingredients but require no such warning. Spices are the most commonly irradiated food sold in the United States, and some natural herb vendors do not irradiate their products. Women should ask their grocers what, if any, irradiated foods they sell. (Food & Water, 1995)

Nutrasweet (aspartame) is a chemical sugar substitute which is found in many foods. It has three ingredients: phenylalanine, aspartic acid, and methanol. Phenylalanine is the amino acid which phenylketonurics cannot metabolize. If the fetus is phenylketonuric, concentrated ingestion of asparatame by the mother may cause brain damage even before birth. There is a larger segment of the population which is sensitive to high levels of phenylalanine. Methanol is a human-specific, highly toxic poison which is converted in the body to formaldehyde and formic acid, both of which have toxic effects on the thymus gland. Toxic side effects include malaise, nausea, recurrent headaches, dizziness, and visual disturbances and symptoms that mimic lupus and multiple sclerosis. It is best to avoid aspartame completely, and this is especially true during pregnancy. (Balch, 1990) (For more details also see the chapter entitled Inborn Errors of Metabolism in Pregnancy

254

in <u>Diagnostic Tests</u>.)

References and further reading:

Balch, J., & Balch, P., <u>Prescription for Nutritional Healing</u>, Avery Pub., Garden City, NY 1990.

<u>Food Safe News</u>, "Study says children at risk from pesticides," report on National Academy of Sciences study: "Pesticides in the Diets of Infants and Children," & "Interview with Arturo Rodriguez," Fall, 1993.

Food & Water, Inc. RR. 1, Box 114, Marshfield, VT, 05658 (802) 426-3700; conversation with a representative regarding current irradiation of foods in US, 6/7/95.

Webb, Tony, <u>Food Irradiation: Who Wants It?</u>, Thorsons Pub., Inc., Rochester, VT, 1987.

Food Preparation

The way in which food is prepared can help to preserve its nutrient content or can significantly reduce it. Of all the food preparation methods, boiling is probably the worst, as it leaches vitamins and minerals into the water, which is usually discarded. Steaming foods preserves the most nutrients because it heats and cooks them without having to leave them in water. While steaming foods, try not to let steam escape, which diminishes nutrients. Salting foods prior to cooking leaches vitamins, especially if foods are to be boiled. Convection cooking helps preserve nutrients, as does baking, broiling and sauteing. Foods cooked at extremely high temperatures are depleted of nutrients. Cooking foods over charcoal can leave carcinogenic residues in the foods. If foods are to be deep-fried, fresh oil should be heated below the smoking point, the food cooked and the oil discarded. Saving oils for frying is not advisable; reheating the oils cause carcinogenic changes to take place. While fried foods are not the best choice, discarding the oil certainly lessens the overall health impact.

When preparing vegetables and fruits for cooking, they should be cut up as close to the time they will be served as possible. Cutting foods causes them to oxidize and destroys valuable nutrients. Never soak vegetables in order to crisp them, as this leaches out vitamins as well.

Avoid the use of aluminum and coated (non-stick) cooking utensils. Aluminum salts are soluble in water and are easily assimilated into the system where they accumulate in the brain and nervous tissues. Foods cooked in aluminum produce a chloride poison which neutralizes digestive juices, and may lead to acidosis and ulcers. Non-stick cookware slowly releases its coating as fumes into the kitchen air and into the food. It is best to avoid it altogether. Cookware made of glass, stainless steel and cast iron fine alternatives.

Food Allergies

An allergy is an inappropriate antibody response to a foreign substance which, in this case, is not really a toxin. If a woman is allergic to a food it will create aggravating symptoms as well as be poorly utilized by her body. Women should find foods to eat that agree with them instead. For example, if milk causes bloating, gas, headaches, or even rashes, these are indications that the woman is having an allergic reaction or is intolerant of it. Allergies will also frequently produce asthma, an irritated cough or tickle in the throat, hay fever or eczema. If a food allergy is suspected, but not proven, the following simple test can help determine if an allergy is the problem: tell the woman to relax for a few minutes, then take her pulse at the wrist, counting for a sixty second period. Then she is to eat the suspect food. Next she should rest quietly and wait fifteen to twenty minutes and then recheck her pulse. If it has increased more than 10 beats per minute, this is highly suggestive of an allergic reaction. (Balch, 1990)

A food intolerance is different from an allergy, because it indicates a lack of the enzymes necessary to digest the food properly. In some cases products are available to provide the missing enzymes such as Bean-O (for beans) and Lactaid (for dairy products). However, if these products do not alleviate the symptoms, other foods should be chosen. Simply eating a food that is on a dietary list doesn't count if the body can't use it! (Balch, 1990) Food intolerances which are chemically based may run in a family. A child can become allergic to a food in the maternal diet while still *in utero*. This is another good reason to track down foods that the mother can't tolerate.

Soy milk: One of the most common food allergies is to lactose, a principle sugar in dairy products. Soy milk can often be used as a substitute, although allergies to soy products are not uncommon (be sure to continue to assess a woman for allergic reactions once she stops eating dairy products). Soy milk is a fine source of protein and calories and there are many acceptable brands on the health food store shelves today (see food lists for a representative sampling). If a woman is drinking commercially prepared unfortified soy milk, the addition of the supplemental items mentioned in the following recipe will almost elevate its nutritional content to equal that of the following recipe. For vegans, vitamin B_{12} can be added as well. As always, the luxury of a processed food is afforded at considerable cost. If a woman is adhering to a diary-restricted diet and hasn't the money to spend on a liter of commercial soy milk a day, then she can make the following milk. This recipe was devised by Cornell University to avoid the bitter taste which often comes with homemade soy milk.

Gail Brewer's Fortified Soy Milk

1 cup whole soybeans (less than 1 year old)
3 cups very cold water
8¼ cups boiling water
2 Tbsp. safflower oil
1 Tbsp. calcium supplement (lactate is good)
25 mcg. B_{12} tablet
½ tsp. salt
¼ tsp. liquid lecithin (holds oil in suspension)
1 Methionine/C-complex tablet finely crushed
4 Tbsp. honey or maple syrup
Flavoring as desired such as vanilla, postum, malt,
 carob, juice or spices

A Blender that can handle boiling water, preferably
 one with a stainless steel container

Sort soybeans, discarding any damaged or broken ones.

Place beans in a colander and run cold water over then for 4-5 minutes turning constantly to wash thoroughly. Transfer beans to a glass container and add very cold water (to prevent fermentation while soaking). Soak 10-12 hours in the refrigerator. Beans should double in bulk.

Rinse beans again under cold water in colander. Drain well. Divide beans into 3 equal portions and place each portion on a paper towel until you are ready to grind them.

Line colander with muslin or open weave linen cloth (too tight a weave will not allow proper drainage of the beans). Place above a large saucepan to catch the soy milk as it drains.

Bring 10 cups of water to a full rolling boil (boiling water deactivates the enzyme that makes soy bitter. Place two cups of boiling water into blender and run it 1 minute to heat blender. The blender container and content must be kept extremely hot (180°F or 82°C), otherwise the milk will be bitter. Discard heating water from the blender.

Transfer the first portion of beans to blender and add 2 cups boiling water. Blend on medium setting for 1 minute, then on high for 1 minute. Pour puréed beans into lined colander. Repeat until all beans are pureed.

Use ¼ cup boiling water to clean last puree from blender container and add to colander.

258

Tie cloth closed or twist tightly, then press down hard with a glass jar, a potato masher, or another pan to squeeze as much soy milk as possible from the beans. Continue until the beans yield no more milk.

Heat milk for 30 minutes in a double boiler, stirring often to prevent scorching. Cover and chill 15 to 20 minutes in refrigerator freezer. Rapid chilling contributes to a more dairy-like taste.

Add the other items as listed above to the entire batch of milk. Return the milk to the blender in two or three portions and blend each for 1 minute. The milk should be smooth and evenly-textured. Yield: 6 cups.

To make a cream substitute, just add half the water called for. (Brewer, 1983)

References and further reading:

Balch, J., & Balch, P., Prescription for Nutritional Healing, Avery Pub., Garden City, NY 1990.
Brewer, Gail, The Brewer Medical Diet for Normal and High Risk Pregnancies, Simon & Schuster, New York, 1983.

Understanding Ethnic Diets

Dietary counseling can be considerably enhanced if you have some ideas about good foods to suggest for dietary changes. Most traditional diets offer high quality foods choices and are an excellent way to direct a woman to eat well and at the same time support her in a manner that is culturally familiar.

Food choices from the Mexican-American diet:

Proteins	Meat (beef, pork, lamb, tripe, sausage [chorizo], bologna, bacon) poultry (chicken), eggs, legumes (Pinto Beans, Pink beans, Garbanzo beans, lentils), nuts (peanuts, peanut butter)
Dairy	Milk, cheese (Monterey Jack, Hoop, Muenster, Cheddar), ice cream
Grains	Rice; tortillas (corn, flour), oatmeal, dry cereals, noodles, bread
Vegetables	Avocado, Cabbage, Carrots, Chilies, Corn, Green beans, Lettuce, Onion, Peas, Potato, Prickly pear, Cactus leaf (nopales), Spinach, Sweet potato, Tomato, Zucchini
Fruit	Apple, Apricot, Banana, Guava, Lemon, Mango, Melon, Orange, Peach, Pear Prickly pear, Cactus fruit (tuna), Zapote (sapote)
Other	Salsa (tomato/pepper & onion relish), Chili sauce

Characteristic food choices of African-Americans:

Proteins	Meat (beef, pork, ham, sausage, pig's feet, ears, etc., bacon, luncheon meats, organ meats; poultry (chicken, turkey); fish (Catfish, Perch, Red Snapper, Tuna, Salmon, Sardines, Shrimp) Eggs, Legumes (kidney beans, red beans, pinto beans, black-eyed peas), Nuts (peanuts & peanut butter)
Dairy	Milk & Buttermilk; Cheese (Cheddar, Cottage), Ice cream (many African-Americans are lactose intolerant)
Grains	Rice, cornbread, hominy grits, biscuits, muffins, bread, dry cereal, cooked cereal, pasta, crackers
Vegetables	Broccoli, Cabbage, Carrots, Corn, Green beans, Greens (Mustard, Collards, Kale, Spinach, Turnip) Lima beans, Okra, Peas, Potato, Pumpkin, Sweet potato, Tomato, Yam
Fruits	Apple, Banana, Grapefruit, Grapes, Nectarine, Orange, Plums, Tangerine, Watermelon
Other	Salt pork (fat back), carbonated beverages, fruit juices, gravies

Food choices familiar to Chinese peoples:

Proteins	Meat (Pork, Beef, Organ meats), poultry (Chicken, Duck), fish (White fish, Shrimp, Lobster, Oysters, Sardines), Eggs, legumes (Soybeans, Tofu (bean curd), Black beans) nuts (peanuts, almonds, cashews)
Dairy	Milk, ice cream (many Oriental peoples are lactose intolerant)
Grains	Rice, noodles, bread, barley, millet
Vegetables	Bamboo shoots, Green & Yellow Beans, Bean sprouts, Bok choy, Broccoli, Cabbage, Carrots, Celery, Chinese cabbage, Corn, Cucumbers, Eggplant, Greens: Collards, Chinese broccoli, Mustard, Kale, Spinach, Leeks, Lettuce, Mushrooms, Peppers, Potato, Scallions, Snow peas, Sweet potato, Taro, Tomato, Water chestnuts, White radish, White turnip, Winter melon
Fruits	Apple, Banana, Fig, Grapes, Kumquat, Loquat, Mango, Melon, Orange, Peach, Pear, Persimmon, Pineapple, Plums, Tangerine
Other	Soy sauce, Sweet & sour sauce, Mustard sauce, Ginger, Plum sauce, Red bean paste, Black bean sauce, Oyster sauce

Characteristic Japanese food choices:

Proteins	Meat (Beef, Pork), poultry (Chicken, Turkey), fish (Tuna, Mackerel, Sardines, Sea bass, Shrimp, Abalone, Squid, Octopus), eggs, legumes: tofu (bean curd), Miso (soybean paste), Soybeans, Red beans (azuki), Lima beans; Nuts: Chestnuts (kuri)
Dairy	Milk, cheese, ice cream (many Japanese people are lactose intolerant)
Grains	Rice, rice crackers, noodles (soba), bread, oatmeal, dry cereal
Vegetables	Bamboo shoots, Bok Choy, Broccoli, Burdock root, Cabbage, Cauliflower, Celery, Cucumbers, Eggplant, Green beans, Gourd (kampyo), Mushrooms, Mustard greens, Napa cabbage, Peas, Peppers, Radishes (white, daikon, pickled), Snow peas, Spinach, Squash, Sweet potato, Taro (Japanese sweet potato), Tomato, Turnips, Water chestnuts, Yam
Fruits	Apple, Apricot, Banana, Cherries, Grapefruit, Grapes, Lemon, Lime, Melons, Orange, Peach, Pear, Persimmon, Pineapple, Pomegranate, Plums (dried, pickled plums called Umeboshi), Strawberries, Tangerine
Other	Soy sauce (tamari), Nori paste (seasoned rice), bead thread (knonyaku), Ginger

Characteristic food choices of Filipinos:

Protein	Meat (pork, beef, goat, deer, rabbit, variety meats) poultry (chicken) fish (Sole, Bonito, Herring, Tuna, Mackerel, crab, Mussels, shrimp, squid); eggs; legumes: Black beans, Chick peas, Black-eyed peas, Lentils, Mung beans, Lima beans, White kidney beans; nuts: cashews, peanuts, Pili nuts
Dairy products	Milk, cheese: Gouda, Cheddar
Grains	rice, cooked cereals (farina, oatmeal), dry cereals, pastas, rice noodles, wheat noodles, macaroni, spaghetti
Vegetables	Bamboo shoots, Beets, Cabbage, Carrots, Cauliflower, Celery, Chinese celery, Eggplant, Endive, Green beans, Leeks, Lettuce, Mushrooms, Okra, Onion, Peppers, Potato, Pumpkin, Radishes, Snow peas, Spinach, Squash, Sweet potato, Tomato, Water chestnuts, Watercress, Yam
Fruits	Apples, Banana, Grapes, Guava, Lemon, Lime, Mango, Melons, Orange, Papaya, Pear, Pineapple, Plums, Pomegranate, Rhubarb, Strawberries, Tangerine
Other	Soy sauce (tamari)

Reference:

Worthington, Bonnie, et. al., Nutrition in Pregnancy and Lactation, C.V. Mosby Co., St. Louis, MO, 1977.

Exercise Before and During Pregnancy

In general, exercise is a very beneficial activity. Aerobic exercise quickens the heart rate and breathing. Twenty minutes of aerobic exercise three times weekly reduces the incidence of heart disease and high blood pressure. It produces HDL, high density lipoproteins, which bind blood cholesterol, and leads to the production of endorphins. Exercise also helps prevent osteoporosis, since weight-bearing stress and movement encourages calcium and other minerals to deposit in the bones.

Intensive exercise can produce significant alterations in menstrual function. Some young women or girls may experience the delayed onset of menstruation. It may also cause amenorrhea or a shortened luteal phase. Physical and emotional stress, poor diet, altered hormonal secretion during exercise, weight loss and decreased percentage of body fat are possible contributing factors to persistently low levels of endogenous estrogen which can be associated with decreased bone mineral density. Common sense dictates that pregnant women should stop exercising when fatigued and not exercise to exhaustion.

Although there has been much rumored concern regarding the possible adverse effects of maternal exercise on the fetus, it appears that any temporary reduction in oxygen is well tolerated by the fetus. Maternal lactic acid levels do rise as the result of muscular fatigue and may cause the baby to be temporarily more active (therefore it is not such a good idea to exercise just before bedtime).

The American College of Obstetricians and Gynecologists has offered the following guidelines for exercise in pregnancy:

*After the first trimester, avoid any type of exercise that requires lying on the back. Lying on the back causes the uterus to occlude the inferior vena cava and laterally displaces the subrenal aorta. This results in the heart pumping less blood in most pregnant women, which can lead to reduced blood flow to the fetus. This can also cause supine hypotension (in 10% of women), shortness of breath or faintness in the mother as pregnancy advances.
*Avoid long periods of sitting still.
*Be prepared for body changes that may throw balance off, especially during the last trimester.
*Any exercise which involves the potential for even mild abdominal trauma should be avoided.
*Exercises which include the Valsalva maneuver (holding the breath and bearing down) should be avoided.
*Caloric intake must be adequate to meet the needs of the exercise as well as the pregnancy.
*Drink plenty of water while exercising and stop before becoming overheated. Pay attention to increasing salt intake appropriately to compensate for sodium loss via sweating.

Generally speaking, any exercise which a woman is accustomed to can be continued with attention to avoiding over-stressing herself and to maintaining a diet which adequately meets her protein and calorie needs. Obsessive concern regarding increased heart rate in a woman accustomed to the activity in question is not necessary, but she should be aware that activities which are normally well within her tolerance limits outside of pregnancy may produce muscle, tendon and ligament stress which can cause damage due to the tissue-softening effects of pregnancy hormones. She should be particularly alert to this possibility as pregnancy advances. Regardless of how accustomed to an activity a woman may be, she should immediately stop any activity which is causing unusual sensations or pain. In the event of bleeding, threatened pre-term labor, loose (incompetent) cervix or evidence of intrauterine growth retardation, activity levels should be carefully monitored until nutritional changes have gotten the problems under control.

Guidelines for a sensible exercise plan during pregnancy:

*Regular exercise (at least 3 times weekly) is preferable to intermittent activity, as it will allow the woman to gradually build her endurance and provide more uniform activity for her system.
*Competitive activities are discouraged.
*Vigorous exercise should not be performed during a fever, when the core body temperature is more easily raised.
*Ballistic (jerky) movements should be avoided, especially as pregnancy advances.
*Any activity which directly stresses the abdominal muscles (such as sit-ups) should be avoided as it will cause the enlarging uterus to put pressure on the abdominal muscles and weaken them, making it harder to regain tone postpartum.)
*Exercise should be performed on a wooden floor or a secure carpet to reduce shock and provide a sure footing.
*Activities requiring jumping, jarring motions or rapid changes in direction should be avoided due to joint instability, which increases as pregnancy advances. Such activities may also aggravate varicosities.
*Vigorous exercise should be proceeded by a five minute warm-up such as slow walking or stationary cycling at low resistance.
*Vigorous exercise should be followed by a period of gradually declining activity that includes gentle stretching.
*Stretching should not be done to maximum resistance due to the tissue relaxation which accompanies the hormonal changes of pregnancy.
*Care should be taken to rise from the floor gradually to avoid orthostatic hypotension. Some form of activity involving the legs

should be continued for a brief period.

*Women who have led sedentary lives should begin with physical activity of very low intensity and increase activity very gradually.

*If in doubt, walking and swimming are excellent exercises for just about anyone, regardless of their level of fitness.

Elizabeth Noble's excellent book <u>Essential Exercises for the Childbearing Year</u>, (Houghton Mifflin, 1983) can be recommended to women for complete information on exercise throughout pregnancy and the postpartum period.

Scuba diving: Of special note is the subject of scuba diving. The increased pressures of submersion have led to speculation that intravascular bubbles may form and obstruct fetal and placental blood flow following maternal decompression; animal studies support this theory. One survey of 208 divers showed a 5.5% rate of anomalies in diver's babies in contrast to no anomalies in the babies of women in a control group who refrained from diving. In spite of this, the study draws no absolute conclusions. However, it is recommended to advise women of the potential risks, limit the depth of dives to 60 feet and to limit the duration of time under water to one-half the limits of the U.S. Navy tables, as well as avoiding strenuous dives, hypoventilation and chilling. (Bolton, 1980)

Pelvic floor (Kegel) exercises: The pelvic floor dilates very quickly as the baby moves toward birth. This makes the pelvic muscles more vulnerable to damage if they are not properly toned. A healthy pelvic floor has both tone and elasticity, which encourage head flexion and stimulation of nerve receptors in the yoni.

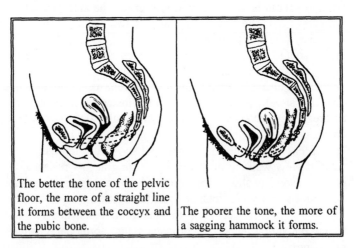

The better the tone of the pelvic floor, the more of a straight line it forms between the coccyx and the pubic bone.

The poorer the tone, the more of a sagging hammock it forms.

Rhythmic tightening and relaxing of the pelvic floor helps build strong, resilient muscles with good genital sphincter control. This, along with perineal stretching encourages elasticity. The muscles should be tightened progressively, layer by layer, in an attempt to exercise each muscle as individually as possible, and then released slowly. This exercise is known as "elevator" Kegels (after the doctor who devised it). Since the muscles are all connected, isolating individual muscles cannot be perfectly accomplished. However, the muscles will be better strengthened with elevator exercises than if simply tightened and relaxed.

Exercise should take place in cycles of 15. The muscles should not be held contracted for longer than five seconds at one time. Progress can be assessed at the toilet by starting and stopping the flow of urine. However, exercises should not be performed on a regular basis during urination, as this may increase the chances of urinary tract infection. Fifty contractions daily can significantly help tone the muscles. (adapted from Noble, 1982)

To isolate the muscles of the pelvic floor, the woman should relax all her other muscles (especially those of the legs and abdomen). The anal sphincter is the strongest muscle in the genital area; if a woman focuses on the muscles around the urethra and yoni instead, she has a much better chance of learning to differentiate them. The woman should note how her perineum feels when she is relaxing and try to exaggerate the relaxation into a bulge (pushing out); this is essentially the action needed for effective pushing. For many women, this instruction is difficult to grasp. Have her cough and note the response of her pelvic muscles as she does so, or imagine ejecting a tampon from her yoni, using only her muscles to assist her.

A woman can tune in to the sensation of involuntary bearing down by being aware of the peristaltic action of her colon when she has a bowel movement. Ask her to notice that her bowels are pushing, and that she can choose to bear down with them or not. The sensations associated with pushing are similar to this but much more intense, and the outward force is centered in the birth passage.

References and further reading

Abrams, Richard, Will It Hurt the Baby?, Addison-Wesley Pub. Co., Inc., 1990.

Bolton, M., "Scuba diving and fetal well-being: A survey of 208 women," Undersea Biomed. Res., Vol. 7, 1984, pp. 183-189.

"Exercise and Pregnancy," Special Delivery, Vol. 17, No. 2, Spring 1994, p. 3.

Noble, Elizabeth, Essential Exercises for the Childbearing Year, 2nd ed., Houghton Miffilin, Boston, MA, 1982.

Tobacco Smoking

You must decide how or even if you will work with women who smoke during their pregnancy, as the harmful effects are many and varied. Not only are there health risks directly incurred by the smoker, but the smoke which comes from the lighted cigarette and the smoke which is exhaled by the smoker can affect the health of anyone breathing the air. Therefore the non-smoking children and partners of smokers are at risk as well. Smoking adversely affects the fetus and newborn. The effects of smoking are lessened if the mother quits smoking before or during early pregnancy.

Cigarette smoke contains 68,000 toxic substances, including nicotine and hydrogen cyanide and toxic heavy metals such as lead and arsenic, all of which readily gain access to the mother's circulation and cross the placenta. Cyanide lowers the fetus's ability to use vitamin B_{12}, which is vital to protein production and the formation of red blood cells. Carbon monoxide, which is produced by cigarette smoke and car exhaust, rapidly enters the bloodstream, firmly attaching itself to red blood cells and preventing the uptake of oxygen. This causes the fetal hemoglobin to be artificially elevated. Carbon monoxide diffuses across the placenta, reaching levels in the fetus that may exceed its mother's by 10 to 15%. Studies show that babies of smokers have carbon monoxide levels that lead to approximately a 20% reduction in their blood levels of oxygen. Cases of birth defects and brain damage have been noted in laboratory animals when carbon monoxide levels are extremely high. It is felt that humans must be exposed to very high levels before these effects would occur; however, there is no known safe limit of carbon monoxide exposure.

Nicotine causes blood vessels to constrict, contributing to hypertension. The body elevates the blood pressure and the heart pumps faster in an effort to counteract the loss of blood volume. This, combined with the decrease in oxygen carrying capacity of the red cells, can lead to mild angina pectoris (chest pain on exertion). The rapid drop in uterine and placental blood flow caused by constriction of maternal vessels causes the baby's heart rate to rise in an effort to maintain oxygen levels. During ultrasound exams, maternal smoking has also been noted to decrease fetal breathing movements. Insufficient oxygen is dangerous for the fetus, especially during labor when the blood flow to the uterus is diminished during contractions.

Cholesterol and platelet adherent properties are both increased in smokers, making hardening of the arteries (arteriosclerosis) and clots more common, as well as aggravating platelet problems in women who have inadequate blood volume expansion. Smoking causes hormonal changes by speeding up the metabolism. Nicotine raises serum glucose and free fatty acid levels as well as elevating adrenal hormone levels; the stress hormones in the mother's and baby's bloodstreams. The nervous system is both stimulated and depressed by nicotine which can slow the transmission of neurologic signals.

Smoking is associated with decreased fetal weight, and an increased risk of miscarriage and stillbirth. In men it causes the sperm to be abnormally shaped. On the average, babies born to smokers are about half a pound lighter than those born to nonsmokers. From 18 weeks on, fetal head diameter is less than average. The more a woman smokes, the greater the reduction in newborn birth weight. However, if she quits by the fourth month the risk of a small-for-dates infant is much reduced. Please note that these studies do not take maternal nutrition into account. When women are truly well-nourished, many of these risks are substantially reduced (Brewer, 1983).

The risk of miscarriage, fetal and neonatal death, placental problems such as abruption, previa and bleeding, and premature rupture of membranes goes up with the number of cigarettes smoked. For example, miscarriages in women who smoke up to 10 cigarettes daily are 46% more common than in nonsmokers. The risk of fetal death or death in early infancy goes up by 20% for parents that smoke less than a pack per day and by 35% at over per pack a day.

During smoking, blood flow to the placenta is reduced, although the better women eat, the less the baby will suffer (Fox, 1991; Brewer, 1983). Acute constriction of maternal vessels beneath the placenta lasts up to 15 minutes after the cigarette is extinguished. A larger placenta relative to fetal weight forms when a woman smokes, probably as an adaption to compensate for fetal hypoxia. However, smokers' placentas are also lighter in weight and have fewer blood vessels than those of nonsmoking women. Smokers have more mineral deposits in their placentas, giving the surface a grainy texture. This mineralization causes the placental tissue to be more friable and decreases the amount of nutrient and oxygen exchange that can take place when coupled with inadequate maternal blood volume. Since mineralization of the placenta generally increases as pregnancy advances and a smoker's blood volume may not expand as much as a non-smoker's because of appetite suppression, smokers are at higher risk if they carry their pregnancies past their due date.

Data suggests that maternal smoking during pregnancy may also have long-term effects on the baby's growth and intellectual development. Small-for-dates infants may have difficulty maintaining body heat and electrolytes immediately after birth, and may have longstanding impairment of growth and intellectual functioning. Newborns of smokers are less responsive to sounds and less easily consoled by soothing sounds. At ages seven and eleven, the children of smoking mothers showed slight but definite lags in growth as well as poor reading and math test scores. Sudden infant death syndrome is increased as well. Older children living in smoking households are subject to more respiratory problems and infections than those in smoke-free households. Even passive smoke (the presence of smoke in the air being breathed) results in higher levels of nicotine metabolite in a child's blood. Childhood cancer risk is increased, especially for non-Hodgkin's lymphoma, acute lymphoblastic leukemia, and Wilm's tumor. In short, the bad news about smoking, both in and out of pregnancy, just keeps rolling in.

Helping women quit:

Smoking is an addiction and, as such, a hard habit to kick. Even though the initial cigarettes that one smokes may make one sick, smoking begins to feel pleasurable as these unpleasant symptoms of toxic intake subside. This is due to a release of endorphins, proteins named from a combination of the words "*endo*genous" (made in your body) and "mor*phine*." These neurotransmitters are produced in the pleasure center of the brain in response to recurrent painful or cell-damaging stimuli. Cigarette smokers literally get high from their habit. Moreover, special times of the day or certain events can become associated with smoking particular cigarettes, which is part of the psychological component of the addiction.

Many methods are used to quit smoking including tapes, programs, hypnosis, etc. I say, use anything that works! Here is one plan which can be used in its entirety or in parts to help a woman develop a program to quit before or during pregnancy. Obviously it makes sense for her to try and quit before conception, when the added stress of the pregnancy is not piled onto the physical and emotional stress of detoxifying from an addiction. Advise her to:

*Make a decision about when to quit. Set a date. This allows psychological adjustment in preparation for the big day.

*Make a 100% commitment to quitting. It is best if she commits because she wants to do it, not to please a relative or because it's best for the baby. If she does it for herself, she won't project anger to the baby or someone else for putting her through withdrawal. Feeling her feelings and telling the truth to herself about why she smokes will help in keeping her commitment. For ideas about how to get at the truth, see the chapter on Working Through Emotional Issues With Clients later in this section.

*Make an honest evaluation of the amount she smokes, when she smokes, and as much as she can get in touch with, why she smokes when she does. When reaching for a cigarette, first, have her close her eyes, breath into her chest and body and ask herself what she is feeling. She should notice any body sensations that arise, and ask herself what they are about. Body sensations are linked to emotions and smoking can effectively distract her from her feelings.

*Evaluate her support system, both professional (does she have a therapist?) and personal. Does she have a friend who is a former smoker that will agree to sponsoring her through the process; that is, agree to offer specific support such as being available for telephone calls or visits when things get rough?

While some people can quit cold turkey once they make up their mind to do so, many will benefit from a gradual program in which they eliminate one-quarter of their cigarettes each week for four weeks. This helps to minimize stress and cravings. She should save the elimination of "favorite" smokes for the last week, after she has three weeks of success behind her.

The good news is that quitting has an almost immediately beneficial effect on the pregnancy. Within 48 hours after stopping smoking, the mother's blood carries 8% more oxygen to the baby!

Dietary/supplemental and herbal suggestions: As smoking is eliminated, stored toxins in tissues and cells will begin to pour into the body. Drinking plenty of water will help the body eliminate them quickly.

Advise women to eat two large and varied servings of fresh vegetables daily. This will help to replace lost nutrients and add roughage so that the bowels can detoxify at their peak efficiency. Whole grains and legumes will help replace depleted B vitamins. Supplementation of B and C vitamins is helpful. Balanced 50 to 75 mg. B-complex tablets are available and 6 grams of C can be taken daily, with dosage built up over a period of a few days. If diarrhea occurs, a woman can cut back slightly on the amount of vitamin C, decreasing the intake in 500 mg. units until she has cut back to a dose her body can handle more easily. Zinc helps maintain healthy mucus membranes and if she has experienced a loss of taste or smell as a smoker, up to 50 mg. of zinc daily can help resolve these symptoms. Whole grains, nutritional yeast and pumpkin seeds are rich in zinc as well.

The amino acid tryptophan is a precursor to the neurotransmitter serotonin, which decreases anxiety and tension inherent during the detoxification process and encourages sleep. It is more optimally absorbed through the blood-brain barrier if taken with something sweet. Tryptophan is found naturally in milk and dairy products. Heating milk will help release its tryptophan and is why warm milk is a traditional aide to sleeping. Tryptophan is also an important precursor to endorphins which improve one's tolerance for pain. Supplemental tryptophan has been linked with some serious although rare side effects and has therefore been removed from the market. However, increasing dietary sources of tryptophan is helpful in the process of quitting an addiction.

Red Clover infusion and lemon juice can be used to detoxify the system. Chamomile, Valerian, and Skullcap infusions can be used safely during pregnancy to calm the nerves. Wintergreen infusion or St. John's Wort tincture can help relieve muscle tension.

Exercise: Light aerobic exercise such as bicycling, swimming or brisk walking are ideal ways of helping the body mobilize toxins. It also provides the body with a healthier stimulus to produce endorphins.

Acupressure points: The stimulation of various accupressure points can assist the body with detoxification. They should be firmly massaged with circular thumb pressure for about 30 seconds. Points should be worked on both the right and left sides of the body.

Large intestine 4: is a deep point located on the back of the hands, in the fleshy web area between the thumb and index finger. Called the Prime Eliminator, this point helps relieve headaches and other toxin related pains and helps in the production of endorphins. (Stimulation of this point is contraindicated during pregnancy.)

Large intestine 11: helpful in decreasing fatigue. It is located at the crease formed when you bend your elbow. Feel for it on the outside of the crease, slightly toward the hand on the inner forearm.

Liver 3: the Prime Detoxifier. It is used to ease headaches, tension, and fluctuations in energy that occur during detoxification. Find the point located at the junction of the first two toes at the top of the foot. Then place your thumb slightly upward from this site toward the ankle.

Triple heater 5: found three finger widths from the flexor (outer) surface of the wrist directly in line with the middle finger. This point balances the autonomic nervous system and helps relieve anxiety, tension, fatigue and depression.

Heart 7: known as the Divine Gate. Turn your palm up. It is at the wrist, near the protruding bone (pisiform) in line with the little finger. It relieves nervousness, depression and irritability.

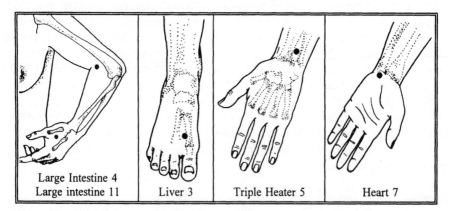

| Large Intestine 4 Large intestine 11 | Liver 3 | Triple Heater 5 | Heart 7 |

Adrenal gland balancing: these points are found one inch to either side of, and then measure one inch above, the umbilicus. These sympathetic drainage points help rid the body of toxins.

Replacing the habit: Since smoking is often a dysfunctional way of attempting to nurture the self, quitting often brings up a sense of loss. It may be important for women to substitute the ritual of smoking with an alternative "thing to do" at those times when a cigarette was the most satisfying. Reading a good book, calling a loved one, taking a hot bath, getting a massage now and then, listening to music and allowing herself to feel her feelings are just a few of the ways that she can reward herself without having to smoke.

Emotional aspects of smoking: Smoking literally sets up a screen between the smoker and other people. It densifies the auric field (psychic space around a person) thus insulating her from the emotional currents in the environment. It also allows her to "stuff" her own emotions, since smoking influences how she breathes, and the breath is very tied into emotional expression. Being aware of these aspects of smoking's "benefits" can help women cope with the emotions which come up during the quitting process.

What if she won't quit?

You must decide if you will work with women who refuse, for whatever reasons, to quit. Having women cut back to 5 cigarettes a day or less could be a goal to shoot for, or smoking only half a cigarette, then putting it out. (The closer one smokes a cigarette down to the butt, the more tar and nicotine become concentrated in the remaining tobacco.) Changing to a brand with less tar may be helpful, as well as watching to see which cigarettes she can most easily eliminate during the day.

If you do choose to work with women who smoke, keep in mind that good nutrition is of paramount importance for pregnant smokers. Part of the problem with smoking is that it dampens the appetite by raising the blood sugar and women will automatically eat less than they need if this is not specifically explained to them. Tom Brewer found that even smokers had babies of adequate weight when the mothers ate an adequate diet (Brewer, 1983).

References and further reading:
Abrams, Richard, Will It Hurt the Baby?, Addison Wesley Pub. Co., Inc., 1990.
Anfang, K., "Before Pregnancy: Help to Quit Cigarettes and Caffeine," Mothering, Summer, 1987, No. 44, pp. 63-68.
Brewer, Gail, The Brewer Medical Diet for Normal and High Risk Pregnancy, Simon & Schuster, New York, NY, 1983.
Enkin, Murray, "Smoking and Pregnancy—A New Look," Birth, Vol. 11, No. 4, Winter, 1984, pp. 225-229
Fox, H., "A contemporary view of the human placenta," Midwifery, Vol. 7, 1991, pp. 31-9.
Samuels, Mike & Samuels, N., The Well-Pregnancy Book, Summit Books, New York, NY, 1986, pp. 125-27

Caffeine and Pregnancy

Caffeine, theobromine, and theophylline are substances found in coffee, black tea, many cola drinks and chocolate. They are all central nervous system stimulants and stressors. They commonly cause anxiety, restlessness, diarrhea, headaches and heartburn, and are implicated in ulcer formation. They also speed metabolic rate, thought, and reaction time, thus aiding concentration. However, they impair the ability to perform skills that require delicate coordination and accurate timing. In large doses these substances cause insomnia, tremor, and tinnitus (ringing in the ears).

To give you an idea of where caffeine comes from in our typical diets, here is a list of some common sources:

Food or Drug	Amount	Caffeine (mg.)
Decaffeinated coffee	1 cup	2
Instant coffee	1 cup	66
Percolated coffee	1 cup	110
Tab	12 oz.	44
Dr. Pepper	12 oz.	38
Pepsi-Cola	12 oz.	37
Coca-Cola	12 oz.	34
Mountain Dew	12 oz.	52
Cocoa drink	12 oz.	10
Milk chocolate	1 oz.	6
Dark chocolate	1 oz.	20
Black tea brewed 12 min.	1 tea bag	40
Black tea bag brewed 5 min.	1 tea bag	21
Iced tea	12 oz.	36
NoDoz	1 tablet	200
Anacin	1 tablet	64
Excedrin	1 tablet	130
Dristan	1 tablet	32
Sinarest	1 tablet	30
Dexatrim	1 tablet	200

Caffeine produces biochemical changes characteristic of a stressful situation or emergency. When faced with stress, the adrenal glands secrete the hormone epinephrine, which increases alertness, shunts blood away from the digestive system toward the muscles, and creates an "all systems go" status which prepares the body for immediate action—the fight or flight response. During the initial stage of this response, the body responds by increasing hormonal production. Next, the adrenal glands enlarge as the body actively resists illness. If the stress is prolonged, the adrenal glands eventually become exhausted, producing great fatigue, chronic illness and symptoms that are difficult to heal spontaneously. Immune function is further impaired by caffeine's ability to decrease the production of mast cells, the white blood cells that specialize in fighting allergens, drugs and toxins.

Caffeine also affects smooth and cardiac muscles, causing an increase in the strength and frequency of cardiac contractions, and has been implicated in causing the irregular beats in cardiac arrhythmia. Caffeine intake is implicated in fibrocystic breast disease; withdrawal has been directly related to a reduction in the size and pain of breast lumps. In addition, it is suspected that caffeine intake may be linked to bladder and pancreatic cancer and to heart attack.

Caffeine may hinder the repair of genetic material. Laboratory animals have a higher rate of birth defects when given large doses. Caffeine crosses the placenta and attains higher levels in the fetal bloodstream than in that of the mother. This is partly because the fetal liver is unable to process caffeine as quickly as the mother's, so caffeine tends to remain in the baby's system for longer periods of time. Caffeine also remains in the pregnant woman's bloodstream much longer than if she were not pregnant. One study correlated very high maternal levels (600 ml. daily or 4 strong cups of coffee) with an increase in fetal death, although other studies have not confirmed this finding. (Samuels, 1986)

Caffeine can also cross into the breastmilk. Its half-life (the rate at which half a dose is neutralized) may be as long as 18 to 20 days in pregnant women, and three to four days in newborns. As a result, caffeine stimulates the nervous system of both mother and newborn for a prolonged period of time.

Caffeine in all forms should be eliminated from the diet during pregnancy. Caffeine consumption can be a hard habit to break; as with cigarettes, it stimulates the production of endorphins. (See chapter on Tobacco Smoking for more details). To assist women in quitting caffeine, you can recommend switching to a Swiss water processed decaffeinated coffee. This process decaffeinates the beans without the use of chemicals (many decaffeination processes use very harsh chemicals). Women can also drink herbal tea, or grain-based coffee substitutes such as Pero or Postum. A plan for quitting caffeine for the more seriously addicted can be formulated using the recommendations outlined in the last chapter for quitting smoking.

References and further reading:

Anfang, K., "Before Pregnancy: Help to Quit Cigarettes and Caffeine," Mothering, Summer, 1987, No. 44, pp. 63-68.
Samuels, Mike & Samuels, N., The Well-Pregnancy Book, Summit Books, New York, NY, 1986, p. 127-29.

Alcohol and Pregnancy

The suspicion that alcohol has an adverse effect on the developing fetus has been with us since ancient times. It was not until 1973, however, that these observations were formally compiled and a clinical term was coined for the characteristic anomalies seen in the offspring of alcoholic mothers: Fetal Alcohol Syndrome (FAS). The amount of alcohol consumed has some bearing on the degree of fetal physical damage it can produce.

MEDICAL CLASSIFICATION OF ALCOHOL CONSUMPTION	
Heavy drinker	More than 45 drinks monthly or more than 5 drinks per occasion
Moderate drinker	1 to 45 drinks monthly, never more than 5 drinks per occasion
Light or rare drinker	Less than 1 drink monthly
One drink is equal to 0.5 ounces of alcohol or *One beer *4 ounces of wine *1.2 ounces of liquor	

Heavy maternal drinking has been associated with an increased rate of the following pregnancy and newborn problems:
*Spontaneous abortion
*Low-birth-weight babies
*Children with learning disabilities
*Infant mortality
*Birth defects known collectively as Fetal Alcohol Syndrome

Ethanol (ethyl alcohol) in its pure form is obtained from fermented grain. Ethanol freely crosses the placenta, however it is not known if it, or acetaldehyde, the breakdown product of alcohol, is cytotoxic and teratogenic at blood levels over 35 μmol/l. Although blood levels in healthy people do not usually exceed 30 μmol/l after alcohol ingestion, those with an inherited or acquired defect of mitochondrial aldehyde dehydrogenase have acetaldehyde levels well over the danger limits even after moderate alcohol intake. This may explain why some women who drink very little have effected babies while others who are heavy drinkers may have perfectly normal babies. The mechanism of damage may also be related to anoxia or to maternal physiological changes peculiar to pregnancy. Most studies suggest that structural damage to the fetus occurs during the first trimester. However other studies show that decreasing alcohol consumption during the third trimester lowers the risk to the baby. This suggests that reducing alcohol consumption enhances the fetus' ability to catch up in its growth, since late pregnancy is when adverse factors have the greatest impact on fetal growth.

Overall, about 43% of the babies born to women who are alcoholic during pregnancy will be affected to some degree. Consumption of more than 3 ounces of absolute alcohol per day around the time of conception greatly increases the risk of fetal damage; there is, however, no minimal level of safety. The most severely affected children have Fetal Alcohol Syndrome (FAS), which manifests with at least one feature from each of the following three criteria:

1. Prenatal or postnatal growth in the child's weight or head circumference is delayed.
2. Certain physical characteristics are present. There is a pattern of abnormal features of the face and head, including at least two of the following: small head, small eyes or short eye openings, a narrow lip without center groove, short upturned nose or flattened midfacial area. Males may also have abnormal testes.
3. Abnormalities of the central nervous system, with signs of brain dysfunction, delays in behavioral development, and/or cognitive impairment.

Those with less severe manifestations of FAS are said to have Fetal Alcohol Effect (FAE). FAE can encompass a wide range of problems such as eye and heart defects, impairment of the lungs, kidneys and other organs, slowed growth, musculoskeletal defects, and behavioral problems such as hyperactivity and extreme irritability. Mental retardation is the most serious and damaging of all alcohol-related birth defects. Other problems have been noted but occur unpredictably—not all characteristics are present in every affected child.

Even very low amounts of alcohol consumption in any given month of pregnancy significantly raise the risk of miscarriage. The odds of spontaneous abortion rise 3% with each additional day alcohol is consumed, beginning with as little as one drink. For women who drink daily, the odds of miscarriage are 2.58 times greater than for the woman who neither drinks nor smokes. For women who drink and smoke a pack of cigarettes daily, the odds of spontaneous abortion go up 4.08 times over that of nonsmoking, nondrinking mothers.

Women should be informed of the risks of drinking alcohol during pregnancy. Risks seem to increase with the amount a woman drinks: babies have about a 10% risk of defects if their mother drinks more than 1 ounce (30 ml.) daily or five or more drinks at once, and a 20% risk if mothers drink more than 2 ounces (50 ml.) per day. Moderate drinking seems less likely to produce visible defects, but these babies still weigh an average of 3 ounces less than those of non-drinking mothers and other symptoms such as tremors and poor neurological response are more common. Lower arousal and slower learning characteristics have also been noted in babies of moderate drinkers. Some researchers believe that "binging" (infrequent but heavy drinking) may have as serious an impact as sustained drinking. Babies of mothers who drink small amounts may show even more subtle effects, but studies indicate that there is no apparent difference between these babies

276

and those of women who do not drink at all. Nevertheless it should be emphasized that there is no known minimum amount of alcohol consumption that can be declared absolutely safe for all pregnant women. If a woman drinks occasionally prior to conception she need not be concerned, but she should avoid all alcohol during the pregnancy to minimize the potential effects on the baby. Women should also be told that stopping consumption at any point during pregnancy may have beneficial results for the fetus.

References and further reading:

Lindor, Elena, et.al., "Fetal Alcohol Syndrome: A review and Case Presentation," JOGN Nursing, July/August, 1980, Vol. 9, p. 222-28.
Samuels, Mike & Samuels, N., The Well-Pregnancy Book, Summit Books, New York, NY, 1986, p. 125-27.

Public Water Supplies

Water makes up approximately 79% of the human body, and it is involved in almost all bodily processes. Clean water is vital to our overall health and well-being. Whenever it is economically feasible, encourage women to purchase a good quality water filter for the tap which they use most often for drinking and cooking (the kitchen is the usual choice) or steam distilled bottled water.

Water is called "hard" when it has a high mineral content, (principally calcium and magnesium). It prevents soap from lathering and deposits a film of sediment on hair, clothing, pipes, dishes and wash tubs. The calcium in hard water can form mineral deposits in the body. Hard water may be treated with sodium to remove the minerals. Soft water may naturally lack calcium and/or magnesium. Artificially softened water tends to dissolve pipe linings. This is obviously a significant threat where lead pipes are used, but plastic and galvanized pipes contain cadmium, posing another risk of toxic poisoning, and copper pipes leach iron, zinc and arsenic; more leaching occurs when soft water is used.

The quality of tap water varies tremendously from city to city. Just because water is clear does not mean it is free of contaminants. Tap water is generally obtained from surface water which runs into a reservoir from ponds, creeks, etc. Rainwater can contain pollutants such as chemical fertilizers and lead from automobile exhaust. Chemicals such as chlorine, carbon, fluorine, lime, phosphates, soda ash, and sodium aluminates are added to kill bacteria during the water treatment process in some areas, while other municipalities do not filter their water or treat it in any way. Calling the local water quality control can help in determining the quality of water in a particular area.

There are 2,100 contaminants which have been identified in public drinking water, but only 89 of these are regulated. Even so, 43% of water supplies are in violation of federal health standards. Out of date equipment, water-borne diseases from raw sewage, organic and inorganic chemical contaminants, pesticides, leakage from underground hazardous waste sites, toxic metals and radioactive particles are among the major problems.

One of the worst and most prevalent contaminants is lead. Estimates are that 98% of the houses in the United States have lead in their plumbing; homes less than 5 years old or greater than 20 years old are at greatest risk. The amount of lead that these pipes leach into the water is determined by how soft and how hot the water. Use only cold tap water for any cooking or drinking purposes and allow the water to run for 30 to 60 seconds before using it first thing in the morning or whenever it has been standing in pipes for awhile will significantly reduce lead contamination. (More on lead poisoning can be found in Diagnostic Tests).

Chemicals such a chorine and fluoride are added to the city water supply in many areas. Chlorine, which is added for the purpose of disinfection, has been linked to increased risks for bladder and rectal cancer. Chlorine interacts with certain organic materials in river water to produce byproducts such as trilalomethanes, which produce cancer in animals. Results of studies done by the Centers for Disease Control and the New Jersey Department of Health which examine the link between chlorine treatment and birth defects are inconclusive, however, higher levels of trihalomethanes have been found in water supplies of women whose babies had increased rates of birth defects and lower birth weights. (U.S. Water News) An alternative treatment is the use of other chemicals, such as chloramine (a combination of ammonia and chlorine), which also kills bacteria but is less likely to produce toxic byproducts. (Maugh, 1992)

Companies which produce bottled water may or may not provide a better alternative. Water is classified in a variety of ways and, due to a lack of strict regulation, labeling or claims can be misleading. Some bottled water is simply local tap water. Many of the toxins to be concerned about are not checked, and federal restrictions of bottled water are no stricter than they are for public water supplies. Bottled water from underground sources may also be contaminated, just as public water supplies have been. Check carefully with local water suppliers to discover what their standards are before ordering bottled water. Try to get it delivered in glass bottles, as some of the large plastic bottles used for home delivery leach methylene chloride, a known carcinogen, into the water.

Bottled steam distilled water is best for ensuring that the water you are buying is indeed contaminant-free (steam distillers can also be purchased for home use). For those who wish to invest in a water filter, the following questions can help evaluate the units being considered:

1. What is the filtration technology used?

Activated carbon is the most effective substance known for removing chemicals from water, and should serve as the primary filtering medium.

2. If the unit contains activated carbon, in what form is the carbon?

Most units use granular activated carbon (GAC) because the granular form is the least expensive and the easiest to obtain. The problem with granular or powdered carbon is that water forms a channel around the carbon and does not have sufficient contact time for removal of most contaminants. Units that have less than one pound of carbon are minimally effective. The larger, more effective units have 20 or more ounces of carbon; but even they will not remove lead or asbestos, and are only partially effective at removing chemicals. GAC units are usually classified as "taste and odor" filters.

The most effective form of carbon is a solid carbon block, which is so densely compacted that the problem of "channeling" does not occur. Most units can filter particles down to submicron levels. Look for a filter with over one pound of carbon that actually screws into the housing of the unit. This unit will remove lead, asbestos fibers, organic chemicals, giardia, pesticides, trihalomethanes and chlorine. "Bacteriostatic" units that contain silver are not recommended. The silver is a health risk and has not been proven effective.

3. Has the unit been tested by the National Science Foundation (NSF)? If yes, ask to see copies of the results.

The NSF is a not-for-profit independent testing organization that conducts very specific laboratory tests on water purification systems. For a unit that will protect from a wide variety of contaminants look for:

Aesthetic effects (NSF standards # 42)- Class 1 rating
Particulate removal down to submicron- Class 1 rating

Health effects (NSF standard #53):
Removal of volatile organic chemicals (VOC) at 95%+ reduction
Removal of Trihalomethanes at 95%+ reduction
Removal of lindane (pesticide) at 95%+ reduction
Removal of lead at 95%+ reduction
Removal of cysts like Giardia at 99%+ reduction

4. What is the size and construction of the unit?

Small faucet mounted units and pour-through units are virtually worthless. The most effective units are larger in size and have replaceable filter cartridges.

5. What is the warranty, and is there a 30 day money back guarantee?

The best units offer a five to ten year warranty and a money back guarantee.

6. What is the cost of the unit including the cost and availability of replacement filters?

A good unit will last a lifetime so $300 to $400 dollars is a fair price. Make sure the company has been in business for several years and is reputable and offers an easy way to purchase replacement filters at a reasonable price ($35 to $45 dollars is a good price for a replacement filter that lasts about 1 year).

One filter system which meets these standards is made by the Multi-Pure Corporation, P.O. Box 4179, Chatsworth, CA 91313-4179 (818) 341-7577 or (800) 622-9206. The standard Multi-Pure filter does not remove fluoride, but one which will do so is available upon special order. For other good filter mechanisms consult your naturopath, chiropractor or local health food store.

References and further reading:

Balch, J., & Balch, P., Prescription for Nutritional Healing, Avery Pub., Garden City, NY, 1990.
Hales, Dianne, "The Silent Health Threat to Children," Family Circle, 8/11/92, pp. 73-78.
Maugh, Thomas, "Experts Downplay Cancer Risk of Chlorinated Water," Los Angles Times, Thursday, July 2, 1992.
Snider, Make, "Fluid intake linked to bladder cancer," USA TODAY, Friday, July 9, 1993.
U.S. Water News, "Birth Defects tied to water," March, 1993.

280

Fluoride

The mineral fluorine is widespread throughout nature, and a small intake of this natural element is practically unavoidable. Fluorine occurs in the body in compounds of calcium fluoride. Sodium fluoride, on the other hand, is an industrial waste byproduct of aluminum and phosphate production, the manufacture of which grew considerably in the 1920s and 30s. At that time fluoride pollution of air from such factories damaged the crops, wildlife and livestock in surrounding areas. Lawsuits and health officials forced the companies to install pollution control devices to trap fluoride waste, which shifted the problem from airborne to solid poisons which had to be disposed of. The companies began to sell sodium fluoride as rat and insect poison; later on it was marketed as a product to prevent tooth decay.

Fluorides are protoplasmic poisons: they have the capacity to modify the metabolism of cells by changing the permeability of cell membranes and by inhibiting certain enzyme systems. (Enzymes are proteins found in all body cells which are responsible for triggering the chemical reactions which make life possible.) Fluoride can also disrupt the hydrogen bonds in amides (proteins), which can lead to DNA molecule disruption. Dr. Ionel Rapaport's research suggests that there is a direct relationship between the incidence of Down syndrome and fluoridated drinking water in areas where fluoride concentrations in the water supply is such that discolored teeth result. (Prevention, 1981)

Fluoride disrupts collagen synthesis. Collagen is a form of protein which acts as cellular "glue" and is the primary substance which attaches the placenta to the uterine wall. Fluoride also interferes with the body's ability to discriminate which collagen to mineralize, (a process which normally only occurs in bones and teeth). Soft tissue mineralization in muscles, ligaments, arteries, etc. starts to occur when the body is exposed to fluoride. Disruption also occurs in normally mineralized tissues. Large amounts of fluoride can lead to mottling of the dental enamel (called dental fluorosis) as well as weakness in the tooth's structure, especially in anyone who is undernourished. Damage to collagen production in the bones can interfere with the normal processes of bone rejuvenation and repair throughout life.

Fluoride affects the immune system by rendering it less able to differentiate foreign matter from the body's own tissues. This causes the immune system to attack its own cells, leading to skin rashes and gastrointestinal disorders. It also inhibits the movement of white blood cells towards foreign matter. Dr. Tateki Tsutsui of the Nippon Dental College of Japan has found that fluoride not only causes genetic damage but is also capable of transforming normal cells into cancer cells (Yiamouyiannis, 1983, p. 57). Other studies have confirmed this finding.

Most of these adverse effects were well recognized before fluoride was being touted as a "cure" for cavities. Both the September 18, 1943 issue of the Journal of the American Medical Association and the October 1, 1944 issue of the

American Dental Association (ADA) carried articles outlining the dangers of fluoride in the environment. The ADA article focused on the risk/benefit ratio for its use as a decay preventative and concluded that the *risk was too great.* However thanks to the promotional efforts of Dr. Gerald Cox of the Mellon Institute (which owns the Aluminum Company of America) in concert with the American Dental Association, the fluoridation of public water supplies "to reduce tooth decay," became a reality in many cities. This was done using data from studies of dubious value, some of which contained erroneous conclusions, which was later admitted by the researchers. (Yiamouyiannis, 1983, p. 101-37)

While the affects already discussed above occur in everyone exposed to fluoride on a subclinical level, there are additional clinical symptoms which may appear in some persons exposed to fluoride in their air, water, toothpaste or at the dentist's office. For example, fluoridated toothpaste contains 1,000 parts per million fluoride, which is enough to kill a 20 pound child if an entire 7 ounce tube is consumed. Other sources of significantly high levels include fluoride mouth rinses and gels used in dental offices. Less common sources of fluoride exposure occur in those who live or work near fluoride-emitting factories such as those producing aluminum, phosphate, steel and frit (the glassy substance used to coat the inside of ovens). These symptoms are as follows:

Black tar-like stools	Unusual excitement
Bloody vomit	Unusual increase in saliva
Diarrhea	Infertility
Faintness	Watery eyes
Nausea and vomiting	Weakness
Shallow breathing	Constipation
Stomach cramps or pain	Loss of appetite
Tremors	Stiffness, pain and aching of bones
Weight loss	Skin rashes
White, brown or black discoloration of teeth	Mouth and lip sores
Reduced thyroid activity	Headaches

It should be obvious that fluoride may not be the best thing to give pregnant women or newborns in the form of infant vitamin drops. Advise women to avoid all fluoride-containing dental hygiene products (toothpaste, mouth wash, etc.) and ask that fluoride not be used when they go to the dentist. This is especially important for anyone who exhibits symptoms suggestive of hypersensitivity to the toxic effects of fluoride.

References and further reading:

Prevention mag. staff, The Complete Book of Minerals for Health, Rodale Press, Emmaus, PA, 1981, pp. 367-370.

Yiamouyiannis, John, Fluoride: The Aging Factor, Health Action Press, 6439 Taggart Rd., Delaware, OH 43015, 1983.

Over-the-Counter Drugs

All substances reach the fetus via the placenta, primarily by passive diffusion across the placental surface. Absorption of a drug is influenced by its fat solubility, ionization, molecular weight and its ability to bind with protein molecules. Absorption of some types of drugs may be delayed due to reduced gastrointestinal mobility, a factor which is primarily important only during labor. Placental pathology such as infarcts (dead areas) and the stage of gestation also impact drug transfer. In most cases it is not understood how the placenta processes drugs before they reach the fetus. Fetal excretion of drugs primarily occurs via the placenta; since the fetus swallows amniotic fluid which contains drug-laden fetal urine, the fetus is exposed to additional amounts.

A **teratogenic (tear-ROT-ah-gin-ick)** agent is one which causes defects or malformations in the embryo. Most teratogenic agents can affect the human embryo only during a short time period, which has elapsed by the eighth week of pregnancy. There is little information concerning the effects of drugs on fetal development from the fifth week on, and the earliest possible teratogenic susceptibility is not known. By 4 to 5 weeks post-conception, cord blood circulation allows drugs to reach the fetus in higher concentrations than earlier in pregnancy. While most of the fetal organs are formed by 8 weeks, the genital tract and nervous system in particular are susceptible to damage throughout the first 4 to 5 months of gestation. Damage *may* occur at any time.

There are between 100,000 and 500,000 over-the-counter products which contain about 200 active ingredients. Single products may contain 1 to 11 substances. No trials or testing protocols are required for these substances. There are many over-the-counter products; an over-the-counter Physician's Desk Reference (PDR) can help you determine if any studies have been done on the remedies that are available. Some of the most common ingredients of over-the-counter agents and their possible effects are described below:

Acetaminophen (Tylenol): Acetaminophen is generally considered the best alternative for pharmacological relief of pain during pregnancy, if taken as recommended. Note that it is a drug which taxes liver function and should be used only when necessary. Ibuprofin and other aduil-based drugs should be entirely avoided; they severely disrupt blood clotting and tax the kidneys.

Acetylsalicylic acid (Aspirin): Salicylates used near term are associated with prolonged gestation, longer labor and increased maternal blood loss at birth. A higher incidence of stillbirth has also been noted. Infants may show increased bleeding times, jaundice, premature closure of the ductus arteriosus, intracranial hemorrhage, cephalhematoma and melena. Significant reductions in intelligence and attention span have been noted in aspirin-exposed children. Aspirin should be avoided throughout pregnancy.

Antacids: No teratogenic effects have been noted, however antacids neutralize natural stomach acids, thus arresting digestion. (See the chapter on Bowel and Digestive Difficulties in the section on Problems That Can Occur at Any Time for more information on the use of antacids.)

Antihistamines: Atropine sulfate is associated with skeletal anomalies in mice, however, there has been no evidence of this in humans. (See anti-nausea drugs below).

Decongestants: Most of these drugs also contain antihistamines. Epinephrine and phenylpropanolamine are both associated with an increased risk of birth defects. Brompheniramine (in Dimetane, Dimetapp, and Drixoral) is associated with a three-fold increase in birth defects in the first trimester and should be avoided. Pseudoephedrine plus triprolidine (Actifed) or pseudoephedrine plus chlorpheniramine (Chlortrimeton or Sudafed Plus) are recommended instead. One of the most widely studied decongestants is Meclizine, which has been shown to be relatively safe.

Anti-nausea drugs: Antihistamines are used to control nausea in pregnancy by mainstream medical providers. Unisom is an over-the-counter antihistamine drug that contains the same agent as Bendectin, a prescription drug removed from the market due to its alleged association with birth defects. The drug companies have down-played the possible connection between Bendectin and fetal damage. Since its removal from the market, some care providers have recommended that women take 25 mg. of Unisom and 25 mg. of vitamin B_6 to control nausea, as this approximates the Bendectin formula. Women should be aware of the possibility of birth defects linked to Bendectin use when deciding to follow this advice.

Folic acid: Inadequate folic acid intake has been shown to increase the risk of neural tube defects. Supplementation may lower serum levels of phenytoin, a prescription drug used for seizure control; blood levels of phenytoin should be followed in women taking this medication and folic acid concurrently.

Iodine: Iodine douches are contraindicated in pregnancy due to easy absorption through the walls of the yoni.

Vitamin A: Excessive vitamin A in the form of retinol (10 mg. or more) can cause malformation of the urogenital tract and central nervous system in early pregnancy. 13-cis-retinoic acid (isotretinoin, Accutane) and its analogue etretinate are synthetic forms of vitamin A used for severe acne and psoriasis. Exposed fetuses have developed small or absent ears, neurologic injuries, cardiac defects and facial malformations; use is contraindicated throughout pregnancy.

Advising women regarding remedies in pregnancy: Whenever a woman asks about taking an over-the-counter preparation, first find out if she is willing to try herbal, homeopathic, Chinese or vitamin therapy for her problem (given your knowledge in these areas and/or the resources available in your community). If she is, recommend appropriate remedies and ask her to keep in touch with you about her progress, especially if she notes no improvement. If she does not want to try non-bio-technical remedies and her condition seems manageable, steer her toward the least noxious bio-technical remedies you can find. Additionally, suggest measures she can take to increase her comfort such as rest, warm drinks, hot baths or other appropriate actions.

If symptoms are severe, consider getting the condition evaluated by a specialist. Referral to an obstetrician, nurse-midwife or naturopath may be appropriate. However, if you feel she has a severe condition which may directly impact her or her baby's health, or that her condition could rapidly turn into a more serious problem, have her evaluated by someone who has expertise in the condition in question.

Recreational Drugs

The use of any "recreational" drugs must be considered with every client, no matter how straight they appear to be. Many upper middle class people use cocaine and some use other drugs as well. Women may assume that occasional or rare use will have no impact on their health or their pregnancy and may therefore fail to tell you unless you ask specifically. It is important to ask open-ended questions in a nonjudgemental manner to elicit the truth from women. If the woman is poorly educated or if for any reason you feel it is warranted, ask her about each specific drug and do not hesitate to use street terms such as crack (cocaine), smack (heroin), and acid (LSD) etc. to find out if she is a user.

Amphetamines (speed): These drugs are central nervous system stimulants that may be snorted, taken orally, or injected. Exposed infants have shown cardiac abnormalities, exencephaly, microcephaly, biliary atresia and withdrawal syndrome. Since use of these drugs is not recorded, there are no studies that accurately reflect risk.

Angel dust, PCP (Phencyclidine): This drug is ingested, taken in intravenous injections or dusted on marijuana joints. Its use during pregnancy has been associated with infants who have extreme sensitivity to touch and environmental sounds, increased muscle tone, tremulousness, and occasional darting eye movements. At two years of age, exposed children commonly exhibit low-normal scores in fine motor, adaptive, and language areas of development. One case of a pregnancy which involved various congenital malformations in the fetus has been documented.

Cocaine: This central nervous system stimulant is highly addictive. It is snorted or injected, or is absorbed in the mouth, rectum or yoni. It is often smoked (free based) in its free alkaloid form, for which the street term is crack. It has a half-life in plasma of about 1 hour, making it a short-acting drug. It produces a rapid euphoria which diminishes in 30 minutes, meaning users are likely to take many doses in quick succession, thus repeatedly exposing the fetus.

Cocaine causes an increase in heart rate, blood pressure and body temperature. It blocks the uptake of catecholamines and sensitizes tissues to their action. Acute heart attack, arrhythmias, seizures, rupture of the aorta and sudden death have all been seen, and anorexia and weight loss are common with chronic use. Pregnant cocaine users are more likely to have spontaneous abortions. Late pregnancy use of cocaine has been reported to induce sudden strong contractions, fetal tachycardia and excessive fetal activity within hours or minutes of ingestion. Abruption of the placenta is also more common. Cocaine's teratogenic effects are not conclusively known at this time. Infants may be shorter, with low-birth-weight and a smaller head circumference. While tremors and irritability are common

286

symptoms assumed to be cocaine related, there is speculation that other variables such as poor maternal nutrition, smoking, alcohol use, and disease exposure may be the major factor contributing to these symptoms. Isolating cocaine use from these factors, which are often present in users, is nearly impossible (Lang, 1992).

Lysergic acid diethylamide (LSD, Acid, Windowpane): This drug can cause hallucinations, paranoia, flashbacks, rapid heart rate, abnormal heart rhythms and a variety of other effects due either to the drug itself or to added impurities such as amphetamines. Although LSD was highly publicized in the 1960s to cause severe birth defects, no clear correlation has ever been proven. There is anecdotal evidence that LSD can enter the breastmilk. LSD should be avoided throughout pregnancy and breastfeeding.

Marijuana: THC (delta-9-tetrahydrocannabinol), the active ingredient in marijuana, has a high affinity for lipids and accumulates in fatty tissues throughout the body, including the brain. Smoking marijuana exposes one to all the dangerous agents found in tobacco but in much higher concentrations. A single dose of cannabis in humans takes as long as 30 days to be excreted, with a half-life in tissues of about 7 days. No data is available on fetal effects. Regular use may be related to low-birth-weight babies; however occasional use does not seem to cause this problem. (See the chapter on Tobacco Smoking in this section for information about how inhaled substances cross the placenta.)

Opiates (Heroin and Methadone): Heroin addicts frequently have irregular menses, amenorrhea and subfertility. Pregnancy usually occurs during withdrawal periods or with irregular use. Maternal risk is related to overdose and septic complications; those who share needles risk contracting hepatitis, syphilis and HIV. Heroin crosses the placenta rapidly and enters the fetus within an hour of administration. Maternal withdrawal causes fetal withdrawal and the risk of intrauterine demise.

Prenatal exposure causes low-birth-weight, impaired growth and behavior, and impaired perceptual and organizational abilities that persist into childhood. Infant withdrawal usually begins within the first two days of life, although it may be delayed until the end of the first week. Hyperactivity, respiratory distress, fever, diarrhea, mucous secretion, sweating, convulsions yawning and face scratching characterize withdrawal in newborns. There is a five to ten-fold increased risk of sudden infant death syndrome (SIDS) in infants born to opiate users.

Testing for drugs: Drug screening tests are discussed in Diagnostic Tests.

References and further reading:
Lang, Heide, "New Hope for Babies Exposed to Cocaine *in Utero*," ADVANCE, 9/14/92, p. 10.
Smith, Judy, "The Dangers of Prenatal Cocaine Use," MCN, May/June, 1988, Vol. 13, p. 174-9.

Prescription Drugs

Virtually all drugs reach the fetus. The only exceptions are pituitary and thyroid hormones, insulin, catecholamines and heparin. It is therefore a good idea to own a relatively recent copy of the Physician's Desk Reference (PDR) where you can look up any drug which a woman may be taking to determine its overall effects, side effects and possible implications for pregnancy. This encyclopedia of drugs categorizes them by brand and generic names and includes information submitted by the manufacturers. Drugs in Pregnancy and Lactation (Gerald Briggs, et al., Williams & Wilkins, Pub. 1994) is the best book specifically addressing drug use in pregnancy. Most large medical centers have access to a nation-wide computerized toxicology hotline for the most current date on drugs in pregnancy.

Keep in mind that, in general, the medical community considers a drug innocent until proven guilty in regard to its effects during pregnancy. There are numerous examples of the folly of this approach, and more attention has been paid to the possibility that certain drugs can be problematic since the uproar that ensued over thalidomide, a drug given to pregnant women in the 1950s which caused severe limb deformities in babies exposed in early pregnancy. In spite of this, many drugs of questionable safety are prescribed to pregnant women all the time. The Food and Drug Administration (FDA) has devised a categorization for drugs according to fetal and neonatal risks:

CATEGORY	INTERPRETATION
A	**Controlled studies show no risk.** Adequate, well-controlled studies in pregnant women have failed to demonstrate fetal risk. No drugs fall into this category.
B	**No evidence of risk in humans.** Animal findings show risk but human findings do not or, if no adequate human studies have been done, animal findings are negative.
C	**Risk cannot be ruled out.** Human studies are lacking, and animal studies are either positive for fetal risk or lacking as well. Potential benefits may, however, justify the possible risk.
D	**Positive evidence of risk.** Investigational or post-marketing data show risk to the fetus. Nevertheless, potential benefits may outweigh the risks.
X	**Contraindicated in pregnancy.** Studies in animals or humans, or investigational or post-marketing reports have shown fetal risk which clearly outweighs any possible benefit to the mother.

Throughout this book and Diagnostic Tests you will find information regarding the best bio-technical drugs to use during pregnancy for a variety of disease conditions and disorders. These recommendations are based upon the best references available at the time of publication. However, since drug technology is always evolving and the effects of drugs during pregnancy are always being reevaluated, it is wise to further research the use of a particular drug for each condition. In this chapter you will find discussion of a few drugs which have not been discussed elsewhere.

Antibiotics: Antibiotics are by far the drugs most commonly prescribed during pregnancy. This is true because an otherwise healthy woman may have a urinary tract or other bacterial infection which cannot be taken care of with non-bio-technical means. Therefore, the question of which antibiotics can be more or less safely used during pregnancy is of great concern to midwives. Broad spectrum antibiotics which have never been associated with adverse fetal risks include Ampicillin, cephalosporins (such as Keflex) Macrodatin, Bactrim, Erythromycin (although Erythromycin estolate is Category D due to a greater likelihood of liver damage) and Penicillin. Streptomycin has been associated with deafness in offspring; tetracycline is associated with discoloration of the teeth in offspring. (Samuels, 1986) All sulfonamides and aminoglycosides are contraindicated in pregnancy; all quinolones are Category C, as they cause degeneration of weight-bearing cartilage.

Metronidazole (Flagyl) in any form should not be used in the first trimester. It falls in category B for use in the second and third trimesters. However, it should be avoided entirely whenever possible, since it has been should in animal studies to have carcinogenic effects. Cleocin (clindomycin) is an acceptable alternative for the treatment of bacterial infections in the yoni.

Tranquilizers: First trimester use of tranquilizers, most commonly Valium (Diazepam), is associated with growth retardation, inguinal hernias, cardiac defects, pyloric stenosis and hemangiomas (birth marks). Cardiac and circulatory defects may also occur with second trimester use. When tranquilizers are used in combination with cigarette smoking, the risk of a malformed infant increases 3.7-fold. Doses of Valium exceeding 30 to 40 mg. daily or prolonged use may cause a decrease in fetal movements and heart rate variability during labor. Newborns exposed *in utero* may show abnormal thermogenesis or may be floppy and lethargic, and have difficulty sucking. They may also experience withdrawal symptoms such as tremors, irritability, hypertonicity, diarrhea, vomiting and vigorous sucking. Valium is contraindicated in nursing mothers because the babies are at risk for lethargy and weight loss.

Benzodiazepines (hypnotic and anxiolytic drugs) include Librium (chlordiazepoxide), Clonopin (clonazapam), Tranxene (chlorazepate), Ativan (iorazepam), Serax (oxazepam) and Centrax (prazepam). Ideally no one should take this category of drugs for more than 5 to 6 weeks; however many take them regularly. All benzodiazepines rapidly cross the placenta and enter fetal circulation. Fetal blood levels equal the mother's within one hour of maternal ingestion. Several studies link their use to first trimester birth defects, especially cleft lip and palate. Near term, use may be associated with lethargy, respiratory problems and withdrawal symptoms in the newborn. These drugs can also cause sedation in the newborn and should be avoided during breastfeeding. Maternal withdrawal from any of these drugs should be encouraged prior to conception to minimize the risk to the fetus and to allow the mother to stabilize without the added stress of pregnancy.

Thalidomide is a sedative which was marketed in 1961; its use resulted in 12,000 babies with characteristic severe limb defects. This was the drug that, once and for all, showed the world that some drugs can and do cause birth defects. It was removed from the market for a while but has made a quiet comeback. It is being used more and more these days to treat complications of leprosy and the side effects of bone marrow surgery. It may also have application in cases of blindness caused by macular degeneration, tuberculosis and even AIDS. In the United States, FDA regulations attempt to ensure that women of childbearing age are informed as to its risks and are monitored closely; however in other parts of the world women are not being adequately informed and babies with defects are once again being born. Thalidomide apparently inhibits the creation of new blood vessels, thus interfering with limb development. (Gorman, 1994)

Neuroleptics (phenothiazines and thioxanthines): These include Thorazine (chlorpromazine), Prolixin (fluphenazine), Trilafon (perphenazine), Compazine (prochlorperazine), Phenergan (promethazine), Mellaril (thioridazine), and Stelazine (trifluoperazine). This class of drugs is only appropriate for psychosis requiring continued medication during pregnancy. Compazine has been associated with fetal defects when taken between the 6th and the 10th week of gestation. Occasional use in low doses seems to be without side effects. Compazine and Phenergan are frequently used as antiemetics which are often prescribed for severe nausea.

Haldol (haloperidol): This tranquilizer is similar to the phenothiazines and is also used for psychotic symptoms. Isolated reports of birth defects with use contraindicates treatment in the first trimester, however use during the second and third trimester appears to be harmless. Preconception treatment should not be discontinued unless close psychological supervision can be maintained and the living environment is well controlled and supervised. Common side effects include sedation, dizziness, dry mouth and a movement disorder called tardive dyskinesia (rapid, jerky yet coordinated movements, slow writhing movements of the hands and facial spasms). While this drug may sedate the baby, breastfeeding is not contraindicated.

Lithium Carbonate: This drug is used for bipolar disorder (manic-depression) and is contraindicated in pregnancy. Malformations of the cardiovascular system are common in fetuses exposed during the first trimester. The overall risk has been shown to be approximately 7%. Toxicity symptoms also noted in newborns include cyanosis, hypotonia, bradycardia, goiter and hypothyroidism. These effects usually

290

reverse themselves.

Motivation is required by the mother to withdraw from lithium and use other means to stabilize her condition. Ideally, withdrawal should occur over a period of 6 to 8 weeks prior to conception; attempts to conceive are best delayed until the mother is reassured that her condition has stabilized. For those who have previously been manic-depressive who successfully withdraw all use, there is a 1 in 5 risk of postpartum psychosis. If postpartum psychosis has been present before, the risk is 1 in 5 for a manic illness and 1 in 10 for a psychotic depressive illness. If a woman has a history of schizophrenia or atypical psychosis, the risk is less.

Those becoming pregnant while taking lithium, should stop treatment immediately. Neuroleptic drugs or tricyclic antidepressants should be prescribed instead. If lithium is felt to be necessary after the first trimester, the level should be maintained as close to .5 mmol/L at 12 hours after ingestion as possible. The mother can be withdrawn from her medication several weeks before she is due. If lithium is continued to term, the mother should stop taking it at the onset of labor and serum levels should be monitored carefully. Renal lithium clearance rises in pregnancy but normalizes shortly after birth. Breastfeeding on lithium is not contraindicated.

References and further reading:

Abrams, Richard, Will It Hurt the Baby?, Addison-Wesley Pub., New York, NY, 1990.
Gorman, Christine, "Thalidomide's Return," Time, June 13, 1994, p. 67.
Samuels, Mike & Nancy, The Well Pregnancy Book, Summit Books, NYC, 1986.

Immunizations During Pregnancy

There is heated debate as to the effectiveness of vaccines and their impact on the immune system. Some of those issues are addressed in Diagnostic Tests, and in Volume III of this book when infant immunization is discussed. You should see those texts for basic details. Here we will review some basic information regarding immunization during pregnancy from the medical perspective. Immunization may be recommended for a few reasons: anticipated travel to an area where a disease is endemic for which a vaccine is available or exposure to a disease or poison (such as a bite or sting) for which an immunoglobulin is available.

The question is, how will vaccination impact the fetus? The fetal immune system is quite immature, gamma globulin suppresses the immune system of young children up to 4 months after administration, how much more severely might it affect the fetus? Induced maternal antibodies may cross the placenta and provide temporary fetal/newborn protection, although such passive immunity may interfere with the development of the baby's own immune response should the parents choose to immunize their newborn. Toxic maternal side effects of the vaccine may affect the fetus by impairing blood flow and transport of oxygen and nutrients to the uterus and placenta or by incapacitating the mother. Side effects from additives and impurities in the vaccine may adversely affect the hypersensitive fetus as well as the mother. Live vaccines harbor the theoretical risk of crossing the placenta and causing fetal infection and damage as well as spontaneous abortion or stillbirth.

Due to these considerations, maternal vaccination is warranted *only* if she has been exposed to a risk which carries significant chances of severe morbidity or death for herself or the fetus. The risk of exposure should be greater than the possible risk of vaccination. Travel to underdeveloped areas may require certain vaccinations such as Yellow Fever (no problem), polio (use killed vaccine) and tetanus, all of which pose less risk than the conditions themselves. Other vaccines, such as cholera and typhoid, are not very effective, have significant side-effects and are best avoided. A certificate can be obtained explaining the circumstances, but some countries may forbid travel without the vaccines even with such a certificate.

If an immunizing agent is unknowingly administered within 3 months of conception or during early pregnancy toxoids are generally considered to pose no particular fetal risk. Live virus vaccines such as polio, measles, mumps and rubella may all theoretically cause fetal infection, although only rubella has been known to do so. Smallpox vaccine may cause fetal infection and is still administered to military personnel; pregnant women should not receive such vaccinations and should avoid those who have until their vaccine lesions are completely healed. If inadvertent immunization or exposure does occur, vaccinia immune globulin (0.3 ml/kg ML) should be given to the mother to minimize possible fetal infection. See Diagnostic Tests for more details regarding vaccines for other disease conditions.

Rayburn & Zuzpan, Drug Therapy in Ob/Gyn, 2nd ed. Appleton, Century, Crofts, Norwalk, 1986.

Toxic Environmental Exposures and Reproductive Risk

There are approximately 25 chemicals known to be teratogenic in humans. Chemical exposure can also cause impaired reproductive potential, mutagenesis and transplacental carcinogenesis. With an estimated 2,000 new chemicals introduced yearly, many of these will undoubtedly be identified as harmful during pregnancy. In reviewing this chapter, the following definitions will be helpful:

Threshold Limit Value (TLV): A recommended concentration at which most workers may be repeatedly exposed without adverse effects.

Short-Term Exposure Limit (STEL): The maximum concentration of a chemical substance to which most workers may be exposed for a continuous period of time, not to exceed 15 minutes. Longer exposure may cause damage or impair function.

Permissible Exposure Limit (PEL): An exposure level set as a legal standard by the Occupational Safety and Heath Administration (OSHA).

Time-Weighed Average (TWA): TLV based on an 8-hour day or 40-hour week.

CHEMICAL PPM=PARTS PER MILLION	DESCRIPTION & USES	REPRODUCTIVE EFFECTS
Bromide (exposure limits not set)	Manufacture of photographic papers & plates	Neonatal bromism
Carbon monoxide TLV 50 ppm STEL 400 ppm PEL 50 ppm	Formed by incomplete combustion of organic fuels used in coke ovens, power plants, foundries, & gasoline or diesel powered engines	Fetal death or neurologic damage
Cellosolve, Methyl TLV (skin) 5 ppm STEL none PEL 25 ppm	Solvent for cellulose esters, dyes, resins, lacquers, varnishes & stains; perfume fixative; jet fuel de-icing additive	Potential embryofetotoxic risk
Dimethylacetamide (DMAC) TLV (skin) 10 ppm STEL 15 ppm PEL 10 ppm	Organic solvent	Potential fetotoxin
Dimethylformamide TLV (skin) 10 ppm STEL 20 ppm PEL (skin) 10 ppm	Solvent for resins & polymers Co-solvent for protective coatings, adhesives, films & printing inks, and a component of many paint removers	Potential fetotoxicity
Hexachlorophene (HCP) TLV/STEL/PEL none	Bactericide in soaps & other cleansing agents	Teratogenic in mammals
Kepone TLV/STEL/PEL none	Insecticide	Potential fetotoxicity
Lead TLV 0.15 mg/m³ (inorganic dust & fumes) STEL 0.45 mg/m³ PEL .05 mg/m³	Major component of many alloys used in paint pigments, storage batteries & ceramics; of metal smelting	Potential neurobehavorial impairment of the fetus

Most pregnant women will come into contact with chemicals at work, although contact in the home should not be overlooked. The chart below correlates typical kinds of chemical exposure in some common occupations.

Occupation	Exposure hazards
Textile operatives Sewers & stitchers, Upholsterers	Raw cotton dust, noise, synthetic fiber dust, asbestos formaldehyde, heat, dyes, flame retardants As above plus organic solvents
RNs, aides, orderlies Dental hygienists Laboratory workers (clinical & research)	Anesthetic gases, ethylene oxide, x-radiation, alcohol, infectious diseases, puncture wounds X-rays, mercury, ultrasound, anesthetic gases Toxic chemicals & x-rays
Electronic assemblers	Lead, tin, antimony, trichloroethylene, methylene chloride, epoxy resins, methylethyl ketone
Farm workers	Numerous insecticides leading to miscarriage & birth defects
Hairdressers & cosmetologists	Hair spray resins (polyvinyl pyrrolidone), aerosol propellants (freons), halogenated hydrocarbons, hair dyes, solvents of nail polish, benzyl alcohol, ethyl alcohol, acetone
Launderers/maids Dry cleaners	Soaps, detergents, enzymes, heat, humidity, industrially contaminated clothing Perchlorethylene, trichloroethylene, naphtha, benzene, industrially contaminated clothing
Photographic processors	Caustics, iron salts, mercuris chloride, bromides, iodides, pyrogallic acid, silver nitrate
Plastic fabricators	Acrylonitrile, phenol formaldehydes, urea formaldehydes, hexamethylenetetramine, acids, alkalies, peroxide, vinyl chloride, polystyrene, vinylidene chloride
Domestic workers	Solvents, hydrocarbons, soaps, detergents, bleaches, alkalies
Transportation operators	Carbon monoxide, polynuclear aromatics, lead & other by-products of gasoline, vibration, microwaves, physical stresses
Sign painters & letterers	Lead oxide, lead chromate pigments, trace metals, epichlorohydrin, titanium dioxide, xylene, toluene
Clerical personnel	Physical stress, poor light, trichloroethylene, carbon tetrachloride & various other cleaners, asbestos in air conditioning; computer terminals
Optician & lens grinders	Coal tar pitch volatiles, iron, oxide, dust, solvents, hydrocarbons
Painters	Lead, titanium, toluene
Plastic workers	Acrylonitrile, formaldehyde, vinyl chloride
Printing operators	Ink mists, 2-nitropropane, methanol, carbon tetrachloride, methylene chloride, lead, noise, hydrocarbon solvents, trichlorethylene, toluene, benzene, trace metals

Jobs requiring shift changes from days to evenings or nights are stressful as they disturb sleep cycles, cause gastrointestinal upsets (especially gastric upset and peptic ulcer) and are associated with an increased incidence of cardiovascular disease. Exposure to antineoplastic (chemotherapy) drugs may lead to an increased incidence of miscarriage as well as fetal malformations. Anesthetic gases may contribute to miscarriage as well as low-birth-weight babies. Leather workers are exposed to chemicals which increase the risk of perinatal death, especially from congenital malformations.

Airline attendants do not have exposure risk, but cabin humidity is low, necessitating increased fluid intake. Pressurized cabins eliminate risks from extremely high altitudes. Physical work may require pushing heavy food carts and lifting which may cause undue stress on joints softened by the hormones of pregnancy.

Waitresses, store clerks or any job requiring lots of standing and lifting stresses the lower extremities, burns lots of calories and will be more difficult to perform as pregnancy advances.

Anyone who is exposed to computers emitting very low frequency radiation are at a tripled risk for miscarriage. Some video display terminals emit much more of this radiation that others; a monitor which meets Swiss or German emission standards will greatly reduce the risk. (Detroit Free Press, 12/15/92)

The following chemicals have adverse effects on male reproductive health:

CHEMICAL	EFFECT
Anesthetic gases	Congenital anomalies in offspring
Carbon disulfide	Impotence, loss of sex drive
Chloroprene	Decreased sperm count and motility, increased miscarriages in women
Dibromochloropropane	Decreased sperm count and infertility
Hydrocarbons	Offspring with higher cancer risk
Kepone	Decreased fertility
Lead	Decreased sperm count and motility, abnormally shaped sperm
Vinyl chloride	Excess fetal loss
Anti-amoeba drugs	Decreased motility of sperm, abnormally shaped sperm
Anticonvulsants	Developmental disabilities in offspring
Iodine	Atrophy of testes
Testosterone enanthate	Sterility

References and further reading:
Samuels, M. & N., The Well-Pregnancy Book, Summit Books, New York, NY, 1986, p. 125-7.

Hyperthermia

Hyperthermia (elevated body temperature) has been suspected of causing birth defects, especially central nervous system damage, when the temperature of the uterus exceeds 104°F (40°C) for at least one day (24 hours) during weeks three to seven of gestation. A link between high core body temperature and miscarriage has also been suggested.

Certain work environments, intensive prolonged exercise, the use of hot tubs, saunas or steam baths, or a prolonged high fever have all been suggested as likely potential sources of hyperthermia which can lead to fetal harm. In one study, when normal, nonpregnant women were tested in hot tubs and saunas in an attempt to raise their body temperature to 102°F (38.9°C), none of the 20 women were able to remain in the sauna long enough to accomplish this. Although it was possible for maternal temperatures to reach 102°F in a hot tub, this occurred no sooner than 10 minutes with a water temperature of 104.2°F (41.1°C) and no sooner than 15 minutes with a water temperature of 102.2°F (39°C). It is extremely unlikely that undrugged, sober women with normal nervous system responses would voluntarily remain in most hot environments long enough to raise their core temperature high enough to cause harm to their babies. When using a hot tub, periodically leaving the water every 10 to 15 minutes to cool off should be an adequate precaution.

A fever with an oral temperature reading of less than 104°F (40°C) is also unlikely to cause any harm. In the absence of severe infection, the natural occurrence of such a high core body temperature is extremely rare. In most cases fever above 102°F (38.9°C) can be reduced with the use of Elder Flower infusion, cool baths, diluted apple cider vinegar sponge baths or acetaminophen (Tylenol).

References and further reading:

Abrams, Richard, Will It Hurt the Baby?, Addison Wesley Pub. Co., Inc., 1990.
Gleicher, Norbert, ed., Principles of Medical Therapy in Pregnancy, Plenum Medical Book Co., New York, NY, 1985.

Psychological Health During Pregnancy

A woman's psychological well-being has a great deal to do with how she will cope with pregnancy, labor, birth and mothering. It is a midwife's job to get to know a mother well enough to help her navigate her particular psychological challenges successfully and have the healthiest birth possible on all levels: physical, emotional, mental and spiritual.

Pregnancy can be considered a rite of passage for the woman, baby, her family and society. The culmination of this passage is the labor and birth of the baby. However, long before a woman reaches that point, many psychological adjustments will take place. How well the woman negotiates and integrates the adjustments required during pregnancy will determine, in part, what inner resources she brings to her labor.

The psychological processes of pregnancy coincide with the physical changes which are taking place in the woman's body. During pregnancy the woman comes to terms with what her life is like before her baby is born and what it may be like after the baby is born. Key elements in this process are an increasing sense of the loss of control of her body, the additional, considerable responsibilities of mothering a newborn and parenting in general, how the pregnancy and birth will impact her relationship with her partner and other children, and how she will maintain her career (if she has one). This can make a woman more dependent or more demanding (a counter response to feeling more out of control). Of course, if she is a first-time mother, she will not really understand how her life will change until after the baby is born!! In reality, her life will never go back to normal, however she defines that for herself.

The emotions of a pregnant woman are extremely changeable. As a woman moves through pregnancy she prepares for the enormous task of opening her body and her whole being to channel the life of another through to this plane of existence. The spiritual openness which pregnancy brings makes women very sensitive and vulnerable to what they feel and what they sense from others, and may result in rapidly changing moods. This openness makes women ripe to share their inner experiences more readily and also more capable of making many life changes (such as changing dietary patterns or quitting abusive behaviors such as cigarette smoking). Women tend to reflect more on their dreams, and the meanings of words, objects and events.

Pregnancy and birth bring a woman into more conscious relationship with the reality of death, mortality, fulfillment and happiness. What these things mean to her and how she would cope with an unexpected occurrence during the pregnancy may weigh heavily on her mind. Fears for her own and her baby's well-being are normal and healthy responses to the increased responsibility pregnancy represents.

Throughout the sections which address prenatal care, you will find chapters pertaining to the unique psychological tasks of each trimester of pregnancy. Generally speaking, pregnancy is a time of slow evolution of the woman's ability to open herself to letting another life into the world, and, as such, requires her to contemplate many levels of what having a baby and parenting will mean for her. In addition to this enormous task, a woman may have to cope with a variety of other stresses and anxiety producing events that can distract her from this process. The chronic stress of anxiety can be wearing on the psychological as well as the physical stamina of a woman and will increase her needs for both physical and emotional support.

The mother's and partner's emotional and psychological state and the baby: Women will experience a range of emotions during pregnancy; fears and concerns as well as joys and anticipations. Women need not feel guilty about this, it is perfectly normal. However, it will be helpful to her developing baby's future emotional health if she acknowledges to her baby that her emotional responses are her own; they are not originating from the baby or the baby's fault (the same is true of her partner in relationship to the baby). This will help the baby differentiate its feelings from those of the parents. As you encourage women to connect and talk to their babies, you can encourage them to think or say something like "I'm feeling pretty afraid right now (or whatever), but this is my fear, not yours, and I will deal with it." (Hendricks, 1995)

The partner's psychological changes: A woman's partner will experience a wide range of feelings as well during pregnancy, and may at times feel they have no place to turn since the focus of attention in on the pregnant mother. Bridge this gap by encouraging the partner to express their feelings, concerns and questions during prenatal visits. Ask straightforward questions about how the relationship is going and how any problems brought up at during the first few visits are being handled.

References and further reading:

Hendricks, Gay, Conscious Relationship Training, Phase II, Colorado Springs, Co, August, 6-12, 1995.
Perez, Polly, "The Emotional Work of Pregnancy," International Journal of Childbirth Education, Vol. 3, No. 3, August 1988, pp. 30-1.
Varney, Helen, Nurse-Midwifery, Blackwell Scientific Pub., Boston, MA 1980.

298

Helping Women Explore Their Dreams

During the nine months of pregnancy a woman's dream world can become a creative forum for many issues in her life: the way she regards her physical appearance, how she feels about her baby, her relationship with her mother, other members of the family and her mate, her opinion of herself in relation to other women, her attitude about labor and birth, and the future she envisions with her child. Openly acknowledging and discussing these universal issues helps increase a woman's personal awareness and emotional growth, helps to strengthen her bonds with her baby and her partner, and helps with the psychological preparation for labor and parenthood.

Male partners may dream about the birth, being pregnant, nursing, giving birth, or fears around fatherhood. Expectant fathers are grappling with their identity and the issues raised about their own parent-child relationships as well as adjusting to their new roles.

While much has been written on the meaning of dream symbols and images, every dreamer is an individual with a unique life that shapes the meaning of symbols which appear in their dreams. In order to tune into patterns from dream to dream it is important, first of all, for a woman to record her dreams. She can use a cassette tape recorder to do so or write them in a dream journal. She should do this upon awakening, when the memory of the dream is still fresh in her mind. If a woman has had a particularly disturbing dream or one which she feels (or you perceive) may be highly significant, or if she has recurring dreams, you might want to delve into the meaning of the dream in more detail. To start, have her tell the dream as though it is happening now, in the present tense. She can refer to her notes if she has them. You can lead her into analyzing the dream by asking:

*What do you think the dream is about?
*What is the mood of the dream?
*What feelings arise during the dream?

As she explores these questions, ask her "What or whom does this remind you of?" The people in the dream should be explored individually with questions such as:

*Who is _____, and what is he or she like?
*Is there a part of you that resembles _____?
*Describe your relationship with this person.
*What or who does this remind you of? How is this familiar?

As she describes each object in the dream, ask her "What is it? What does it mean to you? Is the main action in the dream reminiscent of anything that has happened to you in waking life?"

Another way to approach dream exploration is to go through the dream several times and have the woman discuss the dream from the vantage point of each person and object in the dream. After all, each thing in the dream is coming from her subconscious. This method can be highly enlightening, particularly with disturbing dreams.

If threatening persons appear frequently in dreams, the woman can strongly suggest to herself before going to sleep that she turn and ask them what they want should she encounter them again that night, reminding herself that she is physically safe since she will be dreaming. Such a confrontation means the person is asking their own subconscious about the meaning of the dream. This can be profoundly revealing.

It is also possible to use auto-suggestion to dream an answer to a question about oneself. To do so a woman may:

1. Choose a problem that has been nagging her.
2. Before going to sleep, write down some notes on her day, clearing her mind to concentrate on the problem.
3. Now turn the attention to the problem. Examine its truths and subtleties. Write down apparent facts. What is the cause of the problem? How does it affect her? Does she really want to resolve it? What has she discovered so far about the problem? She is trying to stir her inner emotions on the issue.
4. Next, have her compose a question, in one succinct line, about what she wants to know.
5. She should turn out the lights, assume a relaxed position and repeat the question over and over in her mind. Returning to the question if distracting thoughts intrude. Let the repetition lull her to sleep.
6. When she awakens, morning or night, have her write down whatever images she remembers. She may recall the whole dream or only a fragment. She should not attempt to evaluate it yet, but should be as detailed as possible when recording the dream. She can let the meaning of the dream evolve during the day and write down her thoughts, feelings and reflections on the dream in her journal.

References and further reading:

Stukane, Eileen, "Exploring Pregnancy Emotions and Dreams," Pennypress, Inc., Seattle, WA, 1991.

op. cit., The Dream Worlds of Pregnancy, Station Hill Press, Barrytown, NY, 1995.

Maybruck, Patricia, Pregnancy and Dreams, Putnam Pub., 1989 (out of print).

Understanding Physical and Sexual Abuse Issues

All forms of physical abuse carry with them certain fairly predictable human responses and long term survival mechanisms. It is impossible to rank what abuse is the worst; any type of abuse can be devastating to the mind, body and spirit of the one who is abused. Because of the range and severity of abuse, there may be parts of this chapter that you find upsetting, especially if you have a history of such abuse. Be sure and seek support if this is the case for you.

Humans have a basic set of responses or after-effects which are associated with trauma of any kind. These include: sexual disorders, physical problems, psycho-social problems, and mental problems. These problems may manifest in a variety of ways, depending upon such things as the type of abuse, the length of time the abuse took place, the age at which the abuse started, the closeness of the relationship to the abuser and the personality of the one who was abused. (Davis, 1995)

The types of abuse we will review in this chapter include physical battering, medical abuse, sexual abuse and ritual abuse. Those who have been subjected to one of these types of abuse may have been subjected to one or more of the others. All forms of physical abuse include emotional abuse as well; however, emotional abuse in the form of verbal attacks or deprivation of affection can occur without any physical abuse taking place.

This chapter will not tell you all that you need to know about these types of abuse, but it will provide valuable resource information for identifying abusive situations and helping women cope with previous abuse. Remember you are a midwife, and as such you provide counseling but not full fledged therapy. When women need therapy, they should be referred to the very best people in your area who specialize in helping those from abusive backgrounds.

Physical and emotional battering: It is estimated that 3 to 4 million women in the United States are battered each year by their husbands or partners. In 95% of all physical abuse cases women are hurt by men. However, it is possible for battering to take place between women partners; although far less common, do not overlook this possibility. Battering occurs among people of all races. Most incidents are not isolated events; battering tends to increase and become more violent over time. Even so, most women do not report battering partners, and even if they do, the authorities often cannot or do not respond in a manner which affords the woman protection or removal of the offender from her home.

The psychological milieu of the battering situation is particularly relevant to our work as midwives. *Battering may start or become worse when a woman is pregnant; in fact 25% to 45% of all battering occurs during pregnancy.* Battering can lead to miscarriage or low birth weight babies, or may drive the woman to alcohol or drug abuse. If battering does not occur during a first pregnancy, it is less likely to occur at other times during the relationship (Claypool, 1995).

The following behaviors are typical of partners who have a high potential for becoming physically abusive. Many of them constitute emotional abuse as well; which is more subtle, often goes on more consistently, and is very undermining to the woman's self-esteem. The more signs a person displays, the more likely the person is to become a batterer. As a rule, the last four signs listed are seen exclusively in those who actually batter. Occasionally a batterer will have extremely exaggerated versions of only two or three of these behaviors. At the beginning of the relationship the batterer will often try to explain their behavior as a sign of love and concern and the woman may be flattered at first. As time goes on, the behaviors become more severe and serve to dominate the woman. These behaviors are listed here to alert you to the possibility of abuse:

1. **Jealousy:** At the beginning of the relationship, an abuser will say that their jealousy is a sign of love. The abuser will question the woman about who she talks to, accuse her of flirting, or be jealous of time spent with others. As this pattern progresses, the abuser may call frequently during the day or drop by unexpectedly, check her car milage, restrict where she works, or ask friends to watch her. Rather than being indicative of love, jealousy is a sign of insecurity and possessiveness.

2. **Controlling behavior:** At first, controlling behavior will be explained as concern about the woman's safety or some similar excuse. The abuser will be angry if the woman comes home "late" from the store, or will question her closely regarding where she's been or who she's talked to. As this behavior escalates, the abuser may not let the woman make decisions about the house, her clothing, or where she goes; the batterer may keep all the money or even make her ask permission to leave the house.

3. **Quick involvement:** Many battered women knew their abusive partner for less than six months before they were engaged or living together. Typically the abuser pursued the woman heavily; the batterer needs someone desperately and may have pressured her to make a commitment to him.

4. **Unrealistic expectations:** The abusive partner is very dependent on the woman for all his needs: the batterer expects the perfect partner, mother, lover and friend, both emotionally and in the home.

5. **Isolation:** The abuser tries to cut the woman off from all resources including other friends, family and professional support systems such as therapy. The batterer may want to live out in the country without a phone or may try to keep her from working or attending school.

6. **Blames others for his/her problems:** If chronically unemployed, the abuser will blame someone else; the batterer may blame the woman for his mistakes or

almost anything that goes wrong.

7. Blames others for his/her feelings: An abuser may tell the woman "You make me mad," and blame her for inciting the abuse. Although the abuser clearly makes the decisions about what s/he thinks and how they handle their feelings, s/he will use feelings to manipulate the woman. Harder to catch are the abuser's claims that "You make me happy," or "You control how I feel."

8. Hypersensitivity: The abuser is easily insulted and may rant and rave about common incidents of living which the abuser considers major injustices, such as having to work overtime.

9. Cruelty to animals and children: The abuser may brutally punish animals or children or be insensitive to their pain and suffering. The abuser may expect children to be capable of doing things beyond their age or ability (for example the abuser may spank a two-year old for wetting their diaper) or they may tease children until they cry. Sixty percent of men who beat their partners also beat their children. The abuser may set unreasonable rules, such as expecting the children to stay in their rooms when the abuser comes home from work.

10. "Playful" use of force in sex: The abuser may like to throw the woman down and hold her down during sex. The abuser may want to act out fantasies where the woman is helpless. The abuser is letting her know that the idea of rape is exciting them. The abuser may show little concern about whether the woman wants to have sex, and use sulking or anger to manipulate her into compliance.

11. Verbal abuse: In addition to saying things that are meant to be cruel or hurtful, verbal abuse is present when a partner degrades a woman, cursing her or belittling her accomplishments. The abuser may tell her she is stupid, unable to make it without them, undesirable, ugly, or unworthy. This may involve waking her up at night to verbally abuse her or not letting her sleep at all.

12. Rigid gender roles: The abuser expects the woman to serve them: the abuser will insist she must stay at home, that she must obey him in all things—even those that are criminal in nature. The abuser will see women as inferior to men, more stupid, unable to be a whole person without a relationship.

13. Dr Jekyll and Mr. Hyde: Many woman are confused by their abuser's sudden changes in mood—one minute s/he's nice and the next the abuser explodes. A woman may explain that the abuser has a "mental problem" or the s/he is crazy. Explosiveness and mood swings are typical of those who beat their partners, and these behaviors are related to others such as hypersensitivity.

14. **Past battering:** The abuser may admit to past violence but say the person made them do it. The woman may learn from relatives or ex-partners that the person is abusive. An abuser will beat whoever they are with: situations do not make a person into a batterer.

15. **Threats of violence:** This would include any threat of physical force meant to control the woman such as "I'll slap your mouth off," "I'll kill you," "I'll break your neck." The abuser may try to excuse this behavior with comments like "Everyone talks like that."

16. **Breaking or striking objects:** This can be used as a punishment (breaking beloved possessions) but is generally used to terrorize the woman into submission. The abuser may beat on tables with his fist or throw objects near the woman.

17. **Use of any force during an argument:** This may involve holding the woman down, physically restraining her from leaving the room, or any pushing or shoving. The abuser may hold her against a wall and say "You're going to listen to me."

Spotting abusive relationship dynamics: It is important to know which behaviors are highly associated with abusive personalities so that you will be able to spot trouble in the process of interviewing women and be aware of subtle hints during visits which include both partners. However, it is quite possible for an abusive partner to present a very reasonable face during an appointment and then become a tyrant at home. Unfortunately, an extremely emotionally or physically dominating partner will sometimes push a woman into having midwifery care and a homebirth because the abuser perceives this as a way to maintain more control. Be alert to this possibility in the following situations: the man, not the woman, calls to make the initial contact with you, the partner does all the talking (or tries to) at the appointment, the partner asks about minimizing your role at the birth, catching the baby and his other participation. These must be evaluated *in conjunction with other signs.* Obviously any of these could occur with no underlying problem whatsoever, but midwives have found them to be consistent red flags. When the partner appears to be doing all the talking, direct your questions to the woman as in "And Alice, how do you feel about that?" Watch her facial expressions, her tone of voice and her body language when she responds to try to detect hesitation or fear on her part.

Often as care progresses, women in these situations will want very much to work with midwives while the men do not. This will be especially true in a practice that is woman-oriented rather than family-oriented; if a situation is not good for the woman and her children, the midwife will not hesitate to offer her support in making it different for herself. This may be the first encounter a woman has had with a care system that is primarily advocating for her. Even though a midwife might not verbalize that her practice is "woman-centered" often women pick up on it. At other times you may discover that the woman is afraid of having a homebirth or midwifery care and is being pushed into it by her partner. In those cases, serving as an intermediary to help the woman find the kind of care she truly feels comfortable with is the most supportive course of action.

When you suspect domestic violence: Abused women may not get much support from their relatives or friends, who may be either in denial or too afraid of the abuser to help. The police often can do nothing if they do not see the violence while it is occurring or if the woman has no physical signs of the abuse. Women often fear for their safety and that of their children when confronted with the possibility of leaving the abusive environment. These women can see their situation as hopeless, especially if they lack a means of independent support.

In suspicious situations the midwife needs to decide if she can deal with the circumstances herself. Make every effort to have at least one appointment with the woman alone. You may be able to do this by asking to see her at a time when you know her partner cannot come, saying that it is the only time you have free for that particular appointment. Another tactic would be to ask the partner to leave the room during the physical examination. While this is not usually done in midwifery model care, it is a routine in medically managed care settings and therefore may not be too alarming. This gives you the opportunity to not only talk to the woman but to ask her questions about any marks, scars or bruises you may discover during your examination.

If you discover suspicious injuries during a physical examination in a woman who has not disclosed or has denied abuse, ask her how the injury occurred. In this situation, if she offers an implausible reason for the injury, you might make a comment like "It's unusual that such a injury would occur in this location from that kind of fall (or whatever)." Or alternatively you could say, "I know you have said that your partner has never harmed you physically, but if that were ever to happen, anything you say to me about that would remain confidential. I would be happy to help you learn about the community resources that are available if that should ever be a problem." A statement like this will hopefully help her feel safe enough to tell you the truth if she is being abused. If you feel abuse is likely but no disclosure has taken place so far, ask the assessment questions that follow.

Assessing for the presence of domestic violence in a family: The following questions can help in assessing women who may be experiencing domestic abuse in their home. For some women, answering "sometimes" will be easier than answering merely yes or no. As with all sensitive questions, it is important not to convey an attitude of judgement or condemnation during the interview.

1. Do you know where you could go or who could help you if you were being physically hurt or abused or if you were worried about being abused?
   If yes, ask where she would go or what she would do.

2. Are you or have you ever been in a relationship with a partner who physically hurt you?
3. Has your partner ever threatened to hurt you or done things which make you afraid that they might hurt you?
4. Has your current partner ever hit, slapped, kicked or otherwise hurt you?
   (Ask when, how many times, and examine the areas of attack; make notes in your records)
5. If yes, have they hit you since you were pregnant?
6. If so, did the abuse increase once you became pregnant?
7. Have you been abused by them during any previous pregnancies?
8. Have you ever sought medical attention for any abuse-related injuries?
9. Were you pregnant at the time?

As you conduct this interview, you may find the woman exhibiting behaviors which suggest that she is uncomfortable with the topic. For some women these behaviors may by suggestive of abuse and disclosure of abuse may follow at a later date. Behavior which suggests that the woman may be withholding information:

Laughing or tittering
Avoiding eye contact (not applicable to some
  cultures such as Asian or Arabic)
Crying
Sighing
Minimizing statements
Searching/engaging eye contact (fear)
	Anxious body language (standing to
	  leave, dropped shoulders, appearing
	  depressed)
	Comments about emotional abuse
	Comments about a "friend" who is
	  abused

A woman may be in such an abusive situation that her life is threatened. Based on research done with both abusers and battered women where the woman is eventually killed by her abuser, the following questions were developed to assess the risk of murder. They can be asked in your interview or given to the woman to fill out herself.

1. Has the physical violence increased in frequency over the past year?
2. Has the physical violence increased in severity over the past year and/or has a weapon or threat with a weapon been used?
3. Does your partner ever try to choke you?
4. Is there a gun in the house?
5. Has your partner ever forced you into sex when you did not wish to participate?
6. Does your partner use drugs (uppers or amphetamines, speed, angel dust, cocaine, crack, heroin, mixtures or other street drugs)?
7. Does your partner threaten to kill you and/or do you believe s/he is capable of killing you?
8. Is s/he drunk every day or almost every day (how much does s/he drink?)

9. Does your partner control more of your daily activities than previously? For instance, does s/he tell you who you can be friends with, how much money you can take shopping, or when you can take the car?

10. Is your partner violently and consistently jealous of you? (For instance, does s/he say, "If I can't have you, no one can?")

11. Have you ever threatened or tried to commit suicide?

13. Has your partner ever threatened or tried to commit suicide?

14. Is your partner violent toward your children?

15. Is your partner violent outside the home?

The more yes answers you have to these questions, the more risk of murder exists for the woman. (questions based on Parker & McFarlane, 1991)

When domestic violence is disclosed: If abuse is revealed during this interview, your job is to provide immediate care or referral for any abuse-related injuries the woman may currently have, to assist in reducing emotional stress with any means at your disposal, to document the incidents described to you in as much detail as possible, and to provide referral information for the woman. Talk to the woman honestly about her situation and ask her what kind of help would be most useful to her. As the care provider, you are legally obligated to report child abuse if you suspect it, but you are not obligated to report spousal battering; indeed, there is no legal provision for authorities to intercede in a situation involving two adults.

Be aware that a woman may be in any stage of healing regarding the situation, from total denial or extreme minimizing of the problem to being ready to remove herself from the abusive environment. Being aware of what kinds of services exist in your community such as women's shelters, social service agencies, and local police initiatives can help a woman make a plan using these resources for support. Know the laws in your community. A national, toll free number 1-800-333-SAFE can be called to determine what shelters exist in your community. If possible and with her consent, you could have an abuse counselor from a local women's shelter come to an appointment to assist her in assessing her options.

Leaving a abusive situation during pregnancy may be particularly hard, both emotionally and financially. If a woman *is* ready to leave an abusive situation it is best for her to formulate a plan for leaving her home rather than waiting for a crisis and leaving at that time. She needs to have an idea where she will go; willing friends or relatives may be good people to ask for support in this regard. If a battered women's shelter is her only or best option, she needs to contact them, explain her circumstances and get an idea of what they offer. Typically, there is a waiting list and she will have to ask to be listed. She should plan for her children and what belongings she will take with her. She needs to think this out carefully because the most dangerous time for a woman is after she leaves her abusive partner. (based on Huffman, 1993; Parker & McFarlane, 1991)

Medical abuse: Medical personnel of any kind are in a set-up for recapitulating abusive patterns because they are in a position of authority. Medical abuse occurs when women are "done to" by medical personnel without adequate information about the procedures being performed, or when procedures have *actually* been performed against their will. This happens all the time in hospital settings and can happen in homebirths as well. Sometimes the practitioner may believe that the woman has consented or has been adequately informed, however later the woman does not share this view. In many cases the woman is given partial or incorrect information which serves to frighten her and therefore leads her to make a choice with which the practitioner feels most comfortable.

Medical practitioners can also take sexual advantage of women during care. This can happen not only with those providing reproductive care; even dentists who put women or children under anesthetic have been known to molest them. It is important to be sensitive to the possibility of past abuse and question women about their previous examinations with care providers so that you can be sure of what emotional factors you are dealing with before you proceed with an examination.

Sexual abuse: As many as one in three women are sexually abused, of which 38% are abused before the age of 18; that's almost one out of every 4 women and girls. One-fifth to one-sixth of all men have experienced some form of sexual abuse or molestation in their lives. It is quite likely that these figures grossly underestimate the actual incidence of sexual abuse, since many cases still go unreported. It is inevitable that you will encounter women who have been sexually abused. Sexual abuse occurs in every class of society and in every racial, religious and ethnic group. Although most sexual abuse occurs between males and underage females, women as well as men can be perpetrators of sexual abuse. (Davis & Bass, 1993)

Traumatic amnesia: While there are still many questions about the nature of memory and the influence of trauma on memory, whether traumatic amnesia occurs is not one of them. Traumatic amnesia is a well established psychiatric diagnosis which frequently occurs in response to painful or traumatic experiences such as witnessing violence, war, or experiencing repeated traumas such as sexual, ritual or physical abuse. It involves the following elements: attractions, fears or avoidances unexplained by known history; indications of emerging memories; evidence of disassociation, and time loss or memory blanks. Women can spend much of their adult life unaware of previous abuse which they may have endured for years. (Davis & Bass, 1993)

Memory triggers: While some women may remember their abuse and will have pursued therapy, others will have no recollection until something or someone triggers those memories. There are significant life events which tend to precipitate the unblocking of memories of sexual abuse:

308

1. Pregnancy, birth and the early postpartum period (especially breastfeeding) or the pregnancy and birth of another's child or her own grandchild.
2. The establishment of long-term sexual commitments.
3. When a woman's child (especially a daughter) reaches the age at which she herself was abused (or when a granddaughter reaches that age).
4. When the perpetrator dies or when a parent dies who is being unconsciously protected from knowledge of the abuse.
5. During any time of undue stress.
6. Unknowingly experiencing a situation that is similar in some way to the original abuse. This is a common trigger, but is usually not understood until after the abuse memories begin to surface.
7. The beginning of a new developmental stage, such as puberty or middle age.
8. Confronting a known sexual abuser. The aftermath may trigger the return of memories of abuse by another perpetrator or memories of more severe abuse by the recently confronted perpetrator.
9. Ending an addiction. Addiction may have served to suppress memories.
10. Exposure to the idea of sexual abuse via the media, a friend's disclosure, etc.
11. Feeling safe. Security may create the emotional climate which allows the memories of abuse to surface.
12. Feeling strong. Personal growth may uncover enough strength for the psyche to face the abuse. Often this occurs after recovery from dysfunctional family issues. (Simpkin, 1993)
13. Ritual abuse survivors may have specific triggers programming by their perpetrators; certain colors, words, phrases or images may be involved.

Frequently, pregnancy, and especially labor and birth, causes previously blocked memories to come to consciousness for the first time. The powerful sensations of labor and birth, especially the intense sensations associated with pushing, can trigger the restimulation of body memories. As the body begins to "remember," the mind tries to block what it has protected the woman from for so long. Sometimes the memory of abuse resurfaces so acutely that the woman will flashback as if the abuse is occurring in the present; she may cry out, talk as if she were talking to her abuser, back away, or crawl off in a corner. Be aware that such behaviors may occur during labor and may be related to resurfacing of memories.

The psychological dynamics of sexual abuse: The key element in child/adult sexual abuse or any kind of physical abuse is the power differential that exists between the adult perpetrator and the child. In any adult or older child/younger child interaction the perpetrator *always* has the upper hand and is in the power position. Therefore no matter how cooperative the child may be or how much she may actually find the experience pleasurable (which does sometimes happen) the perpetrator is always responsible and always misusing their power position in relationship to the child. This misuse of power is just as significant to the damage caused by abuse as the actual abuse which takes place.

This power differential is especially significant in cases of incest, "the imposition of sexually inappropriate acts, or acts with sexual overtones, by—or any use of a minor child to meet the sexual or sexual/emotional needs of—one or more persons who derive authority through ongoing emotional bonding with that child." (Blume, 1990) Sexual abuse as a random incident with a stranger as the perpetrator is actually rare. A neighbor or distant relative may be involved; alternately, the perpetrator may be a member of the immediate family. Generally speaking, the more bonded the child is to the adult perpetrator, and the more consistent the abuse, the more damaging the abuse turns out to be. Sibling or parent perpetrators therefore pose the most serious threat to the child's overall well-being.

Sexual abuse of a child involves an adult focusing adult sexual energies directly on the child. Children are in no way prepared to integrate or respond to the psychological or emotional reality of this type of energy. Many different activities can set the stage for subtle forms of sexual abuse. For example, when a baby's diaper is changed by an adult that loves the baby and projects that the baby's body is beautiful, touching the baby with affection and delighting in the baby finding pleasure in her own body, it can be a healthful and esteem enhancing experience for the infant. On the other hand, if the adult involved in the process becomes sexually aroused and continues to use involvement with the child to gratify their own desires, they are engaging the child in their sexual experience; this constitutes abuse, even though the observable behaviors of both diaper-changers may be more or less identical.

Children are often enjoined to keep overt abuse a secret with threats that death or injury may befall themselves or other family members if they tell, or are told that no one will believe their disclosure. If the abuse is subtle, the child may have no reference for why it feels wrong and may therefore feel as if she is imagining it, or she may have no words to articulate the abuse to other adults. The child often forms a self-image of evil, especially if her abuser said it was she who brought on the abuse, or her mother told her that she brought it on herself.

Sexual abuse of any type is likely to be terrifying and confusing to a child. It is common for the child to become quite damaged in their developing ability to maintain appropriate emotional and physical boundaries, not knowing if her body belongs to herself or her abuser. During pregnancy, the body-boundary changes which naturally occur may trigger a resurfacing of this boundary confusion. As a child, a woman learned that she must always be in control and can not depend on anyone else, or that vulnerability was a set-up for getting hurt. As an adult she may project those issues into her relationships with anyone who is in a position of authority or power, since they fill the role that the abuser once did. Trust becomes difficult because it, too, led to hurt. The child cannot truly give consent to sexual abuse, and generally has no choice in the matter. When a woman is subjected to obstetrical procedures without her explicit consent, or when she is convinced to undergo procedures with comments like "We don't want your baby to die," (as often happens in hospital births) this can recreate the feelings of damage or powerlessness which took place during childhood abuse.

Making space for disclosure: As the midwife, it is up to you to provide an open forum in which women will feel safe enough to disclose abuse if they are aware of it. For background, you can read <u>The Courage to Heal</u> by Ellen Bass and Laura Davis, which addresses healing issues for women who have experienced childhood sexual abuse. Asking open-ended questions in such a way that the woman will identify her experience with what you are saying can help bring this information to light (see the chapter on The Initial History for details about how to do so). Many people think that there must be some sort of penetration of the yoni, most typically by a penis, for sexual interaction with an adult to constitute abuse. Therefore, many women will minimize other types of abuse. Yet, even a father looking upon his daughter in a sexually provocative way can terrorize a child.

Since childhood sexual abuse has only come into public scrutiny in the past 10 to 15 years, there are many adult survivors today that never had anyone to turn to, never saw a commercial on TV telling them to tell an adult, or had any reference point that told them they were not entirely alone in their experience. Some may have tried to disclose the abuse as a child, and either weren't believed or had adults ignore the problem while acknowledging that they knew about the abuse. These realities, coupled with the terror from the abuse itself, have caused many women to block their memories of abuse.

The following lists describe some characteristic aftereffects of childhood sexual abuse which you can be alert to during your interviews and interactions with women. *Keep in mind that these lists cannot and should not be used to diagnose a history of abuse.* They are intended to provide a profile of behaviors to look for to enhance your sensitivity to the possibility of traumatic experiences of any type.

PSYCHO-SOCIAL PROBLEMS	MENTAL PROBLEMS

Mistrust of or overdependence on the care-giver
Bonding failure
Fetus or baby perceived as a parasite
Attachment disorders
Post traumatic stress disorder
  (nightmares, high anxiety, minimal feeling of
  safety, panic attacks, flashbacks, preoccupation
  with previous birth experiences)
Eating disorders (85-90% related to sexual abuse)
	Extreme fear of pain
	Depression
	Anxiety
	Phobias of needles, pelvic exams, or other
	  invasive procedures
	Fear of not being a good mother (vigilant
	  attitude toward child; if no memories, may
	  not have sufficient vigilance)
	Dreams and nightmares
	Gender preference for baby (may hate males or
	  fear for a female child's safety)
	Obsessive/compulsive disorders
	Total denial (may be no abuse took place!)
	Mental illnesses
	Dissociative disorders

PSYCHO-SOCIAL PROBLEMS	MENTAL PROBLEMS
Obesity	Repugnance to water on one's face
Desire to change one's name	Alienation from her body
Pattern of ambivalent or intensely conflictive	Phobias
relationships	Limited tolerance for happiness
Substance abuse (dulling pain)	Suicidal thoughts
Fear of being alone	Anger issues
Humorlessness	Rigid control of thought processes
Need to be invisible, perfect or "bad"	Avoidance of mirrors
Childhood hiding or other security seeking	Discomfort with touch
behaviors	Fear of medical procedures
Wearing excessive clothing	Nightmares
Nervousness about being watched	Panic attacks
Requires extreme privacy when using the toilet	Depression
Failure to remove clothes even when appropriate to	Poor self-image
do so (swimming, bathing, sleeping)	Multiple personality disorder (frequently the
Pattern of being a victim	result of severe abuse)
Feeling demand to produce and be loved	Trust issues (inability to trust or total trust)
Abandonment issues	High risk taking or inability to take risks
Aversion to making noise	Boundary and/or control issues
Stealing	Guilt and shame
	Low self-esteem
	Blocking of all early childhood memories
	Feeling of carrying a secret
	Feeling crazy

SEXUAL DISORDERS	PHYSICAL PROBLEMS
Sexual addiction	Chronic untreatable conditions
Inability to achieve orgasm	Infertility
Prostitution (most have been abused)	Migraines or severe headaches
Pregnant teens (66% remember abuse)	Asthma
	Severe PMS
	Chronic constipation
	Swallowing or gagging sensitivity
	Gastrointestinal disorders

Additionally there are some common things which come up during pregnancy, birth and postpartum for women who have been sexually abused:

SEXUAL DISORDERS	PHYSICAL PROBLEMS
Fear of being "ripped apart" during birth	Hyperemesis gravidarum
Inability to breastfeed or difficulty dealing with	Exaggerated symptoms of pregnancy (more
normal behaviors of her baby during nursing	painful, more inconvenient)
(fondling the other breast, etc.)	Threatened premature labor (she may be trying
	to end pregnancy at this point)
	Fear of being out of control or dependent (may
	hold labor at a certain point to protect the
	genital area or the baby)

(Simpkin, 1994)

Even though a woman may display several of these signs, she may not have been abused at all, she may have been abused but not remember it or, if she does, she may not be ready disclose her experience or to deal with it. Nevertheless, you can treat all women with respect and ask yourself why a woman might be acting in a certain way before you react. Ask permission to perform procedures and exams. If a procedure will hurt, you should tell women in advance and be sure you have her clear permission to proceed so that you do not recapitulate or perpetrate any abuse yourself. Even when procedures are designed to be comforting, such as perineal support or massage, make no assumptions; ask before you proceed and get feedback from the woman to be sure what you are doing is comforting to *her*.

As a midwife you must avoid making statements which could be interpreted as convincing a woman that she experienced any kind of abuse. Even a statement like "Often when someone displays these reactions they have experienced some traumatic event but do not remember it; you might want to think about whether that might be true for you," could be construed as leading the client to believe she was abused. During the initial visit, you should ask all women if they recall sexual or physical abuse (see chapter on the Initial History, Contact section) and state your feelings about its relevance to childbearing. Do not belabor the topic without specific requests on the part of the woman to pursue it. When strong emotions or repeated patterns surface, a sincerely curious, open-minded inquiry regarding the elements of the situation *letting the woman lead the inquiry* can help her come to her own conclusions about the meaning of her feelings (see chapter on Working Through Emotional Issues with Clients for more details about how to do this).

Sexual abuse can take many forms, from the perpetrator watching the child to the child being subjected to having guns and other objects thrust into her yoni on a regular, predictable basis, or other forms of systematic torture. When a woman is prepared to disclose abuse, you must be prepared to hear whatever she may have to say. The details of the abuse may be hard or impossible for her to share or she may not remember details. While no woman should be forced to tell you things, you can remind her that pregnancy and birth tend to be strong triggers for sexual abuse issues and that your being aware of whatever details she is willing to share can help you both avoid unwittingly recreating the abusive dynamic during her care. Details can also provide information which can help you both strategize ways to actively counteract abuse-related triggers during labor.

"False" memories? Since about 1860, the dawn of modern psychology, professional recognition of the reality of sexual and physical abuse has surfaced several times, only to be met with an onslaught of denial and ridicule. In 1984, Victims of Child Abuse Laws (VOCAL) was founded in Minneapolis to advocate for the rights of those accused as perpetrators, claiming that children were not credible witnesses. This group was organized after a much publicized sexual abuse trial allegedly involving ritual abuse of dozens of children. Then, in 1992, Pamela and Peter Freyd, the parents of a woman alleging that her father had sexually abused her, were largely responsible for founding the False Memory Syndrome (FMS) Foundation. While the title implies that this is a scientific research group, it is primarily an advocacy group for people who claim that they have been falsely accused of sexual abuse. While false memory syndrome implies that research has been done and a new psychiatric diagnosis has been articulated, such is not the case. The use of the term syndrome serves to validate the cause of a group whose tenants rest on no such research. They cite research involving nontraumatic memories, showing that such memories are frequently unreliable and that people often cannot remember the details of witnessed incidents correctly. These studies do not apply to cases of traumatic amnesia. They contend that one does not block out significant life events either in part or completely and claim that many therapists and treatment centers are convincing people they have been sexually abused and are, in some cases, misusing suggestion, drugs and hypnosis to back up their claims. This, they say, leads women to falsely accuse family members of abuse when none has occurred. While misuse of therapeutic techniques certainly does occur, it is an uncommon practice. (synopsized from Davis & Bass, 1993)

Ritual abuse: Ritual or cult abuse is the type of abuse which has most recently "come out of the closet." As such, there is still a lot of public denial regarding the almost unbelievable claims about these experiences made by those who have been ritually abused. The clinical definition of ritual abuse has not been firmly established; however, the following definition by the Los Angeles County Task Force on Ritual Abuse gives you a good idea of what is being discussed:

> "Ritual abuse is a brutal form of abuse . . . consisting of physical, sexual, and psychological abuse, and involving the use of rituals . . . Mind control is the cornerstone of ritual abuse, the key element in the subjugation and silencing of its victims. Victims of ritual abuse are subjected to a rigorously applied system of mind control designed to rob them of their sense of free will and to impose upon them the will of the cult and its leaders. . . . The mind control is achieved through an elaborate system of brainwashing, programming, indoctrination, hypnosis, and the use of various mind altering drugs. The purpose of the mind control is to compel ritual abuse victims to keep the secret of their abuse, to conform to the beliefs and behaviors of the cult, and to become functional members who serve the cult by carrying out the directives of its leaders without being detected within society at large. . . . A key element of the victims recovery . . . consists of understanding, unraveling, and undoing the mind control which usually persists for a long time, even in victims who no longer participate in the cult. Undoing these controls is critical, for victims may remain unable to disclose their abuse, or vulnerable to cult manipulation if the systematic programming is not dismantled."

In ritual abuse, all forms of abuse (sexual, physical, mental and emotional) are used as means to an end: the total control of the subject. While some satanic or pagan cults are among these groups, there are other cults whose practices are not connected to satanism or paganism that commit similar crimes. Often the abuse includes brainwashing, severe intimidation, extreme humiliation, sensory deprivation, starvation, forced drug experiences, extreme torture, exhaustion, isolation, painful sexual abuse, bright lights used during indoctrinations, and the trauma of witnessing or being forced to participate in the actual or imitated ritual murders or abuse of animals, other children or adults. Whatever horrible types of experiences you can imagine (such as children being put in coffins filled with body parts that are then nailed shut, or being made to witness the birth and murder of a sibling) have all been described by survivors. Drugs and sex are often used together in public rituals.

Pubescent girls may be required to "breed" babies for cult sacrifices. More commonly, ritual abortion is performed. Genital scarring may be present. Most common, however, is the acting out of mock birth rituals in front of children, usually ending with the sacrifice of the "baby." The use of hypnosis and drugs makes these experiences seem very real and the trauma is significant; the survivor may have no idea that the scenes they witnessed were staged. (Roberts, 1990; Stardancer, 1995)

The victims may be told that their participation in the activities is voluntary while being taught that they are evil and have no choice but to join the cult. Many child-victims are born and raised by parents who have themselves been indoctrinated into the cult since childhood. Sometimes the "cult" heritage stretches back through a family for many generations. The parents may have multiple personalities, one of which perpetrates the abuse, leaving the core personality unaware of the abuse.

Typically those who manage to escape the cult have been preprogrammed with post-hypnotic suggestions to commit suicide, "go crazy," or return to the abusive situation rather than talk about their experiences. When survivors do break through this programming and begin to tell their stories, their therapists, the police or whoever is listening will often write off what they are reporting as hallucinations, which adds even more trauma to the situation. As a result of wholesale cultural denial, survivors are understandably sensitive and may be defensive regarding their experiences; it behooves you to be aware of this as a care provider.

Because of the strong programming against disclosure, many ritual abuse survivors have blocked the memories of their experiences. As they begin to remember fragments, such as incidents of sexual or physical abuse, they recognize that these incidents alone do not sufficiently explain their intense feelings. They may continue to have violent nightmares which eventually lead to memories of ritual abuse. Experiences of birth related abuse in one form or another may result in flashbacks or memories resurfacing during pregnancy. When this happens, women need to know that pregnancy and birth are powerful triggers and often bring up memories of abuse, regardless of the type of abuse that occurred.

If memories come up during pregnancy about previous birth related abuse, you can provide valuable support by acknowledging a woman's grief and rage. She may fear that her feelings will make her unable to be a good mother. Regardless of whether the situation was real or staged, it helps to support the woman by accepting her experiences as a woman who has actually borne a child and watched it murdered or whatever she reports. At the same time let her know that she can allow herself to grieve, but that she also has lots of time and can "schedule" time to deal with her past so her feelings won't encroach upon her relationship with her new baby. Supporting women to deal with their feelings while strategizing ways not to be overwhelmed and consumed by them is empowering to many. (Stardancer, 1995)

Sometimes work has already begun on sexual abuse issues when the memories of ritual abuse surface, throwing the survivor back into a full blown emotional crisis of memory reclamation. Healing for ritual abuse survivors may be more multilayered than for other victims of abuse. For further information on ritual abuse issues, read Safe Passage to Healing, by Chrystine Oksana and Ritual Abuse: What it is, Why it Happens, How to Help, by Margaret Smith.

Disassociation as a method of coping with abuse: Survivors of all types of abuse may use drugs, alcohol or others methods of disassociation to cope with the abuse and its psychological aftermath. There are many different degrees of disassociation. At one end is simple "spacing out," such as momentarily losing track of where you are going, or of the conversation you are engaged in, hearing the voice of someone who isn't there, or not knowing how you arrived at your freeway exit. Everyone spaces out like this from time to time. Next comes repression, the purposeful shutting out of the memory of a painful experience. Then comes distancing, removing oneself from the body and seeing the abuse "from across the room." Further along the continuum, there exists the capacity of the human mind to split off into multiple personalities or "alters" to cope with the abuse. This is especially true in cases of ritual or severe sexual abuse. Disassociation has served as a powerful tool for survival; encourage women to see their dissociative abilities as emotional resources while gently encouraging them to remain present and move through their feelings.

If you are working with a woman who is disassociating on any level, try to find out what type of disassociation is going on. Whenever possible, stop the activity that has precipitated the disassociation, and help her reintegrate and talk about her feelings and experience.

Multiple personality disorder is probably the least understood of all dissociative processes. Alters are produced by the child's psyche as a means of compartmentalizing and coping with different aspects of the abuse, thus protecting the primary or core personality of the victim. In ritual abuse, the cult tunes into

316

the development of the alters and may even encourage their development. They program the alters to do things to the victim under certain circumstances, such as kill her if she tells, take her to places where abuse will occur, etc.

Talking to one's inner child or different aspects of oneself does not mean one has multiple personalties. In true multiple personality disorder (or gift as one abuse survivor describes it), the boundaries of the personalities are more distinct. Often some of the alters may not know of the rest, and frequently the core personality does not know of any of the alters at the onset of therapy. The healing process consists of each personality healing individually, as well as communicating with the other alters and having them share their experiences with each other. Each one has played a role in the protection and survival of the core personality and each must be involved in the healing process.

Your response to a woman manifesting multiple personalities will vary depending upon whether she is conscious of her dissociate identities or not. Multiplicity with complete amnesia that is manifested openly during a situation which would normally call on the best dissociative defenses of the survivor indicates a system which may not have the strength to keep a new baby safe and cared for. This is no absolute indication that she *will* be a danger to her child, but the inability to control evidence of multiplicity while the "host" who is seeking care is unaware of the other personalities is a "red flag" that the defense system is breaking down or that the pregnancy is too traumatic to deal with without significant support. To further complicate the situation, the trauma of becoming aware of her alters may greatly impact a woman's ability to deal with her pregnancy. If you clearly see signs that a woman has multiple personalities of which she is not aware, arrange a consult with a mental health professional who has experience with multiples. If they feel that disclosure would be too much to add at that time, at least the realities of the woman's situation can be dealt with through professional support and supervision while the groundwork is being laid to help her accept the diagnosis. If she *can* tolerate the discovery, this is ideal, since it will be essential to get some agreements/contract with the other personalities to keep the baby safe and cared for no matter "who" is the mother. (paraphrased from Stardancer, 1995)

If you are working with a woman who appears to be unconsciously manifesting multiple personalties, and during a visit a completely different person seems to be sitting before you, speak to them as you would anyone else, with respect, interest and consideration. Even if it seems that a child personality is manifesting, continue to speak to the adult, using words the child can understand. Frequently the adult core personality is still listening. Remember that the primary purpose of the development of alters is protection. The alters may be reluctant to speak to a stranger at first, and it may take time to engage their trust. Once the alter has retreated, you might want to talk to the woman more about what therapy she may have had and what, if any, abuse she remembers, keeping in mind that she may have no knowledge of any alters. It is important to understand the potential for unconscious multiplicity to be a danger to a child. Therefore, this is something to take very seriously; search for a counselor who is knowledgeable in this area. Unfortunately, therapists who specialize in the treatment of those with multiple personalties are not very numerous. (Stardancer, 1995)

If you are working with a woman who discloses that she has multiple personalities, the first step is to request more details: is she currently in therapy?, is there a discernable pattern to when the personality shift occurs?, how many alters is she aware of and what are they like? listen to her and find out what she knows about the situation. In women who are aware of their self system, as it is called, when another personality manifests, be sure to acknowledge the alter directly, ask their name; alters distrust those who treat them as though they are not there, when they know you have been told that they *are* there! (Stardancer, 1995)

It is important to talk to her about any fear or concerns she has about how her multiplicity/survivorship might impact her ability to be a mother so she can strategize ahead of time how she might deal with "worst case" scenarios. It is also important to talk to other alters, being aware they each may have very different issues about the pregnancy that they need to discuss and/or talk about. To do so, ask the mother if anyone else inside has any questions or concerns. This gives the alters permission to come forward. Ask how they feel about the pregnancy and if they are making plans about how they can help out with the new baby. Ask the woman if anyone who isn't talking or hasn't yet come forward has any questions (this is important since "hiding" alters are often concrete thinkers). If someone is reluctant to talk, ask if another personality can act as interpreter to help out. Let them know you understand that although *they* may not be pregnant or want a baby, someone they share the body with is going to have a baby and they need to figure out how they are going to handle it in a helpful way. Offer the alter help, even if that means finding a counselor outside of prenatal care. (Stardancer, 1995)

Talking to the alters and getting their cooperation regarding the pregnancy can avoid all the worst potential problems the survivor faces as a new mother. If all the alters find ways to be positive about the coming baby or positive about their ability to have a life for themselves apart from the mothering role of the self system, crisis can be averted. (Stardancer, 1995)

Apart from therapy, women may feel supported to be in contact with another woman who is also a survivor and a mother. Survivorship a newsletter for ritual abuse survivors, has articles on parenting as well as mother/survivors who will be pan pals. Knowing she is not alone in her experiences or her struggle to deal with them can be an enormous help in her healing. Contact them at 3181 Mission St, #139, San Francisco, CA 94110 (707) 279-1209. (Stardancer, 1995)

It is important that you be aware of the varieties of disassociation, including the possibility of multiple personalities, in women you serve; you will find little information about it elsewhere. As more survivors of all types of abuse speak out, (and this is beginning to happen), more victims will feel safer to come forward not only to others but to themselves. This has happened with sexual abuse and we can anticipate that a growing number of people who have been ritually abused will begin to remember their experiences. Ideally, every woman who has been abused can participate in ongoing therapy or at least have access to therapy, during her pregnancy. If the woman is willing, you could either talk to her therapist or participate in a session or two, if that seems appropriate, to determine if you can and should be helping this woman and, if so, how.

Dealing with clients who have been abused: When a woman discloses that she has been sexually or physically abused, there are some affirming things which you can say to help validate her experience and let her know you acknowledge her pain regardless of the extent of the abuse or who the perpetrator may have been:

> *"It was not your fault, you were only a child"
> *"Regardless of what happened, it was horrible and should never have happened; abuse is abuse, no matter what form it takes."
> *If she tells you she felt pleasure during sexual abuse, you can tell her that "You have a normal body and if stimulated in the right way you would feel pleasure. That does not mean you brought on the abuse or that your other feelings of fear, etc. are wrong. It was the adult's responsibility to control themselves, not yours." Acknowledge that the combination of finding abuse pleasurable along with all the other feelings makes it a very confusing experience.

In addition to these supportive statements, you can, if it seems appropriate, create a space in which the woman feels permission to experience the rage, sadness, fear and pain that accompanied the abuse. (See the chapter on Working Through Emotional Issues With Clients, this section, for some ideas about how to do this.)

As you develop your relationship with the woman it may become possible to help her examine how an abuser/victim pattern may play out in her life. At the same time that the statements above are absolutely true, it is also equally true that as adults we are 100% responsible for how we act today based on what happened in the past. Instead of encouraging a "poor me" victim attitude, explain responsibility as noticing the connection between events and help her explore how she functions now based on what happened before. In this way, a woman is empowered while not being blamed, offering her the opportunity to explore her patterns so that abuse does not have to be a repeating drama in her life.

Any woman who has been abused and has begun therapy may be more fragmented emotionally than those who have not. Close scrutiny of the abuse upsets the status quo and begins to break up the way she has functioned in the world to that point. Therapy can bring on a state of emotional chaos as a result. Because of this possibility, some midwives suggest that women postpone beginning therapy until after their birth.

Pregnancy and birth issues: As a result of sexual or physical abuse, a woman may have a variety of responses which manifest during prenatal care or during labor. She may become passive and quiet, having learned as a child that passivity limits the abuse. She may "leave her body." She may be concerned about how she appears in terms of making noises or how her body looks. When therapists address the emotional issues surrounding abuse they may overlook dealing with the physical pain of being sexually abused which directly ties into the birth process. (If there is a Body Centered Therapist to whom you can refer women, they will not overlook this vital piece of the damage that has been done. (See the chapter on Working Through Emotional Issues With Clients, this section.) The same feelings of pressure, stretching and pain which a young child experiences when their genitals are penetrated by an adult finger or penis may be very similar to that which an adult woman experiences as the baby is being pushed out. The birth process itself is as inevitable and may be as painful as was the abuse. If a woman is choosing a homebirth and the abuse occurred in her home as a child, this may set up a safety conflict about letting go enough to actually give birth at home. In fact, the nudity involved in labor, the overwhelming physical sensations, the invasiveness of exams and procedures can all duplicate the milieu of sexual abuse.

On the other hand, some women look forward to the intense, healthy sensations of labor as a force of renewal in their healing process. Even those that start out afraid may be tremendously empowered by their birth experience and still others may find pregnancy and birth rather neutral experiences in relationship to their history of abuse.

To help a woman counter any concerns, have her start by getting things into the home environment that empower her and create a feeling of safety. She can begin thinking of a time when she felt the safest, happiest and most comfortable in her life and recall that time frequently during pregnancy; this can also be used as a visualization tool during labor. Ask her what makes her feel safe. What is her usual coping style for stress and pain (dissociation, withdrawal, etc.)? If the partner will be involved during the labor, ask them to remember a time when the couple was very content together and to use this as a visualization during labor. Other things can be used to harmonize with visualization images such as running water, sounds, voices, etc.

Ask a woman to come up with opening images which are personally meaningful to her. For many survivors, using image metaphors of opening may be much safer than focusing directly on her body. However, especially for ritual abuse survivors, what may seem like a totally benign suggestion (such as the image of a flower opening) may have been a trigger programmed by her perpetrators during her abuse. Offer specific images to a survivor only if requested to do so, explaining that particular images may be helpful to some and very disturbing to others. Watch for signs of distress as you list a few, remembering that abuse survivors can be very adept at hiding their emotions. Assess if the woman seems emotionally stable before you elaborate further. (Stardancer, 1995)

Keep in mind that terms which we often use to help women deal with labor such as "trust your body," "surrender," "yield" and "open up" may communicate that she will be hurt as soon as she does. Actually, this is true; to open to labor means that, in most cases, it will get more painful. Survivors need guidance to focus on the here-and-now healthy pain of labor. She can think of the baby bringing the pain out rather than it being pushed into her as it was during the abuse. You can tell her that the baby's birth is purifying and cleaning the area. Sometimes a survivor is worried that she will hate the baby for causing the pain of labor. You can remind her that since the pain is coming out, the baby becomes her ally in healing, not an enemy. The bottom line is that she is a *survivor*. Continue to affirm that she is a strong, capable person who can use her resources to deal with whatever challenges lie ahead.

Dealing with anger and projection: While the circumstances surrounding abuse will vary, anger is always one component of the after-effects of abuse. This anger can manifest in many ways and is likely to surface during your care-giving relationship with women. Since the advice on how to deal with this is applicable to more than just those women who are identified abuse survivors, it is included it in the chapter entitled When Client/Midwife Relationships are Difficult at the end of this section.

References and further reading:

Claypool, Susan, midwife, San Francisco, CA, editing comments, 3/16/95.
Davis, Laura, editing comments, 3/95.
Fredrickson, Renee, Repressed Memories, Simon and Schuster, New York, 1992.
Huffman, Shay, Healing the Violence, Family Refuge Center, 117 E. Washington St., Lewisburg, WV, 24901, workshop handout, MANA regional conference, West Virginia, 9/93.
Lobel, Kerry, Naming the Violence: Speaking Out About Lesbian Battering, Seal Press, 1986.
Oksana, Chrystine, Safe Passage to Healing: A Guide for Survivors of Ritual Abuse, HarperCollins Pub., New York, 1994.
Parker, Barbara & McFarlane, J., "Identifying and Helping Battered Pregnant Women," MCN, Vol. 16, May/June 1991, pp. 161-164.
Ritual Abuse, Definitions, Glossary, The Use of Mind Control, Order from: Los Angeles County Commission for Women, 383 Hall of Administration, 500 West Temple St., Los Angeles, CA 90012, 31 pages, ($5.00)
Roberts, Sachs, "The Role of Sex and Pregnancy in Satanic Cults," Pre and Post-Natal Psychology, Vol. 5, No. 2, Winter, 1990, p. 105-113.
Simkin, Penny "Childhood Sexual Abuse and Pregnancy," taped workshop presentation from the Midwifery Today conference, Eugene, OR, Spring 1993.
Smith, Margaret, Ritual Abuse: What it Is, Why it Happens, How to Help, HarperSanFranciscso, 1993.
Stardancer, Caryn, editor of Survivorship, a newsletter for ritual abuse survivors, editing comments, June, 1995.
Stratford, Lauren, Stripped Naked, Pelican Pub. Co., 1993.

Working Through Emotional Issues with Clients

There are many ways to help clients work through issues which may impact their birthing experience and many opinions about how involved a midwife should become in this process. Surely a midwife should not expect to take the place of a full-fledged therapist unless she is trained to do so. If not, you can get in over your head. A trained professional whose focus is psychotherapy should work with those who have major, deep seated issues that need intense one-on-one attention. This does not mean, however, that you are incapable of facilitating women in looking at issues which may impact their birth.

With years of personal growth work behind me as well as knowledge of various therapeutic modalities, I would like to introduce you to the most transformative type of therapy I have encountered so far: Body-Centered Therapy. I feel it is appropriate because it takes into account the spiritual level of the human psyche without attaching specific limiting beliefs to this approach. It does not in any way minimize the need to work through, not around, emotional and physical manifestations of dysfunctions. It is a complete system, that is, it does not merely stop at the point where an insight is reached, but offers tools to delve into the feelings and patterns which surround insights. The techniques and theories from various schools of psychology have been put together by Gay and Kathlyn Hendricks, two psychotherapists who have worked with individuals and couples for the past 20 years.

This chapter will give you an overview of Body Centered Therapy with an example of how it might be applied in a typical prenatal setting. If what you see here appeals to you, I strongly encourage you to read the Hendricks books for a more comprehensive presentation (see bibliography at the end of the chapter).

Theory and philosophy: Early in life human beings develop a split between feeling and thinking, which can also be thought of as a split between body and mind. Messages from the body (for example what we are feeling and what we want) become ignored or denied by the mind. There are powerful reasons why we tune out these messages: for approval, for control or even for survival. But ignoring or denying body messages does not make them go away; it distorts their expression instead. Once distorted they express through muscle tension, pain, distorted breathing patterns, gestures and other movements, as well as through dream, fantasy and communication patterns. They are expressed most painfully in actions and patterned behaviors that do not work to get us what we really want. By working with movement, breathing and tension patterns, Body-Centered Therapy assists in healing this mind/body split.

Body Centered Therapy views the human psyche in four different levels or layers. The central core is pure Essence—the part of us that is pure spirit, the clear space within us where consciousness resides in the unconditioned presence of Being. The other levels include feelings, persona or identities and finally projections.

ESSENCE: Pure life, spirit, no conditioning, pure consciousness
FEELINGS: Fear, anger, sadness, sexual feelings, excitement, joy
PERSONA: A way to deal with feelings; a way to make connection; a way to survive
PROJECTIONS: How we view the world and others based on our personas.

In a perfectly healthy world, we would experience feelings and flow from resolving them back into connection with our Essence. However, the connection with Essence can be disturbed in a variety of ways. Deep feelings have two main qualities that make them overwhelming: they feel like they will endure forever, and if we open to them, we will lose control or die. If something happens that triggers overwhelming feelings, such as a loss or a traumatic experience that results in fear, sadness, grief or anger, we look for ways to deal with these feelings. If someone is there to encourage us to be with the truth of what we are experiencing in the moment and work it through to completion, we still have the feelings, but we experience them in the larger context of Essence. If we remain grounded in Essence, we know we are more than our feelings. However, if we are surrounded by people who are not in touch with Essence themselves, we tend to seek whatever tools are at hand to get our needs met and remain connected. We then develop personas as an attempt to deal with the feelings. For example, lets say a little boy experiences a grief which makes him cry. Instead of his father supporting him to feel the sadness fully he says "Chin up, son, be a man, boys don't cry." The child cuts off from his feelings, creating a Little Man persona, to please and gain approval from his father, thus remaining connected. The purpose of a persona is twofold: to gain recognition or approval from those around us, and to protect us from the potential consequences of having feelings. Eventually, the persona filters how we perceive the world around us. Some of the many possible personas which people adopt are:

Little professor	Hard worker	Supercompetent
Get Sick	Jock	Devoted
Have accidents	Delinquent	Rambler
Space Out	Loner	Drama Queen/King
Dependent/Clingy	Victim	Get tough
Caretaker	Peter Pan	Stoic
Emotional roller coaster	Long suffering	Caretaker

And lets not forget one persona close to many of us: Super Midwife!

Created out of the presence of overwhelming feelings, personas "benefit" us in a number of ways:

*There is no need to think creatively; on automatic pilot, we stay locked into a familiar pattern of interaction.

*We do not have to feel. Avoiding or distancing from unpleasant or overwhelming feelings is one of the main purposes of creating personas.

*We get to make others wrong; thus, we avoid taking responsibility for given issues or feelings.

*We get to justify our own position or invalidate someone else's. Justifying a position is easier than doing the inner exploration of the authentic feelings that underlie the position.

The costs of staying locked in persona patterns are high:

*We do not get to think. There is no possibility of creative action when we are living as though we *are* our personas. They are part of a script, written long ago, and have a repetitive, predetermined pattern to them.

*We do not get to feel. Since personas mask feelings, there is a decrease in aliveness. All feelings come from the same source; we cannot selectively block out pain without blocking positive feelings as well.

*We do not get to experience genuine love. When we are locked within a persona, we cannot give or receive the authentic experience of love.

Through the eyes of a persona, we see the world and other people in a distorted way. When a persona is in charge, the world must be shaped to fit it. Instead of seeing things as they are, reality is replaced by our projections. For example, to dependent personas, the world is made up of those to whom they can cling and those they cannot. Our projections interlock with the projections of others, rendering real intimacy or communication impossible. Since personas are our false selves, they call forth the false selves of others. Thus we abandon the world of how we feel inside for the largely visual world of how we appear from the outside. Personas mask Essence, causing a fundamental split within the self. When this split is operating, it shows up as changes in our breathing and body language, as physical symptoms, psychological disturbances and in distortions in our relationships with others. (Hendricks, 1993)

The therapist who can read the language of the body and the breath is in a unique position to help people rapidly and effectively recover their birthright, a deeply felt connection with Essence. Through careful attention and the use of various techniques, the client is guided toward a shift within the self to embrace life the way it is rather than cling to past conditioning and learned behavior. The troublesome symptoms and emotions will then begin to transform. The therapist helps the person open to Essence, the space in which all persona identities reside but not taken seriously—instead of confusing the persona with who she actually is. In Essence a person is connected to herself and others as well as the universe; it is the place she comes home to. When working with clients, the more you are personally grounded in Essence, the more powerful and rapid your work with others will become.

Humans avoid being present with what is true in a variety of familiar ways, such as:

Somaticizing: generating a body pain or problem to take our attention from feelings.

Faulty attribution: blaming something Out There for something that is really In Here. (attributing a headache to someone else's anger rather than seeing that tensing the shoulders is a response to to the anger.)

Explanation: explaining the feeling to distract from feeling it. A good rule of thumb is "you are never upset for the reason you think you are."

Justification: instead of simply feeling the feeling, becoming righteous about the appropriateness of the feeling, thus preventing inquiry as to what the feelings may really be about.

Concepts: creating thoughts that remove us from the immediacy of the feelings.

Soap opera: recycling the life dramas of various personas to avoid discovering the real feelings that lie beneath the act. The drama, which usually involves making others wrong and one's self right, helps the person avoid examining the purpose of the drama and what feeling or truth it is protecting or hiding.

Logic: figuring out feelings (mental analysis) to avoid feeling them and to minimize their importance.

Judgementalness: Judging feelings or those of others to avoid allowing the space to be with them.

The therapist or midwife realizes that those in pain do not know they are acting out of their personas. They do not *have* an act, they *have become* their act. There is no separation between person and persona, no realness.

When grounded in Essence, we become more loosely attached to our personas and can begin to foster the positive aspects of our act and become less needful of the negative parts of it which do not work for us. For example, the positive side of being dependent is devotion, the negative side is clinginess. The loner can encourage independence while dropping the act that pushes others away. Typically, a person operates from two levels of persona: one which seeks positive approval (mother's helper, smart kid, etc.) and one which is used to cope with feelings when the other level doesn't work (delinquent, druggie, getting sick, etc.) This chart depicts the relationships among these two levels and the authentic level on which they are based:

AUTHENTIC	#1 PERSONA	#2 PERSONA
Feelings & needs clearly expressed (I'm scared, I'm angry, I need help)	Seeks approval	Controls feelings & others, blames others, justifies self (I'm right/you're wrong, my reality is the correct one)

Being in touch with Essence allows us to have feelings and persona but not be within their grip. It is easy to give too much weight to feelings when we are out of touch with Essence. Instead of being with them, we run from them, because we have lost touch with the larger, clearer, essential space in which to hold them. By losing touch with Essence and our feelings we become locked into the more superficial persona layer of our psyches. When we identify as if we are our persona, we focus our attention out onto others; we project our persona movie on the universe. The most damaging projections are the ones we have come to believe are the way the world actually is. For example, women who believe that all men are abusive may draw only abusive men into their lives.

A Quantum paradigm for therapy: Body Centered Therapy identifies four components of the human psyche that are key elements of the new paradigm: Essence, feelings, persona, projection. When a person moves from one of these levels to another, a quantum shift occurs in their experience of the world. When a person shifts toward the most superficial layer of the paradigm—projections—they experience less freedom, clarity and aliveness. When they shift toward their center—Essence—greater freedom, clarity and aliveness are the results.

Getting to Essence: The Hendricks have devised a series of questions which can be used during discussions with clients to direct them to look beneath their projections to the persona patterns and the feelings which underlie these beliefs. In doing so, people can rapidly move past their patterns to gain deeper insight, as well as freeing up energy to create their lives in a way that works better for them and those they love. The following questions may come in handy when discussing issues such as why a woman had surgical deliveries, problem relationships, difficult health problems or other events in her life. The key to making this process work is to assume an attitude of genuine curiousness as you proceed. Your curiosity, unhampered by analysis or preconceived notions, opens the space for the woman to feel her feelings and tell her own truth about them. In this work the client truly

326

leads the way, with you as a gentle, nonjudgemental guide.

THE PROJECTION QUESTION:
What are your complaints? or **What's been bothering you?**

Since most people having problems come in with a complaint (my boss is mad at me, my husband is uncommunicative, etc.), it is always useful to let them start from there. Whenever we have a complaint about something, we are operating from projection. When something happens to us more than three times, it is stemming from a persona pattern and warrants examination in that light.

When someone is in the midst of describing their complaint, you can intervene with questions designed to keep her from being stuck at any one level. When you ask a client a powerful question, one that catalyzes a shift of levels, the client's body reacts in a way that reveals crucial information that you can use to help her. When you make such an inquiry, the response may be "I'm angry," or something else more essential, but it is likely to reveal a habitual protective strategy such as defensiveness, suspicion, hostility, etc. Don't let this cause you to become uncentered; when defensiveness is stimulated, you are on to something.

THE PERSONA QUESTIONS:
When did you start experiencing life this way?
What are you experiencing right now?
Exactly what was happening when you started to see the world this way? or
When did the version of you which experiences the world this way emerge?
How is this situation familiar? or
What does this situation remind you of?

If the person has some concept of persona, you can ask: "Given this persona, what kind of people are required to play the other actors in this script?"

One or more of these questions allows the client to explore the possibility that at some point her belief structure had a beginning. It directs her to look beneath the projection to the persona that requires this projection. Thus the client moves from the outermost level of projection to the deeper level of persona. Very often at this point the client will communicate with body language or in some other way that a significant chord has been struck. This "chord" is often a core feeling that the persona is covering or protecting. More on this in a bit.

FEELING QUESTIONS:
What were you feeling when you first experienced the world this way?

Where are you experiencing this feeling in your body? (sometimes
people cannot identify a feeling, then ask)
What are the specific sensations you are experiencing? (have her
point to where she is feeling the sensation; be very specific)

These questions are directed to uncover feelings underlying the persona.
Even if a client says she feels numb or nothing, have her point out where she feels
the most numb, and continue to ask for details about how she experiences the
numbness or nothingness.

REALITY QUESTION: Exactly what happened?

Can she remember exactly what happened when she first felt the feelings that
lead to the persona that created the projection? You are after a statement of what
happened, not an interpretation. Whether the person can remember anything or not
is not as important as her opening the possibility that at some point something
happened. This inquiry disrupts the common belief that problems are pervasive and
permanent. If the client realizes the problems started at some point, she can more
easily imagine herself being free of that issue.

For many, however, nothing specific will ever come to light. It is important
to emphasize that whatever they are feeling is okay. Learning to simply allow the
feelings or sensations to be present with no judgement is essential, especially in a
culture that teaches that we need a "good" or "legitimate" reason to feel what we
feel. The key is to love whatever is coming up.

ESSENCE QUESTIONS:
Can you conceive of yourself completely free of this issue?
Who is the you that was there before this problem occurred?
**Would you be willing to feel and tell the truth about this event or
feeling until it is complete?**

If people are willing to tell the truth about their experiences and to feel their
feelings deeply enough, Essence will spontaneously appear.

The Five Flags: These are signals from the person that a breakdown is occurring
in her persona act. They may appear at any point during an interview and may
occur unconsciously as a habit of daily life. They are evidence of underlying
Essence.

*Breathing: fight or flight breathing is accompanied by tight muscles
which force the breathing up into the chest; this occurs when we
are scared, angry or hurt. Relaxed, centered breathing occurs in

the abdomen.   A shift in breathing pattern signals that an unexpressed emotion is being withheld.

*   **Movement:** any motion the body makes can signal an emotion (leg crossing, picking, squinting, etc.)
*   **Posture:** one side higher than the other, sunken chest, etc. represent ways of holding body tension which are related to persona.
*   **Verbal:** tone of voice, repeated words, emphasis, phrases, a little girl voice, etc. can be integrally related to the persona being manifested.
*   **Attitude:** the overall picture of the persona in question, for example; an angry, hostile manner.

Trying to notice every single little flag is not the point. Repetitive flags are most important and are signals from the unconscious for the person to take note. Pointing out the flag in a nonjudgemental way can help the person become aware of what underlies the flag. A way to do that is to simply say that you notice the behavior, thus bringing it to consciousness.

The nine strategies: There are nine techniques which have proven effective in getting people to tune into and transform their negative emotions. These brief descriptions are taken from the Hendrick's book At the Speed of Life.

Presencing: Problems persist to the extent that we fail to be present with them and with the feelings associated with them. When we can simply be with an issue (rather than judging it or trying to change it), the issue has space to transform in the desired direction. To *presence* means to simply rest the attention on something, without judgement or any attempt to change it. The reason why presencing feelings is so difficult and is so often resisted is that by doing so we are likely to discover why the feeling is there; since it is one that is being blocked, the reason can be pretty potent. However, our feelings are locked into place by resistance to them. Only by fully allowing ourselves to be with feelings can they begin to transform. To accomplish this, invite the person to put their attention on a feeling or sensation as it is experienced in the body. This is a simple report of the sensation or feeling such as "I feel an itchy, crawly sensation on my upper arms and a fluttery feeling in my stomach" or "I feel angry." It is not asking for an analysis of the report. In this work, analysis always follows experience.

Magnification: Many troublesome symptoms and feelings disappear rapidly when a person consciously magnifies their frequency or intensity. Magnification is also a dependable technique for revealing authentic feelings underlying symptoms. You notice something, often a flag, and ask the woman to increase or exaggerate the behavior. Not only does this bring the symptom or feeling to full consciousness and foster presencing, but it removes any sense of judgement from the issue. Further, small repetitive mannerisms cover up feelings. Magnifying the behavior helps bring feelings to the surface. Also, locating the feeling or sensation in time and space tends to reduce the sense that it is overwhelming. For example, the vague feeling of depression is much more threatening than a heavy feeling in the chest.

Breathing: Breath work can help transform emotional and physical symptoms. Breathing shallowly can cause a variety of unpleasant physical sensations. People tend to hold their breath to control unpleasant emotions such as sadness, hurt, anger and fear. Most people breathe into their upper chest with very little abdominal movement. When we breathe this way, only about a half a teacup of blood gets reoxygenated. When we relax and expand our abdomen as we breathe, the diaphragm moves most effectively and the lungs fill with much more air and blood than when the abdominal muscles are held tightly. When we allow our diaphragm to fully expand the lower part of the lungs fill with a liter of blood; no wonder deep abdominal breathing releases so much energy!

To refocus breathing in the abdomen have the client place both hands on her abdomen, just below the navel. Have her tighten, then release her muscles three times. Then have her breathe into her abdomen, feeling the movement of her belly with her hands.

By breathing into the physical sensations of feelings, the feelings will become bigger and then begin to dissipate. Simply have the person breathe into the feeling, attempting to allow it to become larger but not trying to push it away. Conscious use of the breath reduces stress, minimizes or eliminates anxiety and depression, helps control physical pain, can improve health problems and generally improves one's sense of well-being. Just the difference in oxygenation alone is a significant reason why this occurs.

Movement: Movement patterns precisely reflect emotions that need to be addressed. Movement indicates a client's degree of aliveness; it is a bridge to the inner self. Attention to movement is a powerful door to discovery and transformation. A movement may be stopped before completion, which may be evident in incomplete sentences or withholding a desire to reach out. Or, the expression of an impulse can become polarized, as when someone can either have a very productive day or stay in bed all day.

It is important to remember that movement flags are unique to each person. All of us have the same basic emotions, but we learned different ways to cope with them. Therefore, it is important to look openly at what the behavior may mean to an individual rather than analyzing or explaining it based on the experiences of other clients or experts. With this in mind, the following details can serve as a guide to possible connections, but are not intended as a dictionary of body language. Common unconscious movements that signal underlying emotional issues are:

Facial tics: grimacing, pouting, screwing up part of the face.

Scratching: may signal irritation.

Picking: fingernails, cuticles, other body areas, lint from clothes, debris from the rug or furniture; may indicate anger or could be a focusing technique or way to maintain personal boundaries.

Smoothing: hair, face, clothes, the rug, the area around the person; may be a comforting pattern, attempt to smooth things over emotionally, to make presentable.

Holding movements: holding a body part, such as the neck or arm, may carry an emotional charge; the part being held may have to do with the issue being discussed.

Brushing motions: brush off an arm, their hair, imaginary crumbs, or motion in the air during conversation.

Rocking: may signal feelings and sensations arising from early in life.

Self-touching: occurs frequently and often underscores the issues being discussed; may reassure her of being present, stop feelings or ground them.

Cringing: when fearful or avoiding; a person may contract in a cringing movement.

A way to invite inquiry into an unconscious movement is to ask the person to match their feeling with movement or a body posture. This is called the Moving Microscopic Truth. Truth is defined as that which cannot be argued. Once the action or posture has been initiated, ask what feelings or sensations are arising, and ask her to make them bigger; this is magnification through movement. If a polarization has been identified, have her verbalize the two sides of the spilt as she moves to help bring issues regarding the split to consciousness.

Another way to get a person in touch with feelings is to have her sculpt the feeling, such as pain, nausea, headache or tension, in the air with her hands. This bridges the gap between inner and outer experience. Essentially, it is movement that matches feeling, sensation or thought.

Completing: When we have unexpressed emotions, broken agreements, and unexpressed truths, we decrease our aliveness. Encouraging people to be aware of and complete with others in any of these areas can clear up and access a lot of energy for change and growth.

Telling the truth: Problems persist until someone tells a fundamental level of truth about them. When truth is expressed, there is space for the issue to transform in a healing direction. The truth is defined as that which cannot be argued. Most of the time an issue is surrounded by explanations: who's right, who's wrong, a plan about how it could be fixed. These are often directed outwardly at a spouse, a boss or even a child. As long as the feeling (anger, sadness, etc.) is firmly attached to the explanation, it is not possible to inquire about the real source of the feelings. Separating the problem from the pain is the first step to finding out what underlies the pattern which is presenting. How do you recognize the truth?

> *When you hear statements of primary feeling with no blame or justification implied: "I feel sad," not, "I feel really pissed off at that doctor."
> *When you hear statements about the quality of sensations associated with a feeling: "The anger feels like a tight band in my throat."
> *When you hear statements about the exact nature of sensations: " the numbness in my chest feels hollow, empty, as if a large space has been emptied of something."

Many symptoms are signals that a deeper issue is present; as soon as the signal gets attention, it may actually disappear, with a deeper level of the problem being revealed.

Grounding: When a client is be grounded, she can safely leave the appointment and deal with the physical world outside your door. Grounding can often be accomplished by having her stand up, converse and make eye contact until you are satisfied that she is in her body and ready to leave.

Grounding also asks if the person is capable of applying the insights gained to her real life outside the visit. Insights alone are not enough; if she cannot connect them to her feelings and the way she lives her life, there is little possibility for radical transformation.

Thirdly, grounding reflects a balance of feeling and expression. Humans become ungrounded when they have expressed more than they are actually experiencing or when they experience more than they actually express (Hendricks, 1993).

Manifestation: Problems with creating what we want in our lives come from being out of touch with Essence. When we are out of touch, we have no choices about what we want, since our wants arise from our programming. Often our wants are linked to unmet needs in the past. Just as frequently, we are much more in touch with what we don't want rather than what we do. Finally, we cannot get what we want because we have not fully accepted ourselves for being where we are now. *To get somewhere else, we must always start from where we are.*

After dealing with some blocks, getting a clear idea of what is desired can help immensely. You get what you focus on. If all a woman can do is focus on how afraid she is of going to the hospital, chances are that is where she will wind up. *After* confronting the truths beneath those fears head on, she can then start

332

formulating what she does want. She can even create a plan of action to accomplish it.

Love & responsibility: For these purposes, love is defined as the action of being happy in the same space with someone or something else. This means being happy in the presence of fear, anger, or sadness as well as joy and satisfaction. Loving the state in which we find ourselves releases energy and opens up the possibility for change.

Our culture has so interwoven the concept of responsibility with blame, shame and guilt that to suggest that someone is responsible for something can set off a tirade of defensiveness. Responsibility is being fully accountable for your actions. It also involves claiming the fact that you are the source for whatever is occurring. This does not mean you caused past events, such as childhood sexual abuse, but you take responsibility not to allow past traumas to run your life today. *To take responsibility is to notice the connection between events.* The bottom line of all these techniques is to tell the truth about how we are the source of our life's pattern. This gives each individual tremendous power to recreate her life in any way she desires.

<u>Putting the pieces together</u>: Now that you have a capsule review of the different techniques used in Body Centered Therapy, I shall demonstrate how they might be applied in a prenatal setting.

Julie, a first time working mother, is coming in for her third visit at 20 weeks of pregnancy. She is in generally good health, except for some nausea during the first trimester. For the third time she is late for her appointment, which is scheduled to last an hour. She is a pleasant young woman, married 2 years. You have noted that she tends to wear very cute little-girlish clothing and sometimes speaks in a little girl voice, especially when you are recommending things for her to do regarding her pregnancy.

(Julie rushes in, throws her purse down on the couch, strips off her coat)

JULIE: Wow, late again, sorry. Can I go pee first? I have to go real bad.

(Julie rushes off to the bathroom, checks her urine and returns)

JULIE: Everything was fine except some ketones; guess I didn't eat lunch yet.

MIDWIFE: You seem pretty harried. Why don't you just sit down, relax, take a few deep breaths, and get centered before we begin.

(Julie seats herself, closes her eyes, takes a few rapid breaths high in her chest)

JULIE: Okay, I'm fine now.

(Because the midwife has not attempted to work directly with Julie before on any emotional issues, she opens the visit by having Julie center and then introduces the idea before she begins. If they had some background in this kind of interaction, the midwife might have had her tune into feelings as soon as she arrived, without the gap.)

MIDWIFE: I've noticed that the three times I've seen you that you seem to have a pattern of feeling rushed and being late a lot. It's been said that as you live, so shall you birth. I wonder if you'd like to explore a little bit about what those things might mean in your life.

JULIE: Oh, its just traffic. This is a really bad time of day to be getting to this part of town, that's all.

MIDWIFE: Perhaps that is all it is. *(Note that she does not "take the bait" of this slightly defensive stance and get into an argument with Julie about whether this perception is correct. To do so would be nonproductive and distract from where she is trying to go with this inquiry.)* But for now, if your willing, I'd just like you to sit quietly and reconnect to what you were feeling in your body when you came into the room today. Describe whatever physical sensations or feelings you can for me. Point out where they are in your body.

JULIE: This is certainly different than going to the doctor! Okay, let's see *(she closes her eyes and furrows her brow in concentration)* I feel sort of upset, antsy and irritated by the traffic.

MIDWIFE: Good. I notice that as you are tuning in you are frowning, do that a little more.

JULIE: *(slips into little girl voice)* Oh, I didn't know I was doing that, I'm sorry. *(she rearranges her face into an artificially pleasant expression as she tries to tune in again)*

MIDWIFE: You seem to be perceiving that as criticism. What our bodies do at the same time that we are feeling something can be linked. Let your frown be there, be aware of it and exaggerate it as much as you can. Then make yourself look as pleasant as possible and see what that feels like. Switch back and forth several times.

JULIE: *(hesitantly)* Oh, I guess I see how that might be true. *(she begins to frown intently, then switches to her "pleasant" expression)*

MIDWIFE: I also noticed that your tone of voice changed when you said you were sorry. Keep doing that too, as much as you can. What are you experiencing now?

JULIE: Well, I feel kind of put on the spot right now. Like I'm supposed to do it right or come up with the right answer or something.

MIDWIFE: And does that remind you of something or someone else? *(Or she could ask "Is this a familiar situation for you?")*

JULIE: Oh yeah, it sure does. We always had to be totally together as kids when my Dad came home. There was always this big rush to be cleaned up and dressed and everything when he arrived. My parents had a real thing about that. He was an army sergeant and we always had to line up for an inspection. If we didn't pass, we had to eat dinner in the kitchen by ourselves. He was really hard on my brothers, more so than me and my sister, especially when we were younger.

MIDWIFE: So, it sounds like it worked for you to be a little girl for as long as possible when you were growing up.

JULIE: Oh, I never thought of it, but I guess you're right.

MIDWIFE: Lets go back to tuning in to your feelings again. What are you feeling right now?

JULIE: Just remembering that feeling as a child, the hurry and tension and being scared before he got home.

MIDWIFE: Do you see any connection between that childhood experience and your tendency to be late in your adult life?

JULIE: *(looking surprised)* Well, when we were kids we always knew we had to be ready and at the same time we knew we might not be up-to-snuff for the inspection. It made being ready very scary.

MIDWIFE: Just let yourself feel that fear now, Julie. Where exactly do you feel the sensation of fear in your body? *(note that the midwife does not stop at the insight, but proceeds to explore the body/mind/emotional connection to the insight)*

JULIE: *(points to her throat)* Right here mostly, like a tight, gripping sensation.

MIDWIFE: Great. Now breathe into that sensation, just let it get as big as it wants to be.

JULIE: But I don't want to feel afraid, aren't we supposed to take my blood pressure or something?

MIDWIFE: *(another defensive strategy often employed when the mind is protecting us from getting in touch with a truth or feeling that threatens the status quo. Once again the midwife does not take the bait, but gently side-steps the challenge to argue)* We will in a bit, but right now it seems like we may be onto something, lets stick with it a little longer. Just breathe into that feeling in your throat and see what happens.

JULIE: *(breathing shallowly)* It's feeling tighter.

MIDWIFE: Good. Just let the tightness get bigger, breathe deeper or do whatever you need to to make the tightness more.

JULIE: *(beginning to cry)* Every night, we were so scared of my father, but we could never cry because he would get mad. It feels like when I was little, when I was trying not to cry.

MIDWIFE: Just let yourself cry now, Julie. Let yourself feel all the sadness around that. Breathe into it and let the sadness be as big as it wants to be. *(Note she does not try to calm her down at this point, which would cut off the flow of feelings, but encourages her to feel her feeling fully. This is a hallmark of Body Centered Therapy and a big reason why it is so effective.)*

(Julie continues to cry for a few minutes, then looks up at the midwife, who hands her some tissues.)

JULIE: I feel lighter, like something about the sadness has changed, I can't quite explain it. What happened?

MIDWIFE: When we allow ourselves to feel our feelings fully, often they have the space to change into something else. Between now and the next time I see you, which will be in a month, I would like you to start noticing when you get that tight sensation in your throat, and what is going on at those times. When you do, breathe into those sensations, being sure you let your breath go into your belly like this *(demonstrates deep abdominal breathing)*, placing your hands on your upper abdomen if necessary to remind yourself where to take your breath, like this. See what comes up, and if you have time, jot down some notes when you can about those feelings. Then we can talk about it next time you come in. Becoming more conscious of your breathing will also be a great help to you in labor.

(At this point the midwife has Julie demonstrate her understanding of the breathing technique.)

After a bit more conversation the midwife moves along to complete the clinical portion of the appointment, they talk a little more at the end of the appointment and the midwife recommends that Julie read At The Speed of Life.

As you explore these techniques more deeply, you will find that you can integrate many of them into the normal course of appointments and certainly during labor to help women get in touch with feelings and move through them in order to birth. Not every client you see will be open to working with you in this way, and, as always, you will have to use your intuition about how to proceed with each individual woman.   See the following chapter on When Client/Midwife Relationships are Difficult and the one on Physical and Sexual Abuse in this section for some other useful suggestions.

Finding a body-centered therapist in your community: More and more traditional therapists are attending professional training seminars and adding the skills of Body Centered Therapy to their repertoire.   You can find out about training, or whether there is a therapist in your area by calling the Hendricks Institute, 401 E. Carrillo, Santa Barbara, CA 93101, (800) 688-0772. Then you can have someone to whom you can refer those women who need consistent help during their pregnancy that you cannot provide.

Becoming a body-centered counselor yourself: The Hendricks are totally committed to sharing their knowledge and experience with everyone. Training in body-centered techniques is open to all interested parties, regardless of their background or training. This means midwives who so desire can avail themselves of this training which I believe will greatly enhance both individual practice and the health of the midwifery community in general. Two seminars are currently offered, each consisting of two phases or levels: Body Centered Training and Conscious Relationships. All four seminars prepare you to counsel both couples and individuals. Contact the Hendricks Institute for more information.

References and further reading
Hendricks, Gay & Kathlyn, At the Speed of Life, Bantam Book Pub.,NY, 1993. (Most of this chapter was paraphrased from this text. It offers an overview of theory and technique with examples from case histories and explanations about why the techniques work.)
Op. cit., Conscious Loving, Bantam Book, Pub., NY, 1992.
Op. cit., Radiance! Breathwork, Movement and Body-Centered Psychotherapy, Bantam Books, NY, 1994.

When Client/Midwife Relationships are Difficult

Your relationships with clients may be difficult for a variety of reasons. Knowing how to deal with problematic relationships is truly one of your most necessary skills as a midwife. This chapter will focus on emotionally based issues which can arise, and how you can negotiate your way through them with a minimum of trauma. These techniques are particularly useful when the suggestions in the previous chapter do not seem appropriate for an individual woman.

As human beings, we tend to unconsciously reenact traumatic emotional cycles in our lives until we discover a way to heal and thereby break the negative cycle. The care-giving relationship, which includes issues of power, authority, trust, and vulnerability (to name but a few), is a set-up for any control-anger-distrust cycles to replay themselves. If you are not conscious of this possibility, you may unwittingly get caught up in this pattern. In fact, as a woman in an authority role you may find yourself standing in the place of the client's mother.

Remember that people do not behave the way they do by accident. How a woman is behaving now is exactly how she has survived up to this point in her life. Whether or not a woman remembers specific events (such as abuse) which may have "caused" her current reactions is not as relevant as understanding how to deal with her reactions in the here and now without getting sucked into her pattern.

Very often women who "push your buttons" may be unconsciously trying to test you around issues which they have been let down on in the past. This may occur in various ways: the client may present herself as excessively needy and controlling, she may demand "too much," or more rarely she is the perfect client and follows every recommendation to the letter. She may choose you because she projects that you are a "perfect" care-giver who will protect and nurture her through this overwhelmingly vulnerable time.

In response to neediness or to the perfect client who seemingly needs nothing, the midwife may withdraw emotionally. This can occur in the first case because you become fed up with lots of phone calls, overly long appointments when you have other clients as well, and a feeling that you do the woman a disservice if you allow her to depend upon you too much. The "perfect" client may simply appear to need no extra attention.

After the emotional withdrawal by the care-giver the woman will often perceive an action of the care-giver negatively and react with anger. Routine procedures which are perceived as minor or clinically safe by the care provider may be perceived as a big deal by the client. The client may become angry and express this by pointing out the problem and demanding an apology or an admission of guilt or error on the part of the care-giver. If midwives are working in a partnership, the woman may try to play them off against each other. For example, a woman is in early labor and one midwife goes to her home, then calls the other midwife when things start moving along. It was explained prenatally that this was what was going to happen and the woman never expressed her desire to have both midwives present from the onset of labor. Later she says that she is angry and feels neglected due to the fact that both midwives were not there. Your response at this point can help defuse the situation or turn it into an even bigger deal.

The care-giver who becomes sucked into this pattern makes a very bad decision: she becomes defensive, refuses to respond or apologize, and may minimize the incident with comments like "that is routine in our practice," "no one has ever complained about that before," etc. After the tone of the discussion takes this turn the client becomes confused, more angry and feels totally invalidated, leading to a schism or argument between the care-giver and the client. The client then seeks revenge by refusing to pay, litigation, or hurting the midwife's reputation, and may refuse to see the midwife again. The end result is long term hurt on the part of all parties concerned. Thus the client, with her midwife's participation, has "proven" to herself once again that those in power cannot be trusted and will always betray her. Yuk. Perhaps you recognize this pattern working itself out in women you have helped.

How to respond rather than react to the distressed client: You have a needy, controlling or angry client. In response you become respectful, carefully listening to her so that you can validate her wants and needs. And indeed, if some need of hers was unmet or she has felt violated, that feeling is valid for her, regardless of how ordinary or routine the procedure or circumstance may have been. To validate her, you can incorporate a variety of simple communication skills:

> Reflective responses—"Can you tell me more about that?"
> Validation—"That must have been very hard for you."
> Using "I" messages—"I'm surprised to hear how strongly you feel."
> Repeating what she has said back to her "So you felt angry and
>   vulnerable when the strange male resident walked into the room
>   when you were pushing on your hands and knees. I can
>   understand how you felt and I'm so sorry that happened."

In dealing with the situation in this way we acknowledge that what a woman experience is valid for her and that her wants reflect her survival techniques. Frequently it is the woman's "inner child" daring to speak and say that they don't want something. Midwives can be the first people to validate a woman's needs by acknowledging rather than minimizing her feelings. Instead of perpetrating the abusive pattern, this diffuses a woman's anger and distress and creates greater trust. This leads to more reasonable negotiation and a better resolution for all concerned, resulting in a client who is empowered as a woman and a parent.

References and further reading:

Simkin, Penny, "Childhood Sexual Abuse and Pregnancy," taped workshop presentation from the Midwifery Today conference, Eugene, OR, Spring 1993.

BASIC MIDWIFERY SKILLS

This section will discuss the primary skills and procedures used in midwifery care to assess the well-being of the mother and fetus during pregnancy. Phlebotomy, performing a PAP smear, using a microscope and miscellaneous skills regarding fetal assessment and prenatal tests of the mother are covered in <u>Diagnostic Tests</u>.

Using Knowledge and Intuition

Growing up and being educated in a patriarchal culture has led to an overemphasis on rational knowledge while devaluing and often completely ignoring the reality and worth of intuitive perceptions. As midwives practicing holistically, we learn to synthesize academic knowledge, clinical skills, practical experience, intuitive perceptions, and spiritual awareness as we grow in our work. Knowledge can be defined as what we gain from intellectual pursuits such as reading, attending classes and understanding the physical aspects of pregnancy and birth.

The dictionary says intuition is "the immediate apprehension of truth in the absence of rational processes." Intuition is a knowing which is beyond mental understanding and which often seems more real than any mental process. It may be difficult for some to know when a developed intuitive perception has been "arrived" at, for me this grew in conjunction with academic understandings, but in some midwives intuition may be well developed before the knowledge is laid down.

How can you tell if your intuition is talking or if it is just a mental conversation taking place based upon what you know intellectually about a situation? One way to tell is to ask yourself, "how does this feel at a gut level? Am I really concerned about this because I *feel* concerned or is it only that the sum total of the knowledge I have about what this might mean is going off in my head all at once?" These questions, posed to yourself or a client who has presented a concern, will often clarify the feelings involved. The mother or the midwife can have an intuitive sense that everything is fine in spite of worrisome clinical signs. Likewise, the mother or midwife can have a strong intuitive sense of a problem in the face of a totally benign clinical picture. When in doubt, I rely on the mother's sense of well-being or danger; if she is unsure, I go with my own assessment. For techniques to develop your intution see Women's Intuition by Elizabeth Davis.

When you begin primary practice, it will be important for you to err on the side of "better safe than sorry." Clear your mind and psyche prior to your appointment day in order to open yourself to your intuitive side as you see each woman. Note your intuitive perceptions regarding every situation you encounter; does the perception come to you as a voice, a physical sensation, an emotion, or in some other way? If clinical signs point to a problem, act on them and continue to monitor your intuitive feelings. Soon you will accumulate a series of experiences that will tell you whether what appears to be an intuitive assessment can be relied upon. As you gain more experience, your intuitive assessment can take precedence over the clinical picture *when you feel quite sure that your intuition is not being clouded by denial on any level*. This is an important "if" which requires clarity and centeredness; when in doubt, act on the clinical picture.

Denial can interfere with intuition for many reasons. For example, you may want to support nonintervention and ignore your inner sense that she has a problem. In such situations, do not minimize the clinical picture when it correlates with what you intuitively know to be a concern. As you gain experience you will be less tempted to "protect" women in this misguided way.

Equipment to Have On Hand for Prenatal Exams

Prenatal equipment can range from a few simple basics to having more elaborate equipment, such as a microscope, in your office. Having lots of fancy equipment is not necessary; having basic, good quality tools which you feel comfortable using is helpful in providing care. Buy the very best tools you can afford the first time you buy them. Poor quality equipment may do when you have years of experience and are well versed in using the tools in question, however, a student or newly-practicing midwife needs the best tools available to help make up for her lack of experienced skill. If you spend the money when you start your practice, you will have reliable tools for a longer period of time rather than having to struggle through with poor quality tools that do not really do the job.

Carrying your equipment: Many midwives have decided that the most practical way to store and use equipment is in two bags. A bag filled with prenatal equipment can be taken together with a larger bag of birth equipment when it is time to go to a birth. In this way you don't have to duplicate all your purchases and you are still fully equipped at the birth.

Birthing supply houses have prenatal and birth equipment bags which are ready-made for this purpose. These bags work well if you like the idea of putting all your equipment into separate pockets inside the bag. Designate a space for each item and always put it back in the same location. In this way, you will quickly learn your system (as will your helpers or apprentices) and finding things will not be a constant problem.

An alternative approach is to buy a suitcase or fishing tackle box and arrange your supplies in the compartments, with labels. Or, you could buy various sizes of plastic refrigerator storage boxes and fill them with supplies, labeling the tops. You can then ask an assistant to go to your bag, pull out a specifically labeled box and look for a particular item. I use a combination of these ideas, with prenatal equipment in a bag with pockets and birthing equipment in a suitcase in plastic food storage boxes which are appropriately labeled.

Prenatal equipment which you may wish to have on hand includes:

Stethoscope: A stethoscope is a device used to help you hear body sounds. It consists of a binaural or metal piece with two padded ends that insert into your ears, a long tube or tubes and a headpiece. The headpiece usually has two sides, a **diaphragm** and a **bell,** which are designed to amplify and isolate different ranges of sounds. The flat diaphragm may be placed against the body to assist in listening to diffuse physiological sounds, such as lung or bowel sounds. The bell-shaped side is used to isolate sounds or bring distant sounds into sharper focus. You will need a simple nurse's stethoscope for use with your blood pressure cuff. It will have a diaphragm only and is used to listen to the arterial pulse.

It is also nice to have a regular adult stethoscope with a reversible bell and diaphragm headpiece for listening to maternal lung and heart sounds during your initial physical exam. More elaborate styles, for example the Rappaport-Sprague, have interchangeable bells and diaphragms to allow for a range of different uses. Stethoscopes come in adult, pediatric and infant sizes; it is a good idea to have at least an adult and an infant scope on hand.

A note on ear tips: Stethoscopes and fetascopes come with rubber or plastic screw-on ear tips which fit over the ends of the binaural. Be sure these ear tips are the appropriate size for your ears. The wrong ear tips will greatly interfere with your ability to pick up sounds and may cause you to reject a style of stethoscope that would work fine otherwise. Replacement ear tips in various styles and materials are available at medical supply houses. They are inexpensive, making it possible to experiment until you find the right ones for your needs.

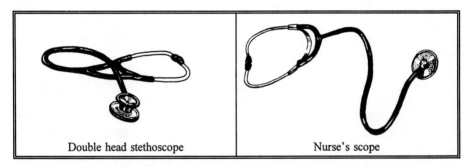

| Double head stethoscope | Nurse's scope |

Fetascopes: This specialized stethoscope is used to listen to the fetal heart through the mother's abdomen. They are available in several different styles. Deciding which works best for you will be very individual, depending upon how you are trained and what you are used to. It will also depend upon how acute your sense of hearing is. Most fetascopes have a bell-shaped head which is designed to isolate low, faint or muffled sounds most clearly. You may want to purchase a fetascope with a long tube leading to the earpieces that allows a mother to hear her baby's heartbeat in addition to the fetascope you will use regularly. Frequently, however, once you find the fetal heart, you can find it again with a regular stethoscope fitted with a long tube to allow the mother to listen.

The **human ear** was the first and still is the most available fetascope. By placing your ear directly on the mother's abdomen and pressing it into the surface firmly you can frequently hear the fetal heart. Traditional midwives in Nicaragua also place their hands on the mother and feel the fetal heartbeat (Vidam, 1990).

The **DeLee** fetascope is distinguished by a metal headpiece which helps conduct sound through the skull. It can be worn with the headpiece in place, leaving the hands free to work; it may be necessary to hold the headpiece in one hand while listening when the mother is in an upright position.

The basic **Allen** fetascope has a smaller forehead rest which also helps to amplify sound waves. It does not leave your hands completely free to work, since it cannot be left in place when you want to move your head. The **Perrell** has a similar design with longer tubing.

The **Series 10 Allen** fetascope looks externally similar to the basic Allen, however, the entire headpiece is internally structured with a special chamber offering maximum sound amplification and resonance. This considerably enhances its ability to pick up faint sounds.

The **Ditmar** or **Sklar Leff** fetascope has an unusual head consisting of a large, round, heavy metal piece. The underside of this bell is slightly concave, with a small hole in the center to conduct sound. While this style fetascope can be cold and rather awkward to position due to its weight, many midwives feel that this instrument offers excellent sound conduction. The sound is lower pitched and more diffuse than with other fetascopes.

The **Pinard** probably represents the oldest of the manufactured fetascopes (with the possible exception of hollow reeds). This simple device has been used in Europe for years. It is a single piece of sculpted wood or metal which has a small flat bell on one end and a larger more funnel-shaped bell on the other. The ear is placed over the smaller end and the funnel shaped end is pressed against the mother's abdomen. The sounds tends to be diffused, but many midwives describe being able to almost feel the vibration of the fetal heart when the sound is very faint. Using only one ear for auscultation means you must learn to ignore sounds with the other ear while listening.

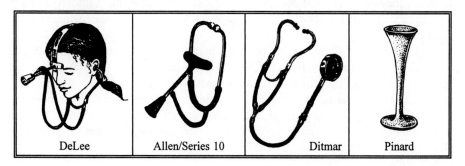

| DeLee | Allen/Series 10 | Ditmar | Pinard |

There are also several types of **Doppler** fetascopes on the market today. Doppler fetascopes produce a continuous wave of high frequency non-ionizing radiation (ultrasound). The waves pass through the body, and their reflections are interpreted by a transducer that displays the information or makes it audible. Some hand-held doppler fetascopes have instantaneous read-out displays which give you the heart rate equivalent per minute, a portable version of fetal heart monitor technology, which might be handy for deaf midwives or in rare emergency situations. However, the trade off in unproven technology may not be worth it. The fact that the doppler ultrasound waves are emitted continuously makes exposure to ultrasound doppler effect considerably more potent than the pulsed ultrasound used for imaging diagnosis—so much so, in fact, that 1 minute of Doppler exposure is equal to 35 minutes of real-time diagnostic ultrasound. Electronic fetal monitors also use doppler wave ultrasound.

Doppler fetascopes can be used to detect the fetal heart as early as 8 weeks of pregnancy. The fact that the small fetus is being exposed to the most intense type of diagnostic ultrasound must be taken into account when you and the mother are assessing the relative merits of one type of fetascope over another. (See the chapter on Ultrasonography and Doppler Diagnostic Techniques in Diagnostic Tests.) I encourage students and practicing midwives to learn to use a fetascope, reserving doppler use for rare emergencies.

Blood pressure cuff: Also called a sphygmomanometer, this device is used to measure the blood pressure. It consists of three parts: an **aneroid** is the hand pump used to inflate the **cuff**. The cuff is a cloth-covered rubber bag or bladder which fits around the arm (in most cases). When inflated, it temporarily occludes blood flow in an artery. The **sphygmomanometer** is the device which measures the pressure within the inflated bladder throughout the reading. Some cuffs have a stethoscope attached; if not, you'll need one with only a flat diaphragm (a nurse's scope).

A variety of blood pressure instruments are available. While sphygmomanometers that use mercury to indicate the pressure range are most accurate, they are bulky and delicate to transport. Therefore, most midwives carry devices which use a clock-face type gauge with a movable dial to indicate the pressure range.

Try several different styles of blood pressure cuffs to see which suits you best. Dial gauges should be certified and have no pin stop (a little pin at the bottom of the dial on which the needle rests). Be sure to have it calibrated periodically at a local surgical supply house, or calibrate it yourself by connecting your dial cuff to a mercury gauge. Remove the cuff from both systems, insert a Y-connector, and then pump the bulb until the mercury reaches 250 mmHg. Deflate, stopping every 10 to 20 mmHg.; compare readings at 140, 90 and 0 points, which should be the same.

You should also have child and large adult sized cuffs available as well as the average sized adult cuff which comes with adult models. Correct cuff size is essential for an accurate reading. If, when in place, the air bladder edges overlap the cuff, it is too large. If the bladder does not fully encircle the arm, then it is too small. Arm size ranges for different cuffs are:

Child 7.24 - 10.51"   Adult 10 - 15.98"   Large adult 13.5 - 20"

Most cuffs which allow you to change from one size to another have only one tube. With these, make sure the hand aneroid feels comfortable to you, since they typically have a metal piece attached to assist in pumping up the bulb which also stabilizes the dial gauge. If it is not designed to suit your hand, this metal piece can make pumping the bulb very uncomfortable.

Urine analysis dip sticks: There are a number of different types of urine analysis dip sticks, each of which includes different tests on the same stick. You will want to use a stick which minimally tests for protein, glucose, ketones and nitrites. Unfortunately no sticks are available which test only for these four things. You will therefore have to choose from among those including several other tests in order to get a stick which will allow you to test for these items. The proper care and use of urine analysis dip sticks is thoroughly reviewed in Diagnostic Tests.

Nitrazine paper or swabs: Nitrazine paper or long handled nitrazine treated swabs can be used to check for amniotic fluid in cases of suspected ruptured membranes. (For more information on their use see Diagnostic Tests.)

Paper cups: It is necessary to provide a clean container for women to use to collect and test their urine at your office or during a home visit. Small 3 ounce Dixie style paper cups are ideal for this purpose. A tin Rumford's baking powder can will hold this size cup perfectly, so you can pack some away in your prenatal bag for use during homevisits.

Centimeter tape measure: A soft cloth or plastic tape measure can be purchased at any fabric store. Retractable ones are nice. You'll be using this primarily to measure fundal height and for measuring the baby during the newborn exam.

Hemoglobinometer: This instrument measures the hemoglobin concentration of whole blood from a finger-prick sample. There are two models widely available, one produced by Buffalo Medical Systems and the HemoCue, produced by HemoCue, Inc., 23263 Madero, Suite C, Mission Viejo, CA 92691 (800) 323-1674 or (714) 859-2630. The HemoCue, which costs $795.00, is the only brand currently waived for use by CLIA, the agency in charge of laboratory regulation (CLIA approval is an important consideration, especially for birthing centers). With the BMS instrument, judgement is required because you must match the color of the sample with the color of a calibrated glass standard. The HemoCue is designed to minimize blood contact and eliminates human error in assessing the hemoglobin value. Although somewhat expensive, these simple-to-use devices are both fairly accurate and a great thing to use to determine a woman's hemoglobin and monitor her response to therapy.

Glucosometer: This is certainly not an essential piece of equipment, but it can come in handy when you are concerned about a woman's blood sugar (either being too high *or* too low); you can also use it postpartum to evaluate neonatal blood glucose if necessary. There are many brands available and they are getting increasingly easy to use. Check out the features of several in your local pharmacy or surgical supply house and choose one that has straight-forward instructions (since you may be sending it home with a client at some point) and readily available reagent sticks. HemoCue also makes a desk-top model which sells for $795.00 and is available from them at the address given in the previous paragraph. If you chose not to purchase a glucosometer, you can still carry blood glucose sticks designed for visual reading in your prenatal bag.

Speculum: This instrument is designed to be placed inside the yoni to hold open the walls of the birth passage. This allows you to see the cervix and the deeper walls of the yoni. There are several styles to choose from, the most popular are the Pederson and the Graves models. These two styles are basically similar, but the Pederson has narrower bills. If you have a large practice, you may find having several sizes useful. Traditional designs have bills which are placed inside the yoni and an adjusting mechanism which forms a 90° angle to the bills which stays outside the yoni during use. A newer pattern has a less acute handle angle which is useful in doing exams which are not being performed on an exam table. The chapter on the Physical Exam will go into detail about speculum structure and use.

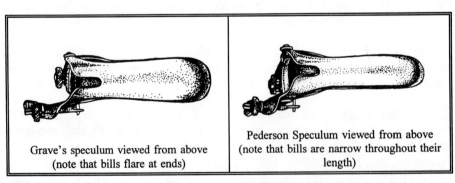

| Grave's speculum viewed from above (note that bills flare at ends) | Pederson Speculum viewed from above (note that bills are narrow throughout their length) |

Exam gloves: Exam gloves are essential these days with the increased risk of contracting blood-borne pathogens; gloves with longer cuffs will provide more protection for you. Latex gloves are the most widely available and come powdered with talc for easy donning. Talc, however, is an irritant in wounds, so be sure none gets scattered into the perineal area. Those who are allergic to talc or latex can get gloves made from hypoallergenic materials that are not powdered. Well-fitting gloves are a real plus; they allow you to feel accurately and do not interfere with delicate finger work during suturing or exams.

70% alcohol: This is used to remove surface dirt from the skin before a puncture for a blood test. Used in this way it does not sterilize anything.

Lancets: A 2.5 mm lancet is a good all-purpose length to use for testing maternal or newborn blood. Spring loaded lancet holders are also available which afford a rapid, less-painful puncture. You may, however, find them a nuisance to clean between tests.

Gestation calculator wheel: Being bad at math, I have relied heavily on a due date calculator over the years. In addition to eliminating the need to figure out gestational age with math, the calculator can be set with a date for conception and instantly give you a due date. This is a big plus when you are trying to date the pregnancy from conception or from when a woman really ovulated if her menstrual cycle is not 28 days. Wheels are produced by many pharmaceutical companies and can usually be obtained free of charge; Cascade Health Products sells them as well. Take a look at as many different types as you can to decide what features are most useful to you. Be sure the indicator is easy to read and calculates the correct date. (Wheels are based on Naegele's rule; see the chapter on Calculating the Due Date in this section for more details).

Reflex hammer: A reflex hammer will help you check a woman's neurological response both at the time of a baseline exam and if a problem is suspected. It will have a triangularly shaped rubber head. The pointed end is used to isolate a small area to elicit a reflex response; the larger, flat side is used to trigger reflexes when isolating a small area is not so critical.

Thermometers: Thermometers come in oral and rectal (or stubby) styles. Both may be used interchangeably; however, rectal thermometers have a thicker glass tip to minimize breakage when placed in the rectum. Since thermometers contain mercury, it is important to protect them from breakage and dispose of them properly should one break. Choose thermometers that meet certification standards— this should be noted on the packaging. They should be hard to shake down and the mercury should not move on its own after you get a reading. Thermometers should be stored at room temperature. Storage in a very hot car can cause a mercury tip to explode!

Most thermometers produced in the United States use the Fahrenheit scale, while those produced in Canada and Europe use the Celsius scale as the standard. Many hospitals also use the Celsius scale. Refer to the explanation of how to take a temperature in the chapter on the Physical Exam in this section for more information about these standards.

There are a number of electronic thermometers on the market. Some are used orally, some place a heat-sensitive probe near the eardrum (tympanic thermometer) and some use a heat-sensitive strip to be placed on an external body part. Tympanic monitors are often used in hospitals and are fast and easy, but nurses frequently comment that they do not trust them if there is any temperature elevation present—and isn't that the reason we would need one? If you chose to use an electronic thermometer, an oral one is probably most accurate. Be sure you know what kind of batteries it takes and always have a glass thermometer on hand as back-up in case your electronic thermometer should fail to work.

Blood drawing equipment: Vacutainer holders, needles, tubes and a tourniquet will be needed to draw blood for various tests. Experiment with different types of tourniquets: I much prefer velcro ones! While you may choose to send women to the lab to have their blood drawn for routine analysis, it is helpful to know how to draw blood in case an unusual need for a blood sample should arise during a prenatal visit, or when a Rh-negative woman needs blood drawn for testing. Among your equipment should be a sharps container for proper disposal of any sharp or potentially sharp item, such as a glass blood tube. Any midwife who hires employees or runs a birthing center will need to be familiar with OSHA (Occupational Safety and Health Administration) regulations regarding the disposal of human body fluids. Check on CLIA (Clinical Laboratory Improvement Amendments) regulations regarding testing in small laboratory facilities as well. OSHA and CLIA rules are federally mandated, but may vary in administration from state to state. Blood drawing procedures are fully detailed in the Appendix of Diagnostic Tests; you should consider this an important midwifery skill.

Culturette specimen collection tubes: There are various culture tubes which are used for detecting herpes, strep-B, chlamydia, bacterial infections of the yoni and the like. Ask your lab exactly what each tube is for and how they are used. Generally, a sterile swab is contained in a larger plastic tube which has a gel-like culture medium in its far end. The swab is used to collect the specimen, then it is inserted into the plastic tube and finger pressure is used to rupture the culture medium; the top is then securely fixed in the tube so that the swab end is immersed in the gel. Read the storage instructions on the tube or ask how the tube should be stored prior to taking it to the lab for analysis.

PAP Smear kits: You may be doing PAP Smears on some women during prenatal care; this test can also be incorporated into your six-week postpartum visit as a routine part of your final exam. PAP smear kits are usually supplied by your lab and contain 2 wooden spatulas used for sample collection, one or two glass slides and a fixative agent. New cell collection devices are being introduced on the market, however. If your kit contains a plastic or brush cell collection device, it may be too abrasive to use on the pregnant cervix. Check with your lab and look in the chapter on the PAP Smear in <u>Diagnostic Tests</u> for more information about appropriate devices for use during pregnancy as well as how to do a PAP smear.

Non-oil based lubricant: Petroleum based lubricants and, to a lesser extent, natural vegetable oils break down latex and certain kinds of plastic. Mineral oil, petroleum jelly and baby oil all fall into this category. K-Y jelly is a water-based lubricant readily available in pharmacies and surgical supply houses. Another non-petroleum, non-oil based lubricant brand-named Astroglide. This stuff is great; it isn't sticky or greasy feeling and does not dry up in gobs, I highly recommend it!

Otoscope and ophthalmoscope: This dual-purpose instrument is used to look into the eyes and ears during a physical examination. While rather expensive, they are good items to have on hand; you might want to save up for them. A Welch-Allen instrument with a halogen light is an excellent choice and should last for your entire career.

Stop watch or watch with a second hand: This is used to count fetal heart tones for 5 second intervals. (This is thoroughly explained in the next chapter).

Additional items: These come in handy to carry in your prenatal bag; some are included simply because you will also be carrying your prenatal bag to home visits during the postpartum period:

        Neonatal Vitamin K.
        Insulin syringes (for injectable Vit. K)
        Ergotrate or Methergine tablets
        Silver Nitrate swabs (to cauterize cord stump if necessary)
        Q-tips
        Ketostix (if ketosis is suspected during labor)
        Plastic cord clamp clipper (handy even if you don't use plastic clamps
            in case a baby is born in the hospital, where they will usually use
            plastic)
        Cotton balls
        Herbs to ease afterbirth contractions
        False Unicorn Root (to stop premature labor)
        Blue Cohosh & Black Cohosh & Ginger (or other herbs to induce labor)
        Client's charts
        Icterometer (for visual estimation of degree of newborn jaundice)
        Baby scale
        PKU forms

There are other things you'll need to have on hand in your office, which you will not be carrying around in your bag (unless you do prenatal homevisits, for which you may wish to carry an adult scale). Some of theses items are listed below.

Adult scale: A balance beam scale is most accurate, but a good quality spring scale with a dial will do. Scales should be placed on a solid surface (not a carpet) and should be moved as little as possible. When making your selection remember that women will be trying to see a dial over or around their belly. Ideally, numbers should be large and the dial big and easy to read. A balance beam scale eliminates these problems, but will be more expensive.

Appointment book: You will want an appointment book that has spaces for every day of the week with plenty of room for notes. Having each day portioned off with time intervals in the left-hand margin is a real advantage as well. It is always a good idea to keep a record of client names, addresses and phone numbers and to have this list taped in your appointment book, allowing you to answer messages and make calls if you must change appointments on the spur of the moment.

Pager: Unless you live down the street from all your clients and never go anywhere, you will want to invest in the luxury of having a pager with the freedom it affords. The cheapest type of pager is a tone-only device which allows someone to call a number, triggering your pager to beep. Most midwives who have this type of service also have an answering machine attached to their phone at home. A client will call the answering machine first, leave a message, then call the beeper. The midwife must call her home phone and retrieve the message from her answering machine.

Another type of pager allows the caller to dial into an "electronic mailbox" where she will be asked to leave a message; then the midwife's pager automatically goes off. The midwife then calls another number, enters a code and retrieves her messages.

Yet another form of pager will beep and then display messages on a digital panel; most pagers like this will only display a phone number. This type of pager is not available everywhere. You can also have an answering service which offers a live message-taker who then pages you from her central office.

Whatever type of pager you choose, be sure to find out such details as "Can it be reached from a rotary dial phone?" (if you are working rurally some of your clients may not have touch tone service); "Do *you* need to be able to find a touch tone phone to retrieve messages?," "What is the range of the pager?," "Are there locations within this range where the pager will not receive messages due to the geographic terrain?"

Answering machine: Regardless of your opinion about how impersonal answering machines can be, they are a real life saver. They allow you to take messages while you finish your dinner. They allow you to forward calls to your midwifery partner or apprentice when you are out of town or unable to deal with calls. They allow you to do such things as leave messages to clients that you have gone to a birth and couldn't reach them before you had to leave. Answering machine technology has improved greatly over the last five years and it is now no trouble to find an affordable machine with these most desirable features:

*Remote message retrieval (usually requires a touch tone phone)

*Ability to change the announcement from another phone

*Choice of number of times the phone rings before the machine picks up. This allows you to set the machine to let the phone ring 1, 2 or 4 times. If you set it for 4, you can leave the machine on all the time and not have to worry whether you turned it on when you left the house; in most cases you will still be able to pick up the phone before the machine does when you are home)

*Voice activated messages (this means callers can leave as long a message as they want, sometimes up to 5 minutes, sometimes longer)

*Time and day notice (a voice comes on to let you know the time and day the call came in)

*Some machines allow you to listen to and delete messages selectively.

Caring for your equipment: Delicate medical instruments should be stored in a way that minimizes jarring and breakage. Unlike medical care providers who are stationed in permanent locations, midwives subject equipment to all manner of transport and use in various settings, which is inevitably harder on it than keeping it in one place. However, a little common sense and care is all it takes for your equipment to last for years. Most of your tools can be cleaned periodically with rubbing alcohol and tissues. If blood should contaminate a piece of equipment, it is best to soak it in rubbing alcohol for at least 10 minutes. Obviously you cannot do this with your blood pressure gauge or similar equipment. In case of blood contamination, simply wipe it down very well with alcohol, let it sit for a day, and then wipe it down again. This should kill every contaminating agent.

Any piece of equipment that enters the body, such as a speculum, should be sterilized between each use. Full instructions on sterilizing equipment may be found in the second volume of this text as well as in Healing Passage.

References and further reading:
McParland, P, et.al., "Time to reinvent the wheel," Brit J. OB/Gyn, Vol. 100, No. 11, 1993, pp. 1061-1062.
Vidam, Donna, midwife, Hartford, CT, editing comment, 1991.

Medical Terminology Relevant to Pregnancy History

While knowing medical terminology does not have anything to do with how competent a midwife you are, it does reflect a level of basic education that will be well received when you interface with the medical community. It also allows you to more easily read medical textbooks and journals as well as a woman's medical records. When venturing into medical terrain, just as in any other foreign situation, knowing the language of the natives helps, even though you may choose not to use any of this language in your own practice.

Throughout this book, basic medical terminology is used and defined; not all those notations will be repeated here. This chapter will go over the medical terms used to discuss a woman's previous pregnancy history, since this is specifically relevant to prenatal care.

Weeks of pregnancy: Traditionally, doctors did not believe that women could know when they got pregnant; as a result, two terms were used to discuss the length of time the baby is inside the mother. Generally speaking, the **weeks of pregnancy** refers to the time from the onset of the last menstrual period until the birth; during the first two "weeks of pregnancy" the woman has not yet ovulated and is not actually pregnant. **Weeks of gestation** refers to the number of weeks from conception; it is typically used when discussing fetal development and maturity, however some textbooks interchange these terms, a point of confusion regardless of how experienced one may be.

There is a standard two week difference between these two measurements, because there are approximately two weeks between the onset of the last period and the next ovulation. Since ovulation occurs 14 days before the onset of the *next* menses, the time from the date of the last period until ovulation is longer in women who have longer cycles.

Mainstream medicine considers pregnancy to be 40 completed weeks (of pregnancy) and mature fetal gestation to be 38 weeks. Pregnancy may actually last longer than this accepted "normal range" and still be healthy when women are well nourished, as well as in those who have longer menstrual cycles (see the chapter on Calculating the Correct Due Date in this section).

During prenatal visits, you will be noting how far along a woman's pregnancy is at each appointment. A precise way to do so is to note the completed weeks of pregnancy, and then the number of days into the next week she may be. For example, if a woman completes her 16th week of pregnancy on Monday and it is now Thursday, she is 16 weeks and 3 days pregnant, or 16.3 weeks pregnant; by the following Monday she would be 16.7 weeks or 17 weeks pregnant.

Menstrual periods: The menstrual period is said to begin on the first day of bleeding and last through the entire cycle until bleeding begins again. The last menstrual period is noted LMP, the last normal menstrual period is noted as LNMP.

Gravida: Literally "the state of being pregnant." (Remember gravity = heavy with child.)

> *A woman's gravidity refers to the total number of pregnancies she has had, regardless of their duration or outcome.
> *A nulligravida is a woman who has never been pregnant.
> *A primigravida is a woman pregnant for the first time.
> *A secundigravida is a woman pregnant for the second time.
> *A multigravida is a woman who has been pregnant more than twice.

Para: This refers to the number of pregnancies before the current one which reached viability; that is, those which lasted long enough for the fetus to have lived. With recent advances in neonatal care, viability is now considered 20 completed weeks gestation or more, or the birth of a baby weighing at least 1 lb. 1.5 oz. (500 g).

> *Parity refers to the number of past pregnancies that have reached viability and have been born. Each pregnancy only adds one unit of parity (i.e., a woman who carried her first pregnancy with triplets to 20 weeks or more would still be considered a para one).
> *A nullipara is a woman who has never given birth to a child that reached viability (e.g., a woman whose first pregnancy ends in a miscarriage at 12 weeks is a nullipara).
> *A primipara is a woman who has had one pregnancy in which the child or children reached viability, whether or not the child was actually alive at the time of birth.
> *A multipara is a woman who has had two or more pregnancies in which the child or children reached viability, whether or not the child was alive at birth.
> *A parturient is a woman in labor.

Here are some examples of how to apply this terminology:

Alice, pregnant for the first time, is a primigravida (gravida 1, para 0).

If Alice miscarries or chooses to abort before 20 weeks gestation, she remains a gravida 1, para 0.

If Alice gives birth at 20 completed weeks gestation or thereafter, regardless of whether her child lives, she becomes a gravida 1, para 1.

While pregnant with a second child, Alice is a gravida 2, para 1. After the birth of her second child past 20 weeks gestation, she becomes a gravida 2, para 2. If

354

she miscarries before 20 weeks gestation, she is said to be a gravida 2, para 1.

Jane's only pregnancies ended in two miscarriages in the first trimester; she is a gravida 2, para 0. When she becomes pregnant for the third time she is a gravida 3, para 0. When she births the third child at or after 20 weeks gestation, she is a gravida 3, para 1.

Remember, multiple births do not affect the number assigned for either parity or gravida. If Nancy has one child during her first pregnancy after 20 weeks gestation and twins during her second pregnancy after 20 weeks is still a gravida 2, para 2.

TPAL(M): Because the system just described does not allow for the inclusion of many useful details in a woman's pregnancy history, it is rarely used by itself these days. A more elaborate system has been devised to discuss a woman's previous pregnancy history. Even though this system uses the term "parity," it consists of a series of digits assigned to the number of children born at different gestational ages, rather than the number of pregnancies, making the use of the term somewhat confusing. Miscarriages and induced abortions that take place prior to viability are also included.

T–Babies born at term (first digit): the number of term babies a woman has birthed. "Term" refers to babies carried past the 36th completed week of gestation or who weighed at least 5 lb. 8.25 oz. (2500 grams). In the event of a multiple birth, each baby gets counted.
P–Babies born prematurely (second digit): the number of premature babies a woman has birthed. "Premature" refers to babies born between the 20th and 36th completed gestational weeks or those that weighed between 1 lb. 1.5 oz. and 5 lb. 8.24 oz. (500 and 2499 grams). In the event of a multiple birth, each baby gets counted.
A–Abortions (third category, one or two digits): the number of pregnancies ending in either miscarriage or induced abortion which occurred prior to the 20th completed week of gestation. (To clarify your notations, you can list "As" for spontaneous miscarriages and "Ae" for elective abortions, meaning this category might, at times, have two digits with letters.)
L–Living children(fourth digit): total number of currently living children.
(M)–Multiples (fifth digit): the number of pregnancies that resulted in multiple births. This is not commonly included, but a useful extra when there is a history of multiple births.

When used in charting, each letter TPAL(M) in the system is replaced with the number relevant to the individual woman's history. Here are some examples:

Julie is pregnant for the first time. She is described as a gravida 1, para 0000. If Julie has a spontaneous miscarriage before 20 gestational weeks, she becomes a gravida 1, para 001s0.

If instead Julie's first pregnancy ends in a premature birth after 20 gestational weeks and before 36 completed gestational weeks, and the child is alive now, she becomes a gravida 1, para 0101.

When Julie becomes pregnant a second time, she is a gravida 2, para 0101.

If Julie miscarries her second pregnancy before 20 weeks gestation, she is a gravida 2, para 011s1. If, however, she gives birth to her second child past 36 weeks gestation and the child is still alive, she becomes a gravida 2, para 111s2.

Diane, has had two first-trimester losses: one elective abortion and one spontaneous miscarriage. She is a gravida 2, para 001s1e0. When Diane becomes pregnant for the third time she is a gravida 3, para 001s1e0. With her third pregnancy, Diane gives birth at term and the child is living now: she is a gravida 3, para 101s1e1.

Ellen carried her first pregnancy to term and gave birth to one child, who is living now. During her second pregnancy, she gave birth to twins at 35 weeks gestation and both children are living now. She is a gravida 2, para 1203(1).

Mary Anne carried her first pregnancy to term, when she birthed a healthy baby girl, who is still living. She carried her second pregnancy to 35 weeks gestation and birthed a stillborn boy. With her third pregnancy, she gave birth to twins at 38 weeks gestation. One twin died, the other is doing well. She has since has two first trimester miscarriages. She is a gravida 5, 312s2(1).

References and further reading

Gilhooly, Joe, Neonatologist, conversation regarding fetal viability, May, 1995.
Oxhorn, Harry, Human Labor and Birth, 5th ed., Appleton-Century-Crofts, Norwalk, Ct., 1986.
Varney, Helen, Varney's Midwifery, 4th ed., Jones and Bartlett Pub., Boston, MA, 2004.

Charting and Record Keeping

Record keeping, although tedious and distracting at times, is an important component of competent care. Records serve as a memory bank, as it is impossible to remember all the physical, medical, emotional and psychological details of each client's history. They serve as a historical file for future health care. They provide an ongoing means of keeping up with what is going on during a process, since in most instances individual findings are of minimal value. You can refresh yourself at a glance as to the particulars of a woman's last visit, thus helping her feel that you are connected with her situation and condition and making it possible for you to practice without having to remember everything. This is particularly true during labor, when time can become very distorted for both you and the family. Accurate charting helps immensely when you must, for whatever reason, transfer care to another care provider. Just think how reassured you would be if a woman, newly moved to your community, presented you with a detailed record of her prenatal care to date. It eliminates a lot of guess work regarding what has occurred so far and thus supports continuous care for the client.

Legal issues: Your charts are a legal record of your interaction with your clients. Your chart is your best and sometimes your only resource to back up your claims should questions regarding your recommendations or how you dealt with a problem come up. While we must all strive to have honest, open relationships with our clients, it is impossible to predict how individuals may respond in the event of a tragic or otherwise unexpected or undesirable outcome. All entries should be legibly entered in black ink to facilitate photocopying. Errors can be corrected by drawing a single line through the error so that it remains legible; obliterating the entry with white-out, scratch outs or markers should not be done. Write "error" above the mistake, initial it, then write the correct information beside or below the error. (Rosenberger, 1995) Each page should contain the woman's name as well as the date, time, and the signature (first initial and last name) of the person charting on that page. In narrative charting, do not leave blank or incomplete lines. Draw a line to the end of the line, then initial it. Do not chart anything until it has been completed. This avoids confusion about whether it was done or not and avoids inaccurate charting in case it is not done at all. Personal notes may legally be recorded on a separate sheet of paper so that you have the option of retaining or including them with the official chart should copies of the records be requested.

Forms: Part of the tedium of charting can be eliminated by using a discussion check sheet to mark off topics which are routinely discussed with each woman you see. The non-routine discussions need more detailed notes in your records.

There are a variety of forms in use and many midwifery practices develop their own. Throughout this book there will be examples of forms to use for every imaginable need; these can be found in the appropriate chapters (for example, history forms are in the initial history chapter). The following sample is from a form I have used to keep track of clients on a monthly basis. Duplicate forms and tape them in the back of your appointment book for easy reference. Include enough rows to accommodate the number of clients you expect to have each month (for example, 5 rows if you think 4 would be your maximum client load).

Month of _____ 19____

#	Client's name, address & directions	Phone #s	EDD	BIRTH	Comments
1					
2					

Other forms to compare and develop for your practice include:

*Prenatal form
*Initial history
*Physical exam
*Diet diary
*Labor chart
*Immediate postpartum monitoring of mother and infant
*Newborn exam
*Intensive care monitoring
*Postpartum form for mother and infant through last visit of your care
*Summary form for prenatal, labor, birth and postpartum information
    (some midwives use their statistics form for this purpose)
*Statistics form
*Transport form
*Financial agreement

Examples of all of these forms will be found in these volumes in the appropriate chapters. Get copies of as many different forms as possible from other midwives and look over the forms you find here for ideas about what to include on yours and how you want them to look.

Charting: Once you have decided upon the various forms you will be using, it can be helpful to have a routine method to record information. This will help you remember to document all pertinent information as well as provide a good future reference. Be sure you are recording the most important details without filling up pages with irrelevant babble. The only way to accomplish this is to know normal parameters inside and out and to develop an understanding of unique aspects of situations which warrant notation. This will come with experience.

358

In some cases, brief notes will suffice for simple problems which you discuss. This is called source oriented charting; it consists of sentences and phrases to describe the situation in a simple storytelling style (Rosenberger, 1995). For more complex situations, a method called SOAP(IER) charting is helpful. While you can use any method which seems to work, SOAP charting provides a simple, logical progression of information so you can organize your thoughts and come up with a plan (this will happen unconsciously as you gain more experience; however, training yourself to think this way will help you become proficient). SOAP charting goes like this:

S: **Subjective:** What the woman says is happening to her, her chief concern or complaint (CC). Record any information the woman gives you regarding the topic at hand as well as information you obtain from her via your questions. You might also note pertinent information that has been noted elsewhere if it is very relevant to your topic (a history of twins in the family of a woman who is reporting that she is large for dates, for example).

O: **Objective:** What you note by examination or observation, as well as any previous test results, diagnoses or procedures.

A: **Assessment:** What you suspect or diagnose or a summary of the available data (i.e. possible urinary tract infection or infection of the yoni)

P: **Plan:** What you recommend be done about the condition in question, any tests you order or if you suggest referral. Record any appointments you set to follow-up on the situation.

I: **Implementation:** How the woman is to proceed with the plan; it may involve such things as giving her the phone number of a referral practitioner, calling a natural foods store to make sure a supplement is in stock or helping her figure out how she will increase her protein intake.

During a follow-up call or visit, the ER part of SOAP(IER) charting comes into play:

E: **Evaluation of plan:** Your evaluation of the plan would cover how realistic the plan turned out to be for the individual woman and whether your recommendations proved effective.

R: **Reassessment of woman's needs:** After reviewing the situation with the woman, both of you decide if the plan worked, and, if not, what needs to be done at this point to further address the situation.

An example of SOAP(IER) charting follows: Rebecca is 25 years old, and is 9 weeks and 3 days pregnant for the first time (or TPALM number code gravida 1 para 0000 [see the previous chapter]). Her first prenatal visit is scheduled for next week. She dropped by at the end of a prenatal day because she has been feeling nauseous and dizzy. Since you have already done her initial, a chart has already been established for her which notes her basic data, you would add the following to her chart:

Date, time, your initials

S-CC: nauseous and dizzy, esp. this morning upon arising, has felt this way on and off for 3 days. Avoiding eating due to fears of becoming more nauseous.

O-9.3 weeks preg., slightly acetone breath, trace of ketones in dark urine, vital signs WNL (within normal limits) BP-110/70, pulse 74, looks somewhat pale and tired, everything else seems normal.

A-Hypoglycemia creating fatigue and dizziness and aggravating nausea

P-Explained that avoiding eating makes nausea worse. Explained hypoglycemia. Rx eat small frequent amounts throughout the day and when waking at night emphasizing protein foods. If she throws up, eat again within 30 minutes. Drink electrolyte balancing fluids such as Third Wind to stabilize nausea. Call in 8 hours to note changes.

I-Will stop by natural foods store on way home and pick up some foods she feels she might keep down. Will call tomorrow am. unless symptoms dramatically worsen during the night.

E-(Date, time, your initials) Called to say the Third Wind helped immensely; ate 2 to 3 Tbsp. cottage cheese every half-hour until bedtime. Vomited about 8 pm. one time, ate again and kept everything down. Ate before rising this am, feeling much better.

R-Helped Rebecca work out a diet plan w/small meals throughout the day; asked her to keep a diet diary & call if she got worse again; will evaluate in detail at prenatal next week

When clients refuse your recommendations: If you recommend a specific procedure and the parents do not want to follow through, make a note in your chart or on a separate form used for this purpose. Have the parents (both, if present) initial the note after reviewing it to make sure it reflects your discussion; you should also initial the note. For example, you can write: "Parents (or mother) decline ultrasound recommended to assess possible multiple gestation." This is purely for legal purposes if, in the future, a question should arise about what was discussed regarding the situation. Some midwives have waivers for parents to sign with lines to fill in the particulars.

<u>**References and further reading**</u>:

Rosenberger, Lani, "Charting Fundamentals," <u>Midwifery Today</u>, Spring 1995, No. 33, p. 23-6.
Styles, D., "Better Charting, Better Care," <u>Midwifery Today</u>, Vol. 1, No. 2, Spring 1987, p. 30-1.

The Signs and Symptoms of Pregnancy

The signs and symptoms of pregnancy are divided into three categories: positive, probable and presumptive.

Positive signs are those which leave no doubt that the changes occurring in the mother's body are indeed due to a pregnancy in progress. Most of the positive signs of pregnancy cannot be detected until the fourth month (week 13 or more).

Probable signs are those which are usually due to pregnancy but may also be present in certain other conditions. They are not absolute indications that a pregnancy is the cause of their appearance.

Presumptive signs are those the woman notes as changes in her body, which are commonly but not exclusively associated with pregnancy.

POSITIVE	PROBABLE	PRESUMPTIVE
Hearing & counting the fetal heart rate	Abdominal enlargement	Mother's sense of pregnancy
Feeling fetal movements on palpation	Changes in the shape, size & consistency of the uterus	Amenorrhea
Ultrasound or X-ray confirmation of pregnancy	Changes in the cervix	Breast changes
	Intermittent uterine contractions	Color changes in mucus membranes of the yoni
	Ballottement of fetus	Increased pigmentation
	Outlining the fetus	Nausea & vomiting
	Positive hormonal test for pregnancy	Quickening
		Pigmentation changes in the skin
		Urinary frequency
		Fatigue

This categorization is based upon a medical model which values the objective signs most highly. However, it is also based upon relying most heavily on those signs which leave no doubt that changes are due to pregnancy and not a pathological condition. Details regarding the signs and symptoms appropriate to each trimester are included in the section on the respective trimester.

Signs of a previous pregnancy: A woman may not always tell you if she has previously been pregnant or given birth. This could be for a variety of reasons such as keeping this fact a secret from her current partner, disassociation regarding a pregnancy which led to adoption, or blocking the memory as might happen in survivors of ritual or sexual abuse. A woman may also withhold information about a previously complicated pregnancy during which the baby died because she does not want to be risked-out for homebirth. It is desirable to know a woman's true medical history, however, and there are physical signs to be aware of that point to a previous pregnancy. The following signs suggest a previous pregnancy. Because these signs are not conclusive, it is important not to rely on a single sign alone.

EXAM	PRIMIGRAVIDA	MULTIGRAVIDA	OTHER CAUSES
Breasts	Firm, nipples do not project excessively	More flabby, soft, nipple pronounced if she breastfed; pigmentation of the areola may still persist in brunettes	
Abdominal muscles	Firm muscles & skin tone	More relaxed; the skin may feel looser	
Uterine wall	Firm with ovoid shape	Less rigid, rounder shape; baby easier to palpate	
Stretch marks	New ones are pinkish	Old are silvery white	Stretch marks can be caused by weight gain & subsequent loss outside of pregnancy
External genitals	Labia tend to lie closed, good muscle tone throughout; hymen partially intact & has a more uniform appearance; no scars present	Vulva may gape & is more open. The labia minora may appear stretched. The yoni orifice is larger & more relaxed; perineal scars may be present	Penetration or laceration of a child during sexual abuse may change the appearance of the external genitals
Internal exam	Yoni muscle tone is good; os is a pinhead opening	Yoni feels more roomy & the cervical os is a transverse slit which admits a fingertip	An IUD or previous abortion can convert the os to a slit shape

Talking to the mother: If you find indications of a previous pregnancy, you may wish to question the woman privately about the possibility. Keep in mind the very real possibility that she has blocked the memory of the previous experience for any number or reasons. You might introduce the subject with a comment such as: "I've asked to meet with you privately because I am puzzled by some things I found during your physical exam which I hope you can clarify. I noticed that (explain signs you discovered). Ordinarily, the only thing that could cause these changes are a late miscarriage or abortion, or a previous birth. It is important that we have an honest relationship for many reasons, but I really need to know what, if anything, you may not have told me about your previous reproductive history." Hopefully this kind of lead-in will get her talking and you can then probe further regarding the relevant history.

References and further reading:
Myles, Margaret, Textbook for Midwives, Churchill Livingstone, New York, NY, 1981.

Calculating the Correct Due Date

The calculation of the expected date of delivery (EDD) or the expected date of birth (EDB), (EDC is the old term meaning expected date of confinement) may at first glance appear to be a simple and straightforward process. This would be true if all women had 28 day menstrual cycles and all women ovulated on the 14th day of their cycles and if the 24 hour period after ovulation was the only time conception could occur. This, however, is not the case. The following things are all factors which must be taken into account when figuring the due date:

*The average length of the menstrual cycle, first day of bleeding to first day of bleeding—usually 28 days, but this can vary.
*The regularity of the menstrual cycle.
*The first day of the last two normal periods. (Was the length, amount of flow, and timing normal for her? If not, how did it differ?) Also, the dates of any other bleeding that may have differed from normal during the last two to three months before she feels she conceived.
*The date she thinks she conceived. If she is unsure, maybe she can recall events (holidays, etc.) when sexual activity was more likely. Did she keep an ovulation chart?)
*Whether she was using contraceptives, and, if so, what kind.
* If the pregnancy is far enough advanced:
    -When she first felt fetal movement (usually 16 to 20 weeks in a primigravida, and 15 to 18 weeks in a multigravida)
    -The date when fetal heart rate could first be heard. (Was a Doppler or a fetascope used at the time?)
    -Fundal height and fetal size
*Ovulation can occur with orgasm, some women ovulate twice, and many have a sense that they got pregnant at a certain time. Delayed implantation has been documented with *in vitro* fertilization. Don't dismiss a woman's experience of her body.

Taking these things into account assures coming up with the most accurate estimate possible, using one of several techniques. You may find that a gestation calculator wheel is a great help in figuring the due date.

Using a gestation calculator wheel: It will help you to have a gestation wheel in hand to go over this explanation. With a little practice, a gestation wheel can be used to assist in figuring a due date using any of the methods described in this chapter. When using the standard Naegele's method of calculation, you place the pointer on the inner wheel on the date of the last normal menstrual period (LNMP). The 40 weeks pointer will automatically fall on the expected date of birth. When compensating for the actual date of conception, the ovulation pointer is placed on the probable date of fertilization; while this allows for variations in the length of the first part of the menstrual cycle, weeks of pregnancy are still counted as usual, making full term the 40th week (not the 38th).

Lunar reckoning: For tens of thousands of years women calculated their menstrual cycles by following the phases of the moon.   When your moon disappears, you are pregnant.   A lunar cycle is just over 29 days (29 days, 12 hours, 44 minutes and 3 seconds); however, women count in terms of whole days. This gives a gestational period of 290 days from the last menstrual period or ten lunar months.

Naegele's rule: In 1709 Hermann Boerhaave, professor of medicine at the University of Leyden in England, proposed a formula for calculating the date of birth. This was later quoted by Dr. Franz Naegele and has since been attributed to him and referred to as Naegele's rule: subtract 3 months from the first day of the last menstrual period, then add 7 days: LMP - 3 months + 7 days = EDD. This is predicated on the assumption that the duration of pregnancy spans ten *regular* menstrual cycles of 28 days each.   It was based on historical rather than observational data.   In the original citations of the rule it was not clear if the calculations should be based upon the first or last day of the LMP, however the first day is the standard used in the United States. (It is interesting to note that when the last day of menstruation is used as the starting point, the expected due date is similar to that derived from using lunar months of 29 days.)

Furthermore, Naegele's rule is not based upon when ovulation occurs, but upon the last menstrual period. It therefore does not account for variations in the length of time between menstruation and ovulation. (van der Kooy, 1994) Since ovulation occurs fairly reliably *14 to 15 days before the first day of bleeding*, women with longer cycles will be ovulating later than those with 28 day cycles. This pushes the date of conception ahead. For those with shorter cycles, the date of conception will be sooner by a few days.

Some midwives use a modified version of Naegele's rule to arrive at the due date from the day of conception: Conception - 3 months - 7 days = EDD. This method eradicates some of the problems inherent in the original formula.

Examples using a modified Naegele's rule: The following examples take into account the length of the menstrual cycle. Examples are given for mathematical calculation and using a gestational wheel:

Beth has regular 32 day cycles. Her last bleeding started December 20th, but was lighter than usual. Her last normal period before that began November 18th. Using a gestation wheel, set the calculator with the first day of the last normal period line pointing to Nov. 18th. The week of December 7th, her husband came home for 4 days and then left to finish some work out of town. She feels sure she got pregnant then. Since she has a 32 day cycle, she most likely ovulated around December 6th (ovulation occurs about 14 days before the onset of bleeding, so subtract 28 from 32 = 4, then move the ovulation (conception) pointer four days ahead to Dec. 6th). The December 20th bleeding was most likely break-through bleeding, not a true period. Therefore, by placing the pointer for probable ovulation (i.e. conception) on December 6th, her due date is August 29th. If you simply place the LMP pointer on November 18th (her last period), per Naegele's rule, the due date would be August 25th, almost one week earlier.

While allowing for variations in cycle length, this method does not make any special distinctions between the length of pregnancy for first time mothers and those who have had other babies.

To modify Naegele's rule without a gestation wheel, calculate the date in the suggested manner, then add any cycle days in excess of 28 or subtract any days of the cycle that are less than 28 to obtain a due date that takes into account individual variations. For example:

The length of Mandy's cycle is 33 days. The first day of her last period was August 12, 1994. Add 9 months + 7 days + 5 days (33 - 28 = 5) = May 24, 1995.

Julie has regular 23 day cycles. Her LNMP began on August 12, 1994 as well. Therefore add 9 months + 7 days - 5 days (28 - 23 = 5) = May 14, 1995.

Wood's method: When Carol Wood Nichols (now simply Carol Wood) was a nurse-midwifery professor at Yale University, she also saw the flaws in the standard method of calculating the due date. She came up with a method which takes into account individual variations in the menstrual cycle as well as the effect of a woman's having had previous pregnancies; it therefore offers the most accurate estimate possible. Calculate as follows:

1. Add 1 year to the first day of the last menstrual period, then:
   -For first time mothers: subtract 2 months and 2 weeks (14 days)
   -For multiparas subtract 2 months and 2.5 weeks (or 18 days)
2. Add or subtract the number of days her cycle varies from 28 days

1st time mothers with 28 day cycles: LMP + 12 mths - 2 mths, 14 days = EDD

Multiparas with 28 day cycles: LMP + 12 months - 2 months, 18 days = EDD

For cycles longer than 28 days: EDD + (Actual length of cycle - 28 days) = EDD

For cycles shorter than 28 days: EDD - (28 days - Actual length of cycle) = EDD

Examples based on Wood's method: Mary, a first time mother, began her last menstrual period June 16th, 1993. She has regular 28 day cycles. Adding one year gives June 16th, 1994; subtracting two months gives us April 15th, 1994, and subtracting two additional weeks gives a final due date of April 1st, 1994. If Mary were a multipara, you would subtract an additional 4 days (i.e. 18 days instead of 2 weeks), making the due date March 28th, 1994. Naegele's rule would have set this due date at March 23rd, 1994. (To use a wheel, set the LMP pointer on June 16th [LMP]; add 9 days to the EDD for primigravidas, or 5 days for multiparas, then add or subtract more days to compensate for variations from a 28 day cycle.)

Sue, also a first time mother, has regular 35 day cycles. Her last period also began on June 16th, 1993. Adding one year gives June 16th, 1994; subtracting two months gives April 15th, 1994, subtracting two additional weeks brings you to April 1st, 1994. But, Sue's cycles are longer than 28 days, which must also be compensated for in our calculation: 35 - 28 = 7. Adding another 7 days to her due date pushes it up to April 8th, 1994. Naegele's rule would have also set this due date at March 23rd, 1994 as it makes no allowances for variations in the length of a woman's cycle.

To use the wheel to figure Sue's due date, set the pointer for the LMP on June 16th. Note that the EDD pointer is now on March 23rd. Count 9 days ahead to get April 1st, then, because she has 35 days cycles, count ahead 7 more days to arrive at April 8th.

Simple addition of days: If the date of conception (ovulation) is known, simply add 266 days to that date (38 weeks X 7 days = 266). This allows for variations in the length of the cycle but does not compensate for how many pregnancies a woman has had. Or, add five months from the date of first definite quickening.

Mittendorf's study: After studying the duration of 31 uncomplicated first time pregnancies and 83 multiparous pregnancies, this research concluded that the length of pregnancy from the first day of the last menstrual period for primiparas was 288 days and the length of pregnancy (from LMP) for multiparas was 283 days. Ovulation was assumed to be on day 14 of a 28 day cycle and was adjusted for longer cycles. Their calculation looks like this:

Primiparas: LMP - 3 months + 15 days (+ or - days more or less than 28)
Multiparas: LMP - 3 months + 10 days (+ or - days more or less than 28)

When formulas just don't work:

Racial and genetic variations: Some studies have indicated that women of African descent tend to have pregnancies that are 8.5 days shorter than white women. While dietary variations may play a role, one study confirming this finding (Henderson, 1967) compared populations of Caucasian and Black women whose environment was essentially the same, presumably eliminating variations due to nutritional differences. A British study (Saunders, 1991) found that maternal height influenced the length of gestation. Such studies show that variations in the length of human gestation are influenced by a variety of factors, the majority of which are not at all understood.

When the menstrual history is skimpy: Sometimes women haven't kept track of their periods and have intercourse frequently enough so that they have no idea when they got pregnant. Backtrack to the last period they remember and evaluate other signs such as the date they first detect fetal movement, fundal growth and when you can first auscultate the fetal heart beat; reevaluate as necessary.

Compare the relationship of the due dates of past pregnancies to previous pregnancy outcomes: In calculating due dates, also consider the length of previous pregnancies and the condition of the babies at birth. Some women, often those with longer cycles, gestate for 10 months. How long were her mother's pregnancies, and what was the condition of her babies at birth? (Adequate birth weight, mature features and reflexes, a plump baby, and a normal quantity of amniotic fluid are good gauges of fetal and placental well-being regardless of the supposed length of pregnancy.) Of course, the situation is muddied if the woman or her mother were induced prior to the onset of natural labor (because you don't know how long she might have carried otherwise). You might take the dates of previous pregnancies and recalculate them based on Wood's method and see if the time of birth more closely matches a revised EDD.

Irregular cycles and the due date: For women whose cycles are very irregular who are unsure of their date of conception, no method will apply accurately. Do the best you can to reconstruct the duration of a woman's cycles for the last several months (6 months would be ideal) and then make the best estimate you can. Pay particular attention to the timing of the last menstrual cycle before she became pregnant, as this will be the cycle that involved the ovulation pertinent to the current pregnancy.

Ultrasound assessment of gestational age: Many mainstream practitioners set great store in an ultrasound exam done early in pregnancy to determine gestational age. While there is a widely held belief that babies are all more or less the same size in early pregnancy, this is not always the case. First trimester estimates may be ±5 days off, second trimester estimates as much as ± 8 days off and third trimester estimates can be up to ± 22 days off! (Otto & Platt, 1991)

The meaning of the due date in Western culture:

The psychological significance of the due date: Remember that the expected date of delivery (EDD) is not a hard and fast certainty. Only about 5% of all women will give birth on the designated day. However, this date is heavily charged in our culture. The medical model has made the due date the hinge on which everything else depends: prior to it women are hassled about prematurity, after it, postmaturity. Friends and relatives will hang on this date as if it were a certainty and may harass a woman to no end if she is unlucky enough to carry beyond it.

Before you declare any specific date, make it clear to the woman that you are only designating a date midway within the *month* (or 30 days) in which she is due. Advise her to tell family and friends that she is due "sometime in May," for example; if she is due late in a given month she can name the following month. Recommend that she think of being due in this way and that she encourage family members to do likewise; tell her not to give a specific date if she can possibly avoid it. If associates won't leave her alone, tell her to name a date two weeks *after* her midway point. This is important groundwork to lay because many women, especially first time mothers (who often think they will go early anyway) may get very depressed if they pass their due date and have not yet given birth.

The significance of the due date: The traditional Naegele's rule is still widely used by doctors and hospitals. You must be clear exactly how you arrived at a woman's due date with any medical practitioner with whom you collaborate. The initial calculation is very important because it may determine the amount of medical intervention a woman is asked to accept in her pregnancy. Because of this, many women will end up attempting to educate other providers regarding new methods of EDD calculation in an effort to avoid being hassled because of an inaccurate date. For example, a collaborating doctor may already be anxious about postmaturity a week ahead of the due date. If there is doubt about when a woman conceived, it is usually best to err on the side of assigning a later due date, not an earlier one, unless placenta-compromising factors are to be considered such as cigarette smoking. Be sure to correlate these results with clinical findings such as the size of the uterus and baby, when the woman first felt fetal movement (this varies, but is usually between 16 and 20 weeks), and when you can first hear the fetal heart with a fetascope.

References and further reading:

Henderson, M., Kay, J., "Differences in Duration of Pregnancy," Archives of Environmental Health, June 14, 1967, pp. 904-11.

Mittendorf, R. et.al., "The length of uncomplicated human gestation," OB/GYN, Vol. 75, No., 6, June, 1990, pp. 929-932.

Nichols, Carol Wood, "Postdate Pregnancy, Part II: Clinical Implications," J. of Nurse-Midwifery, Vol. 30, No. 5, Sept./Oct., 1985, pp. 259-268.

Otto, C, Platt L., "Fetal growth and development," Ob Gyn Clin North Amer, Vol. 18, No. 4, 1991, pp. 907-931.

Saunders, N. & Paterson, C., " Can we abandon Naegele's rule?" Lancet, Vol. 337, No. 8741, 1991, pp. 600-1.

van der Kooy, Brenda, "Calculating expected date of delivery-its accuracy and relevance," Midwifery Matters, Issue 60, Spring 1994, pp. 4-7.

368

Avoiding Contamination from Infectious Agents

Blood may communicate hepatitis, HIV, syphilis, and malaria, as well as other organisms. Although hepatitis B is a larger and far less fragile organism than HIV, concern over possible contamination from body fluids did not really mount until AIDS hit the scene.

Although there is currently much emphasis on contamination by the HIV virus, there is evidence HIV may not be the root cause of AIDS after all. An unpopular, but highly probable theory is that syphilis, not HIV, may be the underlying immune suppressor that precipitates AIDS. HIV may be a virus mutating under the influence of undiagnosed, misdiagnosed, or inadequately treated syphilis. Even if this theory is incorrect, we are currently experiencing a huge resurgence of syphilis infection in the United States. Therefore, HIV and syphilis as well as hepatitis and other blood borne pathogens are all of major concern. Syphilis dies when allowed to air dry, but can be preserved in deep cold (such as that used to preserve blood transfusions) and can be communicated via other blood contact, including needle sticks. Both can be communicated by the same means. Regardless of which agent is the root cause of AIDS, precautions are necessary either way. (See Diagnostic Tests; Chambers, 1969; Coulter 1987; Mitchell, 1990)

As viruses go, HIV is somewhat fragile, but it can live outside the body. Experiments with diluted calve's blood and laboratory concentrations of virus (far higher than biological concentrations) showed that HIV can survive 14 days at room temperature and up to 11 days at 100° F. (37.8° C). Dried HIV loses about 90% to 99% of its infectivity after a few hours at room temperature, with complete inactivity requiring three days. Biological concentrations (i.e. virus in human blood) are far lower with HIV than with hepatitis B, and hep B is about half the size. Thus hepatitis is far easier to transmit from blood contamination than HIV.

Heat inactivates HIV, syphilis, and hepatitis B in liquid human blood solutions: 10 minutes at 140° F (60° C) for HIV (increase the time to 1 hour for hepatitis B). Disinfectants that kill HIV (for sure) and hepatitis B (with longer exposure) include:

*Grain alcohol (ethanol) 50% solution or higher (usually available at 95%)
*Isopropyl (rubbing) alcohol—35% (most is 70%)
*Lysol at 0.5% solution (retails at 2%)
*Household bleach—1 part per 100 parts water (or 1/4 cup to 1 gallon of water). That's right, 1:100, not 1:10. The FDA said this was more than strong enough to kill HIV a few times over.

The alcohols are widely available and the least damaging to rubber and skin. Clean materials with disinfectant soap and water as soon as possible after use and then soak in one of the above solutions for 10 minutes (alcohol is recommended), which should eliminate all HIV virus. Add at least 20 minutes to kill hepatitis B. Tissue proteins quickly neutralize the effectiveness of alcohol, so thorough cleaning prior to soaking is important. (The CDC said this should do it for hepatitis B and syphilis, but the fact is, no real studies have been done on hepatitis in this regard because "people aren't afraid of it. Therefore, there is no research money.")

Freezing has a preservative effect on viruses and syphilis, causing them to go dormant. Although viral infectivity is lost in the freezing process, freezing cannot be thought of as eliminating risk. Therefore, all those interesting placentas in your freezer must be considered potentially contaminated and contagious.

Blood and semen are the most likely sources of body fluid contagion with HIV and syphilis. Saliva contains very small amounts of the HIV virus and is not considered infectious, but may communicate hepatitis. Urine and feces are somewhat problematic with HIV, although it probably requires prolonged exposure (such as caring for a sick person or an infant) before it is transmitted. Hepatitis and polio are highly communicable from fecal contact, and hepatitis via urine as well. Syphilis is usually communicated directly from serum from a chancre, as well as blood or body fluid that enters the mucus membranes, a sore or the blood stream of a non-infected person. Under normal circumstances, syphilis dies within minutes once outside the body, especially when exposed to air and allowed to dry.

In situations where body fluids may splatter, goggles are officially recommended when HIV is the concern. Plain lens glasses can be purchased in many eye wear departments and provide a less obtrusive source of protection. If body fluid contacts skin surfaces, those areas should be washed with an antibacterial agent as soon as possible.

A word about sterile technique: With sterile technique, the basic principle is to only touch sterile things while wearing sterile gloves. In most situations, it is unnecessary to maintain strict sterile technique at home. Exceptions to this might be tropical areas (where infection occurs more easily), or when working with unhealthy women. (Although in the birthing clinic where I trained, women were frequently not very healthy and sterile technique was not used. There were no infections during the 6 months I was in school.) Sterile technique is much more important in hospitals because of the resistant pathogens present. However, it should be strictly observed when dealing with prelabor rupture of membranes.

What I call "clean" technique works just fine at home and does not lead to infection. By clean technique, I mean keeping your washed, gloved hands as clean as possible. However, we often do fundal checks or other necessary procedures with the same gloves we use to suture. If it is necessary to examine deep inside the yoni, a clean glove should be used. Any glove contaminated by rectal contact should be immediately removed and discarded.

Hand-washing procedure: Hand-washing is intended to remove dirt and microorganisms from the skin surface. Thorough washing with soap and running water effectively removes almost all transient organisms from the skin. These are microbes lying freely on the skin surface that are attached by fats, along with dirt. Typically, a high percentage of these organisms are pathogenic. However, their virulence will be determined by where the person has been: far more virulent microbes will be picked up by provision of care in a hospital than in the home.

Thorough hand-washing is sufficient for most purposes. Full lathering with soap followed by 10 to 15 seconds of vigorous rubbing of all hand surfaces and rinsing with running water is sufficient to remove transient contaminants. If the hands are visibly soiled, longer washing is recommended. (CDC, 1985)

However, there may be times when you need to do a full "surgical scrub," which is intended to remove resident organisms from the skin surface. Most resident organisms are not pathogenic and exist at a stable level on the skin surface. However, prolonged exposure to resistant organisms can cause a higher percentage of pathogenic microbes to become resident skin flora. Thorough hand-washing with soap and running water does not effectively remove resident organisms. Therefore, a surgical scrub with an antimicrobial agent is recommended. Either 4% Chlorohexidine gluconate (brand name Hibiclens, ICI Australia, Operations Pty., Ltd., Sydney) or 7.5% povidone iodine agents are good for this purpose. Hexachlorophene acts slowly on resident organisms and is not recommended for use by pregnant women or on newborns. (Amer. College of Surgeons, 1976)

To perform a surgical scrub:

*First rinse the hands and arms under running water. Keep your hands higher than the elbows at all times.
*Pump 2 ml. of antiseptic solution and wash the hands and arms with a circular motion for 30 seconds, stopping 3 cm. past the elbows. Clean beneath your nails under running water with the nail tool supplied with surgical scrub brushes. If no nail tool is available, use a clean toothpick or orange wood stick.
*Rinse hands and arms.
*Pump 2 ml. antiseptic solution onto a scrub brush/sponge. Clean the nails with the brush. Use firm rubbing and circular motions with the sponge to wash your palms and the backs of your hands, paying special attention to the nails and between the fingers. Spend 1 minute on each hand.
*Still using the sponge, scrub up the arms in a circular motion stopping 3 cm. below the elbows.
*Discard the brush and rinse off the solution.
*Use 2 ml. of antiseptic and wash, then rinse the hands thoroughly. Scrub both sides for a total of at least 5 minutes.
*When finished, rinse your arms, starting from the hands down. Hold hands up, allowing water to drip down from the elbows.
*Dry with a sterile (or clean) towel, starting with your hands and

working up to the elbows. Do not touch the faucet as you turn it off. Have someone turn it off for you, turn it with your elbow, or turn it off by first covering the faucet with your towel after you have finished drying your hands. (CDC, 1981; Pereira, 1990)

Exam gloves: Gloves form a protective barrier between you and the client and should be worn for activities requiring exposure to blood or other body fluids. Organisms multiply rapidly in the warm, enclosed environment beneath the glove. If you puncture a glove during use, it should be removed, discarded, and replaced.

Latex weakens when exposed to mineral, petroleum, and vegetable oils. In uncontrolled FDA experiments with condoms, air pressure tests show significant weakening with any oil, while stretch tests showed no discernable change. The FDA has noted that mineral oil causes rapid deterioration, with splits appearing in glove material shortly after exposure. It is not understood how this weakness occurs. Water-soluble lubricants are thus officially recommended for use with latex. Water-based lubricant should be used exclusively with latex gloves.

Another option is to wear vinyl gloves. Vinyl is generally considered impervious to oil of any kind, but it breaks down rapidly in the presence of alcohol. Vinyl is also a good choice when you or the woman are allergic to latex.

Donning sterile gloves: To don sterile gloves, have your assistant peel back the outer wrap of your gloves. If no assistant is there, open the outer wrapper, being careful not to touch the inner wrapper, and prop the package in a convenient place. You can then remove the inner wrapper after you have washed your hands.

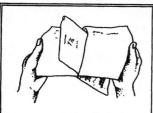	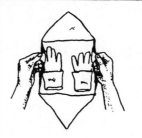	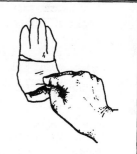
Open the gloves by grasping the flaps on either side of the package with thumb and index fingers. Rolling the hands apart will expose the inner, sterile wrapper. Pull out the inner wrapper.	Open the inner wrap and lay it flat, with the open-end of the gloves pointing toward you. Each glove will have a turned up cuff.	Pick up the first glove by the edge of the cuff with your nondominant hand; lift it up, fingers pointing down.

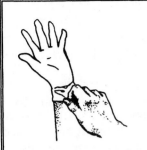 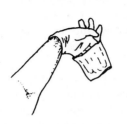 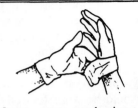

Maneuver it onto your dominant hand without touching the outer surface.	Pick up the other glove by inserting your gloved fingers *inside* the turned up cuff (so as not to touch the *inner* surface).	Insert your nondominant hand into the glove without touching the inner surface with your dominant gloved hand. Now, turn the other cuff right-side out with your non-dominant hand.

In other words, put on the gloves so that your bare hands never touch the glove's outer surface and your gloved hands never touch bare skin or the inner glove surface. (based on Timby, 1989)

To remove a soiled glove, pinch the outer surface of the cuff and draw the glove over the hand by turning it inside out. Do not touch the outer, soiled portion as you do so. Discard the glove. Remove the remaining glove by slipping your fingers beneath the cuff and removing it as before. If the glove is so soiled that you risk skin contamination during removal, get your assistant to turn the water on for you and wash your hands with the gloves still on; then remove them as described.

References and further reading:

American College of Surgeons, <u>Manual on Control of Infection in Surgical Patients</u>, J. B. Lippincott Co., Phil., 1976.

Center for Disease Control, Dr. Walter Bond, Microbiologist, Telephone conversation regarding HIV and HBV contamination, 3/26/90.

op. cit., "Guidelines for the Prevention & Control of Nosocomial Infections: Guidelines for handwashing & Hospital environmental control, 1985," <u>A.J. of Infection Control</u>, Vol. 14, No, 3, 1986, p. 110-2.

Chambers, R.W., et. al., "Transmission of Syphilis by Fresh Blood Components," <u>Transfusion</u>, Vol. 9, 1969, p. 32.

Coulter, Harris, <u>AIDS and Syphilis: The Hidden Link</u>, North Atlantic Books, 1987.

FDA, Dr. Thomas Lowe, HIV research project, Telephone conversation regarding latex permeability to HIV, 3/26/90.

Mitchell, Robert Ben, <u>Syphilis As AIDS</u>, Banned Books, Pub., Austin TX, 1990.

Pereira, Lesley, et. al., "The effect of surgical handwashing routines on the microbial counts of operating room nurses," <u>Amer. J. of Infec. Control</u>, Vol. 18, No. 6, 1990, pp. 354-364.

Timby, Barbara K., <u>Clinical Nursing Procedures</u>, J.B. Lippincott Co., Philadelphia, PA, 1989.

Williams, Vicki, "Sterile (?) Techniques and Home Birth," unpublished paper.

Fetal Heart Rate Assessment and Locating the Placenta

The baby's heartbeat is one of the midwife's primary physical means of determining fetal well-being during pregnancy. Knowing what is normal and under-standing how to detect a problem is an important part of a midwife's assessment skills. The normal fetal heart rate averages 120 to 160 beats per minute throughout pregnancy and labor, although rates of 90 to 180 are not uncommon or always abnormal (Gabbe, 1991, p. 465). Aside from the absolute (beats per minute) baseline rate, there are variations and responses which also indicate well-being; these are known as variability and reactivity.

The fetal heart can often be auscultated before fetal position can be determined, although fetal position becomes increasingly relevant in locating the fetal heart as pregnancy advances. Because of this, fetal heart rate assessment is discussed before the chapter outlining how to determine fetal position.

Basic terms and definitions:

The **baseline** fetal heart rate is defined as that rate present when a healthy fetus is at rest the heart rate is usually between 120 and 160 beats per minute (bpm). It is the result of the intrinsic rate of the heart plus modifications due to sympathetic and parasympathetic nervous responses. A change in the baseline heart rate occurs when a new baseline has been established for 1, 10, or 15 minutes. This wide time variation in definition has to do with the conditions under which changes may occur. For example, maternal oxygen augmentation creates an elevation in fetal heart rate after about 7 to 10 minutes. This response time takes into account maternal circulation, placental transfer of oxygen and fetal response. If the fetus itself initiates activity or rest, the change occurs within only 2 to 3 minutes, and most such changes last 5 to 10 minutes. Since fetal activity is the most frequent reason for a baseline change, using 10 minutes to generally define an alteration in the baseline is reasonable. The baseline tends to change with the fetal state; generally it speeds up when the fetus is breathing, dreaming or moving.

FETAL STATE	1F (QUIET SLEEP)	2F (DREAMING)	3F (AWAKE)	4F (ACTIVE)
Eye movements	Absent	Present	Present	Present
Body & limb movement	Incidental	Periodic	Absent	Continuous
Heart rate accelerations	Isolated	Frequent	Absent	Large, long
Heart rate variability	Low	Increased	Increased	---

(Nijhuis, et.al., 1984)

These activities usually last less that 10 minutes. Such periodic variations are most accurately defined as accelerations rather than a change in the baseline rate. The major baseline changes which occur involve accelerations, decelerations, bradycardia and tachycardia.

Bradycardia occurs when the heart rate falls below 120 bpm. It may occur spontaneously when there is no known reason for it and the fetus is well. In these cases, the heart rate in these cases is rarely less than 100 beats per minutes, as though the baby simply has a lower range of normal. The baseline heart rate is usually less than 100 bpm when bradycardia is due to fetal compromise. A brief period of bradycardia is known as a **deceleration** of the heart rate.

Tachycardia is an elevation of the fetal heart rate over 160 bpm. You may hear transient instances of tachycardia in healthy fetuses during periods of fetal movement, particularly if the baby has a high baseline rate to begin with. Sustained tachycardia may be due to a variety of factors which compromise the fetus. **Acceleration** refers to a transient increase in the heart rate above the normal baseline in response to fetal activity or a temporary, benign stress such as maternal excitement or exercise. Such changes last less than 10 minutes, with the heart rate returning to its normal baseline. See the chapter on Fetal Heart Rate Abnormalities in the section on Problems that Can Occur at any Time for more information about abnormal heart rate variations. (Pauerstein, 1987)

Variability is the normal fluctuation of the fetal heart rate. In a well-oxygenated fetus the time interval between any two successive beats of the heart is seldom the same. This causes the baseline rate to appear irregular. **Short-term** or **beat-to-beat variability**, usually ranges between 3 and 8 bpm around an imaginary average heart rate. **Fluctuation** or **long-term** variability of 3 to 5 bpm usually occurs in a repeating cycle 3 to 5 times per minute. No clinically significant difference between these two forms of variability has been demonstrated. (Gabbe, 1991, p. 466) Good variability reflects the normal interplay between the cardiac regulating centers in the fetal brain stem and the heart; it is one of the best indications of fetal well-being. Overall, normal variability occurs after 28 weeks gestation in a range between 3 and 25 bpm; if beat-to-beat variability is less than 2 beats per minute, variability is defined as absent.

In the healthy fetus, variability is most influenced by the baby's state of consciousness; quiet sleep produces decreased variability, while dreaming produces acceleration. After 36 weeks gestation the fetus moves in and out of these states approximately every 30 to 70 minutes, spending roughly 50% of its time in each state. A fetus usually sleeps for a maximum of 80 minutes, and though variability is reduced, a minor degree should be detectable.

Fetal heart monitoring with machines has refined the assessment of variability. An electronic fetal heart monitor takes the time interval between one heart beat and the next, calculates what the heart rate would be per minute if that rate remained constant, and displays this average on the monitor panel. It is impossible to record beat-to-beat variability without a fetal heart monitor. However, you can get a very good idea of heart rate variability during regular prenatal visits by counting the fetal heart rate successively in the smallest practical interval.

For example, you can count the heart rate for a full minute; let's say you do so and get 144 beats per minute. If you had counted during the same minute but in successive 15 second intervals, you might have heard 34 + 32 + 36 + 42. You would have gotten the same overall total of 144 but would also have more documentable data to judge what variations exist. Had you counted during the same minute at five second intervals, you would have gotten even more information. You may have heard: 12 + 13 + 11 + 11 + 11 + 10 + 11 + 12 + 13 + 13 + 14 + 15. These counts also total 144, but, as you can see, the smaller the time intervals you use to count, the more detailed the information you gather. Five seconds, which is easily counted out using a watch with a second hand, is the smallest practical time interval to use. To arrive at the per minute equivalent of each 5 second count, simply multiply that number by 12. The following chart illustrates this concept:

Count rate: 15 sec.	34		32		36	42						= 144 beats per minute
5 sec.	12	13	11	11	11	10	11	12	13	13	14	15
5 X 12 =	144	156	132	132	132	120	132	144	156	156	168	180

The following table is helpful in calculating per minute equivalents of five second counts:

3 per 5 sec. = 36	11 per 5 sec. = 132
4 per 5 sec. = 48	12 per 5 sec. = 144
5 per 5 sec. = 60	13 per 5 sec. = 156
6 per 5 sec. = 72	14 per 5 sec. = 168
7 per 5 sec. = 84	15 per 5 sec. = 180
8 per 5 sec. = 96	16 per 5 sec. = 192
9 per 5 sec. = 108	17 per 5 sec. = 204
10 per 5 sec. = 120	18 per 5 sec. = 216

As you can see, counts ranging between 10 to 13 beats per five seconds will fall roughly within the normal range of 120 to 160 beats per minute. Although you will be unable to record all the beat-to-beat variability you hear, you will develop a sensitivity for how fast or slow the heart is beating within a given 5 second time period. Assessing the fetal heart rate in this way will allow you to pick up on abnormal patterns. You may have an overall count of 144, but with huge variations, as from 7 to 17, in your 5 second counts. Variability such as this, or, conversely, a lack of variability, can indicate problems. Interpreting fetal heart rate variations is discussed further in the chapter on Fetal Heart Rate Abnormalities in the section on Problems That Can Occur at any Time, in <u>Diagnostic Tests</u>, in Volume II of this textbook and on the following pages.

Reactivity is a type of variability and is defined as how much the heart rate responds to fetal rest or movement as well as to other stress such as that imposed by uterine contractions. Normally, the fetal heart beats faster when the fetus is moving and returns to the normal baseline heart rate when the baby is at rest.

Optimally, the fetal heart rate accelerates at least 15 bpm. above the normal baseline for 15 to 30 seconds at least twice in a 10 minute period, or at least 5 times in a 20 minute period. This frequency reflects fetal health and neurological maturity. It is not always possible to detect reactivity as it is defined above in healthy young fetuses.

REACTIVITY BY GESTATIONAL AGE	
GESTATION	REACTIVITY (AS DEFINED ABOVE)
20-24 weeks	26%
24-28 weeks	55%
28-32 weeks	76%
32-36 weeks	95%
36-40 weeks	99%

(Freeman, 1995)

I have personally heard a slight temporary deceleration with a lag prior to acceleration in early gestation in babies that were normal.

Accelerations are usually associated with fetal movement or excitement. If little or no variability occurs during fetal movement, the baby is said to have a nonreactive heart rate. Although you will often see minimal variability in a normal fetus who is sleeping, if it happens continuously this can reflect a central nervous system which is unable to respond to stress; it indicates a compromised situation for the baby.

Listening to and recording the fetal heart rate:

Listening to the fetal heart is one way we make intimate contact with the baby before birth. Be sure to greet the baby and tell it what you are about to do. Listening with a fetascope or your ear pressed against the mother's abdomen puts you in close psychic touch with the baby; as you become more experienced you will not only be able to sense the fetal heart rate when it is faint (as in early pregnancy), but you will be able to tell if the baby is okay by what you feel intuitively while listening. This emotional and psychic connection is a most helpful addition to your purely clinical assessment of fetal well-being.

Variability and associated reactivity can be detected and recorded during prenatal exams by counting the fetal heart rate successively for 5 second intervals and recording the numbers you get (it is more informative and less work to record 13, 12, 11 than to multiply each number by 12). Often, you will be able to detect fetal movement at some point during auscultation and can then record that the baby was moving as well. If the baby seems quiet during auscultation, talk to the baby and tell it why you want it to wake up. This, along with a bit of palpation or vigorous baby-butt jiggling, will usually elicit a reaction; listening immediately will usually reward you with detectable variability, remembering that a reactive pattern may take between 2 and 3 minutes to become apparent. Fetal movements lasting 3 seconds or longer elicit heart rate accelerations 98.8% of the time. To record these findings you might note something like this: 11, 11, 12, (13, 13 w/palp.). You might also want to draw a belly on your prenatal form and mark where you are hearing fetal heart sounds from visit to visit. You could use an + sign to designate the location of the fetal heart and an o to indicate the location of placental sounds.

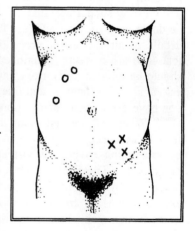

The fetal heart rate is an important clinical link to the well-being of the baby. Your careful records of an individual baby's normal heart rate range and pattern of variability and reactivity will be an enormous help to you in monitoring the fetus as pregnancy advances and particularly during the stress of labor; in many cases this knowledge can avoid an unnecessary transport. While most medical practices assess the rate of the fetal heart beat per minute and record this prenatally, they often pay little or no attention to variability or reactivity until a problem is suspected. At that point, it is impossible to take one-minute intervals from the chart and come up with any meaningful information, unless these intervals are distinctly out of a statistically normal range. Tuning in to the variability and reactivity by counting and recording 5 second counts means you are doing a mini-non-stress test at every prenatal visit (see Diagnostic Tests for details on this test). By doing so, you will have a much better handle on what is truly normal for that baby before any problems arise, and will be more likely to pick up on a real problem sooner. A true baseline normal, not just an average based on statistics, is an incredibly valuable tool.

When to begin listening: It is most valuable to begin listening for the fetal heart as soon as the uterine fundus emerges from behind the pubic bone. This way, you will tune into it as early as it can possibly be heard. Continue to listen throughout prenatal care. You can usually detect the fetal heart sounds with a regular fetascope at approximately the same time the mother can detect fetal movement (sometimes a bit before or after this point). With the Series 10 Allyn fetascope I have frequently heard the fetal heart as early 15 weeks and once at 12 weeks. Most commonly, however, the fetal heart is audible with a fetascope sometime between 16 and 20 weeks of pregnancy. When and where the heart rate is audible varies from woman to woman and is influenced by the weeks of pregnancy, depth of a woman's torso, the size and position of the baby, the amount of amniotic fluid, the position of the uterus in the pelvis, the location of the placenta, and the amount of abdominal tissue between you and the fetus. You may note that the small fetus' heart rate is more rapid, slowing somewhat as pregnancy advances, but remaining within a normal range. I have frequently noted this and it is not a problem.

Finding the fetal heart during an exam: Before you begin, have the mother empty her bladder. This will facilitate your exam, especially in early pregnancy, as the bladder is situated anterior to the uterus. Be sure the head of your fetascope is warm. If it isn't, hold it in your hands or run warm water over it, making sure you do so in such a way that you don't fill the inside with water. Have the mother lie down on a firm surface (see the chapter on palpation in this section for further details about the exam procedure). Check to be sure the binaurals of your fetascope are correctly positioned; when holding them in front of your face, they should be pointed away from you slightly. This lines the earpieces up with your ear canals. Try them on and fine tune this adjustment by tapping on the head until you have good sound conduction. Then proceed with your exam.

When you are first trying to find the fetal heart during early pregnancy, begin by attempting to hear it just above the pubic bone. The faint sounds seem to be amplified by the proximity of the bone and therefore are frequently more easily heard in this area. Press very firmly, the baby is well cushioned by fluid and you will cause no harm. Listen intently; it may help to close your eyes. Move your fetascope around, little by little, until you can detect the heart beat. You must listen for a regular sound behind any overlaying sounds from the mother's circulation or digestive system. Keep trying. It can take a while to find it! Your efforts will be less rewarded if the mother's uterus is

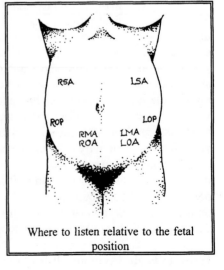

Where to listen relative to the fetal position

retroverted; in early pregnancy the fundus of the retroverted uterus takes longer to rise above the pubic bone and therefore both the fetal heart tones and the true top of the fundus are more difficult to find.

As pregnancy advances, the location of the loudest fetal heart sounds will become somewhat more predictable based upon the fetal position at the time. Traditionally it has been said that the fetal heart is easiest to hear just below the anterior shoulder through the baby's back. Most of the time this will be the case, especially as the baby gets larger. Be sure to assess whether the woman is experiencing a toning contraction while you are trying to listen, which will make finding the fetal heart more difficult. Simply wait a minute or two for the uterus to relax before you continue.

Traditionally it has also been taught that the location of the fetal heart sounds are one way to double check your estimation of the baby's position. Be aware, however, that there is *not* a 100% correlation between the two. This is especially true if you are using a Doppler (another good reason not to!). Should you find fetal heart tones in an unexpected location relative to your estimation of the baby's position by palpation, feel again. If you still feel confident of the baby's position via palpation, give that more weight than where you hear the fetal heart. The fetal heart is often best heard below the mother's navel, even if the baby is breech.

What you are listening for: The fetal heart has a rapid, relatively clear two-beat sound (thu-thump or tick-tock). In early pregnancy it sounds more like a watch ticking under a pillow and more clearly like a rapid heartbeat as pregnancy advances. In very early pregnancy, maternal bowel sounds can momentarily mimic the fetal heart as far as rate and regularity. Keep listening; if the sound changes or disappears, the small baby has either moved away or you are picking up bowel sounds, not the fetal heart.

You may hear other things besides the mother's bowels or the fetal heart as you listen. If you hear a sound which you are unsure of, reach up and feel the mother's radial pulse as you are listening to help distinguish what you are hearing. The mother's uterine arteries can be quite loud. These are soft, diffused sounds which are synchronous with the mother's pulse. They are located in a vertical line on either side of the uterus. These sounds are referred to as the **uterine souffle**.

It is also possible to hear the baby's umbilical cord; a sound which is referred to as the **funic souffle**. This more distinct blowing, almost whistling sound pulses at the same rate as the fetal heart.

Listening for the placenta: Beginning about the 20th week of pregnancy, try to locate the placental implantation site. Start down near the pubic bone, listening over to each side, then over the anterior surface of the uterus and over the fundus. The soft blowing sound of the placenta is referred to as the **placental souffle**. This sound may fall somewhere between the rate of the mother's and baby's heart rate or be almost synchronous with the mother's pulse. It represents the combined sounds of the mother's pulse rate and the faster fetal pulse as blood is pumped on both sides at different rates. It is loud and can easily obscure the sound of the fetal heart when the baby's back is directly beneath the placenta. Hearing the fetal heart may be particularly problematic if the placenta is implanted on the anterior wall of the uterus. If this is the case, listening on the side opposite the baby's back will often afford you a fainter but less obstructed location for listening. You may also be able to pick up fetal heart sounds well over on the side of the baby's back (on the far lateral side of the placenta). The placental souffle sounds similar to the uterine souffle, and can be confusing if you hear placental sounds in the same area where the uterine artery is found. Just remember that the arteries run in a straight line on either side of the uterus and the placenta has a round surface area which will be wider and broader than the artery.

A placenta located near the pubic bone may migrate upwards as the uterus enlarges; the woman can visualize this happening along with her other visualizations. Be especially attentive to placental location in women who have scars in their uterine wall. Implantation over a scarred area could cause the placenta to be abnormally adherent, leading to bleeding problems at the time of birth (see the chapter on Previous Uterine Surgeries in the Special Circumstances section for more details).

References and further reading:

Freeman, Roger, "Update on Antepartum Testing," workshop, Perinatal Care Symposium Strategies for Improving Maternal and Neonatal Outcomes, 6/16/95.

Gabbe, Steven, et. al. ed. Obstetrics: Normal and Problem Pregnancies, 2nd ed., Churchill Livingstone, New York, 1991.

Nijhuis, J. G., et.al., "Behavioral state of the human fetus," in Continuity of Neural Functions from Prenatal to Postnatal Life, H. Prechti, ed., London, SIMP with Blackwell Scientific, Philadelphia, PA, Lippincott, 1984, pp. 65-77.

Pauerstein, Carl, ed., Clinical Obstetrics, John Wiley & Sons, New York, 1987.

Discussing How the Baby is Situated in the Uterus

Palpation of the fetus becomes possible around the 25th week of pregnancy. As pregnancy advances, you will be able to more and more accurately determine fetal position and locate various parts of the fetal anatomy.

In order to intelligently articulate the relationship of the baby's anatomy to that of the mother, it is essential to have an understanding of the universal language used to discuss these parameters. To begin, it is helpful to review the technical terms for various areas of the baby's anatomy:

Acromion or scapula—back of the shoulder; the shoulder blade
Breech—buttocks
Brow—forehead; the area just in front of the anterior fontanelle
Cephalic—to do with the head
Frontum—forehead
Mentum—chin
Occiput—the area directly behind and below the posterior fontanelle to
    the nape of the neck
Sacrum—the central bone in the back of the pelvis
Sinciput—area around the anterior fontanelle
Vertex—area between the anterior and posterior fontanelles

There are six different ways to communicate about how the baby is situated in the uterus: attitude, lie, presentation, presenting part, denominator, and position and variety.

The **attitude** of the baby refers to the position of the baby's head in relationship to its trunk and limbs. This is usually expressed as a degree of head flexion or extension. Full flexion is present when the baby's chin is tucked to its chest (vertex presentation). Full extension is present when the head is fully tipped back so that the baby appears to be looking directly up at the sky (also known as a face presentation).

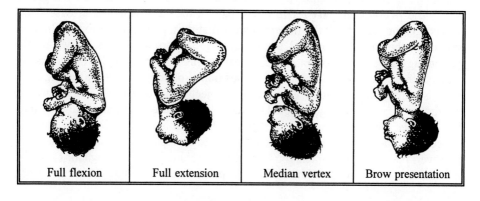

| Full flexion | Full extension | Median vertex | Brow presentation |

382

In a sinciput or median vertex (also called military) attitude, it appears as though the baby is looking straight ahead, chin lifted up. A brow presentation causes the head to be tipped back, as it would be if you were looking at someone taller than yourself. Both the median vertex and brow attitudes represent degrees of extension. The term "deflexion" is sometimes used instead of extension.

The **lie** of the baby refers to the relationship of the baby's spine (long axis) to the spine (long axis) of the mother. In most cases, the baby's spine will be in line with the mother's; this is called a **longitudinal lie**. Both breech and vertex presentations are longitudinal lies. When the baby's spine is positioned at an angle to the mother's spine, it is called an **oblique lie**. When the baby's spine is at a 90^0 angle to the mother's spine, the baby is in a **transverse lie** (sideways).

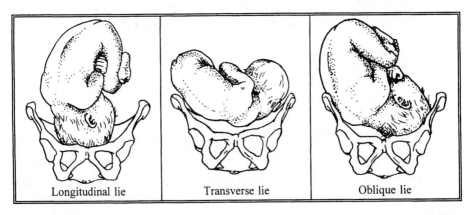

| Longitudinal lie | Transverse lie | Oblique lie |

The **presentation** refers to the part of the fetus which is directly over the inlet of the mother's pelvis. The three possible presentations are **cephalic** (head first), **breech** (pelvis first), and **transverse** (shoulder first). Cephalic presentations are further subdivided into cephalic—vertex, sincipital, brow and face. Breech presentation is further subdivided into breech—frank (legs stretched straight up on body), full (or complete, the legs are crossed Tailor-style) and incomplete, where either one or both feet or knees are extended downward toward the maternal pelvis.

The **presenting part** refers to the part of the baby which is closest to the cervix; i.e. the part which the fingers contact first during an internal exam. In most instances, the presentation and the presenting part are the same; however, the presenting part can also be another fetal part or limb. For example, in the case of a breech baby, a foot or knee could be positioned directly above the cervix. If a baby is transverse, a hand or elbow could project down toward the cervix and be the first fetal part that fingers would contact. In rare cases, the umbilical cord may be contained within the amniotic sac between fetal head, breech or shoulder and the cervix. The presentation is still considered to be cephalic, breech or transverse, however, the small part which you touch first is said to be presenting (for example, a shoulder presentation with the elbow presenting, a double footling breech presentation wherein both feet are presenting extended toward the yoni; or a shoulder presentation with the cord presenting).

The **denominator** is a specific location on the fetus that gives us more information about fetal presentation. It is used to discuss how the baby is positioned in relationship to the mother's pelvis. Each presentation has its own denominator. This point is arbitrarily chosen, but is a universally consistent reference. When an extremity is extended into the yoni (as described in the last paragraph), this does not affect the way the denominator is defined. The locations of the denominators for the various presentations are as follows:

PRESENTATION	DENOMINATOR
Cephalic—vertex (top of head) (Used for sinciput as well)	Occiput (back of skull between the nape of the neck and the posterior fontanelle)
Cephalic—brow	Forehead (frontum)
Cephalic—face	Chin (mentum)
Breech (all variations)	Sacrum
Transverse or oblique lie	Scapula (acromion)

The **position** technically refers to the relationship of the denominator to the right or left sides of the maternal pelvis. Accordingly, with each presentation, there can be two positions, right or left. It is important to keep in mind that all references to position refer to the mother's left or right sides, *not yours or the baby's*. The **variety** is the location of the denominator in relation to the front, back or sides of the mother's pelvis. Starting with the pubic bone at the top and moving posteriorly around the mother's pelvis in a clockwise direction, eight possible relationships for each denominator can be noted. **Position** is commonly, although imprecisely, used to refer to all nuances regarding the fetus's relationship to the mother since this term, more than the others, takes into account the most variables.

1. **Denominator Anterior (DA)**; the denominator is directly under the mother's pubic bone, at 12 o'clock.
2. **Left Denominator Anterior (LDA)**; the denominator is in the anterior or front of the mother's pelvis, 45^0 to the left of her midline (navel point).
3. **Left Denominator Transverse (LDT)**; the denominator is on her left side of her pelvis, 90^0 from her midline, at 3 o'clock.
4. **Left Denominator Posterior (LDP)**; the denominator is now in the back-most segment of the pelvis and is 135^0 to the left of the mother's navel (or 45° to the left of her sacral promontory).
5. **Denominator Posterior (DP)**; the denominator is in the back part of the mother's pelvis, directly in front of or anterior to her sacrum, at 6 o'clock.
6. **Right Denominator Posterior (RDP)**; the denominator is in the posterior part

of the pelvis, 135^0 to the right of the mother's navel (or 45° to the right of the mother's sacrum).

7. **Right Denominator Transverse (RDT)**; the denominator is on the right side of the mother's pelvis, 90^0 from her midline (half-way between her back and her front) at 9 o'clock.

8. **Right Denominator Anterior (RDA)**; the denominator is in the anterior segment of the mother's pelvis, 45^0 to the right of her navel (or her midline).

If you take the above descriptions and replace the generic word "denominator" with the actual denominator for each presentation, you will have the proper abbreviation for each variety of fetal position. For example, if the denominator is the occiput and it is in the anterior portion of the mother's pelvis 45° to the left of her midline, the baby is said to be in the Left Occiput Anterior or LOA position. The following illustration portrays all possible positions of the occiput, looking up into the maternal pelvis from between the mother's legs as she is lying flat on her back.

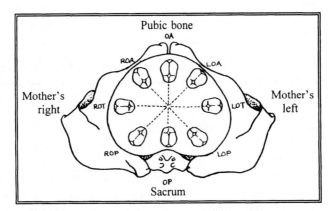

The following chart illustrates all of the fetal positions from the point of view of one looking through the surface of the mother's abdomen. Study it as you review the various terms used to discuss the location of the fetus within the mother's body. (redrawn and adapted by the author from drawings presented in Obstetrics Illustrated.)

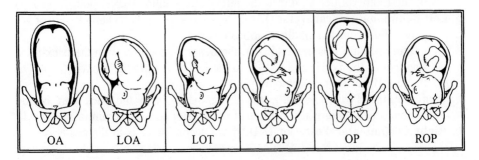

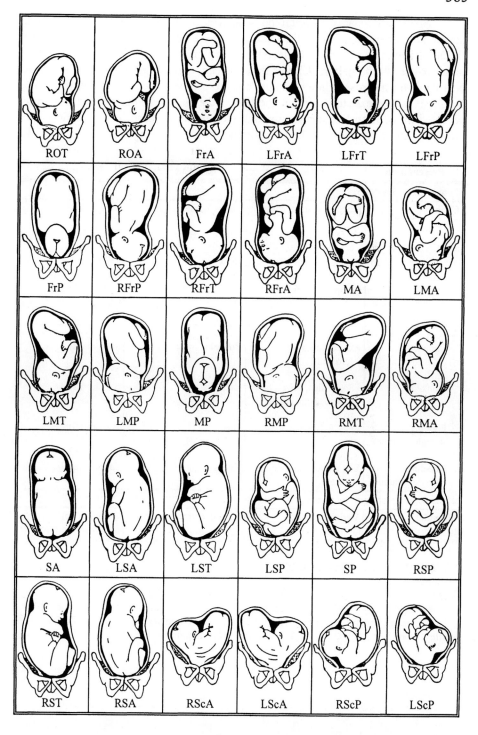

Not every nuance of fetal position can be ascertained from abbreviated notations. For example, from the initials LOP, we do not know if the head is fully flexed or if it is in a partially deflexed (military or median) position. Likewise we do not know if a baby lying LSA is frank breech, if it has a foot or knee extended, or if the legs are crossed in a complete breech fashion, nor do we know if the fetal head is flexed or extended. When and if such details can be determined, they must be noted in addition to those designating the presenting part, lie and variety. The following chart summarizes the points reviewed in this chapter:

Presentation	Attitude	Presenting Part	Denominator
Longitudinal lie (99.5%)			
Cephalic	Flexion (chin to chest)	Vertex (posterior part)	Occiput (O)
	Military (median part)	Vertex (median part)	Occiput (O)
	Partial extension	Brow	Forehead (frontum) (Fr)
	Complete extension	Face	Chin (mentum) (M)
Breech Complete	Flexed knees, legs crossed	Buttocks	Sacrum (S)
Frank	Flexed hips, legs extended up against trunk	Buttocks	Sacrum (S)
Footling (single, double)	Legs fully extended	Feet	Sacrum (S)
Kneeling (single, double)	Leg extended, knee flexed	Knees	Sacrum (S)
Transverse or oblique lie (0.5%)			
Shoulder	Variable	Shoulder, trunk or arm	Scapula (Sc) or Acromion (Ac)

References and further reading:

Garrey, M., et.al., Obstetrics Illustrated, Churchill Livingstone, New York, 1980.
Hellman, L, et.al., William's Obstetrics, 14th ed., Appleton-Century-Crofts, New York, 1971.
Oxhorn, Harry, Human Labor and Birth, 5th ed., Appleton-Century-Crofts, Norwalk, CT, 1986.
Whitley, Nancy, A Manual of Clinical Obstetrics, J.B. Lippincott Co., 1985.

The Fine Art of Palpation

Palpation (pal-PAY-shun) can begin as soon as you start seeing a woman for care. Early in pregnancy, palpation can help you know how the uterus is growing. As you gain more experience you will be able to ascertain whether the amount of amniotic fluid is within a normal range and be able to tell something about the size of the baby relative to the amount of fluid. As pregnancy advances, palpation becomes increasingly more informative regarding fetal size, movement and position. It helps you determine the best location for listening to the fetal heart as well as providing you with the most direct physical contact you can have with the baby prior to birth. All in all, palpation is one of your most important tools as a midwife.

Many newly practicing doctors and even many student nurse-midwives are being taught to depend heavily upon ultrasound to determine the fetal position and to obtain information traditionally gathered through palpation. This dependence on technology is causing practitioners to lose valuable hands-on skills. Therefore, it becomes even more important that we preserve this indispensable tool of our trade. Hands-on skills cannot be replaced by machines. Your intuitive link with the baby and mother are enhanced considerably by the intimate process of feeling the baby within the uterus. Besides, if the power goes out or if there is a disaster, you'll be in much better shape than those who cannot function without a device of some sort or another!

Palpation requires us to use our sight, touch and intuition to gather information about the physical condition of the baby. Even if you cannot pinpoint anything intellectually, palpation can help you tune into the fact that a problem exists. It can help allay fears as well. Palpation is one way we form an emotional link with the baby, so be sure and talk to the baby when feeling for its position.

Preparing a woman to be examined: Have the mother empty her bladder prior to examination. This will not only make palpation more comfortable for her, but more informative for you. Next, have the mother lie down on your chosen examination surface. It should be stable, firm and wide enough for the woman to be comfortable. A soft bed will not do. A carpeted floor is one option, offering a firm, stable surface for her to lie on as well as easy access for you and her family members, especially for small children who wish to listen to the fetal heart during the exam.

Next, have the mother expose her abdomen completely. Keep in mind that modesty is emphasized within certain cultures (e.g. traditional Arab; Amish). The woman may want you to examine her beneath her clothing or she may want all other family members to leave. Be flexible and do all you can to accommodate her wishes. Pants should be pulled down or unbuttoned sufficiently to allow full abdominal exposure. The mother's muscles need to be as relaxed as possible; this can be facilitated by propping her head with a pillow, having her arms by her side or across her chest and having her bend her knees slightly. A small pillow beneath her knees can help. Too much elevation, however, can tip the pelvis and thereby impede your attempts to palpate; have her legs either straight or only slightly propped. Propping a woman in a semi-sitting position, especially as pregnancy advances, is done in an attempt to prevent supine hypotensive syndrome which occurs due to the heavy uterus pressing on her inferior vena cava, which can cause the woman to feel faint or dizzy. However, most women will not experience this during the relatively brief period required for an exam. You will get a better idea of fetal position if you lie a woman flat on a firm surface and then allow her to prop only slightly or roll on her side for a few minutes when necessary during the exam.

Be sure to show the mother what you are doing and why. Guide her hands so that she can learn to feel her baby herself. For example. demonstrate how the head can move independent of the rest of the body by moving your head from side to side and how that motion differs from the way the bottom of the baby might move. The more she understands, the more empowered she becomes and the better able she will be to monitor her own pregnancy. Fine tune that "mother monitor," the most essential expert in the care-giving process. (Loprenzi-Kassel, 1995)

Inspection: A practitioner with a trained eye can readily determine the shape and uniform outline which characterizes the pregnant woman's uterus. The uterus usually lies in or near the midline and is an oval shape with its long axis placed vertically. Especially during early pregnancy, the contents of the ascending or descending large intestine may displace the uterus slightly to one side or the other; this may be more pronounced in a multipara with lax abdominal muscle tone.

Irregularity in the outline of the uterus may be due to fetal position or a fibroid. You may occasionally note a soup-plate sized mass when the placenta is on the anterior wall of the uterus and the woman is exceptionally thin. As you become more experienced you will often have an impression of the fetal position from visual inspection of a mother's belly, especially when she is near term. Use your findings from the manual exam to confirm your initial visual impressions.

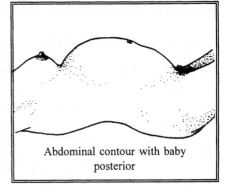

Abdominal contour with baby
posterior

Observation of the shape of the uterus can give you some preliminary clues regarding the position of the baby, as follows:

Observations of uterine contours	Significance
Longitudinal ovoid	Baby is lying longitudinally
Belly is widest from side to side	Baby is lying side to side (transverse)
Long smooth curve to one side of the abdomen	The baby's back is on that side
A saucer-like depression is just below the mother's navel	Baby is lying with its back toward the mother's (posterior)
Small bumps or limb activity can be seen in the center of the mother's abdomen	Baby may be posterior

Developing your hand skills for palpation: Have your nails trimmed short. Long nails interfere with your ability to palpate and may be painful for the mother during some maneuvers. Check the warmth of your hands. If they are freezing cold either rub them together or run warm water over them. Touch her on her arm so she can judge for herself if you are unsure about the temperature of your hands. Hands that are on the cool side are often welcomed by a pregnant woman, whose higher metabolism makes her warmer than usual. Before beginning the exam, rest your hands lightly on the mother's belly. This allows her time to accustom herself to your touch and helps her relax.

When placing your hands on the mother's belly, place your palms on her abdomen first. This helps relax the muscles in your forearm and allows the tactile senses a greater power of perception. Now bring your fingers down on the abdomen. This will ensure that you feel with the flat palmar surface of your fingertips, which are the most sensitive part of the fingers. The flat surface of the fingertips will be more comfortable than the fingertip ends for the mother as well. During most of the exam you will keep the fingers together. Apply smooth deep pressure, moving in slowly but firmly to feel the fetal parts. Be as firm as necessary to do an accurate exam. Palpating too lightly will not be very informative, and often communicates your lack of confidence to the mother. Firm palpation will not hurt the baby, who is well protected in a bag of water. Avoid sudden movements which involve jabbing, poking or prodding. Such palpation will cause tension in the mother and be less informative for you. However, you will find that sharp, flexing movements of the fingers are required at times.

The palpation process is one of dipping into a water bath within a flexible wall and finding a floating solid object. Firm, flexing movements of the fingers quickly displaces amniotic fluid and brings the fingers in contact with the underlying fetal part. Sudden contact can help distinguish the back, head or limbs of the baby. The things you are looking for when palpating the fetus are:

*The back
*The shoulder
*The poles or ends of the baby, i.e. the head and the butt (breech)
*The small parts such as hands, feet and limbs

When to begin palpation: Begin palpating the uterus when you first begin to see a woman for care. Early on, the small fetal size relative to the amount of amniotic fluid allows the tiny baby to easily move away from your examining hand; you will not be able to distinguish fetal poles or small parts except by virtue of the occasional kick or punch. During these early weeks, normal growth can be ascertained by assessing the size of the uterus in relationship to the number of weeks of pregnancy. However, "normal" can vary among individual women and from pregnancy to pregnancy. It is quite common for the amniotic fluid or the baby or both to show a "growth spurt" at any point in pregnancy and then balance out and show a normal size-for-dates relationship later on.

Palpation in early pregnancy: Before a pregnancy reaches the twelve week mark, abdominal palpation will usually afford you little information. However, if there is something unusual about the pregnancy, such as a multiple gestation or a hydatidiform mole, the uterus will often enlarge more rapidly than usual; palpation of the area just above the pubic bone will tip you off to early clues that something unusual might be going on.

Palpation of the uterine shape and size: As pregnancy advances beyond 12 weeks, the fundus, or top of the uterus, can be found by placing the outer edge of your hand around the upper edge of the uterus. Tuck or press the edge of your hand into the belly to demarche the top-most border of the uterine swelling. Once you have established the outline of the uterus, palpate the remainder of the abdomen. Usually nothing abnormal is found, but if the pregnancy is not far advanced, you may discover an enlarged kidney or liver, or possibly a fibroid or other mass.

As pregnancy advances further, if the transverse colon is somewhat bloated or displaced outward, preventing the easy location of the fundus, first place your hands on either side of the uterus and bounce it between them gently to accurately locate its lateral borders. Less commonly, the ascending or descending colon are bloated, which can obscure your findings as well. The uterus will be a distinctly firmer mass between the two lengths of intestine. Then, following the borders of the uterus with the edge of the hands on either side, move them up until the fingers meet at the top. Now remove one hand and allow the other hand to rotate slightly upwards until its lower edge is at right angles to the skin surface. The outer border of the hand then will clearly demarcate the uppermost point of the fundus.

Palpating for fetal position:

In most cases, you will be able to determine fetal lie by 26 weeks. As pregnancy advances, the baby's back and small parts will become increasingly obvious on palpation. The following pages detail various techniques for distinguishing fetal position. For clarity's sake, I make note of the four classic maneuvers of Leopold (a doctor credited with the introduction of these maneuvers). However, because these four maneuvers leave out many nuances of palpation, I do not follow the procedure which he recommended. As you gain experience, you may decide that performing these techniques in a different order suits you better. If you notice that some fetal part feels unusual, keep this in mind as you palpate from visit to visit; you may have discovered a fetal abnormality or a fibroid If you suspect a problem, discuss obtaining more information via an ultrasound imaging exam with the parents.

The baby's back is the broadest expanse of the fetal body and, if the baby is large enough, may be readily identified. Stand, sit or kneel next to the woman (to her right if you are right-hand dominant and to her left if you are left-hand dominant, facing her head). Steady the uterus by placing your non-dominant hand on the nearest lateral wall of the uterus, out toward the side of her abdomen. Place your dominant hand on the woman's opposite side, at the level of the navel. Move your hands across the abdomen, feeling as you go, until they meet in the center of her belly. If the fetus is anterior, a broad, curved resistance will be found to one side of the midline. Sometimes the back can be pushed closer to the surface by applying pressure on the opposite side of the uterus or by pressing the fundus. (This is the second Leopold's maneuver.) The abdominal surface opposite the baby's back should feel more irregular and small parts may even move as you palpate them—these are the baby's arms and legs.

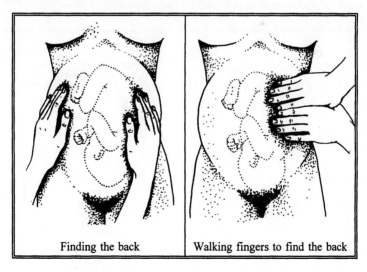

| Finding the back | Walking fingers to find the back |

Another method of determining the location of the baby's back is using both hands simultaneously to "walk your fingers over the abdomen." To do so start with the fingers of both hands on one side of the abdomen, applying deep and firm pressure with the fingers of both hands. Then "walk" your fingers across the abdomen. As you go, your fingers will notice the difference between the firm back and the small, irregular, knobby hands, feet, arms and legs. These will be on the opposite side from the back. This technique will become more informing as you acquire more experience.

You can sometimes determine the baby's position by noting how much of the back is palpable. For instance, if the baby is in an L.O.A. position, the back will be in the anterior left quadrant of the mother's abdomen. The limbs may be somewhat difficult to make out on her right side. If the baby is L.O.T., the back will be along her left side and the fetal limbs will be more easily felt on the right side. However, note that the position of the back does not necessarily indicate the position of the baby's head, especially during labor.

1. What is in the fundus? Once you locate the back, trace it upwards with the appropriate hand until you reach the fundus. Form your hand in a C shape, cupping your fingers around the fetal pole in the fundus. Here you will usually find the breech. The breech can be distinguished from the head as it is both softer and smaller and will not move independently of the rest of the body. However, if the legs are tightly crossed at the knees in a large baby, the breech can assume a sizable form and may be more difficult to distinguish. The head is usually the largest and most distinct object in the uterus and, because it is on the flexible neck, can be moved independently of the baby's trunk, like a ball floating in water. (This quality of movement is referred to as ballotment).

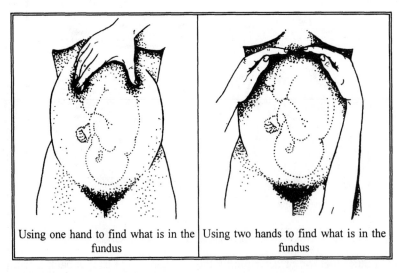

| Using one hand to find what is in the fundus | Using two hands to find what is in the fundus |

Now place your hands on either side of the fundus and curve your fingers around the top. Mold your hands around the contents of the fundus and move them back and forth as one, (i.e. do not flex the fingers as you do so) in order to bounce or ballot the contents of the fundus between your hands This will help you to further distinguish what you are feeling in the fundus. (This is the first maneuver of Leopold.)

FINDINGS ON PALPATION	WHAT THEY SIGNIFY
Part feels round & hard; it is readily moveable independent of the larger body mass	Fetal head
Part feels irregular, bulkier & less firm, poorly delineated & not readily moved independent of body mass	Fetal breech
Nothing appears to be in the fundus	Baby may be lying oblique or transverse or may be very low in the uterus
Firm, convex, consistent, smooth & resistant mass extending from fundus to pelvic brim on one side	Fetal back
Small, knobby, irregular masses that may move	Fetal hands, feet or limbs
Small parts all over the abdomen, back hard to find	Posterior presentation

2. The shoulder may be found next. Turn around to face the mother's feet. Steady the uterus on the side opposite the baby's back with one hand and palpate with the other hand down along the back until the resistance suddenly disappears. Retrace your path about half an inch up. Assuming that the baby is in a vertex presentation, your fingers should be on the shoulder. This may be referred to as the anterior shoulder.

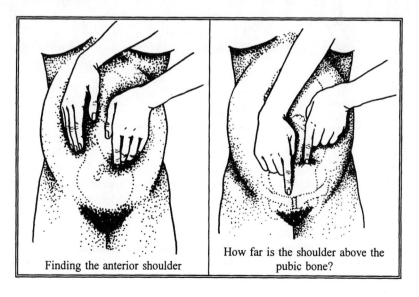

Finding the anterior shoulder

How far is the shoulder above the pubic bone?

394

Note its distance from the mother's midline and its height above her pubic bone. In an LOA or ROA position, the anterior shoulder will be within about 3 inches from the midline. If the head has not descended into the pelvis, the anterior shoulder will be four inches or more above the pubic bone, leaving room for the head between the shoulder and the pubic bone. As the head descends into the brim the height of the anterior shoulder becomes progressively lower on the belly.

3. The head: The head will usually occupy the lower part of the uterus, especially as pregnancy advances. To palpate it, face the mother's feet. Place your hands on either side of the lower abdomen, fingertips pointing downward just above the pubic bone. Press inward gently but firmly. If this proves difficult, have the mother take a deep breath in and begin pressing as she exhales. Now alternate pressure with your hands against the mass in the pelvis to bounce (or ballot) it back and forth. Attempt to outline what is in the pelvis by moving your hands around its borders. The head is harder and rounder than the buttocks. If neither the head nor the breech is found in the lower portion of the uterus, the baby may be lying either transverse or oblique and further palpation of the lower uterus will not be very informative. Feel to either side of midline to find an oblique or transverse lie.

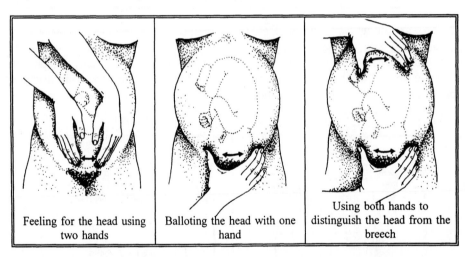

| Feeling for the head using two hands | Balloting the head with one hand | Using both hands to distinguish the head from the breech |

For the next maneuver, some like to remain facing the mother's feet and some prefer to palpate while facing the mother's side, with their dominant arm nearest her feet. Form a "C" shape with the thumb and index/middle fingers of your dominant hand. Grasp the portion of the lower abdomen directly over the largest diameter of the fetal pole in the lower uterus. Gently but firmly press into the abdomen in order to feel the presenting part beneath your hand, between your thumb and fingers. Keeping your entire hand rigid in the C shape, move your hand back and forth in order to ballot the fetal pole between your fingers. If the part in the pelvis is not engaged it will move back and forth freely; if it is the head it will do so more easily. (This is the third maneuver of Leopold; also referred to as Pawlik's maneuver or grip.) You may form the other hand into a C shape and, in the same fashion, simultaneously use it to palpate the pole in the fundus. Using both hands together can help you differentiate the head from the breech. If the fetus is breech, the buttocks will feel less firm than a head and will not ballot independently of the trunk.

If you are still unsure if the head or the breech is in the pelvis, go back and attempt to locate the fetal shoulder again. Although the breech may feel like a head, there will not be a shoulder just above it with the distinct drop-off characteristic of the junction between the shoulder and the fetal neck. Turn yourself around and, using the same shoulder-finding techniques, check for a shoulder in the upper portion of the uterus.

If you have determined that the head is in the lower portion of the uterus, more details may now be gathered.

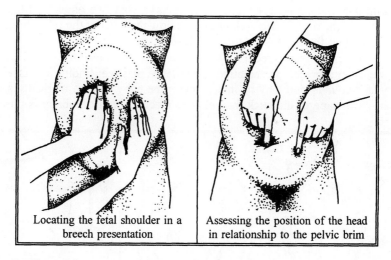

| Locating the fetal shoulder in a breech presentation | Assessing the position of the head in relationship to the pelvic brim |

The diameter of the brim in which the head is lying may be transverse, right or left oblique as well as directly anterior-posterior. Facing the woman's feet, place two forefingers on the lower abdomen, each 1½ inches from midline. Press inward until you contact the head. If the head is lying transverse, both fingers will meet the resistance of the head at an equal distance from the abdominal surface. The same will be true if the baby is lying directly O.A. or O.P.

If, however, the head lies in an oblique diameter, one finger will penetrate more deeply than the other before meeting the head. If the right finger is deeper, the head is lying in the mother's right oblique diameter. If the left finger is deeper, then the head is lying in the left oblique diameter.

The flexion of the head may be assessed by placing your hands on the sides of the uterus with the palms just below the mother's navel and the fingers pointing downwards. Press your fingertips deeply into the lower abdomen as you move them toward the pelvic inlet. One of your hands will contact a hard, round mass while the other will continue in the direction of the pelvis. The mass is the cephalic prominence, the most prominently palpated portion of the head. If it is on the same side as the back, this indicates an extended head; if it is on the same side as the arms and legs, you are feeling the fetal forehead (sinciput); this indicates a well-flexed vertex presentation. If both hands simultaneously encounter a hard, round mass, the head is in a military presentation. If the only cephalic prominence is large and on the same side as the back, the head is quite deflexed.

Flexion may be also determined by using one hand to trace down along the anterior border of the back. Place your index finger in the groove formed by the nape of the neck. Now, with the other hand, palpate the opposite side of the head (the face) from below upwards until the resistance of the face disappears; mark this point with that index finger. Compare the levels of your two fingers. If the finger on the nape of the neck is one inch or more below the level of the other finger, you may assume that the head is reasonably flexed.

By reversing your direction, you can use the same techniques to determine head flexion in a breech presentation. This takes practice; finding the face is not as easy as it sounds, and may be impossible if the baby is in an markedly anterior position. The nape of the neck may also be inaccessible if the baby is posterior.

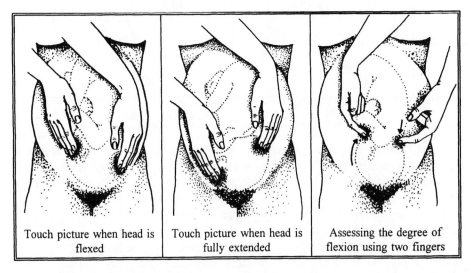

| Touch picture when head is flexed | Touch picture when head is fully extended | Assessing the degree of flexion using two fingers |

After determining the degree of flexion, continue to move your hands towards the pelvic inlet. They will soon come to a halt at the pubic bone. As your fingertips touch in the midline above the pubic bone your hands will enclose the presenting part. The head may then be readily ballottable. (This constitutes the fourth maneuver of Leopold.)

4. Determining the degree of descent into the maternal pelvis: The presenting part is then said to be **floating** when the entire presenting part is at or above the pelvic brim and can freely be balloted from side to side; the examiner's fingers will easily fit between the presenting part and the mother's symphysis pubis.

The baby is said to be **dipping** if the lowermost portion of the presenting part (*not* including the biparietal diameter in cephalic presentations) is below the pelvic inlet. The presenting part is still moveable to some extent, but the examiner's fingers *cannot* fit between the presenting part and the mother's pubic bone.

The presenting part is **fixed** when the plane of the widest diameter of the presenting part (the biparietal diameter in cephalic presentations) has dropped below the mother's pelvic inlet. You will be unable to feel any preeminence in cephalic presentations and your hands *diverge away from the fetal head and maternal midline as you move them down toward the pubic bone.* The presenting part is no longer mobile. Note that the term **fixed** is not the same as engaged: an engaged head will not move, but the presenting part can be immobile (or fixed) without being fully engaged. (Engagement will be further explained in Volume II.)

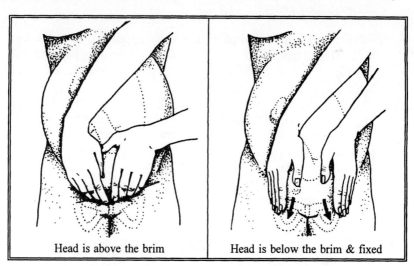

| Head is above the brim | Head is below the brim & fixed |

Things that may interfere with or enhance your ability to palpate:

A variety of things can make palpation either easier or more difficult. The more skilled you become, the quicker you will get at determining if one of these is a contributing factor. Regardless of your skill level, however, situations such as an anterior placenta or a retroverted uterus will continue to make palpation challenging. Keep trying! Factors affecting palpation include:

*Retroverted uterus—when the uterus is tipped backwards in the pelvis the fundus remains sloped backwards in the abdomen until the weight of the pregnancy suddenly brings it forward. The fundus and the fetal heart tones may be difficult if not impossible to locate in early pregnancy. A woman may appear to be earlier in pregnancy than her dates suggest until, all of a sudden between 14 and 16 weeks or so she "has a belly." Your palpation difficulties should largely disappear, after the uterus has come forward. Even though the body of the uterus has tipped forward, the fundus may remain sloped backwards and therefore difficult to identify for some weeks to come.

*A deep pelvis or a deep torso can "hide" the pregnancy, making palpation difficult. This is more true early in pregnancy, but sometimes occurs through until the end. Don't be afraid to reach deeply to feel for the baby and the uterus. A deep pelvis can cause the baby to appear small-for-dates when it is, in fact, growing adequately.

*Small babies are harder to palpate in early pregnancy and may be harder to feel throughout. Always question if there are twins when the woman is eating well, the only fetus you can feel is small, and the uterus is normal to large-for-dates.

*Lots of fluid can make palpation more difficult, especially if combined with other factors listed here. Keep palpating. Try to push the baby against the uterine wall with one hand while you feel with the other.

*Thin women are easier to palpate and the baby may seem to be larger than it actually is.

*Large (obese) women are much more difficult to palpate and the fetal heart tones may be harder to find as well. Press in deeply with your hands and fetascope. If you are unsure of anything, discuss the possibility of an ultrasound diagnosis, a second opinion from another midwife or an internal exam if the question regards the fetal presentation (i.e. is it a head or a butt?).

399

*Fetal position can cause the fetus to be hard to palpate. When the baby is "lying in a lump" have the mother assume a hands and knees position and do pelvic rocks for a few minutes in order to shift the baby around and get it to lift its head. Then have her lie down and recheck. If this does not work, have the mother talk to the baby about letting you know its position during the interval between visits.

*An anterior placenta can pose a problem in palpation and in hearing the fetal heart. Try the pelvic rock mentioned above and then palpate along the sides of the uterus when attempting to feel small parts or locate the fetal heart.

*The mother's torso length can influence how large or small the baby appears. A woman with a long torso can "hide her baby" and seem to have a small fundal height and small fetus, when in fact it only means the uterus is settled back inside her body and everything is perfectly normal. Likewise, the woman with a short torso can appear to have a huge baby and the fundal height can be big for dates, when in reality she just has no place else to put it!! This woman may carry her pregnancy far out in front.

*Toning contractions can obscure your ability to locate and hear the fetal heart as well as your ability to palpate. If the uterus is contracted, wait a few minutes for it to relax before you begin. If the uterus begins to contract during your exam, stop until the contraction is over. If you finish palpation and then note that the uterus looks softer and fetal parts can be seen moving more easily, the uterus was contracted during your exam; try rechecking your findings. The combination of firm muscle tone and toning contractions poses the biggest challenge in obtaining accurate information when you are working with first-time mothers.

References and further reading:

Loprenzi-Kassel, Clarabeth, midwife, Veneta, OR, editing, comments, February, 1995.
Maye's Textbook of Obstetrics, 1953.

Assessing Fetal Size

In addition to fundal height measurements and your visual estimation of the progress of pregnancy, you need to palpate for the size of the fetus. Unfortunately, learning to assess fetal size is quite an art and only an art, since the scientific method of comparing your estimate to some objective measure is impossible during prenatal care. However, you can carefully assess the size of newborns of various weights and then transfer this knowledge to babies that are still *in utero*. You should constantly be palpating women near term and then comparing your last estimated fetal weight to the actual size of the newborn. Is the baby bigger or smaller than you imagined? As you assess yourself for accuracy, be sure to take the many maternal variables into account (weight, height, depth of torso, etc.) as outlined at the end of the chapter on The Fine Art of Palpation and in the chapter on the Overall Assessment of Fetal Size and Growth.

*If you have access to a large number of babies (in a nursery, for example) assess their size visually and palpate them if possible, remembering to make it a pleasant experience for the baby.

*Observe and examine as many premature babies as you can find and compare their body proportions with that of term newborns.

*Finally, study the relative size of the fetus as it grows throughout pregnancy by looking at life-sized pictures in textbooks and handling models of fetuses at various stages of growth.

*Purchase dolls of various sizes which approximate different gestational ages (take measurements and a measuring tape to the toy store, remembering that head size is disproportionately large in earlier pregnancy).

*Palpate models or babies with your eyes closed (you can't see babies *in utero*.)

*Dress and undress babies if you have the opportunity. While doing so, be very conscious of how their little limbs move and flex most easily. This will give you valuable knowledge for use when helping with the birth of babies that are stuck due to shoulder dystocia or breech presentation.

Assessing the Volume of Amniotic Fluid

The amniotic fluid provides cushioning and hydration for the baby, and affords the fetus space to move about and grow normally. The normal volume near term ranges from 1 to 3 pints (550 to 1,650 ml). If the volume of amniotic fluid is abnormal, either by too much or too little, it can spell trouble for the developing fetus.

You should also assess amniotic fluid volume while palpating the uterus for fetal size and position. The volume of fluid will have an impact on your perception of the fetus within the uterus. In early pregnancy, the uterine wall normally feels firm but flexible, indicating that it is full of fluid but not excessively so. Early on, the baby can retreat from your fingers within the uterus because of its small size relative to the volume of amniotic fluid. As pregnancy advances, there is a distinct sense of the baby floating within a body of fluid. Gradually, fetal parts become easier to feel floating freely within the fluid. In first time mothers, the uterine wall remains firm but flexible to your touch; in multiparas the uterine wall becomes decidedly flexible and molds around the fetal contours during palpation. In late pregnancy, the baby fills the uterus, but can still be balloted at each pole. An internal exam reveals forewaters (a spongy, flexible area) behind the closed cervix.

Too much fluid: Polyhydramnios occurs when there is an abnormally large amount of amniotic fluid. The uterus feels tense to the touch, does not indent easily or at all, and the baby feels like it is floating freely within a balloon of fluid. Small parts and even the fetal poles may be hard or impossible to reach; the uterine wall does not give way to your attempts at palpation. Breech or transverse lie are more commonly found because the baby is not being held in position by the uterine walls. Fundal height is larger than it should be for dates and the abdomen takes on a distinctly globular appearance. The woman may report that her belly seems to be growing at a

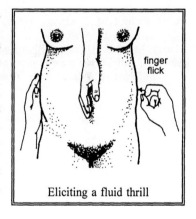

finger flick

Eliciting a fluid thrill

rapid rate and that she notices less fetal movement, a perception fostered by the excessive amount of fluid which prevents fetal movements from reaching the uterine walls. Polyhydramnios produces an abdominal girth in excess of 100 cm at term and may vary a little from visit to visit due to fluid volume fluctuations.

Fluid thrill: This assessment is primarily used to distinguish an abnormal amount of fluid. However, some midwives use it from late pregnancy onward as one way of assessing fluid volume in every woman. A fluid thrill may be elicited with the help of an assistant or the mother herself. The outer edge of someone's hand is pressed into the midline of the woman's belly over the navel point to prevent the transmission of the impulse around the abdominal wall. The examiner then flicks their finger on one side of the uterus while stabilizing the uterus on the other to feel the vibration of the flick. The presence of a distinct fluid vibration with this maneuver supports the suspicion that excessive fluid is present. When used in women who have a normal to low volume of fluid, the thrill will be more subtle. Be sure to check in several locations to detect pockets of fluid.

Too little fluid: Oligohydramnios occurs when there is less than 400 ml. of amniotic fluid. This causes the uterus to mold tightly around the fetal contours, as if the baby is "shrink wrapped" within the uterus. The abdominal wall, on the other hand, may take on a prune-like appearance due to the reduction of tension on stretch marks as the fluid volume drops (Acree, 1995). Fetal movements will be easy to feel and the mother may find them uncomfortable. The fundal height may be small-for-dates. Ballotment of fetal parts will be impossible or nearly so because there is little fluid to allow the small parts to float. There will be no sense that the baby is floating.

References and further reading:

Acree, Kathy, L.M., Louisiana, conversation re: oligohydramnios, Farm Conf, Summertown, TN, August, 20, 1995.

Garrey, M., et.al., Obstetrics Illustrated, Churchill Livingstone, London, Eng., 1980.

Sherman, Patty, "Premature Rupture of Membranes: The apple will drop when it is ripe . . .," Midwifery Today, No. 31, Autumn, 1994, p. 12.

Measuring the Fundal Height and Girth of the Uterus

Assessment of uterine growth in relationship to advancement of the pregnancy has been used for years as a means of determining if fetal growth and amniotic fluid volume are within normal limits. There are a variety of techniques which can be used. Most importantly, everyone you work with should settle on one technique and use it consistently. Midwifery partners should occasionally do duplicate checks at the same appointment as a quality control measure to see if you are getting the same figure. Always double check measurements done by an apprentice. This assessment is very subjective; therefore, consistent technique is an essential component of obtaining accurate results which can be duplicated from midwife to midwife in a clinical situation. The key to consistency in assessing the height of the uterine fundus (top) has to do with determining the location of both the fundus and the point on the pubic bone from which you start your measurement.

Finding the fundus: The fundus is usually below the level of the upper border of the pubic bone prior to twelve weeks of pregnancy, therefore it cannot be palpated directly via an abdominal exam. In most cases, the uterus reaches the level of the upper border of the pubic bone at approximately 12 weeks. A slight swelling can be felt if one presses into this area. By 13 weeks the uterus has risen just above the upper border of the pubic bone and continues to be palpably enlarged throughout the rest of pregnancy.

An exception to this rule is the uterus which is retroflexed or retroverted. Prior to pregnancy, the fundus is tipped back from the abdominal wall. When a woman with this uterine positioning becomes pregnant, the enlarged uterus remains deep within the pelvis until about 14 to 16 weeks, when it tips forward. The woman who previously had no belly suddenly looks quite pregnant. The true top of the fundus is very difficult, and often impossible, to find until the uterus becomes redirected. The retroverted uterus can appear deceptively small and the fetal heart tones more difficult to find before the weight of the pregnancy causes the uterus to tip forward.

As pregnancy advances, finding the fundus may be difficult for a variety of other reasons. Excess abdominal fat or the fetal position may cause the uterine contours to be difficult to discern. Sometimes the uterus pushes the transverse colon up and anterior to the fundus; it may appear to be the top of the uterus. Should this occur, it is possible to distinguish the transverse colon by its rather soft, puffy feel and appearance. There may also be a very slight depression where the lower border of the transverse colon meets the anterior slope of the fundus. Sometimes palpating the walls of the uterus is difficult because of bloating in the ascending or descending colon as well.

To minimize the chance that you will mistake the anterior slope of the fundus for its true top, use the following technique:

Facing the woman's head, place a hand on each side of the uterus at the level of the mother's navel. Ballot the uterus between your hands with gentle pressure to distinguish its contour. While doing so, rearrange your hands as necessary to be sure you are on either side of the body of the uterus. Now, staying to either side, move both hands upward to simultaneously palpate toward the fundus. As you near the top, your hands will begin to come together, and they will meet at the top of the fundus. If the transverse colon is in the way as you do this you will find yourself displacing it to follow the actual contour of the uterus. Staying on the lateral portion of the uterus assures that your hands will meet at the actual top of the uterus.

Another way of making sure you have found the fundus is to palpate for it during a toning contraction. Keep your hand on the fundus; wait for the contraction to subside, and then take the fundal measurement. This can be helpful when the upper fetal pole is not filling the fundus, the transverse colon is prominent, or the fundus is back within the mother's abdomen.

How to measure fundal height: There are four ways to measure fundal height, of which three are most relevant to midwifery practice. The first method is to use your fingers to determine the height of the fundus relative to other maternal landmarks which include the pubic bone, the navel and the xiphoid process. This table describes these relationships:

WEEKS OF PREGNANCY	LOCATION OF FUNDAL HEIGHT	
12	Level of symphysis pubis	
16	Halfway between symphysis pubis & navel	
20	1-2 fingerbreadths below navel	
24	1-2 fingerbreadths above navel	
28-30	3 fingerbreadths above navel	
32	3-4 fingerbreadths below xiphoid process	
36-38	1 fingerbreadth below xiphoid process	
40	2-3 fingerbreadths below xiphoid if baby drops	

Although this method is routinely taught in midwifery schools, it is fraught with problems. There is no standardization of fingerbreadths, nor is there any standardization of the size of women's bodies! In fact, women of different races can have remarkable differences in the location of physical landmarks. While the above chart can be taken as an "average," it cannot be depended upon as a reliable tool in all cases. (See the end of the chapter for other ways to assess fetal growth.)

Method 2: The second method employs a flexible dressmaker's measuring tape marked in centimeters. The end of the tape is placed at the highest bony prominence on the upper anterior border of the pubic bone and the tape is then stretched up the midline of the abdomen, following the curve of the abdomen, placing the tape directly on the skin up to the top of the uterine fundus. The outer edge of the hand is used to demarche the fundal height and a measurement is obtained. This method is said to be accurate after the twenty-second week of pregnancy, when the number of centimeters coincides with the weeks of pregnancy; however this correlation may be seen as early as 15 weeks of pregnancy in many Caucasian women. You may use the table above as a rough estimate of where your measurements should be falling at different weeks of pregnancy.

Method 3: The third method also uses a flexible tape measure. The measurement is started at the upper border of the pubic bone, as above. The hand maintaining the identification of the top of the fundus is placed at right angles to the fundus with the outer edge of the hand pressed against the fundus. The tape is then run through the index and middle fingers at the abdominal midline and the centimeter measurement is read at the point over the top of the fundus. The tape follows the uterine contour only as far as its apex and is then straight to the point where it is held by the fingers (i.e. the tape does not follow the contour of the upper slope of the fundus). With this method some mathematical calculations are necessary:

*Prior to the fundus reaching the level of the navel, add 4 cm. to the measurement. This should approximately equal the weeks of pregnancy.
*After the fundus has reached the level of the navel, add 6 cm. to the measurement. This should total the approximate weeks of pregnancy.

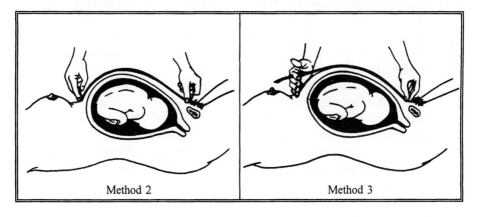

Method 2   Method 3

The most "medical" method involves the use of calipers, a pair of movable, rounded, curved metal chopsticks joined at the top by a measuring device. This awkward and rather intimidating, hard to read, difficult to transport and expensive contraption is probably not something you wish to use in your practice.

Regardless of the method you use, fundal height measurements always have a 2 cm. leeway on either side of the week of pregnancy in question. That is, if a woman is 34 weeks pregnant, her fundal height may fall between 32 and 36 cm. and still be considered within a normal range. If the fundal height is as much as 4 cm. off from what is expected for the gestational age either way, this should alert you to the possibility that the baby is either small or large for dates, or that the volume of amniotic fluid may be abnormal, or that there is a multiple gestation; all of which require further evaluation (see the next chapter).

Toning contractions and the fundal height: Toning contractions begin in early pregnancy and become more noticeable to you and the mother as pregnancy advances. They will become palpable during your examination as well. In fact exams often trigger the onset of contractions. When you are palpating a belly, be sure to keep this in mind. Do not measure the fundus during a contraction, as it will often be artificially altered (usually higher than it would otherwise be). If you realize after the fact that you have taken the fundal height during a contraction, just wait until it is over and recheck.

<u>**Measuring abdominal girth**</u>**:** The measurement of abdominal girth is an additional screening tool which is of limited value. It can only be used after the 34th week of pregnancy in women of average size. It is most useful, perhaps, when an oversized uterus is suspected. Polyhydramnios, multiple gestation or simply a large baby all increase the width as well as the height of the uterus. Polyhydramnios produces an abdominal girth in excess of 100 cm. before term and may vary a little from visit to visit due to fluid volume fluctuations. It is not useful, however, in evaluating fetal size per se.

To measure the abdominal girth, encircle the woman's belly with a tape measure at the level of her navel. The measurement is usually about 2 inches less than the week of pregnancy.

If the abdominal girth remains the same on three or more occasions after 34 weeks or if it decreases by 1 inch or more on two or more occasions, this suggests oligohydramnios, intrauterine growth retardation or fetal demise. A large finding may indicate the need for further evaluation, but should not be used alone. If the woman is quite overweight the results will not be accurate; this may be circumvented by obtaining a baseline measurement on a woman-of-size prior to the 34th week of pregnancy. Just as with fundal height measurements, abdominal girth may be inaccurate due to a woman's body build regardless of her weight.

Weeks of pregnancy	Abdominal girth
34	32 inches (81 cm.)
36	34 inches (86 cm.)
38	36 inches (91 cm.)
40	38 in. (96½ cm.)
Any week after 34	Any measurement greater than 39½ inches (100 cm.) is considered too large

<u>Sometimes fundal height just doesn't apply</u>: The pelvic shape can affect how the uterus is positioned in the mother's torso. There are many women (especially women-of-color) for whom fundal height measurements do not apply, since their pelvic shape is different. When fundal height measurements are just not adding up given the other information you have regarding a woman's due date and how big the baby feels, you must look at other parameters. The following table was inspired by a midwife who had spent time practicing on the Ivory Coast in Western Africa. She said the women's pelvises were so different that fundal height was useless and she had to learn to assess gestational age by the size of the baby's head.

The following table has been devised from a standard chart of biparietal diameters (BPD) used for ultrasound assessment of fetal size. The BPD and the fetal weights, although recognized as normal by mainstream obstetrics, are small compared to the size of term babies in mothers whose nutrition is optimal. Therefore each fetal weight and BPD relationship should be taken as the lower limit of normal for that week of gestation. If the baby seems smaller than this table indicates, the mother probably needs to eat more food!

408

BIPARIETAL DIAMETER (BPD)	EQUIVALENT OBJECT*	CORRESPONDING FETAL WEIGHT FOR BPD	MINIMUM GESTATION** AT GIVEN WT.
3.6 cm	ping pong ball (3.8 cm)	3 oz.	16-17 wks.
4.0 cm	ping pong ball	5 oz.	17-18 wks.
4.3 cm	large egg/US golf ball	7 oz.	18-19 wks.
4.6 cm	paddle ball (4.8 cm)	8 oz.	19-20 wks.
5.0 cm		10 oz.	20-21 wks.
5.3 cm	English billiard ball	13 oz.	21-22 wks.
5.6 cm	US billiard ball (5.7 cm)	15 oz.	22-23 wks.
5.9 cm		1 lb. 2 oz.	23-24 wks.
6.2 cm	tennis ball (6.35-6.67 cm)	1 lb. 5 oz.	24-25 wks.
6.5 cm	tennis ball/orange	1 lb. 9 oz.	25-26 wks.
6.7 cm	tennis ball/orange	1 lb. 12 oz.	26-27 wks.
7.0 cm	baseball	2 lbs.	27-28 wks.
7.2 cm		2 lbs. 4 oz.	28-29 wks.
7.5 cm		2 lbs. 9 oz.	29-30 wks.
7.7 cm		3 lbs.	30-31 wks.
8.0 cm		3 lbs. 11 oz.	31-32 wks.
8.2 cm	polo ball	3 lbs. 11 oz.	32-33 wks.
8.4 cm		4 lbs.	33-34 wks.
8.6 cm		4 lbs. 7 oz.	34-35 wks.
8.8 cm		4 lbs. 12 oz.	35-36 wks.
9.0 cm		5 lbs. 2 oz.	36-37 wks.
9.2 cm	croquet ball	5 lbs. 9 oz.	37-38 wks.
9.3 cm		6 lbs. 2 oz.	38-39 wks.
9.5 cm		6 lbs. 10 oz.	39-40 wks.
9.6 cm		7 lbs. 3 oz.	40-41 wks.
9.8 cm	nerf ball (10 cm)	up to 9 lb. 15 oz.	41-44 wks.

*Ball sizes given unless BPD and ball size are an exact match. Sizes of organic objects are approximate matches and are given as average size unless otherwise noted.

**Remember, gestational age is two weeks less than the weeks of pregnancy (when a woman is considered 12 weeks pregnant her fetus is actually 10 weeks gestation). Since ultrasound is used to assess the fetus, gestational age is the reference used when measuring the biparietal diameter (BPD) and is therefore the reference for the table above.

References and further reading

Garrey, M., et al., Obstetrics Illustrated, Churchill Livingstone, London, Eng., 1980.
Varney, Helen, Nurse-Midwifery, Blackwell Scientific Pub., Inc., Boston, MA, 1980.
Whitley, Nancy, A Manual of Clinical Obstetrics, J.B. Lippincott Co., 1985.

Overall Assessment of Fetal Size and Growth

All women are different and no one parameter is an absolute indication of fetal growth. Careful assessment of several variables is important, with fundal height being used only as a guide to the growth of an individual baby in relationship to all other factors. Always assess the following parameters simultaneously when evaluating fetal size and growth:

*The mother's presumed due date
*The weeks of pregnancy by the calendar
*The weeks of pregnancy by examination
*The fundal height & abdominal girth (if indicated)
*The size of the fetus, noting especially the head and trunk size and the relationship of these parts to each other
*The amount of amniotic fluid
*The mother's body shape, especially the depth of her pelvis, the length of her torso, her height and the thickness of the fatty layer between your hands and the uterus
*Uterine growth patterns from previous pregnancies (per prenatal chart), if applicable
*Maternal impressions of previous fetal growth patterns and size of this baby, if applicable
*Size of previous babies at birth, if applicable
*Rate of fundal growth from visit to visit
*Rate of fetal growth from visit to visit
*Maternal nutrition and stress levels

The presumed due date: Recheck whether the mother feels that the due date you and she previously agreed upon is accurate. If the due date is in question, careful physical exam will often demonstrate this, and the due date can be corrected based on findings from the examination. On the other hand, if the due date is certain, you must scrutinize other factors more closely.

The weeks of pregnancy by the calendar: This will be dependent upon the presumed due date. However, it is possible for a woman to have growth spurts and lags in her uterine and fetal size as the pregnancy progresses. Information regarding her pattern of growth in previous pregnancies can be helpful. Remember that a retroflexed or retroverted uterus is often less obvious in early pregnancy because the uterus is enlarging in its posteriorly tipped position, making the fundus appear quite small-for-dates. A bi-manual exam can often help clarify the situation by giving a more accurate assessment of uterine size.

The weeks of pregnancy by palpation: Even though the uterus may visually appear small or large-for-dates, palpation can reveal a pregnancy which is appropriately sized for dates. Although there can be variations in uterine size in very early pregnancy, the uterus more typically corresponds to a standard size for dates, at this time than later in pregnancy.

Weeks from LMP	Uterine size
6	lemon
7	large hen's egg
8	large orange
10	grapefruit
12	cantaloupe

The fundal height and abdominal girth: Although fundal height is a semi-accurate tool to use as a gauge to decide how a pregnancy is growing, it is important to take into account not only growth spurts or lags but fundal growth in relationship to the woman's pattern of growth in this and previous pregnancies. I have known women to have 8 lb. babies with funduses no bigger than 33 cm., in one case 29 cm.! It is important not to allow fundal height discrepancies to alarm you by themselves. If all other signs point to appropriate fetal growth, fundal height can usually be set aside; it is a good screening tool to alert you to possible problems but not the only deciding factor. Fundal height may be skewed by the following interfering factors:

A low fundal height for dates may be caused by:	A high fundal height for dates may be caused by:
Baby in transverse lie Baby in oblique lie Baby's upper pole leaning over to one side Baby well engaged in mother's pelvis Uterine retroversion in early pregnancy Minimal amniotic fluid Mother carries baby "deep inside" (deep maternal pelvis or torso or long torso) Tall woman Baby small-for-dates	Lots of amniotic fluid Baby carried high in the uterus Baby in a breech position Placenta previa Fibroids, especially in the fundus or obstructing the presenting part in the pelvis Very large baby Multiple gestation Mother carries pregnancy "all in front" Short mother, short torso or shallow pelvis

The size of the fetus: Your assessment of fetal size must be used alongside fundal height measurement to gauge how the baby is growing. Remember that fundal height is irrelevant if the baby appears to be growing well and the amount of amniotic fluid seems normal. The best way to assess fetal growth is by comparing the size of the head to the size of the trunk. The head grows much more rapidly than the rest of the body; it is one of the first things you can distinguish when palpating in early pregnancy. Proper head size and growth give a good indication that the fetus is normal. If the body seems smaller than it should be given the length of gestation, the mother probably needs to increase her dietary intake.

If both the head and body seem abnormally small, something could be wrong with the fetus. However, it is important to assess the overall fetal growth pattern.

This can only be judged through a series of comparative exams. You can certainly encourage a mom to eat more (to increase fetal growth) at the first prenatal where you note the baby is small, but you usually cannot determine that there is a problem until later when better eating does not produce a baby which has "caught up with itself" in terms of its growth pattern. If better nutrition doesn't quickly produce the desired growth spurt and a fetus appropriately sized for dates, a variety of tests can be done in an attempt to determine what the problems may be. Exploration will usually begin with a full examination of the fetus using imaging ultrasound, with other tests being recommended as necessary. If a woman is sure about her dates, a large fundus and a baby which seems small-for-dates could clue you in to a multiple pregnancy, even though you may only be able to palpate one baby or hear one fetal heart at the time.

A baby may appear to be large for dates if you have had a run of smaller babies and all of a sudden have a woman carrying a baby destined to weigh 10 pounds at birth. Popular obstetrical teaching is that the fetal size is fairly uniform early in pregnancy and then individualizes in late pregnancy, but this is by no means always the case. Babies can have tremendous growth spurts and the amniotic fluid can increase in fits and starts as well, only to even out with a plateau in growth later on.

The amount of amniotic fluid: The amount of fluid, if excessive, will make the fetus seem smaller; likewise a scant amount of fluid will often make the baby seem larger. Either can impact your sense of fetal size during palpation. In such cases, carefully find and assess the fetal head size to help distinguish a real problem from the illusion of one based on the volume of fluid.

If you suspect an abnormal amount of amniotic fluid is present, you will need to follow-up on that as well. See the chapter on Amniotic Fluid Abnormalities in the section on Problems That Can Occur at any Time.

The mother's body shape: The size of the mother will impact your perception of fetal growth. A woman with a long torso (the distance from the lower ribs to her iliac crest) has plenty of abdominal room and will carry her enlarged uterus well inside her torso. This woman looks "less pregnant," even near term. The baby can seem exceptionally small, even during palpation, because the uterus has plenty of room to be flexible and stretch as you examine it. Many a woman with a long torso (frequently tall women) has been hassled during a medically-managed pregnancy about her baby being too small, only to give birth to an 8 or 9 pound baby at term!

Likewise, the woman with a very short torso will carry her baby way out front, making her baby and often her fundal height, seem large-for-dates. Because a baby being carried out front will be more accessible to your examination than one deep within the maternal abdomen, the mere fact that you can feel more of the baby will support the illusion of largeness. Her belly may recede within her

412

abdomen somewhat when she lays down and it will then appear to be more appropriately sized for dates. A woman with a short torso carrying her baby high will often appear quite large for dates; once the baby drops into her pelvis, this illusion is altered. Again, check fetal head and body size independent of other factors to discern what is really going on.

The depth of the maternal pelvis will also affect your estimate of a baby's size. A woman with a large or deep pelvis in its anterior-posterior diameter hides an early pregnancy well and will often not have a palpable uterus until the 15th to 18th week of pregnancy, especially if the uterus is also retroverted. Even then, in many cases the anterior slope of the uterus may be just barely felt at the level of the pubic bone. Once uterine size reaches a critical point (which is individual to the woman) it will suddenly pop forward and a big belly will be evident where none was seen before. A deep pelvis combined with a long torso can make a baby practically unreachable until pregnancy is more advanced. If the baby is posterior on top of this combination, you may have trouble feeling much of anything!

A thick abdominal wall will generally dull your ability to palpate accurately and may delay fetal heart auscultation until late in the pregnancy. If you have doubts about the lie of the baby, get another practitioner to check your findings, do an internal exam to assess what is presenting, or get an ultrasound exam early enough to maximize your chances of getting a breech baby to turn.

As you gain experience you will be able to visually assess appropriate size-for-dates in various sized women when they are standing to a certain degree. However, it is always best to withhold comment until you have the woman lay down and feel her belly. Regardless of how big or small, high or low she appears to be carrying when standing, skilled palpation usually reveals a uterus and baby that is at least close to the size it should be for dates.

Mother's abdominal muscle tone: The mother's abdominal muscle tone can hold a pregnancy in tightly and prevent good access to the baby for palpation. This is a problem found almost exclusively in first-time mothers. The abdominal muscles are usually more cooperative, by the time more babies come along. If the mother's tone is very firm, do everything you can to help the mom relax her muscles before you begin to palpate. Prop her head and knees up with pillows, maybe put a small pillow under her lower back and encourage her to take long deep breaths to ease her muscles into relaxation as much as possible; remember to warm your hands!

It can be hard to tell when a woman who has very firm muscles is having a toning contraction. When you first touch her, be sure to lay your hands on her belly firmly but gently and note the uterine muscle tone. If you are unsure, wait a bit to see if the uterus becomes more relaxed.

Uterine growth patterns from previous pregnancies: This information can mean the difference between ordering lots of unnecessary tests to determine if a woman's baby is okay and feeling fine because you know she never got bigger than she is now and always had good-sized babies that were normal. While a recalled history of being hassled about being too small or too large is a good subjective indication that fundal height was probably off in previous pregnancies, a record showing the actual measurements obtained is more helpful. When there is serious doubt and the records are accessible, it makes sense to check what went on during previous pregnancies, keeping in mind the many methods of fundal height measurement.

Maternal impressions of fetal size: Women usually have a very good idea of the size of their baby, especially if they have given birth before. It is helpful to ask the mother how the baby is growing in comparison to her other pregnancies. One study comparing maternal (multipara) estimates of fetal size in late pregnancy with that of the midwife and ultrasound found the mother to be consistently the most accurate predictor and ultrasound to be least accurate. (ref. unknown)

The size of previous babies at birth: This too is revealing and can help you assess apparent problems which may or may not exist in the current pregnancy. A history of having birthed a good-sized baby after a pregnancy involving seemingly small- or large-for-dates growth is a good indication that you can relax about similar findings in this pregnancy. Remember that a history of exceptionally small babies may not necessarily be "normal" for a woman, because small babies are almost always associated with inadequate dietary intake. Likewise very large, edematous (macrosomic) babies may be associated with very poor, empty-calorie dietary choices as well as poorly controlled maternal diabetes.

Rate of fundal growth from visit to visit: Comparative measurements of fundal height can help determine if the fetus is experiencing growth lags and spurts, or is having an abnormal pattern of growth. Steady growth, even if it doesn't match the presumed weeks of pregnancy, is a good sign that a baby is growing, at least to a certain extent. Regular growth which matches an earlier or later due date, especially when dates are in question, may mean the due date is off and should be reevaluated. Keep in mind that fundal growth does not always reflect fetal growth; therefore palpate the baby's size as well and compare your findings.

Maternal nutrition and stress levels: Last but not least, you must always assess maternal dietary intake not only for its basic adequacy in terms of what the mother is eating but also for how much she is eating relative to her activity and stress levels. Always discuss this concept with the mother and err on the side of caution: encourage all women with suspected lags in fetal growth to eat more, focusing on protein and calories from healthy food choices, not to go overboard on exercise and to take steps to reduce undue stress. Have her bring in daily diet diaries until the situation has clearly reversed itself and she feels confident in the dietary and life style changes she needs to make.

Garrey, M., et al., Obstetrics Illustrated, Churchill Livingstone, London, Eng., 1980.

414

The Physical Examination of the Woman

NOTE: Please see the chapter on <u>Equipment to Have On Hand for Prenatals</u> for details regarding the equipment used during the exam that are not covered in this chapter.

The physical exam can be quite thorough, reviewing every organ system and function of the body. However, in midwifery practice, the exam we commonly use is a screening tool. Since we are working primarily with healthy women who have no major medical problems, a detailed exam of every organ system is not usually warranted. Our goal is to catch any obvious abnormalities which may be overlooked by the woman and any changes which may pose a problem during pregnancy. When a suspicious finding turns up, we should discuss the possible implications with the woman and help her find a means of further evaluating the situation so that you may both know how to respond to the new information. Make it clear when you have reached your limits regarding diagnostic skills and knowledge of particular or suspect conditions. With these thoughts in mind, we shall first look over an outline of the general physical exam to be performed at the initial visit:

The Integrated Physical Exam

Observe appearance: gait, general appearance, mental status
Check height, body frame and weight
Assess vital signs: pulse, blood pressure, respirations, temperature (if indicated)
Observe head & palpate lymph nodes of the arms, face and neck
Examine the head: skull, facial features, mouth, eyes and ears
Palpate the thyroid
Check for varicosities of the legs
Assess for edema
Assess reflexes
Examine the torso and listen to the lungs
Examine the back and check for CVA tenderness
Listen to the heart
Perform a breast exam
Perform an abdominal exam: check for rectus diastasis, palpate liver and spleen
Check the lymph nodes in the groin
Perform a pelvic exam

The physical examination can be performed after you complete the history-taking portion of the first prenatal visit. Or, if there is not enough time to proceed with an unhurried exam, you can postpone it until the following visit, unless the presence of problematic symptoms requires an immediate investigation.

Environment and equipment: The light in the room should be diffuse, bright and overhead if possible. Good daylight is a fine choice for lighting as well. Good lighting is important because poor lighting may cause you to miss skin lesions and subtle color differences during your exam which may be significant. The room should be warm and private. Make sure all necessary equipment is on hand and properly prepared for the exam. Depending upon how thorough an exam you plan to do, you may need to gather some or all of the following supplies and equipment:

Stethoscope	Water-based lubricant
Fetascope	Sterilized speculum
Adult scale	Reflex hammer
Watch with a second hand	Flexible tape measure
Thermometer	Hand mirror
Blood pressure cuff and nurse's scope	Mobile light source (flashlight or goose
Penlight	neck light)
Otoscope/ophthalmoscope	Culture tubes
Well-fitting exam gloves	Slides for wet mount preparation
Towel or underpad to put beneath	PAP smear kit & fixative
woman's bottom during pelvic exam	Facial or toilet tissue
Small pillows for propping knees, etc.	

Check to be sure the binaurals of your fetascope and stethoscope are correctly positioned; when holding them in front of your face, they should be pointed away from you slightly. This lines them up with your ear canals. Try them on and fine tune this adjustment by tapping on the head until you have good sound conduction. Look over your other equipment to be sure it is in working order as well. In most circumstances, another party, such as an apprentice or her partner, will be present during the exam. However, if you and the woman find yourselves alone, you might want to ask her if she would like another person present during the exam, if so, this should be arranged; postpone the exam if necessary.

Working with the woman during her exam: Have the woman make herself comfortable by emptying her bladder before you begin. Explain what you are doing and why and that you are checking to discover what is normal for her and to make sure everything seems normal. At each point, assist the woman to assume the appropriate position to facilitate the exam and talk her through relaxing her body as appropriate. This will minimize her discomfort and facilitate obtaining accurate information. While medical model care would have the woman disrobe and don a hospital gown for the exam or use drapes, I have always had the woman remove portions of clothing throughout the exam as I move from area to area on her body. The disadvantage of this is perhaps a less flowing exam, but it gives the woman a better sense of control rather than being completely exposed save for a flimsy little gown. If you do not ask her to disrobe and don a gown, be sure she removes enough clothing so that you can do an adequate exam of each area. Most of the exam can be performed with the woman either sitting or lying down.

Remember that many women have been emotionally or physically traumatized and sometimes they do not remember it. If a woman seems tense, fearful, anxious or hypersensitive during any part of the exam stop and ask her what is coming up for her, what she is feeling and what you can do to make her more comfortable. If she asks you to stop, you will of course respect this and stop at once. No exam is worth damaging a woman's trust in you as her care provider. The exam can be postponed until you can find out what is going on for her and how you can help make her comfortable with continuing the exam, if indeed that part of the exam seems absolutely necessary, at a later time.

As you move through the exam try to do so in a orderly fashion so that, for example, when you examine the back, you listen to the lungs, look at the spine and percuss for kidney tenderness all at once. This avoids having a woman repeatedly removing items of clothing or assuming the same position during the exam.

Now we shall discuss how to perform each portion of the exam. Remember this is not an exhaustive explanation of every possible nuance of a complete and thorough physical exam, which requires a textbook in itself. It is an explanation of normal findings and common problems in a general exam offering a basic review of all the body's systems and emphasizes in more detail those points which are most relevant to pregnancy and gynecological care. If you need further information or wish to perform a more detailed and complete exam, you may refer to the excellent text <u>A Guide to Physical Examination and History Taking</u> by Barbara Bates, which is a good book to have on hand for reference.

Initial observations:

Posture and gait: Observe the woman as she walks into the room. Is her body symmetrical? Are there obvious bony deformities? If so, you need to question her as to their origin and prior treatment. These are especially important if deformities or injuries have involved the pelvis. For example, a limp suggests an obliquely contracted pelvis. If the limp has been present since early childhood, a pelvic deformity on the same side as the *un*affected leg is likely; when the child begins to stand and walk, her body weight is transmitted to her unaffected leg, resulting in an oblique pelvic tilt, higher on the normal side. (Whitley, 1985) A minor difference in the length of the legs does not necessarily denote a serious problem and can often be corrected with chiropractic adjustments.

General appearance: This refers to matters of self-care, personal hygiene and cleanliness. Does she seem to care about her appearance? How are her children dressed and how is their hygiene? This information can tell you a lot about what kind of self-caretaking you can expect, as in the case of early rupture of membranes. While poor hygiene and grooming may occur with the onset of depression, schizophrenia and organic brain syndromes, often it is a product of upbringing. If you do not suspect a physical disorder, take every opportunity to assist her in becoming more aware of her personal hygiene in a supportive rather than a condemning fashion, emphasizing its importance in the context of the pregnancy. Be alert for bruises, physical signs of drug abuse (needle tracks, scars, the smell of alcohol on her breath) or other evidence of substance abuse problems or physical abuse.

Mental status: The mental status refers to the level of consciousness or alertness, attention span, memory, orientation to time and space and coherent thought processes. Deviations from what we consider normal may be due to drug or alcohol use, neurological injury or permanent damage, or circulatory problems such as stroke (uncommon in women of childbearing age). If a woman's mental status seems abnormal, look to reasons in any of these categories, with substance abuse being the first thing to rule out. Keep in mind that a physiologically normal woman may experience varying degrees of disassociation during medical exams (see Physical and Sexual Abuse in the Well-Being section for more details).

Assessing maternal height, body frame size and weight:

Height: Most women know how tall they are and if she does, simply note this on her chart. If she does not, you can take her height yourself. It is handy to have a scale which has a height-measuring gauge attached. Full height balance beam scales often have this feature. However, maternal height can be determined with a steel measuring tape just as easily. Either way, have the mother stand up as straight as possible in her stocking feet on the scale platform. If you are not using a scale with a gauge attached, have her stand with her back next to the wall. Use a flat, straight object such as a ruler or the gauge on the scale. Place it flat and level with the highest point on her skull so that it makes a 90° angle to the wall (or the upright part of the gauge). Now note the height (on a gauge this will often be where the extension rod joins the lower part of the vertical height rod). If you are using a ruler, mark or hold a finger to the wall and have the woman move aside, then measure her height with a tape measure.

Determining body frame size: Body frame is determined by elbow breadth; the distance between the medial and lateral epicondyles of the elbow with the forearm flexed at 90° and held in front of the body. This measurement can be taken from the posterior side of the elbow and is the distance between the most prominent bony projection on one side of the elbow to the most prominent bony projection on the other. (Bend one of your arms at a 90° angle, then grasp your elbow with the opposite hand by placing your hand, palm down, in the bend of your arm. Now reach with your thumb on one side and your ring finger on the other to find the bones which are the most prominent on either side; use these landmarks.

MEDIUM BODY FRAME BY HEIGHT AND ELBOW BREADTH	
HEIGHT WITHOUT SHOES	ELBOW BREADTH
4'-9" - 5' 2"	2 1/4" to 2 1/2"
5'3" - 5'10"	2 3/8" to 2 5/8"
5'11"	2 1/2" to 2 3/4"

Elbow breadths that are larger or smaller than the ranges given above indicate large and small frames respectively.

Determining weight: The above measurement will now help you correlate a woman's frame size to her height and current weight. An adult floor scale should be placed on a flat, level, uncarpeted surface and the needle should point to zero (if it doesn't, check the back of the scale or the instructions to find out how to calibrate it to zero). If

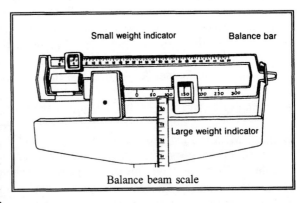

Balance beam scale

the woman is to weigh herself, the light should be sufficient so that she can see to the floor if it is a floor scale. The space behind the scale should also be such that she can pull the scale out from the wall to give herself enough room to bend over to see the dial if a floor scale is being used.

When weighing someone have them remove heavy clothing and shoes and step onto the center of the scale, balancing their weight evenly between their feet. If it is a dial scale, she should stand still while you read it or she should bend over gently until she can see the dial, remain still until the dial stabilizes and then read the weight. A balance beam scale is easier to read. Have the woman stand still to allow the needle to stabilize between each adjustment until it is perfectly poised on center. A balance beam (upright) scale is used as follows:

*First, push all the weights to the zero (far left) side of the balance bar. If the scale is calibrated correctly the needle to the far right will now be freely poised on center.
*The lower bar (large indicator) is marked in increments of 50 pounds and the upper bar (small indicator) is marked in increments of single pounds; the long lines between even numbers indicate odd-

numbered pounds and small lines indicate quarter pounds.
*Have the woman step on the scale. The balance bar will rise to the top of the bar.
*Move the large indicator to the closest estimated weight below what you actually think it will be (for example, if the woman's weight is at least 100 pounds but not more than 150, move the large indicator to the 100 pound mark by placing the point in the center in the 100 pound notch).
*Now gently nudge the small indicator along the bar toward the right until the needle on the far right is freely suspended in the center of the bar once again. Add these two figures together to arrive at the woman's weight.

Values are given for pounds in the table which follows. If your practice uses kilograms, the conversion formula is as follows:

*1 kilogram equals 2.2 pounds: to convert pounds to kilograms, divide the number of pounds by 2.2 (Example: 154 lb. ÷ 2.2 = 70 kg)
*To convert kilograms to pounds, multiply the number of kilograms by 2.2 (Example: 70 kg X 2.2 = 154 pounds)

HEIGHT AND WEIGHT CHART FOR WOMEN AGE 25-59			
HEIGHT WITHOUT SHOES	SMALL FRAME	MEDIUM FRAME	LARGE FRAME
4' 10"	102-111	109-121	118-131
4' 11"	103-113	111-123	120-134
5' 0"	104-115	113-126	122-137
5' 1"	106-118	115-129	125-140
5' 2"	108-121	118-132	128-143
5' 3"	111-124	121-135	131-147
5' 4"	114-127	124-138	134-151
5' 5"	117-130	127-141	137-155
5' 6"	120-133	130-144	140-159
5' 7"	123-136	133-147	143-163
5' 8"	126-139	136-150	146-167
5' 9"	129-142	139-153	149-170
5' 10"	132-145	142-156	152-173
5' 11"	135-148	145-159	155-176
6'	138-151	148-162	158-179

Since a woman's dietary intake is of paramount importance in the clinical assessment of weight fluctuations throughout pregnancy, that issue will be discussed in a separate chapter on Nutrition, Healthy Babies and Maternal Weight Gain in the Well-being section. If a woman has a history of eating disorders or is concerned about gaining weight, it can be most upsetting for her to be weighed on a regular basis. You can offer to note her weight yourself, so that she doesn't have to be confronted with this issue at every visit. (Kolder, 1995)

Assessing the vital signs:

Taking the radial pulse: The pulse may be felt in any artery that lies near the surface of the body over a bone or other firm tissue. For purposes of this exam, the pulse is generally palpated on the inner wrist. With the woman's palm facing upward, feel for a pulse between the tendons and the bone on the side near the thumb, using your index and ring fingers (about 1 to 1½ inches below the thumb joint). Count the pulse for at least 30 seconds. If you note any irregularities, continue to count for a full minute. In any case, always record the pulse for a per minute rate i.e. multiply your 30 second count by 2).

The pulse rate is the same as the heart rate and averages between 60 to 90 beats per minute in the resting state, although it typically rises 10 to 15 points above a woman's personal normal during pregnancy. Intervals between beats should be equal in length. The rate and rhythm of the pulse should feel flowing and regular. If a pulse is missed at intervals, it is said to be irregular, which may point to flow problems in the heart. An irregular rhythm that speeds up on inspiration and slows on expiration can be normal if, when they hold their breath, it disappears. Premature beats may occur occasionally in the normal person but frequent occurrences may be due to heart problems.

The force of the pulse is called the amplitude; each pulse beat should be of equal strength. Irregularities in strength may indicate a lack of muscle tone in the heart or arteries, but are often found in women who have no overt symptoms and do fine in pregnancy. Bounding pulses may be caused by anxiety or exercise as well as heart blockage or other problems, such as anemia and liver failure. A weak or thready pulse is caused by hemorrhage or shock and is noted by fast shallow beats which run into each other so much that you can't count them. The force of the pulse may normally be somewhat diminished on inhalation, but if this is pronounced it could also indicate heart problems. The artery should feel springy. If it does not there may be arteriosclerosis (hardening of the arteries) and accompanying hypertension.

Checking the blood pressure: Blood pressure is the force exerted against the arterial walls when the heart pumps. The beating of the heart has two parts:

    *Contracting—when the heart pumps blood through the arteries to the parts of the body, this is the systolic pressure (top number).
    *Refilling—when the heart relaxes and fills with blood before the next contraction, this is the diastolic pressure (bottom number).

The blood pressure reading is a reflection of how hard the heart must work to adequately circulate the blood. Pathological elevations may represent underlying disease processes or precipitate cerebral hemorrhage, cardiac arrest, headaches, visual problems, etc. In addition, high blood pressure in pregnancy is associated with abruptio placenta, toxemia, and convulsions. But, it cannot be assumed that high blood pressure which appears during pregnancy is always a problem.

The normal, healthy person's blood pressure changes constantly with activity, rest, and anxiety levels. For instance, laughing or talking can elevate the diastolic pressure as much as ten points. In pregnancy, there is generally a drop in blood pressure in the second trimester followed by a rise in the third. This fluctuation is related to normal blood volume expansion and is entirely physiological. In a well nourished woman, the blood pressure may vary a great deal and not reflect any increased risk to mother or baby.

Remember that using the correct cuff size is essential for an accurate reading. The width of the cuff should be half the circumference of the mid-upper arm. If, when in place, the air bladder edges overlap the cuff, it is too large. If the bladder does not fully encircle the arm, then it is too small. Arm size ranges for different width cuffs are: Child 7.24"–10.51" Adult 10"–15.98" Large adult 13.5"–20"

Proper positioning and other considerations: It is best to avoid coffee and smoking at least 30 minutes prior to taking a reading. Have the woman rest quietly at least 5 minutes before you start. Note that tight clothing above the cuff or crossed legs may falsely elevate the reading. The blood pressure should be taken with the person sitting quietly with their back supported and their arm supported at heart level, palm up. If the arm is hanging to the side, the reading could be artificially elevated as much as 8 mmHg. If no resting surface is available, position yourself so that you can support their arm with your arm or leg. Both feet should rest comfortably on the floor. If the woman is lying supine, it is best to place her on her side (left is best) so you do not encourage supine hypotension (the artificial lowering of blood pressure from the uterus pressing into the large vessels in her back). Her arm should rest flat, parallel with her body. Note on the chart how the woman is positioned (this will only be necessary if she is positioned differently than is usual for your practice.)

Position yourself so that you are viewing the dial head-on at eye level, not from above or below.

The sounds you will hear: "Korotkoff's sounds" are what you hear as you take a blood pressure. These sounds are produced by the vibration of the arterial walls produced by blood flow. They are categorized in the following phases:

Phase I: The first clear tapping sound you will hear. This is the systolic reading and lasts about 10 to 15 mmHg.
Phase II: Tapping and murmuring sounds, lasting 10 to 15 mmHg.

Phase III the tapping sounds become sharper and louder.

Phase IV This begins when the sounds first become muffled, The last distinct sound you hear is the diastolic reading in children.

Phase V when Phase IV finishes this is the last sound you hear. This reading represents the diastolic pressure in adults most of the time.

Variations in this sequencing can occur. If the woman is hypertensive, the first few tapping sounds of Phase I may be followed by a period of silence which resumes in Phase III. This is known as an auscultatory gap. A high arterial flow rate may prolong phase IV, which is often seen in children or pregnant women due to the increased cardiac workload. In nonpregnant adults it may indicate a heart or metabolic condition.

If the normal blood pressure is not known and you have little experience with taking readings, the blood pressure can be estimated first as follows:

1. Roll up the sleeve or remove constrictive clothing.
2. Select the proper sized cuff as described above.
3. Squeeze the air out of the air bladder completely.
4. Wrap the cuff smoothly and securely around the arm, level with the heart.
5. Locate the wrist (radial) pulse.
6. Inflate the bladder quickly by closing off the valve and pumping up the bulb. Do so until the wrist pulse disappears and note the number on the gauge at that point—this is your estimate of systolic pressure. This lets you know how high to pump the cuff for the actual reading, because too much constriction can falsely raise the reading.
7. Release air from the bladder quickly, remove the cuff, and wait a few minutes.
8. Repeat this procedure on the other arm.
9. Wait a few minutes before actually checking the blood pressure on the arm with the higher estimated result.

Here are the steps to taking the blood pressure reading: Especially if there is a question about blood pressure readings, take the blood pressure on both arms at the first visit. After that, use the arm which demonstrated the higher reading (usually the right, which is the side opposite the heart).

1. Roll up the sleeve or remove constrictive clothing on the right arm.
2. Locate the pulse point which is just above the bend of the elbow toward the inner, central side between the muscle and bone. You may have to apply pressure to feel it.
3. Place the cuff on the arm smoothly and securely with the center of the air bladder over the pulse point and the bottom of the cuff one inch above the elbow. The cuff should be level with the heart. (To find the center of the air bladder, fold it in half.)

4. Place the diaphragm (flat side) of a stethoscope over the pulse point at the bend in her forearm. (Be sure the head is adjusted so that the sensitive side is against the arm.) Take care that binaural and other tubes are not touching, as this will cause distracting noises. Place binaurals in your ears.
5. Inflate the bladder quickly to 30 mmHg. above the approximate systolic reading (as derived from your estimate), or up to 200 mmHg, which ever is less.
6. Let the air out slowly, at a rate of 2 to 4 mmHg. per pulse.
7. As you do so, you will begin to hear pulsing sounds in the stethoscope. At the first sound, note the number on the gauge. This is your systolic pressure.
8. You will continue to hear pulsing sounds as the needle falls. The last distinct pulse sound you hear is the phase IV diastolic pressure (note number on the dial). Sometimes, this sound will disappear and then return. If it is unclear when the last sound is, note the last distinct sound as well as the very last sound (Phase V) and write it like this: 110/70/50. The Phase V reading is usually the most significant. However, is some pregnant women, you can hear Phase V sounds all the way down to zero. In these cases, take more note of the Phase IV figure.

If you must recheck the blood pressure again quickly, be sure to release the cuff completely, empty the bladder, and wait a minute or so before you proceed. Rechecking immediately without taking these steps may artificially raise the reading. During that time have the woman raise her arm above her head and make a fist, then have her open and close her hand several times to stimulate circulation. (section based on Cooper, 1992; Hill, 1991; Rudy, 1986) The meaning of blood pressure readings will be covered in the section on common problems in pregnancy.

Special considerations for women-of-size: Obesity is often associated with high readings due to an inaccurately sized cuff. This is especially true in those whose arm circumference exceeds 35 cm. If you need a large cuff and do not have one available, take the blood pressure in the forearm. To do so, center the bladder over the radial artery (below the bend of the elbow) and wrap the cuff as you normally would. Position the stethoscope above the radial artery (about 1 inch above the wrist) and then proceed as you normally would. The resulting systolic measurement will be about 7 mmHg. lower than the upper arm and the diastolic will be 14 mmHg. higher than in the upper arm. So add 7 mm to the top number and subtract 14 mm from the bottom to obtain a fairly accurate equivalent to an upper arm reading. Be sure to chart how you took the blood pressure. (Hill, 1991)

<u>Respirations</u>: Normal breathing is quiet and easy, from the diaphragm and barely audible near the open mouth as a faint whoosh. Normal breath sounds have no definite pitch. Note the rate, rhythm, depth and effort involved in breathing. To minimize the possibility of the woman feeling self conscious and altering her breathing, count respirations while the woman is quiet and does not feel observed,

such as when you are taking her pulse. Count the pulse for 15 seconds, then pretend to count it for an additional 15 to 30 seconds but instead count her respirations and multiply your result to get a per minute equivalent. The normal adult respiratory rate is 14 to 20 breaths a minute. The amount of air taken in with each breath should be consistent, and the chest should move symmetrically with expansion. A occasional sigh is normal.

Women frequently report shortness of breath with mild exertion during pregnancy. If there are no other symptoms and this symptom is absent outside of pregnancy, this is usually a benign finding and is due to the extra work being required of the heart from the increased blood volume of pregnancy. Labored breathing using the chest muscles between the ribs (intercostals) and the neck muscles means the person isn't getting enough oxygen and may be due to a heart or lung problem. Noisy breathing indicates some kind of obstruction.

Temperature: Measurement of body temperature may be omitted if there are no signs of problems. Instead you may ask the woman if she knows her normal temperature and make note of that. If she does not, assessing the temperature can give you a normal baseline from which to monitor possible problems later on. The temperature may be measured via the oral, rectal or axillary methods. Most of the time, the temperature is taken orally in adults.

In the United States the fahrenheit temperature scale is generally used, and in Canada and Europe, the celsius scale is used. The fahrenheit thermometer has a scale of degrees divided into tenths, with marks on the thermometer for every two tenths of a degree, with every other degree being numbered.

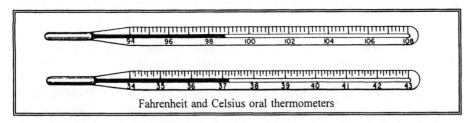
Fahrenheit and Celsius oral thermometers

Depending upon where you take a temperature, you will assess the finding using different ranges of normal as follows:

LOCATION OF READING	FAHRENHEIT		CELSIUS
	AVERAGE	RANGE	RANGE
Oral	98.6°	97.6° to 99.6° F	36.5° to 73.5° C
Rectal	99.6°	98.6° to 100.6° F	36° to 38° C
Axillary (armpit)	97.6°	96.6° to 98.6° F	35° to 37° C

To check the temperature orally: Since eating, drinking smoking, hot or cold baths or exercising can temporarily alter the temperature, wait at least 10 to 15 minutes after any of these activities before assessing the temperature.

1. Hold the thermometer securely in the hand with the red or silver end pointing down. Shake it using a fast, snapping motion until the mercury column reads 96° F (35.6°C) or below. This can be done after each reading.
3. Place the thermometer, colored tip first, against the back of the underside of the tongue and wait 2 to 4 minutes.
4. Read the thermometer by removing it from the mouth and turning it slowly in good light until the column of mercury becomes visible. If it is between two marks on the glass, assess it as the higher reading. Reinsert the thermometer for another minute and read it again. If the temperature is continuing to rise, repeat the reading until it stabilizes.
5. Note the time, date, temperature reading and method (in this case oral).

To check the temperature rectally: Have the person lie on their side or stomach and lubricate the thermometer tip with oil or water based lubricant. Insert the colored thermometer tip about 2 to 4 cm. (1½ inches) into the anal passage, pointing the tip toward the person's navel as you do so. Leave it there 3 to 4 minutes, remove it and read it.

To check the axillary temperature: First, dry the thermometer and the armpit. Then place the colored thermometer tip into deepest center of the armpit, have the woman grasp the opposite shoulder (or hold her arm in position yourself), wait 5 minutes, remove it and read.

Reading the thermometer: A glass thermometer is read as follows:

*Starting with 94°F (34°C) each long line indicates a 1 degree elevation in temperature.
*Only every other degree is marked with a number.
*Between each long line are four shorter lines.
*Each short line equals two-tenths (2/10 or 0.2) of 1 degree.

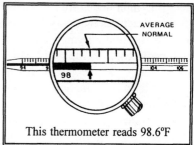

This thermometer reads 98.6°F

*98.6°F (36°C) is marked with an arrow below the gauge.

    Mercury (the solid color line in the thermometer) rises from the bulb of the thermometer within the hollow center of the stem as heat is registered. To read:

*Hold the thermometer horizontal at eye level with the degree markings facing you.
*Turn (rotate) it slightly until the solid column of mercury is visible.
*Look along the edge between the numbers and lines.
*Take the reading at the point where the mercury ends.
*If the mercury stops between two lines, read it to the closest line.

While body temperature is fairly constant, daily variation ranging from 1 to 3°F is normal. The average oral temperature fluctuates throughout the day and must be interpreted accordingly. In the early morning it is at a low point (sometimes as low as 96.4° F or [35.8° C]). In the late afternoon or evening it may be as high as 99.1° F (37.3° C). Rectal temperatures average 0.7° to 0.9° F (0.4° to 0.5° C) higher than oral readings, but this can vary considerably. A rapid respiratory rate tends to increase this discrepancy, therefore rectal temperatures are more reliable in these cases. Basal body temperature refers to when the body is completely at rest and is usually taken in the morning upon awakening but before arising. During pregnancy, basal temperature rises about .5°F. making the normal range 97.9 to 99.2°F (36.65 to 37.05°C) until mid-pregnancy, when it returns to nonpregnant normals (97.4 to 98.2°F/36.15 to 36.55°C).

Hyperpyrexia refers to extreme elevations of body temperature above 106° F (41.1° C). Fever or pyrexia refers to temperature elevated above normal and hypothermia refers to an abnormally low temperature below 95° F (35° C).

Palpate the lymph nodes of the face and neck: Lymph nodes are round, oval or bean shaped structures that vary in size according to their location. Lymph nodes in the face and neck tend to be very small. Only superficially located lymph nodes are accessible to examination. Using the same basic techniques, you can examine the lymph nodes of the face, neck, arm and groin (arms and groin will be included later,

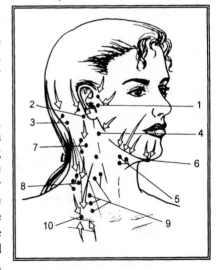

when you are examining those areas). Use the pads of your index and middle fingers to palpate the lymph nodes. Have the woman relax with her neck flexed slightly forward and, if necessary, slightly toward the side for the examination. You can usually examine both sides at once, however it helps to feel the node under the chin with one hand while bracing the top of the head with the other. Firmly apply your fingerpads to the tissue, moving the skin over the underlying tissues in each area (numbers correspond to lymph node locations in the drawing.)

LOCATION	AREA DRAINED BY NODES
1. Preauricular—in front of the ears	Side of face from corner of the eye & the temple
2. Postauricular—behind ears superficial to the mastoid process (jaw bone)	The superficial tissue above & behind the ear
3. Occipital—at the base of the skull	Superficial tissue above the occiput
4. Tonsillar—at the angles of the jaws	Portions of the mouth & throat as well as the more superficial facial tissues
5. Submaxillary—midway between the angles of the jaw & the tip of the chin	
6. Submental—in the midline beneath the chin	
7. Superficial cervical—near the posterior edges of the sternocleidomastoid muscles	Below the ear and the upper neck
8. Posterior cervical—along anterior edges of trapezius muscles	The middle of the neck
9. Deep cervical—around & behind sterno-cleidomastoid muscles (hook fingers around muscle: they may be inaccessible)	The middle of the neck
10. Supraclavicular—deep in angle formed by clavicle & sternomastoid muscle	Enlargement (esp. left) suggests malignancy from a thoracic or abdominal growth

This table describes normal and abnormal findings in any superficial nodes:

FINDING	NORMAL	ABNORMAL FINDINGS & COMMENTS
Size	Nonpalpable or small (5 mm.)	Enlarged from present or past infection, including tuberculosis, syphilis, HIV or cancer. Look for a source of infection in areas drained by the node(s)
Delimitation	Separate (discrete), roll back & forth & side to side	Matted together (neither arteries nor muscles will roll freely, either may be mistaken for a node; a pulsing "tonsillar" node is really the carotid artery)
Mobility	Mobile beneath skin	Fixed (suggests malignancy)
Consistency	Semi-soft	Hard (suggests malignancy)
Sensitivity	Non-tender	Tender (suggests infection)

Examine the head and mouth: Observe the woman for symmetrical facial features and skull structure. Slight asymmetry is normal, but if marked, it could indicate neurological or muscular problems or congenital defects such as hydrocephaly (enlarged skull), microcephaly (small skull), or an injury of some kind. During your exam note the woman's facial features and emotional responses for normalcy. Ask the woman about any moles or other skin lesions which may have appeared or undergone changes during the pregnancy so far. (See separate chapter on Skin and Hair Changes in the section on Problems That Can Occur at

Any Time if you find anything unusual.)

Inspect her mouth by observing the lips for excessive dryness (advise more fluid intake). Look for sores (syphilis?, herpes?, vitamin deficiencies?). Ask the woman to open her mouth and look for the following:

FINDING	NORMAL FINDING	ABNORMAL FINDING
Color of mucous membranes & hard palate	Pink in white women/patchy pink & dark pigmentation in women-of-color	Reddened & inflamed (infection?)
Moisture	Moist	Dry (dehydration?), excessive salivation (associated with excessive vomiting of pregnancy)
Surface	Smooth, glistening and uniform	Cuts, sores, tumors, white spots, small yellow bumps (benign)
Gum color	Smooth mucosal surfaces, sharp margins around teeth with shallow crevices between gums & teeth	Swelling, retraction of gums from teeth, bleeding (most often due to inadequate flossing & vitamin C def.)
Teeth	32 in the adult, including 4 wisdom teeth	Ask about pain, decay, removal of teeth, bridges, dentures, etc.
Tooth color	Creamy white to pale yellow	Chalky white then brownish to grayish color indicates decay, stains indicate food or tobacco intake
Tooth shape & position	Straight and evenly spaced	Crooked, broken teeth, notched & narrow-edged permanent incisors (Hutchinson's teeth) indicate congenital syphilis
Tongue color	Pink or transiently stained by recent food intake (such as blueberries)	Beefy red—inflammation Yellowish—heavy smoking
Tongue surface	Top—moist and roughened Underside—moist and smooth	Dry, smooth or fissured top (suggests def. of B vitamins, niacin or iron) tumors or ulcers. Varicose veins on the underside are benign

Examine the eyes: Observe the eyes for normal appearance. Protruding eyeballs are found in hyperthyroidism, retracted eyeballs are also abnormal. The cornea should appear smooth and clear. To examine the conjunctiva, place your thumbs under the woman's eyes and move the skin downward towards the cheekbones to observe the inner aspects of the lower lids which should appear thick, opaque, pink and highly vascular. Paleness indicates anemia while redness and purulent discharge indicates an infection.

The pupils should be observed for symmetrical dilation. To do so, have the woman look straight ahead. Move a penlight beam into her field of vision from the side. Normally both pupils react equally. The pupils may be fixed and dilated in acute glaucoma, head injury, lesions of the third cranial nerve, sympathetic nerve stimulation or hypoxia. They may be constricted and fixed in narcotic addiction, due to glaucoma medication, with inflammation of the iris and with spasms of the sphincter of the pupil or dilating muscle of the iris.

You may at times also want to perform an examination of the internal eye with an ophthalmoscope. Ask the woman to remove glasses or contact lenses. Darken the room to enhance pupil dilation. Seat yourself directly opposite the woman and have her focus her vision on a distant object directly in front of her. Use a large white light on the ophthalmoscope for dilated pupils and a small white light for constricted pupils. Use your right hand and right eye to examine the woman's right eye, and your left hand and

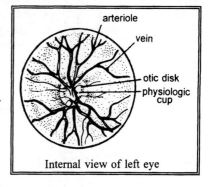

Internal view of left eye

eye to examine her left eye. Set the lens of the ophthalmoscope to -0- diopter (black) initially. Keeping your index finger on the dial, brace the ophthalmoscope against your nose and cheek. Direct the light into the pupil and look for a red light reflex which is a red or orange glow reflected from the fundus of the eye when light is cast on the retina. If there is no red reflex, the pupils could be too small to elicit one or some type of pathology may be present, such as opacity or most seriously detachment of the retina. You may also be performing this portion of the exam imprecisely. If you try several times and cannot elicit a red reflex refer the woman to an ophthalmologist for evaluation immediately. Opacity of the cornea will appear as white spots, those of the lens or vitreous humor appear as dark shadows interrupting the red reflex. Constricted pupils also hinder examination.

Once you have a red reflex, examine the interior of the eye. Approach the woman from 15° from the side while looking into the ophthalmoscope until you touch her forehead. If the optic disc is not immediately visible, follow blood vessels to the center until the disc comes into view. The lens setting you use will depend upon the depth of the eyeball: -0- for a normal eye, -5 to -6 diopters (red numbers) for nearsighted eyes and +1 to +2 diopters (black numbers) for farsighted eyes.

The normal optic disc is regular and round to slightly oval with a sharp outline (the side near the nose may normally be slightly blurred) and appears pinkish yellow with a yellowish white cup.

Observe the blood vessels in all four quadrants by following them from the disc to the perimeter and by looking for signs of occlusion. To do so move your head and the ophthalmoscope together as one, using the woman's pupil as an imaginary fulcrum. Normally the blood vessels are not occluded. Occlusion is suggested by pallor of the background, which is usually light orange in Caucasian women and brownish pink in women of color.

In toxemia the first ocular change which occurs in the retinal vessels is constriction of the arterioles. This may be generalized or localized. Localized changes usually occur in the first half of the arteriole near the nasal edge of the optic disc and appear as a narrowing of a section of the vessel. Retinal edema may occur in eclampsia. This can lead to retinal detachment which appears as a gray fold of tissue and is accompanied by sudden blindness.

The retina should not have any abnormalities such as hemorrhages (which may look like red brush strokes), cloud-like areas or yellowish or flat areas that obscure blood vessels or retinal edema which results in a milky appearance, obscuring the background.

It is normal for a woman's refractive vision to be altered during pregnancy, and women note that their corrective lenses are suddenly not adequate due to the increased fluid volume of pregnancy; this will correct itself after the birth. (See chapter on Eye Problems in Problems That Can Occur at Any Time for details.)

Examining the ears: Ask the woman if her hearing has changed during pregnancy. Hearing loss may first appear during pregnancy or be aggravated by pregnancy (see separate chapter on Hearing Impairment and Loss, which includes examination techniques for hearing acuity). Refer women with diminished hearing or hearing loss to an otologist for evaluation.

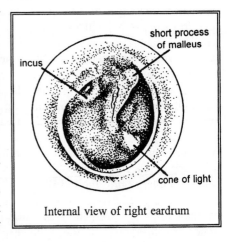

Internal view of right eardrum

There may be times when knowing how to look inside the ear are useful, although if the woman reports no discomfort or other problems it is not routinely necessary. First inspect the outer ears for deformities, lumps or skin lesions. If any ear pain, inflammation or discharge is present, move the auricle up and down and press the tragus. Both of these maneuvers will be painful if there is infection of the outer ear. Press firmly into the groove immediately behind the ear lobe; this will be painful if there is an infection in the middle ear.

To look inside the ear canal, you must use an otoscope. Use the largest ear speculum that the ear canal will comfortably accommodate. Grasp the upper curve of the auricle firmly but gently and pull it upward, back and slightly out. If this does not work to allow painless, easy viewing inside the ear, grasp the middle portion of the auricle and pull straight back and slightly out. Hold the otoscope with the handle pointing up and your hand braced against the woman's head so that you can follow any movements of the woman and avoid injury to the ear canal. Look for normal ear wax (which varies in color from yellow to dark) and any discharge or foreign bodies. In the normal ear, as you advance the speculum slightly downward and forward the ear drum should come into view as a translucent grayish white membrane stretching over the small bones of the inner ear; identify the short process and handle of the malleus and note its position. Find the cone of light. If there is inflammation, the rim may appear inflamed, bulging, or retracted, which is indicated by a prominent short process and a prominent handle that looks more horizontal than usual.

Examining the thyroid gland: First observe the woman's neck. Ask her to tip her head back and to swallow. As she does so, look below the cricoid cartilage for the thyroid gland noting its contour and symmetry. The neck should appear symmetrical with no deviation of the trachea to one side. The thyroid gland, the thyroid cartilage and the cricoid cartilage all normally rise as a person swallows.

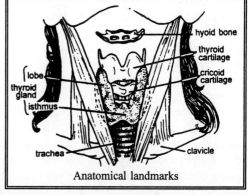

Anatomical landmarks

There are several methods of palpating the thyroid gland, but examining from behind the woman may be the best. From behind, place your fingers on the woman's neck so that the index fingers are just below the cricoid cartilage. The woman's neck should be extended, but not so far as to tighten the muscles. Adjust the degree of extension as necessary. As the woman swallows the thyroid isthmus should rise under your fingers. By rotating your fingers slightly downward and to the side feel as much of the lateral lobes of the thyroid as possible, including their lower borders. Note the size, shape and consistency of the gland and feel for any nodules or tenderness. The anterior lobe is about the size of the end of the thumb and feels somewhat rubbery. The thyroid is easier to feel in a long, slender neck and harder to find in a short, stocky one, in which case further extension of the neck may help. In some people the thyroid gland is partly or completely below the sternum, rendering it inaccessible to palpation.

During pregnancy it is normal for the thyroid to be slightly more palpable than usual. This, by itself, is a byproduct of the changes of pregnancy. An enlarged thyroid is otherwise a sign of hyperthyroidism. An enlarged thyroid, accompanied by signs and symptoms of thyroid problems should be followed up with an evaluation by a specialist. (See the chapter on Thyroid Function in Diagnostic Tests for more information.)

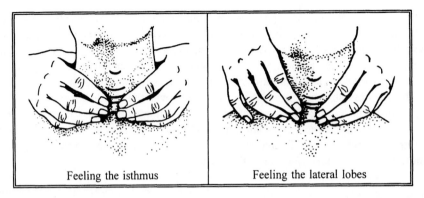

| Feeling the isthmus | Feeling the lateral lobes |

Check for varicosities of the legs: Varicosities are veins whose walls have become prolapsed and dilated and therefore present a tortuous or snake-like appearance rather than being smooth, straight and invisible or nearly so. Varicose veins are most frequently found in the large superficial veins of the legs called the saphenous veins. These veins are relatively poorly supported by surrounding tissue, in contrast to the deep veins of the legs which are well supported and less frequently become varicosed. Ask the woman to stand and then look all around her upper thighs and down her legs for the presence of bumpy, tangled looking veins which may or may not appear darker than the surrounding tissue. If found, look for redness or swelling along the veins and palpate them gently to determine their temperature and if there is a firm cord-like area of clotted blood within. DO NOT massage or press very firmly, as clots may become dislodged in the process. There should not be any difference in temperature along the length of the vein; a vein that is warmer than the surrounding tissue is inflamed. Varicosities may also develop in the genital area or more rarely in the torso or breasts. Hemorrhoids are another common vascular problem. Ask the woman if she has noted any of these and look carefully for varicosities in the genital area when you do a pelvic exam if you have found any in the legs, as many woman are not aware that they have varicose veins in this area.

Any pregnant woman with varicose veins should be encouraged to wear support hose, with heavier hose suggested for the more severe cases of varicosities. (See the chapter on Vascular Problems in the section on Problems That Can Occur at any Time for more details.)

Assessing edema: Observe the extremities for edema before you begin to examine them with your hands. Look for indentations where the tops of socks or hose have been and inquire if the woman's rings are tight, if her face is ever puffy or if other signs of edema have been apparent. Intermittent edema which tends to accumulate more in the extremities is due to the hormonal and fluid volume changes of pregnancy; a sign that the blood volume is expanding. Distended veins may also be apparent when you examine the back of the hands. Generalized edema which does not fluctuate during the day and in which the blood vessels are not prominent is more likely to be due to an abnormal fluid shift from the circulating blood volume into the tissues; dietary review is in order.

Check for pitting: Edema should be measured against a bony prominence such as the ankle or tibia (shin bone). Non-pitting edema gives the appearance of swelling, but when pressure is applied to the area, no indentation is left when the pressure is removed. If edema is so marked that an indentation or pit is left after you apply firm pressure with your thumb to the area for 3 to 5 seconds, it should be assessed as described below.

When recording the degree of edema note if it is pitting or not, and its extent and location, for example: ankle only, ankle and foot; foot to knee; hands, fingers, and face. Edema must be evaluated in conjunction with a woman's nutritional status, laboratory values, and her overall sense of well-being. Clinical evaluation will be discussed throughout the text wherever it seems appropriate.

DEGREE OF PITTING	EXTENT OF EDEMA
Edema present without pitting	Slight (+1)
0 to 0.6 cm. (0 to ¼")	Mild (+2)
.6 to 1.3 cm. (¼ to ½")	Moderate (+3)
1.3 to 2.5 cm. (½ to 1")	Severe (+4)

Check the reflexes: A reflex is an involuntary bodily response involving three basic things: a receiving structure, a nerve center and a responding structure. Deep tendon reflexes are also called muscle stretch reflexes in which the tendon of a partially stretched muscle is briskly tapped. By stretching the muscle's tendon further, a tap stimulates sensory endings in the muscle and generates an impulse that travels up nerve fibers to the spinal cord, causing the muscle to contract briefly, leading to a corresponding brief movement or jerk of the body part affected by the contraction of the muscle.

The main purpose of checking a woman's reflexes is to establish her normal baseline in case any question of hyperreflexia should arise later in the pregnancy. The primary cause of hyperreflexia in the otherwise normal pregnant woman is anxiety. The most common pathological cause is toxemia.

This examination is performed with a reflex hammer which is held by the handle between your thumb and index finger so that it swings freely within the limits set by your palm and other fingers. To elicit a deep tendon reflex have the woman relax, position her limbs properly and symmetrically and strike the tendon briskly, using a wrist motion. Your strike should be quick and direct, not glancing, using no more force than is necessary to provoke a definite response. You may use either the pointed or flat end of your hammer. The pointed end is useful in striking localized areas; the larger end may be less uncomfortable to use for larger areas.

Grading: Reflexes are graded using the following scale:

GRADE	EXPLANATION
5+	Ankle clonus is sometimes graded as 5+
4+	Very brisk, hyperactive, often indicative of anxiety or upper motor neuron or pyramidal tract disease, often associated with clonus (rhythmic oscillations between flexion and extension)
3+	Brisker than average, possibly but not necessarily indicative of disease
2+	Average, normal response
1+	Somewhat diminished, low normal range of response, may be associated with disease
0	No response, may be associated with disease

While there are a number of reflexes that you can elicit, it is not necessary to evaluate all of these in midwifery practice. During pregnancy we generally look at two reflexes as follows:

The knee reflex: The woman may either be sitting or lying down for this exam. Ideally the leg is fully suspended as from the edge of an exam table in the sitting position. However, you can elicit a satisfactory response for our purposes by having the woman sit and cross her legs, as long as her crossed (upper) foot does not touch the floor. Briskly tap the patellar tendon just below the patella (knee cap). To locate the right spot, have the woman slightly tense her thigh and buttocks while you are feeling for a vertical band of tissue just below the lower edge of her kneecap. Once this area is located, have the woman relax her leg completely. Hit the center of that tendon. Note contraction of the thigh (quadriceps) muscle with extension at the knee (the foot kicks outward). If there is no definite response, place your hand on the woman's anterior thigh to feel this reflex. Now examine the other side for comparison.

If the woman is lying down, you may either support one knee at a time or both knees at once. To support one leg at a time, pass your supporting hand under the leg to be examined and brace it just above the woman's opposite knee. Strike the point below the patella as before.

The ankle reflex: Have the woman assume a sitting position and ask her to completely relax her feet. With the leg somewhat flexed at the knee, dorsiflex the woman's foot at the ankle (i.e. push up on the ball of the foot toward the shin). Locate the spot about 2 to 3 inches above the heel along the Achilles' tendon. Now strike this spot on the Achilles tendon. Watch and feel for planter flexion at the ankle, which you will note as the foot presses forward into your supporting hand. This reflex is subtle. Note the speed of relaxation after muscle contraction.

Ankle clonus: If the ankle or knee reflex is hyperactive, test for ankle clonus. Have the woman lie down or cross her legs if she is sitting. If she lies down, support her knee in a partly flexed position. With your other hand, dorsiflex and plantar flex the foot a few times while encouraging the woman to relax and then sharply dorsiflex the foot and maintain its dorsiflexion by keeping your hand in place. Look and feel for rhythmic beats that press against your hand between dorsiflexion and planter flexion. You keep your

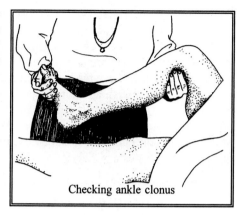

Checking ankle clonus

hand in place because these beats can be very subtle and you may miss them if you let go of her foot. In most normal people, the ankle does not react to this stimulus. A few clonic beats may be seen and felt, especially when the woman is tense or has recently exercised. If the foot reverberates 3 or more beats, this is clonus to be concerned about and should raise your suspicions regarding toxemia.

When you get no response: If there is no reflex response on one or more of these maneuvers, use a technique called reinforcement to see if a reflex can then be elicited. Reinforcement involves the isometric contraction of muscles other than those being tested. For these two reflexes (ankle and knee) have the woman interlock her fingers and pull in opposite directions with her eyes closed. While she is doing that, recheck the reflex. Not only does this distract the woman, thus encouraging relaxation of the muscles being tested, the deliberate contraction of muscles other than those being tested tends to increase the overall physiological reflex response. A reflex is only considered absent if it still cannot be elicited during reinforcement.

Symmetrically diminished or even absent reflexes may be found in normal people. You may not get a response if you have not struck the proper place for the response to be elicited. Always recheck your positioning and try several times before assuming there is no response.

Examine the torso and listen to the lungs: Observe the woman's upper torso for obvious deformities. Palpate along her spinal column to determine if it is straight. Note the slope of her ribs. There should be no marked retraction or bulging of the interspaces between the ribs or impairment of respiratory movement during inspiration.

Listen to the lungs for normal breath sounds, which are clear and unobstructed with no extraneous noises such as wheezing, crackly sounds, etc. Normal breath sounds are similar to those you hear when you brush your finger

436

lightly over the diaphragm of a stethoscope when listening through the binaurals. If you hear nothing in one area it could mean there is fluid in the lungs or it may indicate an undeveloped or damaged section of lung. Less available lung space means less oxygen exchange. While you are listening in each location marked in the drawings below, have the woman breath deeply and slowly through her mouth. Be sure to listen though an entire respiratory cycle of inhaling and exhaling before moving along to the next location. The book and cassette tape set entitled <u>Lung Sounds: A Practical Guide</u>, by Robert Wilkins, John Hodgkin and Brad Lopez, Mosby-Yearbook Pub., 1988, can be used to improve recognition of what to listen for; it even includes a variety of newborn lung sounds.

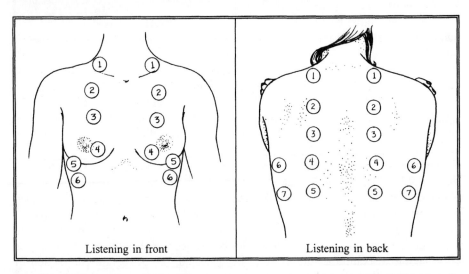

Listening in front   Listening in back

Examine the back and kidneys for tenderness: Look over the back to see if the spine and shoulders appear straight. Percuss the back for kidney tenderness in the costovertebral angle (CVA). This angle is formed by the spine and the lowermost rib in the back. The tip of the lowermost rib usually extends over the center of the kidney. To detect kidney tenderness, press the heel of your examining hand steadily and firmly in the area to the side of the spine at the CVA, then withdraw your hand quickly. The will produce a rebound tenderness if a problem exists. Pain or tenderness

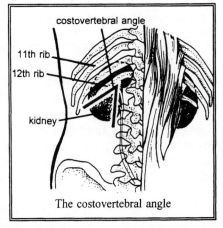

The costovertebral angle

suggests a possible kidney infection; however, this may occur with certain muscle or skeletal problems as well. If the woman is unsure if she felt pain, reexamine her by beginning at a point beneath the shoulder blade to the side of the spine and, using your hand as described above, check successively down the back on one side and then the other, passing over the CVA as you do so to detect any difference in how the CVA area feels, compared to other locations along her spine. True CVA tenderness should elicit an involuntary jolt as the woman reacts to pain when you examine over the kidney (Kolder, 1995). Keep in mind that pain apparently originating from the kidney may be referred pain from more anterior abdominal organs, especially the liver or gall bladder, but rebound tenderness over the CVA will be absent.

Listen to the heart: Ask the woman if she has ever been told she has a heart murmur or other audible heart problems and whether she has been evaluated with an EKG or echo-cardiogram. Has she has ever had any associated problems or symptoms? Next, listen to her heart using the bell of the stethoscope.

The closure of the heart valves is primarily responsible for normal heart sounds. The closure of the mitral valve produces the first heart sound called S1 which means systole 1 (systole is another word for contraction). Aortic valve closure causes the second heart sound or S2. The two other heart sounds, S3 and S4, are usually not heard. (See drawing for where to put your stethoscope to hear these sounds).

If a woman's breasts are large, displace her left breast (or have her do so) to gain access to her chest.

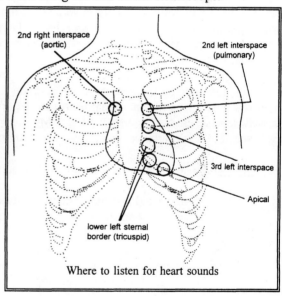

Where to listen for heart sounds

While listening to the heart, concentrate on how the heart sounds when beating, noting any irregularities, extra sounds or swishing sounds (which is blood going in the wrong place). At each location, listen through at least three or four heartbeats, concentrating on the first, then the second heart sound. A galloping beat, which has four distinct sounds instead of the usual two, is associated with heart failure, a rare but dangerous complication of pregnancy. If you detect anything unusual, continue to listen for a few more beats to see if there is a pattern to the irregularity.

Often a woman will develop a benign heart murmur during pregnancy. If you hear anything unusual, such as extra sounds either before, during or after the normal heart sounds, ask her about chest pain, shortness of breath, or unusual heart beat patterns such as palpitations (which occur when the heart beats so rapidly that one beat seems to run into another). If no symptoms are present, murmurs are usually nothing to worry about. However, murmurs accompanied by symptoms often worsen as pregnancy advances and under the stress of labor. If unusual sounds were detected, you should keep an eye out for developing problems as the pregnancy advances, even if the woman appears asymptomatic at the initial exam.

Murmurs associated with mitral valve prolapse, even though asymptomatic, may necessitate the use of prophylactic antibiotics. Prophylaxis is intended to prevent subacute bacterial endocarditis (infection of the heart muscle) which is more likely when bacteria enter the blood stream, as can occur during dental work, surgery or with a normal birth. Women with mitral valve prolapse will probably have been diagnosed before the onset of midwifery care; those that haven't need to be evaluated by a specialist, who will be able to advise her if she needs to consider using antibiotics during labor or postpartum. Current recommendations call for the use of antibiotics only in women with mitral valve prolapse associated with regurgitation as determined by an echo-cardiogram. As a result, many women with mitral valve prolapse do not need antibiotic prophylaxis (Kolder, 1995)

There are many subtle nuances to listening to heart sounds and as a midwife you are not expected to know all of these. When you are learning, there is no substitute for listening to the hearts of other students, family and friends which can help you in knowing how a normal heart sounds. You can also order the book and cassette tape set entitled Heart Sounds and Murmurs: A Practical Guide, by Barbara Erickson, Mosby-Yearbook, Pub., 1991. It is an excellent resource for study.

Breast exam: The breasts are examined for a number of reasons, as follows:

*To determine the shape and erectness of the nipples for breastfeeding
*To instruct the woman in nipple preparation if her nipples are inverted
*To show a woman how to perform a breast exam herself
*To look for any unusual or suspicious masses or other abnormalities of the breasts and make an appropriate referral, if indicated

Check the history: Before you begin a breast exam, check the history for any known masses, tumors, or spontaneous nipple discharge not related to pregnancy or breastfeeding. Note any pain or tenderness in one or both breasts and if the pain is constant, intermittent or if it occurs in relation to the woman's menstrual cycle (which can be normal). The breasts are ideally examined a week or two after the last day of menstrual bleeding to minimize mistaking normal breast changes for pathological findings. If the woman is pregnant, your best baseline will be obtained by performing the exam as early as possible in pregnancy. The following explanation assumes that the woman is either not pregnant or very early in her pregnancy. A list of physiological changes which result from pregnancy follows.

Visual inspection: To begin your exam have the woman sitting so that she is facing you with her body fully exposed to the waist. Full exposure prevents clothing from obstructing your view. First, visually inspect the breasts with the woman holding her arms down at her sides and then raised high over her head. Red circles or marks, or calluses or sores along underwire lines indicate a bra which is too tight. Have her hold each position while you look for any dimpling, bulging, retraction of tissue from one position to another or asymmetry of the breasts (it is normal for one breast to be somewhat larger than the other; asymmetry can be normal if the contour of the breast is smooth and they have always been that way) and the direction in which the nipples are pointing (axis), which is usually slightly away from her midline or directly down if her breasts are pendulous (this can be asymmetrical as well, as long as they have always been that way) (Milan, 1980). While she is in each of these positions, have her press her hands on her hips and look for any of the above signs of problems. Then have her press her palms together at the level of her chin and look again. Cancerous tumors may be present if there is an abnormal elevation of the breast (slight symmetrical elevation is normal), or retraction or flattening of tissue or the nipple during the maneuver, all of which are caused by a tumor attached to the underlying pectoral muscle.

Next have the woman stand and bend forward from the hips with her chin up and her arms and hands extended towards you while you hold her hands for support as you are seated in front of her. The breasts should fall freely away from the chest wall and be symmetrical. Asymmetry and signs of retraction may become evident with this positioning which could be missed with the previous positions. The size of the breasts is an individual variation and as long as the they are symmetrical in contour in relationship to each other they are normal.

The following changes may be abnormal. They may be seen all the time with the woman in any position or may only appear in certain positions during the exam. They should be followed up by a consultation with a specialist.

Asymmetry of contour (bulge or indentation)	Shrunken breast
Retraction signs such as skin dimpling, puckering or furrows	Edema, orange peel skin
Nipple deviation that is not congenital	Prominent superficial veins outside of pregnancy
Nipple retraction that is not congenital	Elevation of skin temperature or redness
Broadening or flattening of a nipple which is not congenital	Excessive breast elevation or asymmetry with contraction of pectoral muscles
Ulcerations	

Accessory breast tissue may be found by itself or in combination with extra (supernumunary) nipples, areola, and glandular tissue. These variations usually

440

occur along the embryological milk lines and are not a problem.

Examine the lymph nodes of the elbow and arm: Next have the woman sitting with her arms at her sides. Palpate the supraclavicular region on both sides for enlarged lymph nodes. These nodes should not be palpable; if they are it could indicate infection or malignancy.

Next support the woman's arm with yours and palpate deep into her armpit

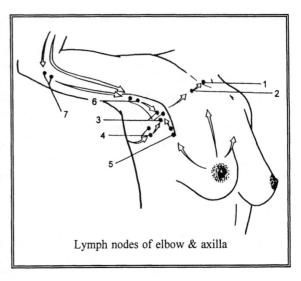

Lymph nodes of elbow & axilla

with your other hand. As you do so, move the woman's arm through a full range of motion to assist you in finding the axillary lymph nodes. If you do find swollen lymph nodes, look at her hand on that side to see if there are any cuts or scrapes which could have caused it. If not, or if you have noted suspicious signs in the breasts, have the woman see a specialist. Palpate the nodes in each elbow as well. The nodes you are examining are described in the following chart (numbers correlate with those in the drawing above):

LOCATION	AREA DRAINED BY NODES
1. Supraclavicular—(& indentations) formed by clavicles & sternocleidomastoid muscles	Right and left upper extremities
2. Infraclavicular—under the outer edge of the clavicle	Arms and breasts
3. Central axillary—deep in the arm pit	Arms
4. Subscapular—along the outside or lateral border of the scapula & are felt deep in the posterior axillary fold	Posterior chest wall & a portion of the arm
5. Pectoral—lower armpit toward the breast	Anterior chest wall and most of the breasts
6. Lateral—along upper armpit toward the arm	Most of the arms
7. Epitrochlear—in the underside of the arm about 3 cm above the elbow	Ulnar surface of the forearm & hand, the little & ring fingers, & the adjacent surface of the middle finger

Palpate the breast tissue: If she has told you she has found a lump during a self exam, always begin with the opposite breast so that you do not overly focus on the "problem," and you get a better idea what her normal breast tissue feels like before you examine the other side.

Have the woman lie down and place her arm above her head on the same side of her body as the breast you will examine first. Place a small pillow under her shoulder on that side if her breasts are large enough to warrant it. Ideally, the breast tissue should be as evenly distributed over the chest wall as possible, so that the nipple appears to be "floating" in the center of the breast tissue.

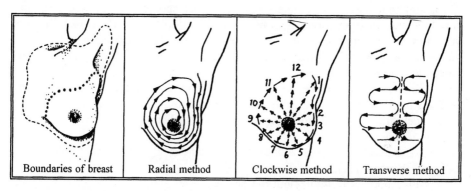

| Boundaries of breast | Radial method | Clockwise method | Transverse method |

It is good to have a routine method of palpation so that you do not overlook examination of any area of the breast. There are several popular methods. The radial method can be performed so it covers all relevant tissue and is the one least likely to cause beginners to cover areas of the breast multiple times, which can increase the chance of traumatizing the tissue. The radial (spiral) method is done by starting at the 12 o'clock point on the outer perimeter of the breasts and proceeding in a circular, clockwise direction, moving in smaller concentric circles until you end up examining beneath the nipple. Start the outer circle far enough out to include the area below the clavicle and down to the lower margin of the breast, which is often felt as a ridge of tissue beneath the lower crease of the portion that protrudes.

Regardless of the method you choose, palpate each area of the breast as follows: begin palpating her breast using the flat portion of the fingers of the examining hand by applying a gentle rotary motion which compresses the breast tissue against the chest wall. At each spot you examine, stop and move the flats of your fingers in three small circles, about the size of a dime. Every inch of breast tissue should be examined. Apply three degrees of pressure at each spot, as follows:

*First, apply light pressure so as to move the skin but not the underlying tissue. Pressing hard at first could cause a lump to move out of the way.
*On the second circle, press midway into the tissue, making sure your finger pads remain flat.

*Lastly, apply deep pressure with the third circle by pressing as firmly
   as possible without causing discomfort; you may feel the woman's
   ribs during this maneuver.

Excessive pressure and rough handling are not necessary and in fact could
cause a cancerous tumor to rupture, thus spreading diseased cells into the
surrounding tissue. Do not lift your fingers except to move along in your exam.
If you stop to make notes it is likely you will miss a spot as you continue. Another
way to ensure that you won't is to have the woman place her fingers on the spot
you examined before you got to where you are now so that she marks you spot as
you make a note. Ideally, however, reserve other activities until your exam is
complete.
   Be sure to palpate the extension of the breast tissue that is located in the
axilla (armpit). To do so, lower the woman's arm to the level of her shoulder. As
you palpate the following findings are within normal limits:

*A transverse ridge, perhaps slightly tender at the lower border
   beneath each breast
*Fine nodularity throughout the breast
*Coarse nodularity generalized throughout the breast which changes
   with the menstrual cycle
*One or both nipples being flat or inverted can be normal if they have
   always been like that (i.e. it is not a new development) and they
   remain inverted in any position (they do not only retract in certain
   positions but are truly flat or inverted all the time).

The following findings suggest cancer and should be checked out by a specialist:

*Coarse, granular nodularity in a localized area
*Loss of elasticity of nipple or breast tissue with increased firmness
   or thickening of the skin texture
*Any mass: if you find a mass, note the following:
   -Location: draw a picture and note the distance from the nipple
   -Size: length and width in centimeters
   -Shape or contour, e.g., round, nodular, smooth, elongated, irregular
   -Consistency, i.e. elastic, tense, firm, soft, hard.
   -Delimitation (demarcation, discreetness, circumscription—this
      means how easy it is to find the edges of the mass, is it well
      defined, or difficult to determine its boundaries?)
   -Mobility or movability: i.e. freely movable, fixed, or movable
      only in certain directions (note which directions)
   -Also note any other unusual findings and the relationship of any
      bulges, dimples, etc. to the mass in question.

*Increased visibility of the superficial blood vessels on the breast of a nonpregnant woman.
*If the woman cannot recall if an unusual, possibly normal, feature has always been present.

Examine the nipples: Look at the nipples themselves. The areola can range from pink to brownish to almost black in some women-of-color. Erosion, ulceration, thickening, redness, shininess, unusual roughness or crusting which appears to be dried discharge may be abnormal, especially if they cannot be accounted for as changes associated with pregnancy or nursing. Next, grasp each areola just below the nipple and pull up. You are feeling for lumps, thickening and looking for discharge. Although many texts recommend that you attempt to express discharge from the nipple during your exam, this is not necessary and may be traumatizing. Leakage of colostrum is normal during pregnancy and milk may leak during or after nursing. Otherwise, spontaneous leakage of discharge from the nipple during the course of your exam may be a problem and requires follow-up by a specialist.

To assess the nipple for breastfeeding, perform the Pinch test. Compress the areola between the forefinger and the thumb just behind the base of the nipple. This simulates the compression that occurs during nursing. If there are adhesions behind the nipple, an apparently erect nipple may retract inward on compression. Likewise, a nipple that looks flat or inverted may pop out on compression.

CLASSIFICATION OF NIPPLE FUNCTION USING THE PINCH TEST	
Protraction	Nipple moves forward, a normal response.
Retraction:	Instead of protracting, the nipple moves inward.
Minimal retraction	A baby with a strong suck exerts enough pressure to pull the nipple forward. A weak or premature baby may have trouble at first.
Moderate to severe	Retracts to a level even with or behind the areola.
Inversion:	All or part of the nipple looks drawn inward within the folds of the areola
Simple	The nipple moves outward to protraction with manual pressure or when cold (pseudo-inversion)
Complete	The nipple does not respond to manual pressure because adhesions behind the nipple pull it inward; rarely there is a congenital absence of the nipple.

As pregnancy progresses, hormonal changes increase the size and protractility of the nipples. Therefore, these changes may cause a nipple that has a tendency to retract to be completely everted by term. (Riordan & Auerbach, 1993)

Normal breast changes during pregnancy: The breasts of a pregnant woman are normally different in several respects from those of a nonpregnant woman. The following are all considered normal physiological changes due to pregnancy which appear during the first trimester unless otherwise noted:

*Both breasts increase in size which may be accompanied by tingling, tenseness, and tenderness.
*There is an increase of generalized nodularity and lobularity of the tissue due to enlargement of the alveoli.
*Spontaneous discharge of colostrum, often beginning as soon as the sixth week of pregnancy as a clear fluid and later becoming more yellow. This may form a crust on the nipples if it is not cleaned with plain water regularly.
*Enlargement of the sebaceous glands in the areola.
*Enlargement and increased erectility of the nipples.
*Broadening and increased pigmentation of the areola.
*Dilated subcutaneous veins usually may be seen beneath the skin as a tracing of bluish veins.
*As the breasts increase in size, striae or stretch marks may appear which look shiny and silver-gray.
*Darkening of the skin around the areola, which is usually mottled, may occur in some women during the second trimester.
*Vascular spider-like vein pattern may appear on the upper chest, upper arms, face and neck in the second trimester. (Varney, 1980)

When you find something: Finding anything of concern during a breast exam is an upsetting and even frightening experience for a woman. Take time to be with her and let her experience her fear, while giving her the names of one or more breast specialists whom she can see for further evaluation. It is important that a practitioner truly expert in breast changes be consulted, not only because she is pregnant but because you want the most useful opinion possible. Due to the normal breast changes which occur during pregnancy, the woman should get another opinion without delay; you might even want to call and make another appointment for her while she is still in your office. Discuss who she might take with her to the appointment for support. Remind her that most suspicious findings in the breast turn out to be benign. (Kolder, 1995)

Examining the augmented breast: In addition to the exam just described, there are several steps that are important to note in examining women with breast implants. Reports of pain may be due to a ruptured implant. Look to see if surgical scars appear normal during visualization. With the woman sitting, palpate the implant for compressibility and mobility. Use one hand to squeeze the implant in the center first from the top, then the bottom, and then each side; simultaneously use your other hand to palpate its opposite edge for contour and irregularities in each position. Next, have the woman place her hands on her hips and lean forward slightly; now examine the superficial breast tissue over the implant by gently and systematically pinching or pulling it away from the implant in both transverse and longitudinal planes. Next, have the woman lay down with her arm relaxed at her side, which renders the implant more mobile. First, palpate as you normally would. Then gently displace the implant away from each quadrant of the breast as you reexamine each quadrant. This may reveal lesions that a soft implant will cushion and thus mask. If the implant is firm or fixed, this type of palpation is possible only in limited areas. Leakage from an implant will produce silicone granulomas that are rock-hard, usually around the edges of the implant or in the axilla. Unusual findings should be evaluated by a specialist knowledgeable about breast implants. (Mann, 1995)

Palpate the abdominal muscles: The rectus abdominous muscles consist of two bands which run from beneath the ribs to the pubic bone. They are joined in the midline by connective tissue. During pregnancy the enlarging uterus presses against these muscles, straining the connective tissue between them and causing the muscles to separate slightly, but normally no more than one-half inch. Unless the abdominal muscles are very weak, undue separation will not be an issue during the first pregnancy. With repeated pregnancies or with too much stress during any pregnancy (from improper exercise, etc.), this separation can become pronounced, producing widely separated muscles. This condition is referred to as rectus diastasis. To assess a woman for this condition, have her lie flat and lift her head up from the examining surface; now look and feel for separation along her abdominal midline above and below the navel using the flats of two fingers.

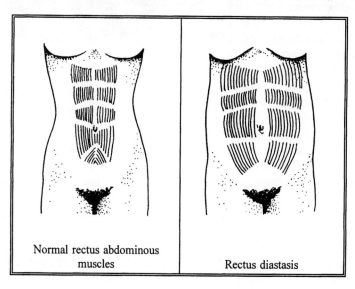

Normal rectus abdominous muscles

Rectus diastasis

If more than a one-half inch separation is discovered, the woman is at risk for more damage during this pregnancy and should consider using some sort of abdominal support device as her pregnancy advances. After birth, she can perform exercises to strengthen these muscles. (See chapter on Exercise in Pregnancy in the Well-being section, and the chapter on Pendulous Abdomen in the Third Trimester Problems section.)

While the mother has her head lifted, also look and feel for any abdominal hernias along her midline, especially in the area of her navel. This will present as a localized bulge, with or without accompanying rectus diastasis. Hernias represent areas of weakness and sometimes pregnancy makes them more pronounced. With or without accompanying rectus diastasis, these women may also benefit from the use of an abdominal support as pregnancy advances.

Palpate the liver and spleen: If the woman's pregnancy is not far advanced it may be possible to get a baseline on the condition of her liver and spleen. This would only be necessary if there was a history of liver or spleen related problems. These techniques can also be attempted if liver or spleen complications arise during pregnancy; however, the enlarged uterus may make them more difficult to perform.

Have the woman lie down with a pillow to support her head and perhaps one beneath her knees. Her arms should be relaxed and across her chest or along her sides. She must be relaxed for you to be able to palpate her abdomen effectively.

First percuss the abdomen to determine the lower border of liver dullness. To do so hyperextend the middle finger of your nondominant hand and press

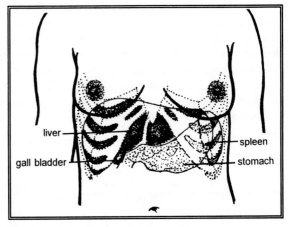

its first joint firmly on the surface to be percussed. Avoid contact by the rest of the hand, since this will dull the vibrations. Position your dominant forearm quite close to the surface with the hand cocked upward. The dominant middle finger should be partially flexed, relaxed and poised to strike at a nearly right angle to the nondominant hand. With a quick relaxed wrist motion use your fingertip to strike the surface of the first joint of your nondominant middle finger. Begin by percussing the entire abdomen to determine areas of tympany (a more hollow or bell-like tone) and dullness. Tympany usually predominates due to gas in the digestive tract; however, feces and normal fluid may also produce a dull sound. To understand what tympany sounds like, perform the percussion maneuver on your own cheek while you fill it with air. Solid organs such as the liver and spleen are also normally dull on percussion.

To palpate the liver place your nondominant hand behind the woman, parallel with and supporting her right eleventh and twelfth ribs. By pressing this hand forward (i.e. upwards into the back) the liver may be felt from the front more easily. Place your examining hand on the woman's right abdomen lateral to the rectus abdominal muscle with your fingertips well below the lower border of liver dullness and pointing toward the lower edge of her right ribs. Press gently inward and upward and ask the woman to take a deep breath. Try to feel the liver edge as it comes down to meet your fingertips. When you can feel it at all, the normal liver edge feels like a firm, sharp and regular ridge with a smooth surface, although sometimes you will only feel an increased resistance when you find it. As your fingers contact the liver edge, release your pressure slightly so that the liver can slip beneath your finger pads and you can feel its anterior surface. Then try to trace its edge to the side and to the center of the woman's abdomen. If the liver feels firm or hard, the edge feels blunt or rounded or the liver seems enlarged, this indicates a possible liver abnormality. An obstructed, distended gallbladder may form an oval mass below the edge of the liver, seemingly merging with it. It will also be dull on percussion.

Another way to palpate the liver is to approach the exam from above the woman's shoulder, reaching over her chest to hook your fingers under the lower ribs below the line of liver dullness. Then, using an inward hooking motion, feel for the liver from this position.

The normal spleen lies in the curve of the diaphragm just posterior to the midaxillary line. If the spleen becomes enlarged, it does so anteriorly, downward and to the center of the body, replacing the normal tympany of the stomach and colon with the dullness of a solid organ on percussion. If you suspect splenic enlargement, have the woman lie on her back with her left arm out to her side slightly. Percuss the lowest interspace of the last two ribs halfway between her armpit and her breast. Then ask her to take a deep breath and percuss again. This area usually remains tympanic if there is no enlargement of the spleen.

To palpate the spleen, use your left hand to reach over and around the woman and press forward and up from the side of her lower rib cage. With your right hand below the left lowermost rib edge, press toward the spleen. Begin palpation low enough to be sure you are below the edge of a possibly enlarged spleen. Ask the woman to take a deep breath. Try to feel the tip or edge of the spleen as it comes down to meet your fingertips. If the spleen is at all palpable in an adult, it is probably considerably enlarged.

Check the lymph nodes in the groin: Using the techniques for examination of the lymph nodes already described, examine the lymph nodes in the groin. Lymph nodes in the inguinal area drain the genital area and may be 1 to 2 cm. in the normal adult. Refer to the chart on page 419 for details regarding your findings.

The pelvic exam: In my practice, I often postponed any pelvic exams until later in the pregnancy. This allows the hormones to relax the muscles of the yoni and thus makes the examination of the pelvic bones easier and more informative; this is especially true of women who have never given birth, since their muscle tone will be quite firm. In many cases, women came to me having already been seen by another care provider who had performed a pelvic exam and a PAP smear, so another exam seemed redundant. If, however, the woman has a history of abnormal PAP results and has not had one within the past

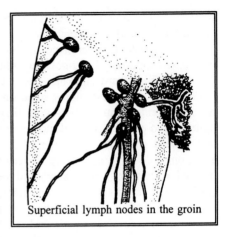

Superficial lymph nodes in the groin

year, the pelvic exam and PAP should be done early in the course of her visits. If a serious change is found, there are more conservative treatment options in the first and early second trimester than there are later in pregnancy. (Kolder, 1995)

When you perform pelvic exams in your practice and how complete an exam you perform will depend upon the individual circumstances, any problematic symptoms a woman may report (such as discharge from the yoni), and whatever your back-up situation may be. It is a good idea to do the pelvic exam last, after the woman has had an opportunity to experience the other parts of the exam with you and hopefully feel more comfortable and relaxed. Even if you want to do a pelvic at the onset of care, it may be best to schedule another appointment soon after the initial exam so that the woman can be fully psychologically prepared, rather than springing it on her when she may have expected just an interview or a belly check. If a woman has had genital mutilation, she may be quite hesitant about showing her genitals to you. Be very gentle and note that even a digital exam may be impossible if she has been tightly infibulated. (See the separate chapter on Previous Clitoridectomy in <u>Healing Passage</u> for more details.)

Before you proceed with any pelvic exam, ask the woman what her previous experiences with such exams has been. As with all components of the physical exam, you will explain what you will be doing and why and showing her any equipment you intend to use, such as the speculum, and how it works. Karen Parker, long time independent midwife who is now a CNM in Portland, Oregon offers her clients a stuffed animal to hold during pelvic exams. One client had expressed the desire for this and she has found many women feel comforted by this as well. The doctors in her practice borrow her teddy bear for the same purpose!

The examination of the woman's internal reproductive organs (the bimanual exam) can be done separately or in combination with an examination of the external genitals and pelvimetry. I will describe the complete pelvic exam, with the exception of pelvimetry, which is covered in a separate chapter because pelvimetry is often done later in pregnancy apart from the rest of the pelvic exam. Pelvimetry can, of course, be integrated into the rest of the pelvic exam if this seems appropriate (as it may be if a woman is coming to you quite late in pregnancy having had no prior prenatal care).

Next, you will want to ask the woman if she wishes to empty her bladder again before you begin. You can perform the exam on an exam table or on a bed with the woman's feet supported by chairs. You would then be seated between her legs on a stool. Or, you can perform a pelvic with the woman lying on the floor, on a blanket or carpet. The problem with using the floor is that it is hard to comfortably manipulate the speculum in this position. If you have the woman lie on large flat furniture cushions, this problem is eliminated since the cushions will elevate her bottom enough to allow the speculum handle to be directed toward the floor when it is inserted into the yoni. Her buttocks should be slightly extended over the edge of the examining surface and a towel or disposable underpad should be placed beneath them.

Wash your hands and put on one or two gloves. The trick is not to touch anything with your gloved hand except the woman or equipment that will not touch anything else either. It is safest for you to glove both hands. You should have all necessary supplies, equipment, lighting, etc. arranged prior to gloving if you plan to glove both hands. A pair of light, clear goggles can also be worn if you do not wear glasses. It is also helpful to have an assistant to hand you things as you proceed through the exam.

When the woman is in position and you are ready to begin, ask her to separate her legs or let her knees fall to the sides. You may want to provide pillows to support her legs. I do not recommend using the phrase "spread your legs," as this may be verbally traumatic for some women given its cultural connotations. Do not attempt to open a woman's legs yourself.

Examine the external genitals: Seat yourself in front of the woman's perineum in such a way that eye contact with her can be maintained. Look at her external genitals and inspect for pattern of hair growth, pubic lice, and normal appearing labia majora and minora. Localized swelling may be due to allergies; if it is in the labia it could be caused by a vestibular gland abscess (painful) or cyst (if not). Small cysts may be sebaceous in origin and are not a concern. Look for inflammation, or skin irritation which could indicate an infection of the yoni. If found, ask the woman if she has noted any itching or other symptoms. Discoloration or tenderness could be from bruising, ask about it and wait until the exam is finished and the woman clothed to further discuss the possibility of physical abuse at home. Varicosities will appear as lumpy distended veins which may or may not show bluish discoloration. Sometimes pregnancy makes otherwise invisible varicose veins stand out due to the pelvic engorgement that takes place.

Any sores, vesicles, crusting, warts or other suspicious lesions should be thoroughly tested as to their cause unless it is an obvious injury for which the woman has an explanation (rare unless she is being abused). Look for scars from old incisions for births and ask about how they healed, any discomfort now or pain with penetration. Unusual scars may also be the result of sexual or ritual abuse or other genital mutilation. Some women shave their pubic hair (Muslims often do). Recommend that she discontinue shaving through the postpartum period, as it actually increases the risk of infection. Separate the labia majora and inspect the labia minora, vestibule, urethral orifice, clitoris and the mouth of the yoni for lesions, bruises, hygiene, etc. and make mental notes. Look for the hymenal ring or tags just inside the yoni, an important landmark when suturing.

Examine the periurethral and vestibular (Bartholin's) glands: At this point examine the paraurethral glands and urethra for abnormal discharge. Insert your examining finger to the second joint. Push upward into the roof of the yoni and milk the paraurethral gland toward the outside on one side of the urethra. Now milk the gland immediately to the other side of the urethra. Now press upwards centrally and milk the urethra. Next, examine the vestibular glands. Sweep your examining finger to the side on the inside of the yoni and use your examining thumb on the outside of the labia majora to bimanually palpate for the vestibular gland on one side. Palpate the entire area paying particular attention to the lower lateral portion of the labia majora behind which the vestibular glands are located. Turn your hand over and palpate the other side in the same fashion. Check for tenderness, swelling, lumps, heat, fluctuation or discharge. There should be none. A painful mass is probably an abscess and could be due to gonorrhea. A nontender mass is probably a cyst which may result from chronic inflammation. Neither of these exams should produce any discharge. If they do, it is most likely due to gonorrhea; obtain a culture immediately.

Look for fistulas: If a woman has reported that she is having foul smelling discharge, or has noted passage of urine or feces from the yoni, look for fistulas throughout the remainder of your exam. A fistula is a healed hole which creates a connecting channel between canals that are normally separated, such as the yoni and the urethra. If you are in doubt about the presence of a fistula, have the woman insert a full size tampon (such as Tampax) and remove it several hours later. Urine or a fecal stain in the tampon indicate the that a fistula exists; the location of the stain shows where to look more closely for the lesion.

Using the speculum: Now you are ready to do a speculum exam, if necessary. The speculum allows you to view the walls of the yoni and the cervix, and allows access to the cervix for cytological (PAP) smears. Explain this to the woman as you show her the instrument and how it works. While there are a number of different styles of speculums, the most available ones and the ones most midwives use are the Pederson and the Graves. These both come in a variety of sizes and in either plastic or metal models. For your purposes, a medium size will be the one you will need the most often. The main difference between the two styles has to do with the bills or blades: the Grave's bills are flared at the end while the Pederson bills are narrow throughout their length. The following chart suggests the use of various size speculums in different circumstances:

CIRCUMSTANCE	RECOMMENDED SPECULUM
Virgin or pregnant teenager	Narrow Pederson
First pelvic exam or First-time mother	Medium Pederson
Woman is extremely sensitive in her yoni	Medium Pederson
Woman has had babies	Medium Graves
Pelvic muscle relaxation	Large Graves
Large woman or very obese	Large Graves

Plastic speculums have no thumbscrew and tend to be less easy to fine tune than the metal variety and can more easily pinch tissue, so be careful. They also make a rather loud and alarming click when the bills are snapped into place on the handle. Warn the woman of this fact before you begin your exam. Due to these drawbacks, it is a good idea to have metal speculums on hand to do your routine exams. Plastic speculum are great, however, for sending home with women so that they can do their own speculum exams.

The parts of the metal speculum are illustrated below:

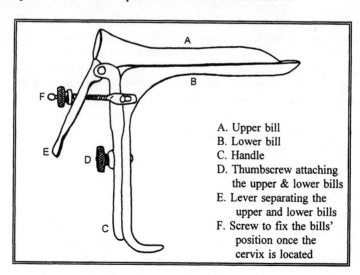

A. Upper bill
B. Lower bill
C. Handle
D. Thumbscrew attaching the upper & lower bills
E. Lever separating the upper and lower bills
F. Screw to fix the bills' position once the cervix is located

Lubricate the speculum with warm water only unless you know, in advance, that no cultures or smears are going to be needed. All lubricants other than warm water may interfere with the accuracy of tests, especially PAP results. If you don't have any warm water, wet the speculum and warm it under a lamp, with a hair dryer or in your gloved hand (then rewet it if necessary). Test the temperature of the speculum with your hand; and again by touching the end near the handle to the junction of the woman's innermost thigh and external genitalia. This way, you are sure she will not be burned when you insert the speculum.

Separate the lower labia with one gloved hand to expose the opening of her yoni. Or, insert one or two fingers just inside the yoni to the first joint and firmly depress the perineal body to hold the introitus open. Hold the speculum in your other hand with your index finger hooked over the top of the near end of the top bill and your other fingers around the handle. This keeps the bills closed during insertion. Insert the speculum very slowly and gently with the bills turned to a sharp oblique angle until just past the hymenal ring. Now, check to be sure you are not dragging labia minora, hair, etc. along as you do so. The oblique angle puts the least amount of stress on the opening of the yoni. Ask the woman how it feels at this point. Slight pressure down once you are past the introitus helps avoid pressure on the anterior structures. Once the speculum is inserted about one-third its length, carefully and gently rotate the speculum bills to a horizontal angle and continue to advance it towards the cervix, directing the bills at about 45° angle downwards until three-quarters of its length is inserted.

Maintain downward pressure by putting downward pressure on the lower end of the speculum handle or by putting your thumb into the near end of the posterior bill and pressing down. Now, slowly begin to open the speculum by putting pressure on the lever and sweep the speculum bills upward until the cervix comes into view. Theoretically, downward pressure during insertion assures that you will find the cervix when you start to sweep the speculum upwards, regardless of the direction in which the cervix is pointing (which varies according to which way the uterus is positioned). However, if you do this and the cervix is not in view, slowly allow the bills to close part way, withdraw the bills about one-third the length of the instrument and then reinsert them, still partly opened. This will often cause the cervix to pop into view when you have missed it with the initial insertion. If the cervix still cannot be visualized, and the woman's yoni seems roomy, try a larger and longer Grave's speculum.

In very large women, or women with relaxed pelvic tissues, you may need some help in holding the lateral walls of the yoni apart so they do not obstruct your view. This can be done by making a tube of latex by cutting one of the fingers off a glove and also cutting off the tip of the finger (or use a condom). Slide the tube over your longest, largest lubricated speculum. Test it by opening it to the extent you anticipate having to open it once it is in place, to make sure the latex will not snap. You will note that a lot more pressure will be necessary to open it, once it is in place. Then close it and insert it as you normally would. (Kolder, 1995)

The cervix and yoni walls may be bluish lavender in pregnancy, the nonpregnant cervix and yoni walls are pink. Cervical size is influenced by childbearing or inflammation. The os, or cervical opening, is a small, round dot or slightly oval in a woman who has never given birth. The os of a woman who has given birth is a slit. In women who have only had IUDs inserted or who have experienced only first trimester induced abortions or miscarriages, the os appears as a slightly larger dot, but is still round. The position of the cervix gives you clues about the position of the uterus:

> *Anterior cervix (os points up from the bottom bill of the speculum) indicates a retroverted uterus.
> *Posterior cervix (os points down from the top bill of the speculum) indicates an antiverted uterus.
> *Midline placement of the cervix indicates the uterus is also in midposition.
> *If the cervix is pushed over to the right or left of the midline this could mean there is some kind of pelvic mass pushing on it. (Feel for masses carefully during the bimanual exam.)

Once you have the cervix in view, move the speculum around slowly and gently until you have as good a view of the cervix as possible. Sometimes one bill of the speculum can get caught in the edge of a cervical lip (particularly in multiparas who have cervical scars), necessitating gently pulling back on the open speculum and then reinserting it. This will usually cause the cervix to rest completely between the bills. Eversion may occur if the speculum is inserted a bit too deeply, pushing the bills deeply into the anterior and posterior fornices; this may force the mouth of the cervix open "peeling back" the opening of the os and thus exposing the rougher and redder looking tissue lining the cervical passage known as columnar epithelium, (i.e. causing tissue that is not normally visible to be seen). Eversion usually appears as a uniform margin of tissue. Ectopy occurs when the cervical lining is visible naturally, which usually appears as an irregular margin. Ectopy may be seen in multiparas or in women taking birth control pills. To differentiate the two, simply pull the speculum out from the yoni slightly and see if the reddish area remains. (Varney, 1980)

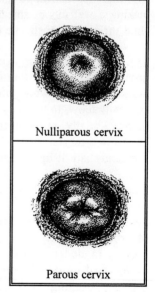

Nulliparous cervix

Parous cervix

Tighten the screw on the lever to hold the speculum open. If more exposure is needed, elevate the anterior bill by releasing the screw and pressing the lever to push the top bill higher for better visualization. If the cervix is covered with discharge, *gently* wipe it off with gauze using a ring forceps or a cotton swab. Try not to cause bleeding as you do so. The use of cotton balls or swabs may interfere with cytologic screening, so take care. Perform any procedures or tests that you need to do now. Assist the woman to see her cervix with a flashlight and a mirror.

Talk to the woman about the condition of her cervix. Note its color, any growths or lesions, the position of the cervix, its size and shape, any swelling, inflammation, discharge, bleeding, the size and shape of the os, scars and any dilation. Areas that look like strawberry spots may be obvious on the cervix or in the fornices or yoni walls in DES daughters and they may have cervical abnormalities as well (see the chapter on Abnormalities of the Female Reproductive System in the Anatomy and Physiology section for more details). If you have found any evidence of problems, such as lesions or inflammation, discuss options for treatment or follow-up care.

Before you are done with your speculum exam, gently rotate the speculum 90 degrees while exerting downward pressure to visualize the yoni walls that have been behind the bills of the instrument. Then return the bills to their horizontal position, release the screw on the lever and partially close the bills by slowly releasing the lever. Keep some pressure on the lever as you do this so you don't "bite" the cervix with the bill tips by closing them prematurely.

Begin to withdraw the speculum until the cervix is released, then stop and slowly allow the bills to close completely, repositioning your index finger over the anterior bill. Watch what you are doing as you close the speculum so you don't pinch the yoni walls or other structures. Slowly withdraw the speculum and begin to rotate it to the oblique angle you used during insertion. You can ask the woman to help by bearing down as you withdraw it. Check the posterior bill of the speculum for discharge and note its odor. If warranted, obtain a specimen for making a wet mount smear for microscopic examination if this was not already done. (See Diagnostic Tests for how to perform a wet mount and PAP smear.)

The bi-manual pelvic exam: While still positioned at the woman's perineum, generously lubricate the index and middle fingers of your examining hand. Separate the labia with your other hand and gently insert one or two fingers, as the yoni will allow, to the second finger joint. Be sure to tell the woman what you are doing. Usually, inserting first one then the other finger gives the woman a chance to get used to your hands. Watch your thumb during the exam so that you don't accidently jam it into the woman's clitoris or anus as you maneuver your hand.

Checking for prolapses: Adjusting yourself so you can see into the yoni easily, exert pressure with your fingers posteriorly against the muscles of the yoni and ask the woman to bear down or cough. (Remember that some women will pass a bit of urine when they have perineal stress of this type, ask her and if she does, prepare to dodge the urine accordingly.) Look at the anterior yoni wall for evidence of prolapse, which would indicate a cystocele. Look next to see if the cervix is "hanging low," that is, if it is placed closer to the introitus than you would expect, and to what degree. If it is, she has some degree of uterine prolapse.

(Advise women with uterine prolapse to assume a knee-chest position for 20 minutes several times daily in early pregnancy to help bring the uterus into a normal position and relieve tension on ligaments.) Keeping your fingers in the same position, spread them as widely as possible and ask the woman to bear down. Look for any bulging of the posterior wall of the yoni for evidence of a rectocele. Now, put your fingers together and ask the woman to tighten her muscles around your fingers to check her muscle tone. (See Healing Passage for more detailed information on muscle tone, herniations of the yoni wall and uterine prolapse.)

Palpating the cervix: Next sweep your fingers around to examine the walls of the yoni as you insert them back to the cervix. As you do so, note any abnormalities or unusual findings. Find the cervix and feel all around its size, shape, consistency (hard like a nose outside of pregnancy, soft like the lip during pregnancy) and how smooth it is. Missing pieces from previous annular detachment (see Healing Passage), or large unrepaired tears may lead to a loose cervix during pregnancy. Roughness may also indicate a problem. If a speculum exam has not been done and your findings are unusual, perform one after your bimanual exam. Remember that a PAP smear will be altered by lubricants other than water. If your findings indicate the need for a PAP, reschedule an appointment for one 2 days later.

Again, note the position of the cervix and if it is dilated by putting a fingertip at the mouth of the os and pressing gently. Next grasp the cervix between your fingers and move it from side to side. This should not be painful; if it is it may indicate a pelvic inflammatory process or an ectopic pregnancy.

Examine the uterus: Recall the position of the uterus from your previous investigations of the cervix. To proceed with palpation you will use both hands; one within the yoni and the other on the woman's abdomen.

If you feel the uterus is antiverted: place your "outside" hand midway between the woman's navel and her symphysis pubis. Use the flats of your fingers up to the first joints to press downward and forward towards the pubic bone and your yoni fingers. At the same time, turn your internal hand palm up and place two fingers on either side of the cervix; bring them around to the front of the cervix (the anterior fornix) and push downward on the cervix with the backs of your fingers and in and upward with the tips of your fingers towards your abdominal hand as though you were trying to touch the fingers of your abdominal hand. When the uterus is anterior or antiflexed, this causes it to slip between the fingers of your two hands as they move towards each other.

If you feel the uterus is retroverted: Place one yoni examining finger on each side of the cervix. Place your abdominal hand immediately above the pubic bone and press downward firmly. Bring your internal fingers together under the cervix (in the posterior fornix) and press against it to follow it inward as far as it goes.

456

If you feel the uterus is located mid-way between: Place your examining fingers on either side of the cervix and press their tips straight inward and feel for the wall of the uterus on either side as far as you can. Then slide your fingers around the uterus until one finger is on top of the cervix and one finger is beneath the cervix. Continue to press inward while moving your fingers to feel as much of the body of the uterus as possible.

If all else fails: Place your examining fingers behind the cervix, press in and curve them upwards. At the same time place your abdominal hand between the woman's navel and her pubic bone and use it to palpate in a dipping motion down and deep to touch the top of the uterus between the fingers of your two hands. If one technique does not allow you to find the uterus, try another, regardless of where you feel the uterus is.

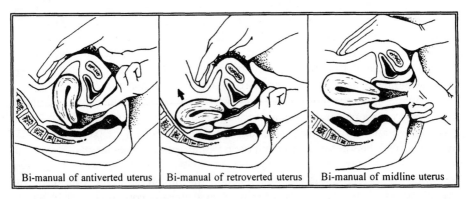

| Bi-manual of antiverted uterus | Bi-manual of retroverted uterus | Bi-manual of midline uterus |

Here is a table of normal and abnormal findings:

FINDING	NORMAL NONPREGNANT		OTHER FINDINGS
	NULLIPARA	MULTIPARA	
Size	5.5-8 cm. long 3.5-4 cm. wide 2-2.5 cm. thick	6.5-12 cm. long 4.5-6.5 cm. wide 2.5-5 cm. thick	Smaller after menopause
Position	Midline		Off-center—growths, scar tissue or adhesions
Consistency	Firm		Soft at the isthmus, body of uterus feels doughy during pregnancy
Mobility	Mobile above cervix from front to back		Immobility may be due to scar adhesions
Shape	Flattened pear		Ovoid; or irregular shape in one coronal area—could be pregnancy Asymmetrical—tumors
Tenderness	None on movement		Pain on movement indicates an infection or could mean an ectopic pregnancy

Examine the ovaries and uterine tubes: Next examine the adnexal area, which is found to either side of the uterus; this is where the ovaries and uterine tubes are located. Place your abdominal hand midway between the hip bone (iliac crest) and the abdominal midline and between the level of the woman's naval and her pubic bone. Using the flats of your fingers to the first joints, press your fingers deeply down and oblique towards the symphysis pubis and your yoni fingers. With your internal palm upward, place both of your yoni exam fingers in the lateral fornix (right or left) on the side that your abdominal hand is positioned to examine. Press your fingers deeply inward and upward towards your abdominal hand as far as possible. Palpate the area between the uterus and the hip bone with a sliding, gentle pressing together motion of your two hands as they move from the highest to the lowest level as you are moving your hand abdominally. Now repeat this procedure on the other side. You are palpating for ovarian shape, tenderness or pain and any other masses (there should be none).

The ovaries will slip between your fingers and feel like small ovoid masses. The ovaries are frequently hard to find even when someone is very experienced. Do not even bother to palpate this area if a woman is past her first trimester of pregnancy, as the ovaries will be carried upwards by the broad ligament with the growth of the uterus and be impossible to find. If you can't find any structures, assume that all is normal and make note that nothing was felt.

The size of the normal ovary of a woman in her menstrual years ranges from 1 to 2 inches long (2.5 to 5 cm.), 5/8 to 11/8" wide (1.5 to 3 cm.) and ¼ to ½" thick (.5 to 1.5 cm.). It is the same shape as a small almond still in its shell. Normal ovaries are somewhat tender upon palpation, which assists in knowing when you have found them. The uterine tubes may be nontender or slightly so. They are normally quite narrow, varying from 2 to 3 mm. at their narrow-most width to 5 to 8 mm. at the widest point. Therefore do not be alarmed if you cannot feel them.

Other than the ovaries, any masses in this area are abnormal and require follow-up evaluation. Ovarian cysts and tumors are usually not painful unless they are about to rupture.

Perform a rectal exam: The final portion of the bimanual exam evaluates the rectal area. Women hate this part of the exam and, indeed, on a young normal woman that has otherwise checked out fine it is not necessary to perform a rectal exam each time a pelvic is done. However, if you discovered masses, or a woman has symptoms such as rectal bleeding or pain, or is over 40 years of age, a rectal exam may give you further information about how to proceed with her care.

At this point you may wish to change to fresh gloves before proceeding to ensure that you do not transfer any organisms from the yoni into the rectum during your exam. Alternatively, you can double glove your examining hand.

Generously lubricate your middle examining finger. Look at the anus first to note any external hemorrhoids, fistulas, skin tags, prolapse or lesions. Next place the tip of your middle examining finger against the anus and ask the woman

458

to bear down, telling her you are about to insert your finger. Gently push your finger past the anal opening. Check for internal hemorrhoids by feeling around the inner mouth of the anus, paying particular attention to two o'clock on the posterior anal canal, five o'clock on the anterior aspect and nine o'clock on the left lateral anal wall. They may be hard to detect because they are very soft. (For more details, see the chapter on Vascular Problems in the general problems section.) Ask the woman to tighten and relax her anal sphincter. If very tight, it could be due to a fissure, lesion or inflammation. A loose sphincter may be related to neurological disease, frequent anal intercourse or a poorly done sphincter repair after a previous birth. If you feel no sphincter this is probably due to an improperly repaired tear from a previous birth. Ask about fecal incontinence if you have not already done so.

Now insert the lubricated index finger of the same hand into the yoni, pushing both your rectal and yoni fingers as far inside as they will reach. Palpate half of the rectal wall by sweeping your rectal finger back and forth, then ask the woman to bear down which will bring more of the wall within your reach.

Use your outside hand to press firmly and deeply downward just above the pubic bone. Place your yoni examining finger in the posterior fornix and press upward firmly against the posterior side of the cervix which will move the uterus to a more posterior position. Now feel as much of the posterior side of the uterus as possible. If you had difficulty locating the ovaries before, use the same techniques already described to try and find them via the rectum. Before you remove your fingers palpate the other half of the rectal wall. Gently remove your fingers being careful not to touch the rectal finger to the opening of the yoni. Give her a tissue or wipe off her genitals yourself so as not to contaminate the yoni with rectal secretions (i.e. wipe from front to back). Any bleeding, roughness or lumps which you palpate during this exam will require further evaluation.

Finishing up: At this point you might leave the room to wash your hands and allow the woman to get dressed. If you are someone who cannot easily explain your findings as you proceed through exams of these types, sit down with the woman and thoroughly discuss your findings at this time. If you have kept her up on what you are finding, use this time to also discuss what to do about any problems you may feel are present.

References and further reading:

Bates, Barbara, A Guide to Physical Examination, 5th ed., J.B. Lippincott, Philadelphia, 1991.
Cooper, K, "Measuring Blood Pressure the Right Way," Nursing92, Vol. 22, No. 4, 1992, p. 75.
Hegner B. & Caldwell, E., Nursing Assistant, 6th ed., Delmar Pub., Albany, NY 1992.
Hill, Martha, & Grim, C., "How to Take a Precise Blood Pressure," American Journals of Nursing, Vol. 91, No. 2, February, 1991, pp. 38-42.
Kolder, Veronika, MD., obstetrician, Iowa City, IO, editing comments, 2/95.
Luce, Judy, R.N., conversation regarding hypertension, MANA regional Conf., Vermont, 1990.

459

Mann, Laurene, "Physical Examination of the augmented breast: description of a displacement technique," <u>OB/GYN</u>, Vol. 85, No. 2, Feb. 1995, pp. 290-2.
Milan, Albert, <u>Breast Self-Examination</u>, Liberty Pub. Co., NY, 1980.
Riordan, J. & Auerbach, K., <u>Breastfeeding and Human Lactation</u>, Jones & Bartlett, Boston, 1993.
Rudy, Susan, "Take a Reading on Your Blood Pressure Techniques," <u>Nursing86</u>, Vol. 16, No. 8, August, 1986, pp. 46-49.
Varney, Helen, <u>Nurse-Midwifery</u>, Blackwell Scientific Pub., Inc., Boston, MA, 1980.
Whitley, Nancy, <u>A Manual of Clinical Obstetrics</u>, J.B. Lippincott Co., Philadelphia, PA, 1985.

Pelvimetry

NOTE: It will be helpful to review the information in the Anatomy & Physiology section on pelvic anatomy before studying this chapter.

Pelvimetry is the art of assessing the size and shape of a woman's pelvis and determining how well suited her pelvis is to childbearing. Knowing a woman's pelvic dimensions can be very informative, for instance it may provide the knowledge you need to help her find the right position to push her baby out. Pelvimetry, however, can be a mixed blessing. For decades doctors have tried in vain to accurately predict which women will be able to birth a baby, and if so what size, by the size and shape of their pelvises. X-rays, ultrasound, manual examination and complicated pelvic measuring tools have all been used in an attempt to make this determination.

The obsession with pelvic capacity was at its height at the turn of the 19th century. In cities, many women had very poor nutrition and worked from childhood on in dark factories with little exposure to sunlight. As a result, many had rickets as children, which permanently deformed their pelvic structures. Adult women giving birth through contracted, deformed pelvises were an enormous problem of the time, especially since surgical birth was still a very risky procedure and only used as a last resort. Naturally, women of small stature with small bones were most at risk. Cesarean surgery was a risky process with a high mortality rate. As a result, doctors sought to hone their skills for assessing pelvic capacity. Unfortunately for today's first world women, most of whom have not suffered from rickets, an underlying prejudice still exists which questions each woman's ability to give birth to a normally sized infant. Therefore many women are judged either prenatally or during labor as being "too small" to birth their babies and wind up with surgical deliveries instead of normal births. Occasionally women get transferred from homebirths for the same reason.

Before we get into the specifics of pelvimetry, it is important to be clear about its limitations. You *cannot tell* if woman can give birth to a particular size baby based on her pelvimetry alone unless her pelvis is grossly abnormal. The pelvis is not made of a solid piece of bone (see anatomy section); it consists of four bones which are joined by flexible cartilage. The cartilage becomes even more flexible under the influence of the hormones of pregnancy. Therefore, the pelvic passage can and does adapt to the size of the baby being born, especially when women change positions during labor. Even if a woman has previously birthed naturally, about all you can say concerning her pelvic capacity in relationship to the size of the present baby is that she has had, say, a 9 lb. baby before with no problem. This does not mean she won't have problems with a smaller baby in an awkward position, nor does it mean she can't have a baby considerably larger than 9 lbs.

I have heard other, experienced midwives tell women they have an "8½ pound pelvis" or whatever they felt the upper limit of fetal size for that woman might be. This is not only impossible to know, but undermines a woman's sense that her body can do what it needs to do and can be one of the most difficult messages for a woman to overcome. It implants fear regarding the size of her baby and may indirectly suggest that she should watch her weight gain, which is downright dangerous. The notion that the size baby a woman can have can be predetermined also influences a midwife's perceptions and affects what kinds of limits she places on the birthing situation. This thinking can sabotage the entire process of normal spontaneous birth. Instead, you should explain the flexibility of the pelvis to the mother and note how remarkable it is that the baby's head molds and the mother's pelvis opens to let the baby out.

I'll finish this lecture with a story. A CNM friend of mine examined a woman's pelvis at her first prenatal visit. As she did so she said to herself "this is the most contracted pelvis I've ever felt." However, to the woman she said, "you have plenty of room in here." This woman birthed an 8 pound baby with no problems. The bottom line is that no one can know what will happen until labor is underway and a woman is completely dilated and pushing effectively with good, strong contractions.

While the original intent of pelvimetry was to divide pelvises into two groups, those that were adequate to birth a baby and those that were not, we shall modify that purpose. Pelvimetry in midwifery is used to familiarize yourself with the nuances and unique aspects of a woman's pelvic contours so that, during labor, you may use that information, if necessary, to help a woman give birth. It is important to be familiar with pelvimetry in cases where pelvic dimensions are most crucial, specifically breech births. How to go about using this information to help women birth will be covered in Volume II of this textbook. For now, the focus will be on understanding the varieties of configurations the female pelvis may assume and knowing how to assess these in clinical practice.

Pelvic anatomy as relevant to pelvimetry assessment:

We will start with a discussion of the different varieties of pelvic shape and present an overview of pelvic assessment. Further details will be covered as we discuss the clinical examination of the pelvis.

The pelvis is divided into two regions, the false pelvis and the true pelvis. The **false pelvis** includes those anatomical features which have no influence on childbearing and mainly refers to the iliac crests (hip bones). The boundaries of the false pelvis are defined by a line drawn beginning at the inferior border of the last lumbar vertebrae in back, around to the upper border of the symphysis pubis in front, following back around on the other side in the same plane, to the lumbar vertebrae in back, where they end. All features of the pelvic bones above this line (called the *linea terminalis* or pelvic brim) are part of the false pelvis. The only birth-related function of the false pelvis is to support the enlarged uterus.

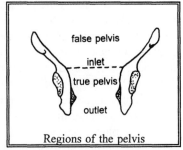

Regions of the pelvis

The **true pelvis** lies below the pelvic brim; it is the bony passage through which the baby passes during birth. It is divided into three regions: the inlet, pelvic cavity, and the outlet.

The **pelvic inlet**, which is defined by the pelvic brim, is the bony entry of the birth passage. Below this plane is the **pelvic cavity**, which forms a curved passage between the inlet and the outlet. The anterior wall of this passage is formed by the inner surface of the pubic bone, which is straight and shallow. The posterior wall is formed by the inner surface of the sacrum and coccyx which is deep and concave. The inner surface of the ischium and part of the body of the ilium are found on either side. The **pelvic outlet** is diamond-shaped and is bounded by the lower border of the pubic bone in front, the ischial tuberosities on either side and by the tip of the sacrum in back.

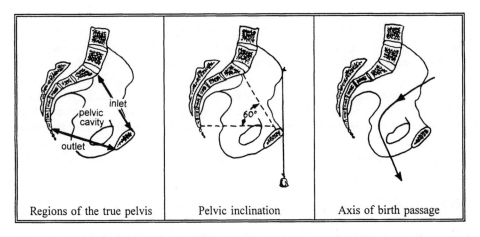

| Regions of the true pelvis | Pelvic inclination | Axis of birth passage |

The pelvis is normally inclined so that the plane of the pelvic brim makes an angle of about 60° with an imaginary horizontal line when the woman is standing. This brings the pubic spine and the anterior superior iliac spine into the same vertical plane (see illustration above).

An axis is a line which passes through the center of a plane. The **axis of the birth passage (the curve of Carus)** is the path of the baby's presenting part as it moves through the pelvis during descent and pushing. It first moves downward and backward to the level of the ischial spines, which is also the level where the pelvic floor muscles attach to the pelvic bones. Here the presenting part meets the resistance of the muscles below and the pubic bone above. At this point, the presenting part begins taking a downward and forward direction as it pivots around and beneath the pubic bone during birth.

The **pelvic planes** represent portions of the pelvis at different levels. They provide us with a way of describing different regions of the pelvis. The most important ones follow. They will be easier to understand if you refer to the illustrations in the tables appearing on the following pages.

1) The **plane of the inlet** is also called the **superior strait** or **pelvic brim**. It is nearly circular, except for the bony projection of the sacral promontory in the back.
2) The circular **pelvic cavity** has several planes; the two most important ones are the **plane of greatest dimensions** and the **plane of least dimensions**.
3) The plane of the **outlet** is also called the **inferior strait**. It is oval or diamond shaped, depending upon the pelvic type.

In order to discuss how the pelvis is shaped, different pelvic diameters have been defined. These are distances between given points on the pelvis. They are:
*Anterior-posterior (front to back)
*Transverse (side to side through the center)
*Oblique (diagonally transecting the center from front to back)
*Sagittal (from the center to the front or back half of the anterior-posterior diameter)

There are four basic pelvic shapes. An individual woman may have a combination of features from two or more of these basic shapes. The gynecoid, or true female pelvis, is ideally suited for childbearing, with the brim, cavity and outlet more nearly circular than in the other pelvic types. A simplified table of the normal diameters for a gynecoid pelvis follows. You can easily remember the diameters by noting that they follow a pattern.

Region of pelvis	Anterior-posterior diameter	Right & Left Oblique Diameter	Transverse Diameter	
Brim	11 cm.	12 cm.	13 cm.	
Cavity	12 cm.	12 cm.	12 cm.	
Outlet	13 cm.	12 cm.	11 cm.	Anterior-posterior view of pelvis

The other types of pelvises are android (male), anthropoid (ape-like) and platypelloid (flat) pelvis. The varieties of pelvises are illustrated and described in the following tables and charts.

Gynecoid	Anthropoid	Android	Platypelloid
Brim	Brim	Brim	Brim
Cavity	Cavity	Cavity	Cavity
Distance between ischial spines			
Sacrum	Sacrum	Sacrum	Sacrum
Side walls of cavity	Side walls of cavity	Side walls of cavity	Side walls of cavity
Outlet	Outlet	Outlet	Outlet
Distance between the ischial tuberosities			

PELVIC FEATURE	GYNECOID (FEMALE)	ANTHROPOID	ANDROID (MALE)	PLATYPELLOID (FLAT)
Incidence among ♀	41%	23.5% white 40.5% ♀ of color	32.5% white 15.7% ♀ of color	<3%
Bone structure	Smooth, light	Smooth, light	Heavy	Medium
Shape of brim	Bowl shaped with dent in back	Egg shaped, with wide end in back	Triangular, wedge shaped, heart shaped (point in front)	Kidney shaped (kidney lying sideways with dent in back)
Anterior pelvis	Well-rounded	Long & deep but rounded	Narrow & sharply angulated	Shallow
Posterior pelvis	Broad, deep & roomy	Long & deep, but narrow	Shallow; sacral promontory indents inlet, reducing capacity	Shallow
Angle of the sacrum	Approximately 100°	Approximately 100°	90° or less	More than 90°
Sacrum/pubic bone relationship	Parallel	Parallel	Convergent (funnel shaped)	Divergent
Length of sacrospinous ligament	2½ to 3 fingers	<3 fingers, runs front to back	>2 fingers or less	<3 fingers, runs from the back to the side
Sacrosciatic notch	Well rounded, shallow, wide	Average height, shallow, wider	High arch, narrow	Wide, shallow
Subpubic arch	At least 85°	More than 80°	Narrowed	More than 85°
Splay angle) of side walls	Parallel or straight	Parallel or straight	Convergent, funneled	Straight or slightly divergent
Ischial spines	Not prominent	Variable, often prominent with blunt end and broad base	Prominent, sharp and projecting into midpelvis	Variable
Anterior/posterior diameter of the outlet	Long	Very long	Shortened	Very long

Clinical examination of the pelvis

With these differences in mind, we can now discuss the clinical procedure for assessing the pelvis. Pelvimetry will be far more revealing if it is postponed until the early third trimester. This allows time for the hormones of pregnancy to affect the soft tissues of the pelvis; your exam will not only be more revealing for you but less uncomfortable for the woman. In a nutshell, here are the different steps in the examination of the pelvis:

The Pelvimetry Exam

Note: height, weight, age, race and largest baby delivered
Skeletal features: note symmetry of shoulders, thoracic & lumbar spine, pelvic crests &
  lower extremities
External pelvic diameters: if indicated
External genitals: note relationship of symphysis to perineum (with woman lying down,
  legs bent & knees spread) Are the genitals at a slight angle posteriorly, do they recede
  sharply, or do they bulge forward below the pubic bone?
Locate & evaluate cervix: is it tipped forward, backwards or displaced to the side? Any
  unusual features?
Check subpubic arch: is it narrow, average or wide?
Inclination of symphysis pubis: is it parallel, anterior, or posterior?
Check inner surface of pubic bone: note depth, thickness and any irregularities.
Assess forepelvis: is it rounded or angular?
Locate & assess ischial spines: are they small, blunt, prominent, encroaching?
  Is one different than the other?
Interspinous diameter: is it average, wide, or narrow?
Angle of the side walls: are they parallel, convergent or flared outward?
Sacral tip & coccyx: is the coccyx movable or fixed? What is its position?
Sacrosciatic notch (sacrospinous ligament): length by fingerbreadths
Level of sacral tip relative to ischial spines: are the spines above, below, or level with the
  sacral tip?
Diagonal conjugate of outlet: is it at least 11.5 cm.?
Width, curvature & inclination of sacrum: is it average, wide or narrow; hollow, flat or
  J-shaped; average, forward or posteriorly inclined?
Compare sacral inclination with that of symphysis: Are they parallel?
Diagonal conjugate of inlet: is it 11.5 cm. or more? Did you account for pubic bone
  findings when measuring?
Check perineal muscles for strength & tone & instruct in yoni stretching
Assess external bituberous diameter: is it 8 cm. or more?

A word to students: It will be helpful to have a model of the pelvis on hand. You can follow the explanations throughout this chapter and practice on the model. This will greatly assist you in identifying landmarks and learning the maneuvers.

How thorough an exam in necessary? Some midwives feel it is adequate to examine only one side of the pelvis, reasoning that, unless a woman has obvious deformities, both sides will be fairly symmetrical. While this is often the case, it is by no means true all of the time. Asymmetries both of bone structure and more commonly muscle tone can be noted in very normal women. Therefore, I recommend examining both sides of the pelvis. If it is very difficult for you to do this with your dominant hand, you may switch hands when examining the opposite side; however this means more inserting of fingers and increases her discomfort.

Measuring your fingers: Before proceeding with this exam, determine the length of the fingers of your examining hand. To do so, hold the index and second fingers of your dominant hand out straight and point your thumb straight up. Now use a centimeter ruler or flexible tape to measure from the web of skin at the juncture where the thumb joins the hand to the tip of your second finger. Press the measuring device first lightly, then firmly into the thumb joint, using the same amount of force you will use when you press against the pubic bone while reaching for deeper pelvis structures such as the diagonal conjugate. When measuring your fingers by yourself, a ruler is easier to use than a tape.

Now, make a fist, and measure from the outside of your index knuckle to the outside of the knuckle of your little finger. If this measures less than 8 cm., position your thumb in line with the index finger's knuckle and remeasure until you come up with at least 8 cm. You can use your fist a guide during exams.

Observations: Clinical estimation of the pelvis begins by observing the woman when she is on her feet and while she is walking. Note her posture, her gait, the symmetry of her stance, the level of the iliac crests relative to each other and the curvature of her spine. From behind, note the diamond-shaped area formed by the dimples of the posterior-superior spines of the ilia, the lines formed by the gluteal muscles and the groove at the end of the spine, which we shall call the Rhomboid of Venus (also known as the Rhomboid of Michaëlis). Asymmetries in any of these features may point to a pelvic abnormality. Minor asymmetries such as one leg being shorter than the other can often be corrected with chiropractic adjustments, as can minor pelvic misalignment. Next, note her height and weight (already recorded on her chart) and her largest baby (if she has had any!). Also visualize the relationship of the genitals and internal soft structures to the bony pelvis; this will assist you in locating landmarks during the exam.

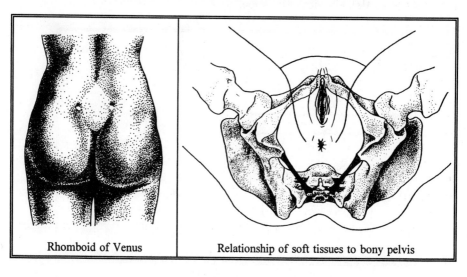

| Rhomboid of Venus | Relationship of soft tissues to bony pelvis |

Before you do the exam: Explain exactly what you will be doing and why before you perform any internal pelvic exam. It is most helpful to have a pelvic model on hand to demonstrate the exam. Using the pelvis and perhaps a doll, show how the baby passes through the true pelvis. Tell the woman that certain parts of the exam will require pressure and will therefore be uncomfortable, especially finding the ischial spines, which necessitates touching the pudendal nerve.

Next, have the woman disrobe from the waist down and position herself for an internal exam. This exam is much easier to perform with the woman on a firm surface such an examining table or a carpeted floor with a firm pillow elevating her buttocks slightly, but it may be done on a bed if necessary. Whatever you use, the woman's bottom should be just over the edge of the exam surface to give you good mobility during the exam. She should be lying on her back with her feet flat on the floor or placed on a firm support such as a phone book to either side, supported by chairs if on a bed, or in stirrups if on a table.

If possible, an assistant can record your findings in the chart as you go through the exam, thus making your task easier. If this is not possible, you'll have to remember your findings and record them after you are done or use a voice activated tape recorder during the exam. Constantly stopping the exam to write is unduly aggravating to the woman and irritating to her tissues.

The external pelvis: Measurement of the external pelvis has fallen by the wayside, primarily because it is recognized that the false pelvis gives no absolute indication of the dimensions of the true pelvis. External measurements are perhaps most useful in populations where pelvic abnormalities secondary to rickets may be more common. It is somewhat difficult to measure the external pelvis if pregnancy is advanced. A pelvimeter helps with this, although the measurements can be taken with a standard flexible measuring tape.

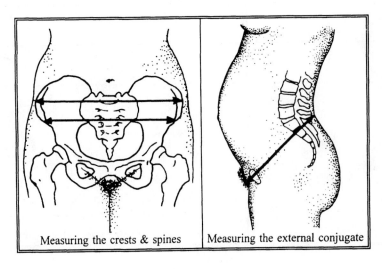

| Measuring the crests & spines | Measuring the external conjugate |

Over the years a number of external measurements have been suggested. We shall review three which have been consistently recommended: the inner aspect of the pelvic crests, the outer aspect of the iliac spines and the external conjugate (Baudelocque's diameter) which is mainly used to differentiate a flat pelvis.

The pelvic crests are measured straight across the abdomen from side to side and should be approximately 28 cm. apart. The iliac spines are located and measured in the same fashion and average 24 cm. apart. The external conjugate is measured from the anterior symphysis pubis to the depression below the spine of the fifth lumbar vertebrae in back. When a pelvimeter is used to take this measurement, the average range falls between 18 to 20 cm. When a tape measure is used it is placed with the zero end on the pubic bone and wrapped around the hip to L5 in back, keeping the tape parallel with the pubic bone as much as possible. Subtract 8 to 8.5 cm. (if the woman is large) from the total tape measurement to arrive at the external conjugate measurement.

The external genitals: As you look at a woman genitals, note any scar tissue from previous cuts or tears, or other unusual findings. If you have performed a previous genital exam, you may want to refer to your notes. Observe the relationship of the symphysis pubis to the perineum. In women with a pronounced anthropoid pelvic shape, the genitals appear to recede at a right angle to the plane of the pubic bone. In an android pelvis, the genitals may appear to bulge out in front of the pubic bone. Gynecoid and platypelloid pelvises show the genitalia sloping off at a gentle angle posteriorly from the angle of the pubic bone; this angle is not pronounced.

Beginning the internal exam: Don two gloves; they need not be sterile but should fit well. This enhances your ability to feel pelvic landmarks and anything unusual that you might find during your exam. Apply lubricant to the index finger of your examining hand. Place the other hand on the woman's leg, and, as you do, tell her you are touching her. Continue talking to her about what you are doing: "I'm touching the opening of your yoni, I'm going to insert one finger, now two, etc . .." Whenever you are performing an exam of any kind always go slowly, continue to discuss your findings and your next step with the woman, and, if she suddenly seems tense, in pain or afraid keep your hand still without removing it and question her as to what she is feeling. Position yourself so that you can maintain eye contact with her throughout the exam.

Finding the cervix: It can be easy to get confused when doing pelvic exams, especially when you are inexperienced. Locating the cervix first can help you navigate through the other soft tissues as you are looking for landmarks. After inserting two fingers into the yoni, follow the birth passage straight up and back until you reach the cervix. Note which direction the os (opening) is pointing and any unusual features, irregularities or growths. (Also see cervical examination details in the chapter on The Physical Examination of the Woman in this section.)

Checking the sub-pubic arch: Next withdraw your fingers slightly, placing their middle joints directly beneath the center of the pubic arch. In the gynecoid pelvis, two fingers will easily fit beneath the arch. If only one finger fits; this is a narrow angle, if three fit, the angle is wide. This arch should be at least 90°. Be sure you are measuring immediately beneath the lower border of the bone itself, not below that point.

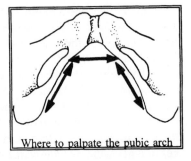

Where to palpate the pubic arch

Checking the inclination of the symphysis pubis: While your fingers are still near the pubic bone, assess its angle in relation to the rest of the pelvis. To do so, straddle your two fingers on either side of the urethra and press them flatly up on the inner surface of the pubic bone. Now note the position of your fingers. Do you feel a slightly inclined surface (parallel), or does the lower border of the pubic bone tip toward you (anterior inclination) or does the lower border of the pubic bone tip inward necessitating your fingers to reach up and around to find the upper border of the bone (i.e. is it tipped posteriorly)? The pubic bone may be inclined in the following ways:

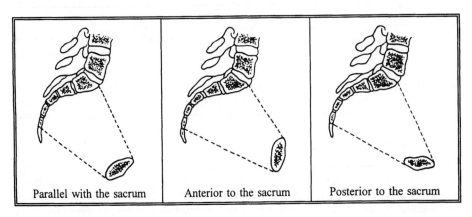

| Parallel with the sacrum | Anterior to the sacrum | Posterior to the sacrum |

The longitudinal axis of the symphysis pubis is normally parallel with the longitudinal axis of the sacrum. If the symphysis pubis is not parallel with the sacrum, the anterior-posterior diameter of the inlet can be reduced significantly.

Check the inner surface of the pubic bone: With your internal fingers still in this position, reach to the top of the symphysis on the inside with your index finger. Use your other index finger to mark the internal depth of the pubic bone from the top edge to the bottom edge. To do so place your other finger at a right-angle in the pubic arch to measure your internal finger. Next using your internal finger, feel to see if any protruding lumps or bumps are present on the inner surface. If the depth of the pubis is 6 cm. or more, it is high. If the upper border of the pubis is quite inwardly inclined, is extremely thick or has lumps on its posterior surface, the actual space at the level of the diagonal conjugate will be reduced. (Greenhill, 1951)

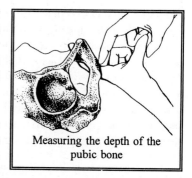

Measuring the depth of the pubic bone

Checking the forepelvis: Before you leave this area, feel either side of the symphysis pubis along the upper inner rami of the pubic bone back toward the sides to determine how round the anterior portion of the pelvis seems to be. The inner curvature of the forepelvis should be rounded. If the forepelvis angles rather than curves towards the sides, this decreases the oblique diameters of the inlet.

Finding the ischial spines: Now, place your fingers in the center of the inner surface of the pubic bone, to one side of the symphysis. Staying in contact with the bone as much as possible, slowly sweep your fingers down and further inside in a wide arch and ask the woman to tell you when she feels you have hit a nerve. You are looking for the ischial spine, which is right beside the pudendal nerve. Once you find the nerve, feel up, down, backward and forward until you find a small bony prominence. This could feel like anything from a sharp spiny projection to a rounded lentil-like bump. Some women have no spines at all. Without removing your hand from the yoni, rotate your thumb down and around so that your palm is facing the opposite direction. Now follow the pubic bone on the other side and locate the other ischial spine.

Another way to locate the spines is to follow the upper rami of the pubic bone on one side to the lateral portion of the pelvic inlet. Then draw your fingers down the pelvic sidewall to the ischial spine. Be sure to get to the lateral portion of the pelvis before moving downwards. If you start moving your fingers down when they are not deep enough, you will come to the tuberosity, not the spine. With this exam you may also note the angle of the pelvic sidewalls.

The interspinous diameter: Now that you know where both spines are located, you can measure the distance between them. Keep your fingers at the level of the spine you just found. Position yourself so that your fingers, wrist and forearm are all in a straight line. Now, keeping them as straight as possible, sweep your fingers across the center of the pelvic cavity to the other ischial spine several times. (This

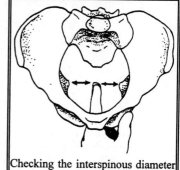

Checking the interspinous diameter

assessment cannot be made if the fingers are allowed to flex.) As you do so, assess how much space appears to be between the two spines; pay attention to bony, not merely soft tissue restriction. A transversely narrowed pelvis will restrict your side-to-side finger motion; this will also occur with firm musculature or if you are doing the exam so early in pregnancy that the tissues have not sufficiently softened to allow palpation of the bones beneath them. The level of the ischial spines is also called the midplane of the pelvis, the plane of least dimensions and the narrowest part of the pelvis the fetus must pass through. It usually measures about 10 cm. across the center (transverse diameter).

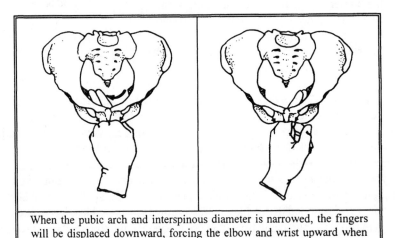

When the pubic arch and interspinous diameter is narrowed, the fingers will be displaced downward, forcing the elbow and wrist upward when sweeping across the cavity.

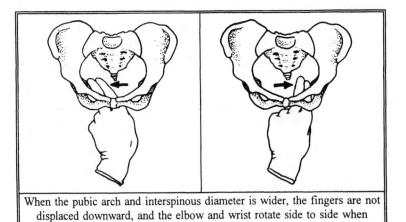

When the pubic arch and interspinous diameter is wider, the fingers are not displaced downward, and the elbow and wrist rotate side to side when sweeping across the cavity.

The angle of the side walls: The angle (or splay) of the internal side walls of the pelvis may be somewhat evident from the last procedure. For further evaluation place your internal fingers as high as possible above one of the obturator foramen areas. Place the thumb of the examining hand externally on the ischial tuberosity on that side. Now press your internal fingers against the pubic ramus and slowly draw them down toward your thumb. Note if the wall feels as if it is converging, straight, or flaring out as you do so. The better the muscle tone, the harder this is to do.

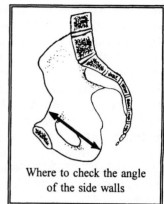

Where to check the angle of the side walls

Another way to evaluate the splay of the walls is to use your internal hand to follow the upper border of the rami of the pubic bone on one side to the lateral portion of the pelvic inlet. Then draw your fingers down the pelvic sidewall to the ischial spine. Be sure to get to the lateral portion of the pelvis before moving downwards. If you start down too early you will come to the tuberosity, not the spine. You may also try to locate the spines during this maneuver, especially if they were hard to find.

Checking the sacral tip and coccyx: Locate the coccyx bimanually. Place your nondominant hand under the woman's buttocks, about 1 inch (2 cm.) above her anus. Now turn your internal hand palm-downward and curve your examining fingers slightly. Making a rubbing motion, press deeply into the posterior wall of the yoni with your fingers inserted about 3 inches. If you run into a soft lumpy mass, this is the colon. Move your fingers to the side and push it aside gently in order to reach the coccyx. Using both your examining hand and your external hand, rock the tissue between your fingers back and forth, moving your fingers up and down until you come to a movable bone; this is the coccyx.

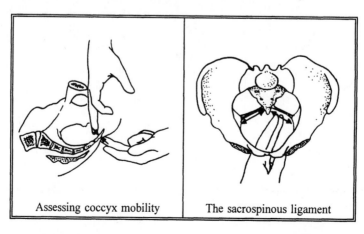

| Assessing coccyx mobility | The sacrospinous ligament |

Note how much mobility there is in the joint. The woman can often tell you when she feels the coccyx being moved. The coccyx may fuse and become immobile if injured. An immobile coccyx may have to be broken during pushing to allow normal birth.

Examine the sacrosciatic ligament: Keep your examining fingers at the tip of the sacrum. Feel to one side for the firm, band-like ligament which attaches there; this is called the sacrospinous ligament. Once you have identified it, follow it anteriorly to the ischial spine on that side and assess its length in fingers. The length of this ligament tells us two things: the angle of the sacrum and the width of the sacrosciatic notch (which cannot be directly examined because it is too deep within the pelvis). Following this ligament to the spines is another way to double check your findings when the spines have been hard or impossible to locate.

SACROSCIATIC LIGAMENT LENGTH (IN FINGERS)	SACRAL TIP POSITION	SACROSCIATIC NOTCH
2 or less	Tipped forward	Narrow
2½ to 3	Average	Average
3 or more	Tipped backward	Wide

Note the level of the sacral tip in relationship to the spines: Now you have an idea of the location of the ischial spines in relationship to the sacral tip (where the sacrococcygeal joint is located). Before moving on, keep one finger on the sacral tip and sweep the other finger over to locate an ischial spine. Note whether the spines are above, below or level with the sacral tip. Be sure you have the tip of the sacrum, where the upper coccyx joins it, not the tip of the coccyx itself. Since the coccyx usually moves back and out of the way during birth, its position is not as relevant.

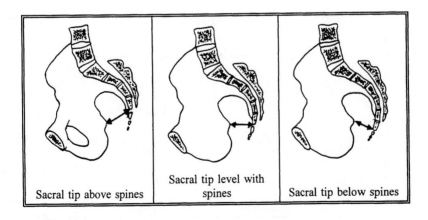

Sacral tip above spines | Sacral tip level with spines | Sacral tip below spines

If the sacrum inclines forward to a marked degree, but is long and extends below the level of the ischial spines this will not affect the descent of the baby during labor. The space in the midpelvis is reduced when the sacral tip is forward or elevated to the same level as the spines.

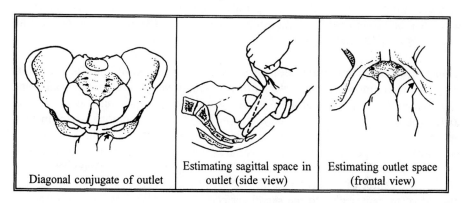

| Diagonal conjugate of outlet | Estimating sagittal space in outlet (side view) | Estimating outlet space (frontal view) |

The diagonal conjugate of the outlet: Place your examining finger on the sacrococcygeal joint and bring your hand upright so that it is in alignment with the bottom border of the symphysis pubis. This measurement should be about 11.5 cm., and is the diagonal conjugate of the outlet. Keep your internal finger on the sacral tip. Now, use the thumb of the examining hand to find the inside curve of the adjacent section of the pubic ramus. Straighten your hand so that it is at a horizontal plane to the pelvic brim. Measure from the tip of the sacrum to your thumb pad. This distance gives you a good idea of the space at the pelvic outlet.

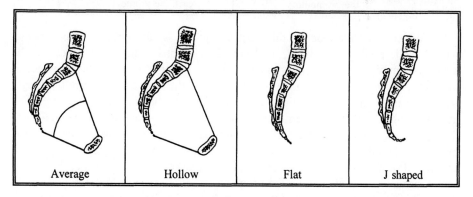

| Average | Hollow | Flat | J shaped |

The width, curvature and inclination of the sacrum: At this point keep your fingers straight, tips against the sacrum. From the sacral tip, slowly follow the center of the sacral bone upwards, noting its depth of concavity (curvature) and its inclination. Spread your fingers as you go to get an impression of its width as well. Curvature is estimated as either average, marked (hollow), straight (flat) or

J shaped. Inclination is noted as either forward, average or backward.

Compare the inclination of the sacrum with that of the symphysis pubis: Also compare the inclination of the sacrum with your findings regarding the inclination of the symphysis pubis. Are they parallel, or is the pubic bone inclined either anteriorly or posteriorly in relationship to the sacrum. (Refer to page 462 for an illustration of this relationship).

Find the sacral promontory and estimate the diagonal conjugate of the inlet: As your fingers move up the center of the sacrum, lower your elbow thus allowing your fingers to be directed at a 45° angle toward the upper sacrum. If you do not lower your elbow, you may think you have found the promontory when, in fact, you are below it. As you place your fingers in the posterior fornix, press your hand against the perineum to afford maximum reach. This exam is also hampered by a full lower bowel, which will feel like a doughy, lumpy, somewhat mobile mass in the center of the sacral surface. Move your fingers to one side and gently displace it to gain access to the sacral surface.

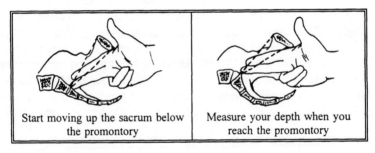

| Start moving up the sacrum below the promontory | Measure your depth when you reach the promontory |

When you have reached the most prominent sacral bone, maintain contact with it while raising your wrist, until your hand contacts the lower border of the symphysis pubis. Use your non-dominant index finger to mark the point which is touching the symphysis. Remove your hand from the yoni and measure the length from your mark to your fingertips. This will give you the diagonal conjugate. The average length is 12 to 12.5 cm. Many midwives with short fingers cannot reach this landmark. If that is true for you, note that the conjugate is greater than the maximum length of your fingers. A promontory which juts forward is often associated with a backward sacral inclination or marked sacral curvature. However, sacral curvature can also make the promontory more difficult to reach.

The diagonal conjugate of the inlet is not really the diameter through which the baby must pass. There are actually three conjugates:

*The **true conjugate** or *conjugata vera* runs from the middle of the uppermost border of the pubic bone to the midpoint of the sacral promontory. It normally measures 11 cm. or more. (V in drawing)

*The **birth (obstetrical) conjugate** extends from the middle of the symphysis pubis on its inner surface a short distance below its upper-most border (i.e. at its uppermost thickest point) to the midpoint of the sacral promontory. This is the narrowest front to back plane through which the baby must pass. It usually measures at least 10 cm. (B in drawing)

*The **diagonal conjugate** extends from the middle of the sacral promontory to the middle of the lower border of the symphysis. It is the only diameter that can be clinically assessed and should be at least 11.5 cm. (D in drawing)

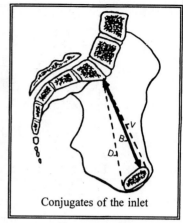

Conjugates of the inlet

The true conjugate is determined by subtracting 1 to 1.5 cm. from the diagonal conjugate measurement. Deduct the higher amount if the pubic bone is thick or wide. If the pubic bone is more than 6 cm. wide from the top to the bottom edge, 2 or 2.5 cm. must be deducted. If the upper border of the pubis inclines more than usual toward the sacrum, or it is extremely thick, or there is a lump on the inner surface of the pubis, 2 or even 3 cm. may have to be deducted to assess the conjugate. (Greenhill, 1951)

Checking the perineal muscles: Position your examining fingers so that the middle joints are in line with the urogenital diaphragm. Now ask the woman to tighten the muscles of her yoni as much as possible. As she does so, identify the muscle group with your fingers and note any areas of unusual tension or relaxation; be sure to check both sides. Show her how to do yoni stretching, using her muscles as a guide. (The next chapter includes a complete discussion of examining the pelvic muscles and instructing women in yoni stretching.)

Measuring the external bituberous diameter: Remove your hand from the yoni. Using the thumbs of both hands, palpate down the pubic rami to the tips of the ischial tuberosities. Measure the transverse diameter of the outlet by placing your fist between the tuberosities. Press your fist into the perineum so that your knuckles are between the tips of the tuberosities. The thickness of the woman's soft tissues may make the actual bony diameter about 1 cm. larger than the measurement of your fist. Do not add this to your measurement but take it into consideration when making your evaluation of the available space, for example, if the woman is very large.

478

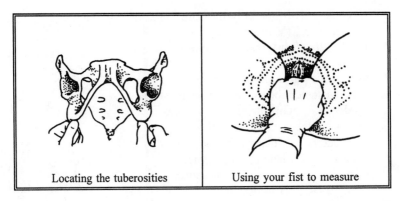

Locating the tuberosities	Using your fist to measure

If you have difficulty locating the tuberosities, have the woman reach around her outer thighs and locate them for you.

When you are through with your exam, hand the woman a few tissues so she can wipe herself (or wipe her yourself), and then go wash your hands while she dresses.

Upon completing this exam you will have some idea of the woman's pelvic dimensions and contours when she is lying down flat with her legs up. Always remember that the pelvis is flexible and that these dimensions change as the woman changes her position.

References and further reading

Greenhill, J., Principles and Practice of Obstetrics, W. B. Saunders, Co., Philadelphia, PA, 1951.
Moloy, Howard, Evaluation of the Pelvis in Obstetrics, 3rd ed., Plenum Medical Book Co., New York, 1975.
Oxhorn, Harry, Human Labor and Birth, 5th ed., Appleton-Century-Crofts, Norwalk, Ct., 1986.
Varney, Helen, Nurse-Midwifery, Blackwell Scientific Pub., Inc., Boston, MA, 1980.
Whitley, Nancy, A Manual of Clinical Obstetrics, J.B. Lippincott Co., Philadelphia, PA, 1985.

Examining the Muscles of the Perineum and Explaining Perineal Stretching

Part of an internal pelvic exam includes assessing the tone of the various muscles of the yoni. This can be done quickly by asking the woman to tighten her muscles around your examining fingers. If the need arises for a more thorough exam, the following techniques can be used:

Palpate the clitoral sponge: To orient yourself, place two fingers inside the opening of the yoni with the pads facing 3 or 9 o'clock. With your thumb, gently palpate the external tissue at the inner junction of the labia majora and minora (along the inside of the pubic rami). Notice the spongy feel? This is the clitoral sponge encased in the bulbocavernosus muscle. Have the woman tighten the mouth of her yoni and note the contraction of the bulbocavernosus muscle as she does so.

Locate the urogenital triangle: Now, using the fingers inside the yoni, palpate the much firmer muscle behind this layer on either side. This is the urogenital diaphragm (the deep transverse perineal muscle).

Identify the hymenal ring or tags: Note the hymenal ring or tags and the location of the muscles in relationship to it. This will vary from woman to woman.

Find the levator ani muscle: Behind the deep transverse muscle (urogenital diaphragm) and wrapping around the middle third of the yoni is the multilayered levator ani muscle. When tone is good, this muscle will be approximately 2 to 3 fingerbreadths deep (4 to 6 cm.). It should offer strong resistance even when relaxed; making the yoni long, cylindrical and snug.

Weak levator ani muscles are indicated by the need to press more deeply into the wall of the yoni to locate them. The depth of firmness from front to back will be less, and the muscle will sag toward the opening of the yoni rather than spanning the middle third.

Have the woman contract her pelvic floor muscles (Kegel). Place the tip of your dominant index finger about 4.5 cm. inside against the yoni wall at 3 or 9 o'clock. Locate the levator ani and follow it up to its attachment behind the pubic bone. Now, locate the more shallow deep transverse muscle just in front of the levator ani and try to insert your fingertip into the angle they form. Lack of tension or inability to locate this angle suggests muscular damage or weakness.

Follow each muscle as it comes to meet the central perineal body located immediately behind the junction of the anal sphincter. Note how far these landmarks are from the perineal surface and the length of the perineum from the introitus of the yoni to the anal opening.

480

The anal sphincter: The muscle just behind the upper center of the perineal skin surface (above the anus) is the sphincter. If the perineum is short, you will also feel it immediately beneath the floor of the yoni. (This is because a short perineum leaves very little perineal body to rest above it.) In a short perineum, note how little of the perineal body there is to allow the muscles to thin during birth.

Next, press down into the sphincter and have the woman constrict the opening of her yoni; note how that feels on your fingers. Have her relax.

The depth and length of the perineal body: When the perineum is short, tears are more likely. To get a sense of the relationship of the perineal muscles to the length and depth of the perineal body, first, place your thumb in the center of the perineum and the index and ring finger of the same hand about 5 cm. inside the yoni at the 6 o'clock point. Now, pull down and forward with your yoni fingers while pressing into the perineum just above the anus with your thumb. Your yoni fingers should run into the deep transverse perineal muscle. You may be able to identify the levator ani meeting horizontal to the more vertical line of the deep transverse perineal muscle (urogenital diaphragm) from behind. At the same time, you will be able to get a good idea of how much perineal body exists between the surface of the floor of the yoni and the top surface of the anal sphincter. Press into the perineum with your thumb and have her contract her muscles. Note the depth of the perineal body in front of the superficial transverse muscle.

Perineal stretching: In my experience, the biggest factor in preventing tears has been a daily, five minute session of perineal stretching, starting six weeks before the due date. Its purpose is to encourage elasticity and help the mother learn to relax and feel comfortable with the sensations of stretching and burning which occur as the head distends the perineum. Pelvic floor exercises should continue through the last six weeks as well, so that elasticity (not laxness) is encouraged.

Perineal stretching should not be started too early in pregnancy. The hormones will not have sufficiently softened the tissue, and it is more traumatic than helpful. Thirty four weeks is a good time to begin with daily sessions, lasting no less than five minutes and no longer than fifteen. You may find it best to postpone this explanation until the prenatal before stretching should begin so the technique is fresh in her mind. Show the partner what needs to be done, unless for religious or other reasons the mother does not want them involved.

To lubricate the fingers, use either a water-based product (such as K-Y, Astrolube or Replens) or a pure vegetable oil. Water-based lubricant is preferred if there is a tendency to develop yeast infections. Petroleum-based products, (mineral oil or petroleum jelly), should not be used. They clog pores and leach vitamins from the tissue.

Rubbing from side to side and massage is painful and irritating to most women. Instead, have the partner place lubricated fingers or thumbs in both sides of the opening of the yoni to the depth of the deep transverse muscle (about 2 to

3 cm. in). The mother then tightens her muscles around the fingers to ensure that the proper landmark is identified. Now the stretcher directs bilateral pressure down and outward toward each ischial tuberosity or "sit bone" (at about 4 and 8 o'clock), while the mother breathes into her abdomen deeply and consciously exaggerates the relaxation of her muscles. When she begins to feel stretching or burning discomfort, or the partner feels an area of resistance, the partner holds the stretch for thirty seconds to a minute while the woman breathes into the tension to consciously relax the area; then the partner slowly applies more pressure, cycling between stretching, breathing and pressure to gradually allow the woman's body to accustom itself to the changes. The stretch can then be held longer and more steadily. To minimize shoulder discomfort for partners doing the stretching with two hands, cross the forearms at the wrists. A hot bath before each session will help soften the tissues. (Loprenzi-Kassel, 1995)

As practice continues and muscles become more elastic, more fingers can be used and the stretch increased until the partner's entire fist can fit inside the band of muscles. This promotes familiarity with the sensations of crowning and really helps women get used to the burning they will experience during birth.

If the partner is unwilling or unavailable, the woman can stretch her yoni herself. Either squatting or lying down with her legs up, she reaches around under her thighs on either side and stretches down and out toward her tuberosities with her index fingers. Or, she can reach between her legs and stretch with her thumbs. Many women find that hot baths are the perfect place to practice.

Occasionally a woman who has herpes will note that yoni stretching causes flare-ups. Should this occur, discontinue stretching and use supportive therapies to heal the lesions. (See Diagnostic Tests for a discussion of herpes in pregnancy.)

Women who have previously had clitorotomies or epidural anesthesia should be warned that they will feel considerably more stretching and burning when no clitorotomy is performed. During pushing, unprepared women are often alarmed by these sensations, insisting that something is wrong. Explain the benefits of an intact birth and what to expect. Prenatal stretching will help them immensely.

Some women have previous scars that are thick or painful. They can massage a mixture of vitamin E and Evening Primrose oil from opened capsules directly into the scar tissue during stretching. This helps make the scar more flexible. Oil from capsules is the most potent because it has been protected from exposure to air and light, which cause oxidation and breakdown of the oils.

All women (especially first-time and YBAC mothers) should visualize the head descending and stretching the yoni when they do their exercises. They need a strong image of birth (always including normal baby and placental delivery, and the uterus clamping down). Birth is a normal process, and they can do it!

References and further reading:
Loprenzi-Kassel, ClaraBeth, lisenced midwife, Veneta, OR, editing comments, 2/95.
Whitley, Nancy, A Manual of Clinical Obstetrics, J.B. Lippincott Co., Philadelphia, PA 1985.

482

Assessing Cervical Changes During Pregnancy

Throughout pregnancy the cervix undergoes various changes in preparation for birth. Knowing what to look for during exams will help in assessing the cervix during miscarriage; distinguishing the breech from the vertex; when determining how well prepared the cervix is for birth in late pregnancy; and when assessing labor, either of premature onset or at term. Some of these factors are mentioned in other parts of the text; we will review changes that occur throughout pregnancy and their assessment in this chapter. More details will be included in Volume II.

Cervical anatomy: In the non-pregnant woman, the lower part of the uterus narrows to form a tight neck which comprises about half the length of the entire uterus in the nullipara, and about one-third its length in a multipara. The uppermost portion of this neck is referred to as the uterine isthmus. Before pregnancy this is a narrowed portion of the uterine wall which begins where the cavity of the uterus and the neck of the cervix start (the inner mouth of the cervix) and ends where the cervical passageway begins. The isthmus divides two regions which are histologically distinguished by the change from endometrial tissue to the tissue lining the cervical passageway. As term approaches, the isthmus softens, then thins and elongates to form the lower uterine segment.

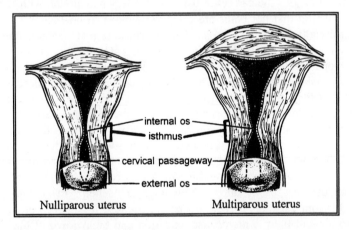

internal os	
isthmus	
cervical passageway	
external os	
Nulliparous uterus	Multiparous uterus

Performing a cervical exam: Do not attempt internal exams with the woman's bottom sinking into a soft bed. Have her urinate, remove her clothing and lie on a firm surface, such as an exam table, carpeted floor or firm mattress. Place a towel or disposable underpad beneath her before you begin. Ask her to allow her knees to fall open. A well-fitting glove will help you feel subtleties during exams.

First trimester: First trimester changes are reviewed in the chapter on Early Signs of Pregnancy in the section on the First Trimester. Aside from a speculum exam to assess if the cervix is normal, your main reason for doing an exam in early pregnancy is to assess changes in relationship to a possible miscarriage, although this is not usually necessary. Don a sterile glove and introduce one and then two fingers into the yoni. Advance your fingers inside, following a yoni wall, until you come to a fornix. Gently move your fingers over the edge of the cervix toward the center until you have identified the os. In a first-time mother the closed os will feel like a small round dimple. In a multipara it may feel like a larger dimple and may even partially admit your fingertip; however, although the outer os will often be open the cervical canal will form a funnel shape and prevent your finger from contacting the amniotic membranes. In early pregnancy the normal cervix is not prepared to open, and effacement will not occur to the degree that it would at term. While the cervix is softer than it is when a woman is not pregnant, it is also not nearly as soft as it would be at term. When checking the cervix for miscarriage, changes are assessed as described below for evaluating the cervix during labor.

Second trimester: The external cervical changes which began in the first trimester are maintained during the second trimester. Normally other changes do not occur until the late second trimester, when minor degrees of dilation may occur in normal women (Gabbe, 1991, p. 859). In women who have a constitutionally loose cervix, painless effacement and dilation may commence undetected by the mother until effacement is nearly complete and 2 to 4 cm. of dilation has already taken place. Typically in these cases the forewaters "hourglass" through the os, and the unequal pressure and preterm conditions cause them to rupture. Therefore, in women who have a history of second trimester miscarriage, known reproductive abnormalities, prior cervical trauma or prenatal DES exposure, it may be prudent to do a gentle internal exam between 12 and 16 weeks to detect any changes. If caught in time, a woman can begin to take False Unicorn Root tincture or consider bed rest or the surgical placement of a cerclage to prevent further cervical changes. If the cervix is quite abnormal, herbs alone will *not* prevent dilation. (See chapter on Loose Cervix the section on Second Trimester Problems for more details.)

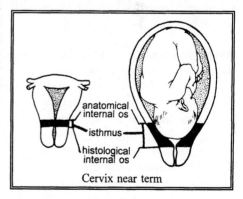

Cervix near term

Third trimester: Starting between 28 to 34 weeks women usually begin to feel twinges in their cervix. These signal that the lower uterine segment is stretching as the baby gets larger and the cervix is becoming increasingly soft or ripe in preparation for birth. Ripening occurs because the structure of the cervix undergoes changes secondary to hormonal influences. Some women will experience slight effacement and the os may more readily admit a fingertip, especially if the woman has given birth before. However, changes are typically slow and slight until the last few weeks prior to the onset of labor. During this time cervical softening becomes more pronounced, progressing to a mushy feel and, in some cases, effacement and dilation begin as well. Cervical softening causes scarred areas to become softer; a multiparous cervix sometimes takes on a ruffled feeling around its edge. The primary reasons you will be checking the cervix in late pregnancy are: to discover if softening or ripening is occurring in a woman who is unsure of her dates or is overdue; to assess whether a baby is lying breech; to see if changes are occurring due to possible premature labor or the onset of normal labor at term. Do not do an exam if placenta previa is suspected as a torrential hemorrhage may be the result. (See chapter on Third Trimester Bleeding for more details.)

Cervical changes during labor: In late pregnancy, the cervical canal is softened and enlarged; it has two ends, referred to as the internal os and external os. Effacement refers to the gradual taking up or thinning of this canal. This usually takes place from the inside out; that is, the internal os dilates first, causing the cervical canal to be gradually "taken up" until finally the passageway disappears when effacement is nearly complete (especially in first-time mothers). Dilation refers to the gradual enlarging or opening of the external os to allow the presenting part of the baby to pass during birth. An easy way to envision this process is to imagine putting on a turtle neck sweater. At the start the long neck approximates the uneffaced and undilated cervix. As you slowly begin to pull the sweater over your head, the length of the neck "effaces" and the hole against your head begins to open as the internal os will do. As the neck is almost taken up, the outer hole begins to enlarge (dilate) to accommodate your head. The cervix changes to allow for birth in much the same fashion.

Assessing cervical changes in late pregnancy: Again, don a glove, and follow the anterior wall of the yoni upward until you stop at the anterior fornix; be sure you have gone far enough to reach the fornix itself and have not been fooled into thinking a fold of the yoni wall anterior to the fornix is, in fact, the cervical lip. Once you reach the anterior fornix, slide your fingers into the center until you find a dimple, depression, or larger opening which will be the cervical os. Insert your fingertip into the os as far as it will go without undue force.

Now assess effacement by estimating the depth of the passage. The uneffaced cervix is 2 to 3 cm. long at the beginning of the third trimester. If the cervix is not effaced at all, this is said to be 0%; it will be maximally long and thick. If it is effaced halfway it is 50% effaced. If it is as thin as possible, it is 100% effaced. Typically the cervix of a first time mother is 70 to 80% effaced prior to dilation beyond 1 or 2 centimeters. In multiparas it is possible for the cervix to be dilated 2 or 3 cm. and sometimes more before much effacement takes place; in most multiparas, 100% effacement never occurs.

To assess dilation, find the cervical opening. In primigravidas, the walls of the cervical passageway usually form a tight tube prior to complete dilation. However, the external cervical os can be loose or even dilated, while the internal os is smaller or closed, forming an inverted funnel (wide end down), particularly in a multipara. In multiparas, when effacement does begin from the internal os downward, the walls of the cervical passageway may also appear funnel-shaped with the internal os forming the wide end (i.e. wide end up). It is the size of the smallest opening that is most important in assessing cervical dilation, regardless of whether that is the internal or external os. Determine this by spreading your index and middle fingers to touch the edges of the os without stretching it. Prior to the onset of active labor, landmarks are sometimes less easy to distinguish; uterine contractions cause the cervical features to tense up and make landmarks more distinct. In addition, the membranes anterior to the presenting part, the forewaters, will also tense up during contractions and will aid in demarcating landmarks. Therefore, go slowly and be sure you have located the correct landmarks before stating your findings. This will greatly increase your accuracy as you are learning.

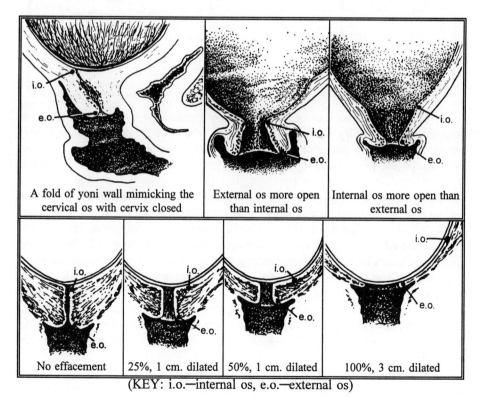

A fold of yoni wall mimicking the cervical os with cervix closed	External os more open than internal os	Internal os more open than external os

No effacement	25%, 1 cm. dilated	50%, 1 cm. dilated	100%, 3 cm. dilated

(KEY: i.o.—internal os, e.o.—external os)

Very rarely, you may discover a rounded, tubular object within the intact membranes; it may or may not be pulsing. This could be the umbilical cord positioned between the presenting part and the membranes (cord previa) rupture of the membranes would likely result in a cord prolapse. Or, it could be due to a cord blood vessel (vasa previa) traversing the membranes distal to its insertion point in the placenta, which is more common in multiple gestations. Should the membranes rupture this vessel could be torn, resulting in fetal bleeding. Visualizing the membranes during a gentle speculum exam may provide more information. The parents should be informed of this possibility and you should discuss the fetal risks and the need for a hospital birth and possibly a surgical delivery.

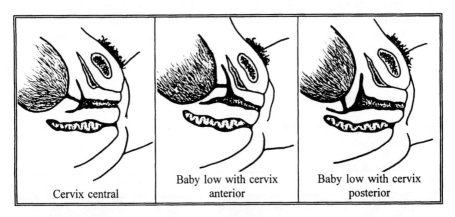

| Cervix central | Baby low with cervix anterior | Baby low with cervix posterior |

The cervical os may not be centrally located at the end of the yoni passageway, especially in a first-time mother whose baby has dropped. It may either be anterior or posterior. Generally when this variation is found it is more pronounced the lower the baby's presenting part is in the pelvis. If the cervix is quite effaced and the os is posterior, it can appear as though the cervix is completely dilated, when, in fact, the os is closed. Have the mother place her fists beneath her buttocks or flex her thighs high on her belly and hold her legs below her knees. Either maneuver will help bring a posterior cervix within easier reach. Feel for the edges of the cervix if you suspect the cervix to be widely dilated, and follow the curve of the baby's presenting part as far as you can toward the pubic bone in front and as far as you can toward the sacrum in back, reaching all the way to the posterior fornix to be sure you haven't missed the os. Assess the feel of the surface within the opening of the cervix; if open with the bag intact it should feel thin and membranous; if the bag is broken you may detect fetal scalp hair, if the "head" is very smooth, think breech or less dilated than you thought; look for the os again.

Distinguishing fetal position during pregnancy: The need to confirm your findings on palpation as to whether the baby is breech or vertex is one reason to do an exam. The fetal parts will be felt through the undilated and usually uneffaced cervix, making your task more difficult and sometimes impossible. Proceed as you would for an internal exam, then use your other hand to press down on the fundus to move the presenting part as low as possible into the pelvis. Reach up with your internal fingers, pressing firmly, and feel around to try and tell what is in the pelvis. Kicks or a bony-feeling pole make the breech likely, although prior to term the fetal skull can feel remarkably irregular in contour.

If the membranes are ruptured: It is unwise to perform any internal yoni exams if the membranes have ruptured without active labor; to do so invites infection. However there may be times when knowing the condition of the cervix will help you in deciding what to do; for example, if there are no contractions, no evidence of infection and the baby is early, it may be advisable to wait to initiate labor until the woman is closer to term. In such cases it is possible to do a rectal exam

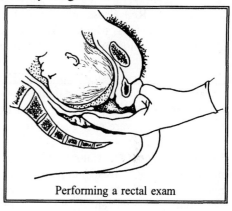

Performing a rectal exam

by inserting fingers into the anus and pressing upward into the anterior rectal wall to feel the cervix. Without practice finding landmarks may be difficult and without active labor, tissues may be so soft that getting any reliable information may be impossible. I mention it only because it is one way to get more information about the condition of the cervix without entering the yoni. *Do not attempt a rectal exam if placenta previa is suspected, it could cause a hemorrhage more severe than when a yoni exam is performed.* In the 1920s, 30s and 40s, rectal exams were used routinely in hospitals to reduce infection rates. They are uncomfortable and you must be very careful not to contaminate the external genitals with fluids or solids from the rectum. Most women will gladly forego such an exam.

If you suspect cord prolapse: If the membranes rupture in late pregnancy and you suspect cord prolapse, rule this out by using a sterile glove to do an internal exam immediately. If found, hold the presenting part up off the cord, place the mother in a knee-chest position, and transport immediately. Tell the mother and baby what is going on, keep communicating the status of the cord to the mother and have her visualize the baby well-oxygenated. Remain with her until a responsible party is ready to take over care in the hospital. (Review the chapter on Cord Prolapse in Volume II for further details.)

Bland, B, & Montgomery, T, <u>Practical Obstetrics</u>, F. A. Davis, Philadelphia, 1935.
Gabbe, ed. <u>Obstetrics: Normal & Problem Pregnancies</u>, 2nd ed., Churchill Livingstone, NY, 1991.
Greenhill, J., <u>Principles and Practice of Obstetrics</u>, W. B. Saunders, Co., Philadelphia, PA, 1951.

Cardiopulmonary Resuscitation and Airway Clearance During Pregnancy

Midwives should be familiar with both adult and newborn CPR. This chapter will review the basics of adult CPR with special emphasis on caring for women during pregnancy. It does not replace classroom study, which is offered through the American Red Cross and the American Heart Association. Check current manuals for details which may have changed since publication of this text. Chapters concerning problems will recommend CPR as appropriate.

Cardiopulmonary resuscitation (CPR): CPR is intended to provide first aid airway and circulatory support until advanced life support measures can be initiated. You are most likely to be called upon to perform adult CPR in rare instances of maternal crisis severe enough to compromise respiratory and/or cardiac function.

Physiologic considerations: As pregnancy advances, maternal blood volume increases with a corresponding increase in cardiac output. Uterine blood flow increases from 2% to up to 30% in late pregnancy and oxygen consumption also rises 20 to 30%. The enlarged uterus presses into the diaphragm and reduces lung capacity by 20%. These changes cause pregnant women to be more susceptible to and less tolerant of major cardiovascular and respiratory insults.

The supine position causes the enlarged uterus to press on the inferior vena cava and the aorta, resulting in a drop in blood pressure and up to a 25% reduction in cardiac output. Performing CPR with the woman flat on her back after 20 weeks of pregnancy severely reduces blood flow to the uterus.

Vomiting and aspiration of gastric contents into the lungs may occur more easily in late pregnancy than in nonpregnant women because stomach emptying is delayed. The enlarged uterus causes the pressure in the stomach to increase, and there is a decrease in the tonicity of the sphincter of the esophagus. Vomiting can be prevented by applying pressure to the cricoid cartilage; this compresses the esophagus against the cervical vertebrae, preventing gastric aspiration and possible vomiting. Although this is a simple technique, it requires two rescuers, and therefore may not be of much use in the rare emergent situation. If a woman vomits during resuscitation, turn her head to the side, take a cloth or gauze and wipe out her mouth, then continue to ventilate. Vomiting is common during CPR.

The effects of maternal cardiopulmonary crisis on the fetus: Prior to 24 weeks of pregnancy, resuscitative measures and life support procedures are aimed at preserving the mother's life; full cardiac arrest is almost always associated with early fetal demise. After 24 weeks, the fetus becomes increasingly viable and support is aimed at the mother, taking the fetus into consideration as well. If the mother has gone into cardiac arrest, effective maternal circulation cannot be restored, and the fetus is mature enough to survive, an emergency surgical delivery should be done, ideally within 4 to 5 minutes of the arrest. Getting the baby out will relieve pressure on the large vessels in the mother's back and maximize the chance of survival for both mother and fetus. While having the baby out within 5 minutes is best, there are documented cases where the fetus has survived when delivered more than 20 minutes after complete maternal arrest with full CPR.

Initial assessment: If you are with a woman who experiences a cardiopulmonary crisis, call the local 911 service without delay. Reassure her and the baby that you will help them and give Rescue Remedy or homeopathic Arnica (30C or 200C) if you have any on hand. Next, position the woman flat on her back on a firm surface. If the uterus has risen out of the pelvis, place a pillow, rolled towel, wedge, other object or your knees under her left hip. Alternately, have an assistant displace the uterus by pushing it over to one side or by using their knees as a wedge under one hip. Open the airway by pressing against the woman's forehead and lifting up on her chin, or by grasping her lower jaw and lifting with both hands, bringing the jaw forward while tilting her head backward. This should move her tongue away from the airway. Check to see if the woman is breathing by watching for respiratory movements and listening and feeling for breath. A mirror can be placed below her nostrils if you are unsure. Reflex gasping efforts may occur early during primary cardiac arrest; do not mistake these for adequate breathing. Wipe away any fluids that may be around her mouth.

Artificial respiration: If there is no respiratory effort, place a mouth-to-mask resuscitation device over her nose and mouth, using the bridge of the nose as a guide; you must have a good seal around the edges or air leakage will occur. If no mask is available, place sterile gauze over the woman's mouth, place your open mouth over hers and pinch her nostrils closed during ventilation. Take a deep breath and seal your lips on the mask or around the woman's mouth, creating an airtight seal. Then give a slow breath lasting 1½ to 2 seconds; take a breath, and give another. Watch to make sure the chest rises. After two breaths, check to see if there is a pulse at the carotid artery (which is found in the groove formed by the trachea and the large muscles of the neck) for 5 to 10 seconds; if so, continue to ventilate at a rate of 12 breaths per minute (one breath every 5 to 6 seconds).

Cardiac compressions: If no pulse is detected, begin cardiac compressions. Locate the notch formed by the edge of the lower rib cage and the end of the sternum. Place the heel of your hand in the center of the lower half of the sternum, and place the heel of your other hand on top of it. The force of your compression should remain on the heel of your hand on the sternum to minimize pressure on the surrounding ribs. The fingers should be elevated off the chest. Lock your elbows and position your shoulders directly over your hands to achieve the most pressure with the least effort. The normal adult chest should be compressed to a depth of 1½ to 2 inches (3.8 to 5.1 cm.) in a smooth, regular, non-jerky rhythm 80 to 100 times a minute. A small woman may require less pressure to maintain a pulse; a very large woman may need more. After each compression, release pressure to allow blood to flow into the chest and heart, but do not lift the hands from their proper position on the chest. When compressions are being done, the ratio of compressions to breaths should be 15 to 2. Perform this cycle 4 times, then check the carotid pulse to see if spontaneous heart action has resumed.

If the woman regains consciousness: If no traumatic injury has taken place, turn the woman on her side and place the hand of her upper arm under her cheek. This will allow fluid to flow from her mouth without choking her. This position can be maintained until help arrives.

If a traumatic injury has occurred (such as a fall, car accident, etc.) do not move the woman to a side-lying position because of possible injury to the spinal column. Movement in such cases can cause broken bones to permanently damage the spinal cord. Stay with her, cover her to keep her warm, displace her uterus to the side with manual pressure on her abdomen and wait for help to arrive.

Clearing the airway: The adult airway typically becomes blocked by food or another foreign object. In such a case the person is likely to be conscious but unable to breathe. The first task is to clear the airway, since ventilation will be impossible otherwise. If a person can breathe, talk or cough, the airway is not completely obstructed; simply encourage her efforts to clear her airway herself and do nothing to interfere. If airway obstruction is complete, or if partial airway obstruction progresses (signaled by a weak, ineffective cough, high-pitched noise during inhalation, increased respiratory difficulty, and possible cyanosis), you should assist the person in clearing her airway.

In early pregnancy, the Heimlich maneuver (subdiaphragmatic abdominal thrusts) can be used as it would be in a nonpregnant person to dislodge an object in the airway. It elevates the diaphragm to force air from the lungs, creating an artificial cough to expel the object. It may be necessary to repeat the thrust several times to accomplish this. To minimize damage to internal organs the hands should never be placed on the xiphoid process of the sternum or on the lower margins of the rib cage; they should be between this area and the navel in the midline.

If the choking victim is standing or seated: You should stand behind the victim, wrap your arms around the victim's waist, and make a fist with one hand. Place the thumb side of your fist against the victim's abdomen slightly above the navel. Grasp this fist with your other hand and press the fist into the abdomen with a quick upward thrust. Repeat and continue until the object is expelled or the woman becomes unconscious. Each new thrust should be a separate, distinct movement.

If victim is lying down: Place the woman in a supine position, face up. Kneel astride her thighs and place the heel of one hand against her abdomen in the midline slightly above the navel and well below the xiphoid. Place the other hand directly on top of the first and press into the abdomen with a quick upward thrust. Also use this technique if you are too short to reach around the waist of a victim, using your body weight to accomplish the thrust.

After 20 weeks or in a woman-of-size who is standing or sitting: Stand behind the victim with your arms directly under her armpits, encircling the chest. Place thumb side of your fist on the middle of the woman's sternum, taking care to avoid the xiphoid process and margins of the rib cage. Grab your fist with the other hand and perform quick, forceful thrusts until the object is expelled or the victim becomes unconscious.

After 20 weeks or in a woman-of-size who is lying down: Place the woman on her back and kneel close to her side. Place the heel of one hand on the lower half of her sternum, and place the heel of your other hand on top of it. The force of thrust should remain on the heel of your hand on the sternum, to minimize pressure on the surrounding ribs. Fingers should be elevated off the chest. Lock your elbows and position your shoulders directly over your hands to achieve the most pressure with the least effort. Apply firm, quick, distinctly individual thrusts.

Finger sweep: Attempt to manually clear the airway only if the woman is unconscious and not convulsing. Open her mouth by grasping both the tongue and lower jaw between the thumb and fingers and lifting the jaw. This may partially relieve an obstruction. Insert the index finger of your other hand along the inside of the cheek, reaching deeply into the throat to the base of the tongue. Use a hooking action to dislodge the object and maneuver it into the mouth for removal. You may have to use your finger to push an object against the opposite side of the throat to dislodge it.

Recommended sequence when encountering an unconscious victim:
* *Open her mouth, look for a foreign object, if one is seen, attempt to remove it.
* *If no foreign object is suspected open the airway and attempt ventilation with 2 breaths. If you cannot ventilate even after repositioning the head, perform the Heimlich maneuver.
* *Open her mouth and perform a finger sweep, then reattempt ventilation. If still unsuccessful, reposition her head and try again.
* *Repeat the sequence for clearing the airway and continue as necessary until the victim begins to breath, you can begin ventilation or emergency help arrives and takes over resuscitation.

Chandra, N., ed., Basic Life Support for Healthcare Providers, Amer. Heart Assoc. 1994.

Assessing Blood Loss

The ability to accurately assess blood loss is an important skill for midwives when giving care during the prenatal period as well as the actual birth. Blood loss can occur for a variety of reasons throughout the prenatal period such as:

*Miscarriage (the pregnancy ends before 20 weeks)
*Placental abruption (the placenta separates from the uterine wall
    before the baby is out)
*Placenta previa (placenta is implanted over the internal cervical os
    and cervical changes cause it to tear and bleed).
*Ruptured ectopic pregnancy
*Hydatidiform mole
*Uterine rupture

Rarely a woman may experience blood loss from any number of causes unrelated to pregnancy and knowing how to assess this loss, should you be on hand for such unhappy events, is helpful. Furthermore, you will often get calls from women who are bleeding and you will be trying to help them figure out how much blood they may be losing. Having a good idea of how to assess such loss will be valuable to you as you advise her what to do next. (Tips on how to question women regarding this are given in the chapter on First Trimester Miscarriage).

In the hospital and in medical textbooks, blood loss is discussed in ccs. (cubic centimeters). In the United States, most of us are used to thinking in terms of ounces and cups. The translation process can be hard on the spur of the moment when more critical things are at stake than mathematics. Lets start with a conversion table which translates ounces into cubic centimeters (ccs). Eight fluid ounces equals 1 cup.

OUNCES	CCS	CUPS	CCS.	CUPS	CCS
1 oz.	28.4	1¼ cups	284.2	3¼ cups	738.4
2 oz.	57	1½ cups	341.2	3½ cups	795.2
3 oz.	85.2	13/4 cups	398.2	33/4 cups	852.0
4 oz.	113.6	2 cups	454.4	4 cups	908.8
5 oz.	142	2¼ cups	511.2	4¼ cups	965.6
6 oz.	170.4	2½ cups	568	4½ cups	1022.4
7 oz.	198.8	23/4 cups	624.8	43/4 cups	1079.4
8 oz. (1 cup)	227.2	3 cups	681.6	5 cups	1136.0

Conventional reckoning estimates that 500 ccs. approximately equals 2 cups, but from the chart above we can see that this is off by more than just a fraction. Measure blood in the clinical situation in whatever units are easiest for you to think in. When you complete your records, you can use this table to convert measurements of ounces to cubic centimeters (leave your notes as they are and in parentheses near or above your figures, insert the proper equivalent amount in ccs.). This table can also be used when translating hospital records. Remember that 1 cup of blood weighs 8 oz. or one-half pound. Clotted blood concentrates the blood lost, therefore a ½ cup sized clot equals 1 liquid cup (Cook, 1995).

Measuring blood loss: In measuring quantities of blood or clots in a home situation, the best method is to catch the blood being lost in a shallow pan, such as a mixing bowl or bed pan, and to transfer it to a measuring device such as a large-mouthed kitchen measuring cup. In order to measure blood like this you must have the equipment at hand and be anticipating the loss of blood, as is the case after a birth while waiting for the placenta.

During prenatal care, such timely anticipation and collection of large quantities of blood will not be the rule. Ask any woman who is bleeding or who you feel is likely to do so to save whatever she passes and to collect blood soaked items for your inspection. In the majority of cases, you will arrive on the scene to be presented with blood soaked articles after the fact or while bleeding is in progress. This makes the estimation of blood loss more complicated.

The reckoning of how much blood has penetrated an article of clothing, a pad or a towel will depend upon many factors: the absorbency of the article, how large it is, how old is the blood soaking it (dry blood will weigh less because its water weight will have evaporated). The most accurate method is to take an identical clean item, weigh it, then weigh the blood soaked item and subtract the difference. This will give you how many ounces of blood are in the item, if the soaked item is still wet.

However, although it could be, all this weighing of blood soaked items is usually not done in the clinical situation. It is important for you to be able to visually estimate blood loss as well. There is no easy way to tell you how to do this in a book. However, I can give you some tips I have gathered over the years in setting up models for you to learn with. It is most convenient to assemble other students so you can all do this together.

Tomato juice, which is red and thicker than water, is a good liquid to use for practice; buy several cans (Cook, 1995). You could even add a bottle of red food coloring to make it darker if you prefer. Fill different containers with varying amounts and note what 1 cup of blood looks like in lots of different containers, then 1½ cups, etc. If you have a special pan that you will use for postpartum blood collection, take special note of what different quantities of blood look like in it, since you will be seeing blood in it most often. Take typical gauze pads, wash cloths, disposable underpads, sanitary napkins, bath towels, etc., and pour varying quantities of juice into these items. Compare the soaked article with an identical dry article to get an idea of the weight difference. Also note how much different quantities wet the fabric. Of course, tomato juice is somewhat thicker than blood and will not soak in quite as readily as blood. Some midwives have used partially jelled red gelatin to simulate blood which is partially clotted. You can also use cow's blood from a butcher which, of course, is the closest you'll come to human blood (if you do, be sure to take precautions, as cattle blood can also carry diseases). Another option is to use fake blood, which is used when training personnel such as Emergency Medical Technicians. Contact a local EMT training center and ask where they get their teaching aides. This will likely be your most expensive option, so you may want to get several midwives together to go in on the investment.

Learn to estimate how much blood loss is going on when a woman is in a tub full of water by filling a tub and then adding whatever you are using for practice in increasing amounts (note what a ½ cup looks like, then 1 cup, etc.) Then do the same thing in a toilet.

References and further reading:

Cook, Barbara, midwife, workshop on "Third Stage Complications," Assoc. of Texas Midwives conf., Arlington, TX, 5/6/95.

A Plan for Dealing With Physical Problems During Pregnancy

Pregnancy gives rise to a number of essentially benign aches and pains as well as other discomforts. The rapid changes which the body undergoes, coupled with a population of women in the developed world who do not do the kind of physical work their foremothers did probably enhances the tendency to some of these symptoms. Lifestyle stress, other children to care for and the need to hold a job during pregnancy also have an impact. Emotional issues can manifest as physical complaints as well, particularly when they are unconscious. The vast majority of the problems women will bring to you during their pregnancy can be temporarily relieved or permanently alleviated with simple home remedies or supportive therapeutics such as a visit to the chiropractors office, more exercise or a change in diet. Otherwise, midwives generally expect women to cope with the physical changes they experience, and do not rush to use drugs in an all-out effort to eliminate symptoms regardless of what it takes.

When a problem is serious, it may require the attention of a bio-technical care provider, in extreme cases drugs or surgery may be required. In some cases, such complications are medical problems presenting alongside pregnancy but are not caused by pregnancy. Their presentation during pregnancy may complicate the clinical picture and delay the recognition of the real problem. Problems, ranging from minor discomforts of pregnancy to rare and potentially dangerous complications such as abdominal pregnancy, will be addressed throughout the text. If a problem is suspected, it is wise for you to have a plan regarding how to proceed. Generally speaking, problems can be approached with a basic, three-step process:

Ensure the mother's and baby's immediate safety: Your first priority is always to determine if the symptoms which the mother is reporting reflect a life-threatening emergency. In early pregnancy, your second priority is to determine if the baby's life is threatened. As pregnancy advances, a life-threatening situation for the baby takes on more significance, because of the increasing likelihood that the baby will survive if it is born. However, in cases where both mother and baby are in jeopardy, the mother is still your first concern. This process includes asking all the questions necessary to determine exactly what is taking place and how rapidly it is progressing. Bleeding and/or pain are the most commonly reported symptoms when a true emergency exists, but both can occur for non-emergent reasons as well. If the mother or baby is in imminent danger, act on the physical situation without delay and discuss emotional issues after the crisis is under control.

When you are assessing the relative danger of the situation, remember to start by ruling out the most likely causes of the problem; as the saying goes "If you hear hoof beats in New England, don't look for giraffes." The same could be said for potential emergencies during pregnancy; rule out gas and indigestion before you send a woman in for evaluation of cramps due to suspected ectopic pregnancy.

Deal with emotional issues: If you have determined that the mother and/or baby are not in immediate danger, a discussion of the psychological and emotional aspects of the situation is appropriate. Specific issues will vary from woman to woman; some general topics which can be universally applied to pregnancy loss will be found in the chapters on problems at the end of the sections covering each trimester. Once you have determined that the woman is clear about her emotional issues (these could include "do I really want this baby?," needing more support at home, an unstable relationship, money matters, fears of parenting, fears of labor at term, "Will baby come out?," "Is the baby okay?") you can proceed to the next step. Be aware, however, that often what she may think is the reason, is not the reason at all. To explore this, start by delving into the feelings and seeing what thoughts or physical sensations accompany the feelings. Asking her to reflect back on the time period just before the problem arose will often help clarify the emotional aspects of the situation. For other ways to explore the possible emotional factors, see the chapter on Working Through Emotional Issues with Clients in the section on Sustaining Health and Well-being During Pregnancy.

What to do next: Discuss both of your intuitive perceptions regarding what is going on. Discuss with the woman what her options are for treatment, beginning with the least interventive options first, bio-technical drugs and surgery are always last resorts but may at times be necessary or even life saving. Is a wait-and-see attitude appropriate, or is transport in order? Even though the problem does not present an immediate threat, symptoms may be such that further evaluation is needed without undue delay.

How far do you go before referring? In my practice, once a woman engaged me for care, in the absence of life-threatening complications, it was very rare for me to recommend, or a client to elect, permanently transferring prenatal care to another practitioner; this book is written with that in mind. However, every client is different. Many women who choose homebirth and midwifery care are willing to work with you via non-bio-technical therapies to maximize their chances of staying at home, even when problems arise. They feel fine about trying herbs, supplements, homeopathy and other modalities, and they welcome a different point of view. Others, although seeking homebirth, will be more conventional when it comes to dealing with complications; they may feel they want to be seen by a mainstream practitioner much sooner. As you gain experience you will get a feel for where your clients are on this continuum. If a woman wants to be seen by someone else, by all means, give her your honest opinion about her condition and then support her to get a second opinion if she would like. In other cases, you will want to refer or suggest more bio-technical interventions sooner than you otherwise might because you are unsure about a client's level of personal responsibility-taking; in these cases you refer to cover yourself as much as cover the situation. When you are really out on a political limb, anticipating a breech or very postdates birth for example, be sure you have a solid relationship with the parents.

Notice the connection between events: Whenever a problem occurs and especially in those that persist or repeat, the chances of unresolved emotional issues being related to the symptom are high. Assess if the woman is open to looking at the issue in this light (see the chapter on Dealing with Emotional Issues with Clients in the section on Sustaining Health and Well-being During Pregnancy). If she is, you might recommend a therapist you know of. Hypnotherapy may be especially helpful for resolving critical issues quickly. If she is not open to exploring the issue, do your best to support her on a physical level and be aware that unresolved emotional issues may resurface as a different symptom later in pregnancy or during the birth.

When transport is necessary: It is important to remain calm and explain to the woman what is going on and what she can anticipate at the hospital when transport is necessary. Continue to talk to her, reassure her and help her to visualize a positive outcome to the current crisis. Accompany her to the hospital or meet her there. Stay with her until the crisis has stabilized. Stay in touch with women who have been temporarily transported to the care of another provider or to the hospital. They will need your help in understanding their options for care as well as your emotional support. When transport is necessary during pregnancy, the situation is often serious, especially for the baby; your support will be vital to her overall well-being. If you or the mother are convinced that a problem exists which is not receiving adequate attention, *insist* that an thorough evaluation be made without delay. I have heard of more than one story where a mother was in a serious condition but her feelings were dismissed by bio-medical care providers.

When surgery is necessary: Be sure to visit the woman often while she is in the hospital, discussing any fears or concerns she may have regarding her or her baby's well-being. Act as an advocate for her with the staff, ensuring that her questions are answered to her satisfaction. Recommend that she take homeopathic Arnica 200C potency immediately before and after surgery, at 30 minute intervals for several hours. She can continue to take the Arnica in conjunction with Ledum, 200C doses at 30 minute intervals for several hours, spacing the doses out to every 2 hours and tapering them off, letting her post-surgical discomfort be your guide (as symptoms diminish, space doses further apart). These remedies speed recovery.

Get another opinion: Whenever there is a problem, particularly one you have never before encountered, don't hesitate to ask another practitioner their opinion of the situation. One our most important skills is knowing when we don't know!!

These basic steps will assist you in remaining centered and in prioritizing your process appropriately.

NOTES:

499

INITIATING CONTACT AND ESTABLISHING CARE

First Contacts

First encounters with women and families with whom you may work can occur in a variety of ways. If you live in a small, close knit community or serve such a community, you may hear of women who need your services by word-of-mouth from neighbor to neighbor. The vast majority of midwives, however, will make first contacts either at public childbirth-related events, such as La Leche League conferences, or with those who have heard of them through the grapevine and call by telephone.

This chapter will address the majority of first contact situations, which are non-emergent (see the next chapter for Crisis First Contacts). In order to cover all bases, I will assume that you do not know anything about the woman inquiring about your services. There are a number of things which you might wish to discover as you have your first discussion in such a case. The answers to many of these questions may come out naturally in the course of the conversation without needing to ask for the information directly.

How can I help you? While many women will contact you who are pregnant and are seeking a homebirth, not everyone will want this. I've received calls for all kinds of problems ranging from infertility and preconception counseling to abortion (which is covered in another volume of this text). Sometimes women are looking for a midwife to provide labor support for a planned hospital birth (this issue is covered in its own chapter in the Special Circumstances section). You have to decide how or if you can help the caller. You may refer them to another provider if you cannot.

Where did you hear about me/get my number? This helps establish a connection regarding who you know mutually. If you work in a very underground situation, you want to know if it sounds as if this is a legitimate call. Some midwives have circles of trusted support people who gather the numbers of interested potential clients and initiate first contacts themselves. This way, the midwife's number isn't given out to people they don't know.

What is your general state of health? You want to know if she has any minor health problems which need attention. You also want to know if she has any major health conditions which may impact where and with whom she gives birth. Most women that are aware of preexisting medical conditions will have made some attempt to determine if they are good candidates for uncomplicated birth prior to talking with you. If a woman has not, she may ask your opinion of her condition in relation to the choice of where to birth. (See the section on Medical Conditions Which May Preexist Pregnancy to see if her condition is discussed.)

Do you smoke, drink alcohol or take drugs of any kind? This can give you a clue about medical conditions as well as lifestyle. Depending upon how and with whom you wish to work, the continued use of any or all of these substances may eliminate the possibility of birthing with you. Be sure she understands you mean over-the-counter items as well as prescriptions or recreational drugs.

If pregnant, when are you due? Of course, some women will be exploring their birthing options before conception and therefore may call you when they are not pregnant (see chapter on Preconception Counseling and Care, this section). If a woman is pregnant, when she is due gives you an idea of how much time you have to work with her and her family before birth, and how quickly you need to schedule an appointment. Some midwives schedule a consultation visit before twelve weeks but put off the initial history-taking visit until after the third month. Knowing the due date can also help you assess any problems or symptoms she may be experiencing. Be sure to discuss the due date in some detail, to ascertain if it seems like a reasonable estimate.

The closer a woman is to term when she begins your care, the more risk you take on as a result. This is not simply due to physical factors which you could have influenced sooner; it also means you have less time to develop a relationship with her and her family which will be solid enough to carry you through the birth, whatever it may bring.

Why do you want to have your baby at home? This will probably get you answers to many of the questions which follow below.

Who have you been seeing so far this pregnancy? Has she had other care prior to contacting you? If she reports that she is seeing another midwife in your community and wishes to change care providers, it is a good idea to contact that midwife to let her know that her client has called you, and to find out her impressions of why the woman is seeking other care. This inquiry of your colleagues can be very revealing. If a woman connects with you late in her pregnancy and has had no prior prenatal care, ask her what she has been waiting for. If she has been receiving care elsewhere, have her obtain a copy of her records to date.

Is this your first baby? If so, she will probably have questions concerning discomforts of pregnancy or want to discuss pregnancy and birth in more detail. If she has had other children, she will probably offer some information about the course and outcome of her previous pregnancies. This is your opportunity to discover why she is making different choices now. If she has had previous homebirths, much of the discussion about the pros and cons of homebirth vs. hospital have already been hashed out, making your job easier, unless her current partner was not involved; in such cases there can sometimes be a big disparity in what each parent feels is best for the pregnancy, a good bit of information to have prior to seeing them in person. A previous difficult birth is often best understood with the help of medical records. You might ask if she has them and, if so, to bring them along. If not, she can begin the process of getting copies. She should always ask for copies of the entire record on file, not merely a summary sheet.

Did you have any problems with your previous pregnancies and births? If you haven't already found this out, ask directly. A very complicated history warrants a request that she gather up her medical records prior to your consultation visit, if at all possible, enabling you to figure out what happened, how much of what happened seemed to be iatrogenic (doctor induced) and how much of it physiological.

Do you plan to breastfeed? You have to decide if you will work with mothers who do not wish to breastfeed. Even if you do so, this is your opportunity to find out how her previous experiences have gone and what her plans are for this pregnancy. You can begin to influence her in a positive direction if necessary, explaining the many benefits of breastfeeding.

What is your diet like? Get more information than "very good." Some people feel that a good diet is food on the table on a daily basis, regardless of what kind of food that may be. This is your first opportunity to influence her feelings regarding weight gain, dietary intake, salt, and related concerns. A discussion of nausea frequently comes up at this point. (See chapter on Nausea and Vomiting in the section on Problems Associated With the First Trimester.)

Do you have a partner? If she has a partner, find out both their name and how (or if) the partner wishes to be involved. Do not assume she is married or even that she has a partner. If she does, do not assume her partner is a man. You may get calls from both single women and lesbians. Encourage both partners to be present at as many appointments as possible, emphasizing the importance of both attending. You may want to insist on this for the consultation visit.

Find out, if appropriate given the conversation, how long they have been together and how they get along as a couple. These types of questions may be more appropriately reserved for the in-person interview, when you will be able to get visual and body language cues as well.

Lesbians may be reluctant to reveal their choice of partner. If a woman mentions that her female friend or roommate will be accompanying her to visits, you can ask point blank, "Are you a lesbian?" This gives her permission to come out to you and gives you a chance to break the ice and let her know that is fine with you. If she does not want to disclose her sexual orientation at that point, she can always say no. If she says yes, and you happen to feel uncomfortable working with her (or with single heterosexual women), you can let her know of your discomfort up front. Better yet, if you know of another midwife who would feel more comfortable, you can suggest that she contact her.

Exchange addresses and phone numbers: This is very important information when you decide to make a consultation appointment. You need to be able to reach her to cancel appointments in case of a birth, and she needs your office number in case she gets lost on her way there; be sure to give good directions.

As the conversation progresses, women may start to ask you many of the things that you usually cover during the consultation visit. If this is the case, you can explain that the consultation visit is designed to cover these very questions; would she like to make an appointment to meet with you and discuss these things in person? Most of the time, women are delighted to hear this. If so, you can then whip out the old appointment book and schedule a time to see both her and her partner. You thus avoid having to go over everything on the phone and then repeating it again when you meet the woman and her partner in person. It is important, however, for both you and her to gather enough information to determine whether a consultation visit is even warranted. Depending upon how the conversation goes, you may need to define the type of midwife you are, your fees, etc. In my practice, it is my policy not to discuss money on the phone unless someone calls very late in pregnancy. In such cases, I touch on all the salient points regarding finances as succinctly as possible to avoid an unnecessary appointment.

Dealing with latecomers: Latecomers can be of three varieties. Some have just moved to your area, come bearing prenatal records and make wonderful clients. In other cases, they live nearby, have been desperately looking for you for most of their pregnancies, finally found you and prove to be very committed to homebirth, or they are fence-sitters who say they have been looking for you, but when they finally find you, after wasting your time and theirs doing a crash initial, chicken out. This has lead many midwives to the practice of never giving latecomers a price break. The client's willingness to pay full price is indicative of their commitment to the choice they are making. In my practice I almost always insist that they go home and discuss the choice to come to me before proceeding with the initial visit. And finally, when the initial visit occurs (sometimes right after the consultation, to save time) I ask for an immediate non-refundable down payment of $150.00. These practices have, for the most part, eliminated the fence-sitters.

Never feel you are getting off easy when you take on latecomers; it means you have less opportunity to allow your relationship to develop. Sometimes women wander in late because they don't have a clue about how different midwifery care can be from medical model care; everything, from the consultation on, becomes a crash course in homebirth and midwifery care. When considering whether you can reasonably take someone on, consider the following factors:

Your current client load when she is due: If you already have a full load of clients or you have one or more clients whom you anticipate will have hard births or special needs, do not compromise their care by spreading yourself too thin.

The season and where she lives: In some areas this won't be relevant, but if it is winter and you are dealing with snow, if she lives far from your other clients or otherwise presents an unusual burden simply in terms of her location, think twice. Perhaps another midwife lives closer or has less clients that month.

Your personal needs: Yes, you are a person too. Do not add additional stress to your already stressful lifestyle by taking on late-comers who are due on a major religious holiday, the day before your daughter's school play or who will birth during the week of your well-earned vacation. Don't be a maniac. Often midwives act the martyr when women contact them late. You are not required to be the personal savior of every birthing woman in the world; don't even try.

Her physical and emotional situation: Has she had a homebirth with midwives before or has she had three surgical births with a history of toxemia and fetal distress, and is currently trying not to gain weight? While you can certainly give such a woman advice, you might not want to take a woman on who has major issues that will require tremendous amounts of energy from you, unless your client load and other factors will truly allow you to give her the quality of care she deserves.

When a partner calls: The previous discussion assumes you are speaking to the pregnant woman who is, in my experience, the person most likely to call and inquire about services. However, fathers sometimes call on behalf of their partners. Sometimes this is because men have a very strict idea about the "role" of their wives and can signal a man who will prove difficult to deal with. You may be able to get a feel for whether this is the case as you talk. Other times, it is a simple matter that he was available to call you first or that it was more culturally appropriate (eg. when working with Arabs, it may always be the man who calls).

Once the appointment for the consultation visit is made, you can usually conclude your conversation with a suggestion to call with any problems which come up in the interim.

After the first contact: It is my practice to send out a cover letter and short list of questions for both partners to consider and write their answers to prior to the consultation visit. I have included examples of these forms. I have kept it simple because I don't want potential clients to be overwhelmed, or so bogged down in my questions that they don't get around to thinking of any of their own. There is also no point in the parents filling out a long list of questions if they are unsure about where they want to give birth. The questions I send help them organize their thoughts, hopefully prompt questions they may have, and give me some basic information. I also request a diet diary with a minimum of three days of meals.

The following form may be useful to keep by the phone. It offers an easy to use record of contacts, as well as a checklist of things to ask. The abbreviations under the "wishes to discuss" section stand for homebirth (HB), labor support (LS) and well-woman care (WWC). There may be other services you want to add as well.

Initial Client Contact

Name_____ Date/time of consult_____

Address_____ Due date_____ # wks now_____

City_____ St_____ZIP_____ Preconsult mailer sent_____

Wishes to discuss:
Phone #_____ __HB __LS __WWC

Where they heard of us_____

Topics discussed: why HB___ # preg.____ # babies____ prev. HB?_____

YBAC?___ #CS___ Smoker?___ # day___ Alcohol___ Drugs___ Diet_____

Plans to breastfeed?____ Current prenatal care provider?_____

Medical risk factors_____ Partner supportive?_____

Other:_____

506

An example of an introductory cover letter which can be sent after your first discussion in preparation for the consultation visit:

We are delighted you want to look into homebirth with us!

At your consultation visit we will be exploring what it means to birth at home. There is much to talk about, so plan to spend about 1 hour with us at that time. It will be helpful for you to complete the enclosed questions and daily diet dairy before we see you. Please also bring questions you have for us concerning any aspect of your birth experience. We feel it is essential for both partners to be present at this interview.

After a consultation visit most parents want to go home and think things over before they make a decision about their place of birth and care providers. Take your time to do this before calling us regarding your next appointment.

An important element of birthing with midwives is the establishment of a warm and open relationship. We look forward to meeting and sharing with you, and to the possibility of working together.

Sincerely,

Before your consultation visit, please keep at least 3 days of dietary history to bring with you. Be sure to include: *Everything you put in your mouth (snacks, vitamins, herbs, drinks, etc.)
      *Approximate amounts of what you eat or drink (8 oz. juice etc.)
      *Is the food fresh, frozen, canned or otherwise processed?
Please give some thought to the following questions. Read all questions before writing your answers in your own words (use the back as necessary).

Why do you want to have this baby at home? _____

_____

Partner: _____

_____

What do you see as the duties and responsibilities of your midwives? _____

_____

Partner:_____

_____

What do you feel your responsibilities are as parents regarding the pregnancy and birth?

_____

Partner:_____

_____

What is your present understanding of problems which may occur during pregnancy or birth?

_____

_____

Partner:_____

_____

Our society does not view homebirth and independent midwifery as "wise" or "safe" choices. What is your current understanding of the political and social ramifications of making such choices?

_____

_____

Partner: _____

_____

The above questions will be discussed at your consultation. Please add any further comments, thoughts or questions which you would like to discuss with us on the back of this sheet.

Crisis First Contacts

As you become better known in your community and gain more experience, your reputation will spread. Eventually you will start receiving first contact calls from women experiencing some sort of pregnancy crisis who are looking for another perspective on their situation. Some of these women will have been planning on seeing you anyway, but an early pregnancy complication has intervened before they got around to calling you. Others will be seeing medical care providers and will be either fed up with the information they have received so far or will feel that their providers are inaccessible. They may have been told of your practice by a friend who was or is your client and decided they were afraid to birth at home; now, in the midst of a crisis, they may be reconsidering. Or, a woman may just want advice on non-medical methods for dealing with her situation while never intending to transfer her care. In any case, here you are on the phone with a woman, often upset or at her wits end with a threatened miscarriage, intractable nausea, poor dietary advice, possible toxemia or any number of other problems. What do you do?

Your response will depend, in part, on your legal status. If you are practicing illegally, you will need to carefully consider what information you give out over the phone. Sometimes sting operations are organized to "get" a midwife, and you could fall into a well-laid trap by innocently trying to help a woman. You must use your intuition and take care. Some midwives simply refuse to deal with such calls and refer the woman to supportive care providers practicing legally in their area.

However, let's assume that you feel okay about talking to this woman. What do you tell her, and how far do you go? First of all, you want to find out who she has been seeing for care, what the problem is, and what recommendations have already been made. Is she calling you for more input because what she has tried so far hasn't helped? Sometimes women who call with a specific problem have had a course of action recommended to them which they do not like, so they haven't done anything. They are seeking a second opinion from you. Knowing these things will help you understand the context in which her questions are arising.

You might start with a brief overview of the difference between midwifery and obstetrical care, emphasizing preventive care and the client responsibility-taking at the core of the care you provide. You can then proceed with "If you were my client, first of all I would . . ." addressing the issue not only from the perspective of what you would do, but also giving her your opinion of what the other provider has recommended as well as your understanding of the problem. It helps to know how the condition has been described to the woman and what she has already tried to do to remedy the situation based on the primary care provider's advice. If she has had no care thus far, you need to know that too; beware of doling out advice freely to a woman who is trying to minimize or is in denial about a potentially serious condition.

If it is a simple case of minor pregnancy discomfort such as nausea or constipation, your practical midwifery-oriented advice will probably help resolve the problems and may even gain you a new client. Helping women generally improve their diet is a major contribution you can make to their overall sense of well-being and will help to minimize many common discomforts.

When a woman calls with a potentially emergent situation underway, your choices get more tricky. How much do you say, and how far do you go with a woman who is in crisis and may be physically compromised, but with whom you have no established relationship? Determine that she is not in a life-threatening situation (which will prompt you to recommend immediate transport), then start pursuing the problem in much the same way that you would with any client, being sure to address emotional aspects of the situation (something her other care provider has probably not even broached). You may want to be more conservative regarding your parameters of referral. (In other words, you are wise to recommend referral sooner than you might if she were a client with whom you felt you had a solid working relationship.) During your conversation you will be able to get a feel for her investment in the medical model of care; this will help you know what to recommend and how to proceed. Refer to the chapter addressing her particular problem for more information.

Preconception Counseling and Care

Although the majority of women you interview will already be pregnant, you will occasionally encounter a woman who is selecting her care provider before becoming pregnant. Some midwives advertize that they are available for a consultation prior to conception. This could be offered as a free consultation visit or, if not, make it clear that you charge a fee. Some women will already be interested in preparing to become pregnant and want to know what dietary changes and other recommendations you have to offer; you can supply valuable input for improving her health prior to pregnancy.

Preconception is the ideal time for a woman to consider all angles of her decision and make changes in her lifestyle that will benefit herself and her baby, since she will not feel the pressure of having to settle upon a care provider immediately. Here are some specific points to discuss with the parents:

*If a woman has a preexisting medical condition, direct her to providers to help her balance her constitution before conceiving.

*Question parents regarding the possibility of inherited disorders (see Genetic Counseling chapter in <u>Diagnostic Tests</u>); if informed, they may want genetic consultation prior to conception.

*Women of Mediterranean, African or other racial or ethnic descent may have an inherited hemoglobin disorder; explain that screening is available to detect such problems.

*Women with a problematic physical health history or a previously difficult pregnancy (due to toxemia, for example) may choose to get a baseline set of lab tests run now. The woman should be well at the time of testing; have her fast for 12 hours (water permitted) before going in for morning tests.

*Even with no identified health problems, some women may want to have screening for sexually transmitted disease such as syphilis, chlamydia, HIV, and gonorrhea, and may want to know if they are immune to Rubella.

*Women who are 15% below their ideal weight can be told the benefits of gaining a few pounds before conception. Providing an extra cushion of calories can take them through the early pregnancy discomforts such as bouts of nausea. (Brewer, 1983)

*Overweight women should be warned not to go on a crash diet before conceiving. This is likely to deplete their bodies of stored nutrients, which could adversely impact a pregnancy. However, they can begin eliminating junk foods and start a program of moderate exercise now. (Brewer, 1983)

*Carefully review a woman's diet and lifestyle habits (smoking, drinking, drugs etc.) and support her to curtail harmful habits and make dietary adjustments now.

*A program of vitamin and mineral supplementation and nutritive herbal infusions such as Alfalfa, Nettles and Red Clover will maximize her health before conception. Be sure a woman knows to begin taking at least .4 mg. of folic acid daily to reduce the likelihood of neural tube defects. This should begin at least one month before trying to conceive.

*Vegetarians who eat no dairy products can be advised to begin taking 3 micrograms of B_{12} 2 to 3 times weekly.

*Ask about the work and environment of both parents and inform them of any associated risks; discuss options for changing jobs or reducing risks if relevant.

*If social services or other community resources are available to a woman, given her income and other factors, make her aware of those now so she can explore when and if she is eligible.

*How emotional factors are impacted by pregnancy and parenting, and explore options if issues need to be dealt with through therapy.

*Family planning; find out if infertility has been an issue; how many children a couple wants to have, and their plans for child spacing.

*Be sure to let women know to avoid taking any over-the-counter or prescription medications; also discuss exposure to environmental hazards which should be avoided before conception.

*Women who have a question about their reproductive organs, breasts or other physical features may want you to do a physical exam. You may want to schedule another visit for this and charge a fee for an additional visit or recommend another care provider who specializes in the problem in question.

*If this is not a first pregnancy, find out if problems such as nausea, miscarriage, pendulous abdomen, varicose veins or other difficulties arose in previous pregnancies. If so, see the chapters concerning the pertinent topics; preventative measures can be discussed prior to conception.

Most of the questions and discussions which are addressed in the rest of the book will apply here as well. Women who approach you prior to pregnancy still need to weigh the pros and cons of a variety of birthing options and care providers and make their own decisions about what is right for them. Discuss those issues in the same way I have suggested for those who are already pregnant.

References and Further Reading:

Brewer, Gail, The Brewer Medical Diet, Simon and Schuster, NY, 1983.

Caring for the Future: The Content of Prenatal Care, A Report of the Public Health Service Expert Panel on the Content of Prenatal Care, Washington, DC, 1989.

The Consultation Visit

The consultation visit is a vital component of good midwifery care. In my practice it has always been free of charge. The offer to sit and discuss an individual family's situation, answering their questions and providing them with thorough documentation of your practice style and statistics, sets midwifery care apart from mainstream medicine. While there are certainly other health care providers who will grant a consultation visit if requested, it is rarely free of charge and rarely even thirty minutes long. Midwives want parents to make responsible, informed choices; we need to offer the information they need in order to do so.

The information contained in the consultation visit can be communicated in a variety of ways. Some midwives hold group visits where they sit down with several potential clients at once, describe their practice and answer questions. There are many advantages to this approach: all the couples hear about the birth experiences of others present; the midwife can often address the same questions all at once, rather than saying the same thing to each couple individually in a private meeting; a sense of community is fostered among those working with you from the onset, and this can be a wonderful benefit for everyone.

Other midwives see each potential client in an individual appointment. This is how my practice has always chosen to provide consultations. My appointments usually last an hour, but sometimes they are considerably longer. The advantages of a private consultation include an opportunity to cater to individual needs rather than managing a group dynamic. It also makes couples feel that you care about them as individuals, and creates an invitation for them to discuss whatever is most important to them, without holding back for fear they will infringe on the time of others. Personal or delicate topics, as well as finances, are more easily discussed in a private meeting of this type.

In my practice, women bring their preconsultation mailers with them to the visit along with the daily diet histories which I have requested. The visit starts out with introductions and launches right into a discussion of their questions and concerns. This is initiated by requesting the answers to the questions they were sent and noting if they have written any questions of their own. Often, they have. If not, I ask what questions they may have and what they would like to know about me, encouraging them to feel free to ask what my training and experience has been.

While most women or couples come with at least a few questions, some are seemingly so astonished by this unconventional approach to establishing a care provider relationship that they are dumbfounded. In this case, I address whatever specifics I can glean from reading their answers to the questions I sent and then present them with my Informed Disclosure statement. If they have had other babies, I ask about their birth experiences. After that, I discuss the diet history, along with any discomforts or complaints the woman may be having at this point in her pregnancy, explaining how I expect her to eat and outlining in simple terms the roles of the liver and blood volume expansion and their relationship to toxemia.

What the answers to the preconsult questionnaire can tell you:

Look over the answers to these questions with an eye for what I call "red flags." Most of the time, the preconsultation mailer questions will be answered with straightforward comments that are fairly universal, such as: "We want to birth at home because it provides us more control, it is where the baby was conceived, it will be more comfortable, it seems natural and right, we hate hospitals." However, some statements may indicate a significant difference of opinion or philosophy regarding respective roles in the care provider/receiver relationship. Here are a few such red flags which may appear anywhere in the responses:

*The midwives are to provide a safe birth/take care of everything/make all the decisions.

My response to this is that there are no guarantees in life or in birth. No one, be they doctor, hospital or anyone else, can guarantee them a particular outcome. You will offer your expertise and skills and try to be as honest as possible about what those consist of, but you want them to make decisions and take responsibility for making them and, most of all, recognize that there are *no guarantees!*

*Do you have malpractice insurance?

My practice never has. If they feel they need to see a care provider that carries malpractice insurance, they may need to be birthing with one in a hospital. The current cultural bias against homebirth and midwifery care does not place you in very good stead if a problem occurs with people who feel the need for insurance back-up.

If you are in a position where malpractice is available and you haven't taken out any insurance, discuss why not (expense is often a big deterrent as well as lack of company support for out-of-hospital births). If you do have insurance, you still need to delve into why they are concerned. Remember, even in birthing situations, people can be out to take advantage of an insured practitioner. If you feel something isn't quite kosher about the answers you get or the vibes from potential clients, *do not ignore your intuition!*

*We want to let nature take its course/obey the will of God as far as complications are concerned.

Does this mean that they will refuse transport even if you feel transport is necessary at the time of labor? Do they want you to do nothing in the event of a complication? If so, I ask them why they are seeking midwifery care in the first place. What will I be doing there if they do not desire to make use of my assistance? Discuss under what circumstances you might recommend transport and be clear about what you need as a care provider regarding this matter.

514

Discussing risks and complications: Answers to the question regarding complications can be very revealing. They not only give you an idea of what the couple has heard described as a complication (such a cord around the neck, which is frequently mentioned in this answer) but an opportunity to clear up any misconceptions. Discussing each complication mentioned and explaining what you would do or how you view it in terms of relative risk can be helpful. For example, you could say that, in general, cord around the neck is very common (about one out of every 5 babies has some nuchal cord) and usually not a problem. Of course, in rare situations, cord around the neck can be life threatening, but in most cases it is a easy matter to correct. You could then describe how you go about doing that. (Cord around the neck has, in recent years, been put forth as a common reason why a surgical birth was done, so many believe it is a major complication.0

Lots of people ask general questions, such as, "What do you do if there is a problem at the birth?" It would seem that many people think midwives just stand there without a clue and do nothing if problems arise during a birth; fathers particularly may have such concerns. Start by trying to discover if they have a specific complication in mind.   You might say, "There are many potential complications. Would you like to know about how we might handle anything in particular?"   Point out that all your transports, the reasons for them, and the outcomes, are listed individually in the statistics found in the Informed Disclosure document. Note that most transports are not life and death emergencies, which they will see as they look over the statistics, and that they may ask any questions they wish regarding any of your cases.

If they want more details about how you handle things, try to simplify the whole specter of complications as much as possible (the medical profession has complicated and mystified problems so much). I explain, "Something can go wrong with the mother or the baby. As long as the mother can eat, drink, sleep or rest, cope and eliminate her wastes, and the membranes are intact, labor go on as long as it needs to. If she becomes compromised, the baby is not far behind."

"The baby must be tolerating labor without problems as well as the mother. As long as the baby is in good shape, which we detect by listening to the fetal heart, noting the color of the amniotic fluid if the membranes have ruptured, asking the mother to stay tuned in to fetal movements, and listening to how the mother feels about the baby's well-being, we feel fine about staying at home. The baby can experience distress due to the strength of contractions in conjunction with a weak placenta or a compromised mother, and the mother can have problems such as bleeding from the placenta. At the time of birth the baby's shoulders may get stuck," and I describe procedures to remedy this problem.

"Once the baby is born the mother may bleed either before or after the placenta is delivered. The baby can be in distress and not start breathing right away. The mother may tear during birth, which can be repaired at home in most cases." And so on . . . As this discussion continues, it often prompts specific questions that the couple couldn't think of before.

I always offer a nutshell review of what I see as the main risks and benefits of having a baby at home versus those of birthing in the hospital. Yes, if a baby is born in an extremely compromised condition, all the machines and drugs and experts at the hospital might save such a baby born there. Likewise, with some very rare maternal complications, a death may be avoided in a hospital setting. However, parents must assess the relative risk of needing all that intervention in the rare emergency and getting more intervention than they need, which happens in almost every case in the hospital setting. I also point out that, although a rare baby may die at home that would not had it been born in the hospital, many babies die daily in hospitals that would have lived had they been born at home. At this point I offer Marjorie Tew's book Safer Childbirth and David Stewart of NAPSAC's book The Five Standards of Safe Childbearing as references and good reading along these lines. Both appeal to skeptical fathers because both deal with statistics in a very matter-of-fact manner.

Discussing local emergency services: At some point it may be appropriate to discuss the specifics of emergency transport in the event of a problem. Calling 911 can be tricky. In many states you get responses from multiple emergency services with fire engines, police and ambulance all arriving with sirens blaring even though you only want an ambulance. Call the local police station and find out if it is possible to ask that only an ambulance respond without a siren if you feel that meets the needs of the emergency. You should have this information ahead of time so you can inform parents whether calling 911 makes sense. Remember that whoever shows up is going to feel that they are somehow responsible to assess the situation and if you have to explain homebirth, the complication, etc. to the police the firemen, the ambulance people and all the neighbors gathered round to see whose house is burning down it will be quite a scene and could spell more risk of legal hassles for you and the parents, not to mention causing undue delay of the transport itself. If 911 personnel refuse to respond with only an ambulance, then the parents need to know that a private ambulance service will be the best choice.

Parenting issues: You might ask first-time parents whether they have ever cared for an infant before and if they have discussed their ideas about parenting in general and discipline in particular. Those who already have children can be asked how they feel about their co-parenting relationship. This will open the topic for their own discussions; frequently people have children without ever having discussed these essential issues.

Review previous births: If a woman has had an extremely difficult, confusing or complicated birth you will want to review her records and try to piece together what happened. Often a woman's memory is different from what you find recorded; she may be correct. Records get altered and things get left out of hospital documentation on a fairly routine basis. The partner's perspective on what occurred may help you fit the picture together as well.

Discussing fees and services: The consultation visit is the time to discuss your fees and the services offered. In my practice, the consultation itself is free of charge. Occasionally, you will have a woman who calls and talks to you for hours on the phone, and then wants an additional consultation visit as well. In such cases it is important to be supportive and at the same time establish some boundaries for yourself. Depending upon the situation, you might ask for a regular prenatal fee to cover the time spent in an additional consultation visit. Such decisions can be made on an individual basis. (See the next chapter for more details.)

Outline your services and be clear with women from the outset exactly what they can expect regarding appointment days and times, how you can be reached, and with whom you work, call schedules, continuity of care issues, etc.

Summing up: Much of what is touched on in conversation during the consultation visit can also be written down in the Informed Disclosure document; review mine in the following chapter to get more ideas about how to answer questions. However, some things are so important that you will want to say them out loud as well. In review, the most important things to discuss are:

*An honest description of your background and experience
*That there are no guarantees in life or in birth
*That there are risks and benefits in every possible birthing environment and the parents must choose which of those sets of risks feel most comfortable for them to take
*A review of the diet diaries and nutritional information
*Answers to the parent's questions and a clarification of their answers to your questions
*Midwifery philosophy and model of care and client responsibility
*Your respective roles regarding responsibility and decision making
*Give out any handouts, your Informed Disclosure Statement, etc.
*Discuss fees and services

Following-up on the consultation visit: In the majority of cases, the woman or couple will call you back to let you know about their decision one way or the other. You can ask them to let you know in two weeks in the usual case, sooner if the woman is due within, say, the next two or three months. If you have not heard from them at all by the end of the allotted time, give them a follow-up call. Lack of follow-up on their part does not always mean they have decided to birth elsewhere. It may simply be that they are early in the pregnancy and have gotten busy with other concerns. In any case, calling resolves the issue and lets you either establish care or stop thinking about whether a woman is going to show up eight months pregnant, surprised that you wanted to see her sooner!

Money Matters

"Spiritual" midwifery: The whole specter of finances can be a very confusing subject for women seeking to provide a service such as midwifery. Fortunately today's student isn't confronted with the notion that the truly "spiritual" midwife offers her services free of charge, which Ina May Gaskin promoted in the first edition of her book, Spiritual Midwifery, in 1975. (When the economics on The Farm changed, her midwifery practice had to begin charging for services too!) However, even without the strong voice of one of the matriarchs of the new midwifery ringing in your ears, it may be very hard to come to terms with how to deal with money in your practice.

Our culture does not value the traditional work of women; that is, nurturing the family. When we expand our nurturing role to encompass midwifery, asking for money in exchange can seem inconsistent; indeed it can feel like prostitution to some women. All this is, of course, usually very subconscious on the part of the midwife, who also feels in some part of her being that her work is valuable and should be compensated. In order to begin to unravel this confusion, it is important to get clear with yourself about what money means to you. When you do, your monetary interactions with clients will be far more trouble free.

Money as energy: There was a time in history when the midwife was respected and supported by her community. While she might not have received money, she often got chickens, wood, her home provided and repaired, or a new horse. Today, we too need an energy flow with the people we serve, and that is usually most conveniently accomplished with currency. Think of money as solidified energy. You put out a lot of energy to assist women in birth; there is nothing wrong with getting some kind of energy that you can really use in return!

In some cases, this exchange can take the form of barter. A cord of wood, chickens, bushels of vegetables or other barter exchanges which you need and with which you feel comfortable may work fine for you. In most cases, however, you will have to buy food, pay for housing, keep your car running smoothly, etc., etc., and all that necessitates a cash flow.

It is important for you to believe that your work is valuable, that you deserve to be compensated. This clarity will be reflected in the attitude you project when you talk with women and their partners about the money issue. When you believe in your worth, you can stop attracting in those clients who never seem to get around to paying you for their birth. This will help your self esteem and make you less frantic about how you're going to afford to fix the car before Betty is due.

Discussing money with clients: In my practice I do not usually discuss money during the first telephone contact unless the woman is very late in her pregnancy. I emphasize that I do not want anyone to chose homebirth because it is cheaper

518

(which it may well be in many areas for those who do not have insurance). Therefore, I postpone the discussion of how much it costs until we can sit down and discuss this in relationship to all the other factors involved in the decision to birth at home.

Working with parents who are only committed to homebirth due to financial considerations is asking for trouble. Often, such people have not explored the others aspects of the choice they are making. Probe their choice with them; you do not want to be stuck working with people whose idea of responsibility-taking in other aspects of birthing leaves a lot to be desired.

May independent midwives do not have the interface of a secretary or receptionist who will be dealing directly with clients around money issues. We are receptionist, accountant and care provider all in one. Therefore, a simple, straightforward attitude backed up by an equally straightforward method of recording keeping and the establishment of a payment plan is a big help.

The financial agreement: A method that has worked well in my practice has been to present a copy of some kind of financial agreement at the consultation visit. I call this a Responsibility Agreement. It includes a statement for the parents to sign regarding their choice of homebirth and independent midwifery care and a sliding scale fee schedule, as well as a place for them to outline a personal payment plan. An example is included at the end of this chapter, which may need to be modified to reflect your particular situation. We do not request to see IRS forms and trust that most clients are honest about where they fall on the scale. Occasionally someone balks at the sliding scale approach and we explain that, for us, this allows people from all economic strata to have a homebirth if they would like. Once the agreement is filled out and signed, you should keep the original in the woman's chart (stapled to the back of the folder is a good place); you may want to give a copy to your clients as well.

Travel expenses: My practice includes a separate fee for gas and phone calls outside a 20 minute driving radius of my office; this pretty much covers all long distance calling areas. If someone lives 45 minutes away, they get the first 20 minutes of distance free, then pay for the second twenty minute increment and another increment for the additional 5 minutes. This is a one time fee, as I don't want mothers to hesitate to call me because they have to come up with a travel fee for every home visit.

One fee or several? With the exception of the travel fee as above, many midwives ask for one fee for all services regardless of the point in pregnancy that care begins. Doing so discourages women from coming late for care just to get a better deal financially, although in fact I have not had this be a problem. I do not want to be thinking of money at every visit, nickel and diming my way to term by charging individually for prenatal care. With one fee you can see a woman as often as her circumstances warrant without any guilt about a woman's individual financial situation. You also know how much you can expect to get from a particular birth. However, there are many midwives who have a set fee for each prenatal visit, with an additional larger fee for the birth itself. Individual fees are charged for postpartum visits as well.

Barter arrangements: If you decide to barter with clients, formalize your agreement early with a clearly written, signed contract as to exactly what you will get in exchange for your services. Give a copy to your clients. Without this, you can run into big problems because your idea of a fair barter and theirs may be very different. If you do not feel comfortable with what they will offer you, do not choose to barter, or barter for only part of your fee.

Collecting insurance: Whether you get reimbursed from insurance companies for your services will depend upon both your legal status in your state and the individual insurance company. Those practicing in illegal states will usually be ineligible for reimbursement, while those practicing in unregulated, legal situations may or may not be reimbursed. Often this depends upon whose desk the claim crosses and how thorough and nitpicky they are about what gets covered and what doesn't. Medicaid will only reimburse licensed practitioners.

If you are legal or unregulated, you can always try for reimbursement. It is best to wait until the birth is over before submitting any bills. That way, if a hospital transport is indicated, you can apply the insurance claim to what will surely be the highest bill. In the meantime, the parents should be clear that insurance is an iffy proposition and they should pay you in full just as if they had no insurance. If insurance pays, it will be a bonus to them.

Filling out the form neatly and having a computer generated billing statement (see pages at the end of this chapter) goes far in getting your claim covered. I have included examples of three different forms which have worked to get insurance reimbursement in my practice. Any of these styles may be requested, depending upon the insurance company. It is also helpful to have the various insurance codes on your billing statement. Ask a friendly practitioner in town if they will assist you in obtaining these codes or buy a copy of the CPT code book yourself or one for the midwifery community to share. Call the American Medical Association at (800) 621-8335.

Payments and refund policy: My practice has always been very flexible about the fee payment schedule with some women paying a prearranged amount per visit, some taking the full amount out of the bank, and some waiting for tax refunds or other payments. These plans should be written clearly on the agreement form. As each appointment draws to a close, check up on the subject of money. Look over their financial agreement, remind them when their payment is due or acknowledge them for paying on time. If they are avoiding the subject of money, ask them frankly why this appears to be the case.

Asking for the entire fee by the thirty-eighth week of pregnancy leaves you free to go to the birth without any left over energy exchange issues to deal with. If unusual events occur during the pregnancy, for example an early miscarriage or a very premature birth, you may wish to offer a refund. If you do and how much you offer all depends on the total demands of the special situation on your time and resources. Some midwives offer a tempting incentive plan by discounting the total fee if it is paid in advance of a certain point in pregnancy.

When you give a refund for services, you can charge a fee for each visit that the woman has already had. These fees are not usually not based on a sliding scale. In my practice as of 1992 I charged $150.00 for an initial and $60.00 for each additional consultation, prenatal or postpartum visit, plus the one-time travel fee, if we have already made home visits. The first consultation visit is generally always free of charge.

What of the woman who is not keeping up with her payments? Ask her how things are going with her monetary situation and what she intends to do. Remind her that the 38 week mark is approaching, and she is about to owe a lot of money at once if she doesn't catch up. Broaching the subject may prompt her to pay. If not, at least an alternative plan can be worked out. Some midwives have found that local banks will give parents family expansion loans for birthing services. Some midwives even take credit cards! If the woman offers to borrow the money from a friend or relative, that is fine. I would much rather have my money and a clear relationship with the families I am working with than to muddy the waters by discouraging a solution they come up with that would work for me as well.

In situations where it is impossible for women to pay the entire fee up front, you may choose to make allowances. Ask for as much as possible (at least half) of the money by term. Then request that the parents give you post-dated checks to cover the balance of the fee at either the 40 week prenatal visit or at a postpartum home visit. If you have no receptionist dealing with bill collection, and it is a task you loathe, this eliminates the need to call and try to politely ask where the payment may be. It also places the responsibility of contact regarding the payment clearly with the parents, who must call you if the check is to be held while money clears the bank or a similar delay in processing occurs. On the whole, this method of dealing with after-the-birth payments works better than anything else I have tried.

My practice does not offer refunds in the event of hospital transport near term, although there are midwives that do. As midwives we often spend more time with women who wind up the hospital, not less, and that time is equally valuable even if the birth or postpartum is not completed at home. After all, if a midwife detects a problem which needs hospital care, she has done her job.

When clients can't afford your fee: Sometimes, even if you offer a sliding scale, clients will say they can't afford your fee. Think out your response carefully and be very clear within yourself and with them regarding what is acceptable in these circumstances. I have found that when people clearly state that they cannot afford the low end of the scale, state what they can afford up front and pay on time things work out well. Those that are vague about what they can afford or are expecting you to offer them care free of charge usually have other issues that are equally problematic; take heed. You are not responsible to take care of everyone just because they ask you to. Don't do them the disservice of agreeing to care for them and then resenting the fact that they are not paying you enough. There are other options in most communities for women who are unable to pay a fee that truly feels fair to you for the work you will do in exchange.

Coping with paperwork: Once the financial agreement is returned (usually at the initial visit) ask how the parents want to make payments and make note of this on the form. This way you can prompt them if they are not forthcoming with the money at the appropriate times. Keep the fee schedule in each client's chart. Refer to it at each visit. If you have somehow failed to write down how and when they intend to pay, ask them now, saying you want to write it down so you are not asking them their plan of payment incessantly at every visit.

I met a midwife who was complaining to me about never getting paid. She kept her fee agreements in a file and never referred to them during the course of care. If you don't make payment a priority and assume you will be paid the agreed upon amount, it is very likely you will be paid less or not at all!

The midwifery community and your fees: There are other issues that arise regarding payment for services. It may be hard to establish a fee schedule or method of payment which varies greatly from those of other midwives in your area. You may choose to discuss money at a local midwifery meeting. How do you respond to potential clients who are shopping around for the best deal as well as for the right midwife? If you have apprentices or childbirth educators within your practice, will they be paid by you? Do you share financial information with other midwives in your community? For example, if a client didn't pay you for a past birth, do you let her present midwife know? The suggestions in this chapter can provide a starting point for such a discussion in your area.

522

RESPONSIBILITY AGREEMENT:

We, _____ are pregnant and have requested the services of independent midwives to assist us during the prenatal period and with the birth of our child in our home. We have read an Informed Disclosure statement which includes information on their philosophy, educational and employment resumes and past birth statistics. We understand that these midwives are not licensed medical professionals of any kind. All our questions regarding their background and experience have been answered to our satisfaction. We understand that we may terminate services at any time. In requesting the services of independent midwives we freely exercise our right to seek the type of maternity services we feel are best for ourselves and our baby. By signing this statement we affirm these things of our own free will and fully accept any and all risks and responsibilities for homebirth and the health of ourselves and our baby. Finally, we agree to reimburse our midwives as indicated below.

Midwife	date	Pregnant client	date

Midwife	date	Partner	date

Suggested reimbursement for services is based on the following income scale:

up to 10,000	$1200.00
10 to 16,000	$1300.00
17 to 19,000	$1400.00
20 to 29,000	$1500.00
30 to 39,000	$1600.00
40 to 50,000	$1700.00
Each +10,000	+$100.00

An additional amount is requested for birth services outside a 20 minute radius of (your town) for extra gas and telephone expenses. The scale is as follows:

$80.00 for the first +20 minute distance
+ $50.00 for each additional 20 minutes

Based on the scales above, we agree to pay a total of $_____ in exchange for birth services with the following provisions: that the final payment is due by the 38th week of pregnancy; should the birth occur in the hospital the agreed upon amount shall be paid in full; should unforeseen events occur during the pregnancy, individual arrangements will be made based upon the situation.

Taking all of the above into consideration, we agree to make payments according to the schedule described on the line below:

RECORD OF PAYMENTS RECEIVED:			
DATE	AMOUNT	DATE	AMOUNT

INSURANCE BILLING EXAMPLE #1:

BABYTIME MIDWIFERY SERVICES
22 Dixie St.
Any Town, NY 01234
(606) 231-1234
Mary Malone SS# 233-44-5566   Betty Lambert SS# 123-45-6789

BILLING STATEMENT:
   Sue Smith   Date of delivery: May 15, 1995
   123 Anywhere Terrace
   Any town, NY 01234

Labor, delivery and immediate postpartum care: $2000.00

   Includes all labor and delivery fees. All checks should be made payable to Mary Malone and Betty Lambert.

   This bill has been paid in full.

_____

INSURANCE BILLING EXAMPLE #2:

BABYTIME MIDWIFERY SERVICES
22 Dixie St.
Any Town, NY 01234
(606) 231-1234
Mary Malone SS# 233-44-5566   Betty Lambert SS# 123-45-6789
BILLING STATEMENT:

Name & address of insured:Date of delivery:_____

_____

_____

_____

Fees for maternity services incl. labor, delivery & imm. postpartum care: _____

____Includes all labor and delivery fees. Checks should be made payable to Mary
      Malone and Betty Lambert.
____This bill has been paid in full, therefore we request that you reimburse the
      insured directly.
               Thank you for your attention to this matter.

524

BABYTIME MIDWIFERY SERVICES
22 Dixie St.
Any Town, NY 01234
(606) 231-1234

Mary Malone SS# 233-44-5566   Betty Lambert SS# 123-45-6789

BILLING STATEMENT:

Name & address of insured: Date of delivery:_____

_____

_____

_____

Date(s)	Services	Fee
TOTAL		

This bill has been paid in full, therefore we request that you reimburse the insured directly.

_____

Statement of Informed Disclosure (Informed Choice Agreement)

This document describes your midwifery practice; it is intended for anyone who may be interested, although it is primarily prepared for prospective clients. In my opinion, presenting such a statement is one of the most important things which the current midwifery movement has prompted in terms of client education, and is a hallmark difference in the care midwives provide. It may be called an Informed Choice or Informed Consent agreement in some areas, but I have always liked the notion of Informed Disclosure the best. Since I am a writer, my practice has a very elaborate document.

Your document should be a reflection of who you are and what you bring to midwifery care. Scrupulous honesty should be the main feature of your presentation; an honest representation of your background and experiences allows parents to truly make an informed decision about their choice of care provider. I have always held that women have the right to choose whichever midwife they wish, but that each midwife has the responsibility to let a woman know if she has only attended five births, has never seen a hemorrhage, has a heavy medical background that colors her perceptions, or whatever nuances she may bring to her work. In the end, neither a midwife nor the parents she works with can be sure exactly what will take place in an emergency situation, but she can try to inform them as much as possible, so that they know what they are getting into and, as much as humanly possible, what to expect.

I present my Informed Disclosure statement at the consultation visit. It is xeroxed front to back and bound in a plastic slip-binding cover. I ask them to take it home, read it, and either return it at the initial visit or in the mail should they decide to birth elsewhere. Some midwives mail out their document with a preconsultation packet, and some give a copy to the parents to keep. In my case, it is rather lengthy, giving out copies to keep becomes an expensive proposition.

My document begins with a cover letter. I am including the substance of the philosophy sections in their entirety, and offer guidelines you can follow in presenting your resumes and statistics. You may not wish to include all this information in your document or you may have other topics you feel are important; formulate your statement accordingly. It is a good idea to make a note on the cover regarding the last revision date. This avoids confusion when updated copies come into use.

<u>Statement of Informed Disclosure</u>

We acknowledge your right and responsibility to be fully informed regarding prospective health care providers. This Statement is intended to provide you with information to assist in choosing a birth attendant. We feel quality care and a trusting relationship are best ensured when an educated public makes an informed decision regarding the care they receive: based on perceived needs and what an individual practitioner can provide. A system of informed disclosure fosters parent responsibility and care giver accountability. We feel this affords optimal protection within the health care relationship for all concerned. In this statement the following topics are addressed:

*Resource list of practitioners and support services in (your state)
*What is an independent midwife?
*The legal status of independent midwifery and homebirth in (your state)
*Our philosophy of care
*Arranging medical back-up and ambulance service
*The political realities of independent midwifery and homebirth
*A few words about safety
*The role of apprentices in our practice
*The role of supervised primary midwives in our practice
*Preparation classes
*Client education
*The participation of family and friends during pregnancy and birth
*The equipment we do and do not carry to births
*Appointments
*Our accessibility
*The services we provide
*Personal resumes of education and employment, including professional certificates
*Birth statistics
*Our statistics in perspective
*An annotated bibliography of the scientific support for midwifery and/or homebirth

As parents, you are ultimately responsible for your birthing experience, regardless of where or with whom you give birth. Therefore we urge you to seriously evaluate the environment for birth and the care givers whose services you engage. In (your state) your choices include (obstetricians, family practice doctors, certified nurse-midwives, and independent, non-regulated midwives). (Explain status of independent midwives in your state). Each has a specific orientation toward birth. Educate yourselves, ask questions and consider the type of information included herein when making an evaluation. Contact childbirth consumer groups and find out what resources they may have to offer. Explore all your options so that your choices will be right for you.

Sincerely,

Revised _____

Resource List of Practitioners and Support Services in (your state)

Members of the (Your State's Midwives Association)

NOTE: Membership includes primary and supervised primary midwives and their apprentices or assistants. In addition some members also offer various classes, homebirth support groups, labor support for hospital bound clients, and YBAC support in their areas.

(If your organization's membership is very small you might offer a list of all members, their practice status, location and phone number. If you have a large state, you may want to just list local midwives that the woman is likely to seek care from in your community. In this way, you all support each other as well as the women you see to make a truly informed choice.)

Consumer Groups in (your state):

Friends of Midwives/contact name & phone number
International Cesarean Awareness Network/contact name & phone number
Homebirth Support Group/contact name & phone number

Childbirth Related Classes:

Siblings at Birth/contact name & phone number
Informed Homebirth/contact name & phone number
etc.

What is an independent midwife?

In the United States there are three different forms of midwifery currently being practiced. Independent midwifery (otherwise known as lay or direct entry midwifery) is a practice which may or may not be legally recognized, regulated, licensed or certified by a particular state. Independent midwives provide health care for pregnant and birthing women. Independent midwives arrive at their practice through a variety of routes: personal study and experience, formal training programs and/or private apprenticeships. Skill levels, experience and educational background as well as practice styles tend to vary widely. Independent midwives exist in every state, although in some they practice covertly and/or illegally.

The most widely recognized group of professional midwives are certified nurse midwives. They are registered nurses (with 2 to 4 years of training) who have gone on for additional training as midwives. In most states they must work under the supervision of a physician; most carry malpractice insurance and do not participate in homebirths. This is primarily because of the adverse climate in the medical community and the accompanying lack of physician back-up.

In some states (such as Arizona, South Carolina, Florida, Washington, New Mexico, New Hampshire and Oregon) there are state educational and licensing programs formally establishing independent midwives as recognized health professionals in the community. In some states, such as Oregon and Massachusetts, private professional organizations offer standards of practice and certification processes for their members. Such organizations may function without formal recognition by state governments.

(You might include a paragraph outlining the situation in your area.)

Midwifery background and training:

(Your path to midwifery could be from a variety of different backgrounds. It is important that this be represented honestly in your statement. Here are a few examples of what you might include based on different backgrounds:)

*(If you are a registered nurse and practice as an independent midwife)
I became a registered nurse in (date) with a focus in obstetrics. I practiced in a hospital setting for # years. During that time I offered labor support, performed internal exams as well as other diagnostic and clinical procedures at a doctor's request and assisted the doctors with normal and surgical births. As a registered nurse I did not make decisions regarding management of cases nor did I carry the full responsibility of the birth outcome as does a primary attendant. In 19-- I became interested in alternative childbirth and began attending birth classes with a local independent midwife. She accepted me for an apprenticeship which was completed in the Fall of 19--. In summary, I have a background as a registered nurse with obstetrical experience and I am now practicing as an independent midwife. This does not make me a nurse-midwife, which would mean I have formal, institutionally based training in midwifery as a certified nursing specialty.

*(if you had gone on the obtain a certified nurse-midwife credential, you might including nursing background as above and then add:)
In 19-- I decided to become a nurse-midwife, and attended the _____ Nurse midwifery program in _____. This training completed the requirements to become a CNM in an institutional setting working with hospital clients. I then returned to the independent midwife I had worked with to get reoriented to homebirth once again before beginning my current practice. I now hold a Masters in nurse midwifery and have passed the certification exam administered by the American College of Nurse Midwives.

*(If you are a state licensed or certified midwife)
I practice as a certified midwife in our state. Procuring this certification involved completing a __ year course of study, passing a __ hour oral and written exam and paying a fee. As a certified midwife I must abide by state regulations which restrict my practice in a number of ways. The certification act is included in its own section in this document. There are other midwives in our state who have chosen to practice as unlicensed practitioners and therefore have broader parameters of care. Their practice is totally self-regulated; however, they may be able to offer you care in certain situations in which I am restricted. If this seems to be the case during the course of your care, I will let you know.

*(If you have taken the NARM Registry Board exam)

I am a NARM registry board listed midwife. To acquire this title I passed an 8 hour written exam which covered the basic academic information which is felt necessary for the entry level practice of independent midwifery. Since it only tests for academic knowledge, my passage of this test does not reflect an evaluation of my clinical skills as a midwife. I took this exam because it was the only objective means available to me for challenging my knowledge of midwifery basics, since our state does not currently have any provisions for such testing.

*(If you are a NARM Certified Professional Midwife)

As a NARM CPM I have passed a written examination of academic knowledge and submitted proof of experiences at births and validation of a wide variety of clinical skills by another CPM. This grants the title of certification. Work is being done on a state by state basis to achieve national recognition of this credential.

*(If you went to a midwifery school or training program)

I attended the (name) training program, completing my studies in 19__. This was a clinically based program which also included didactic classes on a variety of topics. I participated in ## births as either an assistant, labor support person, supervised primary attendant or observer. More detail about my experiences there can be found in the section of this document covering birth statistics.

The legal status of independent midwifery and homebirth in (your state):

*(If the legal status is left vague or undefined)

The legal status of independent midwifery is not defined in (your state). In (date) a new law went into effect which defines and regulates the practice of nurse-midwifery but does not address independent midwifery at all. Therefore the practice of independent midwifery is totally self-regulated by the individual practitioner and is not an endorsement or guarantee of competence. As consumers, you must exercise your own judgement in determining the quality of services and the competence of independent midwives or any other health care provider. As parents you are legally free to choose your birthing environment and care providers.

Although the state of (your state) has no regulations for independent midwifery the (your state) Midwives Association is the professional organization for homebirth practitioners in our state. The membership engages in ongoing education, peer review, and was formed with the intention of maintaining high standards of midwifery care. Complaints about midwifery care in (your state) can be directed in writing to the (state midwifery association, including the address and phone number).

*(Here is a paragraph describing a different state situation)

Our state has a private professional association of independent midwives. All midwives may join the State Midwifery Counsel (SMC) and, at their discretion, take a written and oral examination. These tests examine the basic knowledge and review the skills necessary to attend births on one's own responsibility. The exam does not include direct supervision of the applicant in actual practice settings or at births, although the applicant must show evidence that she has attended ## births and performed ## prenatal and postpartum visits as well. The passage of these exams grants SMC certification. Certified midwives agree to abide by the protocols and peer review processes established by the SMC. SMC certified midwives engage in ongoing peer review and adhere to guidelines which are agreed upon by the organization as acceptable parameters for homebirth practice. These guidelines are periodically reviewed and may be changed if the members feel this is warranted. Depending upon the anticipated risk involved in individual situations, various protocols are recommended. Should your medical history or course of pregnancy, labor or postpartum include any of these problems, you will be informed as to the opinion of the SMC concerning the risks to mother and/or baby. Neither the SMC, its standards nor its certification process are recognized by the state or the medical community.

(Make sure whatever you write about your state situation does not misrepresent the qualifications, credentials or other processes in place for recognizing midwives.)

Philosophy of care statement: (example):

Pregnancy, birth and breastfeeding are natural, normal functions of a woman's mind, body, emotions and spirit, all of which are equally important. As midwives, we seek to nurture a woman's sense of personal strength and self confidence so that she may realize birth as an empowering and enlarging experience. We do not feel we "deliver" babies; we assist and support women to give birth. We believe that women are uniquely suited to attend other women during this life passage. Most of the world's women give birth with midwives who serve as guides to the total pregnancy experience. Birth at home among family members, coupled with continuous care by skilled attendants, can provide an optimal environment for the majority of women. When birth is integrated into life as a family event, the family is strengthened as well.

As care-givers, our clinical skills, intellects and intuitions all serve as valuable tools in our work as guides to understanding the process of pregnancy and birth. We believe the things which matter most in creating a physically healthy pregnancy are those things you have the most control over, including good nutrition, exercise and the elimination of tobacco, alcohol and drugs. On an emotional, psychological and spiritual level, we recognize that birth is not an event which is isolated from the totality of a woman's life. We endeavor to assist women to become as conscious of their personal processes as possible so that they may have a broad base of resources to draw on during their birth experiences. Our responsibility is to make you aware of any concerns we have based on our past experience and current perceptions. We seek to offer informed choice, not merely informed consent. You are our clients, never our patients. Any decisions regarding options are yours to make. At the same time, there are limits to what we are willing to take on as responsible care providers. When and if our limits are reached, we will let you know immediately.

We offer our services as a team working in partnership with clients before, during and after the birth of their child. We feel team practice affords a high standard of care: two perspectives, two sets of skilled hands, and the different perceptions gained from varied backgrounds available at all times. For us, midwifery is a continually evolving process and we are always learning from our experiences. Working in partnership with clients means we are supporting you to create your own experience. You are responsible for the birth and we are assisting you in taking that responsibility. It also means we must all be in agreement regarding the care needed and our ability to provide such care. Complete prenatal care creates the opportunity to develop a relationship before the birth as well as to establish the parameters of well-being unique to each individual client.

Any environment, whether home, hospital or birthing center, presents a distinct set of risk factors for birth. Nothing can guarantee a perfect outcome. We believe each woman has the right to an informed choice of the environment which she perceives as safest for her and her baby. Many women do not appreciate mainstream obstetrics' approach to pregnancy as a problem waiting to happen. Our care reflects their own desire to trust birth and themselves. For such women, homebirth is a logical choice. We endeavor to create an environment which supports women in opening to their own instinctive process rather than imposing artificial interventions or attempting to make labor conform to a specific pattern. When allowed to follow its natural course, pregnancy usually results in the birth of a healthy baby and mother. The range of natural variation is extremely wide. Occasionally, a critical situation arises during pregnancy or labor which necessitates specialized care that cannot be provided in a home setting. In such cases, a previously established medical back-up system is relied upon for appropriate care.

Arranging medical back-up and ambulance service:

An established relationship with medical professionals helps to foster a smooth transition into the medical system should this become necessary. You are responsible for establishing medical back-up with an obstetrician, certified nurse-midwife, family practice physician or in-hospital prenatal clinic who will be available for consultation and/or referral in case of prenatal problems or hospital transport before, during or after birth. It is also your responsibility to find suitable pediatric back-up should the baby require special attention. Pediatricians, family practice physicians, nurse-practitioners or naturopaths will often provide such care.

The majority of transports will take place in private cars, but occasionally use of an ambulance will be more appropriate. It is helpful to notify a nearby ambulance service of your plans to birth at home. This is especially important if your home is rural or otherwise difficult to locate. Provide a map if necessary. Ask details such as what equipment they have on board (oxygen, IV?) and the skill level of their attendants. We have found that notifying ambulance services prior to birth creates more likelihood of cooperation should they be needed. If you call and detect hostility regarding your choice to birth at home it is best to select another service, if possible.

The political realities of choosing independent midwifery and homebirth:

We cannot separate individual circumstances from the social and political contexts in which they occur. As independent midwives we place ourselves outside the mainstream medical framework. We believe in what we do and feel completely committed to serving women and families in birthing as they choose. On a larger scale, we recognize our work as revolutionary: part of a worldwide movement of women and families to reclaim health care, as well as the right to take personal responsibility and make choices. In choosing the care of independent midwives and homebirth it is important to realize that you enter this political arena as well.

Throughout the United States and Canada, independent midwives, other supportive medical professionals and parents are being harassed by those who would seek to deny our right to practice and your right to choose our care. At some point we may be called upon to defend our rights together. To that end we all need to feel clear about our choices and relationship.

In choosing homebirth and independent midwifery care you are going against what our culture expects of responsible adults. It is ironic that the more personal responsibility you assume in this society, the less responsible you are perceived to be. For example: if birth results in death or injury in the hospital, no one will come to you and say "See what happens when you have a baby in the hospital?" People may encourage you to investigate or even sue, but the basic view that the hospital was the best choice will not be questioned. However, if problems arise at home, you will invariably be questioned about the wisdom of homebirth again and again.

In the midst of the personal crisis surrounding the complications, there may be relatives, friends, doctors, lawyers, ambulance attendants and the police demanding information, explanations, and that charges be pressed against your midwives. Your role as responsible parents may be questioned, because many authorities consider homebirth to be child abuse or neglect. We ask you to honestly project yourselves into your worst scenario and examine how you would feel about your original choices after the fact. Would you still clearly feel they were the right choices for you? If not, please let us know, so that we can further discuss and assist in clarifying your decision about the most appropriate birthing situation for you.

We strive to create an open and trusting relationship with you that recognizes the inherent lack of guarantees in life and birth. We depend upon you, our clients, to stand behind us in case of problems in the same way that we place ourselves at personal and political risk so that you may have your choice of care and birthplace in the first place.

A few words about safety:

While we clearly feel it is not our place to "sell" anyone on the idea of homebirth, some insights into our cultural programming about birth may help you to sort out your feelings and facilitate your decision-making process. Furthermore we strongly feel that safety is not the issue (if it were there would be no argument: statistics repeatedly demonstrate that homebirth is safer than hospital). Rather, we feel it is an issue of assuming personal responsibility for your choice. For partners who are puzzled by the desire of women to birth at home, perhaps this discussion will help you to understand more about the underlying motives of such a choice.

Although hospitals are widely believed to be the safest place to give birth, there has never been even one study that shows this belief to be based in fact. In reality, the studies which have been done (most of which attempt to discredit the safety of homebirth and midwifery) have proven overwhelmingly that hospitals and doctor attendance at birth do not result in the best outcomes for mothers or babies. In fact, the United States ranks 23-24th internationally among industrialized nations in infant mortality. Those nations with the lowest infant mortalities have one thing in common—the majority of their births are attended by midwives. If hospitals and doctors are what make birth safe why do we, with 98% hospital births and 94% physician attendance, rank so poorly? Clearly hospitals, physicians and technology do not, in and of themselves, ensure a safer outcome. Nevertheless, our belief is that they do. It is almost impossible for many people to extract themselves from this belief system long enough to look at the matter objectively.

Perhaps an analogy to something we do every day, eating, will shed some light on the current attitudes which surround childbirth safety in our country. Suppose physicians everywhere suddenly decided to focus on eliminating choking deaths resulting from the ingestion of food. The medical focus would become: avoid death by choking. To that end, public eating areas would be set up so that people could be observed by health professionals while dining. Standards of "normal" eating would be established; perhaps times of the day, blood sugar levels, and chewing patterns would all be calculated in relation to the number of people who choked. Some, who had choked before or who were especially at risk (the very young or very old) would be hospitalized during meals to be more carefully monitored. Foods would undoubtedly be chosen to minimize the possibility of choking: most would be mashed or pureed. Eventually, no doubt, doctors would advocate nutritive I.V.s as a solution for the high risk and those who didn't want to risk eating the more careless way. Of course, to completely eliminate this choking problem, everyone could receive nutritive I.V.s. A lot of time, money and effort would be spent developing various nutritive I.V. fluids to meet everyone' needs. People would discover where they stood as far as risk was concerned and those who ate at home unobserved would be seen as reckless and irresponsible.

It is easy for us to see how crazy this idea sounds. Who would want to be hospitalized to eat baby food? Would it really be more comforting to know someone skilled in the Heimlich maneuver was right behind you, knife at the ready, waiting to do a tracheotomy if it didn't work?

It is true that thousands of choking deaths happen every year and we should all be informed about how to assist when a choking accident occurs. But wouldn't so much focus on choking create a lot of unnecessary fear and intervention which might easily result in more choking deaths because everyone was so nervous? And would eliminating all the other pleasures and needs met by dining in a relaxed fashion be worth it? It is easy to see how absurd this would be because we are intimately knowledgeable about the risk/benefit ratio for choking involved in eating. Imposing this kind of fear on eating is something we readily reject as an overreaction to the reality of death by choking. This doesn't sound safe, it sounds ridiculous!

Our society has essentially taken another normal process, childbirth, and done the very same thing. The focus of modern obstetrics is to avoid death at all costs. Technological interventions and the Cesarean rate are soaring; some doctors have advocated 100% Cesarean as a prophylactic measure. People birth in the hospital "just in case something goes wrong." As a result, the myriad other aspects of childbirth have been ignored or simply paid lip service. An event that used to be as much a part of ones' everyday life as eating has been removed to an institution and transformed into a purely medical event. Our focus on and fear of problems prevents us from dealing with childbirth in a rational and balanced way.

Statistically, birth at home with skilled midwives provides the very safest care possible for most women. The few who are better off in a hospital are those who need the technology available there for very specific and relatively uncommon reasons, most of which are medical conditions that have nothing to do with the pregnancy.

The reason why midwifery is safer is very simple: midwives are specialists in normal birth who respect the wisdom of this normal life process. We focus on solutions, not problems. To even suggest we focus on the normal makes everyone rush to ask "Well, it's fine if everything is normal, but what if there are problems?" To focus on the normal does not mean that problems go unrecognized and unattended. It means that the problems are viewed in a different way, one in which imbalances are righted, not expected and not feared.

In our culture today midwifery provides a haven for women who believe that pregnancy can be natural, normal and healthy, and a refuge for parents who want their experience to be seen as more than the sum total of its physical parts. A woman cannot easily relax and give birth with tubes hanging out of her and people standing over her waiting to see if her baby will die, any better than one can relax and enjoy a meal with the knowledge that someone is hovering nearby waiting to see if they will choke. We seek to support families who desire to rise above the culturally imposed terror surrounding birth and come to a more humane and rational approach which puts the medical aspects of birth back into perspective. (For more on safety see the sections on Our Statistics in Perspective and the Bibliography.)

The role of apprentices in our practice:

We feel it is important for skills to be passed on from experienced midwives to those desiring to learn. Therefore we ask interested women to fill the valuable role of assistant/apprentice at births we attend. Apprentices engage in ongoing study, participate in prenatal and postpartum care, and serve as assistants at the birth. Acquiring clinical skills is an essential part of an apprentice's education. In teaching such skills we are always respectful of the mother's feelings. Deciding who actually attends the birth is totally up to the family. You will meet an apprentice during your prenatal care. Feel free at any time to make us aware of concerns regarding this aspect of our care; another apprentice can be chosen or another arrangement made for assistance at your birth if you so desire.

The role of supervised primary midwives in our practice:

We would like to introduce (name of supervised midwife) as a supervised primary attendant. She completed her apprenticeship training with us in (date). She brings extensive educational and experiential background to her work. She if functioning as a newly trained primary attendant at births under our supervision. She is a great asset to our practice. For more details about her, please refer to the resume included.

Preparation classes:

Childbirth preparation classes can be an important aspect of the prenatal experience. Among other benefits, classes create a forum for couples to share emotional, psychological and physical impressions surrounding the experience of pregnancy and birth. We encourage you to attend consumer-oriented classes which emphasize that relaxation, inner confidence and emotional, psychological and physical openness allow birth to take place with the least amount of problems for mother and baby. It is our experience that classes which stress complicated breathing techniques and "stages of labor" artificially represent the nature of birth and tend to hinder, rather than help, the process. We can provide you with a list of appropriate childbirth classes in our area.

Client education:

Education and informed choice are cornerstones of the care we provide. We expect you to take responsibility by informing yourself, and want you feel free at any time to ask questions. You can monitor the care you receive by being aware of what good birth-related care entails. There are numerous childbirth books on the market; a few encourage assuming personal responsibility in this way. If there are concerns which these books do not address, let us know and we will refer you to the proper sources. Our recommendations include:

Right From the Start by Gail Sforza Brewer
A review of pregnancy and birth; physiology, birth environments (home, hospital and birthing center), procedure and interventions; options.

Special Delivery by Rahima Baldwin
A parent's manual, focusing on homebirth and emphasizing personal responsibility.

A Guide to Midwifery: Heart and Hands by Elizabeth Davis
A complete overview of what good independent midwifery care entails; written by an independent midwife.

The Five Standards of Safe Childbearing edited by David Stewart for NAPSAC
Standards focusing on the normal rather than the pathological: skillful midwifery, good nutrition, homebirth, natural childbirth and breastfeeding. Well documented. (Order from NAPSAC, Rt. 1, Box 646, Marble Hill, MI 63764. $11.20 post paid)

Silent Knife: Cesarean Prevention and Vaginal Birth After Cesarean by Nancy Wainer-Cohen and Lois Estner
Examines the current trend toward surgical birth and how to avoid unnecessary

procedures and interventions; excellent review of statistics and safety factors.

The Tentative Pregnancy by Barbara Katz Rothman
Important reading for anyone considering any type of fetal diagnosis.

The Vaginal Birth After Cesarean Experience: Very Beautiful and Courageous by
        Lynn Baptisti Richards
Inspiring stories of women who transformed their relationship to birth and to themselves.

Pregnant Feelings by Rahima Baldwin and Terra Palmarini
A workbook for pregnancy designed to help you explore emotional and psychological issues which may impact your birth experience.

Woman-centered Pregnancy and Birth by the Federation of Feminist Women's
        Health Centers
An excellent and uncompromised reference for birth; good information regarding interventions.

Obstetric Myths versus Research Realities, by Henci Goer
A scathing and intelligent critique of many modern obstetrical practices back-up with their own research using journal abstracts.

The participation of family and friends during pregnancy and birth:

We encourage you to be selective about who is to attend your birth. It is important that the needs of the mother be placed before those of anyone who wants to be present. Friends and relatives with whom you have a close and emotionally clear relationship can be a great asset to you during labor. We will be happy to discuss our perceptions of what is appropriate and assist you in making a decision about who to have with you during birth. Those who are coming need to feel positive about your choice to birth at home and your care providers. If necessary, they also need to be willing to leave during the labor or birth and not take it personally.

Many families want other siblings present at the birth: our experience with this is very positive. Children need prior preparation for the possible noises, faces and concentration their mother will display; bleeding and the birth of the placenta; and the appearance of the newborn. An adult who is willing to miss the birth or remove the children from the home if that becomes appropriate to meet the children's needs should be specifically in charge of overseeing the children. This person should be especially clear of anxiety about your birth choices so as not to communicate discomfort to the children. We feel strongly that children should be allowed to be present or not as they feel most comfortable.

Occasionally partners want to catch the baby. This is fine with us; however, often the partner becomes so involved in giving emotional support that the woman does not want their partner to change positions in order to catch.

The equipment we do and do not carry:

We bring the following equipment to your birth: oxygen, suturing equipment, various herbal and homeopathic remedies, anti-hemorrhagic drugs, DeLee mucus traps for deep suctioning of the newborn (should this be called for), scissors, hemostats, and a variety of other non-medical items which often come in handy such as a heating pad and hot water bottle, plus standard diagnostic instruments such as a blood pressure cuff, stethoscopes of various types, baby scale and urine test strips.

There are some articles which we do not carry or rarely use which other midwives often use more routinely. They are:

Doppler fetascope—An ultrasound device which allows one to hear the fetal heart as early as 10 weeks gestation as well as during labor without moving the mother. We feel the safety of ultrasound is unproven and therefore do not wish to use it routinely in our practice. Doppler effect ultrasound is 35 times stronger than diagnostic (real-time/imaging) ultrasound. Listening to the fetal heart with a Doptone is significantly different that listening with a regular fetascope and many subtleties are lost in the translation of the heartbeat to sound waves filtered through a machine. We strongly feel that our intuitive sense of the baby is enhanced by using a regular fetascope.

Intravenous equipment—We feel a woman in need of IV equipment is most appropriately cared for in a hospital setting; the actual need for an IV is rare. We do not wish to use IV's prophylactically at home. Finally, the cost of IV fluids is high and the shelf life quite short, making it difficult to keep on hand given the actual number of times it would be needed.

Ambu-bag—This device is used to administer a predetermined amount of oxygen via positive pressure to the very depressed newborn. It offers the advantage of being able to deliver a much higher concentration of oxygen than ordinary mouth-to-mouth resuscitation and therefore is especially useful in those rare cases when a newborn has a very slow or absent heart rate at birth. In these cases, a higher concentration of oxygen is needed by the heart in order to maximize the chances of its being able to recover a normal rate of beats. We now carry this device and have been trained in its use. However, we feel that human touch is important to a baby born so depressed it cannot breathe on its own. Therefore we feel we can give all round better and safer care by administering CPR if necessary and reserving the use of an ambu-bag for the most severely depressed infants (so far we have never seen a baby born at home which required the use of an ambu-bag).

Laryngoscope—A device which opens the epiglottis in order to visualize the vocal cords. This would be done in cases of significant meconium staining to detect whether meconium is clinging to the vocal cords. If found, removal of the meconium is attempted prior to beginning resuscitation efforts to avoid forcing it into the lungs. Laryngoscopy requires an extremely high skill level to be done safely; we feel we cannot maintain this due to the very rare occasions when it would be necessary. Our practice is to transport the mother if we perceive fetal distress before birth. If fetal distress occurs when birth is imminent, we use a DeLee to deep suction the upper trachea if meconium is present, evaluate the newborn's respiratory status and transport as necessary.

Local anesthetic for suturing—We carry injectable local anesthetic; however there are several reasons we use it very sparingly. First, it is possible to have a severe, life-threatening drug reaction which we are not equipped to deal with at home; local anesthetic swells and distorts the tissue to the point that reapproximation is difficult; lastly, swelling lasts significantly longer and often makes the first week postpartum much more uncomfortable. Although it is somewhat painful to place stitches near the skin edge when no anesthetic is used (many women do not even feel internal stitches), women most often cannot even feel the sutures the day after birth. Edema is minimized and healing is better. We also have spray anesthetic which minimizes or eliminates some of the problems noted above.

Appointments:

Regular visits are an important part of our care. Prenatal visits establish a means for us to get to know each other. We expect you to make them a top priority in your pregnancy. If you must cancel an appointment, please let us know as soon as possible so another visit can be arranged. If we must go to a birth, we will attempt to reach you at home before you leave for your appointment. If this proves impossible we will leave a message on our door.

Appointments are scheduled Monday through Friday from 8:00 a.m. with the last appointment beginning no later than 4:30 p.m. With the exception of the first two, visits usually last about an hour. We do not schedule appointments in the evenings or on weekends.

Our accessibility:

One (usually all) of us will be accessible to you twenty-four hours a day, seven days a week unless we specifically tell you otherwise. If a situation arises concerning the immediate well-being of mother or baby or you feel your labor has begun, we expect you to call at any time. All of us, full time apprentices included, carry beepers, so you can always find us when you need us. When trying to reach us, first try both of our home numbers and leave messages on the answering machines if you find no one home. Next, call a beeper and be sure to leave your name and phone number (you have only 15 seconds to leave a message). Wait at least 15 minutes (in order to retrieve messages we must find a phone) and call again if there is no response. Please use the beepers only in case of immediate need.

We would appreciate your limiting calls which do not directly concern your well-being (such as changing appointments, finding out about a meeting, etc.) to normal office hours (8 am. to 5 p.m. Monday through Friday). This way we can be available to you when you really need us and still avoid burn-out. Thanks.

We are often asked: what if two women go into labor at once? In reality this rarely happens. Even when it has, we have never had two women giving birth simultaneously.

If this should occur we split up and each take an apprentice with us to the most imminent birth. One birth usually finishes up before the other; the first midwife done would then join the other birth in progress. If we absolutely had to we would ask the woman with the largest house to allow the other woman and family in labor to birth at her home. This is not ideal, of course, but is a better solution than asking one family to go to the hospital should this unfortunate situation ever arise. (So far, it hasn't.)

When any one of us plans a vacation we usually let you know well in advance to avoid any surprises near term.

The services we provide:

The care we provide consists of the following:

*Consultation visit (1 hr. or more) a chance for us to meet and discuss mutual questions and the appropriateness of homebirth for your individual situation. A dietary evaluation is included. There is no charge for this interview.

*Initial visit (2 to 3 hrs.) medical history, physical exam, how to prepare for the birth, dietary review.

*Prenatal visits (1 hr. each) once monthly until the 32nd week, every two weeks until the 36th week and every week thereafter until birth, or as often as necessary for your individual situation. One visit, usually in the last month, will be made to your home.

*Labor and birth care in your home as long as necessary. Attendants stay a minimum of three hours postpartum and longer if warranted.

*Postpartum visits at one and five days in your home, at two weeks and six weeks at our office or as often as necessary. (Visit dates are approximate.)

*Nutritional counseling--throughout your pregnancy.

*Two experienced midwives and one apprentice are usually present at the birth as well as at most prenatal and postpartum visits.

Fees include all the above and are based on a sliding scale according to your income. You are independently responsible for all books, laboratory work, medical back-up, classes, designated disposable medical supplies and any necessary hospitalization for yourself or the baby.

540

(Include resumes of each midwife and apprentice in your practice with the following information:)

Name
Address
Phone number
Beeper number

FORMAL EDUCATION & TRAINING:

(list all education credentials including date completed and title awarded)

INFORMAL EDUCATION: (for example:)

1974-present Personal study and application of herbal and other alternative healing
        methods.

CONTINUING EDUCATION & INVOLVEMENT: (for example:)

3/77   "Choices in Childbirth" Conference, San Francisco, CA
2/78   Lecture by Frederick Le Boyer, MD "Birth Without Violence," San Fran.

(list all relevant activities to date)

WORK EXPERIENCE: (for example:)

2/76-6/78 Coordinator/curriculum consultant, Holistic Childbirth Inst., San Francisco
3/79-11/80 Co-director/founder Rising Moon Birth Place Clinic, El Paso, TX, birthing
        center offering full prenatal, intra- and postpartum care.

(list all relevant activities to date)

AFFILIATIONS: (for example:)

    Midwives Alliance of North America (MANA)
    Informed Homebirth (IH)
    International Cesarean Awareness Network
    Your state Midwives Association

PUBLICATIONS, ARTICLES & REVIEWS:

(list all relevant publications such as articles, books, etc.)

(Follow these pages with xerox copies of any certificates which you may have gotten from various educational pursuits, then proceed to describe your practical experiences:)

<u>**BIRTH EXPERIENCE**</u>:

Personal experiences: (If you have children, you may wish to briefly describe your own birth experiences.)

Informal training: (If you saw births outside a training program or private apprenticeship, you may wish to discuss that experience briefly.)

- -
<u>**FORMAL TRAINING**</u> **(describe any formal midwifery schooling, including apprenticeships)**

Apprenticeship experience at The Birthing Center where you studied or the midwife with whom you worked, city & state:
Observations #
Labor support #
Assistant   #
Postpartum   #

Prenatal exams under observation 6 days weekly for 6 months (average of 4-6 exams daily, including initial intake & postpartum follow-up)

Participated in a total of # births plus # immediate postpartum monitoring.

The next pages should include individual statistics for births done in your various practice settings over the course of your career. I will include one page of my statistics as an example of how you might set this up.

<u>**A guide to reading the statistical information which follows**</u>:

Although most of the statistical information is self explanatory, there may be a few things which are difficult to interpret without a key. The following is a brief explanation of each category. Not every category is covered in all the populations because more complete information began to be recorded as my practice evolved. For this reason and because different populations I have worked with have been vastly different, statistics are given for each practice setting separately.

<u>First time mothers</u>: defined by the medical definition of women who have not given birth to a viable baby (one that can live on its own) in the past.
<u>More than one child</u>: all those who have had one or more viable babies.
<u>Place of birth</u>: homebirths and those transported to the hospital for any reason.
<u>Type of delivery</u>: Yoni births after a previous Cesarean (YBAC) are noted as well as totals of

542

spontaneous births, forceps, vacuum extraction and cesarean deliveries.

<u>Premature</u>: any baby born before the beginning of the 37th week of pregnancy.

<u>Overdue</u>: all those who carried to 42 weeks or beyond.

<u>Presentation at birth</u>:

> Vertex—head down, face down
> Transverse—the baby came out head first but facing to the side
> Posterior—head down, face up at birth
> Breech—baby birthed bottom, feet or knees first
> Nuchal cord—refers to cord around the neck or over the shoulder
>> X1 (etc.) explains how many times the cord was wrapped
> Nuchal hand—a hand was beside or under the chin
>> comp. (compound) means the hand was on top of the head or completely beside the face on or above the cheek at the time of birth

<u>Mother's position at birth</u>: It is typical that women change positions many times during pushing (and sometimes during the birth itself). The position noted is the one the mother assumed for the actual delivery of the head and body of the baby.

<u>Baby's weight</u>: included just to give you some idea of how big our babies typically are.

<u>APGAR scores</u>: A standard newborn assessment made at one and five minutes of age. Each of the following observations are made: grimace response, muscle tone, skin color, respirations and heart beat. Zero, one or two points are given for each item, the highest possible total score being ten. A baby with an APGAR of 6 to 7 needs stimulation to establish good respirations. If the APGAR is 5 or less, resuscitation may be called for.

<u>Complications of pregnancy, labor, birth and postpartum</u>: These are numerous and cannot all be listed in a format of this type. I have selected those which parents may wonder about, especially if they have had experience with them during previous hospital births. Meconium is the baby's first bowel movement. If found in the amniotic fluid it can represent current fetal distress. Heart tones are watched carefully and the baby suctioned after birth to remove debris from the air passages, if necessary—this can be done with a DeLee, a special suction device with a trap for the fluid.

<u>Postpartum maternal bleeding</u>: Most of the women we see do not bleed excessively.

<u>Maternal postpartum problems</u>: This is a tabulation of severe manifestations of the problems indicated. Many minor problems such as breast infections, have not been recorded here.

<u>Newborn problems handled at home</u>: Likewise, this is a tabulation of the most severe problems which were recorded on statistics forms.

<u>Hospital transports</u>: Every transport is listed, divided into those transferred in before term (prior to the beginning of the 37th week) and at term. The reason for transport is given first and the information that follows in parentheses is what transpired at the hospital.

<u>Deaths</u>: all fetal or neonatal deaths and the reasons (if known) are listed separately (if applicable) in the statistics for that population.

<u>Percentages</u>: are the simple percentages of the item for the total population as noted.

<u>Abbreviations used</u>:

AROM—artificial rupture of membranes
DOA—dead on arrival
FHT—fetal heart tones
Gest.—gestation
LLQ—lower left quadrant

ICU—intensive care unit
IM—intramuscular
OP—occiput (back of head) posterior
SGA—small for gestational age
Spon.—spontaneous delivery

Statistics from (dates) in city & state.   Number of clients (number of births):

Cancellation: 8
Miscarriages: 11

First time mothers: 94
More than one child: 294

Place of birth:
home   253
hospital   35

Type of delivery:
spontaneous   277
Cesarean (3.13%)   9
Forceps (0.7%)   2
Primary NBC   9
 (1 NBC CS)

Premature (2.8%):
 25 & 26 wks   2
 28 wks   1
 33 wks   2
 36 wks   1

Overdue: (42+ wk)   29

Presentation at birth:
vertex   271
transverse (vertex)   3
posterior   10
breech (2/term .7%)   4
Nuchal cord X1   57
  X2   10   X3   1
Nuchal hand 1 comp.   23

Mother's position at birth:
semi sitting   65
supported kneel   2
upright kneeling   4
standing   14
standing squat   4
standing to H&K   3
squatting   15
squat to H&K   1
lateral   45
Supine (stirps/C)   44
On chair (1/hosp)   2
w/birthing stool   24
on lap   16
hands & knees   37
not recorded   3

Baby's weights:
 9 + lbs. 48   6- lbs.   14
 Largest   11 lbs.
 Smallest 1 lb. 3 oz. (25 wks)
 Smallest at term   6 lbs.

APGAR SCORES AT BIRTH:
9-10 at 1 min.   163   5-6 at 1 min.   17
9-10 at 5 min.   251   5-6 at 5 min.   2

7-8 at 1 min.   92   3-4 at 1 min.   6
7-8 at 5 min.   23   3-4 at 5 min.   4

1 at 1 min.   3   Unknown (transport) 3
1 at 5 min.   1   Fetal demise   4

Complications of labor, birth & postpartum:
 Midwives missed birth (4.2%) 10
 Meconium staining: Light 33 Medium 24
   Heavy 13
 DeLee suction on perineum   16
    after birth   2
 Unknown due to transport   3
Postpartum maternal bleeding:
 1- cup 91   +4 cups 26   9 cups 2
 Prolonged bleeding   14
Agents used to control bleeding:
 Pitocin IM   20   Pitocin IV (hosp.) 15
 Methergine IM 9   Ergotrate tablets   6
 Pit & Met. IM 3   Herbs   43

Lacerations: no tears (9%)   26
 Superficial (no sutures req./38%) 112
 Peri-urethral involvement   61
 Tears requiring sutures: (44%)
   1° 106   2° 7   3° 10   4° 3
 Mother refused sutures: 11

 Episiotomies (2.7%): Home 2 Hospital 6
                          (1 hymen)

Maternal postpartum problems:
 Kidney infection 1 Uterine infection 1
 Breast infection   21   (man. removal)
 Severe hemorrhoids 5

Newborn problems handled at home:
 Eye infections 1   Down syndrome 2

Hospital transports: Total transport rate prior to birth: 11.1%

Transports due to prematurity (37- wks--3.13% of 288 total births):

#Placenta previa (CS at 33 wks)	2
#Major abruption (CS at 25 wks/baby died 5 hrs pp)	1
Variable FHT in labor w/PROM for 6 days from 35 wks (Vag/APGARS 6/8)	1
Mother's request--36 wks (NBC)	1
Labor at 33 wks--(SGA/anencephalic baby/stillborn)	1
#Abruption at 26 wks (CS w/breech/baby in ICU 2 mths)	1
Labor at 34 wks (birth in route to hospital)	1
*Rupture of membranes 36 wks, breech choose hospital birth w/out our support(CS)	1
	1

Transports of mother at term in labor (8.7% of 279 birthing at home):

Low FHT w/contractions (O²/incised hymen)	1
Ineffective contractions/poor pushing urge (Pitocin)	2
Exhausted, dehydrated from vomiting (IV/Pitocin w/PP hemorrhage)	1
Unprepared for homebirth/began care @ 37 wks (spon. birth)	1
*Psychological dystocia (Pitocin/epis./forceps)	2
Psychological dystocia (spon. birth)	1
Psychological dystocia (IV sedative/spon. birth)	1
Bloody amniotic fluid/abruption (spon. birth)	1
Bright red bleeding in early labor (cervical tears)	1
Difficult pushing w/thick perineum/new meconium (epis.)	1
Difficult pushing w/hypoglycemia & thick perineum (epis.)	1
#Poor FHT in active labor, attempted NBC (CS/APGARS 1 & 1)	1
Arrested labor 8 cm. (Epidural/Pitocin/Mag. Sulfate)	1
Fresh meconium bef. pushing (spon. birth)	1
#Cord prolapse (CS/APGARS 5 & 7)	1
Contractions stopped at 6 cm. (Pitocin)	1
LLQ pain prenatally & in labor (pain med/epis)	1
#Undiagnosed breech/FHT good/fetus DOA at hosp. (choose CS)	1
Thick meconium/low FHT w/head compression (O2/epis)	1
Ineffective contractions (Pitocin/manual removal of placenta)	1
Meconium and slow progress at 8 cm. (NBC)	1
#Ineffective contx./OP/arrested labor (Pitocin/epidural/CS)	1
Hospital induction at 37½ wks w/fetal demise (mother's choice)	1

First time mothers transported in labor at term: 18 (72%)
Multiparas transported in labor at term: 7 (28%)
    * Forceps births   # Cesarean deliveries

Postpartum transports of mother (1.3% of 253 birthing at home)

Hemorrhage w/retained placental fragment	1
Hemorrhage w/adhered placenta (Manual removal/IV)	1
4th deg. laceration w/extensive peri-ureteral involvement (sutured)	1
4th degree laceration (sutured)	2
Adhered placenta (manual removal & sutures for labial laceration)	1

Newborn transports (Total 3.1%, Born at home 0.4%)

Myelomeningocele (surgery/baby survived)	1
Baby remained in hospital after birth	6

Fetal deaths   4   Neonatal deaths 1 (abruption/CS in hospital at 25 wks)

Our statistics in perspective:

It is nice to know our record regarding previous births, but unless you have something to compare it to it may be difficult to assess whether you should be impressed or distressed. Unfortunately what makes our results better than mainstream medicine is something hard to quantify and therefore hard to represent in a statistical system which focuses primarily on outcome. However, the good news is that our difference in process is reflected in our results which can be seen when examining our statistics. The two outcomes most statistics concern themselves with are mortality (death) and morbidity (damage or illness resulting from birth). We shall examine both.

First, lets look at our mortality statistics. One problem in examining our statistics is that we have done relatively few births when considering that fetal/infant/neonatal mortality is counted per 1000 births and maternal mortality is counted per 100,000 births. In taking this into account we have presented our total combined number of births attended as primary practitioners as well as those we have attended in partnership, both in New York and Connecticut (name the states you in which you have practiced). We have done this because, statistically speaking, very few births are not as relevant. Mortality statistics are calculated by taking the number of births and the number of deaths and projecting the death rate per 1000. This must be kept in mind when looking at these figures.

The total deaths we have seen in our practices:

First, we can review the total deaths we have had and the circumstances surrounding them. The fetal deaths (babies that died before birth) include:

Anencephalic baby born spontaneously after transport at 33 weeks
gest./defect incompatible with life   1

Fetal demise at 28 wks gest./medically confirmed/chose
homebirth/no apparent cause/autopsy refused   1

The babies that were born alive and subsequently died include:
Incompetent cervix due to abnormality/began dilation at 21 1/2 wks
gest./breech birth in hospital/baby lived approx. 1 hour   1

Placental aburption at 25 wks gest./CS/baby lived 5 hours   1

In addition to these deaths, since 6/83 we have seen 11 miscarriages, all before 12 weeks (although some mothers thought they were farther along). Prior to practicing in (relevant states), early miscarriages were not consistently recorded and were few, due to women coming for care later in their pregnancy than they tend to currently.

To translate these deaths into mortality statistics we must first define the population that our care has covered.

International infant mortality statistics:

The most universally established definition of baby deaths is the infant mortality rate (the number of deaths during the first year of life, regardless of gestational age, per 1000 live births). Here is the data from the 1987 World Population Data Sheet:

1.	Japan	5.5		15.	Singapore	9.3
2.	Iceland	5.7		16-17.	Belgium	9.4
3.	Finland	6.5		16-17.	United Kingdom	9.4
4.	Sweden	6.8		18.	West Germany	9.5
5.	Switzerland	6.9		19.	East Germany	9.6
6.	Hong Kong	7.5		20.	Australia	9.9
7.	Canada	7.9		21-22.	Antigua &	10.0
8.	Denmark	7.9		21.22.	Barbuda	10.0
9.	Netherlands	8.0		23-24.	Netherlands Ant.	10.5
10.	France	8.1		23-24.	Spain	10.5
11.	Norway	8.3		25-26.	United States	10.8
12-13.	Ireland	8.9		25-26.	New Zealand	10.8
12-13.	Taiwan	8.9				
14.	Luxembourg	9.0				

Our infant mortality rates:
  Grand total of all live births: ###
  Infant mortality rate: # per 1000

Live births attended in partnership: ### Infant mortality rate: # per 1000

In (your state) the infant mortality rate for 19## was ## per 1000 live births.

As you can see, the United States ranks very poorly. Not only that, but our current ranking of 25-26th place is a drop from 16th place since 1979!

Perinatal mortality statistics:

Perinatal mortality is estimated by calculating all fetal and infant deaths per 1000 total births from a certain point in gestation until a specified amount of time (days or weeks) after birth. There are several definitions of perinatal mortality:

Def. 1: Infant deaths of less than 7 days and fetal deaths with stated or presumed gestation of 28 weeks or more.
Def. 2: Infant deaths of less than 28 days and fetal deaths with stated or presumed gestation of 20 weeks or more.
Def. 3: Infant deaths of less than 7 days and fetal deaths with stated or presumed gestation of 20 weeks or more

The following table looks at various perinatal mortality rates:

Definition	YOUR STATE	United States	Your births ###	The Farm
1	N/A	12.6	##	N/A
2	N/A	17	##	N/A
3	13.6	15.7	##	11

Notes: Source of state data.

United States rates were taken from the **Monthly Vital Statistics Report: Perinatal Mortality in the United States: 1950-81,** Vol. 34, No. 12, Supplement, March 1986, p. 9.

The Farm in Summertown, TN is an independent homebirth practice organized by Ina May Gaskin (author of Spiritual Midwifery). They have some intensive care facilities in their clinic and an excellent back-up system with a local M.D. Their data is included to compare statistics with another homebirth practice. This figure was taken from a tabulation of 1682 births from 10/70 through 1988.

N/A indicates the rates for this definition were not available.

Maternal mortality rate: Maternal mortality is defined as the deaths of women that result from the reproductive process per 100,000 live births. Most maternal deaths are caused by infection and hemorrhage (approx. 50%) with toxemia and anesthesia as the next two leading factors. Sometimes preexisting medical conditions precipitate maternal deaths as do internal malfunctions (such as an amniotic fluid embolism). The exact number of maternal deaths per year is not known because a birth-related death can be hidden in another category if the woman has prolonged problems originally resulting from birth trauma.

Maternal mortality has been reduced since the turn of the century primarily due do to better general nutrition and sanitation, antibiotics, aseptic technique, improved surgical technique, transfusion and more recently the legalization of abortion. Not very much can be attributed to safer obstetrical technique per se.

Since 1977 the maternal mortality rate has once again started to climb because of the rapid increase in Cesarean deliveries, for which mortality is 4 to 5 times higher than with normal birth. In 1977 the U.S. maternal mortality rate for board certified obstetricians was 10 per 100,000. In 1978 it went up to 30 per 100,000. In 1985 the rate for all practitioners was 7.8 per 100,000. I have had no maternal deaths in my practice.
(If there has been a maternal death in your practice, explain as per neonatal deaths.)

An annotated bibliography of the scientific support for midwifery and/or homebirth:

Jour. Reproductive Medicine, 1977. Vol. 19, pp. 281-290. Mehl, L. Peterson, G., Whitt, M., et al., Outcomes of Elective Home Births: A Series of 1146 Cases.
Gives data showing safety of homebirths attended by independent midwives.

Birth & the Family Jour., 1977. Vol 4, No. 1, pp. 47-58. Devitt, N., The Transition From Home to Hospital Birth, U.S..
An historical review of available scientific & statistical data showing that hospitals have never been proven to be the safest place to give birth.

Jour. Amer. Medical Assoc., May 2, 1980. Vol. 243, No. 17, pp. 1732-1736. Adamson, G. & Gare, D. Home or Hospital Births?.
A review of homebirth data by two physicians, neither of whom believe in homebirth, but who conclude that no valid data exist that prove hospitals are safer than home.

Jour. Amer. Medical Assoc., Dec. 19, 1980. Vol. 244, No. 24, pp. 2741-2745. Burnett, et.al., Home Delivery & Neonatal Mortality In North Carolina.
Shows safety of planned, attended homebirths with midwives or family physicians.

J. Am Public Health Assoc., June 1983. Vol. 73, No. 6, pp. 641-645. Sullivan, D., & Beeman, R., Four Years Experience With HomeBirth by Licensed Midwives in Arizona.
Data showing safety of new state licensing program for independent midwives.

U.S. Gov't Center for Health Statistics, 1984. Pub. (PHS) 84-1918, Series 21, No. 40, 43 pgs, Taffel, S., Midwife & Out-of-Hospital Deliveries in the United States.
Gives data showing that, both in the hospital and at home, midwives get better outcomes as measured by lower rates of prematurity and low-birth-weight babies.

Jour. Amer. Medical Assoc., Mar. 15, 1985. Vol. 253, No. 11, pp. 1578-1582. Hinds, M., etla., Neonatal Outcome of Planned vs.Unplanned Home Births in Kentucky.
Gives data showing safety of homebirth attended by independent midwives.

World Health Organization, The Lancet 1985. August 24, pp. 436-437. Appropriate Technology for Birth.
Recommends training & use of direct-entry (non-nurse) midwives as best way to help improve pregnancy outcomes worldwide, including in developed nations.

British Medical Journal, Sept., 6, 1986. Vol. 293, pp. 606-8. London, I. Obstetric Care, Social Class and Maternal Mortality.
Reviews published data, (1785 to present), showing that improvement in pregnancy outcome since 1900 cannot be due to increased obstetric intervention, nor hospitals; that these factors are more closely correlated with bad outcomes than good.

NOTE: This is a sample of reports supporting homebirth and midwifery. Complete Bibliographies are included in The Five Standards of Safe Childbearing by NAPSAC.

The Initial Visit and Medical History

The visit which follows the consultation will usually include the a general review of the medical history and a physical examination. The initial history is handled in various ways by different midwives. Some prefer to have a woman fill out a form at home, then bring it in for discussion, in this way, she has thought about each question and may have more to offer when the interview rolls around. However, a woman will not understand a question's purpose and either answer it inappropriately or not at all. Many clinicians have clients fill out forms in a waiting room; to some women this can seem impersonal.

Other midwives ask the woman each question in person and fill in the form themselves. Not only does the midwife engage with the woman in documenting the information, the midwife can determine if the woman understands each question and can probe for more information if significant facts are brought to light during the interview. Also, if a partner has anything to add or has a different perception of what happened, they can let you know . Still, other midwives will have a woman fill out her form and then ask every question again during an interview.

There are probably almost as many different forms for documenting the initial history as there are midwives. As you go through this chapter and gain some experience, you will learn the order in which topics are addressed which feels most comfortable to you. The form you like best will depend upon what you are used to and what information you deem important to gather. I have included the four page form from my practice as an example. It is important that your forms have enough room to document important data without being unwieldy. While many of the questions regarding medical history will not be relevant for most women, it is important to question every woman about each individual condition or category of conditions. In this way, something which may be significant or which happened long ago and has been forgotten may be recalled. If you discover a pregnancy related problem or preexisting medical condition that has not been mentioned prior to this visit, consult the appropriate chapter or section elsewhere in the text.

Reference materials: It is always a good idea to have your library close at hand. You will find it helpful to have the following reference books handy: <u>Diagnostic Tests</u>, a medical dictionary, a book describing the effects of prescription drugs such as a recent edition of the Physician's Desk Reference, perhaps a booklet of medical abbreviations (to use when reviewing medical records) and any other textbooks you find particularly useful.

Be observant and listen carefully: If you are carefully observant your initial interview can tell you a lot about the woman and her family circumstances. Be aware of her tone of voice, her body language and her willingness to discuss various issues. During the interview, be aware of hostility, guilt, lack of eye contact, and curt replies. Notice if she rubs her nose (cocaine use?), seems belligerent, smells of alcohol or cigarettes and if you notice any bruises or scars on her face or other exposed areas of her body. Watch her and listen carefully as you inquire about potentially problematic topics. See the chapters on Physical Abuse and those on various types of substance abuse as well as the chapter on Working Through Emotional Issues With Clients in the section on Sustaining Health and Well-being During Pregnancy for more information about what to look for or how to proceed if you feel you have uncovered a problem.

How to ask questions: When conducting any interview, it is important to try and elicit as much information as possible by asking open-ended questions. Try not to include an answer within the question you are asking, as you would be doing if you asked "Did you have a reddish rash that itched?" Instead ask "What color was the rash? Were there any other symptoms or discomforts that accompanied the rash?," If the woman is having trouble understanding your question or it seems appropriate to ask a more directive question after you have elicited some information on a problem, you can offer a list of choices such as: "Was the pain aching, burning, cutting, stabbing or what?" or "Is your hearing worse in one or both ears?."

We will review the rational for each question using the forms included as examples at the end of this chapter.

Date of initial History (Hx): It is a good idea to record this, since pertinent information that is date-specific will be recorded during this interview. It also documents when your formal care relationship begins.

Due date: It is good to have this date recorded in several places, as a reminder. When you have 20 to 30 clients, it is not easy to remember the details of each chart!

LNMP: This stands for Last Normal Menstrual Period. This provides a quick-check location to record the date. More details, such as if it was normal and what the next-to-the-last period was like will be recorded later in the form.

Blood type and Rh factor: Again, this is pertinent information that needs to be readily accessible in more than one location.

Mother's name, age, birth date and occupation: Having the correct spelling of the mother's name is important, as well as the name she most likes to use, which isn't always her first name, her nickname or her married name! A woman's birth date is necessary so that you can pass this along, when required, to hospital staff, and/or insurance and other pertinent forms, etc.

Her age will give you clues about possible age-related risk factors and which prenatal tests would be suggested by mainstream care providers. It is also important to know the mother's age so you can dispel some of the myths surrounding maternal age and its impact on birth.

Studies document that maternal age (over 35) does not adversely affect the process of pregnancy or birth. However, there may be psychological issues for these women, especially those who are becoming first-time mothers. Their lives are in order in a different way than women who are in their twenties. Therefore, control issues, letting go in labor and concerns about how having a baby will impact their lives may loom larger than for younger women. After age 35, the risk of genetic defects does rise, however, and women need to know what tests are available to detect a problem, how accurate they are, what they can tell her and when they must be performed (see Diagnostic Tests for details and the chapter on Ordering Baseline Laboratory Tests in this section.)

A woman's occupation helps you determine her general level of activity and stress. Question her further to find out if she works with any potentially harmful equipment or chemicals or is exposed to other environmental or work-related hazards. Advise women to request transfer to work areas which pose minimal risk from air, noise and chemical pollution. Jobs requiring strenuous labor, heavy lifting and other physical stress should be temporarily transferred as well. As pregnancy alters a woman's center of gravity and ability to balance, her risk will increase in work situations where she relies on these abilities and she is at more risk for injury as a result. Knowledge of a woman's specific work environment can help you formulate a plan regarding what you can recommend to her employer as her care provider. A friendly letter from you advising work-related changes may have significant impact; it is one time you can use your power as a care provider appropriately and to great advantage. (See chapter in this section on Helping Women Deal With Work and Activity Concerns.)

Address and telephone numbers: This information is important to obtain and to keep current. If she has no phone, get the name of a friend, relative or neighbor with whom you can leave messages. A telephone has always been a requirement for homebirth in my practice. In some populations, this may be unrealistic (in Amish communities, for example), but at least you can have the parents locate the closest phone which would be available for your use in case of an emergency. Ask her to bring in a map or directions to her home for you to file in her chart.

Partner's name, age, birth date and occupation: You want this information on the partner as well for some of the same reasons cited above. This is also an opportunity to distinguish between the biological father and the current partner, should they be different, if this information hasn't already come to light.

Have you had any prenatal care? With whom?: While you may have gotten the answers to these questions on the telephone and during the consultation, it is a good idea to write them down now. The less prenatal care a woman has had and

552

the closer she is to term both increase the amount of work you must do to educate her and the amount of risk you take in accepting her as a client.

Do you plan to breastfeed? Midwives vary regarding their feelings about working with women who do and do not choose to breastfeed. Breastfeeding for the first six weeks has always been a bottom line requirement in my practice. The physical benefits to both mother and baby are so important and protective (from preventing infection in the baby to preventing hemorrhage in the mother) that I have never felt comfortable caring for women physically capable of breastfeeding who choose not to. There will be some women who cannot breastfeed, either due to physical abnormalities of the breast (which is very rare), or to previous surgery (for breast reduction or enhancement or cancer). Many women who have had surgery have already questioned their doctors about breastfeeding and will have a good idea of their chances of success. If a woman has not questioned her doctor before, a visit or phone call is in order to find out the surgeon's opinion about her chances, as well as how to deal with lactating breast tissue if, in fact, she cannot nurse.

PRIOR PREGNANCIES: Total, Live, Stillbirths, Abortions, Miscarriages: These figures should indicate the grand total and the total in each category, regardless of the weeks of pregnancy.

Record of pregnancies ending ≥20 wks preg.: The questions you will ask about pregnancies carried beyond 20 weeks are different than those you will ask about those which ended earlier, so I have divided these questions into two categories. The first set of questions asks about any pregnancies which ended at 20 weeks or thereafter; the section reviewing pregnancies ending prior to 20 weeks will follow; gather this information on each pregnancy. An additional form is included at the end of the chapter to use for women who have more pregnancies than space on the standard form allows.

Child's name/pregnancy number: Even if a child was stillborn, it is important to be able to refer to all children by name. The sequence of the pregnancy in relationship to others is important, because miscarriage or other losses prior to 20 weeks may be interspersed with pregnancies which were carried longer.

Birth date/place/care-giver: How closely spaced were her pregnancies? The birth dates will tell you. Where and with whom she gave birth will record who she has chosen for care in the past; her impressions of the care she received can be linked to her choices. This information will also help you in discussing such things as acquiring the charts from previous births.

Planned/using contraception: Unplanned pregnancies are not always unwanted, but this question will open the subject of how she has accepted her pregnancies. If she was using contraception at the time, be sure to ask what type. You can discuss her success rates with various forms of contraception and whether she simply failed to use one form correctly this time, or if contraception failure is a repeating problem. Be sure to discuss, both now and after the birth, various forms of contraception and their proper use, as appropriate.

Weeks gestation/pregnancy at birth: This refers to the number of weeks pregnant the mother thought she was, either from conception (which would be weeks of gestation) or her last menstrual period (which would be weeks of pregnancy). To clarify this, it is best to pull out a gestation wheel and calculate the due date for the pregnancy in question if you are at all unsure about what she is telling you. The weeks gestation can then be compared to other parameters such as the amount of amniotic fluid and the apparent gestational age, weight and condition of the baby. This will give you an idea how she carries her pregnancies; for example, if she previously gave birth at 42 of weeks of pregnancy (from LMP) or later and was sure of her dates, but she had plenty of amniotic fluid and a plump well-grown baby, she was not postmature, even though she was post-term. Likewise, if she has lost pregnancies in the second trimester without being aware of early labor, this should alert you to the possibility of cervical abnormalities (see the chapter on Loose Cervix in the section on Problems Associated With the Second Trimester).

Type of birth: This refers to normal, spontaneous birth or those assisted with forceps, vacuum extraction or cesarean section. If the midwife asked her to assume a particular position or used pressure on the pelvic bones to open the pelvis, this should be noted as well. Women who have had forceps or vacuum extractors used during previous births may be somewhat intimidated by the prospect of giving birth naturally, but not so much so as the woman who has had a surgical delivery. Please see the chapter on Yoni Birth after Cesarean, Special Circumstances section, for more details.

Total weight gain: This is asked not because there is any magic number of pounds to gain, but because comparing the maternal weight gain to the weight of the baby can help you discuss why diet is so very important. You can also find out if she was advised to gain a certain amount or if she has feelings about the amount of weight she gained. This is your opportunity to praise her if she gained a lot and had a healthy baby and to remind her that a small weight gain is not anything to strive for; she should focus on eating good foods to appetite (as described in the chapter on Maternal Nutrition and Weight Gain), not on how much she gains!

Prenatal problems: What did she perceive as a problem? What did her care provider see as a problem? What was done to deal with any problems in that pregnancy? Did it help or make things worse? And finally, in your opinion, was there really a problem? This is your chance to dispel myths about swelling, high blood pressure or other signs and symptoms which may have appeared during a previous pregnancy. Other questions to ask: Was there any drug, alcohol or tobacco use during that pregnancy? Were any drugs prescribed? For what?

Early labor history: How did labor begin (water broke, contractions, lost mucus plug)? What was early labor like? Did she have a few contractions, rush to the hospital and find herself to be two centimeters or almost fully dilated? Did she perceive herself to be in hard labor for hours and hours, only to be told she had failure to progress at three centimeters? In such cases you can discuss the realities of prodromal (very early) labor. On the other hand, you need to have a different discussion if a rapid labor has occurred previously.

Active labor: What happened once she got to 4 to 5 centimeters? How fast did labor progress? Were there any points where she got hung up, and if so, when? Did any particular fears, concerns or other emotions arise at those times? How does she feel she handled labor, and how does she feel about how she was treated?

Pushing phase: Did she have a spontaneous urge to push, or was she forced into pushing without one? How long did she push? In what positions did she push? Some women have no trouble with the passive part of labor but are not very good at the active part; pushing. Likewise, the reverse can also be true. Question women to find out what came up for them if pushing was difficult and what worked if pushing was easy.

Placental birth: After the baby came out, how long did it take for the placenta to deliver? Did the care provider "do anything," for instance cord traction, to assist this process? Was the placenta intact? (If the birth occurred in the hospital, the placenta may have been left in the pan, unexamined.) Does she have any questions about the birth of the placenta? If getting the placenta out has been hard in the past, she might need a step by step review of placental detachment and delivery. Show her a picture of a placenta, a fresh one (remember to use gloves), or a model (such as those made by Childbirth Graphics) to refresh her memory at some point during prenatal care.

IV/drugs used: Did she have any drugs at any time during her labor, birth or postpartum? Did she have an intravenous line? (In this case she may be unaware of having been given drugs.) Does she know what drugs she had? If not, ask questions like, "Did your contractions suddenly get stronger after they gave you something in your IV?" (This would indicate that she got oxytocin to strengthen her labor. If no IV was hung during labor, she had no oxytocin augmentation in hospital). "Did they give you a spinal anesthetic or a shot in the back?" (a spinal anesthetic of some kind would numb her from the upper waist or hips down). Did she have any adverse or severe reactions to any of the drugs used? Were the drugs effective or did they further complicate the situation?

Experience of birth: How did she feel, overall, about this birth experience? What would she want to have been different? What was the best thing about her experience? The worst?

Complications: Were there any specific diagnoses given for any problems she experienced during this birth? If nothing was defined medically, did she feel her birth was complicated in any way and, if so, how?

Perineal trauma: Did she tear, or did she receive a clitorotomy (episiotomy)? If so, does she know where and how the damage occurred (was it a median or a mediolateral incision)? Was it sutured, and how did it heal? How long did it take for her perineum to feel normal? (If it never has, what problems is she experiencing now?) Excessive swelling, itching, suture breakdown and the like may have been related to an allergy to the suture material itself, local anesthetic, or secondary to an infection. Get details!!

Baby's position at birth: Did her care providers discuss fetal position during labor? What does she remember about what was said? Was the baby born breech, posterior, vertex? One way to ask this is: "Was the baby head down, face down (toward your back) when it came out or was it facing up?" Usually, if she doesn't know this, the partner will remember.

Weight/length of baby: The baby's weight gives you a good idea of whether the diet was adequate during that pregnancy. A woman who has been diagnosed as toxemic due to high blood pressure who has a 9 lb. 8 oz. baby clearly had a well expanded blood volume and was not toxemic unless she was starving her last few weeks of pregnancy. Connecting things like this helps support your theories regarding the medical interpretation of a woman's symptoms.

An exceptionally small baby (less than 5 lbs. 8 oz.) may indicate an early birth, poor nutrition or inadequate absorption of nutrients. Likewise a large baby may simply be due to a good diet but can indicate uncontrolled diabetes, especially if the baby was puffy with a lot of watery fat (macrosomic) or was born early.

APGAR scores at 1 and 5 minutes: This assessment of newborn well-being checks for grimace response, respirations, heart rate, color and muscle tone. It can help you determine whether a baby that may have been hurried along to birth because of supposed fetal compromise was really distressed. Keep in mind that standard practice in many areas is to use the hands to compress the chest and suppress breathing in a baby with meconium stained amniotic fluid. In many cases this could artificially lower the one minute APGAR score.

Problems with baby: Again, you want to find out what was said about the condition of the baby and draw your own conclusions. This is a good time to discuss alternative management of jaundice, meconium staining and other relevant newborn problems. Difficulty with nursing counts as a problem as well; get as many details as you can about any problems which occurred.

Postpartum experience/breastfed?:   How did the weeks after the birth go? How did she adjust to mothering, going back to work, nursing, integrating another child, etc.? How helpful (or unhelpful) was her partner? Did she get depressed? Were there any delayed bleeding problems or breast infections? Note if she breastfed her other babies and for how long. Ask if nursing was easy or difficult and get details.

If this child was placed for adoption, ask how the mother dealt with her grief. Did she receive counseling, and, if so, for how long? How did she say goodbye to the baby? Was it an open or a closed adoption? See the chapter on Working with Women Who Have Had Difficult Yoni Births or Pregnancy Losses in the Special Circumstances section for more details.

Child's health now: It is important to know if the child is still alive and if not, why. The general health of the child can be discussed: Are there any particular problems? Learning disabilities? Hyperactivity? How likely is it that these problems may have a genetic origin (some of which do not appear until a child is older; see the Genetics Counseling chapter in <u>Diagnostic Tests</u> for more details). Are they attributed to birth complications? Be sure to compare the history of any drug or substance abuse with problems in any of her children now. If the child is dead, find out how she dealt with her grief, if she got counseling, etc.

<u>**Record of all pregnancies which ended before (≤) 20 weeks pregnancy:**</u>

This section records all miscarriages, stillbirths or induced abortions which occurred at or before 20 weeks of pregnancy.

Date ended/weeks of pregnancy/pregnancy number: These bits of data are important because you want to know when pregnancy losses have occurred in relation to a woman's total pregnancy picture. At what age did these losses occur?

Location/care-giver: Where and with whom a woman gets care is important and will impact her experience of the pregnancy loss. Was she, for example, left alone in a room to have a saline abortion at 18 weeks of pregnancy?

Drugs used: Often women will have received some kind of drugs for either an induced abortion or a problematic miscarriage. Was she sedated for any procedure? If she was, her feelings about the procedure were numbed as well, and this may have impacted her emotional processing of the experience. Did she have any adverse reactions to the drugs given?

Complications: Was there any infection or hemorrhaging following the pregnancy? Was the fetus normal or were there obvious genetic or other defects? If so, were they identified? If it was a spontaneous pregnancy loss, was there any preexisting condition or infection which may have prompted it? Did the water break early? Was there a loose (incompetent) cervix? (especially likely with spontaneous miscarriage after 12 weeks but before 20)

Experience: What was her experience like? How has she resolved her feelings now? How does she feel about this pregnancy given her past experience?

Counseling: Did she have any counseling before, during or after the abortion or miscarriage to help her make her decisions or work out her feelings? If so, how did she feel about it? If not, does she feel that she needs counseling now? Does she feel resolved about that experience now?

<u>**Contraceptive history**</u>:

Remember that lesbians have no need for contraception, but may have used it in the past with male partners before coming out.

Oral contraceptives: Birth control pills significantly alter a woman's hormonal balance. Women may experience a range of symptoms when taking them such as weight gain, water retention, headaches, internal clots and hemorrhages, liver and gallbladder problems, nausea and vomiting, breast tenderness and depression. While studies show no increased risk of heart or limb defects from inadvertent use during early pregnancy, nevertheless, oral contraceptives are categorized as X class drugs and should be discontinued as soon as pregnancy is suspected (PDR, 1991, p. 2191). The pill places significant demands on a woman's nutritional status, depleting vitamins and minerals. Any woman who has been on the Pill should begin taking a multi-vitamin/mineral supplement as soon as she begins care. The artificial hormones in the Pill simulate those of early pregnancy, thus fooling the body into not releasing an ovum each month. Long term exposure to hormone based birth control of any type can lead to cervical rigidity in some women, oils containing prostaglandin precursors, such as Evening Primrose oil, can be taken in the last 6 weeks to help soften the cervix.

IUD: The use of an intrauterine device (IUD) for contraception has been fraught with problems, and some have been taken off the market. Ask how long she had the IUD, what type it was, and if she had any problems with it in place. Get details. Did she have uterine puncture, scarring or infection from the device or was surgery necessary to remove the IUD? Did she ever conceive or carry a pregnancy with an IUD still in place? Progesterone releasing IUDs can also cause cervical rigidity (see comment above). If an IUD is in place at conception it should be left in place; miscarriage or infection are a risk whether is left in place or not, but removal is felt to increase the risk of losing the pregnancy.

Morning after pill: Diethylstilbestrol (DES) was used for a short period of time in the 1970s as a deterrent to the implantation of the fertilized egg. It was often given out at college clinics at that time. It is, of course, cancer-producing and highly toxic. It was later shown not to prevent pregnancy and its use was discontinued.

Other forms of contraception: To be sure you cover all the possibilities, contraceptive methods can be divided into three categories:

HORMONAL METHODS	BARRIER METHODS	NATURAL FAMILY PLANNING
Depo-Provera (hormonal injection which suppresses ovulation) levonorgestrel inserts (needle shaped hormone-releasing implants which are inserted in upper, inner arm)	Spermacides (foam, gell) Diaphragm Cervical cap Condom Sponges	Rhythm Lunation cycle Mucus ovulation Astrological birth control

If were in place at conception, they should be removed as soon as possible.
Condoms (now available in male and female versions), diaphragms, foam, contraceptive sponges, Norplant (progesterone-releasing tubes inserted in a fan pattern beneath the skin in the upper, inner arm), hormone injections and cervical caps are the most widely available "other" forms of contraception. How has she liked or disliked using them? Did she experience problems such as allergies to creams or materials? Was there partner acceptance? Were they effective? How long did she use each method, and why did she discontinue use? Hormone-based contraceptives of any kind may make the cervix more rigid (see comments in section on the Pill, above)

Menstrual history:

Age of onset: This gives you a clue about her hormonal balance. For example, if she started menstruating at a very young age, her body may have been overstimulated by hormones from meat and dairy products. If she started in her late teens, her hormonal system may not be working as well as it could.

Average length of: cycle_____days, flow_____ days: The length of her cycle is the time from the first day of bleeding to the next first day of bleeding. Note whether she counts her first day of spotting as the first day of bleeding, if the two are not the same. Although the average length is 28 days, many women have longer or shorter cycles and this will often impact how long they carry their pregnancy. Long cycles mean that a woman ovulates late in her cycle, so *the due date should be figured from the 14th day before the expected onset of bleeding*, not the 14th day from the beginning of the last period.

Are you regular: Irregular or skipped periods must be taken into account when you are trying to determine when a woman conceived and how advanced her pregnancy may be.

What is your usual amount of flow: This gives you a clue to how debilitated she may or may not be from her menses. It is said that women with heavy periods bleed more after birth; however, this is strictly anecdotal information. Heavy bleeding may also be associated with endometriosis or fibroids, as well as anemia.

Problems: Does she have cramps, premenstrual syndrome, endometriosis, fibroids or any other symptoms or conditions which may affect her menstrual cycles? Has she been treated for these and, if so, how?

First day of last normal period: It is important emphasize that you are asking for the date of the last *normal* period. If there is any doubt, get the date of the last two periods. If either of these was abnormal in any way, get her to describe exactly how it was abnormal (scant, early, late, etc.).

Probable date of conception: Ask women if they know when they might have conceived; many of them will be able to tell you the approximate date. Reviewing calendars and special occasions can help her to recall when the date may have been. If a woman knows her date of conception, take this into consideration when calculating the due date. This is particularly relevant for the woman who has long or short cycles; her due date will not match the 28 day cycle on which the gestation wheel is based.

Date of 1st fetal motion: When the due date is uncertain, the date of the first fetal motion can be helpful in determining how far along a pregnancy is. Fetal motion is usually felt between 16 and 18 weeks of pregnancy and usually no later than the 20th week.

Contraception at time of conception: If any type of contraception was being used (either topical chemicals such as foam, or a hormonal agent such as birth control pills), it could affect a woman's sense of when she conceived. If an IUD is still in place this presents a real danger of uterine perforation or entanglement with the products of conception. She should be sent to an obstetrical practitioner for evaluation and removal.

Due date: See the separate chapter on Calculating the Due Date in the Basic Skills section for complete information. Be sure to record which method of calculation you use in the method space.

Woman's mother's birth-related history: The information gathered in this section is similar in content to the information gathered for your new client (see corresponding sections above); however, the rationale behind the questions is different. You are looking for how her mother gave birth to discover several things about the woman you are working with:

*Are there any genetic or physiological predispositions such as long pregnancies, twins on her mother's side of the family, long labors or anything else which may carry over into her pregnancy?
*What is her "programming" about birth from her mother's experiences; what did her mother and family tell her about pregnancy, birth and newborns when she was a child?
*Where was she in the sibling order? If she was born before other siblings, she will have her own impressions of her mother's other pregnancies and births, whether she remembers these impressions from childhood or not.
*What was her birth weight and the weight of her siblings? This may influence her impressions of how big babies should or shouldn't be and the difficulty of labor.
*Was she thrust into a parenting role for her siblings? At what age? Under what circumstances?
*Did her mother breastfeed? If not, what did she learn about how difficult, easy, unseemly, etc. breastfeeding was considered to be?

Comments/DES exposure: From 1948 to 1971, a potent synthetic nonsteroidal estrogen called diethylstilbestrol was widely prescribed for 4 to 6 million women in the United States as a preventative measure for complications of pregnancy such as threatened miscarriage, a history of repeated miscarriage, toxemia, prematurity, postmaturity and fetal death *in utero*. In addition, it was given to women with special risk factors such as diabetes. Typically treatment began in the first trimester and continued throughout pregnancy. Sometimes, women were not told what they were being given or why (one friend's mother thought she was receiving vitamin injections). Any woman born between 1946 and 1972 who is unsure of her status should ask their mother if they were given any drugs or other agents during pregnancy and, if so, why. DES daughters are at increased risk for the development of clear cell adenocarcinoma of the yoni, usually an uncommon form of cancer found in women over the age of 50; this risk warrants yearly PAP smears and careful gynecological examination. A colposcopy exam, which uses magnification to aide visual exam, should also be performed if cervical dysplasia is found. (Mittendorf & Herbst, 1994) This type of cancer is a relatively rare outcome of exposure; reproductive organ anomalies are much more common. Women with a history of this cancer may be reassured to know that there is no difference in the 5-year survival rate of pregnant women compared to nonpregnant women with a positive history. Conception is generally reported to be possible among those affected, however, the rate of pregnancy loss is relatively high. (For more details, see the chapter on Variations and Abnormalities of the Female Reproductive Tract in the Anatomy and Physiology section.)

Personal lifestyle & habits: Does the woman or her partner:

Smoke?: Smoking places both the woman and fetus at higher risk for a variety of complications and problems. Read the section of smoking for more complete information. Here are some things you should consider when presented with a smoking client: smoking dampens the appetite and makes it harder for women to get what they need nutritionally; smoking uses up valuable nutrients; as a rule smokers have more friable, calcified placentas which means an overdue smoker is something to be very concerned about; smoking diminishes oxygen flow to the fetus and leads to the formation of constricted blood vessels in the cord. On the other hand, if a smoker does eat well, she can give birth to a good-sized healthy baby in spite of the constriction in the placental vessels. You need to be clear about how you feel about working with smokers so that you do not communicate mixed messages to the mother.

A smoking partner's side stream smoke also affects the mother and fetus/baby in much the same way that the woman's own smoking would. Smoking partners should smoke outside or, preferably, quit!

Drink alcohol?: Alcohol consumption can be problematic during pregnancy for several reasons. It does its worst damage by producing Fetal Alcohol Syndrome, a characteristic set of facial and mental deformities which can have a wide range of severity. No one knows the minimum amount of alcohol it takes to cause Fetal Alcohol Syndrome (FAS). Daily drinking is usually related to alcoholism. Ask your clients how much they drink and, if it seems regular or excessive, then ask if they feel they have a problem with alcohol. Many times, a women will feel alcohol is a problem for her partner, but the partner is in denial about their addiction. It is important for you to be aware of such problems and of how the woman or her partner may react in case of stress or tension, especially at the birth. The following questions are helpful when exploring possible alcoholism:

*Have you felt you should cut down on your drinking?
*Have you been annoyed by others criticizing your drinking?
*Have your felt guilty about drinking?
*Have you taken a drink in the morning to steady your nerves or get rid of a hangover?

A "yes" answer to any of these questions suggests an alcohol problem. (See chapter on Alcohol in the Well-being section for more details.)

Use medications (over-the-counter/prescription)? Any drug must be explored for its possible damaging or compromising effects during pregnancy. No drugs have been shown to be absolutely safe during pregnancy, but some have proven to be apparently benign as far as fetal and maternal effects; there are definitely some drugs that are more desirable to take during pregnancy than others. Be sure to ask about inhalers for asthma or sinus congestion. The use of these may lead to prolonged labors and start-and-stop contraction patterns, as well as dependence.

Have a history of recreational drug use (IV?)?: Is the woman or her partner using recreational drugs now, or have they in the past? If so, how long past? What have they taken, how frequently, and have they had a problem with addiction? Watch carefully as she responds to this question. Do not hesitate to ask about each drug by name (see the chapter on Recreational Drugs) and ask her to agree to stop using *now*! Intravenous (IV) drug use brings up the question of exposure to blood borne diseases such as hepatitis, syphilis and HIV. Anyone with a history of IV drug use should be tested for all these conditions.

Have religious beliefs that effect her health care?: While some midwives may want to discuss religious beliefs in more depth, this is the minimum you need to know about someone's religious convictions. The main religions which have restrictions impacting the use of bio-technical medical technologies are Jehovah's Witnesses (who refuse transfusion with blood products, including RhD(o) immunoglobulin) and Christian Scientists, who avoid the use of physical means of healing whenever possible. Some sects of fundamental Christians may object to the use of any kind of intervention. Roman Catholic families may want you to baptize a distressed or stillborn infant at birth; ask. Orthodox Jewish men may not touch their wives once the membranes have ruptured. (See the chapter on Cultural and Religious Practices in this section for more information.)

Use chemicals or harmful substances at work or home?: Just as with drugs, the use of or exposure to any chemicals or other substances must be explored for their potentially damaging effects on the pregnancy. Ask about such things as hair coloring, permanent wave products, acrylic nails, what they use to clean house. All types of highly chemicalized cosmetic products should be avoided unless she is willing to use a natural alternative (she can ask her hair dresser or check at the health food store). Strong household cleaners, paint removers etc. should be avoided entirely or only used with gloves in an extremely well ventilated area. They should not be used on a daily basis. Latex paint fumes are okay, but exposure should not be prolonged to any such substances. For more information, see the chapter on Environmental Exposures, Well-being section.

Use or work with/near microwave ovens?: Microwaves produce non-ionizing radiation. They heat food by causing the water molecules in the food to vibrate rapidly. The fetus is surrounded by water, which places it at particular risk from leaky microwave devices. Microwave ovens can leak; they also destroy the nutritive qualities of food. Encourage women to avoid the use of microwave ovens and, if they must, to stay clear of them (preferably out of the kitchen) while in use.

Use computers/radiation?: Computers produce very low frequency radiation. Radiation output is strongest from the back and sides of the monitor; therefore women should request that they not be seated with their back facing the back of another monitor in an office environment. Many newer monitors are being produced with reduced radiation output; if a woman is considering buying a new computer, she should be encouraged to get one that poses as little risk as possible (the Sony Trinitron monitor is shielded and has excellent resolution for a relatively low price). Older monitors can be shielded with radiation minimizing glare screens. Such screens can be obtained from MISCO, Box 399, W9-CL, Holmdel, NJ 07733-9980 (800) 876-4726; in NJ dial (201) 264-1000.

Get regular exercise?: Knowing the type and amount of exercise a woman is accustomed to will help you advise her about the kind of exercise she can continue during pregnancy. Women can usually continue with any type of exercise that they are comfortable with, provided it does not put direct pressure or tension on the abdominal muscles (for example belly rocking and sit-ups). Women who have a high metabolism may have to reduce their activity level to spare calories for the pregnancy. Be sure all women are getting adequate calories to compensate for their activity level.

Drink caffeinated/sugared beverages?: This includes black tea, coffee and sodas (remember that many sodas and chocolate also contain caffeine). Both caffeine and sugar have profound effects on the appetite, blood glucose levels, and the adrenal glands. Encourage women to gradually reduce their caffeine and sugar intake, recommending appropriate alternative foods. Caffeine addiction signals a weakened adrenal system and someone who needs that artificial kick to get going. Eliminating caffeine will cause a person to feel more sluggish, possibly depressed and irritable, and may produce headaches. Frequent meals and reducing other stresses as much as possible will help women cope with this withdrawal period. For those who feel the taste of coffee or tea will ease their symptoms, recommend Swiss water processed decaffeinated coffee or tea.

Have pets?: Bird and cat feces can carry toxoplasmosis (see <u>Diagnostic Tests</u>). Women owning birds or cats should assign someone else to clean cages and litter boxes. Gardening should be done using gloves. Women who have never owned a bird or cat should postpone getting any until after the birth. Big dogs which require strenuous exercise may also pose a problem if there is a time when the woman feels she cannot do the dog walking herself.

Type of diet? (omnivore/ovo-lacto/vegan/macrobiotic/other): Although you may have already gone over a diet diary by this time, this provides a formal place to enter details about a woman's dietary choices and restrictions.

Discuss: Seat belts, Fluoride, Deodorant, Bras, Talc, Tap water: Advise women to use seat belts when riding or driving a car. The use of a shoulder harness and a lap belt together is safest. The shoulder harness should be arranged up and over the belly with the strap between the breasts and the lap belt should be placed snugly below the belly. (Pearce, 1992) Most deodorants contain toxic substances which are absorbed directly into the axillary lymph nodes and make their way to breast tissue and milk as well. Shaving the armpits, (thus abrading of the skin), and wearing bras (which reduce lymph flow) are contributing factors. (The area of the breast most prone to the development of cancerous tumors is the upper outer quadrant, the area nearest the armpit!) Natural deodorants which do not contain aluminum are good alternatives to standard drug-store brands. Also advise women to reduce the time that they wear a bra (or stop entirely), eliminate underwires, and to massage around their breasts when the take it off to help circulate lymph fluids. Using talcum powder in the genital area has been found to be associated with ovarian cancer and should be avoided (Rinehardt, Heidi, M.D. 1995). See section on Sustaining Health & Well-being for discussions regarding fluoride and tap water.

<u>**MEDICAL HISTORY:**</u> The medical history usually does not turn up problems, but it can occasionally prove valuable in helping you discover if a woman is constitutionally weak in a certain area. For example, if many of her relatives have diabetes, you can assume her pancreas is fairly weak as well. This does not mean she will get the condition in question; however, if she does become chronically ill, the weakest parts of her body will usually feel the effects first. You may also discover that she has a condition or has had one in the past which she has forgotten but which may be of concern during the pregnancy. To learn more about how to

evaluate disease conditions in pregnancy, see the opening chapter in the section Medical Conditions Which Preexist Pregnancy. The following codes will help in making intelligible, notes about what family members have specific conditions.

MM—maternal mother	MA, MU—maternal aunt/uncle	PS—paternal sibling
MF—maternal father	PM—paternal mother	PGM—paternal grandmother
MS—maternal sibling	PF—paternal father	PA, PU—paternal aunt/uncle
MGM—maternal grandmother		

Have the pregnant woman, biological father or any immediate relatives had any of these health conditions? The medical history is divided into three subsections. The first deals with those conditions that are relevant in the woman, biological father and their immediate family.

Heart/circulation/blood pressure: All circulatory conditions fall in this category. Ask if she has ever been told she has a heart murmur or other heart condition and especially note any history of high blood pressure in the family. Mitral value prolapse is perhaps the most frequent heart condition in otherwise healthy women of childbearing age; it is usually benign. For more details, see the chapter on Heart Conditions in the section on Medical Conditions Which May Preexist Pregnancy.

Anemia/blood disorders: Any hereditary anemias? Has she ever bled excessively or clotted abnormally? Any bleeding problems during surgery, dental work or with an injury? Any babies with clotting or bleeding problems in either family? What treatments have been used to correct any problems? Have the problems recurred? Women from specific ethnic or racial backgrounds should be made aware of screening programs for hereditary anemias (see Diagnostic Tests, Anemia chapter).

Diabetes: Any history of diabetes? If so, was it with age (adult onset) or during childhood? Is it insulin dependent or controlled by diet alone?

Thyroid disorders: Any problems with growth or development in the family? Weight problems? If thyroid disease has been found, how severe has it been and how has it been treated? If she has had her thyroid removed, when was this done? How stable are her thyroid levels now? Is she currently taking thyroid medication?

Respiratory disease: This includes TB, asthma, pneumonia or bronchitis (especially if chronic) and other respiratory problems. If respiratory problems have appeared in relatives, find out if they smoke or if they live with a smoker.

Convulsive/Central Nervous System disorders: Convulsions may be caused by epilepsy, but its not always the causative factor. An injury, such as a blow to the head, IUD removal (due to triggering nerves in the cervix), and sometimes drugs

566

or allergies can cause severe nervous system responses. Get the details of any convulsive disorders that exist and any drugs used for treatment now or in the past (several popular anticonvulsant drugs can increase the chances of birth defects). Generally speaking, unless the convulsions interfere with oxygen exchange (such as with Grand Mal convulsions of epilepsy) they pose no particular risk in pregnancy. A number of herbs can help control seizures; refer her to a naturopath for guidance. If there is a history of seizures, be sure to tell her to let you know immediately if she starts to have any neurological symptoms during the pregnancy.

Cancer/growths: A history of cancers or growths should be explored for related factors such as living near a nuclear power plant, toxic waste dump, electrical power station, or radio or microwave tower. Smoking (either by the person or via side stream smoke), poor dietary choices, alcohol and drug use could also be contributory factors. Did the person serve time in the military where Agent Orange or other toxic chemicals were in use? Were there occupational exposures? Get details of treatments and research their impact on reproductive health.

Varicose veins: Varicosities are primarily relevant for the woman and her female relatives. Varicose (prolapsed) veins can appear in the genital area as well as the thighs and lower legs. Hemorrhoids are prolapsed cushions of rectal mucosa containing blood vessels. Liver congestion is a primary aggravator of varicose veins. The liver can be assisted with various herbs. (see the chapter on Varicosities in the section on Problems That Can Occur at any Time).

Genetic disorders: What is her racial and ethnic background? Does she know of any familial genetic problems? Have there been any babies that died? If so, does she know why? Are there any relatives with Down syndrome or other mental retardation disorders? If so, get as many details as possible. Are there other problems such a persons with extra fingers or toes, heart problems or any other organ malfunctions? Is there any hearing loss in the family? See the chapter on Genetic Counseling in <u>Diagnostic Tests</u> for how to conduct a full genetic interview.

Has the pregnant woman, biological father or current partner had (or been exposed to) any of the following? NOTE: Ask about risk factors and all previous partners when discussing sexually transmitted diseases.

DES/steroid therapy: Steroids include injections sometimes used by weight lifters, birth control pills or any hormonal therapy. While there is nothing that can be done about past intake, you can discuss specific hormonal therapies that the woman has taken and suggest they be discontinued, if possible, during the pregnancy.

Genital herpes: Has either partner ever had genital herpes? Was it cultured and positively identified as such? How frequent and severe are outbreaks now? Have any therapies been used to try and control outbreaks and, if so, what? When did the first outbreak occur?

Genital warts: Does either partner have or have they had genital warts? Were they removed and if so, what was used? Have they recurred? In women, how often are PAP smears being done? Are there any genital warts present now? If they are present in the woman, examine them during the physical exam. Ask if they were rough or smooth; smooth genital warts may have been due to syphilis, but may have been mistaken for common venereal warts. Follow-up testing is advisable (see chapter on Syphilis in Diagnostic Tests for details).

Gonorrhea: Has either partner or any previous partner had gonorrhea? Was it a penicillin resistant strain? How was it diagnosed and treated? Were there any complications? If so, what were they? Chlamydia is a closely related infection and frequently accompanies gonorrhea. In many areas chlamydia testing is now routine.

Syphilis: Discuss the problems with the diagnosis and treatment of syphilis (see Diagnostic Tests). Has syphilis ever been diagnosed in either partner or any previous partners? Has either partner or a previous partner ever served in South East Asia? Sexual contact, broken skin or mucus membrane contact with a chancre, IV drug use involving the sharing of needles and contaminated blood transfusion are the principal ways that venereal syphilis is spread. Other forms of nonvenereal syphilis are prevalent in various parts of Africa, the tropics and Arabia. (For details, see the Syphilis chapter in Diagnostic Tests.)

HIV: The same types of behaviors which expose one to syphilis expose one to HIV. Be sure the woman and her partner are aware of them (see Diagnostic Tests). If either partner is high risk for having contracted HIV, discuss testing with them and the possible connection between HIV and syphilis (see Diagnostic Tests and the chapter on Ordering Baseline Laboratory Tests, Contact section). Many cities have anonymous testing programs available.

Excess X-rays/Ultrasound: While it could be argued that any X-rays or ultrasound exams are excessive, by this I mean X-rays over and above a few dental X-rays (such as a digestive tract study or broken bone). Document all exposures. Were any X-rays taken during the first eight weeks of this pregnancy? If so, was she properly shielded? If not, she is at high risk for damage to the fetus.

Has the pregnant woman had any of the following prior to this pregnancy:
These conditions are only relevant to the mother's health. Emphasize that these are questions regarding her past history only. There is another place on this form to enter those conditions that are currently problematic during this pregnancy.

Severe illnesses: Has she had any severe or prolonged illnesses such as hepatitis, polio, or mononucleosis? Has she had any chronic conditions such as recurring rashes or colds (reconsider syphilis exposure) or other ailments? This gives you an idea of what damage her body may have suffered in relationship to the conditions in question. Check in Diagnostic Tests for details regarding any of the conditions she may mention.

Anorexia/bulimia: Just about every woman in our culture has had concerns about her weight at one time or another. However, full blown anorexia (starving oneself) and bulimia (gorging on foods and intentionally throwing up) can wreak havoc with the digestive system, interfering with assimilation of nutrients and the biochemical balance of the entire body. To broach this subject, you might ask "Have you ever tried to limit the amount of food you eat to control your weight?" Many women will say yes; then you can move on to what form this takes. If there is a history of eating disorders, find out exactly how long it lasted, what was done for treatment and how she feels about her body now. If the woman is currently anorectic or bulimic it will be an uphill battle for her to allow herself to get bigger as the pregnancy advances. Either way, she will need careful monitoring so that she does not develop toxemia. You must speak frankly to her regarding the importance of her nutrition, issues regarding changing body image and weight gain, and may need to outline exactly what she needs to eat daily. (Also see the chapter on Helping Women Get the Foods They Need in Sustaining Health and Well-being.)

Stomach/GI: Stomach or bowel problems can interfere with nutrient assimilation as well as digestion in general. Some problems necessitate eliminating certain foods from the diet. Get as much information as you can about any problems she may have had, treatments given and how her digestive system is doing now.

Severe headaches: Women who experience severe headaches could have several things going on: emotional stress (the headaches allows her to take a break), hypoglycemia (low blood sugar can cause severe headaches), high blood pressure, or disorders involving the vasculature in the brain. Find out as much as you can about the frequency, character, symptoms, and treatment for her headaches. This will give you an important baseline when you need to assess if headaches occurring during pregnancy are typical for her or resulting from the pregnancy itself. Women with severe headaches and migraines often have drugs that they take routinely; determine exactly what those drugs are and research them to discover their impact on pregnancy. Sedative and relaxing herbs can be recommended instead.

Allergies: Is she aware of any food, environmental or drug allergies? Write down exactly which ones and what her reaction has been. If she is a highly allergic person, you might consider using only undyed, synthetic suture if she needs perineal repair. Some women are also allergic to the latex or talc used in gloves or even the gel used for ultrasound exams. Vinyl gloves are available which are less allergenic and are also impermeable to oil.

General surgery: Any surgery, such as the removal of wisdom teeth, can give you information about how she responds to anesthesia and if she bleeds excessively. With any previous abdominal or reproductive surgery, scar tissue adhesions may be disrupted as the uterus enlarges. They can cause pain and pulling sensations.

GYN surgery: Any breast or reproductive surgery? When and why? Did she ask her care provider how it may impact her current pregnancy or her ability to breastfeed? If not, she should contact them to find out. If a woman has had extensive abdominal surgery, there is a possibility that she has scar tissue adhesions (bands of scar tissue which are connected to other structures). These can stretch during pregnancy as the uterus enlarges, causing pain. Providing there are no cervical anomalies, these women can take one 500 mg. capsule of Black Currant or Evening Primrose oil every other day throughout pregnancy to assist in softening the scar tissue, thus making it more elastic.

Transfusions: Has she ever had a transfusion? For what reason? When? Any adverse reactions? Keep in mind that even a cross-matched transfusion can occasionally lead to blood sensitization. The antibody screen done with the regular prenatal blood type and factor tests should pick this up. Blood borne diseases such as syphilis, HIV, and hepatitis can be transmitted via transfusions. Ask her if any symptoms occurred immediately after transfusion and what, if any, tests were done.

Back problems: Any scoliosis or back injuries which cause her pain now? Has she ever been to a chiropractor and, if not, would she consider seeing one? What other treatments has she had? Does this condition limit her activity in any way? Does she know if or how it may impact her pregnancy or birth?

Severe accident: Has she ever had a severe accident or fall that broke bones or left her permanently injured? If so, find out when, exactly which bones were broken, and what any long term disabilities from the accident entail.

Arthritis/Rheumatism: Has she ever been diagnosed with arthritis or rheumatism? Does she experience stiffness or swelling in her joints? What kinds of treatments and medications has she taken for her condition? Aspirin and other drugs containing salicylic acid are often prescribed, but are contraindicated during pregnancy due to their effect on platelet function. Arthritis can be a secondary symptom of syphilis; review her history in that regard (See Syphilis chapter in Diagnostic Tests for details).

Insomnia: Inability to sleep can be due to emotional or mental anxiety, frequent urination, hypoglycemia (hunger), or physical pain. Is it every night or only in certain situations? Find out her daily routine regarding sleeping. Coffee, chocolate, black tea, and sugar intake may all contribute to insomnia. Suggest relaxing activities such as a warm bath, drinking hot milk (which releases tryptophan, a calming amino-acid), Skullcap tincture or Hops infusion (after the first 20 weeks of pregnancy) to help her get to sleep more easily. Being sure she does not go to bed hungry and eating when she does wake will also help.

Urinary tract (UT)/kidney infections: Any history of urinary tract or kidney infections? When, under what circumstances and how were they treated? Does she know if any permanent kidney damage resulted? If so, has she had any kidney tests recently? A liver profile/chem panel/SMAC test can help determine how her kidneys are functioning. Has she had kidney problems with any prior pregnancies? Recommend that any woman with a history of urinary tract infections drink Nettle infusion, 1 cup daily throughout pregnancy. It will help rebuild damaged kidneys.

Infections of the yoni: Does she have a history of infections? If so, when, what kinds, and how were they treated? Are they currently a problem? If not, can she identify when they stopped appearing? Get more details about specific infections in Diagnostic Tests.

Pelvic infections: Any history of pelvic infections? When, what organism and how was it treated? Did she have an IUD at the time? Does she know if any damage was done to her uterus or tubes by the infection? How severe was the infection? Does she experience any problems now that she thinks might be related? Scar tissue adhesions can be pulled and cause pain during pregnancy as the uterus enlarges; note that she may be at more risk for ectopic pregnancy. Ask if she has ever had pelvic inflammatory disease (PID), and test carefully for syphilis (see Diagnostic Tests).

Other: Ask if there are any additional health conditions which have not been addressed. Ask specifically if the woman wears contact lenses or dentures of any kind and make note of either on the front of her chart. This information will be important in the event of certain complications or if transport is necessary.

Health profile of biological father: This health profile can offer valuable information about how the father's genes may impact the fetus. It can also uncover useful information about the father's current state of health, which may affect his ability to assist during the birth.

Body build: Is he large, small, medium? If the father is much larger than the mother, be sure NOT to communicate to the woman that this will create a problem with having a big baby. There is no absolute correlation between the two.

Blood type/factor: If the father and mother are Rh-, then Rh sensitization is almost impossible (about 1 in 100,000 babies will have a genetic mutation leading to Rh+ blood). You can explain this to the parents so they can choose whether they want routine antibody screens during pregnancy. Remember that if a woman has been previously sensitized to a minor blood factor and the father is positive for that factor, the baby could also be positive and the possibility of a blood incompatibility problem would then exist. Therefore, if the mother knows herself to have been sensitized via a previous transfusion or pregnancy, the first step is to get the blood type of the father to determine if he is positive for that factor. Read the chapter on Blood incompatibilities in Diagnostic Tests for more information.

Relationship to mother: Is the biological father merely a sperm donor? If not, how are they related? If married, for how long? How long were they in relationship prior to marriage? This gives you some idea of the level of commitment between the two of them. If the woman is single or has a female partner, ask the same questions regarding her current significant other.

Health problems: Are there any health problems of which the biological father is aware? Do they sound like they may be genetic in origin? If so, what does he know about this? If not, do they cause him any problems now? Is he taking any medications or receiving any treatments for the conditions in question? If these facts are not known of the biological father, they might be obtained from a sperm bank, if one was involved. You can also ask the current partner if they have any health concerns which may affect his ability to assist during or after pregnancy.

What do they know about their own birth or the birth of siblings?
The fears and concerns a partner brings to the experience of pregnancy and birth can have a powerful influence as well. What messages did they get about pregnancy and birth when they were children? Encourage the partner to question their mother regarding details of their birth so that you all can be aware of any potentially fearful aspects of the experience before you are in the midst of a similar experience. For example, if a partner is afraid of the woman bleeding or the pain of labor the woman may unconsciously try to protect them by altering her labor pattern accordingly. The more cards you can get out on the table about all types of concerns and previous programming, the better off you will be.

Psychological profile: In some ways the entire initial exam is a psychological profile, in that you are observing how the woman responds to your questions and how forthcoming she is with details, emotional experiences and the like. The following questions offer a very basic review of specific psychological issues. Many more questions could be added to this list, but these have proven to be a good starting point for the initial exam. As you get to know a woman throughout her care, these topics may be elaborated upon and other questions frequently arise.

Try to get answers from both partners, but be sensitive to the woman who may not be telling you the whole story because her partner is present.

How do you handle emotional issues in your life? Most people understand this question and answer truthfully about how they respond emotionally to difficult issues. Get a full answer from the woman, then turn to the partner and ask the question again. Make a mental note of what is said and what you have already learned about substance abuse and how this may impact emotional responses.

Have you ever been raped or molested? If asked this question directly, many women will say no. However, if asked "Have you, as a child or an adult, had uncomfortable physical contact with another person?" many more women will say yes. Get her age at the time of the incident(s) and as many details of the experience as possible. Whenever someone is disclosing sexual abuse it is important to validate the fear they may have about the experience and acknowledge that, while they may feel embarrassed about the experience, it was not their fault. It is important that you remain as open, nonjudgmental and as neutral as possible so that she will not feel she has offended you with what she says. Validate her experience as abuse, and affirm that it should not have happened. Many women will try to trivialize or minimize their experiences, especially if limited to looks, touching or other more vague kinds of abuse. Ask if she has received counseling for the experience. Has she confronted her abuser? Has she revealed this to her partner? Did she try to tell anyone at the time, and what was their reaction? (See chapter on Abuse Issues, Well-being section, for more information)

How do you feel about the way your parents related to you as a child? This can tell you something about their ideas regarding parenting. If they do not feel their parenting models were desirable, find out as much as you can about why they feel that way. Note any tendency toward physical abuse in their history.

Was there domestic violence in your family (physical or emotional)? This is a different question than the one about sexual abuse, above, but sometimes it will reveal sexual abuse in the partner's history as well as physical or emotional abuse. It is good to ask this question directly, in addition to the question above, because some details will not come out otherwise. If there was physical or emotional abuse, try to find out exactly what form it took and how frequently. Ask if she has received any counseling for these issues.

What are your intuitions about the pregnancy, birth or the baby? This can be a very informative question. It will bring up both positive and negative comments. Make note of any specific fears mentioned. If misinformation is the basis of the fear, provide correct information. If personal issues seem to be at the core (these two categories can overlap) see the chapter on Working Through Emotional Issues

With Clients, Well-being section, for ideas about how to help them work through these fears. Ask if the fears seem to be thoughts running around in their head due to intellectual knowledge from books, films or stories, or if there is a gut level instinct that something is not right. One way to deal with fears is to ask "What is the worst thing that could happen?" Then ask them to visualize themselves dealing with this worst case scenario. Invite her to experience the fear fully, without resistance, breathe into it and inquire as to what is familiar about this fear. After she has worked through her fear, encourage them to put the intellectual concerns attached to the fear aside and visualize the experience she wants to create, in every detail. Remind them that it is important to be in touch with fear and concerns, but it is equally important to focus on what they *do* want to happen.

Comments: Write your general impressions of this interview and any further concerns or questions you feel need to be addressed at a later time.

Problems which may have arisen during the current pregnancy: These problems many be present during this pregnancy or may have shown up during previous pregnancies. Try to elicit both types of information with an emphasis on current conditions. If the problem appeared earlier in this pregnancy but has now subsided, note the approximate weeks of pregnancy that it occurred. If it is a current problem you want to know:

*When and how often it occurs
*Under what circumstances does it occur or get worse
*What has she tried to do to correct the problem?
*Do other symptoms seem to be associated with the problem?
*How severe is the problem?
*How is it interfering with her lifestyle or eating habits?
*How is she feeling about the problem?
*Are there any psychological or emotional needs which she has right
    now that are not being met? (Physical problems are often signals
    that things are also out of balance on other levels)

See specific chapters on all the common discomforts of pregnancy for more details regarding what to ask and how to treat them. The discomforts as listed in the forms should all be discussed. How to deal with each of these topics will be found in chapters throughout the book.

References and Further reading:
Lichtman, R, & Papera, S., Gynecology: Well-woman Care, Appleton & Lance, Norwalk, 1990.
Mittendorf, R., Herbst, A., "Managing the DES-exposed woman: an update," Contemp.OB/GYN, Vol. 37, No. 9, September, 1994, p. 62.
Pearce, Malcolm, "Seat Belts in Pregnancy," Br. Med. J., Vol. 304 No. 6827, 3/7/92, pp. 586-7.

MEDICAL HISTORY

Date of initial Hx_____ Due date_____ LMP_____ Blood type & factor_____

Mother_____ Age____ Birth date_____ Occupation_____

Partner/support_____ Age____ Birth date_____ Occupation_____

Address_____ Telephone #s:_____ _____
        street   apt. no.   city   state   zip   home   work

Have you had any prenatal care? ____ With whom? _____ Do you plan to breastfeed? _____ Comments:_____

PRIOR PREGNANCIES: Total___ Live___ Stillbirths___ Abortions___ Miscarriages___ Record of those ending ≥20 wks preg.:

Child's name/Preg. #					
Birth date/place/care-giver					
Planned/using contraception					
Weeks gest. at birth					
Type of birth					
Total weight gain					
Prenatal problems					
Early labor history					
Active labor					
Pushing phase					
Placental birth/blood loss					
Drugs/IV used					
Experience of birth					
Complications					
Perineal trauma					
Baby's position at birth					
Weight/length of baby					
APGAR 1/5 minutes					
Problems w/baby					
Postpartum exp./breastfed?					
Child's health now					

Record of all pregnancies which ended before 20 weeks of pregnancy:

Date ended?/Wks gest./Preg. #									
Location/care-giver									
Drugs used									
Procedures used									
Complications									
Experience									
Counseling									

CONTRACEPTIVE HX:

METHOD	TYPE	WHEN & HOW LONG	COMMENTS/PROBLEMS
Oral contraceptives			
IUD			
Morning after pill			

MENSTRUAL Hx: Age of onset:_____ Average length of: cycle_____days, flow_____ days Are you regular?_____

What is your usual amount of flow?_____ Problems?_____ First day of last normal period _____ Probable date of

conception ____ Date of 1st fetal motion ____ Contraception at time of conception?_____ Method_____ Due date_____

♀ **MOTHER'S OB HISTORY:** Total Pregnancies____ Live____ Stillbirths____ Abortions____ Miscarriages____

Sibling order:				
Weeks gest. at birth				
Labor history				
Drugs used				
Type of birth				
Complications				
Breastfeeding				
Comments (DES/drug exp):				

PERSONAL LIFESTYLE & HABITS:

DO YOU OR YOUR PARTNER:	PREG. ♀	PARTNER	WHEN & HOW OFTEN/COMMENTS:
Smoke			
Drink alcohol			
Use medications (over-the-counter/prescription)			
Have a Hx of recreational drug use (IV?)			
Have religious beliefs that affect your health care?			
Use chemicals or harmful substances at work or home?			
Use or work with/near microwave ovens?			
Use computers/radiation?			
Get regular exercise?			
Drink caffeinated/sugared beverages?			
Have pets?			
Type of diet (omnivore/ovo-lacto/vegan/macrobiotic/other)			

Discuss: Seat belts___ Fluoride___ Commercial deodorant___ Bras___ Talc___ Tap water___

MEDICAL HISTORY: Has the preg. ♀, biological father or any immediate relatives had any of these health conditions?

PROBLEM	NO	PREG. ♀	FATHER	RELATIVES	COMMENTS
Heart/circ/BP					
Anemia/blood dis.					
Diabetes					
Thyroid disorders					
Respiratory dis.					
Convulsive/CNS dis.					
Cancer/growths					
Varicose veins					
Genetic disorders					

Key to codes: MM--maternal mother MF--maternal father MS--maternal sibling MGM--maternal grand mother MA, MU--maternal
aunt/uncle, use P for paternal before each designation for the biological father

Has the pregnant ♀, biological father or current partner had (or been exposed to) any of the following:

PROBLEM	NO	Preg. ♀	FATHER	COMMENTS:
DES/steroid therapy				
Genital herpes				
Genital warts				
Chlamydia				
Gonorrhea				
Syphilis				
HIV				
Excess X-rays/Ultrasd.				

COMMENTS:_____

Has the pregnant ♀ had any of the following prior to this pregnancy:

PROBLEM	NO	COMMENTS	PROBLEM	NO	COMMENTS
Severe illnesses			Back problems		
Anorexia/Bulimia			Severe accident		
Stomach/GI			Arthritis/Rheumatism		
Severe headaches			Insomnia		
Allergies			UT/kidney infections		
General surgery			Yoni infections		
GYN surgery			Pelvic infections		
Transfusions					

<u>PROFILE OF BIOLOGICAL FATHER:</u> Body build _____ Blood type/factor_____ Relationship to mother _____

Health problems_____

<u>PSYCHOLOGICAL PROFILE:</u> How do you handle emotional issues in your life?

Preg. ♀ _____ Partner_____

Have you ever been raped or molested?

Preg. ♀ _____

How do you feel about the way your parents related to you as children?

Preg. ♀_____ Partner_____

Was there domestic violence in your family (physical or emotional)?

Preg. ♀_____ Partner_____

What are your intuitions about the pregnancy, birth or the baby?

Preg. ♀_____ Partner_____

Comments:_____

_____

PROBLEMS WHICH MAY HAVE ARISEN DURING THE CURRENT PREGNANCY:

PROBLEM	NO	IF SO, WHEN/COMMENTS	PROBLEM	NO	IF SO, WHEN/COMMENTS
Nausea/vomiting			Drug use		
Heartburn			Spotting/Bleeding		
Poor appetite			Colds/virus infec.		
Bruising easily			Yoni infec./herpes		
Bleeding gums			UT pain/infec.		
Backache			Abdominal pain		
Muscle cramps			Headaches		
Itching			Dizziness		
Rashes			Blurred vision		
Constipation			Swelling		
Diarrhea			Pigment changes		
Hemorrhoids			Insomnia		
Varicose veins			Radiation/US		
Fainting/black outs			Excessive fatigue		

Today's date_____ Due_____
Gravida_____ Parity___
Abortions____ Miscarriages____
Weeks pregnant_____ Age_____

Height____ft. _____in.
Pre preg. wt._____lbs.
Present wt. _____lbs.
Radial pulse___/min.
Blood pressure___/____
Hemoglobin_____grams

EYES: Reaction_____
Membranes_____
Retinas L_____ R_____

LUNGS: L_____ R_____

HEART: Rate_____/min.
Sounds_____

HANDS: Size_____
Swelling_____

MOUTH: _____
Lips_____
Tongue_____
Teeth_____

GLANDS: Lymph_____
Thyroid_____

LEGS: Veins_____
Swelling_____
Reflexes L_____ R____

FEET: Swelling_____
Reflexes:
Knee L____ R____
Ankle L____ R_____
Ankle clonus L___ R____

SKIN:_____

HAIR:_____

BREAST EXAMINATION:
Masses: L_____ R_____
Nipples: L_____ R_____

Reaction to exam_____

ABDOMINAL EXAM:
Fundal height _____ cm.
Stretch marks_____
Tone: Skin_____ Muscle_____
Scars_____ Placental sounds (o)
Fetal motion_____ Position___
FHT_____/per 5 sec. (+)

PHYSICAL EXAMINATION

Draw in findings from general physical exam:

External genitals:

URINE ANALYSIS:

Color_____ Glucose_____

Clarity_____ Ketones_____

Protein_____ pH_____

EXTERNAL GENITALS:
(draw in findings)

Perineum:
Scar tissue_____
Stretchiness_____
Length_____
Instructions in stretching___

Internal yoni exam:
Scar tissue_____
Muscle tone_____
Varicosities_____
Abnormalities_____

INTERNAL EXAMINATION:
Date___ Weeks pregnant ____
Midwife_____

CERVICAL FINDINGS:
Placement_____
Scar tissue_____
Growths_____
Dilation_____
Effacement_____

PELVIC ASSESSMENT:
Ischial spines: R_____ L_____
Interspinous diameter:
__narrow __average __wide

Subpubic arch:
__narrow __average __(90°) __wide
Inclination of pubic bone:
__ant. __straight __post.
Thickness of pubic bone:_____
Angle of side walls:
__convergent __straight __divergent

Sacral tip & coccyx:
Mobility_____
Diagonal conjugate of outlet: ____cm.
Sacrospinous ligament:
R_____cm. L_____cm.
Ischial spines: __above __level with
__below: sacral tip

SACRUM:
Curvature of sacrum:
__average __marked __straight

Inclination:
__forward __average __backward

Diagonal conjugate____cm.

External bituberous diameter_____cm.

CONTINUATION OF PREVIOUS PREGNANCY HISTORY

Mother _____

Continuation of records for those ending ≥ 20 weeks of pregnancy:

Child's name/Preg. #						
Birth date/place/care-giver						
Planned/using contraception						
Weeks gest. at birth						
Type of birth						
Total weight gain						
Prenatal problems						
Early labor history						
Active labor						
Pushing phase						
Placental birth						
Drugs/IV used						
Experience of birth						
Complications						
Perineal trauma						
Baby's position at birth						
Wt/lgth of baby						
APGAR 1/5 min.						
Problems w/baby						
Postpartum exp./breastfed?						
Child's health now						

Continuation of records for all pregnancies which ended before 20 weeks of pregnancy:

Date ended?/Wks preg./Preg. #									
Location/care-giver									
Drugs used?									
Procedures used									
Complications?									
Experience?									
Counseling?									

Comments:

_____

_____

_____

_____

Ordering Baseline Laboratory Tests

I've written a huge book on the use of laboratory tests in pregnancy and do not plan to repeat all that information in this book as well. This chapter will give an overview of what tests to order when a woman is basically healthy with no underlying medical conditions which need to be monitored in conjunction with her pregnancy. It is only intended as a reminder about what to order and why; further elaboration on all of these tests and the conditions they look for is readily available in Diagnostic Tests. If you are confused by the information given here because it is incomplete, rest assured that your questions will be answered when you go to Diagnostic Tests for more details. (If a woman does have underlying medical conditions, see chapters in this book and Diagnostic Tests concerning other tests and a discussion of the condition in question.)

This chapter will discuss the baseline laboratory work-up for pregnancy. Baseline results are exactly that: a basis established while the mother is in a presumably healthy state. Such testing offers a starting point from which to judge any potentially problematic conditions which develop later as well as the opportunity to catch any hidden problems such as anemia or subclinical infection. Ideally, baseline lab results are obtained prior to the 8th week of pregnancy, or at least by the 12th week if the 8th week proves impossible. If a woman comes to you after 12 weeks, draw blood for her tests as soon as possible if no results are available for this pregnancy from a previous care provider.

Basic laboratory workups for first-time clients can be more or less elaborate. Generally speaking, you want to order at least the following blood tests on all clients for whom you have no previous laboratory records:

*Pregnancy test, if necessary (see the last chapter for a brief review).
*Complete blood count—which should include:
  -Red blood count
  -White blood count
  -Differential (counts the different kinds of white blood cells)
  -Hemoglobin and hematocrit
  -Platelet count
*Blood type and factor with an antibody screen
*Rubella titer
*Hepatitis B surface antigen
*Urine analysis
*Syphilis screening (ideally a VDRL *and* an FTA-ABS)
*HIV testing, if desired after discussion
*Liver or Chem profile
*Tuberculosis screening

The following reviews indications for each test and what the results can tell you:

Complete blood count (CBC): This gives you information on the general health of the blood stream and the immune system:

> ***Total Red Cell Count (RBC):** gauges how well the bone marrow is functioning to produce blood cells and gives an overall impression of the health of the blood stream.
>
> ***Total White Cell Count (WBC):** the number of all types of white cells together in one figure; this test also gives information about bone marrow health, and indicates if the immune system is being stimulated for any reason. Since the WBC normally rises in late pregnancy, the baseline is of limited value in following a potential problem (for example, with prelabor rupture of membranes.)
>
> ***Differential:** an analysis of the number of each type of white cell, giving specific information to help track down the cause of any problems. Because the total WBC can be normal in the presence of abnormal levels of one or more types of white cells, Differential results always provide important additional information. Changes in some values normally occur in late pregnancy (see above).
>
> ***The Hemoglobin:** a gauge of the oxygen-carrying capacity of the RBCs; if low, the cause needs to be investigated further. Normally this value is 33% of the hematocrit.
>
> ***Hematocrit:** represents the amount of red blood cells packed by centrifuge in a given volume of blood.
>
> ***Platelets:** only one factor in a complex blood clotting system; however, this value can give you a rough idea of the woman's clotting status. A good count reflects bone marrow health.

Blood type and factor and antibody screen: Every woman needs a blood type and factor test if she does not already know what they are. Even if she does, it is a good idea to have these retested at least once, as sometimes the lab will make a mistake, with potentially serious consequences for the woman and her baby.

The blood type will tell her which major blood group she is in: A, B, AB or O. The blood factor will tell her if she has the Rh(o)D factor, which is the strongest minor factor among some 400 thus far identified on the red blood cell. If a woman lacks the Rh factor (i.e. she is Rh negative) she will need further testing with additional antibody screens to determine if antibodies are being developed in her system during the course of the pregnancy. Rh negative mothers who are not sensitized to the Rh factor do not require additional tests during the first trimester, but will need another test at 28 and 36 weeks.

Whenever a type and factor are ordered, an **antibody screen** is routinely done, regardless of the Rh factor. The screen looks for any kind of minor blood factor related antibodies which may be present in the woman's system. If any are found, further, more specific testing must be done using an **Antibody ID** to determine exactly what type and quantity of antibodies are present. The lab should do this test automatically upon getting a positive antibody screen, without your having to order an additional test separately.

If a woman is sensitized to a particular antibody, test the biological father whenever possible to determine if he is positive for that factor. If he too is negative, the baby is not at risk except in the very rare instance of a new genetic mutation (1 in 100,000) (Brawn, 1994). A woman will only form antibodies when exposed to a foreign factor; that is, one for which she is negative.

If the father is positive for the factor to which the mother is sensitized, consultation with an obstetrical specialist knowledgeable about blood incompatibilities may be advisable, depending upon which factor is in question. (See Diagnostic Tests for more background concerning blood incompatibilities.)

Rubella antibody titer: The rubella titer tells us if a woman has been previously exposed to Rubella and, if so, if she is now immune to Rubella. An antibody titer can form in response to natural infection or vaccination. If a woman is negative for Rubella, she should be advised to steer clear of small children who have been exposed to the disease. Maternal infection can cause serious fetal damage throughout pregnancy; this is especially true during the first trimester. A woman who is immune from natural infection is immune for life and does not require additional tests with each pregnancy. Those with vaccine-induced immunity may become susceptible in the future and should be retested during each pregnancy.

Hepatitis-B surface antigen screen: Of the many Hepatitis B tests available, this is the best for screening purposes. The presence of antigen indicates a current infection or a chronic carrier state, which are the most dangerous manifestations of Hepatitis B during pregnancy for both the mother and baby. If positive, a full Hep B profile should be ordered to determine if the woman is currently infected or a chronic Hep B carrier; either would make her contagious to you and her baby.

Urine analysis: You will be checking the urine at each prenatal with dip stick tests. Therefore, laboratory urine analysis is somewhat optional unless there are signs of problems now or a history of urinary or kidney problems in the past. Bacteria can be detected upon microscopic examination of the urine. The lab should be told to perform a culture and drug sensitivity routinely if a significant number of bacteria are discovered. To help rule out any false results, the urine sent to the lab should be collected with a clean catch.

Syphilis screening: Twenty seven states no longer require routine syphilis screening prior to marriage or during pregnancy (McKenna, 1993). In spite of this complacent attitude on the part of health department officials, syphilis is epidemic in the United States, with an estimated 40 million current cases, many of which have never been diagnosed as such. With this in mind, syphilis screening is imperative for all pregnant women, regardless of their presumed risk status. (McKenna, 1994) The following situations make a person high risk for having contracted syphilis at some point during their life:

*Multiple sexual partners or partners with numerous sexual partners
*Recalling associates talking of syphilis diagnosis or treatment (no talking about it won't spread syphilis, but this indicates the possibility of active infection in her sphere of associates, which may mean a sexual partner of hers was exposed)
*A sexual contact being treated for syphilis
*A known, untreated exposure
*A partner had diagnosed syphilis, but when the woman was tested, her tests were negative
*Diagnosis and treatment with no follow-up tests
*Chronic or unexplained skin conditions, including non-recurrent or recurrent genital herpes, persistent unexplained illnesses, ARC or AIDS
*Anyone who was stationed or has visited Asia, Southeast Asia, Africa, or the Caribbean, (particularly note if a sexually transmitted disease or reproductive tract infection was contracted while there, regardless of the diagnosis)
*IV drug use with needle sharing, past or present, in the woman or a partner
*HIV positive test results (likely to have seronegative, atypical presentation of syphilis)

The screening tests which are routinely done look for non-treponemal antibodies that are known to show up with syphilis and a number of other conditions. These tests are notoriously inaccurate, especially in cases of syphilis which have advanced beyond the primary stage (which many undiagnosed cases have). Therefore, it is ideal to order a FTA-ABS in addition to a screening test such as the VDRL or the RPR.

The FTA-ABS is one of two confirmatory tests which are normally done only after a VDRL or an RPR shows up positive. If finances do not allow for the use of both tests, order only the FTA-ABS. It looks for treponemal-specific antibodies and is positive for life if a person has ever been infected with the more common form of syphilis (but could be negative in the presence of infection with Black [Nylon] syphilis, which is seronegative in many cases). In spite of this complicating factor, the FTA-ABS is still more accurate than a screening test by itself. You will have to talk to the lab specifically about running this test without a positive VDRL. They may think you are crazy, but they will probably go along with it once you are very clear that you have your reasons and want to use it as a *screening* test. (Read the chapter on Syphilis in <u>Diagnostic Tests</u>).

HIV testing: The notion that the HIV virus causes AIDS has gone largely unchallenged since this hypothesis was introduced in the 1980s. The symptoms of AIDS and those of syphilis are identical in every respect. Internationally, there are some highly respected researchers who believe there is a link between AIDS and syphilis infection. Other correlations with the development of AIDS include heavy drug use and even the toxic therapies recommended for treating HIV.

What the HIV virus might be or whether it can cause illness are topics of debate among a growing number of researchers. Counsel everyone regarding their risk factors for HIV and syphilis exposure (which are identical). Explain to them that there is a growing scientific controversy regarding exactly what HIV is, whether it is a problem, and what HIV antibody titers mean. Anyone who is HIV positive should review these issues carefully, and consider having laboratory work evaluated for a possible hidden syphilis infection through the BASIS Project, 2811 Martin Luther King Jr. Way, Berkeley CA, 94703 (510) 548-4000. (McKenna, 1993) This is a private research project set up to investigate unusual forms of syphilis. See Diagnostic Tests, 6th ed. for more details concerning HIV and syphilis.

Liver profile/chem panel/SMA-12/SMA-24: These names are used in various areas to refer to a group of tests which give you values from which to judge any liver- or kidney-related changes which may appear in pregnancy. This group of tests is especially important if you suspect that a woman is becoming toxemic. Be sure the profile includes at least the following tests: BUN (blood urea nitrogen), creatinine, uric acid, albumin, total protein, and the liver enzymes (alkaline phosphatase, LDH, SGOT, and SGPT).

Tuberculosis screening test: Screening may not be necessary for all your clients, but should be considered for women coming from any of the following risk groups:

*Those from Asia, Africa, Latin America and the inner city
*Those in recent contact with someone known or suspected to have TB
*Those with signs and symptoms of TB
*Those who have a diagnosed condition that make them at higher risk
 for TB (HIV, syphilis)

The tine test is inaccurate and a poor screening test to use in high-risk populations. The Mantoux test is the most accurate screen for those at real risk. It is a skin test which involves injecting weak TB solution under the skin and waiting 48 to 72 hours to evaluate the result. It is most accurate three months after infection. Chest X-rays are an inappropriate screening tool to use in pregnancy.

584

Anyone found to have TB should be evaluated carefully for both HIV and syphilis.

Other types of prenatal testing: While the tests listed above are the basic ones used for all pregnancies, you will also need to discuss certain other tests which are widely recommended by the medical model. You will do this for two reasons: women need to know what is available so that they can make informed decisions about their care, and because you need to make clear how your practice differs from the medical model. Because of the need to inform women of these tests before they would be done (so the woman has time to think about them) they are discussed in this section.

All women: In many areas, the medical model routinely recommends the following tests for all women:

> *Alpha*-fetoprotein testing
> *Ultrasound scan for dating and general fetal exam
> *Gestational diabetes screening

Maternal Serum *Alpha*-fetoprotein testing (MsAFP): In medical model practices, blood for *Alpha*-fetoprotein tests is often drawn along with that taken for routine initial lab work. It is therefore important to discuss this test with women as soon as possible after they contact you for care. AFP screening used by itself is not particularly accurate and, if positive, leads to more testing, often in the form of an amniocentesis. Ultimately, if a problem is found, the choice is to carry the baby or have a second trimester abortion. Here is a review of the pertinent points regarding this test (details in <u>Diagnostic Tests</u>).

> *AFP is produced by the fetal liver
> *Small quantities pass into the maternal bloodstream where the concentration gradually rises until late in pregnancy
> *A blood test determines if the level is abnormally high or low
> *MsAFP alone is not very accurate and leads to more invasive testing such as amniocentesis for a definitive diagnosis
> *The best time to draw a MsAFP is between 15 to 18 weeks
> *The Triple screen tests for MsAFP, hCG & estriol and is more accurate, reducing the number of women referred for amniocentesis to 5% of those tested; it should be requested if AFP testing is desired (details in <u>Diagnostic Tests</u>).

However, new research shows that the triple screen detects only 60 to 70% of all Down syndrome in women over 35 *if* all those with abnormal tests go on to have amniocentesis. Some feel that all women over 35 who want testing should forego any blood screening in favor of amniocentesis. (Kolder, 1995)

Ultrasound exam: Imaging ultrasound exams are now used routinely in most obstetrical practices. Your palpation skills and ability to hear the fetal heart should be better than ultrasound in determining the status of the normal fetus. Be sure women understand that they can refuse routine ultrasounds if they do not want their fetus exposed to unproven technology without good reason.

Imaging ultrasound can be used in an attempt to determine if fetal growth and development are within normal limits. Parents may desire such an exam if they have had a previous baby with defects that were not genetic. The ideal time to perform the exam is at 20 weeks of pregnancy. The biophysical profile can be used after 34 weeks to evaluate general fetal well-being when there is cause for concern. Also advise women to count fetal movements at home if there is a question regarding fetal movement patterns.

Gestational diabetes screening: Depending upon where you live, gestational diabetes tests may be done only for those who are high risk or for everyone. Gestational diabetes is a controversial topic; some practitioners feel that the alterations in insulin use that occur during pregnancy are a healthy adaptation to the presence of the fetus and are designed to meet the growth needs of the pregnancy. Be sure women understand this controversy before they decide whether or not to undergo testing. Once a woman is labeled as gestational diabetic, her pregnancy will be considered high risk.

Toxoplasmosis screening: Toxoplasmosis is an organism carried in the feces of infected cats and birds; maternal infection can cause fetal damage. This test is not done routinely in most practices. It may be desired by a woman who has had recent exposure to cats or birds if she has no previous history of exposure.

In addition to the above tests, specific tests should be discussed with women who fall into the following categories. Remember that this chapter only provides a reminder and a summary of what to discuss; complete details for each of these tests can be found in Diagnostic Tests.

For women with a known history of a detectable birth defect in a previous baby or in her family, racial or ethnic group: Discuss genetic counseling and testing to determine if the genes are present in either biological parent. Chorionic Villus Sampling (CVS) can be done between 9.5 and 11 weeks of pregnancy for some conditions. Amniocentesis can be used if it is too late for CVS or when the defects in question cannot be found via CVS.

For women 35 or older: Chorionic Villi Sampling (CVS) before 12 weeks, amniocentesis before 18 weeks, or an ultrasound exam around 20 weeks can look for evidence of Down syndrome, the most common birth defect in this age group.

Always discuss that the only option for "correcting" a genetic problem is a

586

therapeutic abortion, which is not an option for many women. In some cases fetal surgery is being used to correct defects, but this is a costly and still largely experimental medicine which is fraught with risks for both mother and fetus.

Sickle cell prep: This test should be discussed with African-American women and their partners if they have never been screened for Sickle cell anemia.

Hemoglobin electrophoresis: This test looks for normal hemoglobin. It should be performed on anemic women of Mediterranean descent or from other ethnic backgrounds that have a high rate of inherited anemias.

The following tests are done using samples and cultures from the yoni: These tests should be discussed with all women seeking your care. They are routinely performed in many medical practices on every woman, regardless of risk status:

*PAP Smear
*Gonorrhea screening
*Chlamydia screening
*Strep-B screening in late pregnancy

The **PAP smear** can be done at the initial pelvic examination. However, unless the condition of the cervix warrants testing, it may be best postpone the PAP smear until the six week postpartum visit because of the tendency of the pregnant cervix to bleed during sample collection. Blood will cause inaccurate results.

Both **Chlamydia** and **Gonorrhea** can exist asymptomatically in the yoni, therefore both of these cultures are obtained during the initial pelvic exam in most practices. Many monogamous women have been found to carry chlamydia, making testing important, even if a woman considers herself low risk.

Beta-Strep is an elusive bacteria which can come and go at whim, regardless of test results. Therefore, it has not been routinely screened for in many areas. However, *Beta*-strep has been receiving more attention in recent years, and screening may be a standard of care in your community. If testing is done, it should be done late in pregnancy or only in the event of membrane rupture prior to the onset of contractions.

References and further reading:
Brawn, Jennifer, midwife, workshop at Colorado Midwifery Assoc. conf., August, 1994.
Frye, Anne, Understanding Diagnostic Tests, 4th ed., Labrys Press, Portland, OR, 1993.
Kolder, Veronika, editing notes, 7/95.
McKenna, Joan, letter to the editor, Policy Review, Fall, 1992.
op. cit., "Syphilis and AIDS," (notes taken from taped workshop), MANA conference, San Francisco, CA, Nov. 1993.

Prenatal Concerns Regarding the Breasts and Breastfeeding

The chapter on the physical exam covers the general examination of the breasts. This chapter will cover some specific concerns women may have regarding breastfeeding and offer suggestions about what can be done to minimize or alleviate these conditions during pregnancy, when possible.

Nursing in Western culture: Our culture is removed from our physical and emotional beings in so many ways that breastfeeding has become a real challenge for many first world women. Deprogramming women who feel bad about their breasts (too big, too small, too droopy, etc.) and helping them come to an understanding of how wonderful breastfeeding is for their own health as well as that of their babies can be a healing experience for many women.

Benefits of breastfeeding: The details of breastfeeding will be covered in the third volume of this text. For right now, you need to communicate to women that breast milk is the best milk for any baby. The mother's body tailors the milk to the age of the baby and offers a thoroughly digestible and nutritious source of nourishment. Breastfeeding also offers the closeness which young babies need. The baby goes from being nourished by the mother's body inside via the umbilical cord to being nourished by equally living food from the breast once he is outside. The milk contains the perfect balance of proteins, fat and calories as well as valuable antibodies, beneficial bacteria and the life energy of the mother. While it is true that many chemicals can pass through the milk, this does not negate the other benefits of breastmilk for the baby. For the mother, nursing provides a means of maintaining hormone levels so that she gradually becomes reaccustomed to life outside of pregnancy; it fosters emotional attachment to her newborn and lets her body know that the baby is out and safe, speeding the involution of her reproductive organs to their nonpregnant state. The hormones which support breastfeeding also contract the uterus, minimizing postpartum blood loss.

Previous breast surgery: A special circumstance is the woman with a history of previous breast surgery. These women are often anxious to know how their surgery may impact their ability to nurse. Surgery may have been done for breast enlargement or reduction, or because of a disease such as breast cancer.

Breast reduction or augmentation: An incision in the vicinity of the cutaneous branch of the fourth intercostal nerve (on the left breast at 5 o'clock or on the right breast at the 7 o'clock position) may have severed nerves supplying the nipple and areola. Any surgery along the edge of the areola is likely to interfere with milk production to some degree. However, breastfeeding is possible for the majority of these mothers. Techniques for breast reduction surgery have improved over the years, and it is now possible to maintain the anatomical and physiological

588

relationship of the nipple and the underlying breast tissue to some degree. The degree to which this is accomplished is directly proportional to how successful breastfeeding will be. The woman should ask her surgeon the details of her surgery if she has not already done so.

Leakage of silicone breast implants has been well documented, and may cause a variety of problems for women who have had them placed such as scleroderma, an autoimmune rheumatic disease. Less well known are studies which suggest that nursing infants of these mothers are likely to develop decreased motility and reduced peristalsis in the lower esophagus due to exposure to silicone in the mother's milk. Why this occurs is not clear; factors include changes in the immune response and increased macromolecular uptake in the newborn intestinal tract (silicone is a macromolecule). Onset of disease in affected women is typically delayed 2 to 20 years after the surgery, so more severe delayed disease in newborns is not out of the question. Therefore, it is advisable for any woman who wishes to become pregnant to have her implants removed before doing so. She may want to pump her breasts for the first two weeks after birth and discard the milk in an attempt to remove any residual silicone from the tissue before beginning to breastfeed (this suggestion seems to be a reasonable precaution; there is no data to back up this recommendation). (Levine & Ilowite, 1994)

Variations in breast anatomy: Here are the main anatomical features about which the mother may need reassurance or assistance in correcting:

Are my breasts normal? Some women may have this concern, especially if they were told that their mother could not nurse due to lack of milk. There was an epidemic of women who "could not nurse" from the nineteen thirties through the sixties. This had much more to do with obstetrical drugs and incorrect protocols regarding breastfeeding than any anatomical abnormality in the mothers. Ask a woman if she is experiencing normal breast changes such as enlargement, tenderness and soreness. Normal breast changes usually indicate adequate development of breast tissue responsive to changing hormonal levels. Colostrum (the first milk) is produced throughout pregnancy and is more easily expressed from the breasts of some women than others. If a woman is still worried later on, you can try to express colostrum yourself by grasping the areola from above and below and pressing it between your fingers. This will milk colostrum from the ampulla behind the areola, much to the delight and sometimes the amazement of the woman.

Small nipples: The size of the nipples does not significantly affect a woman's ability to breastfeed, although small nipples may sometimes make it harder for the baby to latch on (more true with flat nipples than small, erect ones).

Scaring from burns: While the tissue over a severe burn scar will be less elastic, burns rarely extend deeply enough to damage lactation tissues, even if the burns occurred during adulthood. Significant scars may result in reduced sensation during nursing, lessened elasticity of the breast necessitating the mother to alter the baby's nursing position, and reduced milk ejection if the nipple was surgically reconstructed. Scar tissue on the breast or nipple does not, by itself, preclude breastfeeding. One 500 mg. Evening Primrose oil, Borage oil or Black Currant oil capsule can be taken every other day throughout pregnancy to soften scar tissue, provided the mother is not a DES daughter. Capsules can also be opened and massaged directly into scar tissue. Vitamin E, 400 IUs daily, may also help.

Preparation for breastfeeding: For most women, there is no need for any specific preparation for breastfeeding. For those with flat nipples, there are techniques to help bring the nipple out, which follow below. Answering questions or loaning out a video tape on breastfeeding basics may be all you need to do in most cases. Some general tips you can give every woman are to go without a bra at home to expose the nipples to the air and to involve the breasts in lovemaking when the mother desires (tender breasts will not want to participate!)

For women who have never handled their breasts these suggestions are harmless and may, in fact, help them become more comfortable with their breasts and thus facilitate breastfeeding. However, it has been determined that, in most cases, problems with sore nipples are not avoided through prenatal preparation but with the proper positioning of the baby during nursing. Washing or rubbing the nipples with a towel to toughen them actually removes valuable oils which keep the nipple soft and may do more harm than good.

Flat nipples: In addition to the simple measures already described, there are several steps a woman can take during pregnancy to try and remedy flat or inverted nipples. These include rubbing with the fingers to cause the nipple to become as erect as possible, then grasping the nipple, gently pulling it out and rolling it between the fingers; using a breast pump to apply suction to the nipple just enough to cause the nipple to become erect, then leaving the pump in place for a few minutes on each side; and the use of breast shells.

Breast shells consist of a hollow plastic dome that is placed over a base through which the nipple protrudes. They can be held in place by a bra. The dome may have one or several ventilation holes, depending upon the brand. Several vents provide better air circulation and are preferable. If a particular device with few vent holes otherwise fits the nipples, additional vent holes can be drilled into the dome. Advise a woman using breast shells for flat nipples as follows:

*Wear the shells for 1 to 2 hours daily, gradually increasing the time
15 minutes each day until they are worn all day; remove the shells

590

before going to bed, wash them well, rinse and air dry overnight.
*In hot weather, or if moisture build-up occurs, remove the shells for
20 minutes at a time, 2 or 3 times daily and dry the shells well.
*If the nipple does not fit completely through the hole in the base, use
a brand with a larger opening or a less sloping base.
*If soreness or irritation develop, call the midwife promptly
(recommend that she temporarily discontinue use and expose her
nipples to the air and apply an herbal salve if appropriate)

If an absorbent pad is used with the shells, it should be changed as often as necessary to maintain fairly dry contact with the breast surface. A clammy, moist or wet pad should not be left in place for the entire wearing time, as this will promote bacteria growth and the possibility of a yeast infection on the nipples.

Breast support: Bras interfere with superficial lymph drainage, encouraging the accumulation of toxins in breast fatty tissue as well as in the milk. Advise women to go without support as much as they can and massage their breasts upon bra removal. When necessary, advise a well-fitting but not constricting bra with no underwires, preferably in a cotton fabric. The breasts will enlarge throughout pregnancy and more so when the milk comes in. She needs to purchase bras of different sizes to accommodate these changes. (Singer & Grismaijer, 1995)

Nursing while pregnant: Some women want to continue nursing an older child once they become pregnant. In a healthy woman, continued nursing during pregnancy is not a problem, as long as she compensates for the additional nutrient requirements by altering her diet; basically she needs to eat as though she is carrying twins, adding the equivalent of an additional quart of milk daily in calories and protein. As she gets closer to term, her milk will naturally transform into colostrum. The nursing sibling may at this point decide that the milk tastes "funny" and will often self-wean. The mother can explain that her body is getting ready to feed the new baby "real baby milk," not big girl or big boy milk.

Potential problems with nursing during pregnancy include increased uterine stimulation, fatigue, and decreased milk supply. Uterine stimulation is not a concern unless threatened miscarriage or premature labor should develop. The breast changes of early pregnancy, particularly nipple tenderness, may make nursing quite uncomfortable for the mother. If this occurs, the mother and her child will have to work out a nursing relationship that meets both their needs.

Brewer, Gail, The Brewer Medical Diet, Simon & Schuster, Pub., New York, 1983.
Levine, J., & Ilowite, N., "Sderoderma-like Esophageal Disease in Children Breast-fed by Mothers With Silicone Breast Implants," JAMA, Jan. 19, 1994, Vol. 271, No. 3, p. 213.
Riordan, J. & K. Auerbach, Breastfeeding and Human Lactation, Jones & Bartlett, Boston, 1993.
Singer & Grismaijer, Dressed to Kill: the Link Between Breast Cancer & Bras, Avery Pub, 1995.

Helping Women Deal With Work and Activity Concerns

You may have cause to use your authority as a health care provider to help a woman deal with her work environment or negotiate the rules of some public service, such as public transportation. Employers are not always quick to allow women snacks at their desk, time off their feet or the privilege of moving around or taking more frequent bathroom breaks that they otherwise might require. As a midwife, you can call or write to employers with a list of specific requests in an attempt to enlist their cooperation. Often, with the requests in writing from a care provider an employer will feel compelled to comply, for fear of liability if something goes wrong. Just a few of the issues your client might face are as follows:

*Working with toxic chemicals, fumes or other substances
*Working around dangerous machinery which her changing center of gravity may cause it to be more unsafe than usual
*Being on her feet constantly (waitresses, store clerks, factory workers)
*Having a job which requires wearing certain types of clothing or shoes which may be uncomfortable or ill-advised during pregnancy (high heels, nylon stockings, etc.)
*Working in an environment which prohibits employees from snacking at their desks or work areas
*Working in a room full of computer terminals or other electronic equipment
*Working with drugs, anesthetic gases, infectious agents, or around radiation (nurses, doctors or lab technicians)
*Working near a microwave oven

The kinds of responses you will be called upon to make in such circumstances may vary widely. For example, an employer may be more likely to grant a request that a woman be allowed food at her desk than one to remove her to another type of work while she is pregnant. Sometimes a woman may have to make the choice to remain at a job which poses potential danger to herself or her unborn baby. (See the chapter on Harmful Environmental Exposures in the section on Sustaining Health and Well-being as well as the chapter on X-rays, Radiation and Pregnancy in Diagnostic Tests for more information.)

You may also have to write letters stating that a woman may participate in exercise classes, that it is okay to take an airline flight, or for her to otherwise engage in activities which the provider considers may create a libelous situation. The next two pages give examples of letters for two types of situations.

BABYTIME MIDWIFERY SERVICES
22 Francis St.
Hamden, CT 06517
(203) 281-0811

Sue Jones   Mary Lambert

September 24, 1994

Dear Mrs. Smith,

Your employee, Madaline Hamilton, is our new client for maternity services. Her expected date of birth is on or near March 30, 1995. We asked Madaline to give us detailed information regarding her work environment as we do with every woman we care for. In order to avoid any miscommunication, we are writing you directly to let you know the things we have recommended to her which impact her activities at work based upon her current health status and previous health history.

We recommend that all of our clients wear flat shoes during pregnancy. As the center of gravity changes throughout pregnancy, heels can cause a woman to become imbalanced and increase the likelihood of falling. In addition, flat shoes assist with circulation in the lower legs and the equal distribution of weight.

We have informed Madaline of the possible dangers of exposure to computer display terminals and have suggested she request transfer to duties which require a maximum of 3 hours of exposure a day or less. If that is impossible, placing her on a low emissions terminal or at least getting a shield which reduces emissions has been recommended. We have also recommended that she not sit so that she is exposed to the rear of other terminals (much of the radiation from computers is emitted through the back of the equipment).

Lastly, we have recommended that she eat small amounts of foods frequently during the day to stabilize her blood sugar and avoid nausea. To do so, we have suggested that she keep snack foods at her desk.

We trust that these requests will not prove a problem. If you have questions regarding them, please let us know. Feel free to call or write us at the address above. Thank you in advance for your assistance.

Sincerely,

Sue Jones, Midwife

BABYTIME MIDWIFERY SERVICES
22 Francis St.
Hamden, CT 06517
(203) 281-0811

Sue Jones   Mary Lambert

August 20, 1992

To Whom It May Concern:

   We have been asked to confirm the health of our client, Catherine Smith, who has sought our care during her pregnancy for prenatal and delivery services. As per her request, three original copies of this letter have been prepared.

   Please be advised that we have examined Catherine Smith today and have found her physically fit to travel by air from New York to San Francisco on August 21, 1990 and to return from San Francisco to New York via airline on August 28, 1990. Her estimated date of birth is September 24, 1990. She is in excellent health and we have no reason to suspect that she will go into labor prematurely.

Sincerely,

Sue Jones, Midwife

Cultural and Religious Practices

Culture can be defined as that complex whole that includes knowledge, belief, art, law, morals, customs and any other capabilities and habits acquired by humans as members of society (Paul, 1955). A woman's cultural background is important to her. It becomes more important if a woman has just moved to your area from another country, if she doesn't speak English or if there are very few people in your area with the same background with whom she has any relationship. Knowing which things make a woman most comfortable and her cultural attitudes regarding pregnancy, birth and parenting can help you provide appropriate, empathetic care.

Even though a woman may be from the same cultural background as you, her religious beliefs can strongly influence her care choices and perceptions. This chapter will also focus on those religious beliefs that have a direct impact upon health or health care.

When a woman's cultural and religious background are unfamiliar to you, knowing where to begin to connect with her will be vital to establishing a solid relationship. Remember that background and cultural practices are influenced by many factors, such as the length of time a person has been away from her native culture, level of education (especially education acquired outside the native culture), occupation, family origin and extent of travel. When you are already familiar with the customs and beliefs of the people with whom you are working, do not hesitate to put your recommendations in terms with which they are familiar.

Understanding people and birth in a cultural context:

This book cannot provide a complete discussion of every culture that exists. Therefore a discussion of the concepts of cultural norms and how they can be applied to any given culture will help fill in the gaps when you encounter a woman from a culture with which you are unfamiliar and for which no resource materials exist.

Humans live in a physical environment of climate, terrain and natural resources, and an inner environment of emotions and thoughts filtered through a cultural context that mediates and helps them to interpret the outer world and interact with other human beings. Since cultures vary, so do our perceptions of how the world works; what is valuable and what is not. Culture provides a framework which infuses life's experiences with order and predictability, thus freeing the psyche from constant turmoil about how to respond and what may happen next. Cultures are subject to constant change; any process which introduces new ideas to a group of people is subject to their acceptance, interpretation and modification. These are not random reactions, but are dependent upon how the people perceive the new ideas as harmonizing with their current values and assumptions and whether the ideas fit into their system of social relationships. Each culture has its own health and healing system. Generally speaking nowhere in a culture are there more prescribed rituals and ways of behaving than are found surrounding the experience of pregnancy and birth. The white Western world is not excluded from this definition; our worship of the scientific process is just as much a product of our cultural climate as is VooDoo in Brazil.

When we examine the role of childbearing within any given culture, we focus on four aspects of the cultural system:

1. The moral and value system, which articulates conduct involving duty, desirability and obligation.
2. The kinship system, which refers to categories of reciprocal rights, duties and obligations of role behavior for relationships among family members.
3. The knowledge and belief system, which defines the processes of conception, labor and birth.
4. The ceremonial and ritual system, which provides the means for the reenactment of the relationship of the symbolic elements in the culture and allows for the incorporation of their symbolic meaning into daily life.

When trying to understand another culture, we want to ask ourselves, "What processes related to birth can be linked to the concepts listed above? What are the obligations of individuals to one another? What is believed to be true? What ritual forms are available for human behavior? How is birth honored as a rite of passage for the mother, the infant, the family and the community?" Seeking answers to the following questions will be useful in understanding the other person's frame of reference for the experience of childbirth:

Prenatally:
　　*Who may have a child? At what age?
　　*By whom may one have a child?
　　*How many children can/should one have?
　　*Can one space pregnancies, and if so, how?
　　*What are the beliefs regarding conception?
　　*How is the fetus formed? When is the fetus considered fully human?
　　*What should be the behavior during pregnancy? (i.e. should certain activities, foods, persons, places or things be avoided or sought out?)
　　*Are there any restrictions on or specific requirements of the father?
　　*Are there any rules regarding sexual activity during pregnancy?
　　*Who may see or touch certain body parts and when is this appropriate?

*How is the mother prepared for the experience of birth? What form (if any) does prenatal care take?

During labor and birth:
*What causes labor?
*How does one behave during labor? Should certain activities, foods, persons, places or things be avoided or sought out?
*How should one respond to pain?
*Should one take medication or other substances during labor?
*Where should labor take place?
*Who should attend the woman in labor?
*How should the attendants behave and what is expected of them during the labor?
*At what point is the woman expected to begin pushing?
*Is the father welcome at the labor? During the birth?
*What behaviors are expected of the father? Other family members?
*What are other children told about the birth?
*Are children welcome at the birth?
*How should the woman be touched or otherwise cared for during labor? During birth? By whom?

Postpartum:
*In general, what behavior is expected of the mother? The father? Other family members?
*Are there special rules regarding food, drink, activity, persons, places or things?
*What is expected of the birth attendants?
*Are there special rules regarding the placenta? The mother's blood and body fluids?
*Is birth control or family planning permissible?

Care of the newborn:
*After birth, how is the newborn to be treated?
*Are there specific rituals, verbal or physical, used to welcome the child? When?
*When is the child recognized? By the family? By the community? In what manner?
*When is the child named?
*Are there special rules regarding exposure of the baby to particular people, activities, things, places or events?
*What are the beliefs regarding breastfeeding, colostrum and when the baby can begin nursing? Other rules regarding infant feeding?
*How is the baby's cord cared for?

*Who cares for the baby after birth?
*What is the relationship of the father to the baby? Other family
   members?
*What differences exist between caring for a male and female infant?

Remember that a person's cultural practices are influenced by the reality in which those practices grew up. For example, if the infant mortality rate is high and children are expected to work family land as well as function as the primary care providers for their aging parents, the cultural norm may be to have as many children as possible, and birth control may not be permitted.

When trying to understand a person's cultural context, always keep in mind that people from a culture other than your own are still individuals. Depending upon their own feelings, the other cultures they have been exposed to, and their sense of self-determination, they may or may not adhere to all the cultural "norms" which will be described below for specific groups. It is just as patronizing to assume that everyone from a certain background is the same as it is to assume that all people act and think like you or that they believe and adhere to the same "truths" as you do. It is equally imperialistic to assume that your way (whatever way that is) is the factual, correct way and that everyone else's views are merely cultural beliefs. Your cultural background, (including white Western scientific belief) is just as much a cultural phenomenon, in every sense of the word, as anyone else's.

The following notes have been gleaned from my own experiences as well as several articles addressing the cultural practices of those areas listed. It is by no means complete. Use the general discussion given here as a guide to expanding your knowledge in necessary areas when information is lacking. All aspects of the cultural practices of the various locations mentioned regarding prenatal, intrapartum and postpartum customs are included here for ease of reference, and because it is important to have a broad overview from the onset of care.

Chinese culture: The customs related to childbearing among Chinese peoples vary widely according to the length of time the parent's families have lived outside of China and their level of Western education. Belief in the value of maintaining physical and spiritual balance during pregnancy and the postpartum period may be strong. Herbal teas may be used as tonics during pregnancy and certain foods may be avoided.

The custom of "doing the mother" postpartum for a period of 40 days is part of this balancing belief. During this time, the mother stays in the house resting and avoids unnecessary activity. She may also avoid contact with water, reflecting a belief that she has excess cold from the birth and will be vulnerable to arthritis and other problems later in life if she becomes chilled during this time. (Neeson, 1987)

Southeast asian cultures: These cultures include Cambodian, Laotian, Vietnamese and Hmong peoples. While all of these cultures have subtle variations in their practices, there are many similarities between them as well.

Buddhism and Hinduism are the primary religions in Cambodia and Laos. However, some people also believe in animism, that spirits exist who can exercise power over the destinies of humans.

Educational opportunities in these countries are limited, especially for girls, and illiteracy is high. Most women coming out of these countries are of childbearing age and have been subjected to a traumatic early childhood filled with war and the loss of friends, relatives and personal belongings. They may have never encountered Western culture or medicine before and may be ill prepared for the culture shock it entails, especially if they come from a rural area. As the result of losing many family members to war, some women may desire large families.

Relatives of several generations may live in one household, men are the wage earners and women care for the home and children. Parents discipline by setting a good example, so sharp words and physical punishments are avoided. Restraint in gestures and quiet speech are considered desirable in children as well as adults.

General health: Health care in Cambodia, Laos and Vietnam is crisis-oriented with symptom relief as the main goal. Infectious disease, malnutrition and dental caries are common among Southeast Asians. Medicines or herbs are usually self-prescribed and might only be taken until symptoms subside, then stopped. Therefore, having to come to a care provider for certain types of treatment will be a new idea. As in the West, many people have but a superficial understanding of drug effects and may think doubling the dose will get them well twice as fast or that if a dose is forgotten, a double dose will make up for it. There also may be confusion over taking several things simultaneously; be sure to assume nothing when making recommendations. In addition, many Chinese healing methods such as acupuncture, cupping and the use of various herbs, have been incorporated by traditional healers in these countries.

There is widespread belief that illness may be caused by evil spirits or departure of the soul. Illness may be believed to be caused by supernatural forces, as punishment for faults or for breaking religious codes. These peoples also recognize that natural causes, such a poor sanitation, contribute to illness.

Fertility/contraception/abortion: Southeast Asian women's fertility rate is about three times that of Western women. They may wish to have information on contraception, but may be reluctant to ask for it directly.

Pregnancy outside of marriage is considered a family disgrace and abortion does occur. These abortions are often accomplished using herbs supplied by a local woman healer, who also may be called upon to administer herbs and perform traditional healing dances during a wanted pregnancy.

Pregnancy: Heavy lifting and strenuous work are to be avoided. Raising the arms over the head pulls on the placenta and may cause it to break. Respiratory distress in the infant may be caused by sexual relations late in pregnancy, which are thought to thicken the amniotic fluid. Avoiding sex is felt to make a prettier baby with little vernix, which is believed to be accumulated sperm.

Prenatal care is not the norm in Southeast Asia. Southeast Asians may not seek prenatal care until they are late in their pregnancy due to financial constraints, fear, or lack of perceived need. At the same time Southeast Asian women may also believe that Western maternity care is safer for mother and baby than what they grew up with. Be aware that Southeast Asia has epidemic levels of intestinal parasites, anemia, hemoglobinopathies, active tuberculosis, hepatitis and antibiotic resistant syphilis and gonorrhea. Studies indicate that Cambodian and Laotian women are least likely to receive prenatal care and that Hmong women are at the highest risk for the problems listed above.

Diagnostic tests are frequently frightening to these women who may fear invasive procedures such as drawing blood because they do not understand that blood is continuously being formed, or they may suspect it will be sold. In their native country they may have found that giving personal information to authorities was dangerous and may therefore be reluctant to share their medical or personal histories with you. In addition, they may not know the names of conditions they have had or the types of drugs or herbs used to treat them. Be aware that children who have been abandoned or who are the offspring of other relatives may be incorporated into a household; do not make assumptions about the children of the woman seeking care. Some may believe that any kind of surgical cutting such as clitorotomy, cesarean section or circumcision allows an exit point for the spirit to leave the body and that rupturing the membranes prolongs labor.

Recommending additional prenatal calcium in the form of milk products may be inappropriate for these women due to lack a of familiarity with milk or a deficiency of the enzyme lactase causing bloating, cramping and diarrhea after ingestion of milk products.

Modesty: Southeast Asian women are very modest, especially regarding exposure of the area between the waist and the knees, and may therefore find pelvic exams especially humiliating. This area is rarely seen and then only by their husbands or other women. Women may wish to wear a sarong during labor to maintain their modesty and often want to birth squatting. A woman care provider is their provider of choice.

Communicating: Women are often isolated at home without extended family around. It may be that they speak little English, even after having lived away from their homeland for some years. Translators are ideally women, since most Southeast Asian women will be reluctant to reveal intimate information to a man. Family members may be helpful, but the woman may carefully select the information she reveals in front of others to save face. Therefore, history-taking is best done privately with a female translator. Be aware that family elders are usually consulted for important decisions; addressing the woman directly may be perceived as insulting to any elders present.

While Vietnamese women are often the primary decision-makers for family health care concerns, Cambodian and Laotian women tend to be more shy, deferring to the decisions of men in the family. The cultural norm is subservience to husbands and grown sons. Women may be reluctant to discuss sex, childbearing or contraception in the presence of male relatives and may show this by giggling, shrugging their shoulders or averting their eyes. They may try to anticipate the "right" answer to questions to please you as the care-giver and to avoid conflict and save face. Women are taught to yield to the wishes of authority figures. There may also be an effort to avoid confusion and cultural conflict between herself and those she feels are her social superiors. Deference is shown by avoiding eye contact as well as social and physical contact. (Neeson, 1987)

Southeast Asians may be reluctant to admit they are in pain, and relief may not be sought until the pain is unbearable. Crying out or complaining in labor is seen as shameful, especially if men are present. Likewise, other things may be tolerated to avoid conflict. Do not assume that what you propose to do is okay simply because a woman is not protesting. Offer her specific options in an unbiased manner so that she may feel at ease in choosing what she really wants most. Keep this in mind during the entire care cycle.

Father's role: The role of the father at birth varies; some Southeast Asians believe that the presence of the baby's father will complicate the birth. Vietnamese women often prefer a female friend to be present, or if Chinese-Vietnamese, she may prefer her mother-in-law. Laotian women often want their husbands with them. In rural Laos, the husband traditionally supports the woman's shoulders, catches the baby, cuts the cord and ritually buries the placenta under the house or in the dirt floor under the bed.

Sacredness of the head: The head is considered the seat of life and the most sacred and honorable part of the body. The head is not to be touched except by close intimates, so touching a woman's head in labor may be distressing to her. Touching the baby's head is also to be avoided which means that inserting an internal fetal monitor electrode, intubation equipment or wiping away vernix may meet with family disapproval. Tubes and IV lines may be seen as possible points of exit for the child's spirit. The mother may refuse to wash her baby's hair after birth. Parents may prefer that the back of the infant's head be flattened and may encourage this by propping the baby's head between pillows. Encourage the parents to play with the baby and feed it in different positions.

Birth defects: Birth defects may be blamed on the mother having eaten the wrong foods or the mother or baby having engaged in harmful activities in a previous life. Southeast Asian parents may give up on sick babies because the child may die and suffer less in its next life. Birthmarks are believed to be marks placed at the child's death in a previous life so that relatives will recognize him in the next incarnation. If the death of a mother or baby should occur, loud wailing is the cultural norm.

Amulets: Many believe that wearing strings around the wrist or ankles or amulets as necklaces prevent the soul from being lost and causing subsequent illness. After a baby is born, elders may want to place such items on the infant to signify spiritual wholeness and family support. Every effort must be made to keep these strings in place if the baby needs to be transported. If they must be removed, this should be thoroughly explained to the family. It is believed that praising the baby or making positive comments about it is dangerous, since jealous spirits may make the baby sick.

Postpartum practices: Most women will restrict their activity for 1 to 2 months after the birth. Women are not expected to perform household duties and are taken care of by elders or others who assume the tasks of cooking, cleaning, and caring for the baby. They fear that too much activity on the mother's part will make her susceptible to arthritis, headache or weakness in old age. Childbirth is seen as a cold condition which, if not properly attended to, can lead to illness. Traditionally, Vietnamese women lie on cots placed about 2 feet above smoldering coal fires, sweating profusely. Laotian and Cambodian women usually lie next to the fire. Cambodian woman also cover their heads with blankets or towels. This practice of raising the body temperature may serve to kill infectious organisms. Without access to a fire, women can use hot water bottles, heating pads, electric blankets and down comforters to keep themselves warm. Hot foods are sought postpartum to strengthen the blood and to prevent later illness. They avoid juices and cold drinks but want to eat meats and soups made from chilies and black peppers, and sweets. Fruit may or may not be considered too cold a food. Many Asians eat steamed rice at every meal. Drinking wine steeped with herbs is a common postpartum practice.

Infant feeding: Colostrum is considered old milk and is discarded. The baby is fed rice paste or boiled sugar water for several days while waiting for the milk to come in. Once nursing begins, it is believed that the maternal diet of hot foods benefits both mother and baby, but after that a conflict arises. Continuing hot foods is considered best for the mother, but cold foods are believed to best ensure an adequate milk supply. Those who have moved to the West may solve this dilemma by switching to formula, since it is readily available.

Since there is much malnutrition in Southeast Asia, a fat baby is considered a healthy baby and many believe that American babies are taller and heavier because they are fed formula, which is not dependent on the mother's health. Be aware that if they cannot afford formula, parents may feed their babies rice boiled with water or fresh milk, which can result in anemia and growth retardation.

Dietary considerations: Vegetables and meats are mixed together to balance the "hot" (yang) and "cold" (yin) elements. Cold foods such as poultry, fish and most fruits and vegetables are acceptable during pregnancy and are believed to ensure healthy babies. Eating or drinking foods considered hot such as red peppers, spicy soups, red meat, garlic, ginger, onion, coffee, and sweets is considered good after the birth. If hot foods are eaten during pregnancy, they are believed to cause abortion or premature labor. (D'Avanzo, 1992)

Hmong customs: In addition to many of the practices described above which overlap among Southeast Asian cultures, the Hmong have specific practices unique to their culture. Historically, the woman's spouse was traditionally considered her main source of support during labor and birth. Midwives, per se, were not very prevalent. Most of the time, nothing was done to accelerate labor or relieve pain. A technique of massage and pressure might be used to bring the baby down into the pelvis and external version may be used to convert a baby to a vertex presentation. Generally an upright position is considered best for birth. The placenta is always buried in the house; a girl's goes under the bed and a boy's goes under the center post in the house. The placenta has to be protected from any disturbance such as insect infestation, which might cause a rash or eye problem in the baby. Incineration is an acceptable alternative for the disposal of the placenta to many Hmong women.

There are no specific prenatal taboos regarding diet. The mother may change clothes after birth and lay down by a fire to sleep. The first meal may be an egg cooked in water, all of which is eaten. Following this meal the postpartum diet consists of rice and chicken served in its cooking broth with coarsely ground pepper (finely ground pepper has unacceptable white specks). Some women eat only the chicken and rice diet and forego the egg.

After birth the baby was traditionally taken, usually by the father, to be washed in warm water and dressed. The baby was allowed to sleep and nurse when it cried. Some women may want a friend or relative to nurse the baby until her milk comes in. A ritual necklace is put around the baby at any time after birth (unless the baby has a nuchal cord, in which case the necklace is placed immediately). After three days a birthday celebration is held, during which the child is named and the child's head shaved. (Bjorkman, 1985)

Vietnamese customs: Refer to the section above regarding Southeast Asian peoples in general; then read this section for more specifics about Vietnamese customs in particular.

General health: Modern Vietnamese health practices have been influenced by three traditions: Southern medicine, *thuoc nam*, the true folk medicine of South Vietnam; *thuoc bac*, the more formalized Northern medicine based on Chinese principles; and Western medicine, brought there by the French and US Americans. Most Vietnamese practice a combination of these medicines, choosing the treatment that seems to work best.

The Vietnamese theory of *Am/Doung* corresponds to the Chinese theory of yin and yang and to the principles of hot and cold as used by other Asian cultures. Good health results from the balance of these two elements. Certain conditions are attributable to excesses of hot or cold and treatment consists of balancing the body with food or drugs possessing the opposite properties. Western drugs are considered hot, while Oriental herbal medicine is usually considered cold. *Phong* or *gío*, is a noxious element that can enter a person and cause respiratory tract infections, epilepsy, strokes or skin disorders. *Cao gío*, the Vietnamese practice of coin rubbing literally means "rubbing out the wind" and is used for a number of problems such as colds, headaches and abdominal pain.

Pregnancy: A principle caretaking activity in Vietnam is the choice of the appropriate foods during pregnancy and the postpartum period. The first trimester is considered cold; therefore hot foods are taken to balance this condition. The second trimester is considered neutral, and cold foods are allowed as well. Tonic foods are taken in the first and second trimesters, but avoided in the third to prevent a large baby and a difficult birth. The third trimester is considered hot and tonic, therefore cold foods are encouraged. Anti-tonic foods are also to be avoided in the third trimester and postpartum. Raw foods, leafy vegetables and fruit can also be classified as "windy" as well as cold and may cause wind illnesses such as arthritis, flatulence or diarrhea. Certain foods may be considered dangerous because of their magical properties, but which foods these might be varies among individuals. Soups and water may be avoided to prevent stretching of the stomach.

COLD FOODS	HOT FOODS	TONIC FOODS	ANTI-TONIC FOODS
Gourd type plants such as squash, melons, leafy vegetables & most fruit	Meat, condiments, alcohol and fatty foods	Increases the amount of blood & are high in energy. High fat, sugar & carbohydrate foods High protein foods & Medicines	Sour, sometimes raw or cold. These foods deplete the volume of blood

Labor: Traditionally, a special bed was used for birth to protect the mother and baby from wind, which might carry evil spirits. The mother may want her mother with her, or no relatives at all. In Vietnam, fathers are not usually included in the

604

birth, but many immigrant families wish to include fathers. Some believe that the woman is "dirty" at the time of birth and may feel that children will be adversely affected by viewing birth, resulting in a lowered intelligence.

Postpartum practices: The most distinctive and consistent information regarding pregnancy has to do with postpartum practices. These mostly involve dietary and activity limitations. They are considered very important for first time mothers in particular; although these practices are also considered important after the birth of subsequent babies, the time period for these practices may be shorter. Postpartum, women may not want to walk, leave their home, have sexual intercourse, bathe or wash their hair for up to two months. The mother stays in bed as much as possible for one week of this time and then stays in the home for up to 3 months. A type of facial steam bath (*xong*) may be allowed during this time period, but showers and baths, particularly with cold water, are usually avoided for a period of one week to three months. Scrubbing the skin during the postpartum period is believed to cause prominent hand veins at an early age. These restrictions are imposed because the woman is considered open after birth; if not kept warm, cold will enter her body and make her ill in old age. The involvement of family members in the care of the mother should be welcomed.

After birth the mother has an excess of cold and a hot diet is preferred. Salty hot foods are eaten, consisting of meat, fish or rice cooked with salt or fish sauce and lots of black pepper. Boiled green cabbage and soup may also be taken in some cases. Salt helps the stomach to contract after birth and causes the mother to desire more water, thus increasing her milk supply. Cold drinks, vegetables, raw foods, fat and citrus or sour foods are often prohibited after birth. Some women may avoid fish, beef, bananas, watermelon or fish. Food restrictions may last from one to three months. Cold drinks cause the bleeding to stop too soon and lead to a "fat stomach." Citrus fruits or sour foods lead to incontinence in old age. Raw foods cause the stomach to move too much, which is to be avoided due to stretching from the pregnancy.

Infant feeding: Traditionally, babies are breastfed up to four months with the gradual introduction of neutral foods. However Western influences have lead many mothers to bottle feed. A good breastfeeding diet includes pork cooked with vinegar, milk, soup made with animal bones, potatoes, papaya, fruit and juices. (Wadd, 1983)

Japanese culture: The Japanese highly value deference and politeness, emotional reserve, conformity and allegiance to family. Traditional families may show strong male dominance and the extended family may be an important part of daily life. Pregnancy is viewed as a state of health that requires little change in normal activities. Prenatal childbirth education is not widely utilized in Japan. Birth of a male child generally confers high status on the mother. Postpartum the mother is expected to satisfy infant needs immediately and to maintain very close contact with the baby. Since Japan has become quite Westernized, many Japanese women will be familiar with modern Western birth-related practices. (Neeson, 1987)

A traditional Japanese practice involves binding the abdomen during pregnancy and after the birth. This binder could be used by any woman wanting more abdominal support in late pregnancy. The cloth used for the binder should be 6 yards of 13 inch wide cotton material with both edges bound or hemmed. This is exactly the amount of cloth used in a kimono, so it is readily available throughout Japan. The *sarashi* (binder) is folded lengthwise and wrapped around the body (as illustrated). The folded side is placed superiorly, the bound edges to the bottom. The first lap is tight with a corner sticking out, which gets folded down in the second wrap to prevent loosening. From the third wrap, the "gaiter" wrap is done several times, either in the middle or at the side. The end of the cloth is then folded in, to adjust the length, so that it can be safety pinned in place. Looseness that allows two fingers beneath the finished wrap is recommended. (Ishida, 1977)

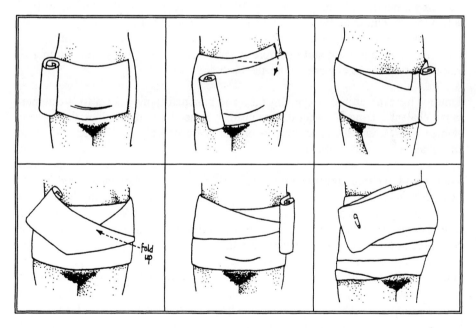

Arab cultures: Arab peoples include those from Lebanon, Palestine, Jordan, Syria, Iraq, Egypt, Yemen and the countries of the Arabian Gulf. The principle religion of these areas is Islamic (Muslim), with some practicing Christianity. However, Arab cultural practices transcend religion per se. For example, all Arab women can be expected to be extremely modest, regardless of their religious beliefs.

Affiliation: The need for association with others is dominant in Arab cultures. Family relationships fulfill many of these needs, and in Arab families there is a very close unity of individuals tied together by blood relationship. Most families include extended family members who stay in close touch. Visiting among members is a social obligation during illness and on happy or sad occasions. It may occur on a weekly basis to provide structure and social control, reinforcement of norms, development of values and a mechanism for change. During gatherings, families discuss daily events and their reactions to them. However, those who offer this support or service must share religion, country of origin and language in common with those seeking advice. One way to communicate with Arab clients is to offer to help, for example, by enlisting another Arab woman to act as an interpreter and inviting the extended family to visits. Although the woman may refuse help at first because she fears she is imposing, continuing to offer help will be seen as sincere by Arab peoples.

Planning ahead: Planning is a very Western practice; Arabs often view it as potentially defiant to God's will and therefore as bringing about the evil eye. Also, to plan ahead only to have those plans not work out is disappointing. Arab society is oriented in the present and therefore women may not have any baby clothes or a space set up for baby care before the birth.

Time: The Arab attitude regarding time and punctuality may seem to Westerners as nonchalant. Time does not dictate need, it is need that determines time. Arab women may be late for appointments or skip them entirely, and schedules of any kind may be foreign to them.

Verbal and written agreements: Arabs respect verbal agreements and have a basic mistrust of the written word. The signing of any paperwork may be a source of considerable distrust. Women may also be reluctant to make decisions on their own responsibility; care should be taken when discussing anything with a woman who does not also have her spouse present.

Women's roles: In many families, roles are divided on the basis of gender. A woman's power is derived from careful management of the home. In the Middle East, all family members are expected to help achieve family goals. Immigrants, however, are often isolated from the resources of the extended family, and their husbands, who are earning a living, are often unable or unwilling to help share in managing the household. This leaves many women feeling very isolated; they may prefer smaller families as a result.

Modesty: Arabs value female modesty. One interpretation of Islamic law requires that women cover their head and body to the ankles and their arms to the wrists. Care providers need to respect, preserve and protect a woman's modesty by making sure no one with whom the woman does not feel comfortable is in the room during exams and draping her so as to expose as little of her body as possible. Women are expected to display bashfulness, humility, diffidence, and shyness when interacting with men or strangers. Sex and reproduction are topics which are discussed with other women relatives and friends, but not with men or with strangers. Care must be taken when introducing such topics so that the woman will discuss them, and not merely give the answers she thinks you want to hear in order to change the subject.

In some parts of the Arab world and in Africa, clitoridectomy and infibulation are still practiced. See the section later in this chapter for details.

Pregnancy: Traditional Arab women have few means of increasing their self-esteem. Their domain and primary source of identity are in bearing and rearing children. Pregnancy is considered the greatest opportunity for women to actualize their potential. Much attention is directed toward the capacity of women to bear children, particularly sons, which improves their status and acceptance by the husband's family. In fact, the sex of the child may be even more of a focus of concern than the child's health. The woman who bears only girls is considered almost as worthless as the woman who has no children at all. The ability to bear children is considered miraculous. Because women feel compelled to demonstrate her fertility, births occur early in Arab marriages. In some areas, infertility is considered grounds for divorce.

The evil eye: Much attention is given to the concept of the evil eye and the influences of jealous, envious or wicked women. Expressions of congratulations may be perceived in this light. Appropriate Arab compliments may take a form that Westerners would interpret as a put down, such as "For nine months work, couldn't you do better than this?" The mother understands this to be complimentary and also an attempt to displace the power of the evil eye. Her feeling is that a negative statement will convert the possibility of evil and misfortune into a positive blessing. It is better to comment on the mother and her difficult labor and to congratulate her on her achievement or as the future mother of many healthy children. Compliments to the baby should be accompanied by touching wood or mentioning God's blessings.

Customs regarding menstruation: Women do not shower or bathe during menstruation. Many believe pregnancy will not occur as long as they are breastfeeding or for as long as they have not resumed menstruation.

Perceptions and reactions to pain: Pain is not tolerated well and is expressed vocally. Pain seems to be experienced in a diffuse and generalized way, i.e. it

608

affects their whole being and is not separated from their total well-being. To ask a woman to describe the pain or where it hurts may be fruitless, as it is often felt that the care provider should be able to figure this out without assistance. Arab women typically moan, cry and scream during labor, especially if members of their family are present. However, if transported, they may also refuse medication during labor, as there is a great deal of fear regarding epidural and spinal anesthesia. Touch and distraction techniques may be well received methods of assisting women to cope with pain during labor.

Contraception: Due to the primary importance of childbearing in the Arab culture, many women will resist the notion of birth control under any circumstances. Methods such as rhythm or birth control pills require planning, which is contrary to the Arab culture. An IUD, on the other hand, seen as tangible and more interventive, is in keeping with the Arab concept that intrusive treatments are more effective. While vasectomy for men may be rejected, tubal ligation is an alternative for Arab women. Abortion is also common in the Middle Eastern Arab countries.

Children: Children are expected to be part of all important family events; therefore discussing when the children will be welcomed after the birth (probably not at the birth for modesty reasons) is important.

Mexican culture: Many women along the United States/Mexican border will be accepting of white Western Bio-technical medical norms during birth as "the better way." However, generally speaking, traditional Mexican women view pregnancy as a natural event that requires no medical care under normal circumstances.

Views about pregnancy: Women from traditional backgrounds who have lived within the interior of Mexico or who have not been exposed to or have actively resisted indoctrination into Western cultural standards may hold some of the following beliefs. The woman and fetus are considered vulnerable to outside bad influences. During pregnancy women may wear a *cinta* (a belt with keys attached) or a *muñeco* (a knotted cord around the abdomen) to prevent birth complications. A baby born at 7 months of pregnancy is considered to have a better chance of surviving than one born at 8 months. A mother experiencing *susto* (shock or fright) can suddenly become diabetic, have her milk turn sour, or give birth to an ill baby. Vitamin pills are believed to make people fat (or cause weight gain). Weight-conscious pregnant women may avoid them. Dizzy spells or feelings of faintness are caused by abrupt *bajadas* (sudden dips) in blood pressure. During a solar eclipse women will wear a key, coin, safety pin, or other metal object preferably tied on or a sash of red ribbon over their belly to protect the baby from potential death, deformation, or retardation which could ensue if exposed to the eclipse unprotected. Pregnant women are referred to as *gorda* (fat), or *enferma* (sick), or *embarasala* (pregnant).

A woman who carries her baby "wide", i.e. whose belly and hips become fuller and wider, is believed to be carrying a girl, while the woman whose uterus protrudes straight out in a manner more compact and in front (*picudo*) is said to be carrying a boy. The most essential part of prenatal care consists of *sobadas* or prenatal massage of the baby *in utero* performed by a midwife or healer to ensure that the baby is in a good position. Massage may also include external version for breech or transverse positioning. Women may avoid drinking milk and stay physically active to avoid having a large baby and a difficult birth.

Birth: The laboring woman may want to be attended by her mother, mother-in-law (*suegra*), sister or other female relatives and friends rather than her male partner or other male relatives. In traditional families the men are rarely involved in the labor process. This is because women are seen as healers and helpers of the sick in Mexico. Women will also feel most comfortable with women as birth attendants. The traditional midwife encourages women to birth in a squatting or other upright position; however, due to government training many now believe that lying down is easier and minimizes tearing. The most appropriate time for the father to see the mother and greet the newborn may be postpartum, after the mother is cleaned up and rested.

Postpartum: Mexican women spend 40 days in bed with their baby postpartum (*la cuarentina*) eating certain foods, which are usually prepared by their mother and following certain guidelines. To encourage abundant milk, a hot beverage (*atole*) is made from ground corn, cornstarch or oatmeal, milk and sugar. Women are encouraged to eat hot and warm foods, nothing cold, after birth. Teas for milk flow include star anise (*estrella*), fennel (*hinojo*) and *ixbud*. During this time sexual intercourse is forbidden. The mother often wears a *faja,* a large bandage or cloth or type of girdle around her waist to keep in the heat and help her organs get back into place. A homemade liniment may be used the first week postpartum as a belly rub to prevent heat loss and keep it from remaining flabby. This consists of Rosemary (*romero*), camphor and ether dissolved into a liter of grain alcohol and left to steep for several weeks prior to birth. Other plants may be added depending upon the region the woman is from.

Newborn care: Babies are kept well wrapped and have their faces covered by a light blanket on their first outings to protect from the *aires* (bad winds, drafts, dirt) and *mal ojo* (overly admiring gaze of others).

Breastfeeding practices differ; some women may believe that colostrum is unclean and refuse to breastfeed until the second day after birth. An abdominal binder made of flannel or cotton gauze may be used on the baby, sometimes with a bean placed on the navel before wrapping, to assist in preventing herniation of

610

the naval and to prevent "bad air" from reaching the navel; therefore the mother may resist suggestions to allow the cord to air dry. Camomile tea may be given to fussy or colicky babies after the birth, and you must emphasize that the tea cannot be given as a substitute for breastmilk. (Neeson, 1987, Parra, 1993)

Filipino culture: During pregnancy the mother may observe traditional dietary patterns; avoiding hot, spicy or salty foods. Satisfying food cravings may be seen as important in preventing premature birth. Pregnant and postpartum women are encouraged to decrease their activity level. Filipino peoples are generally polite and show deference to family authority while displaying a relatively easy social interaction. The mother may smile and agree to recommendations which she later does not follow, but will instead follow traditional practices as instructed by her mother. Women are socialized towards motherhood at an early age and the extended family may play an important role in child care. (Neeson, 1987)

Navajo culture: There are, of course, many different indigenous tribes in North America. Those who live on reservations in the Untied States have supreme domain within the property limits of the reservation land. Therefore, regardless of the state laws regarding midwifery, Native American midwives can practice unharrassed. While some tribes were traditionally more peaceful than others, all had a strong cultural consciousness which was infused with an intense concern for the spiritual aspects of life. Native American peoples traditionally viewed the land as their mother and the animals as brother and sister spirits, all of which deserved honor and respect. All aspects of life were associated with ceremony, celebration, or condemnation if they were thought to be contrary to the health and well-being of the individual or the tribe. Some of these practices continue to this day.

In the Navajo tradition good health means being in harmonious balance with the total physical, social and spiritual aspects of life. Healers use a form of hand trembling (a diagnostic technique), head-sweating and sandpainting as therapeutic techniques. Sweats (a type of sauna) and prayers at dawn are commonly used spiritual practices as well. Women view childbearing as a natural process. The pregnant woman becomes one with Mother Earth, Father Sky and the Universe of Holy People as she physically relives the creation plan of humankind. It is, therefore, very important for her to attune herself to the divine events of conception, fetal development, and birth.

Prenatal: Keeping the peace is important during pregnancy and the mother is admonished to think good thoughts, say morning prayers daily and have a shielding ceremony if she has nightmares. Arguing and scolding children are to be avoided, as well as letting bad thoughts occupy the mind for long periods of time. The mother is not to talk negatively or with criticism.

The mother is to eat good foods for the baby, get up early and walk, and may have a Blessingway ceremony for a safe delivery. She is not to drink milk or eat salt or those foods taken away in ceremonies. She is not to lay around, tie knots, weave rugs, make pottery or lift heavy things. She may not attend funerals or look at the body of a dead person, animals or taxidermic trophies; she must not kill things. She is forbidden to be with sick people too long, to go to crowded places or attend ceremonies for the sick. She must not look at the eclipse of the moon or sun. She must not make plans for the baby or prepare clothes until after the birth.

Labor: The mother is to think about having a good birth and the medicine person is asked to sing "baby out" chants and unraveling songs, if necessary. Only those assisting the birth are to observe the labor. The woman may want to loosen her hair, drink corn meal mush, wear juniper seed beads, hold onto a sash belt when ready to push, have someone apply gentle fundal pressure during pushing, get in a squatting position to push, or drink herbal teas to help her relax or to strengthen contractions if necessary. Tying knots or braiding the hair are both forbidden.

After the birth: Burying the placenta is customary. The mother may want to drink juniper ash tea for internal cleansing and blue cornmeal mush to increase her milk production. The mother may smear meconium on her face to show her love for the baby. Breastfeeding is supported. A sash belt is worn around the waist for four days after delivery. The mother may not drink cold fluids or be in a cold draft, smell afterbirth blood for too long, or show signs of displeasure if the baby soils on her during a diaper change. The placenta and blood may not be burned. Intercourse is forbidden for three months after delivery.

Infant care: The umbilical cord is buried in a sheep corral, near a rug loom or in another special place. Infant massage is done soon after the birth. Corn pollen and juniper ash tea are given to the baby to cleanse its insides. The baby is greeted with a hand shake and called by its Navajo name. A cradle board is made soon after the birth, marked with the direction of the growth of the tree it was made from. A "first laugh" ceremony is held as well as a Shielding ceremony. The baby's hair may not be cut until the baby talks; the anterior fontanelle is not to be covered with the fingers. The head may not be covered with a bowl or a basket. (Goldstein, 1993)

Northeast Zaire (Central Africa): It is believed that when the frenulum is attached toward the front of the tongue (tongue-tied) the baby will have difficulties with speech; any variation in the attachment of the frenulum is considered damaging. Therefore, mothers may request that the frenulum be snipped in early infancy.

Ugandan influence has promoted the belief that when the gums of the newborn have a pearly appearance (a normal variation), there are teeth underneath pushing to the surface. These "teeth" are felt to be a curse which will destine the child to an early death when it is a toddler. Some parents become so concerned that they have a traditional healer lance the gums to remove the pearly areas.

The Wahema people believe that twins are a curse on the entire family, and in the past they killed the weaker twin so the surviving twin would have a better life. The Wibira people view twin birth as a blessing and believe twins have special powers that can influence the prosperity of the village. Villagers will bring gifts to the parents in hope of gaining their favor. (Nyirjesy, 1991)

Female genital mutilation: Since more women are immigrating to North America from various parts of the world, as a midwife, you must be prepared to assist women who have had genital mutilation. In industrialized countries, female genital mutilation takes the form of routine clitorotomy. In less than half the African nations and in parts of the Middle East, it takes a much more severe form because genital structures are removed. It is estimated that at least 90 million women world-wide have been subjected to some form of severe genital mutilation.

COMMUNITIES THAT PRACTICE SOME FORM OF SEVERE FEMALE GENITAL MUTILATION						
COUNTRY	%	COUNTRY	%	COUNTRY	%
Somalia	100%	Kenya	60%	Niger	20%
Djibouti	100%	Senegal	50%	Chad	20%
Ethiopia/Eritrea	90%	Egypt	50%	Benin	20%
Mali	90%	Guinea Conakry	50%	Togo	20%
Sudan (North/Central)	90%	Guinea Bissau	50%	Ghana	20%
Sierra Leone	90%	Nigeria	50%	Tanzania	10%
Burkina Faso	70%	Mauritania	25%	Uganda	5%
Gambia	60%	Central Africa	20%	Zaire	5%
Ivory Coast	60%				

(Hedley & Darkenoo, 1992)

There are three degrees of severity: **Sunna (traditional) circumcision**; the removal of the foreskin and tip of the clitoris. **Excision** or **clitoridectomy** (KLIH-toe-rid-ECK-toe-me) is the most used form in Africa. It involves removal of the entire clitoral shaft and glans, together with adjacent parts of the labia minora. Sometimes the external genitalia (with the exception of parts of the labia majora) are removed or additional incisions are made to enlarge the opening of the yoni; a practice which produces more scar tissue but is believed to ease childbirth.

Infibulation (in-fib-you-LAY-shun) means to clasp or pin. **Pharaonic circumcision** (excision with infibulation) is currently practiced in the Sudan, throughout Somalia, parts of Ethiopia, southern Egypt, northern Kenya, and some parts of West Africa, mostly by Muslims. Infibulation involves removal of the entire clitoris and labia minora. The inner surfaces of the labia majora are partially sliced off or scraped raw and then sewn together with catgut. (A remote white western relative is the "husband's stitch," intended to give the yoni a virginal tightness after birth.) In Sudan and Somalia thorns or a paste of gum arabic, sugar, and egg are used to hold the sides together. This operation obliterates the yoni opening except for a tiny hole created by a splinter of wood or bamboo which, when healed, allows the passage of menstrual blood and urine. This opening is often located at the level of the yoni, thus the normal urethral orifice is not exposed.

Any of these mutilations are typically performed using knives or bits of glass on the unanesthetized child who is held down by female relatives. The girl's legs are tied together afterward and she is kept immobile from several days to several weeks to ensure that the wound closes. Typically, bandages are not changed or removed to clean away excrement. Hemorrhage or infection which may result in more scarring or even death are common complications. The scar is cut open when she is married and opened wider for childbirth. Should unattended birth occur, both mother and baby may die because the tissue will frequently resist both stretching and tearing, making delivery impossible. The routine procedure is to sew the woman tightly after each childbirth. When their baby is weaned, the scar is again cut open enough to allow intercourse.

Female genital mutilation is a male-dictated practice perpetrated by a girl's female relatives. The myths which surround it function to maintain male control over women as a group. Don't be fooled by the fact that women generally request and perform these procedures. These practices ensure the only possible life choice as perceived by extremely oppressed women: marriage.

Clitoridectomy is traditionally done to prepare girls for marriage. Theoretically, the strength of female sexual passion is such that, if the clitoris is not removed, women will be unfaithful. Male social injunction dictates that intact women are undesirable. In reality, clitoridectomy removes the purely female organ of sexual pleasure. As such, it "purifies" the purpose of female sexuality; to provide men with sexual gratification and reproduce their sons. Although traditionally performed on pre-pubescent girls, these operations are now being done on younger children because fathers fear resistance once their daughters enter school. Since he will lose the bride price if his daughters aren't "done," he ensures that they are mutilated at an early age. Many educated families that have abandoned all traditional customs may still adhere to this one alone.

The real purpose of infibulation is to make intercourse impossible. Men that demand it highly value virginity and this guarantees that a bride is intact. A virgin bride means that succession rights and inheritance of property cannot be questioned. A small opening demands a higher bride price. Frequently, women are inspected by a man's relatives before they will agree to marriage.

Other reasons given for these operations include: the ancestors decreed it

(Africa), excision is believed to increase fertility (widely accepted), to treat hypertrophy (unusual enlargement) of the clitoris (Ethiopia, parts of Nigeria), to remove "ugly" female genitals (Egypt and others parts of Africa), as well as to promote health and cleanliness (middle class urban women in Cairo and Bamako).

Local women's groups and midwives in these countries are campaigning against these barbaric practices and have requested that they be officially known as female genital mutilation. Their influence has, so far, barely made a dent in the number of girls being mutilated.

Assisting women who have been severely mutilated: Urinary tract and yoni infections, difficulty with hygiene, impaired flow of urine and menstrual blood, endometriosis, adhesions from scar tissue, inability to obtain PAP smear samples and pain with yoni penetration are the main problems common to women who have had such procedures. Because of the small opening and its lack of elasticity, pelvic exam is exceptionally painful to these women. Culturally they are taught not to express their fears or pain. Therefore, ask her to tell you how your exam feels and encourage her throughout her care to express her needs. During pelvic exams go slowly, explain everything, and use a liberal amount of lubricant to help minimize discomfort and anxiety. Supplying the woman with drapes to maintain her modesty and privacy during the exam will also relieve some of her tension. A pediatric speculum should be used if necessary. A bi-manual exam may be done using a single finger within the yoni and palpating the uterus and ovaries via a rectal exam. If manual exam is difficult, ultrasound may be helpful in determining if the pelvic organs are normal (Lightfoot-Klein & Shaw, 1991). In England, a special prenatal clinic has been established to care for women who have been severely mutilated. Reversal surgery is being performed successfully in the 7th month of pregnancy, which allows the tissues time to heal before birth (Eaton, 1993). At the time of birth a clitorotomy may be necessary, depending upon the extent of the scarring and the elasticity of the tissue.

Many cultures which incorporate female circumcision dictate that the woman must have permission from a male family member before she receives medical care. It is important to gain the trust and respect of any male relatives who accompany her to appointments. If male care providers are involved, her family may prevent her from being examined or treated. Be aware of this if transport is necessary.

Many of these women are afraid that western practitioners will not know how to care for them. Frequently, they find themselves in hospital situations where they are stared at or worse. You can help alleviate some anxiety be letting her know you have an idea of what has been done, what her health concerns may be, and how to care for her genital area during birth. Prenatally, discuss the need to cut, and the possibility of suturing so that the tissues are more open, if that seems feasible at the time of repair (her male partner will have to agree to this as well). To enlist his support, *do not* take a feminist stance, instead emphasize the health benefits and how he stands to gain as well. It is also a good time to discuss her feelings about clitoridectomy and what she and her partner intend to do if she has a girl. (As a midwife, examine how you feel about these practices versus your attitudes regarding male circumcision. If you feel parents should not mutilate their girls [you might well be horrified by the idea] but if they really want to, they should circumcise their boys, ask yourself why? What's the difference?)

The psychological ramifications of these practices are beginning to be explored, but it is obvious that these women have experienced intense sexual abuse from their female relatives and friends. This betrayal may be reflected in her relationship with you. Her connection with her genital area holds deep-seated pain and suffering, which may come up for her during labor. To survive the torture of the mutilation, she may have become very disconnected from her body. (Chapter based on Daly, 1978; El Saadawi, 1982; Hosken, 1990) (For more information on these procedures, see the chapter on Clitoridectomy and Infibulation in Healing Passage.)

Amish: The Amish and Mennonite communities in North America maintain a separate lifestyle and thus form a subculture within the larger society. Founded in Switzerland in the 1500s, these tightly knit, closed communities are made up of two religious groups of German descent which moved to North America to maintain their way of life. Although small communities can be found throughout the United States and Canada, some of the largest communities of Amish reside in Pennsylvania and upstate New York. While their practices, beliefs and lifestyle choices will vary to a certain extent from place to place, there are some general things that can be said about these peoples.

General beliefs: The Amish and Mennonite philosophy is to be in the world but not of the world. The founder envisioned a community set apart that would have simple ways, that would dress alike so that the world could recognize them as different, and that would center around strong Christian faith. Old order Amish follow these teachings to the letter. The Amish and Mennonites refer to themselves as Plain and to all those that are not Amish as English.

Meetings: The Amish use each others' homes for group religious services held every other Sunday which may last from 9 a.m. until 1 or 2 p.m. Women and men sit separately at church. They have visiting in the afternoon.. A church district typically includes 80 to 100 families. On alternate Sundays they have private family devotions at home.

Frolics are large community gatherings where specific work, such as a barn raising, is done, and are held instead of parties. Because of the hard physical labor within these communities, serious injuries are not uncommon.

Diet: Dietary choices tend to include meats, carbohydrates and sweets.

Communities are largely self supporting and use very little technology. Their gardens and livestock are, by default, largely organic. Cooking methods may not be the best for preserving the nutritive content of foods; much homegrown food is home canned to last through the winter. Some communities may be open to learning ways to can which preserve the maximum amount of nutrients. You will need to encourage women to eat green vegetables and cut down on sweets; however, since most meals include meat, protein intake is usually not a problem and neither are calories. There are no self-imposed dietary restrictions during pregnancy, birth or postpartum.

Attitudes toward technology and education: German or a combination of German and Dutch is the community language and Bibles are often in German. Amish children typically do not learn English until just before they enter school at the age of six. Schooling only goes through the eighth grade, the government imposed minimum. Mennonites tend to be more open to higher education and more willing to go out into the world to attend conferences.

The Amish do not have phones, electricity or running water in their homes. Mennonites tend to accept more "modern" conveniences than do the Amish; however this, too, may vary among different locales. Horse and buggy is the main form of Amish transportation. Some communities allow for turn signals on the buggies and glass to keep rain out. Mennonites sometimes own old black cars. Amish and Mennonites tend to have little money but will barter, often very generously. Sometimes the church will have a fund for medical bills; insurance is not used.

Relationships: On church-going Sunday the youth get together for a social gathering called a Sing. It is one of the only times that young, unmarried people can mingle openly together. Most get married between 20 and 22 years of age.

Courting is a private affair and "special friendships" are kept a secret until a couple publishes their intentions to wed, usually two weeks prior to the marriage. Courtship takes two to four years and is done surreptitiously with boys sneaking into the homes of their girlfriends. The grapevine in the Amish community is very active and the whole community may be aware that something is going on, but no one will say anything except to make subtle, indirect, teasing remarks. Weddings take place in the spring, fall or winter, when the work load is not so heavy. The bride's family provides all the kitchen articles and other things appropriate to her new role as a wife and the groom's family does the same for him. Most come into marriage as virgins. Babies born outside of marriage are rare.

In general, compliments focus on activities and proficiencies and not on physical attractiveness; to compliment appearances is to judge by the world's standards. They try not to be "one up" on their neighbor and, although colors may be used for clothing fabric, they tend to choose dull tones.

The father is the head of the household and the authority figure. However, men may not want to make independent decisions, even in the case of an emergency. The father may want to confer with his own father or the community Bishop before deciding on a course of action.

Pregnancy: Large families are desired and women often consider it a blessing to get pregnant during the first week of marriage. Infertility is seen as God's will. Some women are willing to use basal body temperature to monitor their ovulation but most seek no outside help. An Amish community that accepts an "English" midwife will send along a lot of repeat clients.

The Amish are very reserved and shy about discussing issues of sexuality, pregnancy and birth. Mothers do not tell their daughters anything about childbearing; however, pregnant women are often very receptive to the midwife teaching them the basics in simple language. They are very modest and do not talk publicly about their pregnancies. Typically word will come to you through the Amish grapevine or a letter will be sent saying something like "Hi, how are you, praises to the Lord above, you better put me on your list as I seem to be in that way again." The Amish do not announce to the rest of the community or even to other family members other than their husband, that they are pregnant. Sometimes a sister or sister-in-law may know of a conception and pass the word along at a prenatal visit. The woman's mother might be told as well. It is not so much a secret as a private matter. However, women may tease each other when they start to show. In order to respect their privacy, you should refrain from discussing other women's pregnancies or births within the Amish or Mennonite communities.

Due to the limited forms of transportation acceptable to the community as well as the large families, many midwives offer prenatals in the form of home visits. Women will be most comfortable being visited when men and hired helpers are not there, primarily because they wish to keep their affairs private. It is respectful to enter the home and ask if it is okay to talk. This way the mother can remove unwanted parties, such as older children, before the prenatal visit begins. Physical components of prenatal exams can be done by placing a blanket or sheet over the mother, pulling up her dress and performing the exam beneath the covering to preserve her modesty. Grand multiparity is common, with few associated complications due to the hard work, lack of substance abuse and trust in birth which characterizes women in these communities.

Women may choose not to attend church for the six weeks prior to their due date for fear they will go into labor or rupture membranes in public, a highly embarrassing event.

Labor and birth: Women typically work until they go into labor. The husband may be sent to a neighbor's house or a public phone to call to tell you labor has begun. Women may be reluctant to write down what is happening for fear someone else will read it. A caller may tell you she just started her period (has bloody show), can't hold her water (broke her membranes), or is having terrible stomach aches (is having contractions). Prenatally, request that the woman tell the father exactly what is going on and then agree that you will ask the questions and he can just say yes or no. This preserves their privacy. Women tend not to make noise during labor and do not whine or resist labor. Births tend to be easy and uncomplicated. Women may wear an old dress for laboring but do not labor nude.

Men at births: Husbands do attend births. Men will sit in a chair by the bed or behind their wives and will often translate what the mother needs to do into German or Dutch. First time mothers may want their mother or older sister with them during labor.

Postpartum: Women take six weeks off after the birth to give the baby time to adjust. Women's roles are well defined and focus on household chores, cooking, baking, sewing and harvesting. The mother will rest for the first three weeks postpartum while a helper comes in to do the household work. The helper stays for an additional three weeks while the mother resumes light work; then she goes back to her full work load. Amish and Mennonite women will often nurse, but the liberal use of pacifiers and the use of formula to supplement the baby contribute to the prompt return of the menstrual cycle and closely spaced pregnancies. Babies may come as often as every 13 to 18 months.

Children: Typically the Amish are loving, kind parents that rarely raise their voices to their children. Formal entry into the community usually occurs at the age of 18, with baptism, when children can fully understand the commitment they are making.

Children are not told another baby is on the way. They are usually removed from the home during labor. Older children help in naming the new baby, and names tend to be used repeatedly in the same extended family. Siblings are presented with the baby by being told "look what Jesus has brought us." Parents often prefer the firstborn to be a boy. Community tradition is that the lazy parent gets the most helpers, that is, same-sex children!

Old order Amish: Old order, or, as they are called in some areas, Swartzentruber Amish, are even less "of the world" than other Amish. They tend to be less attentive to personal hygiene, have babies closer together, and have many health problems. Old Order Amish may not come for prenatal care until very late in their pregnancy and are less open to advice from outsiders than are other communities.

Family planning: Some families may be open to the concept of child spacing (do not use the term birth control) in the form of abstinence until a woman's cycles return postpartum and then the rhythm method. The best approach is to speak to the husband regarding the wife's health and the necessity for giving her body a break with longer intervals between children.

Problems due to intermarriage: To preserve their separateness, intermarriage among first cousins has been historically commonplace among Amish and Mennonite communities. This brings with it a higher incidence of genetically related birth defects. Down syndrome is common, as are other types of genetic syndromes, some of which are peculiar to certain Amish communities. When communities really began to notice this pattern they changed the rules and now only marriage as close as second cousins. Parents tend to move around to try and bring fresh blood into their community for children of marriageable age. Special children are loved and accepted as gifts from God, and the weak, old and ill members of a community are well cared for.

Death: The Amish have a matter-of-fact attitude regarding death. Babies that die are dressed and laid out, and may or may not be embalmed. The bishops look over the body and a death certificate may or may not be filed. The baby is buried within two days. The children are allowed to see the body. (Cooper, 1994)

Christian science: Christian Scientists believe that prayer and faith are the best and most primary means of affecting healing. While they subscribe to the notion that good foods and the avoidance of alcohol, tobacco, caffeine and drugs are health promoting, they look to spiritual principles as their primary source of treatment. There are Christian Science practitioners whose job it is to pray regarding specific health problems. Such a practitioner will be engaged during the pregnancy and the mother may wish for them to attend the birth as well.

The separation between the mind and the body inherent in this belief system can leave the first-time mother poorly prepared for the task of labor. This is primarily because she is not ready for the hard, very physical work of getting the baby out. Of course some Christian Scientists have had some contact with medical care providers, but don't be surprised if new clients have never had their blood pressure taken, a blood draw or any kind of standard Western health care. Their doctrine specifies that they are never to break the law, so if you live in an illegal state you will probably be approached by few, if any, Christian Scientists. Typically, Christian Scientists seek homebirth and midwifery care to avoid the hassle of refusing interventions and therapies in a more medical setting.

In the extreme case, Christian Scientists will absolutely refuse any kind of intervention; however, official doctrine states that once someone has been engaged as a care provider, the believer should respect their work in their sphere of expertise. That is, in the event of a problem they should not put up too much of a fuss if you want to do something that ordinarily they might rather not have done. You should discuss this issue during prenatal care, and decide if you can work with those who might refuse what you view as life-saving treatment. If transport is necessary, hospitals do have wavers for Christian Scientists to sign for refusing drugs, surgery or prophylactic treatments for the newborn.

620

Fundamental Christian: There are many denominations and sects of Christians in North America today. The majority of Christians seek homebirth for the same reasons as anyone else in our culture; to foster family bonding, have control over their births and eliminate unnecessary interventions. Specifically, fundamental Christians interpret the Bible very literally and adhere to strict rules regarding personal conduct, concepts of right and wrong, and may have strict views regarding family hierarchy. However such rules vary somewhat from sect to sect. There are many small, local groups of fundamental Christians (some of whom may also refer to themselves as Born Again Christians). The best thing to do is to try and find out as much as you can about the beliefs of any groups with which you might be working as they present themselves to you as potential clients.

There are many reasons why fundamental Christians seek homebirth and independent midwifery care, among them: they do not want to patronize a care provider who does abortions, they feel they will have more control over any interventions that might be recommended if they are at home, they feel God created their bodies to birth, and to keep the birth within the family.

Feelings about the use of drugs, surgery, herbs and other treatment modalities vary widely from group to group. While many Christians feel fine about the use of a variety of healing modalities, some are intensely distrustful of herbs because they are associated with witchcraft; others feel herbs were put on earth by God for our use. However, there are some fundamental Christians that feel the use of any form of healing other than the laying on of hands and prayer is contrary to trusting in the will of God. As with Christian Scientists, it behooves you to ask specific questions of fundamental Christians regarding what is and is not acceptable to them in terms of treatments and procedures which you might use during pregnancy and birth. You must decide for yourself as a care provider if their wishes coincide with your ethics about what you will and will not do. I have told families who want nothing done in the event of an emergency that perhaps they do not need a birth attendant, explaining that I could not stand by and do nothing knowing I could help in an emergency situation.

Some fundamental Christians adhere to a more or less rigid patriarchal family structure, with the man seen as the head of the household and the decision-maker. If you find this to be the case, direct your questions to the woman and get her opinion, while at the same time acknowledging the man by asking his opinion as well. This can be tricky and requires tact on your part so as not to alienate him.

Others will not use birth control, believing that God opens their wombs to give them as many children as he desires. The majority will breastfeed.

Jehovah's Witness: Jehovah's Witnesses are a unique Christian sect which highly respects Old Testament laws. In the Jewish dietary laws there is mention that one should not eat the blood of an animal. The Jehovah's Witnesses interpret this to forbid not only the dietary ingestion of blood but the use of blood or any blood products or derivatives for any form of treatment. Most strictly, this is applied to the use of blood and blood products (such as red cells, platelets, etc.) during transfusion, but it is also applied to the use of Rho(D) immunoglobulin for prenatal and postpartum maternal prophylaxis against Rh sensitization. While the use of immunoglobulins is considered a matter of personal conscience which individuals can interpret for themselves, the vast majority of Jehovah's Witnesses will refuse the use of any blood-derived products for any reason, even preferring death of themselves or a child to the use of such products. Otherwise, Jehovah's Witnesses generally have no problem with the use of any other healing modalities. Jehovah's Witnesses, more so than other Christian couples, may seek circumcision for their infant sons, feeling it too is desirable, having been put forth in the Old Testament.

Jehovah's Witnesses do not celebrate Christian holidays, recognizing that these holidays were originally pagan festivals. Birthday celebrations are also forbidden and felt to be idolatrous and violating of the first commandment, "Thou shalt have not other Gods before me."

Jewish law and culture: Judaism is based on the observance of the Torah laws which were given to Moses by God on Mt. Sinai. There are many denominations of Judaism: Hasidic and Orthodox Jews follow a strict, traditional interpretation of the laws; Conservative Jews take a more moderate approach; Reformed and Reconstructionist Jews tend to identify more with Jewish cultural than religious beliefs. What is acceptable in practice varies widely among these groups; however Hasidic and Orthodox Jews will follow the letter of the laws described below.

Traditional (Orthodox) Judaism views humans as individuals created in God's image with a soul that will survive eternally and be returned to God after death. Observant Jews accept the Torah laws that teach them how to emulate Godlike behaviors in their day to day lives, making them better human beings. Jewish law details every aspect of life, from diet to burial rituals. Even though all laws are not fully understood, they are followed as a manifestation of faith.

The family is seen as the only appropriate environment for sexual expression and the best place for the practice of Judaism. Children are a necessary extension of marriage, and having children is incumbent upon married couples as a means of providing continuity to the Jewish people. Birth control, abortion and sterilization are not permitted unless the mother's physical or psychological health is at risk and rabbinic counsel has been sought by the concerned couple; therefore grand multiparity is common in orthodox communities. The rabbi must okay any variation from the routine observance of Jewish law. This is usually done in writing. Women are considered the cornerstone of family spiritual life and therefore women may be very concerned about adhering to Jewish law.

Jews also highly value mental acuity. Therefore the birth of a retarded baby or one with birth defects may be especially hard on the family, who may consider it a curse or believe that someone has given the mother the evil eye while pregnant.

622

Ease this struggle by pointing out the beautiful aspects of the baby and encourage the mother to know that the baby's needs are not basically any different than any other baby; she needs her love.

The following summarizes the major categories of Jewish law with which you may want to be familiar:

Tsniut: These laws address modesty, which is felt to maintain the dignity of the body. Orthodox women generally choose clothing that covers the elbows and knees and married women cover their hair with a wig, hat, or scarf; single women may wear the hair exposed. Orthodox men do not directly observe their wives while the are immodestly exposed. To respect these laws, the woman may wish to be covered throughout labor, including their hair covering. Give the father opportunity to leave the room by informing him before you will perform body-exposing exams. Or, if they feel okay about it, drape the mother carefully to avoid exposure. Suggest that the father remain at the head of the bed during the birth if he desires to do so. Ask if the mother wants to watch the birth; don't make any assumptions.

Niddah: These laws define the time of physical separateness between married partners. Men and women do not touch, and they will sleep separately from the onset of any non-traumatic uterine bleeding; for this reason, they will most likely have twin beds. Once the last trace of bleeding is gone the woman bathes in a ritual bath called the *mikvah* and can then resume physical contact and sexual relations.

In labor, some rabbis interpret Niddah to apply at the onset of contractions, others at the appearance of bloody show, at membrane rupture, at full dilation, or when the mother finds if difficult to walk unassisted. Ask when they wish to begin observing the Niddah laws. Encourage the father's nonphysical supportive efforts such as eye contact, verbal support and prayer. Female friends or relatives or the midwife can provide physical support if the woman so desires.

Laws concerning food and drink: Kosher dietary laws are meant to elevate the act of eating to a context of holiness, and not primarily observed because of health or hygiene considerations. Kashrut or kosher laws govern the types of foods eaten and methods of preparation. Handwashing & blessings are observed at mealtime, especially before a meal which includes bread. Observant Jews do not eat meat and dairy products during the same meal. Fish and eggs are neutral foods which may be eaten with either dairy or meat meals. Leafy vegetables may be avoided because the cook must be certain no insects which could be eaten have been accidently left in the leaves. Most processed foods must be certified Kosher to assure that they have not been improperly prepared. Pork and shellfish are forbidden foods.

Separate dishes and utensils are maintained for dairy and meat preparation and eating. Be sure not to barge into the kitchen and "make yourself at home" during labor. If you need something for yourself or the mother, have a relative or someone else who is familiar with the kitchen prepare the food.

Sabbath (pronounced SHA-bis) and holiday laws: The Jewish Sabbath begins at sundown on Friday and lasts until dark on Saturday. This is a day of rest, signifying that God rested after having created the world in six days. Women usually prepare all the food for the Sabbath the day before. Observant Jews will abstain from labors that display human's mastery over nature. This means they will not ride in cars (walking is okay), use the phone or other electrical devices (a light may be left on Friday afternoon, but not turned on or off during the Sabbath or a holiday), write, handle money, or do anything which requires the use of something which humans have invented. How strictly this is interpreted varies among communities.

Yom Kippur, the Day of Atonement, is the most significant Jewish holiday. This holiday includes fasting. Most rabbis waive the fast for pregnant women from the onset of labor until at least 72 hours (30 days for nursing mothers) after birth. Some will waive fasting requirements during pregnancy as well. Try to plan your visits (home or prenatal) so that they do not fall on Jewish holidays. Do not expect women to sign papers or ride in a car on a holiday or the Sabbath unless it is an absolute emergency.

It is important to discuss how willing your clients are to breach Sabbath or holiday observances in the event that the woman goes into labor. If they will not call you, how will they contact you? All Jewish laws are waived in the event that a true health crisis exists. Some observant Jews will push this to the limit; it is a good thing to remind them of this if things are really critical and people are refusing to assist because of the day.

B'rith Milah: The covenant of circumcision began as a pact between Abraham and God and was first performed on Abraham's son Issac. Early circumcision consisted of a ritual nick in the foreskin to draw blood, the blood of the covenant. As the Jewish culture evolved, Jewish youth began to scrape the sides of the scar to heal it back up so they could participate in the Greek games. The rabbis then mandated that the incision become larger, until it finally entailed removal of some or all of the foreskin.

Most observant Jews will adhere strictly to the performance of circumcision and even those who observe no other aspect of the Jewish religion will often have the *bris* ceremony. The *bris* is performed no sooner than the eighth day of life by a mohel (pronounced moil) chosen by the family. The mohel is a religious specialist trained in the art of circumcision and is usually very good at it, with a fast, almost bloodless technique. If the baby is compromised for any reason, such as prematurity, jaundice or illness, the *bris* is postponed. The rabbi examines the baby himself to check for jaundice if the baby isn't hospitalized.

At the *bris*, the ceremony of circumcision, the male baby is officially named and welcomed into the family. Parents may be reluctant to disclose the baby's name until after the naming ceremony. Men gather round the baby for the procedure and the women stand in the back of the room. The baby is usually given a few drops of wine prior to the circumcision. Afterwards, the mother nurses the baby privately. The care of the circumcised penis is overseen by the mohel.

Girls are named by the father at a Torah reading ceremony. The Sabbath after the birth of a daughter is an ideal time for the naming ceremony so that the parents can sponsor a kiddush (ceremonial blessing) in her honor. The mother may be eager to attend Sabbath services as soon as possible after birth so that she can give thanks for her recovery and for the birth of the baby.

Muslim (Islam): Islam was founded by Mohommad, whose teachings have been passed down in the Qur'an and Hadiths. It is widely practiced in the Middle East, Africa and Asia. Five times a day, prayers are said on a prayer mat facing Mecca, the sacred city of Islam. Fasting takes place during the month of Ramadan, although menstruating, pregnant and nursing women are not required to do so. The status of men and women is equal, but their roles are different. Men are required to provide total financial support; women are not obliged to work. In many Islamic countries local customs may overlay religious mandates from the Qur'an, including arranged marriage, preferring a male child, and female genital mutilation. Male circumcision is traditionally performed at age 7, but some perform it in infancy. Cleanliness is highly valued and some women may shave their pubic hair. Muslim women are extremely modest and some cover their bodies from head to toe with a garment called a hijab, leaving only their hands and faces exposed. They prefer female health care providers and will want their modesty maintained throughout exams. No men should be in the room when a woman is examined; abdominal and yoni exams should take place under a cover or beneath her clothing. Mixed sex childbirth classes may be unacceptable as well. Dietary restrictions include avoiding alcohol and pork; other meats should be slain using lawful Islamic rules.

Motherhood is a powerful role and very respected. Pregnancy and birth are normal events and midwives are well respected. Support people are usually the woman's mother and female family members. The mother may pray during labor, asking for help and protection. Suffering in labor is expected and an important part of motherhood. At birth the "call to prayer" is whispered in the baby's right ear and a mixture of crushed dates and rosewater is touched to its tongue. A metal may be pinned to the clothing to remind others to pray for the baby. Women typically breastfeed for two years. (Aust. Newsletter, 1990)

Scientology: Scientology is a belief system which is largely based upon the idea that past traumatic experiences influence how we act in the present. It offers a theory about the link between body, mind and spirit. By understanding this relationship, a person can alleviate unwanted sensations and emotions, accidents, injuries and psychosomatic illnesses. There are various techniques used in special sessions for adults to deprogram themselves from past traumas to clear the way for creating a healthy life in the present.

Scientology believes that what happens in the womb during pregnancy and during birth affect the child for a lifetime. Recognizing that the unborn baby is a feeling, aware and remembering being, intrauterine experiences affect the personality, drives and ambitions of the person after birth in important ways. Any physical experience (such as mother bumping into a table) and anything which the baby hears is recorded in the baby's unconscious mind. Normally many such events occur throughout pregnancy, all of them potentially harmful because the fetus may interpret them as personally traumatic. Later in life, these experiences may be reactivated by specific circumstances which cause the person to act in irrational ways, or limit their abilities and intelligence all without knowing the real reason. The reactive powers of traumatic intrauterine events can be reduced by keeping silent in connection to and immediately after the unborn child may have interpreted an experience as traumatic. The following precautions are recommended for the mother during pregnancy:

*Be careful with your body movements. A fetus is more easily injured than you may think. Picking up heavy objects and even bending over could affect the child. Have someone help you to avoid physical pressure or strain on the unborn baby.

*Be quiet if injured. If you know that your baby is under physical stress or possibly injured, stay quiet. A fetus not only hears the sounds outside the womb, but makes a detailed recording of them, when under physical stress. The words you may say have an unconscious influence on the child later in life. If you bump the baby, stay quiet; even saying "shhh" to quiet those around you may make the baby grow up to be a stutterer.

(Abdominal palpation to determine fetal position and the pressure applied to use a fetascope qualify as bumping the baby. Silence may be requested from the onset of the abdominal exam until the parents leave the appointment; therefore, postpone palpation so it is the very last thing before they leave.)

*Stay calm. The fetus, particularly in late pregnancy, is aware of the sound and rhythms of its mother's voice. Fetuses have been known to respond to this if their mother is under stress or upset. Don't argue in the presence of your unborn child!

*Don't drink alcohol. Alcohol puts the fetus in a state of mental unconsciousness, just as if s/he were injured. Everything said at that time is recorded and can later cause irrational behaviors. An alcoholic parent who makes such comments as "I'm only happy when I drink" will definitely influence the child's later behavior.

*Avoid drugs. All drugs stay in the fetal body long after they are
gone from the mother's. Find out what effects stimulants or
depressants could have on the unborn child before you take them.

During the labor and birth itself it is recommended that, because of the pain
and trauma involved, all parties present should be as quiet as possible.

The practices described above are "pure scientology" taken almost verbatim
from a Dianetics publication. They are not strictly adhered to by everyone and are
offered for reference when you interview prospective clients who are scientologists.

Sikhs: In the 1970's several East Indian teachers came to North America to spread
their teachings among the hippie generation. One such teacher was Yogi Bajan, the
founder of the 3-H-O Organization, a mystical Sikh movement in the United States.
Note that there are thousands of native East Indian sikhs in North America that *do
not* subscribe to the practices outlined here. The primary spiritual practices of 3HO
Sikhs involve an early morning meditation, Kundilini yogi exercises, reading and
chanting passages from their scriptures, living and working in close knit sikh
communities, and fostering strong family systems within which children are reared
to understand Sikh ways. Kundilini yoga and special breathing techniques are used
to raise the spiritual energy focused within the spinal system. Most 3HO Sikhs
have adapted their lifestyle after growing up in Western culture, so they will be
thoroughly familiar with Western medical practices. Sikh's tend to use a variety
of healing modalities and prefer to try herbal, chiropractic or homeopathic remedies
prior to resorting to Western medicine. The Sikh tradition includes many remedial
recipes for foods used for a variety of health conditions.

Some 3HO Sikh women wear modest clothing, often preferring gold, blue
and white fabrics of natural fibers. Hot baths are felt to drain one's energy and ice
cold showering while still wearing special undergarments intended to keep the
sacrum warm are encouraged. Cutting the hair, as well as eating meat and eggs are
forbidden, as is the use of alcohol, tobacco and recreational drugs. Marriage is
considered a lifetime commitment and the partner may have been selected by the
spiritual teacher. Abortion is permitted during the first 120 days of pregnancy,
before the spirit of the child has entered the fetal body. Sikhs often prefer
midwifery care and homebirth, feeling trusting of the birth process and wishing to
avoid hospital intervention.

After the birth, the mother will remain secluded in her home for 40 days,
attended by personal women friends in her community. The mother's task at this
time is to meet all the needs of the infant, the belief being that when a person's
needs are met completely after birth, a solid foundation is established for future
independence and trust in the universe. During this period visitors are severely
restricted to allow both the baby and the mother to adapt to their relationship and
the baby to adapt to life outside the womb without being bombarded by a variety

of difficult to integrate energies.

References and further reading:

Homebirth Australia Newsletter, "Towards and understanding: Muslim women in childbirth," No. 26, Spring, 1990, pp. 7-10.

Bjorkman, E., "Childbirth Care for Hmong Families," MCN, Nov./Dec. 1985, Vol. 10, pp. 382-5.

Cooper, Mary, workshop in "Cultural Birthing: Working with Amish Women," Midwifery Today Conference, Eugene, OR, March, 1994.

Daly, Mary, Gyn/ecology: the Metaethics of Radical Feminism, Beacon Press, Boston, 1978.

D'Avanzo, Carolyn, "Bridging the Cultural Gap with Southeast Asians," MCN, Vol 17 No. 4, July/Aug. 1992, pp. 204-8.

Eaton, L., "Going Forward," Nursing Times, Vol. 89, No. 46, Nov. 17, 1993, pp. 14-15.

El Saadawi, N., The Hidden Face of Eve: Women in the Arab World, Beacon, Boston, 1982.

Hedley, & Darkenoo, Child Protection and Female Genital Mutilation, London, Forward, 1992.

Hosken, Fran, "Female Genital Mutilation," Woman of Power, Issue 18, Fall, 1990, pp. 42-5.

Goldstein, Deborah, Navajo traditions, handouts given at MANA conf., San Francisco, 1993.

Griffith, S, "Childbearing & the Concept of Culture," JOGN Nursing, Vol. 11, 1982, pp. 181-4.

"How to Safeguard Your Future Child's Well-being," pub. by the Hubbard Dianetics Foundation & Bridge, Inc., 1992.

Ishida, Yasuo, "Innovations: the Sarashi," JOGN Nursing, Vol. 6, Jan/Feb. 1977, p. 53.

Kushi, Aveline, Infertility and Reproductive Disorders, Japan Pub., 1988.

Leyn, Rita, "The Challenge of Caring for Child Refugees from Southeast Asia," The American Journal of Maternal Child Health, Vol. 3, May/June 1978, pp. 178-82.

Lightfoot-Klein, Hanny, & Evelyn Shaw, "Special Needs of Ritually Circumcised Women Patients," JOGNN, March/April Vol. 20, No. 2, pp. 102-7, 1991.

Lutwak, R., et.al., "Maternity Nursing and Jewish Law," MCN, Vol. 13, Jan/Feb 1988, pp. 44-6.

Meleis, Afaf & Sorrell, L., "Arab American Women and Their Birth Experiences," MCN, Vol. 6, May/June 1981, pp. 171-6.

Neeson, Jean, Clinical Manual of Maternity Nursing, J.B. Lippincott Co., Philadelphia, PA, 1987.

Nyirjesy, Karen & Paul, "Neonatal Care in Northeast Zaire," JOGNN, Vol. 20, No. 5, September/October, 1991, pp. 362-6.

Parra, Alison, "Mexico," in Rothman, B. Katz, ed., Encyclopedia of Childbearing, Oryx Press, Phoenix, 1993.

Paul, B., ed., Health, Culture and Community, NY: Russell Sage Foundation, 1955, pp. 462-74.

Wadd, Lois, "Vietnamese Postpartum Practices; Implications for Nursing in the Hospital Setting," JOGN Nursing, July/August, 1983, Vol. 12, No. 252-8.

628

Unique Birthing Practices and Philosophies

There are a few practices that cannot be classified as either cultural or religious which will be discussed in this chapter. Parents may come to you requesting these practices; this chapter will give you some background on them.

Leboyer birth: In the mid 1970's Frederick Leboyer, a French obstetrician, made the startling discovery that the newborn is a sentient, sensitive being. He became aware that the noise, low temperature, bright lights, separation from the mother and isolation common to delivery rooms and newborn nurseries were upsetting to the infant, producing fear, tension, and excessive grimacing and crying. He viewed labor as a violent, assaultive experience for the fetus, and therefore came up with a "method" of birth focusing on the baby's needs for warmth, quiet, and a slow adjustment to breathing, gravity and an air environment. After an initial period of adjustment, ideally taking place on the mother's abdomen, the baby is placed in a body-temperature bath, where it relaxes, opens its eyes and looks around. His book Birth Without Violence, published in 1976, outlined this attitude toward the newborn.

This book entered into a revolution that was occurring on many fronts in our attitudes about birth in general and the newborn's needs in particular. It urged hospitals to treat the newborn with the respect it deserves rather than as a piece of meat to be processed. Some parents may come in requesting a "Leboyer birth." However, the mothers of home born babies will usually not go through the same kind of traumatic labor that occurs in hospitals and neither mothers nor babies are drugged. Most of the newborns I've seen seemed to prefer to stay with their mother rather than be separated even for the short time it takes to bathe the baby in a separate basin. The recommendations for lowered lights, warmth, and silence at the time of birth are easily accommodated in the home setting.

Lotus Birthing: The practice of Lotus birthing (also called Whole birthing) was originated by a woman named Clair Day of California in the mid-1970s. It consists of allowing the baby and placenta to remain attached, leaving the umbilical cord untouched until it atrophies and falls off at the navel base naturally. The cord is never clamped, tied or cut. The baby, placenta, amniotic membranes and cord are seen as a whole birth unit; to sever this unit prematurely is felt to be traumatic and unnecessary.

When the placenta is born it is wrapped in sterile cotton gauze, cloth or disposable (chux) pads. The cord and placenta are kept clean and wrapped in natural fabrics. They are placed level with the child's body for the first day and at night thereafter. Keeping the placenta under a pyramid built to the dimensions of the Cheops pyramid in Egypt is thought to help keep it from rotting and smelling during the period before the cord detaches.

This practice stems in part from an adverse attitude regarding the use of any cutting instruments. It is advised to keep all such instruments away from the mother and the baby during and after birth. Further, only those with whom the mother feels comfortable and trusting are allowed to visit during the breaking forth time (the period between the birth and when the umbilical cord spontaneously detaches). This practice is said to be least traumatic for the infant in making the transition from intrauterine to extrauterine life and makes for calm, peaceful and contented babies and children. In reality, lugging the placenta around for several days is a hassle, but if the parents want to do it, it causes no harm to the baby.

Waterbirth: Native Americans, traditional Hawaiians and other cultures around the world have used water for laboring and sometimes for the actual birth. Perhaps the "father" of modern day waterbirth is Igor Charkovsky, a Russian obstetrician who has overseen the births of hundreds of babies under water. Western women, chief among them Rima Beth Star, visited Russia and observed first hand the benefits of waterbirth for both mothers and babies. Today, there are a fair number couples who seek homebirth so that they too can birth their babies under water.

For those unfamiliar with the concept of waterbirth, this request gives understandable pause. Humans are not, after all, aquatic creatures. Since we don't live in water, what could be the rationale for birthing our babies under water? Simply put, the baby is surrounded by amniotic fluid *in utero,* and it is felt that the transition from a watery to a dry environment is eased considerably if the baby is slowly introduced to gravity by being gently removed from water rather than instantly thrust from intrauterine water to extrauterine air.

Waterbirth is said to reduce oxygen consumption right after birth and thus provides more oxygen to the brain, kidneys and liver, to the lifelong benefit of the baby. Psychologically, waterbirth is seen as less traumatic than air birth. Some advocate leaving the baby under water for a period of time after it emerges, confident that the umbilical cord will continue to provide oxygen to the baby during this time and that the infant that has never been exposed to air will not try to take a breath. Only after adjusting to the new freedom from the confines of the uterus is the baby slowly brought to the surface and then slowly removed bit by bit to allow the baby to adjust to gravity. Of course, many women benefit greatly from laboring in water; dilation is shortened and pushing is made less painful, as the perineal tissues relax well in warm water.

Arguments against waterbirth include the belief that a woman, left to her own devices, may labor in water but would rarely choose to remain in water for the birth of the baby. No other land mammal gives birth in water. Even whales and dolphins bring their babies to the surface as quickly as possible after birth. While it may be true that some waterbirth babies are calmer than their hospital born counterparts, almost every home born baby I and many other midwives have seen has been absolutely content after birth in air.

Some questions and topics you might wish to consider for yourself and then discuss with the women seeking waterbirth are:

630

Why do you want an underwater birth? It seems that many women are very well read and have an intellectual notion that this is a "better way" to birth. However these same women may often seem far removed from their instincts regarding their birth experience.

Some women are under the impression that the water will take all the pain away, which is just not true. These women may or may not want to get in the water and stay there. It is good to discuss the need to get out, move around, use the toilet and change positions early on. Women sweat in labor, even when they are in warm water. Staying in the water too long may lead to dehydration and overheating. Choosing any birthing method with the primary goal of avoiding pain generally blocks labor energy and is counterproductive.

It seems that many women prefer the idea of waterbirth because they are under the impression that birth is difficult for the baby. They may have read traumatizing birth stories describing labor as violent and scary (as Leboyer recounts in his book). It is important that the mother not perceive the labor as frightening, harmful or otherwise damaging to the baby. (Of course, if she feels it is, the baby is more likely to perceive it that way too.) While there is certainly no guarantee how any person will react to a particular experience, home born babies do not often appear traumatized by their birth. If her own birth was traumatic, counseling may help her to separate her experience from the coming birth.

Michel Odent, who provides shallow pools of water for laboring women, comments that he never encourages women to get into the water to labor or birth. Many women seek the water to ease labor pain and a few wind up remaining in the water to birth. This is not a premeditated plan and therefore is probably most in sync with the mother's instincts of the moment. Once the baby is born no effort is made to keep the baby under water, it is brought immediately to the surface. It has been erroneously assumed that Michele Odent "advocates" waterbirth, but he emphatically denies this, stating that only if the mother's gut instincts tell her to stay in the water does it seem appropriate for her to do so.

Do you wish to keep the baby under water or bring it immediately to the surface? I had a waterbirth candidate ask me if it was normal for babies not to breathe and to be blue for 10 to 15 minutes after birth!! I told her certainly not. Later, upon viewing a video tape she had of several underwater births, I saw that all but one of these babies came out of the water floppy, blue and not breathing very well. Encourage mothers to envision their babies pink, well oxygenated and breathing easily after birth once they are above the surface of the water.

It has been my practice to bring the baby to the water's surface immediately upon delivery. You will have to decide what you feel most comfortable with as you gain experience. Some waterbirth experts feel that no newborn will take a breath while still under water if the cord is intact and continues to pulse. There are many anecdotal incidents of babies born into water who remain under for as long as 15 minutes and who experience no distress.

Emergencies and changes of plans: In the event of an emergency, such as the need for the mother to assume a hands and knees position in order to deal with a shoulder dystocia, the baby may not actually come out under water. It is important to clarify that if anyone attending the birth feels that it is inadvisable for the birth to occur in the water, that it will not. For example, I had a woman who wanted a waterbirth, but every time she entered the water during labor her contractions stopped. Another woman had a long, difficult labor and a hard time pushing her baby out. At the last minute she did not enter the water, and after the birth had a massive, rapid hemorrhage. Still another woman had a beautiful and trouble-free birth under water, and remained there until the placenta was delivered.

Should an emergency arise, fetal heart tones drop, or meconium suddenly appear in the fluid, for example, it may be advisable to get the woman out of the water before the birth, especially if you are unfamiliar with waterbirths. One midwife, very experienced in waterbirths, always got the mother out of the water for the placental delivery to prevent a water embolism in the tub. It would also seem ill advised to assist a breech birth underwater, because gravity is a primary factor in getting the baby out without problems. Likewise, the normal birth of twins is greatly facilitated by the force of gravity which helps to bring the second twin down into the pelvis; there is also a greater likelihood that one or both twins will be breech.

What kind of tub does she plan to use? Does she have an adequate water source? It is best to use a light colored or white tub or hot tub with a light source inside the unit. Ideally, the tub is deep enough to allow the mother to submerge her torso, but not so deep as to necessitate complete submergence of the midwife to assist the birth. That way, you can most easily assist, assess progress and see the color of the baby and any fluids. The water will need to be changed every couple of days as labor nears. An alternative is to leave the tub empty until early labor begins, thus reducing the possibility of the growth of harmful bacteria. The water should be maintained at a constant body temperature of 99 to 100°F (37.2 to 37.8°C) and the room in which the tub is located should also be very warm. An inflatable birthing tub can be purchased or rented from the Global Maternal/Child Health Assoc., P.O. Box 1400, Wilsonville, OR 97070, (503) 682-3600. A tub should be reserved at least 6 to 8 weeks before the due date.

Universal precautions and waterbirth: Whether or not you will enter the tub to assist with the birth must be weighed against your greater exposure to any blood borne pathogens which the mother may be carrying. Another potential problem is fecal contamination. It is not unusual for a small amount of stool to be pressed out during pushing. Because of this possibility, you might discuss whether or not an enema is acceptable to the woman at some point during active labor.

Discuss priorities for the birth: Assess whether the woman agrees to follow what seems right in the moment and not to press for a waterbirth regardless of the situation.

Try to find out who wants the waterbirth more, the woman or her partner. Do this by discussing each one's feelings about waterbirth separately. If the partner wants the waterbirth more than the pregnant woman, it is important to try to find out just how committed she really is. It is a set-up for problems if a woman is doing anything in her birth to please anyone else, especially if she is really frightened or feels the practice unsafe for herself or the baby.

While the above considerations may seem harshly put to the staunch advocate of waterbirth, they are well considered for those who have little or no experience with waterbirths. In fact, most statistics for waterbirths show that both mother and baby fare very well. The most important thing is for you to have a clear understanding with the parents regarding what they want and what you feel comfortable with as a care provider. Details regarding how to assist at waterbirths will be found in Volume II of Holistic Midwifery.

References and further reading:

Harper, Barbara, "Waterbirth: The Hows, Whys and What Ifs," Midwifery Today conf. workshop, Spring 1992, Eugene, OR.
Lotus Birth, descriptive pamphlet.

AN OVERVIEW OF PRENATAL CARE

634

Prenatal Visits

Midwifery care begins with the first contact you make with a potential client and continues throughout pregnancy. Prenatal care consists of everything the woman does for herself during pregnancy, punctuated by a series of visits with you. These visits allow you to get to know the woman and establish an emotional connection with her and her baby and family; the foundation of midwifery caregiving. You will follow the progress of the pregnancy, establish the parameters of maternal and fetal well-being in this particular case, and troubleshoot any problems, minor or major, which may arise. Prenatal visits can be a time to discuss many aspects of pregnancy. You can help a woman prepare for birth; exploring with her ways that she can best work though any issues from her past that may impede the full use of her resources, both physical and emotional, during the challenging work of labor and help prepare her for the mothering experience that lies ahead. Visits will also give you the opportunity to get to know her family and significant others, creating a solid relationship for the birth experience to come.

However, prenatal visits serve much more purpose than merely monitoring the course of a pregnancy. Given the incredible level of fear around birth in North America, prenatal care with midwives can provide a safe haven, a sub-culture in which women can reclaim trust in themselves and the birthing process. In Europe, where women are far less terrorized about birth, midwives report that they see women infrequently during their pregnancy. The midwife's job during the prenatal period is much more important in North America, where the midwife must stand between the women she serves and the larger society. Counter this undermining societal attitude by empowering the mother to realize that she is the only real care provider for her unborn baby. Show her that you value her sense of well-being or danger regarding her health and that of her baby; the baby is in her body, after all, and who should know better than she if something is not right? Your support of her intuitive perceptions about the pregnancy will go far in helping to distinguish real problems from imaginary ones throughout her care.

Individual or group visits? In our practice, and in most practices I have been acquainted with, prenatal visits are privately arranged for individual clients. However, there are some midwives who do group prenatal visits. An extension of the childbirth class, group visits afford women time to create community among themselves and hear the problems and fears of other women. However, some things are more difficult to discuss in a public arena. Weigh the pros and cons carefully when considering group vs. individual visits; a combination may be best.

Frequency of visits: There are different opinions about how frequently prenatal visits should take place. It is important to remember the totality of what prenatal visits can accomplish, as discussed above. When all of these benefits are considered, it becomes obvious that reducing the number of prenatal visits because a woman is physically healthy does not really make much sense. In the past, the midwife was often a woman well known to the mother; usually a relative or close family friend. Create an environment where such a relationship of trust can be approximated with as many leisurely visits as your life will allow.

Most midwives begin care in early pregnancy, seeing women at least once monthly and sometimes every three weeks until the 28th to 32nd week of pregnancy. At that point, visits are scheduled every two weeks until the 36th week, then weekly until birth. One of these late pregnancy visits usually takes place in the woman's home. Additional visits are scheduled as the situation warrants.

Supporting responsibility-taking during your care: Prenatal care is only as useful to a woman as she allows it to be. The real prenatal care in any pregnancy is what the woman does for herself between visits: how she eats, if she avoids harmful substances, when she exercises and rests as needed, and whether she works to resolve psychological issues that she knows of which may interfere with her birthing process. Your job is to guide, monitor her health and well-being and offer your expertise and experience as a midwife. Many midwives encourage women to take on specific responsibilities such as checking their own urine during care, weighing themselves, learning how to palpate and generally understanding everything you are doing and why, as well as making them responsible for following up on appointments with other practitioners when needed.

Time: In order to accomplish all of the above, a primary, necessary ingredient is enough time. Planning your prenatal schedule so that women do not feel rushed in and out of appointments underscores your invitation to discuss whatever they need to at every visit. During the first months of care, you may only be seeing women once monthly. As pregnancy advances, you will see them more often and sometimes, these visits will be somewhat shorter because of their frequency.

I routinely allot an hour for each prenatal whenever possible. Other midwives find they can comfortably address needs in 45 minutes or even a half-hour. Occasionally I get so backed up that I select some women to see for a shorter appointment, always considering each case on an individual basis, and evaluating what a particular woman needs at that time in her pregnancy. Those visits which will include pelvic exams, general physicals or other, non-routine procedures, should be given a full time allotment whenever possible.

Before each visit: Prior to the appointment, it is a good idea to prepare for the visit by looking over the woman's chart to review her history, previous visits, and to figure out her current week of pregnancy. Take a moment to review her financial agreement so that you can deal with that topic appropriately as well. While this will be less necessary the better you know your clients and the fewer clients you have, when you are seeing several women in a day it is a good idea to double check your memory in this fashion. Chart review will remind you what is unique about this woman (is she approaching the week she discovered her last baby was dead? is she a sexual abuse survivor?); it reminds you to try to obtain any information which may have been overlooked or purposely put off until another visit, and it helps you discern if previous recommendations for specific problems or circumstances have been effective by reminding you to ask about them at the upcoming visit. If phone conversations have occurred between this visit and your last, look to see if any procedures, tests or consultations were suggested to refresh yourself about follow-up at this visit. In order to have time to review each chart, it is most helpful to anticipate spending a short time between each visit for this purpose.

What to do during prenatals: Each prenatal visit may include any or all of the following observations and evaluations, with considerations as to which are appropriate to the weeks of pregnancy, your relationship with the woman, knowledge of her body and the way you practice (how technical you wish to be):

> *Greetings and getting any accompanying children settled
> *Discuss and assess general sense of well-being (fatigue?, etc.)
> *Nutritional assessment and counseling, review of diet diaries as indicated
> *Discussion of and follow-up on any problems found during a previous visit
> *Discussion of any new concerns, problems or symptoms such as:
> -Swelling
> -Headaches
> -Dizziness
> -Visual disturbances
> -Illness
> -Nausea
> -Bowel difficulties (constipation/diarrhea?)
> -Problematic yoni discharge or odor
> -Back pain or pain during urination
> -Pains, cramps and other physical complaints
> *For each problem noted discuss frequency, duration, what makes symptoms better or worse, remedies she may have tried and a plan of action to deal with it
> *Reference to and discussion of topics as outlined in the prenatal discussion checklist (see chapter on Books, Handouts and Forms later in this section for an explanation and example)
> *Maternal exercise & activity level
> *Maternal weight gain or loss
> *Maternal blood pressure, pulse (and temperature as indicated)
> *Maternal hemoglobin check as indicated

*Determination of fetal lie, attitude, variety, position & presentation
*Measurement of fundal height (and girth if indicated)
*Estimated fetal weight and size
*Assessment of amniotic fluid volume
*Observation or palpation of fetal movement
*Auscultation of fetal heart tones
*Assisting mother & family in feeling & hearing the baby, if desired
*Discussion with the mother regarding fetal movement: frequency, quality, quantity and any changes
*Discussion of uterine activity/toning contractions and cervical sensations with mother
*Urine analysis using a dip-stick which minimally tests for protein, glucose and preferably ketones
*Be alert to the presence of any wounds, bruises, scars or other indications that the woman may be being physically or sexually abused
*Be alert for signs of emotional distress and invite her to talk about them
*Instruction regarding the stage of pregnancy, the process of labor, birth, placental delivery or breastfeeding, visualizing the birth or other topics to review by way of education
*Discussion of and collection of fee payments as appropriate

One midwife I know gives each woman a massage at every visit past the 20th week of pregnancy. What you actually provide for each woman will depend upon your style and what she needs at the time. The problems listed above will be discussed, in detail, either in relation to the trimester in which they most commonly appear or in the section entitled Problems That Can Occur at any Time. Basic information about each of them can be obtained by looking them up in the appropriate chapter elsewhere in this book. The skills are covered in the section on Basic Midwifery Skills for Pregnancy.

Language: It is important to remember the exquisite sensitivity of the pregnant woman. What you say and how you say it can have a profound impact on the attitudes and beliefs she brings to her birth experience. Be sure to praise her, letting her know at every step how well she is doing and how ideally suited she is to birth her baby. For example, instead of telling a woman her pelvis is adequate, you might say "Wow, you have a wonderful pelvis; its perfect." Instead of referring to risk factors, you could call them special circumstances. Instead of telling a woman what she is doing wrong, tell her what she is doing right first and then, when appropriate, direct her toward the healthier choice, i.e., "I see are drinking more water and less sodas, wonderful. Also, you ate salad on Tuesday, and that's really great. It would be fantastic if you ate a salad like that every day."

Remember too, that the subconscious does not hear negatives such as not, don't, etc. So instead of telling a woman to focus on not tearing or not bleeding after birth (which the subconscious understands as an instruction to tear and bleed!!), frame it in positive language "see your perineum stretching as the baby is born and returning to its original shape like a piece of strong elastic. You can get huge, as big as you need to stretch to let your baby out. Your uterus will continue to contract after the birth, the placenta will be born and there will be very little blood," and so on. In short, think before you speak! (Whitridge; Klaus, 1995)

Keeping an eye out for toxemia: In an otherwise healthy young woman, one of the primary purposes of prenatal care is preventing and detecting toxemia. Read the chapter on How Pregnancy Impacts Maternal Anatomy and Physiology in the A & P section for an understanding of the etiology of toxemia. The following things place a woman at higher risk for developing toxemia:

*History of drug or oral contraceptive use before pregnancy. Either places extra nutritional demands on the body and depletes vitamins and minerals. One survey of women who had been toxemic showed 79% had been on oral contraceptives prior to conceiving (Kuse, 1990)

*Severe nausea or vomiting for an extended time in early pregnancy. (Offset this by forcing easily digested protein rich foods frequently—low blood sugar is usually the problem.) Nausea and vomiting may reappear as the liver becomes more compromised and toxemia severe.

*It is a myth that toxemia is primarily a disease of first-time mothers. (Brewer, 1982, p. 5) A woman with many mouths to feed and little money to do it is just as much at risk.

*Poor appetite (explain that eating is always a life or death must!)

*Teenagers (because they often have poor diets and are still growing, especially those 16 or younger.)

*Poor women (suggest they apply for food subsidy programs such as WIC and food stamps and buy cheap, nutritious foods).

*Multiple gestation (increase the dietary intake as soon as multiples are suspected).

*Digestive or eating disorders (colitis, anorexia, etc.). Be sure not to confuse simple heartburn, indigestion or gall bladder irritability with the much more serious epigastric (upper right-quadrant) pain and sometimes tenderness that signals liver impairment and severe toxemia. If a woman is seriously ill, there will be other clues.

*Previous liver-related disease (hepatitis, mononucleosis, history of jaundice, etc.). Recommend Dandelion root tincture and choline supplementation to strengthen the liver. Spring Dandelion is a most more liver tonic than roots gathered in the fall, which produce a gentler tonic and can be used in cases of previous liver compromise. Choline (500 mg. daily) can be taken along with a B-complex vitamin to prevent B^{12} deficiency, which can result from taking choline alone. Note that generalized itching in pregnancy may indicate a compromised liver.

*Any woman on a low salt or low calorie diet (i.e., Scarsdale, etc.)

*Watch out for the trim, exercise-conscious woman who eats a basically good diet. She often has a high metabolism that increases even more in pregnancy. She may not be getting enough calories to meet her energy needs. Frequently she needs to cut her activity back and eat more to compensate. If a woman eats just one third fewer calories than she needs, she burns half her protein intake in their place!

In short, anything interfering with the liver's work or with digestion may lead to a problem. Note that liver supporting herbs and vitamins may help the liver do its job but are no substitute for the amino acids needed to manufacture blood; these can only come from adequate dietary intake.

Charting: Information should be recorded on a standard form used for prenatal visits which makes locating information after the fact easier. There are many different types of forms in use by midwives; the ones on the next two pages are the front and back of the one I have used in my practice. Except for unusual cases, this double-sided form allows you to keep the entire prenatal record on one piece of paper while allowing you space to write about specifics for each visit. An additional page consisting of lines could be used to note down any extensive discussions that take place. The checklist described in the chapter on handouts in this section will serve as a record for most topics that are routinely discussed.

Separate sheets should be included in the chart to record non-routine visits or telephone calls regarding questions or problems. You may want to design a form for this purpose and keep a few by your phone in case you get calls from women when their chart is inaccessible for some reason.

For reference and further reading:

Brewer, T, Metabolic Toxemia of Late Pregnancy, Keats Pub., New Canaan, CT, 1982.

Klaus, Phyllis, "Psyco-social etiology of symptoms of pregnancy," Midwifery Today conf., workshop, Eugene, OR, 6/18/95.

Kuse, Sabine, paper presented at National German Gyn. Congress, Hamburg, Germany, 9/11/90.

James, Dawn, "New Thoughts About Pre-eclampsia," presentation 9/15/89, Royal College of Medicine, London Eng. President, Pre-eclamptic Toxemia Society, Ty Iago, Carmel, Caernarvon, Gwynedd, LL54 7AB, Wales, England.

Whitridge, Candice, ""Prenatal care is what she does between visits," workshop, Midwifery Today conf., Eugene, OR, 6/18/95.

PRENATAL RECORD OF _____   DUE DATE _____   BLOOD TYPE/FACTOR _____

DATE/WKS. PREG.							
WEIGHT/Hemoglobin							
BP/PULSE							
U — Color/Clarity							
R — Protein/Glucose							
I — pH/Ketones							
N — Blood/Pain							
E							
EDEMA							
HEADACHES							
DIZZY/VISION?							
ILLNESS/NAUSEA							
CRAMPS/PAIN/BH							
BOWELS?							
YONI DISCHARGE							
DIET							
SLEEPING?							
EXERCISE?							
FUNDAL HT.							
FETAL POSITION							
FETAL MOTION							
EST. FETAL WT.							
FHT (+) PLACENTA Sound (O)	(·)	(·)	(·)	(·)	(·)	(·)	(·)
COMMENTS & RECOMMENDATIONS							

WEIGHT/Hemoglobin									
BP/PULSE									
U R I N E — Color/Clarity									
Protein/Glucose									
pH/Ketones									
Blood/Pain									
EDEMA									
HEADACHES									
DIZZY/VISION?									
ILLNESS/NAUSEA									
CRAMPS/PAIN/BH									
BOWELS?									
YONI DISCHARGE									
DIET									
SLEEPING?									
EXERCISE?									
FUNDAL HT.									
FETAL POSITION									
FETAL MOTION									
EST. FETAL WT.									
FHT (+) PLACENTA Sound (O)	(·)	(·)	(·)	(·)	(·)	(·)	(·)		
COMMENTS & RECOMMENDATIONS									

Childbirth Education

Educational materials:

There is a list of some of the best childbirth books in the chapter covering the Informed Disclosure/Informed Choice document. In addition to these, you may want to have some videos and a library of other books on hand in order to send women home with materials they cannot afford to buy. A good core library would start out with the books listed in the Informed Disclosure, and would also include magazines which publish midwifery and homebirth related articles such as Mothering, Midwifery Today and The Birth Gazette. Other subjects to include would be circumcision, postpartum care, immunization, a medical dictionary, as well as introductory books on herbology, homeopathy, Chinese medicine or whatever other healing modalities you may use or recommend in your practice. Cascade Health Care Products publishes a quarterly review newsletter, Imprints, which lists the most current books on many of these topics.

To set up your library, place a card in each book and invest in a date stamp or write in the due date for each book checked out. Ask the woman to give you a check for the cost of each book or video which you will hold in the chart until the items are returned. This system has worked well for many midwives—they tend to have more books returned and are able to replace any which are forgotten.

It is a good idea to invest in a few teaching aides, even if you do not plan to teach your own childbirth classes. Beautiful models of the pelvis, baby, uterus and placenta are available from Childbirth Graphics, PO Box 21207, Waco, TX 76702, (800) 299-3366. These models help tremendously in explaining the physiology of pregnancy and any procedures that might be done.

Should you encourage women to read about birth? Women vary greatly in how eager they are to read about pregnancy and birth. Generally speaking, the more well-read a woman is when she begins care, the less she needs to read more. In fact, she often needs to set aside her desire to have an intellectual grasp of the process and tune into what she is feeling about her pregnancy.

While a basic knowledge of the anatomy and physiology of pregnancy is worthwhile, too much knowledge can be a dangerous thing. Some women believe that if they only understand what will happen with their head, their fears and anxieties will somehow disappear or become less significant. This thought process hinders getting in touch with internal emotional realities regarding the pregnancy and upcoming birth. Troubleshoot this early by encouraging women to listen to guided meditation tapes, work in their garden, do yoga, pray or whatever they feel comfortable with to get in touch with their inner selves as well as their physical bodies.

Additional information can be invaluable, however, when women are faced with making choices during their pregnancy. Encourage women to utilize your library and any other resources to the fullest when deciding on any course of action—midwifery care is based on fully informed clients making their own decisions.

Prenatal childbirth classes:

As a midwife, you must decide if you feel classes are a necessary requirement for your clients and if so, where they should go for these classes. My one hour prenatals and my general dissatisfaction with all immediately local childbirth educators led me, in my practice, to leave the issue entirely up to the parents. I emphasized that, if they chose to attend, I wanted them to take classes that focused on the emotional and psychological aspects of giving birth, feeling that they could easily get the physiology background from books and from me during prenatals. In fact, prenatals often included teaching clients about various aspects of birth and discussing their personal fears, concerns and questions.

The good news about *good* classes is that each couple or woman will interact with other pregnant women and their partners and get a feel for the commonality of questions, concerns and feelings about pregnancy. It gives them an opportunity to discuss issues purely as parents with parents and to hear the previous birthing stories of other women. This can make attending classes very worthwhile. However, a bad class (one that does not support alternatives or personal responsibility-taking, or one that only reviews the most basic anatomy and breathing techniques and does not encourage interaction among class members) can be worse than no classes at all. One way to solve this dilemma is for you to teach classes to your own clients; this of course means more time, effort, and the need to round up a place to teach. Some midwives have apprentices teach childbirth classes, providing them more opportunity to form a relationship with your clients.

What kind of classes should I teach or recommend? While the traditional Lamaze classes of the 1950s are still with us in some parts of the country, the options have broadened considerably since Lamaze was first introduced to the United States. One resource for teaching your own classes (particularly appealing for Christian midwives), Teaching Natural Birth by Jan Whitcomb, could be used as a reference, along with the other recommended reading listed in the next chapter on Books, Handouts and Forms. This section will provide an overview of different educational philosophies.

Lamaze: Traditional Lamaze, also known as the psychoprophylactic method of training for childbirth, is based on developing a conditioned response during pregnancy which the woman can use during labor to deal with pain. Women will learn specific breathing techniques which become increasingly complicated as labor progresses. Much of this breathing consists of various styles of panting, puffing, blowing out and deep breathing. In conjunction with the breathing, women are taught to use light abdominal massage (effleurage) intended to send a competing, pleasurable message to the brain to inhibit the pain message the cervix is sending during a contraction.

The theory is that these techniques, plus the use of a visual focal point to be mounted on the wall at eye level, will distract the woman from her contractions, causing them to be painless (although most teachers today do not teach that labor will be entirely without pain). She is taught to push by holding her breath and bearing down on command by her care provider. While the physiological mechanism of birth is described in classes, there is no effort made to help a woman learn to tune into her body during pregnancy or labor. Rather, focus is on teaching the woman to control her behavior, but not the situation or the medical decisions being made for her. Relaxation reminders, timing of contractions and helping women remember how to breathe are jobs given to the partner. Lamaze classes are also famous for teaching women to be "good patients," with advice about how to breathe during clitorotomies, etc. Many women come out of such classes feeling that they have failed if they run out of breathing techniques and still feel pain. Lamaze teaches women to rely on techniques and does not help her get in touch with her own inner resources to cope with labor.

Lamaze classes are still the most widely available hospital-sponsored classes; they most commonly limit their discussions to birth in a hospital or birthing center with doctors or nurse-midwives. Today, many Lamaze teachers have tried to modify their approach to the breathing techniques, but most still emphasize a stylized form of breathing.

Bradley: Bradley education is the second most well-known style of childbirth education in the United States. Robert Bradley was an enthusiastic supporter of Grantly Dick-Read's ideas that fear and tension produce and enhance pain. He disagreed with the types of breath work promoted in Lamaze classes, pointing out that only animals which do not sweat pant during labor. He advocates darkness, quiet, solitude, physical comfort, relaxation, controlled deep breathing and closed eyes as important elements of coping for women in labor. The partner is taught to assist the woman in relaxing and maintaining steady, deep breaths throughout contractions as well as offering pleasant visualizations to assist her in getting through contractions. Bradley educators strongly emphasize good nutrition a-la the Brewer diet during pregnancy.

Bradley classes are sometimes offered through hospitals but are most frequently taught independently. A list of local teachers can be obtained through the American Academy of Husband Coached Childbirth, P.O. Box 5224, Sherman Oaks, CA 91413.

HypnoBirthing: This technique uses four two-hour sessions where the mother is guided to replace her fears with confidence, understand the interplay between baby and mother during birth, how to assist rather than resist birthing energy including breathing and relaxation exercises and tips for the birth partner in how to maintain a relaxed atmosphere during the birth. HypnoBirthing classes are taught by a hypnotherapist who has had additional training in these methods. Midwives whom I have talked with whose clients have used this method are enthusiastic about the results. For East coast referrals, contact HypnoBirthing Foundation, Marie Mongan, 146 Sheep Davis Rd., Pembroke, NH 03275 (603) 225-3441; for West coast referrals contact Debbie Wagner, Continental Office Park, 13333 Bel Red Road, Suite, 109, Bellevue, WA 98005-2332.

ICEA (International Childbirth Educators Association): There are ICEA teachers throughout the United States who teach an eclectic brand of childbirth education that is founded on "freedom of choice based on knowledge of alternatives." ICEA teachers vary widely in their knowledge of different alternatives in their area, although the aim of ICEA is to offer a well-rounded knowledge of all options available. ICEA has a position paper that explicitly supports homebirth with a "trained attendant" as a viable option. ICEA does not promote any particular "method" of preparation for labor (as does Lamaze); this is left to the discretion of the instructor who strives to individualize her teaching to the needs of the students. For details regarding ICEA certification or an instructor in your area, contact ICEA P.O. Box 20048, Minneapolis, MN 55420 (612) 854-8660.

Informed Homebirth/Informed Birth & Parenting: These classes focus on responsibility-taking by the parents and informed choices. The teachers are well informed about the risks and benefits of various bio-technical medical procedures and discuss them in classes. Psychological processes which accompany pregnancy are a focus of the classes, and women are encouraged to get in touch with their own inner resources as a preparation for coping with labor. Call or write Informed Homebirth/Informed Birth and Parenting, P.O. Box 3675, Ann Arbor, MI 48106, (313) 662-6857, for referrals, or contact ALACE (Association of Labor Assistants and Childbirth Educators), P.O. Box 382724, Cambridge, MA 02238 (617) 441-2500 (this is the branch that sets up training workshops) to find teachers near you.

Birth Works: This childbirth education is offered by the International Cesarean Awareness Network. The philosophy is that birth is a safe and normal life force and that women can learn to trust and believe in the body's ability to give birth. Birth Works is not a method, it recognizes that there is no one right way to labor and birth. Classes offer support to integrate mind, body and spirit, working from the belief that everyone is always doing the best that they can. By examining belief systems in a supportive environment, blocks to having healthier births can be overcome and women can learn to feel good about themselves, regardless of their birth outcome. Emphasis is placed on understanding the risks, benefits and

646

alternatives to routine medical procedures. Women learn to decrease their chances of having a surgical delivery by developing confidence in decision making skills and learning about the effects on birth of factors such as nutrition, exercise, drugs and smoking cigarettes. To locate instructors in your area contact Birth Works, 42 Tallowwood Dr., Medford, NJ, 08055 (609) 953-9380.

What to look for in a childbirth educator: There are pros and cons to having clients attend childbirth classes outside of your practice. The biggest benefit is that it is one less thing for you to be responsible for, and, believe me, a full time midwifery practice is a BIG responsibility! On the down side, you need to find out if the teacher's philosophy of childbirth education is anywhere near your own, so that your clients are not hearing one thing from you and another in class. This is especially important when you need clients to be prepared for homebirth. This preparation is different in many respects than that which prepares clients for hospital birth. If the instructor has little or no knowledge of homebirth or independent midwifery practices, she may have little to offer your clients. Also ask if she has experience in teaching women who have disabilities (are teaching space and bathroom facilities accessible?), women planning to put their babies up for adoption, teenagers, lesbians, or women from different cultural backgrounds.

One way to find out more about a specific instructor is to interview her. Get her to go over what she covers in classes and ask honest questions about her feelings regarding homebirth and midwifery care outside the medical model. You surely don't want your clients attending classes taught by someone who really feels they are making a dangerous choice for themselves.

Nutrition	Prenatal testing
Emotional and psychological issues	When to do internal exams
Exercise	Sexually transmitted diseases
Fears	Sexuality during pregnancy/postpartum
Death of the mother/baby	Breastfeeding
Partner's fears	Baby care
Intuition	Newborn exam and appearance
Anatomy & physiology of pregnancy & birth	Cord care
	Circumcision
Normal changes and discomforts of pregnancy and postpartum	Immunization
	Breathing methods for labor (if any)
Conception and fetal development	Cesarean prevention
Complications of pregnancy, labor & birth	Making a birth plan
Minor discomforts of pregnancy	Partner's role during labor/birth/postpartum
Feelings regarding possible transport	Birth of the baby
Coping with labor	Birth of the placenta
Interventions during pregnancy, labor & birth	Pushing: how and when
	Impact of pregnancy and new baby on couples' relationship
Ultrasound and Doppler fetascopes	
X-rays	Parenting

Ask their views on these topics and the relative importance of each one. For instance, how do they teach nutrition? How often is it mentioned during classes? (Of course, the more something is mentioned the more important it is. Ideally, nutrition should come up frequently in the context of its impact on every physical aspect of pregnancy and birth). The same could be said for emotional factors, fears, and other concerns. Is death discussed, or does she avoid such topics to keep from upsetting the students? Ask the teacher to give you an example of how they might teach certain topics, for instance cord prolapse or pushing.

In general it is a good plan to avoid hospital-based classes all together. In some rural areas, they may be your only choice, in which case you have no options for classes other than your own. The same holds true for any childbirth educator who is hired to teach by a private physician, birthing center, or other third party, unless that third party is a group of other midwives. The reason is that the content of such classes is often (usually) strictly controlled by the sponsoring institution or physician. Your clients, with their different choices and needs, do not need to be lulled into "good patienthood" according to the institution in question. Such classes very selectively explore "options" and these are usually presented as two or more choices that are entirely acceptable to the institutional staff and not necessarily what is in the client's or baby's best interest.

If you have narrowed down your choices of who you will recommend but still have concerns about class content, attend a few classes which you feel will offer some of the most sensitive material, such as the complications in labor class or the one that deals with death (is there a class which deals with death at all?). Do not necessarily dismiss a class because it is not comprehensive in the conventional sense of the word. The best classes focus almost entirely on feelings, thoughts and fears related to pregnancy, with clients reading about the basics on their own time. Most clients who choose homebirth are very well informed and need to "get out of their head" and deal with some of their emotional issues to be fully prepared for labor.

Sibling classes: Some areas have teachers who offer classes geared to children, perhaps offering different classes for different ages. Childbirth educators you interview should have an idea of who might be offering these, or they might do so themselves. Such classes should explain birth in simple terms and realistically describe the hard work, noises and facial expressions the children will see their mother experiencing. A discussion should cover the birth, the amniotic fluid, the placenta and the normal bleeding afterwards, as well as the children's fears and concerns.

Siblings can also be prepared by watching videos or slides of births (preferably some which show other children at birth) as well as reading books written especially for children such as Mom and Dad and I are Having a Baby by Marianne Maleki, which prepares children to be present at a birth.

<u>Books and Handouts</u>

Books: I always have clients buy a copy of <u>Special Delivery</u> by Rahima Baldwin to use as their standard reference text and resource. This way, it is not necessary to copy handouts covering general information that is already reviewed in the book. Another excellent book for this purpose is <u>Woman Centered Pregnancy and Birth</u> by Ginny Cassidy-Brinn, Francis Hornstein and Carol Downer. Both books take an honest look at medical interventions; the information is generally complete, well written and highly supportive of women taking responsibility for their decisions. However, <u>Woman Centered Pregnancy</u> is more feminist and radical than <u>Special Delivery</u> and therefore may be less well-received by some clients. <u>Essential Exercises for the Childbearing Year</u> by Elizabeth Noble is an excellent book to recommend for all types of activity-related questions arising throughout the childbearing year. Women with a history of back labor, posterior births or a family history of either will do well to read <u>Back labor No More</u> by Janie McCoy King (order from Plenary Systems, Inc. P.O. Box 181629, Dallas, TX, 75218-8629 800-841-1070, $22.85 per copy incl. post.) Women carrying twins (or more!) need to read Elizabeth Noble's excellent book <u>Having Twins</u>, which fully supports women in eating an adequate diet for multiple gestation. Rahima Baldwin and Terra Palmarini co-authored <u>Pregnant Feelings</u>, which addresses the emotional process of pregnancy and preparing for birth and Suzanne Arm's <u>Seasons of Change</u> can also help women explore their feelings and the emotional impact of their choices. (For any topics you want to emphasize, additional handouts serve to underscore your verbal advice.)

Handouts: Handouts for clients can be more or less elaborate. Some handouts you might want to consider providing for your clients are (some of these topics can be addressed in your Informed Disclosure document):

*Pre-consultation handouts (see chapter on First Contacts, Contact section)
*Fee schedule, appointment days, phone numbers, how to reach you
*Childbirth educators in your area of whom you approve
*Other midwives in your area (to support truly informed choice)
*Information from your state organization or local government regarding what credentials are offered and how clients might file complementary comments, suggestions or complaints
*Possible warning/danger signs which may show up during pregnancy
*An outline of your childbirth classes and what will be covered (if you teach your own) and additional fees for classes (if applicable)
*How to use herbs, homeopathic remedies or other remedies you might prescribe or recommend
*Diet diaries and nutrition information (for example, I recommend you enlarge and xerox the portion tables given in this book so they can

be posted in the client's kitchen)

*A drawing of a baby head down and flexed (LOA). Be sure the umbilical cord and the baby's hands are not up near the head in this drawing. You might include several copies of the same drawing to cut out and post around the house to help the mother visualize how the baby is ideally positioned during pregnancy.

*Recipes for special food items you might recommend for women who restrict their diet

*Responsibility agreement (see chapter on Money Matters, Contact section)

*A copy of the prenatal record form so that women may record their care as they go. Another alternative is to give women their own charts to bring to each visit, or to copy their chart for them at the last postpartum visit.

*A supply list for the birth

*A discussion checklist

*A form to record all lab results so you can easily compare results from one series of tests to the next

Birthing kits: A list of what you expect clients to have on hand for the birth is very important. You'll want them to have it soon after care begins so they have plenty of time to gather these things before the birth. Each midwife has her own preferences for the content of such lists, and yours will in part depend upon your resources in time and money. For example, you can pay for sterile exam gloves out of your own pocket, or you can have parents pick up the tab by including exam gloves on your list of supplies for them to order. Some midwives buy items wholesale and make up their own birthing kits which they sell separately or include in the cost of the birth. If you run a birthing center, have lots of help or just feel that you have the resources to assemble your own birthing kits, great. If not, Cascade HealthCare Products will gladly assemble custom kits for you. Here is a list of things you might want to consider including in such a kit:

Disposable underpads (number & size?) or old or cheap new towels & washcloths	Breast pump (esp. first-time mothers)
Cotton baby hat (1 or 2)	Sterile exam gloves (number, size, singles or pairs?)
Oral thermometer	Plastic or metal cord clamp
Infant rectal thermometer	Herbal tinctures
4 X 4 sterile gauze pads (#?)	Homeopathic remedies
2 oz. sterile bulb syringe	Flexible drinking straw
8 oz. to 1 qt. Peri bottle	Herbal sitz bath packs (number?)
Antiseptic scrub	Sanitary belt
Maternity sanitary pads (2 or 3 doz.)	Textbooks
Plastic mattress cover	

Of course, the more you include in your kit, the more expensive it will be for your clients to purchase. If finances are tight, you could have a streamlined kit and provide such things as gloves and delete such things as textbooks and the breast pump (an expensive item). In addition to what should be ordered, the parents will also need a checklist of what to gather from around the house and a reminder list of things to have for the birth (foods, film for the camera, etc.). An example list is included at the end of this chapter.

Things to discuss: You will be greatly assisted by designing a discussion checklist for your practice. A form like this can be placed in each chart and be checked off as pregnancy advances. An example follows at the end of this chapter. Many of the topics which need to be addressed prenatally will be discussed either in this volume or in the other volumes of this text. For example, infant circumcision, vaccinations, details about labor, placental delivery and so forth are all covered in the other volumes. Due to the scope of this text, it is impossible to include details of all the relevant topics in this text as well. As you move through your study of the sections on each trimester, you will note that a few pertinent topics for discussion are listed at the end of each overview chapter. However, you should always review the discussion checklist for more ideas about relevant topics which should be addressed.

<u>Medical supplies</u>: can be gathered separately or ordered in a kit (see separate sheet).

<u>Herbal remedies</u>: if desired, may be ordered from either of these locations:

Equinox Botanicals, Rt. 1, Box 71, Rutland, OH 45775
Herb Pharm, Box 116, Williams, OR 97554

<u>Miscellaneous supplies</u>: be sure to have on hand the following for the birth:
small bottle olive oil (baby care)
cotton balls & Q tips (cord care)
Bulb of garlic & sea salt (for herbal bath)
1 bottle of echinacea tincture (cord care)
plastic garbage bags
white, unscented toilet paper & facial tissue
cornstarch, arrowroot (or other non-talc baby powder)
abrasive cleanser (Comet, etc. for cleaning tub)
sanitary belt (if desired)
film (if photos are desired)
Vitamin E, 400 IU capsules
30C arnica, 30C bellis perennis
Astrolube, K-Y or similar oil-free product for perineal massage
Hypoallergenic lanolin (nipple care)

If you like you may also
get extra herbal sitz packs
in your birth kit or comfrey
leaf from the health food
store to make more herbal
baths after yours run out for
after the birth.

<u>Other necessary things to prepare, borrow or gather from your home</u>:
old cloth diapers (for meconium)
loose gowns, heavy socks etc. (for labor)
humidifier or vaporizer (for baby, esp. in cold weather)
baby clothes, hats & socks—cotton, wool or silk (wash everything)
8 cotton receiving blankets (for immediately after birth)
6 to 12 old washcloths & bath towels
bright flashlight
list of pertinent phone numbers by phones/in wallet (Ob/Ped. backup, hospital, private ambulance service)
very firm mattress (place board underneath or mattress on floor if necessary)
enough food for at least 4 days postpartum for your family
food for midwives (vegetarian)
full tank of gas in a car in good condition (for transport)
crock pot (for hot compresses at birth)
2 cookie sheets, large shallow baking pans or trays (for instruments)
lots of ice, juices and light food for labor
sibling support person for labor, birth & postpartum
postpartum help/meals from family & friends
clock that keeps exact time
old wool blankets or plastic felt-backed table cloth (to protect carpet in birthing room)
1 bottle peroxide (for blood spot removal, if necessary)

<u>The house where you birth needs to have</u>:
working stove
heat & hot water
running water
telephone
places for midwives to
 sleep

<u>To make bed for the birth</u>:
-place fitted & flat sheet on bed, tuck in
 edges all around
-cover these with one of the following:
 plastic drop cloth, shower curtain, split
 garbage bags, fitted plastic sheet--secure
-make bed again using old fitted and flat sheets

652   <u>Discussion/Handout Checklist</u>

Name_____   Due date_____

Handouts:
__Responsibility form
__Informed Disclosure/returned__
__Birth supply catalogue
__herb prep. chart
__Circumcision info.
__Mothering form
__Birthing kit order form
__Misc. birth items list
__Information handout
__Diet info.
__Diet diary sheets
__Brewer diet article
__Vegan protein sources
__Soy or Almond milk recipe

8-16 weeks:
__Responsibility form returned
__Explain __BP __FHT __Fundal Ht.
__Nutrition __vitamins
__Prenatal fetal testing
__Activity & exercise
__Pelvic floor exercises
__Body mechanics
__Minor discomforts
__Deodorant/fluoride
__Call schedule/backup
__Beeper & phone numbers
__Lab work ordered
__Discuss birth kit
__tinc. __H bath __ Breast pump
__Visualize __vtx __birth
__Sex during pregnancy
__Back-up situation

16-24 weeks:
__Childbirth classes
__Work/job
__Toning contractions
__Labor support
__Glucose testing Y N
__28 wk Rhogam Y N
__Discuss cultures for chlam/strep
__RH antibody screen
__Lab results

24-32 weeks:
__Siblings at birth
__Recheck hemoglobin
__Breastfeeding
__Circumcision __Moyel's #
__Immunizations
__Directions to house
__Danger signs cntx/bld/H2O/cord
__Backup? __Ped. __OB

__Discuss Evening Primrose oil
__Discuss vit. K supplements
__Birth kit ordered?
__Gathering birth supplies?

34-38 weeks:
__Internal exam
__Birth certificate
__Start EP oil (36 wks)
__Start vit. K sup. (36 wks)
__Recheck hemoglobin
__Schedule homevisit
__Rh antibody screen
__Discuss labor/food/rest
__PP procedures/uterine cks.
__When to call in labor
__Help after baby comes
__Newborn care/diapers
__Jaundice
__Newborn vit. K
__Newborn eye prophylaxis
__Newborn screening tests (PKU, etc.)
__Childhood vaccinations
__Rh- cord blood tests arranged?
__Rhogam arrangements?

Homevisit:
__Food
__Midwife sleeping space?
__Help after birth
__Siblings
__Check birth room
__Check birth supplies
__Baby clothes/blankets/hat
__Phone list
__Route to hospital
__Visualizing birth?

38-41 weeks:
__Carbohydrate loading
__PKU test ordered?
__Review dates
__Fetal well-being
__Tests/fetal well-being

42+ weeks:
__Fetal well-being
__Due date review
__Tests/fetal well-being
__Induction techniques

Other topics discussed:
__ _____
__ _____
__ _____

Books/handouts borrowed:
__ _____
__ _____
__ _____

After birth:
__Temp. mom/baby
__Bleeding mom/baby
__"Sick baby" signs
__RDS (mec./preemie)
__Infant feeding
__Cord care
__Perineal care
__Breast care
__Hemorrhoid care
__Milk supply/demand
__Maternal diet/rest
__"Sick mom" signs
__Vitamin E
__Afterbirth pains
__Ped. visit pp?
__Delayed onset heart prob.
__Urate deposits in diaper
__Yoni bleeding in girls
__Baby breast engorgement
__Birth certificate
__Blood drawn mom/baby if Rh-
__Rh- blood to lab

Postnatal visits:
__Work/job
__Ped. care
__$?
__Postdated cks.
__Needs bill? amt._____
__Discuss gyn. care
__Rh- lab results/Tel#_____
__Rhogam administered

Postpartum choices of parents:
Circumcision: Y N (religious other)
Vit. K: Y N oral__ injec.__
        __mw advice __parent's choice
Eye Prophylaxis Y N type_____
        __mw advice __parent's choice
PKU test Y N Retest Y N
Rhogam Y N Reason refused_____

Other topics discussed:
__ _____
__ _____
__ _____

The Family, Friends and Prenatal Care

Partners: A woman's partner is usually her primary support person throughout her pregnancy and birth. Ideally the partner will attend all prenatal visits so that a relationship can develop with both parents; some midwives insist on this. For some people this presents a hardship, since fitting appointments in around job responsibilities is not always easy. However, co-parenting can begin during pregnancy and helping the partner to feel involved and valuable to the process can pave the way for it to continue after the birth. Attendance at prenatal exams, in my opinion, becomes essential if the partner has misgivings or is hesitant about the care you may provide. Any decisions that must be made, as well as normal variations, can be discussed with both parents on the spot, thus minimizing the possibility that the partner will feel left out of important choices. This also allows the partner the opportunity to see first hand the type of care you provide. If the woman is also receiving care from a bio-technical physician, the partner should accompany the woman to those visits as well so that the quality of care can be compared and mutual decisions discussed with the physician. If you suspect domestic violence, this is one situation where arranging a visit with the mother alone is helpful. She may be willing to disclose her circumstances in a private visit. (See the chapter on Physical, Sexual and Ritual Abuse Issues in the section on Sustaining Health and Well-being for more information.)

Siblings: Most parents who have other children will initiate a conversation about their children's relationship to the birth. If not, you should open this discussion with questions regarding whether the parents want their children involved during the prenatal period. Regardless of their wishes in that regard, encourage them to bring their other children to at least one prenatal appointment so that you can meet them in your setting. Then, at the home visit, you can meet them again. While some parents will want to bring their other children to consultation or initial visits, most will agree that waiting to bring them when care is established and visits are shorter is best. Having child-proof furniture and a toy box in your office or waiting area will make children feel more welcome and also eliminate your worries about the furniture. Also, be sure lancets, urine test strips, paper cups, facial tissues and other interesting objects that are potentially harmful or destructible are out of reach.

The behavior of children varies a great deal, and you will find that some will be quite unruly during appointments and others will play quietly or even ask questions. If a woman has many children, she may try to come alone, since prenatals may be one of the few times someone is focusing exclusively on her. If she hasn't thought of this and her children are very demanding, you might suggest this to her as an option.

Even in families choosing homebirth, sometimes children are abused. Be aware of any unusual behavior or injuries in children or comments from parents

654

which suggest abusive attitudes. This delicate issue is addressed in detail in Volume III of this text.

Different ages: The age of the children will impact how and whether they want to be involved in learning about the pregnancy or be present at the birth. Typically, children toddler age and younger are still emotionally and psychologically fused with their mother. Many may still be nursing. Mom's mood and desire (or lack thereof) to have them present during appointments will greatly influence their own responses. Young children often react to what is being done to their mothers, especially if they perceive that it will be harmful or it seems threatening in any way; for example, a child may burst into tears when you take her mother's blood pressure. Having old equipment in the toy box for the child to examine is helpful in this regard, although many children are mistrustful of you and the equipment in general. In addition, small children frequently want to empty the contents of your prenatal bag as well, so be careful to keep it out of reach. As pregnancy advances, small children know that babyhood for them is about to end and often become clingy and needy. Talking to the mother about how young children are adapting to the idea of a baby is an important part of prenatal care.

Children between the ages of 4 and 10 are usually quite interested in the goings-on at prenatal visits and will be most enthusiastic about listening to the baby, feeling the position and other curiosities. Be sure to use language they can understand and point out the things that are normal about the changes their mother is going through. Parents often get their children dolls so they can have a baby of their own. Dolls which depict birth and a number of books describing birth for children, such as How You Were Born by Joanna Cole. (A local women's book store or Cascade HealthProduct's Birth and Life book catalogue will have others.) The response of older children who are approaching puberty can be a very mixed bag. Some will, of course, be interested, but they may be shy about asking questions and at times embarrassed by their mother's exposure during exams. Be sensitive to this and talk to the child during appointments about any questions they may have. Boys in particular may not want to have much to do with the whole affair. However, letting boys see for themselves the result of sexual interactions can be very worthwhile. Likewise, girls will know exactly what they are in for if they choose to be sexually irresponsible. Many older children may want to be involved right from the start, as they will be taking a fair amount of responsibility for the new baby.

Children at birth: Talk to the parents about whether they feel comfortable with the idea of the children being present at the birth. Some parents will not want their children present; even so, it is a good idea to encourage all parents to educate their children regarding the birth process. It is helpful to have videos and picture books on birth in your lending library that parents can share with their children at home. If the parents are open to the idea, the children should be asked if they want to be present, and their wishes should be respected. Children can be given jobs such as being in charge of snacks and drinks, choosing baby's first outfit, making signs for after the birth. Many parents buy each child a present from the new baby, to be opened after the birth; this is especially nice for young siblings. (See the chapter on Childbirth Education in this section and the chapter on The Home Visit in the Third Trimester section for more suggestions.)

Asking older children about their feelings or concerns regarding family expansion can help them feel included when the family dynamic is about to undergo a tremendous change which will impact them. Helping children feel valuable to the process, while not pushing them into adult level responsibilities, is often the best way that you, as a midwife, can support family expansion.

Relatives and friends: Sometimes women bring relatives or friends with them to appointments. In most cases this is not a problem as long as the woman feels comfortable with their participation. However, when the accompanying relative is the woman's mother and especially if there is never a time to see the woman privately, this can be a problem, because the mother/daughter relationship and how the daughter really feels about her mother's presence may not come to light. In such cases, tactfully arrange a time to see the woman alone or with her partner so that you can find out more about the mother/daughter dynamic and in what ways it does or does not support the woman. Depending upon what you find out, support the woman in being truthful with her mother about the level of participation she would like.

656

Using Technological Diagnostic Techniques and Routine Remedies

Our connection with the women and the babies we care for during the process of pregnancy and our intuitive sense of what is going on with individual women are essential components of competent midwifery care. The use of technology undermines this connection in several ways. For the inexperienced midwife, it can seem that machines, Doppler fetascopes and the like, know more than she does. She does not learn to trust or hone her own skills as finely; not learning this early on in practice will make it harder to learn them well and trust them later on. The liberal use and recommendation of technology encourages women to focus outside themselves on experts and machines for the health of their pregnancy and the well-being of their baby. *The mother is the only real care provider for her unborn baby; with the right kind of support to tune in to her baby and her body, her intuitive sense of fetal well-being can be trusted in most cases.* As midwives, we constantly underscore this vitally empowering piece of wisdom by focusing on preventive care and sustaining maternal well-being with advice about how women can stay emotionally, psychologically and spiritually connected to the process taking place in their bodies, to maintain good nutrition and exercise patterns and to eliminate the use of drugs and substance abuse. These are the only factors which really make a difference in most cases regardless of what tests reveal.

Since none of the technology being used on pregnant women has been conclusively proven safe for either mother or baby, it will be prudent for you to resort to the use of technology only when clearly indicated. No directly applied electronic or invasive technology (other than drawing blood) should be routinely used to aid in the diagnosis of problems. If all manual and nontechnological means have been exhausted and the cause of a problem is still unclear, technology may then be reasonably resorted to. The parents should understand why you are taking this conservative approach in the face of the larger medical community which uses technology wantonly, and implicitly or outright declares it as safe. While each midwife and mother will have to decide for themselves exactly how technology can be appropriately applied in any given situation, here are the guidelines I've used in my practice for years.

Ultrasound: Today the most commonly applied technology is the use of ultrasound for auscultating the fetal heart and providing images of the fetus *in utero*. The mother should be clearly informed that Doppler ultrasound is used in electronic fetascopes and exposes the baby to a continuous ultrasound beam. Prenatally:

*a Doppler may be used to detect a fetal heart beat if no movement has been felt/no fetal heart heard by 22 weeks and fundal growth is questionable.

*a Doppler may be used to evaluate a suspected intrauterine death

Even though using a Doppler may be quick and easy, a woman who understands that they put out more intense ultrasound can make an informed decision to go ahead or forego this in favor of less intense exposure via an imaging ultrasound. While many physicians are enthusiastic about using ultrasound imaging routinely in pregnancy, there is no evidence that this is of any benefit whatsoever (Wagner, 1994). Diagnostic (imaging) ultrasound can be considered to further evaluate the possibilities of:

*Suspected fetal abnormalities
*The presence of twins and their position near term, if unclear
*Suspected breech presentation if unclear with palpation alone
*Suspected cervical or pelvic obstruction (previa, tumors, etc.) or other intrauterine abnormalities, especially if accompanied by bright red bleeding
*Suspected missed abortion
*Suspected fetal demise
*Suspected size/dates discrepancies that have not responded to nutritional adjustments

In addition, ultrasound is used in the following testing situations:

*A Biophysical Profile ultrasound exam, may be recommended in pregnancies carried past 42 wks. This test evaluates fetal well-being using five parameters: movement, heart rate, respiratory efforts and volume of amniotic fluid. Placental well-being is also included at some testing sites. For women with a history of postdatism and healthy babies this need not be routinely recommended.
*Non-stress tests which correlate fetal heart rate variability with fetal movement may be recommended whenever there is a question about fetal well-being due to maternal history or current observations which cannot be cleared up with office procedures

It should be recognized by the midwife and explained to the parents in no uncertain terms that there is a known risk with x-ray diagnosis in pregnancy and an unknown risk to mother and fetus with diagnostic ultrasound. In choosing ultrasound examination this unknown risk must be carefully weighed against the anticipated benefit to the immediate situation. Recommend that the mother discuss her safety concerns with the technician (who will not be likely to share her concerns at all), and that she allow ultrasound exposure only long enough to evaluate the conditions in question. All the tests mentioned above are covered in

658

detail in Diagnostic Tests.

Refusing tests and technology: If medical personnel are assuring a woman of the safety of some technology which she does not want to use, she can say "I refuse to give my consent," which legally binds them to stop what they are doing. She can also politely ask them to put their assurances of safety in writing and sign it before she proceeds: that should cause them to reconsider their statements.

Other diagnostic techniques: These tests commonly include amniocentesis and chorionic villi sampling (CVS). Less commonly, percutaneous umbilical cord sampling, fetoscopy, home uterine activity monitoring, vibroacoustic stimulation (used in conjunction with ultrasound) and the contraction stress test may be recommended by medical model providers. As a midwife you need to understand the implications of these tests, their relevance to genetic and other problems and to whom the tests are normally recommended. All this information can be found in Diagnostic Tests. Other laboratory procedures are covered in the chapter Ordering Baseline Laboratory Tests included in the Initiating Contact and Establishing Care section.

Using remedies routinely in practice: Another area of debate is the routine use of any therapeutic modality. For some midwives this means routinely recommending anything, such as vitamins, herbs, homeopathic remedies or other substances. This school of thought adheres to the principle that pregnancy is a natural process and need not be subjected to routine interference, regardless of how benign it is thought to be. To routinely recommend remedies is to undermine a woman's belief in her own body and ability to give birth without outside interference. Other midwives regularly recommend that women begin taking certain supplements, herbs or homeopathic remedies at various points, with the intent of providing optimal physical support for the pregnancy and upcoming birth. This school of thought takes into account the fact that women are usually not eating organic foods, live in a polluted environment and are surrounded by a culture that is fearful of birth. Herbs and supplements are seen as a way to provide the body with the raw materials it needs to meet the increased demands of pregnancy. Homeopathic remedies are used by some midwives as a way of centering and strengthening the mind, body, emotions and spirit of the birthing woman. You will have to decide for yourself what seems appropriate in each case. Various remedies routinely recommended by some midwives are included in the text as examples of how remedies can be used for these purposes.

References and further reading:
Wagner, Marsden, Pursuing the Birth Machine, ACE Graphics, Australia, 1994.

659

Relating to the Baby During the Prenatal Period

While I fully support the philosophy that the baby and mother are physiologically one being, there are still two consciousnesses to consider when you provide care. As the baby moves from the spiritual world into its physical body it becomes more and more aware of external influences as the pregnancy advances. This is reflected by the baby's increasing ability to see, hear and respond to outside stimuli. As the midwife, you will be one of the people with whom the baby will develop a consistent relationship prior to birth.

From the onset of care, whenever I come into contact with the baby, I talk to the baby about what I am doing, how it is growing, what position it needs to be in, etc. I give the baby positive verbal feedback to get it used to the sound of my voice, to let it know what is happening, and so that, in the event of a problem during the birth, we have already established a relationship. This lets the baby know that such activities as palpation and listening for heart tones are not just random pokes from the big world outside but are due to the care and interest of a particular individual. If a problem arises during prenatal care, I tell the baby what is needed (for example, it is easiest to come out head first). If the baby won't cooperate, I consider that the baby may be trying to tell me something and proceed from there (perhaps the cord is around the neck, making it, in fact, easier to be breech).

I have found that it sets up a psychic connection with the baby to relate to it as a sentient and sensitive being right from the start. I feel much more in tune throughout the pregnancy, the labor and the birth, and have had experiences which bear this out. Try it and explore your own experiences in this light.

References and further reading:

Church, Dawson, Communing With the Spirit of Your Unborn Child, Aslan Pub.,San Leandro, CA, 1988.
Noble, Elizabeth, Primal Connections, Simon & Schuster, 1993.
Schwartz, Leni, The World of the Unborn, Richard Marek, Pub., New York, 1980.

Maintaining Continuity of Care

Full continuity of care benefits everyone concerned in the care-giving process. For you, it provides uninterrupted intuitive connection with the mother and baby so that you are maximally tuned in during pregnancy and prepared to continue this connection at the time of birth. For the woman, it provides the same kind of connection and eliminates her concerns about who will attend her birth. This describes an ideal situation from the point of view of the practice. However, we must balance our personal needs with our needs to connect with our clients. Most of us, at some point or another, need to take a break. It is healthy and desirable to take vacations and mental health days, and you may occasionally be sick. If you have established a group practice, continuity of care will be even more of a concern, for the more people you work with, the more likely it is that at least two or more midwives will be seeing a woman at various points during her care.

The organization of your practice should be made clear to women at the onset of care. She should be told outright if she will have any say in selecting the midwife with whom she feels most comfortable, or if she will have to take whoever is on call for her prenatal exams, pregnancy emergency or birth. Some midwives in group practice minimize this issue by assigning at least one primary care midwife to each woman. In this case another midwife or apprentice may also attend prenatals or the birth, but at least the woman knows she can depend upon one stable member of her birth team. Often an apprentice can be assigned as well, giving the woman two attendants she can count on. Other midwives inform women that they have a call rotation, which means one of several midwives may attend her birth based on who is on call at that time. In this case, each midwife who may attend a woman should make every effort to be involved in at least one prenatal visit before the woman is due. Your policy regarding special requests a woman may make for a particular midwife should be included in your Informed Disclosure document or somewhere else in writing as well as in your verbal discussions upon initiation of the care relationship. That way, the woman knows what the policy is and doesn't feel personally rejected if your practice makes no allowances for special requests of this nature.

One way to bridge the gap between total continuous care and rotating call is for the woman to write a Prenatal and Birth Choice Plan to place in her chart. For example, she might state that she wants someone else to weigh her at every visit and not tell her the result. This would be discussed beforehand, along with other requests. A written Birth Plan should include all relevant details (who will be at the birth, a bath for the baby or herself afterwards, how does she feel about the timing of cord clamping and cutting, does she have position preferences, hospital-related issues should transport be necessary, etc.). This saves each midwife from having to ask the same questions; it not only fosters the mother's sense that she is getting consistent care from midwife to midwife, but will also help in not loosing track of her individual needs in the shifting of midwives' schedules.

661

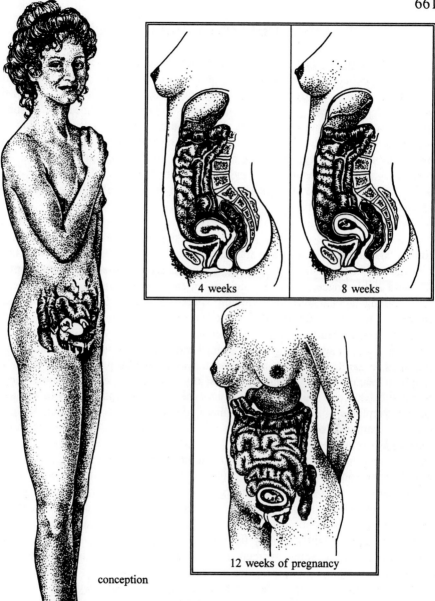

conception

4 weeks

8 weeks

12 weeks of pregnancy

PRENATAL CARE: The First Trimester
(From the first day of the last menstrual period
through the 14th week of pregnancy)

Prenatal Care During Weeks 1 Through 14

An Overview of the First Trimester: Although on the surface, it doesn't appear that much is changing during the first 14 weeks of pregnancy, a lot *is* happening within the mother's body to accommodate new life at this time. A woman may want to know if she is pregnant the day after she ovulates, especially if she has been consciously trying to conceive. (This is a bit early to tell, so she will have to wait a week or two.) After the first day of her next period is missed she may either try a home pregnancy test or come to you for testing. Order a *Beta*-pregnancy blood test, as it will be the most sensitive to use at this very early stage. This test is positive 8 to 10 days after conception or 4 days after the expected onset of menstruation.

As the conceptus implants and early growth continues, the cells which will become the placenta are already sending out signals to the mother's body in the form of hormones. The most dramatic change she will experience will be the cessation of her menstrual periods, an event charged with excitement, happiness, fear and ambivalence. Morning sickness, increased urination, breast changes and food cravings appear over the following weeks. By the eighth week of pregnancy (6 weeks gestation), the mother's blood volume is just beginning to expand in response to the need to support the placenta (which is still very tiny at this point). She may also be experiencing mood swings and a general unsettledness about being pregnant, regardless of how much she may want to be pregnant. Fatigue is a common complaint in the early months; my midwifery partner commented that when she felt tired she *had* to lie down wherever she was and go to sleep. At times, symptoms of early pregnancy may make her feel like she is sick or that she is on an emotional roller coaster. Your advice during these early weeks can help her work through her feelings as well as make appropriate nutritional choices so that these symptoms are minimally bothersome.

From conception onward the uterus undergoes dramatic changes in size, shape and tissue volume; from an organ weighing just a few ounces to one that weighs about two pounds near term. The increase in uterine muscle mass accounts for most of this weight. Uterine changes prompt benign, usually painless toning contractions and slightly crampy ligament stretching, both of which begin even at this early stage. Some women may also note some light spotting which accompanies implantation; therefore it is important for women to realize that mild cramps and a little bleeding can, in fact, be a sign of pregnancy and occur often. In most cases the uterus will begin to make an appearance just over the horizon of her pubic bone at the end of this twelve week period. Even before this occurs, most women will have begun to feel "different," as the uterus enlarges, displacing the abdominal contents upwards. You can point out even more subtle changes such as those which occur in the color of the cervix and yoni which you might note during your initial physical exam. These changes are discussed in the chapter on Early Signs of Pregnancy later in this section.

Spacing visits during the first trimester: Generally, most women do not begin to seek care until they have missed a period. Many factors can interfere with a woman seeking care early on, and you won't hear from some women until late in their first trimester. This seems to be more true of women who have already had at least one baby.

Ideally, the consultation visit takes place sometime during the first six weeks, the initial visit around 8 weeks (drawing blood for initial lab tests at that time), with the next visit at 12 weeks of pregnancy. Some midwives do the consultation visit and then postpone the initial visit and physical exam until the woman reaches her twelfth week of pregnancy. This is to better ensure that the pregnancy is well established (i.e. that no early miscarriage will occur) before undertaking care. If a woman has a history of early pregnancy complications (especially ectopic pregnancy) her initial exam should be done as soon as she decides to come to you for care. If a woman waits until 12 weeks for her initial, make sure nutritional information and exercise during pregnancy have been thoroughly discussed at the consultation visit. If a medical condition exists which makes lab values more critical, be sure baseline lab tests are done prior to the eighth week of pregnancy. When full prenatal care is begun during the first trimester, visits are normally scheduled every three to four weeks.

Early pregnancy care: Midwifery care during the first trimester of pregnancy should ideally encompass the following points and activities:

> *Having the consultation visit
> *Establishing if the woman is truly pregnant via testing if she feels unsure or if there are questions regarding possible pathological processes taking place and this has not already been done (see Diagnostic Tests for test options)
> *Performing the initial history-taking visit and physical exam
> *Obtaining baseline laboratory values
> *Establishing a nutrition plan for pregnancy which meets the woman's specific needs (see separate chapters in the section on Sustaining Health and Well-being During Pregnancy)
> *Discussing vitamin supplements, especially folic acid (see separate chapter on Supplements in Sustaining Maternal and Fetal Well-being)
> *Giving the mother informational handouts, as indicated
> *Having the mother obtain textbooks

Here are some details of early pregnancy visits:

From conception until week 12: Apart from the physical exam done at the time of the initial visit and the baseline lab work, there isn't much to check pertaining to the mother's pregnant condition during these weeks unless a problem should arise. Unless you use a doppler, the fetal heart can not be heard and unless you do bi-manual yoni exams at each visit, uterine enlargement cannot usually be detected abdominally until the 13th or 14th week of pregnancy. Early visits can be useful in establishing a series of baseline vital signs, but this is really not necessary in healthy young women; the baselines you obtain at the initial visit will suffice in most cases.

Regardless of when you begin full prenatal care, the woman should always know how you can be reached in the event of an emergency. At this stage, the most frequent emergency is a threatened miscarriage, which will be covered in a separate chapter in the First Trimester Problems section.

Weeks 13 to 14: Between the 12th to 14th week of pregnancy the uterus enlarges to the point where the fundus can just begin to be palpated above the pubic bone. In a woman whose uterus is very retroflexed (tipped backwards) this may be delayed until as late as the 16th week, although some uterine swelling should be detectable just above the pubic bone even in such cases. Uterine enlargement often triggers sharp crampy pains from stretching of the round ligaments; this can occur at any time from here on out. Note that symptoms of ectopic pregnancy may appear about now in women who have an interstitial implantation; severe symptoms should be thoroughly investigated before they are assumed to be benign.

At this point, women often begin to experience relief from early pregnancy nausea. They feel more "on their feet" as their blood volume begins to expand and take some of the concentrated metabolic load off the liver. Urinary frequency subsides as the uterus lifts itself up off the bladder. Appetite returns and women may find themselves very hungry. Most women are delighted at the first signs of their belly beginning to show. If you choose to use a Doppler fetascope, you should be able to hear the fetal heart easily at this point.

If you previously discussed factors regarding her work environment that need to be modified, this is a good time to find out if those changes have been made. It is also time to explore how she is feeling about her work as pregnancy advances.

Women who have a history of long, slow labors or postpartum hemorrhage can begin to drink 1 or 2 cups of Red Raspberry leaf infusion daily to provide nutrients for optimal uterine tone at term. Some midwives recommend Red Raspberry to all the women they see, as it is a nutritive, rather than strictly medicinal herb. (see the Appendix of Diagnostic Tests, for a discussion of the use of Red Raspberry during early pregnancy.)

Nutrition for early pregnancy: Now is the time to look over a woman's diet to see how she is dealing with any recommendations you made during the consultation visit. Reiterate the basic physiology of blood volume expansion and how good nutrition provides what her body needs to build more blood, which stimulates placental growth as well as transports nourishment to the baby.

Review the chapters on nutrition, give her nutrition handouts and go over her exercise and activity levels. Although the blood volume is beginning to expand after about the eighth week of pregnancy, there are less physical demands on a woman in early pregnancy than there will be later on. At this point the pregnancy itself is supported by a minimal quantity of nutrients. However, getting a good diet with adequate food intake throughout the day is important to help prevent or at least minimize the side effects of rising hormone levels from the placenta, one of which is nausea. These hormones must be metabolized by the liver; high hormonal blood levels without the benefit of an expanded blood volume (which dilutes the hormones) causes additional stress. Women are advised to follow the recommended diet as closely as possible as well as to:

*Eat to appetite
*Drink to thirst
*Salt to taste
*Eat small, frequent meals as needed
*Make sure all foods are of high nutritional value

Reassure women that their appetite will increase as pregnancy advances and not to worry too much if she can't eat all the foods on the charts now. They should use the list as a guide to make the best choices possible and as an inspiration to help select a balanced diet, emphasizing protein, fresh vegetables and calories from whole foods.

Recommendations to optimize normal birth: Beginning now, all women can be advised to begin to communicate with their baby. Visualize the baby and placenta as healthy and well oxygenated with a free floating cord. It is early to ask women to visualize the birth process, but if they ask, you can tell them to see themselves coping confidently with whatever labor brings them, the specifics of normal birth with the baby head down, facing the mother's back and flexed for delivery, the baby pink and breathing at birth, good perineal stretching and normal placental delivery with minimal bleeding, uterine contractions after the birth, and an easy postpartum and nursing experience. Affirmations can be formulated to address the woman's specific needs or beliefs about birth, either to reinforce positive ones or change those that may be unhelpful (such as women are supposed to bleed a lot after birth). Word affirmations positively and using present tense, i.e. "My body is perfectly designed to birth my baby," "My uterus clamps down after the placenta is born."

Other things to discuss:

Be sure all relevant handouts have been given to the woman and that any questions she or her partner had as a result of reading your Informed Disclosure have been answered to their satisfaction. Other things you may want to talk to her about over the course of the first couple of visits:

*Firm up financial arrangements and get back a signed financial agreement

*Explain the basics of each component of your exam, if you have not already done so

*Continue to assess her nutrition

*Remember that any symptoms she may experience such as constipation or nausea may be caused or aggravated by vitamin supplements—be sure to check this out when making a evaluation

*Discuss prenatal fetal genetic testing such as *Alpha*-fetal Protein, Chorionic Villi Sampling (CVS), and amniocentesis.

*Activity and exercise levels may need to be adjusted; be sure calorie intake is adequate for her stress level

*Pelvic floor exercises can begin now (see chapter on Exercise in the section on Sustaining Health and Well-being)

*The changes which take place in body mechanics should be explained (see chapter on Exercise, Well-being section)

*Minor discomforts need not be itemized for the woman, but should be explained as they come up. (Those problems and discomforts not covered in a particular trimester section can be found in the section entitled Problems That Can Occur at Any Time)

*Be sure each woman has your call schedule, beeper numbers, and other means of contacting you and that back-up consultation arrangements have been discussed, preferably with a practitioner who has hospital privileges

*Whenever possible, order lab work in the first trimester to obtain the most accurate baseline for future reference

*Discuss the items on the birth kit list; those which you absolutely must have her purchase and those which are not essential (if money is a problem). This can be discussed again later in pregnancy as a reminder.

Early Signs of Pregnancy

Clinical evidence of pregnancy begins to appear during the second week of gestation (the fourth week from the last menstrual period). Knowledge of these signs receives less emphasis than it used to due to the advent of better pregnancy tests and the increased use of ultrasound in early pregnancy. Since midwives are interested in preserving clinical skills regardless of technological advances, these signs are important to know. They are given here in order of appearance, keeping in mind that there is a normal variation from woman to woman as to when each sign actually appears. Almost all the signs have the name of a male doctor assigned to them; while I highly object to male names being attached to functions within the female body, for the sake of historical consistency from text to text I mention these names in parentheses. All time frames refer to weeks of pregnancy from the last menstrual period unless stated otherwise.

FIRST APPEARANCE:	SIGN/SYMPTOM	COMMENTS/OTHER POSSIBLE CAUSES
Conception & after	Basal temperature remains elevated	The corpus luteum continues to produce progesterone until the placenta can take over this function.
As early as 8 to 10 days after conception (4 days after 1st missed period)	*Beta*-pregnancy test positive	Blood test to detect level of hCG is positive.
3rd-4th week	Spotting	Implantation may result in benign bleeding.
4th week	Amenorrhoea	Other causes such as ovarian-pituitary imbalance, emotional upset, travel, fatigue, extreme weight fluctuation, going off oral contraceptives, breastfeeding or local infection must be considered. Ovulation may have occurred earlier or later than usual, delaying the onset of menses.
4th week	Morning sickness	May be due to hypoglycemia, increased circulating hormones w/out blood volume expansion having occurred yet; may also be due to food poisoning, tension, infection & a variety of diseases.
5th week	Longitudinal division of the uterine body	The uterus is divided into two parts of different size & consistency. One side becomes more elastic & may feel enlarged with a longitudinal groove between the soft & firm sides (Braun von Fernwald's sign).

FIRST APPEARANCE:	SIGN/SYMPTOM	COMMENTS/OTHER POSSIBLE CAUSES
6 weeks	Bladder symptoms	Increased frequency through the 3rd month is due to increased vascularity & pressure; usually subsides during 2nd trimester & reoccurs near term. May also be due to urinary tract infection, diuretics (herbal as well as pharmacological), tension, or diabetes.
6-8 weeks	Breast changes	Increased vascularity/heavy feeling/tingling—1st 8 weeks (also caused by oral contraceptives; may also occur just prior to menses) Nipple & areola darken—8 weeks Oil glands on areola become prominent—8 weeks (nipple changes may also be due to hormonal imbalance or prior pregnancy)
6-10 weeks (sometimes later)	Cervical & uterine softening	Cervix goes from feeling like the tip of the nose to as soft as the lips. Also seen just before onset of menses; (Goodell's Sign). Softening of the thin areas on the sides of the cervix can also be found in some women.
6 through 12 weeks	Softening of the lower uterine segment	When two fingers are inserted into the anterior fornix of the yoni & the other hand is placed behind the uterus abdominally, the fingers of both hands almost meet due to the softness of the isthmus (neck of the cervix) (Hegar's Sign). This sign is highly suggestive of pregnancy. The ease of pressing the fundus toward the cervix depends upon this softening (MacDonald's sign).
7 weeks	Palpable uterine enlargement	The uterus feels enlarged during an internal exam. At 7 weeks, its the size of an egg & tends to be globular rather than pear shaped. May also be due to tumor or fibroid growth.
8 weeks	Increased pulsation in lateral fornices of the yoni	Due to increased vascularity. May be present in other conditions. (Osiander's sign)
8 weeks	Violet-blue coloration of yoni mucus membranes	May be due to impending menstruation or pelvic engorgement of pregnancy. (Jacquemier's Sign, also called Chadwick's Sign)
8-10 weeks	Irregular uterine contour	Caused by non-central implantation; detectable on bi-manual exam. One side of the uterus is thicker than the other (Piskacek's Sign) or either the anterior or posterior wall of the uterus bulges out.
10 weeks	Vulval varicosities	If present these become apparent about now.

FIRST APPEARANCE:	SIGN/SYMPTOM	COMMENTS/OTHER POSSIBLE CAUSES
10-12 weeks	Fetal heart heard with Doppler	A fetascope can be used at about 15 weeks at the earliest.
12 weeks	Skin changes	Pigmentation changes may occur in dark skinned women such as the dark line down the abdomen called the *lina negra*. May also be caused by hormonal imbalance or effect of prior pregnancy. As the woman gains weight and her breasts enlarge, stretch marks may also appear.
12-14 weeks	Uterus can be palpated abdominally	The uterus reaches the top of the pubic bone by 12 weeks and is felt as a gentle swelling above it by approximately 14 weeks.

Some of the most important signs and symptoms of early pregnancy will be discussed below.

Cessation of Menstruation: Women rely on the disappearance of the menses to signal that they are pregnant more than any other sign. In a woman who has reliable and regular menstrual cycles and who has regular heterosexual intercourse, cessation of the menses is indeed a very good indication of pregnancy. It is important to recognize, however, that pregnancy can occur in the absence of menstrual bleeding. This might be the case in a girl prior to puberty, during lactation, with tuberculosis, stress, after curettage and after menopause.

Menstruation may also continue after conception in a few women (about 5%). Usually this bleeding is less in quantity and duration than the normal menstrual flow and happens only once. If a woman is in denial about being pregnant, the continuation of the menses can confuse the matter and result in a delay in seeking care. However, a bloody discharge can also be due to a pathologic condition such as threatened miscarriage, ectopic pregnancy, polyps, fibroids, cervical erosion, rupture of a blood vessel or diseases such as uterine cancer; such causes need to be ruled out. Other things that may also lead to amenorrhea include:

1) Variations in climate or environment
2) Fear of conception
3) Low fat-to-body weight ratio (seen most often in very slim, very active women)
4) Anorexia
5) Pathologic conditions
6) Irregular menstrual cycles (some women may become confused regarding whether they are pregnant)

Because there are many reasons why the menses may cease, it is only a presumptive sign of pregnancy, but it is certainly one of the most compelling.

Basal body temperature: It is possible to make an educated guess that a woman is pregnant if her basal temperature remains elevated for more than 16 days after ovulation if she has kept track of her basal body temperature during several previous menstrual cycles. A sustained rise of 98.8 to 99.9°F (37.1 to 37.7°C) with slight fluctuations not exceeding 0.4°F (0.2°C) in either direction is compatible with pregnancy. The diagnosis of pregnancy based on a consistently elevated basal body temperature is correct in about 97% of cases.

Pregnancy tests: The first trimester is the most likely time when a woman would appear to be pregnant but in reality have a medical condition other than pregnancy that is mimicking its symptoms. If there are any questions, a pregnancy test should be ordered to determine whether physical changes are related to pregnancy or to some other underlying problem.

Blood testing primarily refers to the *Beta*-pregnancy test which detects the presence of the *Beta* subunit of human Chorionic Gonadotropin, hCG in maternal serum. Although urine tests for hCG are fairly accurate and readily available in any drug store, blood tests are valid sooner and are more precise. HCG rises progressively from conception. To simply determine pregnancy, order a qualitative test which will detect the presence of hCG. When assessing the viability of the pregnancy it will be more informative to order two successive quantitative tests, which determine the actual level of hCG. These tests should be spaced 5 to 7 days apart. Blood pregnancy tests are thoroughly discussed in <u>Diagnostic Tests</u>.

Implantation bleeding: Implantation begins approximately 6 days post-conception and continues during the following week. Spotting is often a by-product of this process, occurring during the 3rd to 4th week of pregnancy. If implantation occurs high in the uterus (as it typically does) such spotting may be delayed a bit as it works its way down to the cervix. This is not an absolute indication of pregnancy, nor does it happen consistently; many other conditions can cause bleeding.

Morning sickness: About one-third to one-half of all pregnant women experience some nausea with or without vomiting. Due to the many and varied reasons why nausea may occur, it too is only a presumptive sign of pregnancy.

Frequency of urination: The extreme anteversion of the uterus presses on the bladder and tends to elongate its base, leading to an increased urge to urinate. This symptom disappears as the uterus rises into the abdomen at about 12 weeks.

Breast changes: The woman may notice breast changes such as tingling or burning and enlargement as early as four weeks of pregnancy. Enlargement progresses from the outer borders of the breasts toward the center and continues throughout pregnancy, although not always evenly. Stretch marks may begin to appear on the breasts as they get bigger. New stretch marks look like purplish blue lines. Old ones are silvery. Nipples darken and become more sensitive. In nursing mothers, pregnancy may reduce the quantity of milk due to the additional nutritional demands of pregnancy. Breast tissue in the axillary area (under the arms) may also become tender.

Bluish coloration of the vulva, vestibule and yoni: This is usually seen most clearly around the meatus and in the vestibule, extending up the anterior wall of the yoni, and is an opaque bluish or violet tint. It appears between the 8th and 12th weeks and becomes more pronounced as pregnancy advances. It is more definite in multigravidas than in primigravidas, and in women with diseases of the genitals. It may not appear until late in pregnancy and rarely will not appear at all. Any pathologic conditions that cause pelvic congestion such as tumors or obesity as well as heart disease may also produce this sign.

Softening of the cervix, yoni and uterus: The yoni and cervix become noticeably softer starting the 6th week in primigravidas and even earlier in multigravidas. The upper and lower portions of the cervix soften first, followed by the yoni. An increase in discharge from the yoni may also be noted in some women.

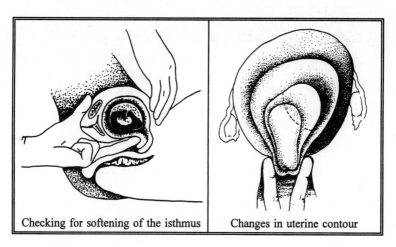

| Checking for softening of the isthmus | Changes in uterine contour |

The neck of the uterus (isthmus) becomes noticeably softened as well, by the 8th week of pregnancy in primigravidas and by the 6th week in multigravidas. When two fingers are inserted into the anterior fornix of the yoni and the other hand is placed behind the uterus abdominally, the fingers of both hands almost meet due to the softness of the isthmus (neck of the cervix) as illustrated (this is Hegar's Sign). This softening is seldom fully developed until the 10th week of

672

pregnancy, however. Since this sign is also commonly seen months after abortion or labor and usually just before menstruation, it too is only a presumptive sign.

Changes in uterine form, size, consistency and position: The change from the thin pear shape of the nulliparous uterus to the rounded plump form of the pregnant uterus is very noticeable on bimanual exam. If the conceptus is implanted near the entrance to a tube, that side of the uterus will be asymmetrical by palpation early on. As the pregnancy advances, symmetry is reestablished. Bulges may be felt during a bi-manual exam by placing one finger in each of the lateral fornices and pressing upwards.

The size of the uterus will gradually increase as pregnancy advances, and while other conditions may cause it to enlarge, nothing causes it to grow at the same rate as pregnancy. Too much palpation during an exam can cause the uterus to contract, thus making it seem deceptively small. If this occurs, wait a few minutes and recheck. Gentle handling will help prevent this from occurring.

The consistency of the pregnant uterus is tonic, spongy and soft, resembling dough. The uterus may contract as a whole or just in certain spots during an exam. The weight of the pregnant uterus may cause it to tip forward and lie "like a lump" on the bladder.

References and further reading:

Greenhill, J. Principles and Practice of Obstetrics, 10th ed., William Saunders Co., Philadelphia, PA, 1951.

Conception and Growth of the Baby and Placenta During the First 14 Weeks (First 12 Weeks of Gestation)

The menstruation and ovulation cycles without fertilization are discussed in the Anatomy and Physiology section. This chapter will focus on what takes place prior to and through conception and the first weeks of pregnancy.

A human baby develops from a single cell into a whole human being, a miraculous process at least! The most dramatic growth and development takes place during the first trimester, which is also the time when the baby is most susceptible to damage from outside influences.

Why embryology is important: Even though the developing baby is an embryo for only a very short period early in its growth, the study of its development throughout gestation is called **embryology (EM-bree-OL-o-gee).** The study of embryology gives information which you can then provide to the parents about the development of their unborn baby. It helps us determine the gestational age of the baby and thus facilitates making informed choices in many situations. Should a woman miscarry, knowing how the conceptus looks at specific weeks helps you determine how far along the pregnancy was at the time the baby died.

The embryo's organ systems develop primarily during the fourth to eighth week and exposure at this time to drugs, chemicals, viruses, radiation and other substances which can damage the cells may lead to congenital defects. These harmful agents, known as **teratogens**, do the most damage when fetal tissue is actively differentiating. Since many agents can cause harm to the developing baby, knowing when a woman took or was exposed to an agent can help you give her an idea whether her baby was susceptible to damage at that time from the agent in question. This can help her make better decisions about the option of abortion, fetal diagnosis, the place of birth, possible needs for specific pediatric care and what she might expect about the condition of her baby at birth.

A word about dates: When considering the development of the unborn baby, always keep in mind that conception occurs two weeks after the first day of the last menstrual period in a woman with a 28 day cycle. Although pregnancy will be counted from the first day of her last menstrual period (two weeks before she got pregnant), embryology discusses development counting day one as the day of conception. Therefore, embryologic dating is always two weeks less than the number of weeks a woman is considered to be pregnant. For example, a woman who is in her 8th week of pregnancy is in her 6th week of gestation.

An overview of gestation: Human development may be divided into three essential phases, which overlap to some extent:

> ***Growth** (increase in size) involves cell division and the development of cell products.
> ***Morphogenesis** includes mass cell movements to create the form of the embryo.
> ***Differentiation** is the maturation of physical processes, resulting in the formation of tissues and organs that perform specialized functions.

During most of pregnancy, the fetus grows in a fluid filled environment which is contained within a double layer sac called the fetal membranes. This sac is made up of an outer layer, the chorion, and an inner layer, the amnion. A good way to visualize this is to imagine the fetus floating by a cord within a double layered inflated balloon. Now imagine the placenta as a flat, thick, meaty organ shaped and sized more or less like a dinner plate, the surface of which is adherent to the surface of the balloon. The outer surface of the placenta is dusky red and meaty looking, the inner surface (facing the baby) is smooth and a milky bluish color because it is fused to the membranes. The umbilical cord attaches to the center of the inner surface of the placenta and extends to attach to the navel of the baby. The conceptus has developed to the point described here by the end of the first trimester. Yet the very early development process which takes place, leading to this configuration, is very complicated, and is hard to describe and to visualize. (Refer to the summarized pictorial description at the end of the chapter to help with this.)

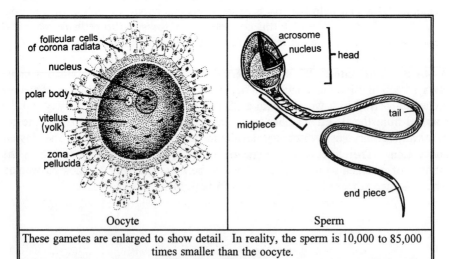

Oocyte   Sperm

These gametes are enlarged to show detail. In reality, the sperm is 10,000 to 85,000 times smaller than the oocyte.

Two cells evolve to become the fetus described above. We'll start with a brief review of the gametes or specialized cells which come together to create a new human being: the **oocyte** and the **sperm**. After ovulation the oocyte is surrounded by a ragged halo called the **corona radiata**, which is made up of follicular cells. Beneath this is a uniform coating called the **zona pellucida**, a clear glycoprotein layer. Under this layer lies the cell membrane of the ovum, which contains the cytoplasm and genetic material to be contributed by the mother.

The sperm consists of a **head**, which contains the genetic material to be contributed by the father and a **tail**, which propels the sperm along its path to the ovum. The junction between the head and tail is called the neck. The **acrosome** forms a cap on the head; it contains more than ten different enzymes to facilitate the sperm's penetration of the layers around the ovum.

The pre-embryonic period: conception and early pregnancy day by day:

Day 1: The **pre-embryonic period** begins when an oocyte is fertilized by a sperm. **Fertilization** takes about 24 hours and usually occurs in the ampulla of the uterine tube. (While it may occasionally take place further down the tube, fertilization does not occur in the uterus itself.) The sperm releases substances which assist in penetrating the corona radiata and the zona pellucida of the oocyte. Mucosal enzymes secreted by the uterine tube and the motion of the sperm's tail also appear to assist this process. Once the first sperm penetrates the zona pellucida, a reaction occurs which makes the zona impenetrable to any other sperm.

After the sperm is inside, the oocyte completes its second meiotic division, forming a mature oocyte whose nucleus is known as the **female pronucleus**. The **male pronucleus** forms when the head of the sperm enlarges. During the growth of the pronuclei, both replicate their DNA.

Next, the pronuclei lose their nuclear membranes and fuse with each other to form a new cell called the **zygote**. Within 24 to 48 hours after fertilization, an immunosuppressant maternal serum protein known as **early pregnancy factor (EPF)** appears in the maternal bloodstream, providing the basis of pregnancy tests during the first week of gestation (although such tests are not commonly available).

Day 2: Division or **cleavage** of the zygote into first two, then four, then eight, etc., cells called **blastomeres** begins about 30 hours after fertilization. The zygote travels along the uterine tube toward the uterus as it divides. Subsequent exponential divisions follow one another forming successively smaller blastomere cells. The blastomere cells change shape and tightly align themselves against each other to form a compact ball of cells resembling a raspberry and known as the **morula (MORE-uh-luh)**.

Day 3: By now the morula is a solid ball of 12 cells. It has completed its four-inch (10-cm) journey down the uterine tube, and now enters the uterus.

Day 4 and 5: The morula develops into a fluid-filled hollow sphere called a **blastocyst (BLASS-toh-see)**, with an inner cavity called the **blastocoel (BLASS-toh-sist)**. As the fluid increases, it separates the blastomere into two parts. A thin, outer layer called the **trophectoderm**, made up of **trophoblast cells**, forms the spherical wall of the blastocyst; this will later develop into the chorion. A group of centrally located blastomeres, known as the inner cell mass or **embryoblast** projects into the blastocoel; this will develop into the embryo. Trophoblastic cells secrete human Chorionic Gonadotropin (hCG), a hormone which maintains the corpus luteum (which would continue its usual cycle if the woman were not pregnant). The corpus luteum is supported so it will continue secreting estrogen and progesterone, preventing menstruation.

The blastocyst floats in the uterine cavity for about two days. The zona pellucida gradually degenerates and disappears to allow the blastocyst to increase in size. During this time, the blastocyst is nourished by secretions from glands in the walls of the uterus.

Day 6: The blastocyst attaches to the endometrial epithelium. Attachment usually takes place in the upper endometrium, more often on the posterior than the anterior wall of the uterus. As soon as this occurs, the trophoblast starts multiplying rapidly and gradually differentiates into two layers: an inner **cytotrophoblast** and an outer **syncytiotrophoblast**. Finger-like projections of the syncytiotrophoblast extend through the underlying endometrial epithelium and attach themselves to the endometrial connective tissue of the uterine lining, thus begins the process of becoming anchored to the uterine wall. Up until implantation begins, all embryonic cells are identical. When implantation starts, all cell division temporarily stops. When it begins again, the cells will begin to differentiate into different types: they will no longer be alike.

Day 7: The blastocyst is now superficially implanted in the compact layer of the endometrium and is deriving nourishment from maternal tissues.

Day 8 and 9: As implantation of the blastocyst progresses, the inner cell mass changes shape, and the blastocyst assumes a flattened disk shape to form the **bilaminar** (two layered) **embryonic disk**. As the bilaminar disk is forming, several supporting membranes and other structures also develop. A small cavity appears at the embryonic pole between the embryoblast and the trophoblast. This space will become the **amniotic cavity**. Cells from the cytotrophoblast organize to form the amniotic membrane that lines the amniotic cavity. Cells from this membrane become modified to form the **primary or primitive yolk sac**. This fluid-filled yolk sac is a primitive respiratory and digestive system which transports nutrients to the embryo during the second and third weeks of life before placental transfer is fully developed. It is also the first place that fetal blood cells are formed.

The embryonic disc now lies between the amniotic cavity and the primary yolk sac. A loose tissue layer surrounds the amnion and primary yolk sac. Simultaneously, isolated spaces (lacunae) which fill with maternal blood appear in the syncytiotrophoblast. This is the beginning of the uteroplacental circulation.

Day 10 and 11: The conceptus is completely embedded in the endometrium. A closing plug of clotted blood covers the exposed edge of the implanted blastocyst for about two days.

Day 12: The epithelium overlying the blastocyst has now completely regenerated. Adjacent syncotiotrophoblastic lacunae have fused to form networks, the beginnings of the intervillous space of the placenta. A large isolated cavity called the **extraembryonic coelom** (early chorionic cavity) forms. This fluid-filled cavity surrounds the amnion and yolk sac except where they are attached to the chorion by the connecting stalk, which develops into the umbilical cord. As this occurs, the primary yolk sac decreases in size and a smaller, secondary yolk sac forms, which later plays a part in the formation of the gut.

Day 13 and 14: At the end of the second week the primitive **chorionic villi** of the early placenta appear. The amniotic sac and the yolk sac look like two balloons pressed together, where they make contact is the site of the 14-day embryo; a flat, two layered disc. These structures are suspended by a cord from the inside of a larger balloon; the chorionic sac. Cells at one end of the embryonic disk now form a thickened circular region call the prochordal plate, the future site of the mouth.

The Embryonic period:

The third to the eighth weeks of gestation constitute most of the **embryonic period**. The beginnings of all major internal and external structures are established during this time. At the end of this period all the main organs have begun to develop but the function of most of them is minimal.

Days 15: This marks the first missed day of the expected menstrual period. The formation of three germ tissue layers, from which all tissue specialization will arise, begins; the endoderm, the mesoderm and the ectoderm. This process is called **gastrulation** and during this time the embryo is known as a **gastrula**. Ectoderm development begins with the formation of the **primitive streak** down the center of the embryonic disk. This will become the site of the neural tube (primitive spinal cord). The three layers and the other structures they differentiate into are:

ENDODERM	MESODERM	ECTODERM
Epithelium of: 　Pharynx, larynx, trachea, 　lungs, tonsils, adenoids, 　thymus, parathyroids, 　esophagus, stomach, 　intestines, liver, pancreas, 　gallbladder, glands of 　alimentary canal (except 　salivary), bladder (except 　trigone), urethra, (except 　terminal male portion), 　prostate, bulbourethral 　glands, yoni (partial), 　vestibule, inner ear & 　auditory tubes.	All muscle tissue except in 　iris & sweat glands All connective tissue Synovial & serous 　membranes Lymphoid tissue Spleen Blood cells Reticuloendothelial system Dermis of skin Teeth (except enamel) Endothelium of heart, blood 　vessels, lymphatics Epithelium of: 　gonads, reproductive ducts 　adrenal cortex 　kidneys, ureters 　coelom, joint cavities	All nerve tissue Epidermis of skin, hair 　follicles, nails Epithelium & myoepithelial 　cells of sweat, sebaceous 　& mammary glands Lens of the eye Receptor cells of sense 　organs Enamel of teeth Adrenal medulla Anterior pituitary Epithelium of: salivary 　glands, lips, cheeks, gums, 　hard palate, nasal cavity 　sinuses Lower third of anal canal Terminal portion of male 　urethra Vestibule of yoni & 　vestibular glands Plain muscle of iris

Days 16-21: Early in the third week, the **allantois (uh-LAN-toh-ihz)** forms. It is a small finger-shaped pocket in the wall of the yolk sac that is involved with the formation of blood cells and the development of the urinary bladder. Its blood vessels will become the vein and arteries of the umbilical cord. Continued development of the chorion also occurs, with formation of chorionic villi, which exchange nutrients and wastes with the maternal system.

Day 19: The neural tube develops by a process of folding in of tissues. This tube will become the spinal cord. During this third week if something goes wrong in this process, the spine or brain may not develop properly and the baby could be born with a defect along its neural tube.

Day 20: Blood circulation begins. The heart has developed into a pair of tubes joined to blood vessels in the embryo, the connecting stalk (primitive umbilical cord) and the yolk sac.

Day 21: At this point, the embryo is almost straight. Approximately now, somite formation begins. **Somites** are paired block-shaped structures which appear on each side of the developing neural tube. During the third week, the number of somites is a reliable indicator of the age of the embryo. Somites appear from the head end of the embryo downward and give rise to various structures such as skeletal, muscle and skin tissues, depending upon their tissue composition and their location along the path of the neural tube.

The heart begins to beat on the 21st or 22nd day; thus, the cardiovascular system is the first to reach a functional state. By now the primitive placental structures necessary for physiological exchanges between the mother and embryo are present. The kidneys and endocrine system have also begun to form within these first three weeks. A droplet of amniotic fluid appears at the dorsal end of the embryonic disk at about 3 weeks.

Day 22: This begins the fourth week of development, a time when the shape of the embryo changes rapidly due to a complex process whereby the various layers already formed fold inward. This happens both longitudinally, along the sides of the embryo as the disc-like embryo's edges roll to its "abdominal" side, and at each end, causing the previously straight embryo to gradually become curved in a C-shape during the coming days. The result is the rapid growth of the embryo.

Day 24: By now, the neural tube is widely open, forming neuropores at both the head (rostral) and tail (caudal) ends, and its length is marked by rows of somites on either side. The first (mandibular) and second (hyloid) arches appear as folds in the head region "under the chin." The first, or mandibular arch will give rise to the lower jaw, and an extension of it will become the upper jaw. The embryo is now slightly curved due to head and tail folds, and the heart produces a large protrusion in the "chest."

Day 26 & 27: Three pairs of pharyngeal or branchial arches are visible by 26 days and the tail-end of the neural tube has closed. The forebrain produces a prominent elevation of the head and the embryo is now curved in a C-shape. Upper limb buds become visible on day 26 or 27 as small swellings on the sides of the body; the otic pits (primitive ears) are also seen. The connecting stalk narrows and is transformed into the umbilical cord.

Day 28: The fourth pair of branchial arches and the lower limb buds are now visible. Thickened areas which will become the eye lenses are seen on the side of the head. At this point the embryo has an attenuated (small) tail. The oral cavity of the mouth has formed, Primitive jaws are present and the longitudinal esophagotracheal septum begins to divide the esophagus and trachea. The stomach has formed, and the esophagus and intestine have become tubular. Ducts to the pancreas and liver are forming and liver function is starting.

Fifth week (days 29-35): Changes in body form are minor during this week compared with the fourth week. Growth of the head exceeds that of other regions due to rapid development of the brain. The brain has differentiated and cranial nerves are present; developing muscles also have innervation. The heart's atrial division has occurred. The facial area bends so far forward that it contacts the heart prominence. The hyoid arch grows, forming the cervical sinus. The upper limbs begin to show some regionalization as the elbows and hand plates develop. The primitive fingers, called digital rays, begin to develop at 33 days. Spontaneous twitching of the trunk and limbs may begin.

Sixth week (days 36-42): The upper limbs continue to develop rapidly during this week. The elbows and wrists are clearly seen, as are the digital rays, which will become the fingers. Small swellings develop around the branchial groove, which will become the auricle of the external ear. Retinal pigment makes the eye obvious. The head is now larger than the trunk and is curved more forward over the heart, which results from bending of the brain in the neck region. The trunk and neck then begin to straighten. The embryo will now show reflex response to touch. The liver begins to produce red blood cells. Rudimentary bones are present and a skeletal shape is forming. Muscles mass increases. Chambers are present in the heart and groups of red blood cells can be identified. The oral and nasal cavities and upper lip have formed. The trachea and bronchi are present and lung buds appear. Embryonic sex glands appear.

Seventh week (days 43-49): The communication between the primitive gut and the yolk sac is now reduced to a small duct, the yolk stalk. The intestines enter the extraembryonic coelom, causing them to be outside the body; a normal occurrence for the embryo. The limbs continue to develop rapidly. Notches appear between the digital rays in the hand plates, clearly indicating the site of the future fingers. The heart beat can be detected. The palate folds this week, and the tongue separates. The stomach attains its final form. The bladder and urethra separate from the rectum, and the diaphragm separates the abdominal and thoracic cavities. Sex glands begin to differentiate into ovaries or testes.

Eighth week (days 50-57): Up until now chorionic villi have covered the entire chorionic sac. As the sac grows, the villi associated with the decidua capsularis are compressed. Their blood supply is reduced and they soon degenerate, leaving part of the chorion bare and smooth. Simultaneously, those villi implanted over the decidua basalis rapidly increase in number, branch profusely and enlarge. There are now about 7 ml. of amniotic fluid.

The fingers are now short and webbed. Notches are visible between the digital rays of the toes and the tail is still present, but stubby. The blood vessels of the scalp now form a band around the head. The eyelids are open. Muscle development proceeds in the limbs, trunk and head. Heart development is essentially complete. Fetal blood still circulates into the yolk sac as well as within the body. The lips completely fuse this week. The midgut rotates into position and the membrane over the anal opening disappears.

By the end of the eighth week all regions of the limbs are seen; the fingers and toes have lengthened and separated; purposeful limb movement begins. All evidence of the tail disappears. The embryo has distinctly human characteristics, but the head is still disproportionately large, making up almost half of the body. The neck region is established, and the eyelids are more obvious. The intestines still protrude into the base of the umbilical cord. At the end of the week the eyelids begin to fuse. The ears begin to look mature, but are still set low on the head. The middle and inner ear are also almost complete. External genital differentiation is beginning, but is not distinct enough to tell what sex the baby is. At this point the beginnings of all the main organ systems have been established.

The fetal period:

The end of the eighth week marks the beginning of the **fetal period**, so-called because the developing baby now looks quite human. Development focuses on rapid growth of the body and differentiation of tissues and organs that started to develop during the embryonic period. During the fetal period there is a relative slowdown in the growth of the head compared to the rest of the body.

Ninth week: At the beginning of the ninth week the head constitutes half of the crown-rump length of the fetus (the distance between the top of the head and the buttocks). The face is broad, the eyes widely separated, the ears low-set, and the eyelids fused. Early in the ninth week the legs are short and the thighs relatively small. The external genitals of the fetus still appear unisexual at the end of the ninth week. The fetal liver is now the major site of red blood cell production.

Ten weeks: Neurons appear at the tail end of the spinal cord, and the basic divisions of the brain are present. The lips separate from the jaw this week and the folds of the palate fuse. The lacrimal sacs of the eyes develop now. Muscles appear in the gut region. Coils of intestines are still clearly visible at the base of the umbilical cord until the middle of the tenth week. Finger and toe nails begin to develop. The islets of Langerhans in the pancreas have developed. The bladder sac has formed and urine formation begins; urine is discharged into the amniotic fluid. The baby also swallows amniotic fluid at this point. Amniotic fluid volume has increased to about 32 ml..

Eleventh week: The intestines have usually returned to the abdomen by the middle of the 11th week.

Twelfth week: By the end of 12 weeks, body growth has been so rapid that the crown-rump length has more than doubled. The genitals are now distinctly male or female in appearance. The spleen largely assumes the work of red cell production. The neck is well defined. The skin is pink, translucent and delicate. Bile secretion begins. The thyroid secretes hormones and lymphoid tissue appears in the fetal thymus gland.

Primary ossification centers appear in the skeleton, especially in the skull and long bones. The upper limbs have almost reached their final relative lengths, but the lower limbs are still not as well developed and are slightly shorter than their final relative lengths. Involuntary muscles appear in vital organs. The lungs acquire definite shape at this time.

Early placental development:

The developing baby has no functional circulatory system during the first two weeks of life. During the implantation process, enzymes released by the trophoblastic cells destroy tiny capillaries in the endometrium beneath them. Blood from these capillaries comes into direct contact with trophoblastic cells, providing a temporary source of nutrition. As the trophoblast grows, it branches and extends into the tissue of the uterus. Small chorionic villi grow outward into the maternal tissue from the protective sac around the embryo. Two kinds of tissue, embryonic and maternal, grow until there is sufficient surface contact to ensure the adequate passage of nourishment and oxygen from the mother, as well as the removal of metabolic wastes from the embryo. By the end of the third week, the anatomical arrangements necessary for physiological exchanges between the mother and embryo are established. Trophoblastic cells have entered underlying maternal vessels, gradually transforming them from thick-walled muscular, spiral arteries into wide-mouthed, flaccid, sac-like uteroplacental vessels, a process completed by the 16th week of gestation (Fox, 1991). The chorion makes up most of the placenta. The fetal part of the placenta and the fetal membranes separate the fetus from the endometrial lining of the mother's uterus, thus there is no direct interchange of blood. The vessels of the umbilical cord connect the placental circulation with the fetal circulation. The chorion, amnion, yolk sac and allantois constitute the fetal membranes, which develop from the zygote; the chorion and amnion do not become part of the embryo or fetus, however the yolk sac and allantois are eventually incorporated into the baby's developing body. The fetal membranes and placenta perform the following functions and activities: protection, nutrition, respiration, excretion, and production of hormones which maintain the pregnancy.

Decidua (which means a falling off) is the term applied to the pregnant woman's uterine lining (technically known as the gravid endometrium), so called because the endometrium separates from the remainder of the uterine wall and is discharged after the birth. Endometrial cells enlarge and form decidual cells in response to increased levels of progesterone. Cellular and vascular changes occurring within the endometrium in response to pregnancy are called the **decidual reaction**. Decidual cells contain large amounts of glycogen and lipids. It is thought that decidual cells may protect the maternal tissue from uncontrolled growth of syncytiotrophoblastic cells, and that they are involved in hormone production.   Three regions of the decidua are identified according to their relationship to the implantation site:

1. The **decidua basalis** is the part of the decidua beneath the conceptus which forms the maternal component of the placenta.
2. The **decidua capsularis** is the superficial portion of decidua which overlies the very early conceptus.
3. The **decidua partietalis** or the **decidua vera** is the remaining endometrium lining the rest of the uterus.

Until the 8th week, chorionic villi cover the entire chorionic sac, forming a bushy covering known as the **villous chorion**. As the sac enlarges, the villi which were associated with the decidua capsularis are compressed and their blood supply is reduced, causing them to degenerate. This leaves a relatively bare, avascular area on the chorion. As this occurs, the villi next to the **decidua basalis** increase in number, enlarge and begin to branch out. This causes the placenta to thicken. As the fetus grows, the uterus and placenta enlarge.

From early in conception, the placenta is the source of several hormones which help to support the pregnancy:

*Human chorionic gonadotropin (hCG)** is a protein hormone first produced in the 2nd week of gestation by the syncytiotrophoblast. It supports the corpus luteum and thus the endometrial lining of the uterus, preventing menstruation. Maternal blood concentrations rise to a maximum at 8 weeks and then gradually decline.
*Human placental lactogen (hPL)** is a protein hormone produced early in pregnancy, most likely by the syncytiotrophoblast. It is involved in milk production and metabolic processes. It has an anti-insulin effect, which serves to spare maternal glucose for the pregnancy and maintain nutrition for the fetus during maternal fasting (as when she is sleeping). It has also been called chorionic growth hormone and chorionic somatomammotropin (hCS).
*Human chorionic thyrotropin (hCT)** and **human chorionic adrenocorticotropin (hCACTH)** are also formed by the placenta; their functions are not well understood.
*Estrogens** are steroid hormones. The placental contribution produces a high level of estrogens in the mother. The adrenal cortex of both mother and baby provide precursors for their production.
*Progesterone** is also a steroid hormone. The placenta uses blood cholesterol as a precursor when making this hormone and continues production throughout pregnancy.

The timing of teratogenic effects:

The stage of development determines an embryo's susceptibility to given agents: the most critical periods are when cell division, differentiation and morphogenesis are at their peak for various parts of the baby. Development is most easily deranged when tissues and organs are forming. Each type of tissue, organ and body system has a critical period during which its development may be disrupted. The congenital defects which occur depend upon which parts and organs are most susceptible at the time the agent is active. Some parts of the baby, such as the brain, bones and teeth, continue to develop significantly after birth, so teratogens may affect these areas both before and after birth.

While a timetable of critical periods can give us a general idea which parts and organs are susceptible to damage, it is incorrect to assume that defects always result from a single exposure to an agent during the critical periods or that we can determine from such tables the exact day the anomaly was produced. All we can know is that the agent would have had to disrupt development before the end of the critical periods for the part or organ concerned. (For example, the critical period for limb development would be 24 to 36 days after fertilization.)

During the first two weeks after fertilization the pre-embryo is usually not susceptible to teratogens. When damage does occur, it usually disrupts most or all of the cells, resulting in death. Or, it may damage only a few cells, from which the conceptus can recover and go on to develop defect-free. It is during the first eight weeks of gestation that the baby is most sensitive to major damage.

The following chart gives some of the more common defects which can occur at specific times during gestation. A timeline for sensitive periods of teratogenic effects is also given at the end of this chapter.

WEEKS GESTATION	POTENTIAL MALFORMATION
3	Ectopia cordis (heart forms outside thoracic cavity), Omphalocele, Absence of arms, Ectromelia (poor development of long bones in limbs), Anotia (absence of ears), facial nerve paralysis, Ear malformations, Duodenal atresia, Phocomelia of arms (hands are attached close to body)
4	Absence of arms or legs, Ectromelia, Tracheoesophageal fistula, Hemivertebra (absence of half of a vertebra), Ear malformations, Heart defects, Duodenal atresia, Phocomelia of arms or legs
5	Tracheoesophageal fistula, Hemivertebra, Nuclear cataract, Microphthalmia (small eyes), Facial clefts, Carpal or pedal ablation
6	Microphthalmia, Carpal or pedal ablation, Hairlip, agnathia (absence of lower jaw), Lenticular cataract, Heart defects
7	Heart defects, Digital ablation, Cleft palate, Micrognathia (small jaw), Epicanthus, Brachycephaly (short head)
8	Heart defects, Epicanthus, Brachycephaly, Persistent ostium primum, Nasal bone ablation, Digital stunting

Terminology can be confusing. Here is a list of current definitions:

Anomaly: A structural abnormality of any type.

Association: A nonrandom occurrence in two or more individuals of multiple anomalies not known to be a polytopic field defect, sequence or syndrome.

Birth defects, congenital malformations and congenital anomalies: All-purpose terms used to describe developmental defects present at birth. These may be structural, functional, metabolic, behavioral or hereditary.

Deformation: An abnormal shape, form, or position of a body part which results from mechanical forces, such as compression due to lack of amniotic fluid.

Disruption: A morphological defect of an organ, part of an organ or larger region that results from the extrinsic breakdown of, or an interference with, an originally normal developmental process, as would occur after an exposure to a teratogen. This problem cannot be inherited.

Dysmorphology: The area of clinical genetics that is concerned with the diagnosis and interpretation of patterns of structural defects.

Dysplasia: An abnormal organization of cells into tissues and its morphological result; the process and consequence of abnormal tissue formation.

Malformation: A morphologic defect of an organ, part of an organ, or larger region that results from an intrinsically abnormal developmental process. Being intrinsic implies that the developmental potential was abnormal from the beginning, such as chromosomal abnormalities occurring at fertilization.

Polytopic field defect: A pattern of anomalies derived from the disturbance of a single developmental field (or area).

Sequence: A pattern of multiple anomalies derived from a single known or presumed structural defect or mechanical factor.

Syndrome: A pattern of multiple anomalies thought to be pathogenetically related and not known to represent a single sequence or a polytopic field defect.

Fox, H., "A contemporary view of the human placenta," Midwifery, Vol. 7, No. 1, 1991, p. 31.
Moore, Keith, & T. Persaud, The Developing Human: Clinically Oriented Embryology, 5th ed., W. B. Saunders Co., Philadelphia, PA, 1993.
Olds, Sally, et al., Obstetric Nursing, Addison-Wesley, Pub., Menlo Park, CA, 1980.
Samuels, Mike & Nancy, The Well Pregnancy Book, Summit Books, NY, 1986, p. 119.

Days of Gest. Age	Length (mm)*	Main External Characteristics
20-21 (3 weeks)	1.5-3	Flat embryonic disc. Deep neural groove & prominent neural folds. Head fold evident
22-23 (3 wks & 3 days)	2-3.5	Embryo straight or slightly curved. Neural tube forming but widely open at both ends. First & second pair of branchial arches visible as deep wrinkles in the curve of the "neck."
24-25	2.5-4.5	Embryo curved due to head & tail folds. Head end of neural tube closing. Primitive eye parts present.
26-27	3-5	Upper limb buds appear. Head end of neural tube closed. Tail end closing. Three pair of branchial arches visible. Heart protrudes from upper embryo, primitive ear pits present.
28-30 (4 weeks)	4-6	Embryo is C-shaped. End of neural tube closed, tail present. Upper limb buds are flipper-like. Lower limb buds appear. Ear vesicles & eye lenses present.
31-32	5-7	Upper limbs are paddle shaped. Eye lens pits & nasal pits visible. Optic cups present.
33-36 (5 weeks)	7-9	Hand plates formed, fingers rays present; lower limbs paddle shaped. Lens vesicles present; nasal pits prominent. Cervical sinuses visible.
37-40	8-11	Foot plates formed. Pigment visible in retina. External ear begins to develop.
41-43 (6 weeks)	11-14	Finger rays clearly visible. External ear more developed. Trunk beginning to straighten. Cerebral vesicles prominent.
44-46	13-17	Digital rays clearly visible in foot plates. Elbow region visible. Eyelids forming. Notches between digital rays in hand. Nipple visible.
47-48	16-18	Limbs extend ventrally. Trunk elongating & straightening. Midgut herniation prominent.
49-51 (7 weeks)	18-22	Upper limbs longer & bent at elbows. Fingers distinct but webbed. Notches between the toe rays in the feet. Scalp vascular system appears.
52-53	22-24	Hands & feet approach each other. Fingers are free & longer. Toes distinct but webbed. Stubby tail present.
54-55	23-28	Toes free & longer. Eyelids & auricles of external ears more developed.
56 (8 weeks)	27-31	Head more rounded w/human characteristics. Genitals still sexless. Distinct bulge still in umbilical cord, caused by herniation of intestines. Tail is gone.

*There are 10 millimeters to 1 centimeter. Through week 25 the greatest length is noted; after that the crown-rump length is given (i.e. from the top of the head to the area where the buttocks will eventually develop).

687

SUMMARY OF HUMAN PRENATAL DEVELOPMENT: 1 to 2 weeks gestation

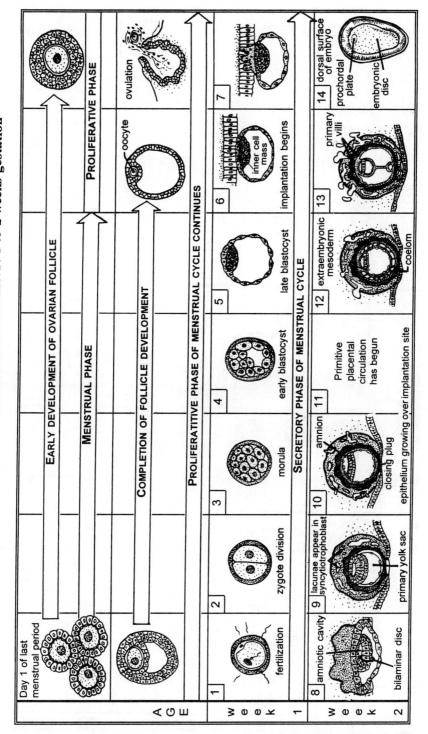

EARLY DEVELOPMENT OF OVARIAN FOLLICLE

MENSTRUAL PHASE

PROLIFERATIVE PHASE

COMPLETION OF FOLLICLE DEVELOPMENT

PROLIFERATITIVE PHASE OF MENSTRUAL CYCLE CONTINUES

SECRETORY PHASE OF MENSTRUAL CYCLE

ovulation

oocyte

Day 1 of last menstrual period

AGE

week 1

1 — fertilization

2 — zygote division

3 — morula

4 — early blastocyst

5 — late blastocyst

6 — inner cell mass — implantation begins

7

week 2

8 — amniotic cavity — bilaminar disc

9 — lacunae appear in syncytiotrophoblast — primary yolk sac

10 — closing plug — epithelium growing over implantation site

11 — amnion — Primitive placental circulation has begun

12 — extraembryonic mesoderm — coelom

13 — primary villi

14 — dorsal surface of embryo — prochordal plate — embryonic disc

SUMMARY OF HUMAN PRENATAL DEVELOPMENT: 3 to 6 weeks gestation

week 3

15 — 1st day of missed menses; primitive streak

16 — notochordal process

17 — intraembryonic mesoderm; cross-section of trilaminar embryo

18 — neural plate; primitive streak; Length: 1.5 mm

19 — neural fold; notochord; embryonic coelom

20 — brain; neural groove; somite; thyroid development begins

21 — neural groove; somite; heart tubes begin to fuse

week 4

22 — heart starts beating; primitive streak

23 — rostral neuropore; very early eye & ear present; caudal neuropore

24 — heart bulge; rostral neuropore closes; 2 pairs of branchial arches

25 — otic pit; 3 pairs of branchial arches

26 — forebrain prominence; upper limb bud; tail

27 — 4 pairs of branchial arches; upper & lower limb buds present; CR= crown-rump length

28 — CR: 4.0 mm

week 5

29 — neural folds fusing; four branchial arches; CR: 5.0 mm

30 — lens pits optic cups & nasal pits developing

31 — developing eye; nasal pit; primitive mouth

32 — cervical flexure of brain; paddle-shaped upper limb bud

33 — hand plate; CR: 7.0 mm

34 — head larger relative to trunk; primordia of cerebral hemispheres distinct; foot plates present

35 — CR: 8.0 mm

week 6

36 — oral & nasal cavities forming

37 — paddle-shaped lower limb; elbow; hand plate; CR: 9.0 mm

38 — upper lip formed

39 — CR: 1 cm

40 — arms bent at elbow; digital rays, palate & external ears forming

41 — fingers forming; ventral view

42 — CR: 1.3 cm

SUMMARY OF HUMAN PRENATAL DEVELOPMENT: 7 to 10 weeks gestation

week						
7	**43** CR: 1.6 cm	**44** eyelids forming	**45** tip of nose distinct; Digital rays appear in foot plates; CR: 1.7 cm	**46** loss of villi; smooth chorion forms	**47** genital tubercle; urogenital membrane; anal membrane; ♂ or ♀	**48** eyelid; trunk becoming longer & straighter / **49** notches between digital rays; CR: 1.8 cm
8	**50** fingers distinct; upper limbs longer & bent at elbows	**51** Anal membrane perforated; urogenital membrane degenerating; testicles & ovaries distinguishable	**52** fingers separated; fan-shaped webbed toes	**53**	**54** genital tubercle; urethral groove; anus; ♀ or ♂♀; external genitals have begun to differentiate	**55** Beginnings of all essential external & internal structures are present / **56**
9	**57** FETAL PERIOD BEGINS	**58**	**59** genitalia show some distinct features but ♀ & ♂ still easily confused	**60** phallus; urogenital fold; labioscrotal fold; perineum ♀	**61** Genitalia show fusion of urethral folds; Urethral groove extends into phallus	**62** phallus; urogenital fold; labioscrotal fold; perineum ♂ / **63** CR: 5 cm
10	**64** face has human profile; note growth of chin compared to day 44	**65**	**66** baby now looks human	**67** clitoris; labia minora; urogenital groove; labia majora ♀	**68** genitalia have ♀ or ♂ characteristics but still not fully formed	**69** glans penis; urethral groove; scrotum ♂ / **70** CR: 6.1 cm

PERIODS OF CRITICAL TERATOGENIC SUSCEPTIBILITY DURING PRENATAL DEVELOPMENT

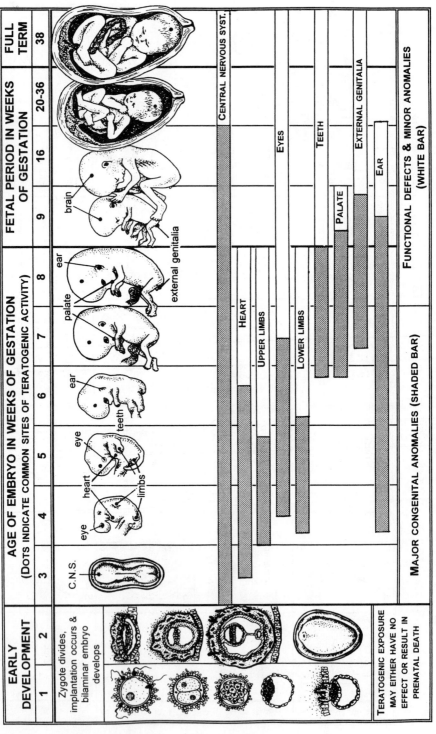

(these four charts were adapted from charts presented in Moore & Persaud, 1993, p. 156)

Emotional and Psychological Changes in Early Pregnancy

During the first trimester of pregnancy the primary psychological, emotional and spiritual task for the mother is incorporating the reality of the pregnancy into her psyche. At this point, the "reality" may in fact seem abstract, since she cannot yet see her belly or feel any fetal movement. At this time she integrates the concept and feelings of being pregnant by perceiving herself at one with the pregnancy due to its relative physical invisibility; the baby is not yet perceived as a separate entity. Because she will be looking for signs that she is pregnant, she will be watching closely for changes in her abdomen and breasts. When you find evidence of pregnancy via a pelvic exam, make sure that your findings are thoroughly explained. If a woman is trying to hide her pregnancy or has a history of eating disorders, be aware that she may attempt to starve herself to "keep from showing."

Perhaps the first response to the discovery of conception by any woman, regardless of how wanted the pregnancy may be, is ambivalence. Women who have been trying to get pregnant for some time or who have been telling friends how excited they are about the prospect of becoming pregnant may be especially uncomfortable with these feelings, and feel they have no forum to express their mixed emotions. On the one hand they feel elated, on the other they know that pregnancy, happening as it does within their very body, is a huge unknown and carries with it the weight of being responsible for another human being for many years to come. Women commonly feel rejection, anxiety, depression and unhappiness at this point. It is your job to make sure a woman knows these are normal and common feelings. Besides reducing anxiety, you can help minimize the chance that she will blame herself should she later miscarry or if the baby dies or has defects at birth. These ambivalent feelings are usually resolved by the fourth month of pregnancy. If they persist beyond this point, the woman may be in need of special counseling.

The sense of oneness with the pregnancy can be disrupted for women choosing to undergo prenatal fetal testing. In these cases, the woman's relationship to the pregnancy and her baby are often put on hold until test results return; in some cases this disrupts normal adjustment well into the second trimester, depending upon the tests that are done and when results are obtained. Acknowledge that this commonly occurs when women seek testing, thus giving the woman permission to discuss this dilemma. Barbara Katz Rothman's excellent book The Tentative Pregnancy can be recommended as a resource for helping the woman sort out her feelings about testing and her baby.

While these issues may come up, they will often be overshadowed by the more immediate questions of where and with whom the woman will seek prenatal care. Where and how will she give birth? Many women are quite concerned about selecting their care provider early in pregnancy. Once these decisions are out of the way, they can settle down to dealing more directly with their feelings about the

692

pregnancy. On the other hand, strongly ambivalent feelings may prevent a woman from seeking care until these feelings have resolved. Women who have miscarried in the past may postpone care to avoid emotional attachment, or they may be overly anxious to begin care at once.

Dreams: Dreams are one way that humans do emotional work. An intense dream life is common among pregnant women. Issues that they may feel ill-prepared to deal with consciously are dealt with unconsciously in their dreams. First trimester dreams tend to be about strangers, injuries to the self, and a woman's relationship to her own mother. (See the chapter on Helping Women Explore Their Dreams for more details).

Sexuality: A cardinal point to convey to pregnant women and their partners is that anything is normal regarding their sexual feelings. Frequently women do not feel like engaging in sexual activity during the first trimester. As they adjust to the concept of pregnancy, as well as its emotional and physical realities, they may need more time to themselves. In addition, early pregnancy complaints such as nausea will tend to dampen their mood for closeness. Others will feel that they are finally relieved of concerns regarding becoming pregnant, resulting in a heightened desire for sexual relationship. Encourage women to understand that every woman is different and that whatever an individual is feeling is perfectly normal, whether she suddenly wants a lot of sex, none at all, or physical closeness with no sexual demands. Partners need to hear this and be encouraged to be supportive while expressing their feelings as well. Suggest that both partners read Sheila Kitzinger's book Women's Experience of Sex or Elizabeth Bing and Libby Coleman's book Making Love During Pregnancy for more information. If she and her partner are shy about discussing sexual issues openly, having them both read either book will provide a starting point to open dialogue.

References and further reading:

Perez, Polly, "The Emotional Work of Pregnancy," International Journal of Childbirth Education, Vol. 3, No. 3, August 1988, pp. 30-1.
Varney, Helen, Nurse-Midwifery, Blackwell Scientific Pub., Boston, MA 1980.

PROBLEMS ASSOCIATED WITH THE FIRST TRIMESTER

Problems of all types can occur at any time during pregnancy. There are, however, certain problems or symptoms which are more likely to make an appearance during one part of pregnancy than another. There are also some things which occur at certain times during pregnancy that cannot occur at others. Many of the possible problems that can occur have been grouped in their own section of the book. The chapters in the sections on each trimester will point to conditions or symptoms which are closely associated with that particular trimester.

The first trimester symptoms you are most likely to encounter, and the range of most likely causes are:

*Nausea and vomiting
-Response to increased hormones of pregnancy
-Hypoglycemia
-Secondary symptoms of a serious abdominal condition related to pregnancy (such as a ruptured ectopic pregnancy)
-Secondary symptoms of a serious abdominal condition unrelated to pregnancy (such as a ruptured ovarian cyst or appendicitis)

*Bleeding
-Onset of menses (woman is not pregnant)
-Breakthrough uterine bleeding due to slight hormonal fluctuations with a normal pregnancy
-Implantation bleeding
-Threatened miscarriage of an intrauterine pregnancy
-Ectopic pregnancy
-Cervical erosion, injury, or cancer
-Yoni infection
-Hydatidiform mole
-Polyps

*Cramps
-Round ligament spasm or stretching
-Miscarriage of an intrauterine pregnancy (with bleeding)
-Digestive upsets
-Ectopic pregnancy
-Hydatidiform mole
-Serious abdominal condition unrelated to pregnancy

*Excessively large-for-dates uterine growth
- Inaccurate dates
- Multiple gestation
- Mother's physique (making the uterus appear large)
- Multiparity (is often a normal variation)
- Hydatidiform mole
- Uterine tumor (especially fibroids)

Remember that other, less likely conditions could cause any of the above symptoms. This list summarizes those things to rule out first.

Nausea and Vomiting of Early Pregnancy

By far, one of the most common and annoying complaints of early pregnancy is nausea, with or without some vomiting. Nausea and vomiting occur most frequently between the 6th and 14th weeks of pregnancy, and may be due to a variety of factors which work together, such as:

*The rapidly rising hormone levels of early pregnancy
*Hypoglycemia (low blood sugar)
*Inadequate dietary adjustments to pregnancy
*Psychological ambivalence regarding the pregnancy

The demands from the growing conceptus are minimal in the first trimester; nevertheless, changes associated with pregnancy are occurring, chiefly the increased influx of hormones and greater metabolic demands. Although hormonal levels are higher, the blood volume of early pregnancy is not much different than when a woman is not pregnant. This combination results in a concentrated amount of hormones in the blood stream; some women are more sensitive to this than others. As the blood volume expands, although the hormones levels remain high, they become more diluted. This eases the stress on the liver and the mother.

It is typical for women to enter pregnancy with a pattern of skimping or eliminating some meals throughout the day since most women in our "skinny is beautiful" culture have issues with eating. Often coffee or non-nutritious food choices such as doughnuts will make up one or more snacks or meals. While a nonpregnant person can exist on a minimal intake of nutritious foods, pregnant women cannot do so without paying for it dearly in the form of low blood sugar. Headaches, dizziness and fainting can also all be related to hypoglycemia. While the volume that women will feel like eating will increase as pregnancy advances, in early pregnancy they still need to eat small frequent meals of nutritious foods throughout the day.

Some women will automatically curtail their dietary intake upon becoming nauseous in the hope of staving off further nausea. As distasteful as eating may be at this point, women must eat. Even if they throw up, they must eat again in an attempt to stabilize their blood sugar. Various strategies have been recommended by experienced practitioners to curtail and reverse the nausea cycle; what works varies from woman to woman. Here are some general suggestions:

*Eat small amounts throughout the day, before you feel hungry (this
    keeps the blood sugar from dropping too low before eating)
*Do not take supplements on an empty stomach
*Eating before arising from bed each morning may help.
*Eat something every two to three hours
*Eat foods you know will settle the stomach; yogurt, cottage cheese,

cereal, toast, and crackers are a few suggestions. Sharp cheddar cheese may be well tolerated by some women as the sharp smell and taste increases salivation and digestion, placing less burden on the stomach (El Halta, 1989).

*Be sure to include many high protein foods

*Beverages such as carbonated drinks may help initially to settle the stomach but should not be taken regularly or "lived on." Nutritious foods are really needed to turn the pattern around.

*Eat a high protein snack before going to bed and whenever you wake in the night (often waking signifies that your blood sugar is low, even if you don't feel hungry)

*Drink to a healthy thirst, avoid dehydration. Women may find plain water more tolerable if they add lemon or if they drink it very cold (El Halta, 1989)

*Moderate exercise will assist the body in mobilizing toxins and high levels of hormones through the liver and out of the body.

*Avoid constipation with plenty of fluids and high fiber foods such as fruits, vegetables and whole grains

*Multiple gestation can cause more nausea because of the larger amount of hormones from two placentas as well as the increased metabolic and nutritional demands; if suspected, investigate thoroughly so the diet can be adjusted accordingly (see separate chapter on Multiple Gestation in Special Circumstances section)

*Avoid spicy or greasy foods

*Eat a high complex-carbohydrate food such as crackers followed by a high protein food 20 minutes later

*Eat an unrefined sweet food (such as fruit) followed by a high protein food shortly afterwards (the sweet will begin to bring the blood sugar up and the protein will help to stabilize it)

*Inadequate dietary intake quickly leads to burning stored fat for energy needs. This causes ketones to appear in the urine (ketonuria). This process can lead to more nausea.

*Dizziness may accompany morning sickness. Have the woman lie back down with a very cold cloth across her eyes and breathe evenly and deeply until the dizziness passes. Darkening the room may also help. (El Halta, 1989)

When questioning women regarding nausea, be sure to find out if other digestive upsets such as gas, bloating, bowel irregularities, abdominal pains, etc. are present. These symptoms can be related to food allergies (see chapter on Food Allergies, Well-being section). Also, take women off all supplements for the time being and add them back slowly once the nausea is more under control. Sometimes one brand of supplements will contribute significantly to nausea in early pregnancy;

it may be necessary to switch brands in some cases.

Constipation slows the movement of feces through the colon. The longer that feces remain in the colon, the more toxins are reabsorbed through the colon walls, further taxing the liver. Vitamins can cause constipation, especially iron supplements, although anemia may also make some women nauseous; try herbal iron sources rather than supplements. (See the chapter on Bowel and Digestive Difficulties in the section on Problems That Can Occur at Any Time for more information. See the chapter on Anemia in Pregnancy in Diagnostic Tests for suggestions on natural iron supplementation.)

Also find out if any environmental factors may be playing a part. Things to ask about include household or locally applied insecticides (crop spraying?), nearby factories, or other sources of toxic fumes. Is she sick only when she is at home or in a certain location? This can be a clue that some environmental factor is the culprit. In addition, some women are adversely affected by sleeping on a water bed, a firm mattress may work better until the nausea is under control (El Halta, 1989). Due to changes in the contour of the eyeball, reading or watching television may make nausea more severe, if the woman complains that she feels seasick, she should have her vision checked. (El Halta, 1989)

In some cases, more specific measures are needed to turn nausea around. Some suggestions which have worked for various women are:

*If the vomitus looks like bile, have the woman drink a cup of water with 2 tsp. of salt added upon arising. Usually this will cause vomiting once, then stabilize the stomach.

*Drink Third Wind, Recharge or another natural foods brand electrolyte balanced liquid before eating or when nauseous (Gatoraide should be avoided since it and similar brands are full of chemicals).

*Eat a boiled egg. While this may sound awful, eggs are perfectly balanced protein and can calm the nausea quickly in some cases.

*Take powered ginger in 00 size capsules throughout the day, up to 60 daily if necessary.

*Take Ginger root tea in tablespoon doses at the onset of nausea.

*Use Wild Yam root tincture by the dropperful in mint tea or water.

*Drink Peach leaf tea

*Drink Peppermint or Spearmint leaf infusion first thing in the morning

*Drink Anise or Fennel seed tea on rising or chew either of these seeds during the day

*Take 1 tsp. apple cider vinegar in 8 oz. warm water first thing in the morning

*Rub lobelia tincture on the feet, under the arms and on the abdomen to sooth tension and spasms which trigger vomiting. (Block, 1984)

698

*Take B complex and try extra B_1 and B_6 for 2 weeks (long term use of isolated B vitamins can cause deficiencies of the others).
*Bee pollen in teaspoon doses has helped some women.
*Raspberry leaf tea or infusion—drink 1 to 2 cups daily before rising or suck on ice cubes made from the infusion.
*Figure out a homeopathic remedy for the specific case. Often this works when nothing else will!
*Accupressure wrist bands can be purchased which put pressure on the anti-nausea point at the inner wrist. These work wonderfully for some women. (They may be sold as "seabands," and are often available at health food stores or at your local American Automobile Association office)
*Give 50 mg. of B_6 twice daily, once 20 minutes before arising and once at night (Auerbach, 1983)
*Take small sips of the following tea throughout the day, but no more than 1 cup in a 24 hour period: 1 part cinnamon, 5 parts Blackberry leaves, 5 parts Yarrow, 10 parts Red Raspberry leaves; mix and steep 1 tsp. in ½ cup boiling water for ½ an hour (Auerbach, 1983).
*Consult a naturopath or doctor of oriental medicine

The role of B_6: Many women have dramatic improvements when they supplement with B_6 (which is involved in maintaining normal blood sugar levels). Deficiencies result in an inability to use glucose or release glycogen, thus wreaking havoc with a woman's ability to maintain her glucose levels. On top of that, if glucose is unavailable for the cells, the body burns fat, which produces ketones, which can lead to more nausea. As much as 50 milligrams of B_6 can be taken every 4 hours, along with 400 milligrams of magnesium each morning. In extreme cases, intramuscular injections of B_6 have been found to stop vomiting long enough for the woman to begin eating again; give 1 cc. or more on alternating days for one week, then every third day after that if the nausea returns, once stabilized she can switch to an oral supplement. (El Halta, 1989)

Most nausea subsides by the fourth month of pregnancy. Severe nausea which persists may be associated with inadequate amounts of foods (especially in multiple gestations), pre-existing hypoglycemia, hydatidiform mole, or severe emotional problems. Remember that any digestive upset points to self-nurturing issues as underlying psychological factors. Also, be sure to also rule out possible metabolic imbalances.

Hyperemesis gravidarum:

When the usual tricks do not work and women are nauseous and vomiting all the time to the point of nutritional compromise and dehydration, hyperemesis gravidarum or excessive vomiting of pregnancy exists. This is a serious problem which must be stabilized or the woman may not only lose the pregnancy but severely compromise her health as well. Signs that a woman is moving into hyperemesis are:

*Pernicious vomiting (ceaseless, uncontrollable vomiting)
*Poor appetite
*Weight loss
*Dehydration (dry, coated tongue, ketonuria, rising pulse, falling blood
   pressure, acetone breath, and concentrated urine. Emaciation
   follows, and the urine may then contain protein and bile.
   Epigastric tenderness may occur as well as mental confusion, nerve
   sensitivity and ultimately coma and death)
*Electrolyte imbalance
*Acidosis (low blood pH) due to starvation
*Alkalosis (high blood pH) from loss of stomach acid during vomiting
*Hypokalemia (low blood potassium)
*Severe ketonuria as fat is burned for energy (over +2 on dip stick)

When nothing can be kept in the system, other measures must be taken to stabilize the blood sugar and turn the situation around. Keep in mind that some underlying cause such as vitamin B malabsorption, liver compromise or active disease (such as hepatitis), kidney infection, pancreas or gall bladder problems, hydatidiform mole (see that chapter) or multiple gestation may be influencing the symptom picture. Psychological factors such as extreme fear should be explored; remember that a woman may not be consciously aware that she is afraid or may have other emotions coming up. Dietary practices which encourage women not to gain weight, to eliminate salt, or to eat very little protein could also be at fault. Underweight women or those who are very thin are at more risk for severe vomiting because they have no fat stores to draw on and will become compromised that much quicker.

Nutritive enemas are a good first step to see if hospitalization for IV parenteral nutrition therapy can be avoided. An enema made up of wheat grass juice or a combination of liquid chlorophyll and herbal infusions and tinctures which settle the stomach may be helpful. This should be mixed with an electrolyte IV solution such as Ringers Lactate or unflavored Pedialyte, which is sold in pharmacies. Have the woman lay on her left side and infuse the solution slowly into her colon. Have her retain as much of it as she can as long as she can. If dehydration is significant, the body will make use of the fluid and little will be

700

expelled; the colon will absorb the fluid right into the system. (Also see the section on Ketonuria in <u>Diagnostic Tests</u>.) Once nausea stabilizes, she must immediately begin to take nourishment orally.

If this and everything else you can think of does not quickly turn the situation around, get the woman to a hospital without delay. Wernicke's encephalopathy due to thiamine deficiency may result from extreme hyperemesis. Consciousness clouding, constant movement of the eyeball, double vision, and poor muscle coordination are some symptoms which should prompt immediate treatment with thiamine. (Gleicher, 1985) Nutritive IV's and anti-nausea drugs will help nourish the pregnancy and stabilize nausea so that a woman can feel better; you can then talk to her about any emotional factors which may be influencing the situation. See the chapter on Nausea and Vomiting in the section on Problems That Can Occur in the Second Trimester for a discussion of drugs used for nausea.

References and further reading:

Auerbach, Tami, Informed Homebirth childbirth teacher, personal correspondence, 6/13/83.
El Halta, Valerie <u>Moving Midwifery Forward</u>, Garden of Life, Pub., Aug. 1989.
Gabbe, Steven, et.al., <u>Obstetrics: Normal and Problem Pregnancies</u>, 2nd ed., Churchill, Livingstone, New York, NY, 1991.
Gleicher, N. <u>Principles of Medical Therapy in Pregnancy</u>, Plenum Pub., NY, 1985, p. 1028.
Varney, Helen, <u>Nurse-Midwifery</u>, Blackwell Scientific Pub., Boston, MA 1980.

When a Baby Dies in Early Pregnancy

  The following chapters describe various complications which may lead to the loss of a pregnancy. Whenever this occurs, regardless of the reason, the psychological impact on the mother is that her baby has died. Even in cases where the mother was uncertain of her desire to be pregnant, losing the baby can be a devastating experience. Losing a pregnancy in the first trimester is usually heralded by a series of symptoms which suggest that the pregnancy is threatened and may or may not lead to the actual death of the baby. The explanations and psychological support you actually offer will vary from woman to woman; this chapter will cover some general topics and things to consider doing in relation to maternal psychological, emotional and spiritual well-being as you proceed to deal with the physical factors as well.

Why some pregnancies don't make it: The reasons why pregnancies don't go to term are varied, and may be too technical for parents to grasp in the midst of a crisis. This is not to say that you shouldn't explain things to parents, but to suggest that you keep your explanation simple and straightforward. An analogy to plant growth may help. Soil conditions and the condition of seeds must be ideal for seeds to grow well. If a seed is planted in a way that it cannot receive proper nourishment, it will not make it. If something goes wrong with its development, it will not grow healthy and strong. This straightforward explanation can be applied to early conception, implantation and fetal growth. Often this analogy eases a woman's conscience when she considers that a miscarriage may indicate that something wasn't right with the pregnancy to begin with. (PatKelly, 1995)

Hold on or let go? If a seemingly normal pregnancy is threatened due to miscarriage, it may reflect a psychological ambivalence on the part of the mother concerning pregnancy or the responsibility of parenting. In these cases, the mother's clear intention to let go of the baby or hold on to the pregnancy can help her then decide what to do next. Ask the mother to contemplate the reality of the situation, whether the pregnancy feels right to her or whether it needs to be released. Naturally, if the pregnancy threatens the mother's life, as is often the case in ectopic pregnancy, you will want to encourage the mother to let go of her pregnancy, since its progress will jeopardize her well-being. (PatKelly, 1995)

Seeing the baby: In any grieving process, dealing with the physical reality of the loss is an important step in healing. Some women will want to see what they have passed. Others may be reluctant or outright refuse. You should gently encourage women to look at whatever they pass with you present for support and explanation. Seeing that there was no fetus, or that the fetus was well formed or deformed, or whatever the truth of the matter, will eventually assist a woman in coming to terms with her experience. If the mother refuses to view the remains, respect her wishes but be clear with her that many women feel as she does and later regret their decision. This will be her only opportunity to deal with the physical loss in this way. If she still can't bring herself to do this, make every effort to photograph what was passed, especially if there is a recognizable fetus. You can also encourage the partner to see what was passed so that he can describe it to the mother at a later date.

Having a ceremony: If the baby dies and the parents are encouraged to relate to the loss, a ceremony and cremation or burial of the remains can help them complete the healing process. Although this is not usually done with an early miscarriage, you can suggest that the parents might want to honor the loss in this way. By bringing it up you give the parents permission to formally acknowledge their loss, and you show respect for their process as well.

Dealing with family and friends: Women who were early in their pregnancy may not have many friends that knew they were going to have a baby. If they had started to tell people, it can be very difficult to face those who may unknowingly make cheerful comments or minimize the loss because the pregnancy was not far advanced. You can help bridge that gap.

Pain and guilt: Women often feel intensely guilty after the loss of an early pregnancy, particularly if they were ambivalent about proceeding with the pregnancy in the first place. At the same time, if the pregnancy was unwelcome, a woman may feel relief as well, which may heighten her feelings of guilt. Feelings of failure, shame, and loss of faith in the physical body are commonly reflected in relationship difficulties such as poor communication and sexual disharmony. Talking to the woman during the process about her feelings, having the mother complete the process at home whenever it is safe to do so, and continuing your dialogue with her will go a long way in helping to resolve these feelings. Just making her aware that these feelings and problems are common after an early pregnancy loss and acknowledging to her how totally blind our culture is to the enormity of the experience will assist her in dealing with her pain. Encourage her to feel her feelings; remind her that anything she is feeling, including anger, is okay. Elizabeth Kubler-Ross says "It's okay to be angry at God, God can take it." You might also recommend that she take homeopathic Ignatia, 30C or 200C doses three times daily. Ignatia helps a person move through grief without suppressing necessary emotional release.

Physical changes: Women who find themselves suddenly unpregnant will experience a rapid hormonal shift very unlike the shift that occurs after the birth of a baby at term who goes on to nurse. This hormonal let down will often exaggerate a woman's emotional responses and make her feel quite depressed. Physical reactions such as hot flashes, uterine cramps as the uterus recovers its nonpregnant size, and breast tenderness may also occur. Make sure that the woman continues to eat well (which can be difficult during grieving) and encourage her to take vitamin and mineral supplements, particularly vitamins C, E and zinc. Blood loss as well as poor diet may leave such women anemic, which can aggravate emotional swings and depression. If bleeding has been heavy, check the hemoglobin after 36 hours have passed to determine if this is a factor; otherwise check the hemoglobin at a two week visit.

Follow-up visits: Encourage women to have one or two more appointments to discuss how they are feeling and to acknowledge their grieving process. A good all-purpose question to ask anyone experiencing a death is to ask "What can I do for you?" or "What do you need at this point?" and then help her figure out ways to get that support. Penetration of the yoni during sex should be avoided until any discharge has stopped, signalling that the cervix is fully closed.

The partner: While women's pain around early pregnancy loss is not well supported in our culture, the pain and bewilderment a partner might feel is usually not even addressed. A man especially, may feel that the pregnancy was only a mental concept to him, now he must cope with a grieving woman who was physically bonded to a baby that died. To avoid being overwhelmed by his partner's grief, a man may try to minimize the loss and encourage his partner to get over it. It is important for men to acknowledge and feel their loss as well. Most of all, both partners need to keep the lines of communication between them open and allow each other to feel their feelings through to completion. While physical and sexual intimacy often feels comforting at these times, there may be mixed feelings about being intimate due to both the fear of getting pregnant and the guilt of enjoying sex in the midst of grief. This aspect of grieving needs to be discussed. As the midwife, you can bring up these issues, hopefully opening the space for better communication between the parents.

When can I get pregnant again? This is many women's first question once the initial shock of the loss has subsided. Menstruation should resume shortly after a miscarriage, and pregnancy is possible at any time. However, both physical and emotional healing can take some time. It is wise to remind women that if they get pregnant right away they may not give themselves the opportunity to fully grieve this loss. For this reason, my general recommendation after a first trimester loss is to wait at least 6 months and preferably a year before conceiving again. This will also help to separate one experience from the other.

References and further reading:
Panuthos, Claudia & Romero, C., Ended Beginnings, Bergin & Garvey, Pub., Boston, MA, 1984.
Patkelly, MARI, midwife, New Hampshire, editing comments, 2/22/95.

704

Miscarriage in the First Trimester

Under the medical model, a miscarriage is called a spontaneous abortion. It is the natural end of a pregnancy before the fetus can live outside the womb. Even though miscarriage may be considered to occur as late as 20 to 24 weeks of pregnancy, the vast majority will occur during the first trimester. Indeed, 30% of women that miscarry are unaware that they are pregnant, losing the pregnancy very early with a delayed, heavy period. Another 15% miscarry sometime during the first 2 months; thus miscarriage commonly occurs although women may not be aware of this fact (Rubin & Farber, 1988).

There are many things to consider when evaluating a woman for the possibility of miscarriage. Frequently, women have symptoms, even fairly severe symptoms, and go on to carry a healthy pregnancy to term. As midwives, we must remember that a few symptoms suggesting miscarriage do not mean that losing the baby is inevitable. We must also keep in mind that a woman can have cramping and/or bleeding which indicates a serious medical emergency such as ectopic pregnancy. Differentiating between a common miscarriage and a more serious disorder which requires immediate medical intervention is important and sometimes life saving. Remember your basic care plan: ensure the mother's safety, discuss emotional issues (see chapter on When a Baby Dies in Early Pregnancy), then decide what to do.

What's happening? When a woman first lets you know that she fears she may be miscarrying (usually by phone), there are some questions you will want to ask her. If possible, pull her file before you start.

*What symptoms are you having? When did they start?
*How long have they been going on?
*When was the last time you had intercourse or penetration of the yoni?
*Is there any bleeding or spotting? What color and what amount?
*Are there any cramps or pains? Where are they located?
*Have you passed anything other than blood?
*How do you feel otherwise? What other pregnancy symptoms are still present?
*At what point in gestation is the pregnancy? (check your records)
*Are you a DES daughter? (check your records)
*Have you recently been exposed to any environmental contaminants?
*Do you have a history of miscarriage? (check your records)
*What is your blood type and factor? (Rh-negative women may need RhD(o) immunoglobulin).

Maintaining a calm, centered attitude yourself will go a long way in helping the mother center herself and relay all that is happening. Women who want their pregnancies are generally quite anxious about the prospect of miscarriage and will be understandably upset if they are showing symptoms which suggest they might be miscarrying. Women often assume that cramps or bleeding mean that miscarriage is inevitable; they feel overwhelmed and frightened. When you remind women that bleeding and cramping can occur for many reasons and begin to ask them questions regarding other possible causes for their symptoms, they almost always calm down, as they realize that the issue is not as black and white as they feared. First, you want to offer assurance that many women who experience symptoms of threatened miscarriage go on to carry their pregnancies to term. In addition, remind them that mild cramping and slight bleeding from implantation are associated with normal pregnancy. Tell a woman that you want to review with her exactly what is going on so you can both figure out what to do next. While it may not be necessary to ask all the above questions of every woman, for the sake of consistency they will be discussed in series.

What symptoms are you having? When did they start? While this is an important question to ask, some women may be so upset that they cannot organize their thoughts to give a coherent answer. Therefore, regardless of what a woman says at this point, you will still ask the specific questions that follow regarding bleeding and cramping, the two primary symptoms associated with miscarriage.

How long have the symptoms been going on? Often, but not always, women will call at the first sign of a problem. A woman who has had significant bleeding but who has been sitting at home denying the possibility of miscarriage should be seen quickly, or should be told to go directly to a hospital or obstetrical care provider. Remember, a woman in early pregnancy does not have an expanded blood volume, and what would amount to normal bleeding postpartum can cause her to become shocky much more quickly. Prolonged bleeding over the course of several days may leave a woman weak and debilitated; however a reduction in coagulation ability leading to disseminated intravascular coagulation (DIC) is exceedingly unlikely during the first trimester (Kolder, 1995).

When was the last time you had intercourse or penetration of the yoni? It is often the case that pressure on the cervix during sexual activity will cause a minor amount of discharge ranging from brown spotting to bright red bleeding. (Brown spotting is most common because the bleeding will have stopped and the blood will have turned from red to brown before being discharged.) If cervical stimulation is the cause, the bleeding should not continue and will usually be limited to some spotting on the sheets the next morning or a sudden spot appearing when the woman sits up in bed, stands or first uses the toilet; however heavier bleeding from the cervix can occur and is often benign. In addition, the pregnant uterus sometimes has stronger contractions than usual during orgasm. The combination

706

of spotting and cramping may cause a woman to fear she is miscarrying.

Of course, if the pregnancy is not very healthy, orgasm and cervical stimulation can jar the uterus and cause symptoms of a miscarriage that would have been inevitable anyway. Intercourse, other cervical stimulation, or even vigorous exercise such as horse-back riding will not, by themselves, precipitate miscarriage in the healthy, well-nourished woman with a normal cervix and uterus who has a viable pregnancy.

Is there any bleeding or spotting? What color and what quantity? Bleeding may be defined as the passage of bright red to dark red fluid blood or clots in trickles, gushes or streams. Spotting may be defined as the appearance of small stains of blood which may be bright red to dark brown on a woman's sheets, underpants, sanitary pad or toilet paper. Generally speaking, when a woman who is spotting tries to find more blood by wiping or cleaning herself, no more is present at that time, although more spotting may appear at some later point in the day.

The color of the blood indicates how recently the bleeding occurred. Bright red bleeding has just occurred; it becomes progressively darker as time goes on. Brownish bleeding or spotting or stained fluid that is streaked with clear serum is old. That is, it occurred at some previous time. Such brown spotting may have occurred high in the uterus and worked its way down to the cervical opening to be expelled. In that process it can become diluted with other fluids, and the blood changes from red to brown in the process of clotting and deterioration.

It can be very hard to gauge the amount of spotting or bleeding over the phone, because what looks like a lot to the woman may, in fact, be very little, or vice versa. Here are some helpful questions to ask in trying to discern how much bleeding is taking place:

*Does it soak through your underwear? Your outer wear? Is it only on the sheet or does it soak through to the mattress?
*Is the area very wet or just damp? Can you blot up blood by pressing into the spot?
*What is the diameter of the spot? (compare to common objects such as a dime, a quarter, a lemon; how many such spots?)
*Does bleeding occur only when you wipe at the toilet? Does it saturate the toilet paper or just stain or moisten the surface?
*Are you wearing a pad? How large a pad? Is it being soaked? How often are you changing it?
*Are you bleeding continuously, or does it start and stop? (Remember, a continuous discharge of black, brown or darkly stained fluid is still old blood. However, if continuing, this discharge is likely to be classified as heavy spotting. Fresh bleeding will be brighter; fresh bleeding from high in the uterus

may be somewhat darker but still red and clotted. Blood darkens whenever there is a delay between the bleeding and when you see it.)

*Ask the woman to save all stained articles such as pads, clothing, sheets and towels in a plastic bag for you to see before she lauders them if you still have questions about the amount she is bleeding. A bowl or plastic bag can be placed under the toilet seat to catch anything that may be passed on the toilet; better yet, she can squat over a wide-mouthed bowl.

Are there any cramps or pains? Where are they located? It is quite common for women to have cramping by itself; various sensations may feel like cramps that are perfectly normal, such as indigestion (gas). Cramps can be caused by the enlarging of the uterus in early pregnancy. Those located to either side of the pubic bone are usually due to stretching of the round ligaments. As the pregnancy advances, these sensations will shift and be found somewhere between the woman's abdominal midline and the iliac crests, running in two distinct lines up the sides of the uterus. A woman who has had any kind of lower abdominal surgery (appendectomy, ovarian cyst removal, etc.) may have scar tissue adhesions which can be stretched and cause pain and pulling sensations as the uterus enlarges. Pains can occur from the enlarging uterus putting pressure on an ovarian cyst.

The uterus will cramp and bleed if it is trying to expel its contents in a miscarriage; the further along the pregnancy, the more cramping must occur to force the products of conception through the cervix in order to empty the uterus. Occasionally a woman will only feel pain in her lower back during a miscarriage. Lower back pain could also be related to a urinary tract or kidney infection.

Pain may also be present in an ectopic pregnancy which is about to rupture. (See that chapter for complete information.) An appendicitis attack will also cause pain, but bleeding from the yoni will not accompany this emergency. A urinary tract infection is another common cause of pelvic pain, and blood in the urine may be confused with bleeding from the yoni.

The location of the pain provides important clues as to the possible origin of the problem. Ask the woman specifically if it is off to one side; sharp pains off to one side or the other may be caused by ligament spasm but also suggest an ectopic pregnancy, which should be ruled out with an ultrasound exam. Intrauterine as well as urinary tract upsets will be characterized by centrally located lower abdominal pain with or without backache in some women.

Have you passed anything other than blood? Ask her to save everything she passes in a glass jar in the refrigerator so that you (or her referral practitioner) can examine it before disposal. If she does miscarry you want to identify a fetus and placenta if possible to determine if all the products of conception have been passed. In addition, a distressed woman who flushes her fetus down the toilet or throws it

708

away may forever feel haunted. If any masses are passed into the toilet, have her cover her hand with a plastic kitchen bag or a glove and fish them out for your inspection, have someone who is with her do this, or tell her not to flush the toilet and do it yourself when you arrive. One-sided pain and the passage of only white or pinkish tissue is usually endometrial lining and should alert you to the possibility of an ectopic pregnancy.

How do you feel otherwise? Emotional reactions to the possibility of miscarriage are normal. However, while comforting the woman on that level, you want to know if she feels weak, dizzy, light headed, faint, or nauseous. Has she noticed a rapid pulse? If you are unsure of her condition, have her or her partner count her pulse. Any of these could be symptoms indicating that she has lost too much blood or has hidden internal bleeding from an ectopic pregnancy or other emergency.

If she is calling you some days after the fact, ask if she still has any other symptoms of early pregnancy such as breast tenderness or enlargement, nausea, or urinary frequency. Does she still "feel" pregnant? If she has lost the pregnancy, the hormonal levels will drop and the symptoms of early pregnancy will gradually disappear.

At what point in gestation is the pregnancy? Check your records to find out how far along her pregnancy is (remembering that the actual gestational age of the fetus lags two weeks behind the weeks of pregnancy). The larger the conceptus is at the time of miscarriage, the more her uterus will have to work to expel its contents.

Are there known uterine abnormalities or is she a DES daughter? A number of cervical and uterine abnormalities predispose some affected women to miscarriage. A miscarriage from a loose (incompetent) cervix will usually take place once the fetus is heavy enough to cause the cervix to open from increased pressure, which is usually past the 12th week of pregnancy and is typically painless until dilation is well underway, when uterine contractions may begin to be felt.

Have you recently been exposed to any environmental contaminants? Depending upon where a woman lives, she may be exposed to agricultural sprays, insecticides, chemical plant exhaust fumes, radioactive substances or other toxic substances which could increase her chances of miscarriage. If she feels such an exposure has taken place, be sure to notify your local agency which tracks teratogenic agents. You can call your local health department for such a number or see Diagnostic Tests to find the agency nearest you. Let them know the specific agent, if known, and find out if other reports of pregnancy related complications have come in recently or been reported in the past. They may also have some recommendations about how to proceed with care.

Is there a history of miscarriage? A woman with a history of miscarriage may be especially fearful in this situation. Repeated miscarriage in the first trimester can be due to poor maternal nutrition, teratogenic environmental effects, hormonal abnormalities, lethal genetic problems, substance abuse, or maternal disease or infection, to name some of the most common reasons. After one miscarriage the chances of having a second are the same as for the general population. After two consecutive miscarriages the chance of a third goes up to 33%, and after three consecutive miscarriages the chance of a fourth goes up to 50%. These statistics are reassuring to many women. (Kolder, 1995)

Is there a history which increases the likelihood of an ectopic pregnancy? The importance of ruling out ectopic pregnancy cannot be overemphasized. Check your records and review details in the next chapter.

What is her blood type and factor? Remind yourself if the woman is Rh-negative by checking her lab results. If so, you want to be sure she makes an informed choice regarding RhD(o) immunoglobulin if a miscarriage does take place.

<u>**Differential diagnosis of symptoms suggesting miscarriage:**</u>

Benign bleeding: In review, bleeding can occur due to a variety of reasons which do not threaten the pregnancy. These reasons include:

Implantation bleeding: This is caused by erosion of maternal blood vessels at the implantation site in the uterus. This usually occurs by 7 to 10 days post-conception but may be delayed a little longer if the blood is working its way down the uterine wall. This painless spotting or bleeding may occur any time during or even throughout the week when implantation takes place, but it then stops.

Cervical bleeding: This may be due to softening, stimulation during sexual activity, increased vascularity, lesions or infection of the cervix. If a lesion or infection is suspected, the cervix should be visualized with a speculum exam and cultures taken as appropriate. Bleeding may also be due to the presence of polyps, benign growths which hang on a stem from the inner cervical passageway. If the stem is narrow, they can be removed by simply snipping them off at the stem. If polyps seem to be the source of bleeding, get them evaluated before you attempt to remove them.

Stretching of decidual capillaries: As the uterus grows, stretching combined with minor decidual necrosis can cause some harmless bleeding.

Menstrual breakthrough bleeding: During the first few months of pregnancy some women have slight bleeding at the time they would normally menstruate. In rare cases this continues throughout gestation.

False pregnancy: A woman who believes herself to be pregnant when she really is not will often continue to have some monthly bleeding, even though in some cases it will be less than she would normally have. (See separate chapter in the Second Trimester Section)

Delayed menstruation: *Metrophathia hemorrhagia* is a period of cessation of menses followed by excessive bleeding from accumulated layers of endometrial tissue in a woman who is not pregnant. Pain is usually not a feature except for cramping associated with the passage of huge clots. (Donald, 1979) I have seen this in a woman who was on prednisone.

Benign cramping/pain by itself: Various normal processes may cause some cramping and pain in early pregnancy:

Normal response of the uterus to pregnancy: As the uterus enlarges and gains muscle mass it begins to have toning contractions and stretching sensations which are intermittently apparent to many women.

Indigestion/gas: Be sure to ask about this obvious, benign reason for abdominal pain before moving along to more serious considerations.

Stretching of the round ligaments: This can cause cramping along either side of the pubic bone in early pregnancy and further up as the uterus enlarges.

Orgasm: Cramps can be precipitated by orgasm as the uterus contracts more strongly due to the changes of pregnancy.

Vulval engorgement: Some women find the vulval engorgement which begins in early pregnancy to be painful at times. In some cases, this can be confused with more serious causes of pain in some cases. Many women find that orgasm temporarily relieves engorgement (at least to a certain extent).

Other causes of bleeding and cramping may include:

Poor nutrition: This is a major cause of otherwise normal pregnancy loss not related to genetic anomalies. Always review the dietary intake whenever a problem occurs that indicates poor placental attachment.

Urinary tract infection: Cramping, lower pelvic pain and achiness can be due to a urinary tract infection which needs attention.

Scar tissue adhesions in the lower abdomen: Although occasionally severely stretched adhesions may have to be released surgically if they begin to tear and bleed internally, this is rare. Have the woman take Evening Primrose oil or Black Currant oil (1 capsule every other day in the first trimester) to assist in softening the scars and reducing the pain (contraindicated for DES daughters).

Adhesions within the uterus: Fifteen to 30% of women with intrauterine scar tissue adhesions (synechiae) miscarry. Adhesions may form after invasive procedures such as curettage postpartum, intrauterine surgery, or endometritis. Pain, bleeding and miscarriage occur as the uterus enlarges. (Adhesions can be severed if discovered, but 50% of these women will continue to miscarry). (Gabbe, 1991) See recommendations for softening scar tissue above.

Ovarian cysts: Pressure from the enlarging uterus can cause ovarian cysts to become painful.

Hydatidiform or vesicular mole: This is an abnormality of the placenta which can mimic a more typical threatened miscarriage. (See separate chapter in this section for more details.)

Fibroids: Fibroids often cause quite a bit of uterine pain on and off throughout pregnancy. They can also cause bleeding and pain, especially if they become twisted. Submucosal and intramural fibroids are the two types most commonly associated with miscarriage. (See the chapter on Fibroids in the section on Problems That Can Occur At Any Time for more details.)

Uterine scars: Many women who have had a surgical delivery or other uterine surgery report that the scar can be painful at times as the uterus enlarges. As long as the discomfort does not persist and increase, it does not mean the scar will rupture; in a normal pregnancy rupture virtually unheard of in the first trimester. (See chapter on Uterine Rupture and also the one on YBACs.)

Cervical or uterine cancer: These will cause painless bleeding.

Preexisting maternal disease: Some conditions such as severe kidney or heart disease will make carriage of a pregnancy unlikely, impossible or dangerous.

Torn hymenal vessel: May be caused by penetration of the yoni and may bleed, sometimes to the point of being life threatening (rare).

Inevitable miscarriage of an intrauterine pregnancy: If the pregnancy is no longer viable, cramps and bleeding will usually increase until the uterine contents have been expelled. The larger the conceptus, the more the uterus will have to work to push the baby and placenta through the cervix, which is not ready to open as it would be at term. Inevitable abortion is the term used in the medical model when the cervix is open but the conceptus has not been passed.

Fifty to sixty percent of first trimester miscarriages are due to verifiable abnormalities of the baby or placenta. In these cases the baby usually dies before bleeding begins. The average amount of time between the death of the fetus and expulsion is 6 weeks and the average time for the actual miscarriage to occur is 10 weeks from the LMP.

Ectopic pregnancy: As the conceptus gets too large for its implantation site, cramping and bleeding occur, increasing just prior to rupture. Classically, symptoms begin with pain and are followed by bleeding, however rupture and internal bleeding can occur without any blood being passed. Multiple gestation can result in simultaneous intrauterine and ectopic pregnancies. (See the next chapter for more details).

Loss of an intrauterine multiple gestation: Bleeding, even passage of tissue, can accompany the loss of one baby and the retention of another normal baby which will go to term. Such miscarriages usually occur quite early in pregnancy. In this case *Beta*-pregnancy blood test values may fall but remain within a range which indicates viable placental tissue still exists. This is also a reason why you should be cautious in telling a woman that she has lost her pregnancy, even if some tissue has been passed. This is especially true if her uterus remains enlarged and signs of pregnancy persist.

Emotional issues: Unless an emergency such as profuse bleeding or suspected rupture of an ectopic pregnancy is underway, now is the time to deal with the emotional aspects of the situation. Discuss particulars as appropriate to each individual woman, whatever is in the mother's mind and heart. Try to find out what specific stresses, fears, concerns or interfering factors she is currently grappling with and assist her family or support network in understanding how they can ease those stresses whenever possible. Threatened miscarriage and premature labor often signal cries of help from the mother regarding her needs. Have the "letting go or holding on" conversation (see the chapter on When a Baby Dies in Early Pregnancy). Once that is done, proceed with the next step: what to do.

Dealing with different miscarriage symptoms:

In the otherwise normal circumstance, bleeding from the pregnant uterus is due to a partial or complete detachment of the placenta. If you feel the pregnancy is intrauterine, proceed as follows:

Threatened miscarriage: Typically this *begins with bleeding,* which may or may not be followed by accompanying cramps and lower backache within the next few hours or days. If you do an internal exam the cervix will be found closed and the size of the uterus appropriate for the weeks the woman is pregnant (an internal exam is rarely necessary). Bleeding alone, even though heavy, is often transitory and frequently does not end in miscarriage. One out of every five women will have some bleeding (including spotting) in the first half of pregnancy. If a woman who is bleeding in the first trimester has a verifiable living baby, her chances of carrying the baby to viability are 90%. (Kolder, 1995)

Options for treatment: Most women will have made the decision that they want to keep a pregnancy. Have the mother rest in bed and focus on the baby and placenta; have her see the baby surrounded with white light and the placenta strong and healthy, firmly attached to the uterine wall. Be sure she is getting adequate protein, salt and calories in her diet and plenty of fluids. Avoid doing an internal exam. Have the mother take 2000 IU of vitamin E and 500 mg. of Vitamin C with bioflavinoids daily to help strengthen the placental bed. This dosage of vitamin E should be continued for 2 to 3 weeks and then tapered off.

One of the following herbal combinations can help to prevent a miscarriage if the mother is weak but the baby is healthy. Herbs are said not to stop a miscarriage if the conceptus is damaged or defective.

> *1 oz. Cramp Bark and 2 oz. Wild Yam root (Colic root) to equal 2 oz. total herb material. Boil 20 minutes in 1½ quarts of water. Take 1 tsp. in water 3 to 4 times daily between meals.

714

*2 to 4 ozs. of Wild Yam root infusion every half hour, results should be evident by the second dose. (Or, take 10 drops of Wild Yam root tincture every half-hour until cramps stop, then taper off as for False Unicorn Root, described below.)
*1 part Black Haw, 3 parts False Unicorn Root, 1 part Lobelia. Boil a total of 3 oz. of herb material in 1½ quarts of water for 20 minutes. Take 1 Tablespoon in water 3 to 4 times daily.
*Take 5 drops of False Unicorn Root tincture and 5 drops of Lobelia tincture every 15 minutes until cramps cease, then space doses out over the next four days unless cramps resume, then go back to 1 dose every 15 minutes. Dosage can be spaced out to every 30 minutes for 2 hours, then every hour until she falls asleep, then 6 times the next day, tapering it off in this manner over the course of several days.
*Take 15 drops of Lobelia tincture in a little water as often as every 15 minutes for several days, if necessary, until symptoms disappear.
*Combine 1 Tbsp. dried Black Haw Root Bark or Cramp Bark, 3 Tbsp. dried Red Raspberry leaves, 10 drops Wild Yam root tincture, 10 drops False Unicorn root tincture and 60 drops Lobelia herb tincture. Put dried herbs in a quart jar and fill with boiling water. Steep until cold enough to drink. Add Wild Yam and False Unicorn tinctures to 1 cup and drink. If cramps continue for more than 30 minutes add 60 drops Lobelia to another cup of tea and drink. Drink 1 cup every 3 hours, adding tinctures as needed until symptoms subside.

When using herbs, be alert for side effects such as nausea or low blood pressure (especially when using Lobelia). Discontinue the herb or cut back the dose if side effects are noted; fortunately side effects are rare.

Inevitable miscarriage: If bleeding steadily increases and is joined by cramps and pain, and especially if it is accompanied by cervical softening and dilation, the inevitable loss of the pregnancy is much more likely. In the majority of cases, an internal exam is not necessary. However, should you decide to do one, the cervix may be felt to be shorter and more in line with the body of the uterus or bulging (see illustration on next page; the dotted lines show changes in contour of the cervix and lower uterine segment when miscarriage is inevitable) (Bald & Montgomery, 1935). If the conceptus has been dead for a length of time, the uterus will be small-for-dates. If the miscarriage seems to be inevitable, the woman still has some options. While some women will want to go right in and have their uterus emptied by either a dilation and curettage (D&C) or a vacuum procedure, many others will want to avoid surgical intervention whenever possible. There are good reasons why women who are not experiencing excessive bleeding should be supported in letting nature take its course, as long as problems do not arise which make a watch-and-wait plan unwise. Surgical intervention can damage the cervix or perforate the uterus, may introduce infection, and is often a traumatic experience. If a woman feels that she wants to just go to the hospital

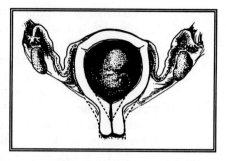

and get it over with, you might remind her that it will not lessen the pain to wind up in the hospital with a lot of interventions. Transport can distract her from the emotional experience of the process and may therefore prolong her grieving.

Those women who can focus their attention enough to attempt it can support the completion of the process with the aid of visualization. Encourage the woman to see her body releasing the placenta completely and letting go of the pregnancy. Ask her to imagine her uterus contracting with a rhythmic wave-like pattern; she can visualize the ocean waves coming and going, or use whatever other effective image she can conjure up. In addition, labor support measures including the use of a heating pad over the pubic area, massage, pacing, position changes, and tightly holding small combs so that the teeth are pressed into the mounds at the base of the fingers (which stimulates pressure points to facilitate the uterine contractions) can be used to help deal with the pain.

Have the woman keep in close touch with you and consider going to her house to support and monitor her yourself. Do not let a woman miscarry without any support people present, as she could become shocky and pass out; she will also need emotional support. The mother should be kept warm, the amount of bleeding should be monitored closely and she should be watched for other signs of shock such as pallor, dizziness and spaciness. If symptoms are severe, she should not be allowed to sleep until the miscarriage is complete and bleeding has subsided; the desire to sleep can also be a symptom of shock. Encourage her to drink freely, at least a cup of clear fluids every 2 hours. She can take 20 drops each of Blue and Black Cohosh tinctures every 30 to 60 minutes to help stimulate contractions. If the mother is not hypertensive, another option is to give 0.2 mg. Methergine tablets by mouth, one every 6 to 8 hours. Some reasonable guidelines regarding the progress of a miscarriage are:

> *Expect bleeding and cramping to increase until the bleeding is very heavy (soaking a sanitary pad every 30 minutes to 1 hour) and cramping is severe (usually worse than any menstrual cramps).
> *In most cases severe symptoms (as above) should not last for more than 1½ hours; almost all women will have a complete miscarriage in this amount of time. If symptoms are less severe, a miscarriage

can take longer, sometimes the fetus will be passed at one point, the placenta a few days later. The amount of bleeding, the mother's overall condition and signs of infection should be monitored throughout a prolonged miscarriage; if signs of infection become apparent or symptoms increase in severity without completing the miscarriage, transport is appropriate.

*If heavy bleeding or severe cramping persist beyond 1½ hours, the woman should be examined by you, her back-up care provider or in the Emergency Room. (Kolder, 1995)

If bleeding continues and is more than slight or if pain is prolonged or severe, referral to a consulting physician is advised. The physician will be looking for the following information with an internal exam. If you practice rurally or if for any other reason (such as bad whether) you are unable to reach medical assistance, you may opt to do an internal exam using sterile gloves and a sterile speculum. If the woman refuses transport at this time and is still stable, plan to stay with her until the miscarriage is complete and bleeding has almost stopped or until you both decide it is time to transport. At this point, you might find one of two clinical pictures:

*The uterus is enlarged, the cervix is open, but no products of conception are visible on speculum exam. More bleeding and cramping can be expected. If no products have been passed or tissue is high in the uterus, monitor the mother and wait to see if the miscarriage will complete itself before intervening. If the woman has already experienced heavy bleeding (soaking more than a pad every 45 minutes for more than 1½ hours) or has other worrisome signs such as light-headedness or rapid pulse, surgical intervention to complete the miscarriage is warranted. Or,

*The fundus feels only slightly enlarged and appears to be sitting on top of a widely dilated lower segment and cervical passageway from which products of conception can be easily felt as they protrude or rest just inside the os or in the posterior fornix (Donald, 1979; Kolder, 1995). In this case, the miscarriage is in process and the woman can be reassured. Generally speaking, it is best to avoid pulling out tissues felt at the os; allow them to continue to be expelled on their own to avoid retention of tissue.

If you have opted to stay home, have waited another hour or so, and the miscarriage has still not completed itself, you might consider doing an exam to see if you can feel or see tissue protruding from or just inside the os. If you are far from medical assistance you might insert a sterile speculum, if you haven't already done so, and gently remove the remaining tissue with a sterile sponge forceps.

Remember that any invasive procedures carry the risk of uterine perforation and infection. This should not be attempted by an inexperienced midwife who has no training in invasive procedures; in that case transport is your safest alternative. Give vitamin C with bioflavinoids (1000 mg daily) and Echinacea tincture (½ dropperful 6 times daily) for one week to minimize infection.

Charting: Whenever you are present at a miscarriage keep a chart of the mother's condition, recording vital signs such as temperature (to check for infection) blood pressure and pulse, blood loss, fluid intake, options discussed, supplements or herbs given and any procedures performed.

Determining if a complete miscarriage has occurred: Three hours after it appears that everything has passed and bleeding has slowed to staining an internal exam should reveal a closed cervix. While such an exam might be warranted if you live far from the mother's home, it can almost always be postponed until a two week follow-up visit. Pain and cramps will steadily decrease or cease but slight tenderness may persist for a few days. If tenderness is more than slight or accompanied by a fever or foul smelling discharge, further assessment for a possible infection is warranted. Bleeding may continue as it would during a normal postpartum; however, since the placental site is small at this point, it should only be a light flow.

Dealing with an incomplete miscarriage: A miscarriage is incomplete when bleeding and pain persist, signaling that even though some products of conception have been passed, tissue is still retained. The cervix will usually remain open and the uterus may or may not feel smaller than the number of weeks of pregnancy. In this case, portions of the placenta have usually been retained (most often this occurs after twelve weeks gestation when the slender cord can easily break, allowing the fetus to be expelled and the placenta to remain inside; however this can also occur in the late first trimester). During the first trimester the uterus is not that large and the placenta may be firmly implanted (since it is not ready to release), making for a difficult placental detachment.

If you suspect an incomplete miscarriage, first work with the mother to visualize the release and passage of the tissue. If this does not work, it is an appropriate time to recommend transport for a Dilation and Curettage to reduce the chances of infection in the mother. For those who refuse transport, another option is to try taking herbs such as equal parts Blue and Black Cohosh tinctures, 20 to 30 drops total every 2 to 4 hours or one Ergotrate or Methergine (0.2 mg.) tablet every 8 hours until the remaining products of conception have passed and perhaps for a few days beyond. This will cause uterine contractions, reduce bleeding and assist the passage of tissue. If the clinical picture remains the same, advise transport.

Missed abortion: A missed abortion occurs when the baby dies but the products of conception are not expelled from the uterus for two months or longer. Often a missed abortion is assumed to exist after the onset and subsequent subsidal of miscarriage symptoms, only to find that the pregnancy is intact and growing. In a genuine case of missed abortion, bleeding and pain subside, uterine growth stops and the uterus gradually reduces in size but the menses do not resume. Other signs of pregnancy, such as breast changes, revert to non-pregnant status. *Beta-*pregnancy tests reveal falling hCG values which finally revert to nonpregnant levels. A brownish discharge is the only indication that the products are retained. Typically the cervix is closed.

This can be quickly remedied by evacuating the uterus with a dilation and curettage or a vacuum procedure. Do not attempt invasive procedures if dealing with this at home, as infection with anaerobic organisms may occur and can be fatal. Many women may want to allow the pregnancy to pass naturally. Waiting also allows a still viable pregnancy to make itself known. It can take up to 14 months for the conceptus to pass, but typically takes only 1 to 2 months in first trimester situations. In these cases, a clotting panel should be done immediately as a baseline, then repeated every two weeks until the uterus empties itself, although the disruption of maternal clotting status is highly unlikely. In the past, many cases of actual clotting failure leading to disseminated intravascular coagulation were associated with retained hydropic fetuses due to Rh sensitization (Donald, 1979), a rare occurrence today with the advent of RhD(o) immunoglobulin. Have the mother monitor for signs of infection by taking her temperature daily, and making sure her discharge does not smell foul.

Examining what is passed: If you have the opportunity to examine what a woman has passed during a miscarriage you may be able to determine if the miscarriage is complete. Remember to do this with an attitude of respect; a woman's baby has died. Look at all stained articles to get an idea of how much blood has been lost. Wearing gloves, gently pull apart clots to see if any products of conception can be found. Remember that clots will be dark red or purple and may have fibrous stringy areas. These are fibrinogen fibers, not pieces of placenta.

You may be able to identify a placenta and fetus (or an empty sac which would indicate no fetal development or early death of the embryo). However, a discernable fetus is often not found prior to 8 to 10 weeks, either because it is too small or because no baby ever developed (a "blighted ovum"). The membranes appear whitish and the placental and fetal tissue are pink, as opposed to red blood and deep wine colored clots.

When the products of conception can be distinguished in the first six to eight weeks of pregnancy the whole conceptus is usually passed and may be covered with a portion of the decidua. Prior to 40 days gestation (that's 9.5 weeks of pregnancy) the baby will be less than 1 centimeter in length. At 2 weeks of pregnancy the gestational sac is about the size of a pea, at 2 weeks the size of a fat fava bean and at 4 weeks, it is the size of a walnut. By 6 weeks of pregnancy, it is about 1 3/4" or 4.5 cm across. Up until 8 to 10 weeks of pregnancy, chorionic villi will still cover most of the gestational sac and will appear as a soft, fluffy white to light pink or bushy covering on the sac, reminiscent of fine short tentacles of a sea anemone. Portions of this fluffy tissue may detach and be expelled separately during the miscarriage. From 10 weeks of pregnancy on, more and more of the gestational sac will be smooth and will appear white, the villus chorion (early placenta) will continue to look fluffy and white, gradually becoming denser and more defined as gestation advances. If products of conception are retained, it is much more common for the placenta to remain in the uterus and the fetus to be expelled. If you discover grape-like cysts on all or part of the placenta, save the tissue in a glass container in the refrigerator and refer to the chapter on Hydatidiform or Vesicular Mole later in this section.

See the chapter on embryology (this section) and the chart describing the size and appearance of the embryo in early pregnancy to tract down the approximate age of the embryo or fetus, if one is found. Since the gestational sac is larger than the embryo it contains, it is possible to find a sac and not find an embryo early on, even when one was present. If timing the weeks of pregnancy is possible, it will assist the woman in reexamining what she felt at different points as she tries to come to terms with her experience.

Encourage the mother to examine what has been passed as well, offering your assistance and support. Seeing it will help her deal with what has taken place, will help ground her in reality (rather than remaining in a dreamy nightmarish fantasy that it will go away) and will ultimately assist her grieving process.

Decidual cast: A decidual cast results when the entire uterine lining (the decidua) detaches from the uterine wall intact. The cast is expelled in one piece and is the shape of the uterine cavity; usually a flat triangular reddish brown or brownish pink shaggy, very soft mass of tissue. The passage of a decidual cast is a hormonal reaction to pregnancy and does not always mean that an intrauterine pregnancy existed. There are several conditions that may result in the passage of a decidual cast:

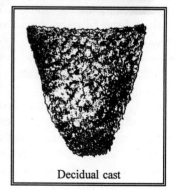

Decidual cast

  *Hormonal influences from an ectopic
     pregnancy can cause a decidual cast
         to be shed, and the passage of one should alert you to the possibility that an ectopic pregnancy may be the cause of the symptoms of an apparent intrauterine miscarriage. If this is the case, other presenting symptoms will not subside.

*A decidual cast may be the end result of an intrauterine miscarriage with the conceptus contained within it. Cutting the cast open reveals the tiny conceptus inside. (Myles, 1968)

*A decidual cast may also be passed at the time of normal menstruation in the absence of pregnancy.

Blood mole: In some cases of missed abortion a blood mole forms. This forms when the products of conception are surrounded by a capsule of clotted blood. The capsule is of varying thickness, with degenerated chorionic villi scattered through it. It presents as a reddish, brown mass about as big as a medium-sized orange with a small, fluid-containing cavity within it which appears compressed and distorted by the thick wall of old blood. Blood moles occur when the conceptus dies and the placenta separates slowly, allowing blood to collect between the decidua and the chorion to coagulate and form layers. (Hellman & Pritchard, 1971)

The blood mole forms before the twelfth week of pregnancy and is retained *in utero*, sometimes for months. During this time the fluid separates from the blood and a fleshy, firm, hard mass known as a **carneous mole** results. When cut, it resembles a miniature placenta at first, but what appear to be cotyledons are raised areas of amnion with blood underneath. A tiny embryo may be found within the mole. (Myles, 1968) A carneous mole may calcify and become a **stone mole**. (Hughes, 1972). These formations are not the same as a molar pregnancy, which is caused by an abnormal growth of the chorionic villi (see separate chapter on Hydatidiform or Vesicular Mole, this section.)

Tuberous mole, ovum tuberculosum, tuberous subchorial hematoma: These three terms describe a type of blood mole, which is characterized by a bumpy looking amnion, the result of localized elevations from hematomas of varying size which form between the amnion and chorionic membrane.

Follow-up on miscarriage:

You will often hear from a woman after she feels she may have miscarried. For example, she may call you the following morning. It may not always be clear if the miscarriage has been complete or even if one has occurred at all. Women may not think to save what they pass; you then have no way of knowing what was discharged. Ask the woman all the usual questions to try and determine has transpired. You and she have several options:

Beta-pregnancy blood tests: Two quantitative tests done 5 days apart can help determine if the pregnancy is still viable. (See Diagnostic Tests for more details). This is an accurate and minimally invasive means of determining pregnancy status. *Beta*-pregnancy tests may be unreliable in cases of ectopic pregnancy and should not be used alone to rule them out (see chapter on Ectopic Pregnancy, this section).

Listening for the fetal heart with a Doppler: An on-the-spot means of determining viability is to use a doppler if the pregnancy is thought to be past 10 weeks. However, a woman needs to understand that a doppler exposes the fetus to more intense ultrasound than an imaging exam. She therefore may want to wait and have an imaging exam if she feels that ultrasound is an option for her.

Imaging ultrasound scan: In cases where an ectopic pregnancy is suspected or when it is unclear if a woman has miscarried and the mother doesn't mind exposing herself and her fetus to ultrasound, an exam can usually determine if the pregnancy is intrauterine and if the fetus is viable. The yoni probe ultrasound wand can confirm an intrauterine pregnancy as early as 5.5 weeks or when the *Beta*-hCG level is at least 1,000. Viability with visualization of the fetal heart can be confirmed as early as 6 weeks or when the *Beta*-hCG level is between 5,000 and 10,000. (Kolder, 1995)

Examining cervical mucus: British obstetrician Ian Donald reports that the following technique is helpful in determining the viability of a pregnancy (I have no personal experience with this technique and could find no one that did; I offer it for those who want one more means of low-tech diagnosis). Once bleeding has settled down, cervical mucus can be examined to determine whether hormonal levels indicate that the pregnancy is viable. The quantity and appearance of cervical mucus depends upon estrogen and progesterone activity; ferning is absent during normal pregnancy.

Obtain a specimen by inserting a speculum. Gently mop the surface of the cervix with a tissue held in a sponge forceps, then use the wooden end of a long-handled cotton swab to gather mucus from the cervical passageway. Spread the specimen thickly and as evenly as possible on a clean slide. Allow it to dry without a coverslip.

Examine the specimen 20 minutes later using a microscope set on low power, or with The Lens (a magnifying device for fertility assessment). A complete absence of any ferning patterns and the presence of endocervical cells (cells only visible with a microscope) indicates a good prognosis for the pregnancy to continue (or that the woman is premenstrual). Any ferning probably means the woman is not pregnant or that her pregnancy is no longer viable. Note that ferning has been seen in cases of hydatidiform mole (see that chapter, this section).

Atypical ferning appears as broken, scarce or fragmented portions of fronds and may be seen some days before the onset of inevitable miscarriage. (Donald, 1979)

When bleeding continues: Mild bleeding which persists for more than 4 or 5 days should be followed up with an internal yoni exam using a speculum to determine if something else, such as a cervical lesion, is causing the bleeding. Likewise, if a miscarriage has occurred, any woman who continues to bleed more than enough to stain a pad every few hours should be examined for possible retained products of conception. Herbs which cause uterine contractions such as a combination of equal parts Blue and Back Cohosh tinctures can be given in 20 to 30 drop doses every 4 hours. Or, Methergine tablets can be given in doses of one 0.2 mg. tablets every 4 to 8 hours, depending upon the severity of the symptoms (the pharmacology and use of bio-technical agents to stimulate the uterus will be covered in Volume II).

After a complete miscarriage: If a complete miscarriage has indeed taken place, Vitamin C with bioflavinoids (1200 mg. daily) and Vitamin E (1000 IU daily) can be taken to help heal the uterus.

The Rh- woman: The incidence of transplacental hemorrhage in truly spontaneous miscarriage with no accompanying intervention is approximately 6%. About 25% of miscarriages which include medical intervention have some transplacental bleeding. Rhesus antigens have been found on fetal red cells as early as the 38th day of pregnancy but the general recommendation is to provide 50 µg. of Rho(D) immunoglobulin prophylaxis for those women who were 8 weeks pregnant or more. (Donald, 1979) Some women may want to have Rho(D) immunoglobulin regardless of the duration of the pregnancy.

For women who have a history of miscarriage:

When a woman has three or more miscarriages in a row, the medical model calls this **habitual abortion**. Often, this is due to stress, poor nutrition or ambivalence about pregnancy, birth and parenting. However, be sure to discuss other underlying causes which predispose women to miscarriage:
> *Genetic factors (see Genetic Counseling chapter in <u>Diagnostic Tests)</u>
> *Blood incompatibilities
> *Maternal disease (syphilis, Listeria, etc.)
> *Substance abuse (including cigarettes and alcohol)
> *Congenital anomalies of the mother's reproductive tract such as those frequently found in DES daughters (see separate chapter in Anatomy and Physiology section.)
> *Previous severe cervical damage that may make the cervix unable to hold the pregnancy. Most often such miscarriages will wait until the conceptus is sufficiently heavy to push the cervix open from

the inside, and therefore occur during the second trimester.

*Hormonal imbalances or insufficient production (especially luteal phase defects and more rarely thyroid problems)

*Fibroids

*Undiagnosed medical conditions, such as lupus

If, upon exploring the possibilities, it seems to be a simple case of needing to strengthen the mother so she can carry a pregnancy, there are a number of things which can be used to assist in the process. These can be used if medical evaluation has failed to discover any specific problem, if the mother is under treatment, and in women who have only experienced one or two miscarriages as well.

*If the mother is underweight, she should gain enough weight to be within the normal range for her height and body frame before conception

*Increase folic acid and other B vitamins, vitamin C and E supplements (see nutrition section)

*Drink Red Raspberry leaf infusion daily (see controversy over types of raspberry leaves in appendix of Diagnostic Tests)

*Improve nutrition in general

*Stop smoking, drinking caffeinated or alcoholic beverages and other substance abuse

*Drink 1 or 2 cups of Black haw root bark tea or ½ cup of infusion daily. Black Haw may be used throughout pregnancy, if desired.

*Begin taking 3 drops of False Unicorn root tincture 4 to 5 times daily one month before conception through the entire first trimester

*Acupuncture treatments and constitutional homeopathic remedies may have a positive impact on a woman's ability to carry a pregnancy.

Reference and further reading:

Bland, P. & Montgomery, T., Practical Obstetrics for Students and Practitioners, F.A. Davis, Pub., Philadelphia, PA, 1925.

DeLee, J, & Carmon, M., Obstetrics for Nurses, W.B. Saunders Co., Phil., PA, 1940.

Donald, Ian, Practical Obstetric Problems, Lloyd-Luke Lt.d, London, Eng., 1979.

Gabbe, Steven, et.al., Obstetrics: Normal and Problem Pregnancies, 2nd ed., Churchill, Livingstone, New York, NY, 1991.

Greenhill, J. Principles and Practice of Obstetrics, 10th ed., William Saunders Co., Phil., 1951.

Hafer, E.S., ed. Advances in Reproductive Health Care: Spontaneous Abortion, MTP Press, Ltd., Boston, MA, 1984.

Kolder, Veronika, Obstetrician, Iowa City, IO, editing comments, 1995.

Moore, Keith, & Persaud, T., The Developing Human: Clinically Oriented Embryology, 5th ed., W. B. Saunders Co., Philadelphia, PA, 1993.

Myles, Margaret, Textbook for Midwives, 6th ed., E. & E. Livingstone, Ltd., London, 1968.

Rubin E. & Farber, J., Pathology, J.B. Lippincott, Philadelphia, PA, 1988.

Weed, S., Wise Woman Herbal for the Childbearing Year, Ash Tree Pub., Woodstock, NY, 1985.

Ectopic Pregnancy

When the blastocyst implants anywhere outside the uterine cavity, the result is an ectopic pregnancy. The incidence of ectopic pregnancy varies from one in 80 to 1 in 250 pregnancies, (approximately 1% of all births), and is highest in women aged 35 or older and in women of color. In the past decade alone the incidence has risen five-fold. This can be attributed to the rising incidence of sexually transmitted diseases and the use of antibiotics (see below). Ectopic pregnancy can occur alone or simultaneously with another pregnancy (itself either intrauterine or extrauterine) and it can occur even after the uterus has been removed via hysterectomy.

Predisposing factors: Factors which increase the chances of ectopic pregnancy include blockage in the tubes caused by scarring due to previous pelvic infection (multiple infections increase the risk even more) and abnormalities of the reproductive tract. While the use of any form of contraceptive decreases the general incidence of ectopic pregnancy, having an Intrauterine Device (IUD) in place can create a hostile enough environment in the uterus that implantation occurs elsewhere. IUD users seem to be at greatest risk immediately after the IUD is removed, and pregnancy is best avoided for two to three months after removal. Progesterone-only oral contraceptives also increase the risk, which is thought to be secondary to their minimal propulsive effect on the uterine tube at the junction of the ampulla and the isthmus, increasing the chances of the fertilized ovum becoming trapped. (Gabbe, 1991) Any variation in the normal hormonal cycle may cause menstrual irregularities which lead to poor function of the various mechanisms which ensure the transport of the ovum to the uterine cavity. Tubal spasm may occur and prevent normal passage of the ovum as well.

Abnormalities in tubal structure or function contribute to tubal implantation. The normal passage of the zygote into the uterus can be impeded as a result of partial occlusion of the uterine tube. This can be caused by infection or scar adhesions which result from damage to the tubes from infection (especially likely in neglected cases of gonorrhea, chlamydia or other forms of pelvic inflammatory disease [PID]). Arresting the progress of infections with antibiotics often prevents complete occlusion of the tubes by scar tissue, leaving them open enough to allow for conception but not wide enough for the conceptus to pass into the uterus. The result is that about 25% of ectopic pregnancies are associated with past or concurrent pelvic infection. Inflammation can cause impairment of the ciliary and muscular activity of the uterine tubes, which further interferes with movement of the ovum. Women who have a history of ectopic pregnancy have 10 to 20% chance of a reoccurrence in a subsequent pregnancy. (Danforth & Scott, 1986)

The progression of ectopic pregnancy: When transportation of the zygote is delayed 6 to 8 days, the trophoblast may develop while still in the tube. At the same time, areas in the tube resembling endometrium may develop decidua and provide an implantation site. As the trophoblastic cells burrow into the tubal wall, the chorion secretes gonadotropin, triggering the usual hormonal changes that cause a pregnancy test to be positive. Hormones are also responsible for some uterine enlargement and the cessation of menstruation.

The fate of the zygote will depend on its placement. Ninety-six percent of ectopic pregnancies occur in the uterine tube, 2% are interstitial and the remaining 2% include cervical, abdominal and ovarian pregnancies. (Gabbe, 1991)

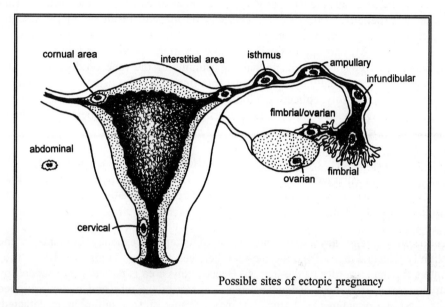

Possible sites of ectopic pregnancy

Signs and symptoms: A woman carrying an ectopic pregnancy has all the usual signs and symptoms of very early pregnancy, even though 33% of ectopic pregnancies produce false negative *Beta*-pregnancy tests. Depending upon where the pregnancy is implanted, she will usually begin to have lower abdominal pain and tenderness due to the enlarging conceptus stretching the tissues in a location which cannot accommodate its growth. Stretching plus the fact that the underlying location of placental attachment is not designed for this causes the wall to thin, weaken and eventually rupture. The onset of pain depends upon where the pregnancy is implanted and therefore how much room it has to grow before increasing pressure results in pain. (Gabbe, 1991) Symptoms usually begin between five and ten weeks of pregnancy but may appear later (14 to 16 weeks) if the implantation site is sufficiently accommodating. Some ampulla implantations resolve on their own in one way or another without problems, often by simple death and reabsorption. In rare cases, a multiple gestation is entirely ectopic. Typical symptom pictures are as follows:

Symptoms of an enlarging tubal pregnancy: Amenorrhea, a vague, crampy lower abdominal pain (often on one side only) and slight brownish bleeding from the yoni are the rule. In cases where menstruation has stopped, *pain usually precedes bleeding*, which is often not the case in an intrauterine miscarriage. However, with an ectopic pregnancy, bleeding varies from normal monthly menses to highly irregular spotting. Periodic spotting may cause women to think they are having monthly periods and not realize they are pregnant. A bimanual internal exam reveals a normal or slightly softened uterus and a unilateral tender adnexal mass. In some cases, the woman will pass a decidual cast (when the entire uterine lining is expelled as one piece). This can be the end result of an intrauterine miscarriage, however, in an ectopic pregnancy other symptoms will persist. (See the chapter on Miscarriage in the First Trimester in this section for more details on decidual casts.) Those implanted in the isthmus of the tube produce early and dramatic rupture, usually due to the placenta burrowing through the tubal wall or distention and rapidly collecting blood. Rupture commonly occurs toward the peritoneal cavity but in some cases it takes place between the fibers of the broad ligaments. (Danforth & Scott, 1986)

Ovarian pregnancy: Symptoms are similar for those of a tubal pregnancy. The ovary will feel enlarged or have a mass attached to it. Earlier pregnancies may grossly resemble the corpus luteum and microscopic examination may be necessary to distinguish the two.

Interstitial pregnancy: This rare form of ectopic pregnancy implants in the slightly widened area of the uterine tube between the ampulla and where the tube enters the upper corner of the uterus. Because this area is partially surrounded by myometrium, it is more distendable than the rest of the tube and better equipped for placental attachment. Pregnancy may advance further before it is detected; rupture occurs between 12 and 14 weeks of pregnancy but may be delayed as late as 16 weeks with cornual implantations. They are often very hard to diagnose, even with ultrasound exams. They produce a distinctly asymmetrical uterine contour with a tender mass at the junction of the tube and the upper uterine cavity. If diagnosis is delayed beyond 12 weeks of pregnancy the risk of rupture is great, often followed by a rapid and profound collapse which is often fatal. (Danforth & Scott, 1986) If the placenta is implanted closer to the uterine cavity, in the coronal area of the tube, the pregnancy may grow somewhat larger before detection, however rupture in this area is also rapidly fatal if not dealt with immediately. In cases where the fetus and placenta are situated so that they grow inside the uterine cavity an essentially normal pregnancy may result, however placental detachment after birth may be problematic since that area of myometrium is not an ideal location for placental detachment.

Cervical pregnancy: These very rare pregnancies present with profuse painless bleeding in the cervical passageway between the internal and the external os soon after implantation and rarely go past the 22nd week of pregnancy (Varney, 1980). An internal exam reveals a cervical mass with distention and thinning of the cervical wall, partial dilation of the external os and a slightly enlarged uterine fundus. They can easily be confused with cervical cancer or an incomplete or septic miscarriage. Because of the depth of placental attachment, hysterectomy is sometimes necessary. If implantation occurs in the upper cervix, the pregnancy may advance to term and be able to be delivered with surgery. (Danforth & Scott, 1986)

Rudimentary uterine horn: If a woman has an abnormally small uterus or a communicating rudimentary uterine horn, implantation can take place there and produce symptoms similar to ectopic pregnancy. Be especially alert for this possibility in DES daughters.

Differentiating an ectopic pregnancy from an intrauterine miscarriage can be tricky; this chart compares the symptom pictures of both:

INTRAUTERINE MISCARRIAGE	ECTOPIC PREGNANCY
Onset quiet, with gradually intensifying and regular pain in the lower abdomen, resembling labor.	Onset stormy, with irregular, colicky & sometimes excruciating pain which is localized on one side.
External hemorrhage profuse or moderate, with clots	External hemorrhage slight, continuous, dark & fluid or absent
Symptoms of shock proportionate to visible blood loss	Symptoms of shock not proportionate to visible blood loss
Discharge of products of conception	Only uterine decidua can be identified, no villi are found
Bimanual reveals an enlarged uterus and normal pelvis	Bimanual reveals a tender mass alongside the uterus
Uterine size appropriate for dates	Uterus smaller than dates suggest
The mass is soft, feels like a pregnancy, and is movable as part of the uterus	The mass is harder, lies to the side of the uterus or in the cul-de-sac and is not movable within the body of the uterus

(Greenhill, 1951)

Signs and symptoms of ruptured or imminent-to-rupture tubal pregnancy:

*Acute sharp stabbing, tearing lower abdominal pain (may be generalized over the entire abdomen, only on the side of the implantation, or on the opposite side)
*Referred pain may be felt in the shoulder, back, chest or rarely the

yoni due to bleeding into the peritoneal cavity.

*Fainting, dizziness and shock may accompany rupture.

*Bleeding or spotting may be scanty or dark brown, continuous or intermittent, or infrequently profuse. As long as the placenta is functional there will be no bleeding, unless tissues are being torn due to the enlarging conceptus.

*Upon internal exam:

-The uterus may feel non-pregnant, may be slightly softened or enlargement may be consistent with normal pregnancy throughout the first trimester, due to hormonal effects. (Remember that an ectopic pregnancy may also co-exist with a normal intrauterine pregnancy.)

-Movement of the cervix causes increased abdominal pain, which may be excruciating. Cervical motion may also cause shoulder pain. In other cases movement of the cervix is painless.

-Bulging of the posterior fornix may be felt due to pooled blood behind the uterus (in the cul-de-sac).

-In about 75% of cases, a soft, pliable mass is felt to one side behind or beside the uterus on bimanual exam (such exams are extremely painful and must be done gently so as not to encourage a pregnancy that is about to rupture to burst). If ruptured, this mass may feel boggy or mushy; if distended with blood, it may feel firm.

*Low blood pressure and a rapid pulse signify internal bleeding, although vital signs may remain normal.

*Commonly diarrhea and less commonly nausea and vomiting are present.

*The white blood count may be normal or reach as high as 30,000.

*A rare sign is a bluish tint beneath the mother's umbilicus, indicating intraperitoneal hemorrhage (Cullen's sign).

Further evaluation: If the history and physical exam do not rule out ectopic pregnancy, and if rupture does not appear to be imminent or to have occurred, there are lab tests which can be done to further diagnose the situation. A quantitative *Beta*-subunit human Chorionic Gonadotropin (hCG) blood test with a sensitivity of 5 mU/mL can be used to determine if the woman is pregnant. This sensitive test avoids the false-negative results which can occur with other pregnancy tests. Serum levels of hCG normally double every 2 to 3 days through the first six weeks of gestation (8 weeks from last menstrual period), after which they level off. At 6.5 weeks the average hCG level is 10,000 mlU/mL. Failure to reach this level by this time or failure of the level to double within 48 hours suggests ectopic pregnancy. In most ectopic pregnancies, serum hCG remains below 6,000 mlU/mL..

Ultrasound exam can be used to identify the location of the gestational sac six weeks after the last menstrual period or when the *Beta*-hCG level has reached 6,000 to 6,5000 mlU/mL or higher. Standard sonograms are unreliable in detecting ectopic pregnancy prior to this point, however transyoni ultrasound is more sensitive and can aid earlier detection of ectopic or intrauterine gestation. Definite evidence exists for the location of the conceptus when a gestational sac containing a fetus with a heartbeat is seen. While absence of an intrauterine pregnancy and the presence of an adnexal mass with a gestational sac and fluid behind the uterus suggests ectopic pregnancy, such a finding is not conclusive.

If the above tests raise suspicions of ectopic pregnancy, culdocentesis may be done to discover whether free blood is present in the pelvis. This procedure involves inserting a needle into the peritoneal space and withdrawing fluid. Since bleeding can be from other sources such as a ruptured ovarian cyst, this technique is not conclusive; it has been used less in recent years.

Dilation and curettage (D&C) or suction may be done if the woman is willing to risk aborting a normal pregnancy. Retrieval of decidua and villi confirm intrauterine pregnancy, although there may rarely be a coexisting ectopic pregnancy as well. An empty gestational sac suggests a blighted ovum. If a D & C or suction procedure does not recover pregnancy tissue from the uterine cavity in the presence of positive *Beta*-hCG tests and nothing is seen in the uterus on ultrasound, ectopic pregnancy is diagnosed. (Nichols, 1995)

In laparoscopy a tiny periscope-like device is introduced through a small abdominal incision to look at the pelvic organs. An unruptured tubal pregnancy is smooth, egg-shaped, and dusky blue. Combined false negative and positive results total 3%; however this procedure carries with it the risks of surgery and anesthesia.

If an ectopic pregnancy is discovered early (gestational sac less than 3 cm. to 3.5 cm. and no fetal cardiac activity evident on ultrasound) the chemotherapy drug methotrexate is being given as an intramuscular injection in selected cases to kill the pregnancy and thus avoid surgery. This drug is highly toxic, but may spare the woman the loss of reproductive organs. It seems to be relatively safe when used for this purpose and has been shown to be 92% effective; the remaining 8% experience a rupture despite treatment. Anemic women should receive iron supplements and all should have normal liver and kidney function tests prior to treatment with follow-up assessment and for hCG titers at 4 and 7 days. (Slaughter & Grimes, 1995; Nichols, 1995) Intercourse, alcohol use and folic acid supplements should be avoided until the hCG tests is negative.

An imminent-to-rupture or ruptured ectopic pregnancy with resulting hemorrhage and shock is a medical emergency requiring surgery. If you suspect an ectopic pregnancy, advise immediate medical evaluation. If the woman is calling you from home, you should meet her in the hospital. If rupture appears to be imminent or to have occurred, do not delay transport by having her wait for your arrival at her home before she leaves. She should be brought to the hospital by a relative or friend; if she is imminent to rupture she should not attempt to drive

730

herself. If a rupture has occurred, it will be necessary to repair if possible and remove if necessary the area that has burst in order to stop the bleeding. In most cases a salpingostomy can be performed, consisting of a small incision in the tube at the site of the pregnancy through which the conceptus is removed. This is allowed to heal without stitches. (Kolder, 1995) Rh negative women will need to receive Rho(D) immunoglobulin.

Differential diagnosis: The lack of a specific symptom picture in ectopic pregnancy means that similar symptoms may be present in a variety of other situations:

*Normal intrauterine pregnancy with implantation bleeding
*Intrauterine pregnancy with associated abdominal pain from:
    -Round ligament pain or spasm
    -Painful, but normal corpus luteum
    -Ruptured, bleeding corpus luteum
    -Ovarian cyst
    -Torsion (twisting) of the ovary containing the corpus luteum
    -Torsion of the uterine tube
    -Degeneration or torsion of a pedunculated fibroid
    -Threatened miscarriage
    -Missed or incomplete miscarriage
*Urinary tract or kidney infection
*Kidney stone
*Sacculation of the uterus (see separate chapter, Second Trimester section)
*Appendicitis (lower right quadrant)
*Endometriosis
*Pelvic inflammatory disease
*Ovarian tumors or cysts
*Pedunculated fibroids or tumors of the uterine tube
*Tubo-ovarian abscess
*Diverticular abscess (Lichtman & Papera, 1990)

Other possible outcomes of ectopic pregnancy: Apart from rupture of the area surrounding the implantation site, there are several other possible outcomes of ectopic pregnancy:

Tubal abortion: The lining of the uterine tube ruptures releasing the ovum and blood into the tubal passage. This causes the ovum to be expelled into the peritoneal cavity through the fimbriated end.

Tubal mole: The conceptus dies and becomes encased by layers of clotted blood.

Primary abdominal pregnancy: If an intact gestational sac is expelled from the tube, the placenta can implant in the abdominal cavity. The pregnancy may then proceed as a primary abdominal pregnancy (see separate chapter on Abdominal Pregnancy in the section in Problems That Can Occur in the Second Trimester).

Secondary abdominal pregnancy: An ectopic pregnancy may rupture such that the fetus and membranes escape into the abdominal cavity, leaving the placenta attached where it is implanted (usually the tube or ovary). This is called a secondary abdominal pregnancy. The baby may be located in the broad ligament or peritoneal cavity depending upon the site of rupture. If the fetus escapes alive, it may continue to develop among the intestines or in the broad ligament. It may or may not be contained within the membranes. If not, a new sac can form made up of fibrin, adherent intestines and other surrounding tissues. If the baby is not enclosed in a normal amniotic membrane, the lack of fluid may lead to poor development of the lungs.

If rupture of the implantation site does not take place but the tube or ovary distends, a large swelling forms made up of the original surrounding tissue, fibrin and muscle fibers from adjacent organs; this swelling adheres to all the surfaces it touches. The placenta spreads from its first point of attachment, and tends to be thin but otherwise is like a uterine placenta. Left alone, the baby may even go to term, when hormones will trigger uterine contractions and the uterus will release a decidual cast with minimal bleeding. Surgery would be necessary to accomplish the birth. The intraabdominal baby is likely to die as a result of placental disruption and subsequent hemorrhage. (Greenhill, 1951)

The mother is at higher risk as well. When the placenta attaches itself outside the uterus, it tends to grow more deeply into the underlying tissue in order to establish proper nutritive exchange. Therefore, removal of the placenta becomes impossible. In these cases, it must be left in place for the mother's body to reabsorb, with the accompanying risk of infection.

References and further reading:

Greenhill, J., Principles and Practice of Obstetrics, W. B. Saunders, Co., Philadelphia, PA, 1951.
Danforth, D., Scott, J., eds. Obstetrics & Gynecology, 5th ed., J. B. Lippincott, Phil., PA, 1986.
Gabbe, S, Obstetrics: Normal & Problem Pregnancies, 2nd ed., Churchill, Livingstone, NY, 1991.
Kolder, Veronika, editing comments, 7/95.
Lichtman, R,, Papera, S., Gynecology: Well-Woman Care, Appleton-Lange, Norwalk, Ct, 1990.
Nichols, Mark, MD, conversation re: methotrexate use, 7/10/95.
Slaughter, J, & Grimes, D., "Methotrexate therapy, nonsurgical management of ectopic pregnancy," Western J of Med, Vol. 162, No. 3, March 1995, pp. 225-8.
Varney, Helen, Nurse-Midwifery, Blackwell Scientific Pub., Boston, MA 1980.

Hydatidiform or Vesicular Mole

A **hydatidiform (hi-dah-TID-eh-form)** or **vesicular mole** is a genetic abnormality of the placenta. It may either result from the fertilization of one ovum by one or two sperm where the nucleus of the ovum is absent or inactive. The subsequent growth is the result of the single sperm reproducing itself or the interaction of the two sperms. Chorionic villi transport nutrients to the placenta. In the absence of a vascular system within the villi, they proliferate and the center of each one swells, producing an abundance of avascular fluid-filled cysts which vary in size from that of a pin-head to a small grape. The placenta is transformed into a mass of pale, grape-like clusters which are connected by narrow strands. The excessive growth of the chorionic villi causes an overproduction of human Chorionic Gonadotropin (hCG), resulting in large amounts being excreted in the urine and high blood levels in *Beta*-hCG blood pregnancy tests. The hCG levels are often 200% higher than their peak high in normal pregnancy. These extremely high levels of hCG increase the metabolic burden on the liver and give rise to those secondary symptoms of molar pregnancy, such as high blood pressure, which mimic toxemia. High hCG levels may also be responsible for the formation of multiple lutein cysts which often appear on the ovaries.

The process of molar formation typically begins about the sixth week of pregnancy. Sometimes only a portion of the placenta will appear to have hydatidiform villi with an accompanying viable fetus. This is a result of a triple set of chromosomes; commonly two from the father and one from the mother. Such babies may be small for gestational age or have various anomalies. Such partial apparent molar formations are only rarely persistent trophoblastic tissue. In the case of multiple gestation, it is possible for one twin to survive in the presence of a hydatidiform twin placenta.

Signs and symptoms: Hydatidiform moles are often obvious within the first trimester of pregnancy and present the following signs and symptoms:

*Bleeding from the yoni, beginning about the 12th week, is the earliest sign. Discharge may be bright or watery red and profuse, or brown due to the presence of old blood. In a few cases, a few vesicles, which look like white currants or grapes in red currant juice may be passed.
*Excessive vomiting and nausea are usually seen.
*If the mole is still attached to the uterine wall, the uterus is large for dates, often reaching the level of the navel by 12 weeks of pregnancy.
*If the mole has detached from the uterine wall, the uterus may be normally sized for dates or even smaller than expected.
*Multiple lutein cysts cause the ovaries to enlarge. They sometimes

become almost as big as the uterus, adding to the abdominal distention.

*In spite of the large uterus, no fetal movement is felt by the mother or is seen when you observe her abdomen, a tip that wrong dates are not the explanation.

*No fetal heart can be heard and no small parts palpated (as might be expected if large-for-dates uterine growth is due to miscalculated dates).

*Hypertension and proteinuria are frequently present.

*The uterus may have an elastic or doughy consistency, with pain and tenderness due to the excessive distention by the mole or blood clot.

*Uterine infection is sometimes present, causing tenderness or pain.

*Both blood and urinary hCG pregnancy tests will show exceptionally high levels of hCG for dates (this could cause you to confuse a molar pregnancy with a multiple gestation; be sure to evaluate the total picture).

*Thyroid tests will reveal elevated thyroid stimulating hormone and sometimes high T_3 and T_4 levels.

*Anemia may be apparent in tests and in the mother's appearance.

*Minor degrees of intravascular coagulation may occur.

*Platelets are reduced and fibrin degeneration products are increased.

Differential diagnosis: Be sure to rule out the following more common causes of some of these symptoms:

*Threatened miscarriage of a normal pregnancy
*Inaccurate dates
*Multiple gestation
*Uterine fibroids or ovarian tumors (causing enlarged ovaries, however lutein cysts are often associated with molar placentas)
*Hyperemesis gravidarum (excessive vomiting of pregnancy)

It is important to note that swollen villi are not a disease by themselves and any tissue with this appearance must be microscopically examined so that its true cellular structure can be distinguished.

What to do: If you suspect a hydatidiform mole, get an ultrasound exam without delay. An ultrasound should be able to detect if the placental tissue has vesicular formations and whether there is a viable fetus. It should also be able to diagnose a multiple gestation or uterine growths.

If a molar formation is discovered, the uterus should be emptied in hospital.

This is accomplished by softening the cervix with prostaglandin suppositories and inducing contractions with an oxytocin IV drip, by dilation and curettage, or by using suction and then curettage. Molar placentas sometimes erode through the uterine wall. The uterus may also be so thinned from distention that it is easily perforated with a curette. These factors plus possible coagulation disturbances make for a significant risk of sudden and profuse hemorrhage either before or after the uterus is emptied, this makes home care a dangerous option.

Possible complications: If remnants of the mole become invasive, the trophoblast can retain its villus structure but invade the myometrium. This is called **chorio-adenoma destruens** or invasive mole. Neoplastic cells may spread to other parts of the body, even the lungs and brain.

Invasive mole usually dies within nine months, and even though the villus tissue can spread, this is not considered a cancerous condition. Tissue obtained from the uterine wall should be examined for the presence of malignant cells. However, histologic examination may not be very helpful and differentiation from carcinoma is often impossible. The risks of severe hemorrhage, either intraabdominal, uterine or pulmonary, as well as metastatic spread, and possible conversion to choriocarcinoma, make removal of a molar placenta important. (Garrey, et.al., 1980)

More rarely, molar pregnancy is a precursor to the development of cancerous trophoblastic tissue called **choriocarcinoma**. Trophoblastic cells invade the surrounding muscle and blood vessels, causing gross hemorrhage. The tumor can spread anywhere, and may arise from fragments of the chorionic epithelium which have traveled outside the uterus. Choriocarcinoma occurs about once in every 40,000 Caucasian pregnancies, it is somewhat more common in Asian peoples. It follows hydatidiform moles in about 40% of cases, abortion in 40% and term pregnancy in 20% of cases. It is occasionally found to originate from the ovaries. While hydatidiform mole rarely reappears, choriocarcinoma does much more often. (Garrey, et.al., 1980) Symptoms of chorioadenoma destruens and choriocarcinoma are similar and include:

*Continued bleeding
*Symptoms which may subside for weeks or months, with bleeding subsequently recurring and hCG reappearing in the urine
*Anemia may be present
*Pelvic pain, painful urination, headache or visual disturbance, spitting up blood, cough, or pulmonary embolism, or other presenting symptoms may be due to metastases.
*Elevated urinary hCG

Follow-up care: Because of the risk of malignancy, women who have had a vesicular mole on part or all of their placenta should have repeated quantitative hCG blood tests performed on the following schedule:

*Every 2 weeks for the first month
    -hCG should return to non-pregnant levels by the 4th week
*Every month thereafter for the next 6 months
*Every 3 months thereafter for the next 18 months

These women should not plan to get pregnant until they have had negative urinary hCG tests for at least 12 months. Delaying conception will minimize the chances of normal levels due to pregnancy masking rising levels from abnormal trophoblastic tissue (Donald, 1979). Some practitioners recommend waiting two years to conceive in all cases. A rise in hCG or any bleeding other than regular menstrual bleeding are cause for further examination. An endometrial biopsy can be done to determine if there are any trophoblastic cells in the uterus. A lung x-ray may be suggested to determine if metastasis has migrated to the lung field, especially if respiratory symptoms are present. In invasive mole, curettage of the uterine lining recovers friable material which proves to be benign villous tissue. In choriocarcinoma, the tumor consists of masses of abnormal trophoblastic cells. Sometimes these symptoms are present but no histological evidence of a tumor can be found. Bio-technical recommendations will include chemotherapy or hysterectomy or both.

If no problems are noticed during the period of supervision, the chances of a recurrence are low.

References and further reading:

Donald, Ian, Practical Obstetric Problems, Lloyd-Luke, Ltd., London, Eng. 1979.
Gabbe, Steven, et.al., Obstetrics: Normal and Problem Pregnancies, 2nd ed., Churchill, Livingstone, New York, NY, 1991.
Garrey, M., et.al., Obstetrics Illustrated, Churchill Livingstone, New York, 1980.
Myles, Margaret, A Textbook for Midwives, 9th ed., E. & S. Livingstone, Ltd., London, 1981.

736

NOTES:

737

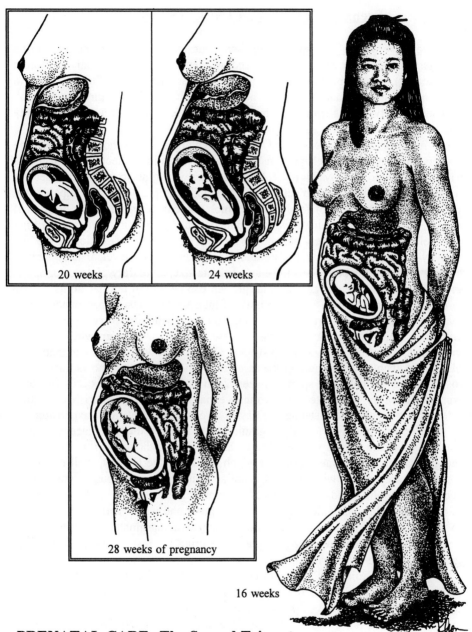

20 weeks

24 weeks

28 weeks of pregnancy

16 weeks

**PRENATAL CARE: The Second Trimester
(From the 15th through the 28th
week of pregnancy)**

Prenatal Care During Weeks 15 through 28

An Overview of the Second Trimester: During the second trimester uterine enlargement becomes more apparent and women begin to feel fetal movement (quickening). Early pregnancy complaints such as nausea and fatigue begin to subside and the woman generally becomes excited about beginning to look pregnant. Early in this trimester, the mother will begin to perceive fetal activity and the heart rate will be audible with a fetascope.

As weight gain increases and the uterus enlarges, hemorrhoids may become bothersome (see separate chapter on Vascular Problems in the section on Problems That Can Occur at Any Time). Appetite usually begins to climb mid-second trimester as the baby starts to get larger. As small fetal parts become palpable you will have a better gauge of fetal growth which you can compare to her nutritional intake. Watch for plateaus in weight gain or fetal growth in women with high metabolisms or who are very active; nip intrauterine growth retardation in the bud now by having the mother eat more and reduce her activity level, if necessary.

As long as the baby feels to be an adequate size, temporary plateaus or spurts in either maternal weight gain or fetal growth can be within normal limits. Keep in mind that some women may gain most of their weight in early pregnancy, some may wait until now to start really gaining, and those who are overweight to begin with may gain little or actually lose a few pounds. As in growing children, growing fetuses may have an inconsistent pattern of growth; babies can also have obvious, palpable weight gain at the same time that the mother shows none. A 5 to 10 pound weight gain spurt between 24 and 28 weeks may occur in some women, reflecting adequate blood volume expansion in a well-nourished mother. Intermittent edema and distended veins are also indicative of good expansion.

Blood volume is gradually beginning to climb now that the placenta is well established as the baby's source of nourishment. Throughout this important time, the gradual blood volume expansion which occurs in the healthy, well-nourished woman corresponds with the placenta's need to continuously enlarge to accommodate the needs of the fetus. Remember, it is the amount of blood perfusing the placenta which stimulates it to grow and which carries the nutrients to the fetus. Inadequate nutrition now leads to a marginally expanded blood volume and an inadequately grown placenta during the last trimester, when fetal growth needs are most critical.

Some first-time mothers and many second-time mothers will start to notice painless toning contractions of the uterus in this trimester, sometimes as early as the 18th or 19th week. As the pregnancy advances, painless toning contractions, and lots of them, are a sign of health. Unless the diet is suffering or cervical or uterine abnormalities are a problem, don't worry; they don't mean premature labor is just around the bend. Some women experience an increase in normal yoni discharge during this trimester, if no accompanying symptoms such as itching, foul smell etc. indicate an infection, this is perfectly normal.

Frequency of visits: Visits during this trimester are typically spaced four weeks apart, unless women are having problems which necessitate more frequent visits. However, in recent years many midwives have started to increase the frequency of visits, beginning at the 24th week, to every two or three weeks to allow for more time to develop a relationship. You will have to judge what seems appropriate as well as what you can realistically offer as a practitioner.

Care during the second trimester: The pregnancy will become increasingly more evident and therefore more easily monitored during this time. Here are the highlights that will be relevant during each week of pregnancy:

Weeks 15 to 17: In most cases, you will be able to hear the fetal heart with a fetascope for the first time during this period. Do not be afraid to press firmly into the mother's abdomen to listen, as the baby is well protected. While doing so, you may feel slight bumps as the fetus pushes or kicks against the pressure. The mother will often begin to feel fetal movement during these weeks. Usually the mother's first awareness of fetal movement correlates with your first success at hearing the heart with a fetascope. Even this early, once located, the fetal heart can usually be auscultated with a regular stethoscope so the mother can hear as well, or have a fetascope with long tubing on hand for this purpose. Although you can begin to palpate the uterus abdominally for size, symmetry, and fluid volume, you won't be able to feel fetal parts for a while. Encourage the mother's awareness of fetal movement by asking her how the baby is moving at every prenatal visit.

By now the uterus can be measured for a fundal height assessment, but remember that fundal height does not necessarily match the weeks of pregnancy in this early stage. Again, a very retroverted uterus will delay your ability to find a well-defined fundus until after the uterus has completely "popped up" out of the pelvis. Women with a retroverted uterus that has not yet tipped forward will often feel a lot of pressure on their bowel, as the uterus is becoming heaver. Assuming a hands-and-knees position and doing pelvic rocks (slowing swaying the back, then straightening it) will relieve

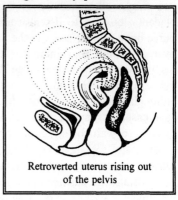

Retroverted uterus rising out of the pelvis

pressure and assist the uterus to find it's way forward. (See separate chapter on Incarceration of the Pregnant Uterus in the Second Trimester Problems section.)

The uterus may be starting to enlarge rapidly if the woman is carrying a multiple gestation. Alert women to the possibility of toning contractions before they begin so they are not alarmed. Multiparas may begin to feel toning contractions even before they note fetal movement.

If anemia was discovered with the initial lab work, another hemoglobin should be checked between 15 and 20 weeks to be sure the situation is resolving, keeping in mind that a slight rise or stabilization of the count usually reflects good therapeutic response in the presence of an expanding blood volume.

If a woman is a DES daughter or has known reproductive abnormalities, it might be a good idea to do a gentle internal exam at this visit to see if her cervix is undergoing any quiet changes. If effacement or dilation is discovered, a cerclage can be placed or she can choose to go on bed rest to minimize any further changes. If she chooses bed rest, another exam should be performed in one to two weeks to see if further changes have been arrested. If not, a cerclage should be considered.

Weeks 18 to 20: The uterus should be well above the pubic bone by now and in many cases uterine height will correlate with the weeks of pregnancy (make note of exceptions in the chapter on Fundal Height, Skills section). Even in cases where the uterus is retroverted, the body should have popped forward, although the fundus may remain sloped backwards and hard to distinguish for a few weeks yet.

The fetal heart tones are usually heard easily with a fetascope. One exception is when the placenta is implanted on the anterior wall of the uterus. In this case, it can be difficult to hear the fetal heart in the usual locations throughout pregnancy. Try listening along either side until the swishing sound of the placenta is faintest. Once you cross over the edge of the placenta, you can often pick up the heart on the side where the fetal back is positioned. Press against the opposite side to help move the small fetus against the wall of the uterus. It may be difficult to locate the fetal heart in women-of-size. Try listening higher on the abdomen than you might otherwise do at this point in gestation. If you haven't heard the placenta, be sure to listen around for its location as well, particularly above the pubic bone or over scars in the uterus; note its location on your chart. Implantation over a uterine scar increases the risk of abnormal adhesion which should be discussed with the parents (see Bleeding in the Third Trimester chapter for details).

Almost all women can feel movement by the 20th week of pregnancy, although small parts still not distinct on palpation. If viability has been a concern, as in cases of suspected missed abortion or false pregnancy, this is usually the limit of time to wait for signs of normal pregnancy to appear. If you are not seeing, hearing and feeling what should be normal at this point, it is time to suggest an ultrasound exam to determine what is going on.

If anemia has been a concern, recheck the hemoglobin to see if therapies are working. A slight rise or stabilization of the count is a good indication that therapy is being effective, given the fact that the blood volume is expanding.

Weeks 21 to 24: The mother perceives fetal movements as more vigorous during these weeks, and fetal heart tones become louder and easier to locate. The uterus can be palpated easily and the amniotic fluid can be identified, but the ratio of fluid to the size of the baby is still such that palpation of small parts remains difficult. It is possible to ballot the fetal head between your fingers by the 24th week in some multiparas. This is true because the uterus has been previously stretched and is therefore less firm than in a primigravida. Primigravidas usually feel at least occasional toning contractions by this point, often identified as a sudden tightening or hardness of the uterus which then relaxes. These contractions are painless and do not dilate the normal cervix at this point.

There is frequently a spurt of weight gain in the neighborhood of 5 to 10 pounds sometime between the 24th and 28th week, reflecting good blood volume expansion. For Rh-negative moms, discuss performing another antibody screen and give the mother information about the pros and cons of 28 week RhD(o) immunoglobulin. Also discuss the controversies around the concept of gestational diabetes and local protocols for diagnosis and treatment, and recheck the hemoglobin at the 28 week visit.

Weeks 25 to 27: These weeks are characterized by the excitement for both you and the mother of being able to determine with more certainty the position of the baby. By now the ratio of baby's body to amniotic fluid is such that you can begin to feel small parts and fetal position in more detail. Heart tones are increasingly easy to find and easier for the mother to hear.

Now is the time to get a handle on small-for-dates fetal growth, if that seems to be a problem. Remember that small-for-dates growth is most likely due to inadequate nutritional intake. Don't monitor the situation for visit after visit before alerting the mother to your concerns! Don't send her in for an ultrasound right off the bat either, as that will not make the baby grow any bigger and will suggest to the mother that tests are more important than what she can do to impact the situation. Attend to this now with diet diary and activity review. Fetal growth should respond quickly if an underlying disease or defect is not causative.

By now most women are noticing at least a few uterine toning contractions during the day. This important uterine activity helps prepare the cervix for birth. If a woman still isn't sure she is having them (common in first time mothers) try to palpate to see if she is having any during your appointments. When she does, point them out. These contractions can feel like the baby making a big movement, painless tightening, or the uterus becoming hard for a few seconds up to several minutes. Sometimes they make a woman catch her breath, but most of the time they are not at all painful. A few women only experience uterine activity as sensations in their lower back. Note that as pregnancy advances into the late second trimester, detectable cervical changes become less predictive of problems as they are quite common among women with a normal cervix (Gabbe, 1991, p. 859), particularly in women who have previously given birth. Therefore, assessment of any cervical changes must be evaluated relative to the overall symptom picture such as the amount of uterine activity, sensations of pressure down, etc., as well as individual history. However, it is *not* normal for the membranes to bulge through a partially open cervix at this point (See the chapter on Loose Cervix should you discover bulging membranes during an exam.)

742

Continue to monitor fetal movement patterns by asking the mother about this at every visit. (Read the chapter on Assessment of Fetal Movement in <u>Diagnostic Tests</u>.) Fetal position becomes increasingly significant as the weeks go by. If the baby is not vertex, see the chapter on Ensuring a Vertex Presentation at Term, Third Trimester section for suggestions about how to proceed.

Anyone wishing to be screened for gestational diabetes should also have that test run between 26 and 28 weeks. (See Diabetes and Pregnancy chapter in <u>Diagnostic Tests</u> for more details.)

Week 28: Inadequate fetal growth which you detected at the last visit should have corrected itself in the majority of cases, if your nutritional advice has been followed. You might check a woman's hemoglobin now, especially if her dietary changes have been slow, (otherwise it can wait until the next visit). Checking now will catch any otherwise undetectable problems with blood volume expansion early enough to do something *before* secondary symptoms of toxemia are apparent. Rh-negative mothers will need to have another antibody screen done at this time. An antibody ID should also be done to detect any changes in titer levels in women known to be sensitized to any minor blood factor. Those women who want Rho(D) immunoglobulin for prenatal prophylaxis should receive it at the 28 week visit. (See chapter in Special Circumstances for more details; also see chapters on Blood Types and Incompatibilities and Diabetes and Pregnancy in <u>Diagnostic Tests</u>.)

Fetal position and heart tones should be fairly easy to discern by now, unless the mother is a woman-of-size. You can now feel the different parts of the baby distinctly enough so that you can begin to show the mother how to find the fetal parts herself (if she hasn't already figured it out on her own).

Nutrition: With early pregnancy nausea out of the way, most women experience an increase in appetite. Severely malnourished women and those carrying multiple gestations with inadequate nutrition are at high risk from the 24th week on to manifest secondary symptoms of toxemia and premature labor.

Things to discuss: Now that the pregnancy is more obvious, you can begin to discuss some of the preparations a woman will need to make for the birth.

   *Now is a good time to discuss childbirth classes
   *Discuss how she is adapting to the pregnancy
   *Talk over her lab results and explain each finding
   *Discuss labor support and who will be at the birth
   *Pediatric and obstetric collaboration arrangements

References and further reading:
Gabbe, S., <u>Obstetrics: Normal & Problem Pregnancies</u>, 2nd ed., Churchill Livingstone, NY, 1991.

Signs of Pregnancy in the Second Trimester

The following signs appear during the second trimester of pregnancy. It is during these weeks that positive signs can be detected which confirm the pregnancy without the use of high-tech diagnostic techniques. As with signs in early pregnancy, the timing of the appearance of each sign varies from woman to woman (weeks of pregnancy are indicated).

1ST APPEARS:	SIGN/SYMPTOM	COMMENTS
14 weeks	Internal ballotment	During an internal exam, gently tapping upwards on the cervix causes the fetus to be displaced up & then sink, producing a gentle tap on your examining finger.
15 weeks	Abdominal enlargement	The uterus becomes palpable abdominally.
16 weeks	Colostrum	Clear fluid can be expressed & is naturally secreted from the nipple.
16 weeks	Uterine souffle	Soft blowing sound synchronous with mother's pulse can be heard. Also heard with fibroids in the absence of pregnancy.
16-18 weeks	Quickening	The mother can feel fetal movement.
16-20 weeks	Auscultate fetal heart	Depending upon your skill with a fetascope, in some cases the fetal heart can be heard as early as 15 weeks.
20 weeks	Palpable fetal movement	Fetal movements can be felt through the abdominal wall. As pregnancy advances, you will be able to see the fetus moving as well.
20 weeks	Secondary Areola	Area around the areola & the nipple become darker.
20 weeks	Palpable uterine contractions	The uterus begins toning contractions during the 9th or 10th week; they can often be palpated by the 20th week.
24 weeks	External ballotment	The fetus can be "bounced from side to side" in the uterus during abdominal palpation.

References and further reading:

McLennan, C, Synopsis of Obstetrics, 8th ed., C.V. Mosby Co., St. Louis, MO, 1970.

Fetal and Placental Development in the Second Trimester

All the fetal organ systems are basically formed, but much maturing must take place before the fetus can live outside the mother's uterus. Dating refers to weeks of gestation.

Thirteen through fifteen weeks: The 13th through the end of the 15th week of gestation marks a time of rapid fetal growth. The lower limbs are well-developed and the toenails are developing. Limb movements become coordinated but are still too slight to be felt by most mothers. Slow eye movements occur and scalp hair patterning is also beginning. The head is now erect. The fetus appears more human because the eyes are now in position on the face and the external ears are close to their term position on the sides of the head.

16 weeks: The head is relatively small compared with that of the 12-week fetus and the lower limbs are longer. The skeleton continues to ossify, and bones are clearly visible on x-ray by the beginning of the 16th week. The ovaries are differentiated and contain primordial follicles that have oogonia (immature eggs). The ears now stand out from the head. The crown rump length is 4½ inches and the fetus weighs 3½ to 4 ounces at the end of the 16th week. There is about 200 to 250 ml. of amniotic fluid at this point.

17 weeks: From 17 to 20 weeks fetal growth slows, but crown-rump length increases by about 50 mm. (2 inches). Brown fat which is the site of heat production, particularly in the newborn baby, forms from the 17th to the 20th week. This specialized adipose (fat) tissues produces heat by oxidizing fatty acids. It is found mainly at the base of the neck, behind the sternum and in the area surrounding the kidneys. It has a high mitochondria content, giving it a distinctly brown hue.

18 weeks: Vernix caseosa covers the skin. It consists of a fatty secretion from the fetal sebaceous glands of the skin and dead epidermal cells. Vernix protects the delicate skin from abrasions, chapping and hardening that could result from unprotected exposure to the amniotic fluid. The mother probably feels fetal movement by now. The uterus of the female fetus is formed and canalization of the yoni has begun. Many primordial ovarian follicles containing oogonia have formed. In males the testes have begun to descend but are still located on the posterior abdominal wall, the site of the ovaries in the female fetus.

20 weeks: The baby is covered with fine, downy hair called lanugo, which helps to hold vernix on the skin. Eyebrows and scalp hair are also seen at this point. The baby begins to hear sounds. At the end of this week the crown-rump length is 6½ inches and the average weight is 12 ounces and amniotic fluid volume has reached about 350 ml..

21 weeks: Rapid eye movements begin (the fetus is starting to dream).

21 to 25 weeks: There is substantial weight gain during this period. As pregnancy advances, fetal size becomes more individual. Although lean, the fetus is proportioned more like a full-term baby.

22-23 weeks: Blink-startle responses have been reported following application of vibroacoustic noise on the mother's abdomen. The skin is usually wrinkled, particularly during the early part of this period, and is more translucent. It is pink to red in babies born at this gestation because the blood is visible in the capillaries.

24 weeks: The secretory epithelial cells in the walls of the lungs begin to secrete surfactant, a surface-active lipid that maintains the patency of the developing alveoli of the lungs. Fingernails are also present by 24 weeks.

Babies born between 22 and 25 weeks may survive if given very high-tech intensive care. The earlier the baby is, the more likely it will suffer long term disabilities such as cerebral palsy if it does survive. Due to the immature development of its lungs, those that do survive early infancy may die during the first year or so of life from respiratory complications.

Placental development and function through the second trimester to term:

Growth in the thickness of the placenta continues until the 18th week of gestation. The fully developed placenta covers 15 to 30% of the decidual lining of the uterus. The fetal circulation is contained within each villus projection which look like branches of a tree. These branches are contained within several sacs which make up the surface of the placenta that faces the uterine wall. These sacs make up the cytotrophoblastic shell which contacts the decidua basalis. Specialized stem villi anchor the placenta to the decidua through the cytotrophoblastic shell. During early placental formation, endometrial tissue is scooped out, leaving wedge-shaped projections of decidual tissue known as placental septa that project toward the chorionic plate. These projections divide the maternal surface of the placenta into irregular convex areas called cotyledons, each of which contain two or more stem villi and their many branches.

In fetal placental circulation, fetal blood passes from the fetus through the umbilical arteries to the placenta. The arteries branch and subdivide at the site of the cord's attachment to the placenta until the blood reaches the extensive arteriocapillary-venous system within the villi where nutrients and wastes are exchanged with the mother's blood. This blood then passes into tiny veins that run parallel to the placental arteries and finally converge into the umbilical vein, which carries the blood back to the fetus.

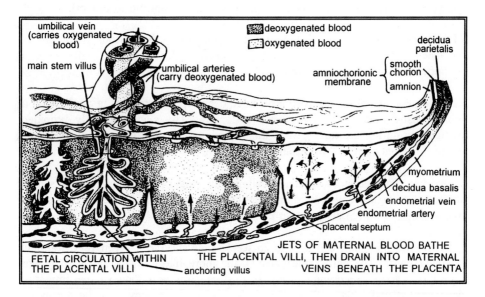

On the maternal side of placental circulation, the mother's blood is temporarily outside the maternal circulatory system as it bathes the placental capillaries. It enters the intervillous space through 80 to 100 spiral arteries in the decidua basalis which have been transformed into wide mouthed, sac-like, open uteroplacental vessels throughout the first 16 weeks of gestation. The uteroplacental vessels can passively dilates in order to deliver the greatly expanded blood flow which is required as pregnancy advances. These maternal arteries and veins pass through gaps in the cytotrophoblastic shell and open beneath the placenta. Blood from these open ended maternal vessels forms a lake beneath the placenta. This nutrient-rich maternal blood showers the placental villi in jet-like fountains with each maternal heartbeat, bathing the villi with nutrients. Waste products from the fetal circulation cross the cellular membranes of the villi and exchange with maternal nutrients. The blood then pools below the placenta and drains into maternal veins. These pulsed jets are at a higher pressure than that in the intervillous space. The amount of blood which is projected with each maternal heartbeat is what stimulates placental growth. In a normal, well-nourished pregnancy, the blood volume steadily increases until 28 to 30 weeks and then remains more or less constant until birth. The intervillous spaces of the mature placenta contain about 150 ml. of blood that is replenished 3 to 4 times per minute.

The physical health of the fetus and placenta is dependent upon the adequate bathing of the villi with maternal blood more than any other factor. Recent research shows that the placenta does *not* age with advancing gestation, as is commonly believed. In fact, there is a continuous expansion of the villous surface up to and beyond the expected date of birth. Problems traditionally attributed to placental insufficiency are really caused by restricted flow of maternal blood to the placenta. Even a large dead area of the placenta (an infraction) and visible calcifications are not clinically significant *if* the placenta is adequately perfused with maternal blood. (Fox, 1991) Reductions in uteroplacental circulation result in fetal malnutrition and hypoxia (lack of oxygen). Inadequate maternal nutrition, leading to an inadequately expanded blood volume and resulting in a poorly profused placenta is the leading cause of fetal and placental growth problems.

The placental membrane or "barrier" which encases the cotyledons consists of extrafetal tissue separating the maternal and fetal bloodstreams. It is made up of four layers until 20 weeks, after that, in most places only three layers remain. The placental membranes rarely function as a true barrier to foreign substances; only compounds of a certain size, configuration and electrical charge are unable to pass through this membrane. As pregnancy advances, the placental membrane becomes progressively thinner, and the blood of many fetal capillaries is extremely close to the maternal blood in the intervillous space. This facilitates the passage of substances from the mother to the fetus. The chart below lists those substances which are known to cross the placenta from the maternal to the fetal bloodstream. The last column lists those few things which cannot cross the placenta.

NUTRIENTS	HARMFUL SUBSTANCES	OTHER SUBSTANCES	NONTRANSFERABLE SUBSTANCES
Oxygen	Drugs & poisons	IgG antibodies	Transferrin
Water	Carbon monoxide	Unconjugated	Bacteria
Carbohydrates	Viruses	steroid hormones	Heparin (drug)
Amino acids	Strontium-90	Vitamins	IgM antibodies
Lipids	Toxoplasma gondi	Intravenous fluids	
Electrolytes	Syphilis		

Note that this does not necessarily mean that the chorioamniotic membranes are impermeable to these substances; for example, some bacteria can penetrate the intact membranes.

During early pregnancy there is a fluid-filled space between the two layers of membranes which surround the baby. The amniotic sac enlarges faster than the chorionic sac, which leads to the fusion of the surfaces of both membranes by the 22nd week. (In some cases this fusion does not occur perfectly, and some fluid remains trapped between the chorion and the amnion.) The composite membrane fuses with the decidua capsularis and, after the disappearance of this part of the decidua, the decidua parietalis.

748

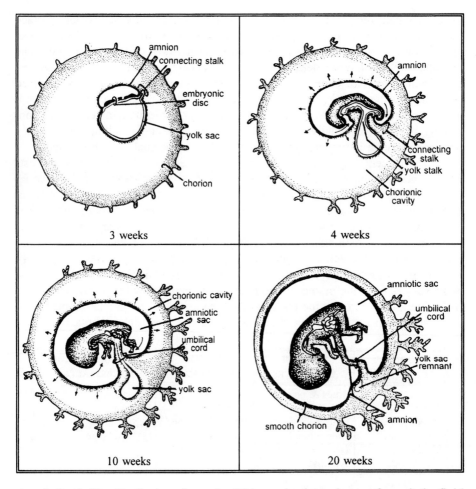

3 weeks

4 weeks

10 weeks

20 weeks

Amniotic fluid: Beginning about the 25th week, the volume of amniotic fluid increases an average of 50 ml. per week, peaking at 900 to 1000 ml. at 37 weeks, then deceasing slightly until term. While there is a wide normal range of volume, on the average it remains stable at 800 ml. until 39 weeks of pregnancy, then it declines to about 500 ml. near term. (Danforth, 1986)

At this time, researchers are still unsure exactly where all the amniotic fluid comes from. It appears that fetal urine and alveolar fluid contribute the majority of water. The fetal lungs secrete 300 to 400 ml. of fluid daily. Fetal urine output varies widely between 400 ml. daily to three times this much. Between 20 and 40 weeks gestation fetal urine output rises 10-fold. Water is removed via fetal swallowing and through the membranes in contact with the uterine wall. Indirect sources of fluid exchange include the intervillous spaces within the placenta. Removal of fluid from the amniotic space occurs primarily due to fetal swallowing, which may account for volumes up to 1,500 ml. daily. In contrast, water removal through the membranes to the uterus is only estimated to be 80 ml. daily. At term the total exchange of water between mother and fetus, mother and amniotic fluid and fetus and amniotic fluid reaches 4 liters per hour (Danforth, 1986). In addition, adequate maternal fluid intake helps maintain normal levels of amniotic fluid throughout pregnancy (Kilpatrick, 1993).

References and further reading:

Danforth, D. & Scott, J. eds., Obstetrics and Gynecology, 5th ed., Philadelphia, PA, Lippincott, 1986.

Fox, H., "A Contemporary View of the Human Placenta," Midwifery, Vol 7, No. 1, March 1991, p. 31-39.

Gabbe, Steven, et. al. ed. Obstetrics: Normal and Problem Pregnancies, 2nd ed., Churchill Livingstone, New York, 1991.

Kilpatrick, Sarah, et.al., "Maternal Hydration increases amniotic fluid index in women with normal amniotic fluid," OB/GYN, Vol. 81, No. 1, January 1993, pp. 49-52.

Moore, Keith, & Persaud, T., The Developing Human, 5th ed., W. B. Saunders Co., Philadelphia, PA 1993.

Emotional and Psychological Changes of Mid-Pregnancy

The second trimester is marked by an absence of annoying symptoms for many women and is therefore often a period of radiance. It can be divided into two periods: quickening (first feeling the baby move) and thereafter. Quickening signals that the physiological changes a woman is experiencing are due to a part of her that is also distinct from her: the separate life of the baby. This event often marks the beginning of a primary psychological task of pregnancy, the development of her own sense of mothering distinct from her own mother's. This is especially true for first-time mothers.

Prior to quickening, a woman may begin to minutely examine her relationship with her own mother; how she feels about her mother, and how she was mothered herself. The potential inherent in the mother-child relationship is examined. She seeks to integrate those qualities which she admires or respects and reject those she perceives as negative. Conflicts may emerge over whether she or her mother is a good mother or over who is the better mother. This may cause her to feel guilt and inner conflict unless she is helped to understand the normalcy of this process, and to realize that rejection of what her mother has done is not a rejection of her mother as an individual. Part of this process is the transition the woman makes from being a care receiver to a care giver. At the same time, the pregnant woman needs nurturing in order to have the psychic energy to overflow to her baby.

Quickening marks the verification of the pregnancy in the woman's mind. She may increasingly seek the company of other pregnant women whose discussions focus on pregnancy, childbearing and preparing for their new role. Letting go of her life "as it is," her one-on-one relationship with her partner or the expansion of her life to shift her relationships with other children to allow for the coming of another baby, career and other changes all mark losses which will precipitate a normal grieving process. Much of this new role identity is worked out in the form of fantasy and daydreaming.

Quickening also allows the woman to relate to the baby as a separate entity. She may spend time thinking about what her child may look like. She starts to refocus her attention from herself to her baby, and begins to attach to her baby as a part of herself, yet separate. Women also begin to think about plans for the upcoming birth. This is prime time for women to begin to communicate with the baby more consciously.

For women choosing mid-trimester fetal diagnostic techniques (such as amniocentesis or even ultrasound examination of the fetus to see if it is normal) this process of attachment can continue to be severely disrupted. It is often the case that women do not perceive fetal motion until test results have come back. This shuts the mother off from the reality of the baby as a person separate from herself until she decides if she will continue with the pregnancy. Knowing the fetus is not normal, even if she chooses to keep the pregnancy, can also cause excessive anxiety and worry and continue to interfere with her unconditional attachment to the baby.

If a woman is having problems attaching to her baby for any reason, try drawing her baby on her belly with a washable marker. This can work dramatically to connect a woman with her baby within her body; quite different than the abstract "relationship" that is fostered by ultrasound scans on a TV screen. (Whitridge, 1995)

Dreams: The woman's integration of the fact of a separate life within her own may cause her to dream of strangers or of her partner being injured, which may be due to fears of harm to the baby. She may also dream of small living things, or her competency as a mother.

Sexuality: Many women feel more erotic during the second trimester. The size of the abdomen is still not cumbersome, lubrication of the yoni is greater, and many woman have relaxed into their pregnancies and are relatively free of worries at this time. However, whatever level of sexual desire a woman does feel is perfectly normal. Women should be encouraged to tune into what they need and not feel pressured by partners into activities they do not feel they want. Refer women to Sheila Kitzinger's book Women's Experience of Sex or Bing and Coleman's book Making Love During Pregnancy for more information.

References and further reading:

Perez, Polly, "The Emotional Work of Pregnancy," International Journal of Childbirth Education, Vol. 3, No. 3, August 1988, pp. 30-1.
Varney, Helen, Nurse-Midwifery, Blackwell Scientific Pub., Boston, MA 1980.
Whitridge, Candace, workshop on prenatal care, Midwifery Today conf., Eugene, OR, June, 1995.

Laboratory Tests in the Second Trimester

Normally baseline blood values are not rechecked in the second trimester. However, most fetal diagnostic techniques are done during the 13th through 24th weeks of pregnancy. The exception is Chorionic Villus Sampling (CVS), which must take place between 9.5 and 11 weeks of pregnancy.

Fetal diagnostic techniques are most relevant for women who are over the age of 35, those who have a history of congenital defects in their families and those who are at risk due to their ethnicity or other relevant background data. Second trimester tests include:

*Alpha-Feto-protein blood tests (ideally 15 to 18 weeks)
*Amniocentesis (12 to 18 weeks)
*Ultrasound exam to detect fetal anatomical problems (20 weeks)
*Hemoglobin recheck to make sure it is falling appropriately or
      stabilizing if the woman was anemic to begin with

These tests should have been discussed during a visit in the first trimester, so that the woman can now announce her decision as to whether or not she wants testing. Women may choose one or more of these tests, depending upon their individual risk factors and how much they wish to know about the condition of the fetus. They may also choose to forego any testing, regardless of their presumed risk factors, because they would not have an abortion in any case and do not wish to expose their baby to possible harm from the tests themselves. All fetal diagnostic tests as well as genetic counseling are discussed at length in individual chapters of Diagnostic Tests. Women seeking such tests should be encouraged to read The Tentative Pregnancy by Barbara Katz-Rothman.

Who Should Be at the Birth?

Now is a good time to discuss who will be at the birth. While it may seem early to begin this discussion, many friends and relatives may have already made their desire to be present known, and the woman will have to be dealing with these requests as they come up. Paramount in these considerations are the mother's needs and desires. She is the one having the baby, after all, and birth is not a spectator sport. Family and friends are typically both nervous and excited about the prospect of homebirth. They may be skeptical of the care you will be giving her and question the safety of the choices she is making. On the other hand, the irresistibility of being so closely involved in the event may have a number of people requesting that they be present, or even worse, assuming they are welcome. This can be especially problematic with family members.

While each situation will be different, here are some cardinal points to impress upon the parents as they grapple with these decisions:

*The mother's needs *must* come first. She should not invite people she feels would benefit from seeing a birth, for whom it would be healing, etc. over her own needs and desires. Don't try to do any favors, mend old relationships or otherwise work things out with other people through the birth experience: this usually will not work and will often lead to a hospital transport because it is the only way the mother can get the emotional space she needs in order to get on with the labor.

*All those who *are* invited must recognize the final decision of who will be present rests with the parent's along with input from the midwives. They must realize that, at the last minute, they may not be called at all or may be asked to leave. This has to be okay and not taken as a personal affront; the mother's needs must come before anyone else's.

*Ideally, only those with whom the mother (and preferably both partners) have a clear and emotionally clean relationship should be invited. The more entangled the relationship, the more likely it is that it will interfere with the birthing energy.

*It is usually unwise to invite a large group of people for a party atmosphere. Birth is a private, intimate and sexual experience. Those who come should have assigned roles (cook, child care, etc.)

*If there are people the parents want to involve but are hesitant to invite to the birth, they can ask them to bring over food afterwards or to do laundry or other chores which are needed but which will not involve them directly with caring for the mother or baby.

*Be careful when considering the wisdom of having the mother's mother present at the birth. Mother/daughter relationships which carry a lot of unresolved emotional baggage may cause a complete stalemate during labor and the labor will stop as well. No matter how clear a woman is prior to labor that she can and will ask her mother to leave if necessary, this is impossible for most women when it comes right down to it. This is because on an emotional level a woman needs mothering, which she hopes to get from her own mother (that is why she wanted her there in the first place). As midwives, we often stand in the place of a nurturing mother; therefore the woman knows that by asking her mother to leave she is telling her she cannot meet her needs and the midwives can. This prevents her from taking any action, and you get saddled with the unpleasant and sometimes nearly impossible task of asking her to leave yourself.

This may be a problem if the mother is under 18, as her mother has a legal right to demand to be present. In these cases you can use your culturally derived authority as a care provider to set limits on the number of people based on concerns about infection or whatever you need to conjure up. How this situation might be dealt with should be discussed with the parents prenatally.

If the mother/daughter relationship is a good one, having the mother there can be a real asset. I have seen labors where the mother's mother's presence was the only thing that got a woman through her labor at home. You must evaluate each situation individually.

*Unless a great deal of healing between *both parties* has taken place, it would be equally unwise for any relative who has been abusive to the woman to be present, as she will feel most vulnerable during labor.

If the mother's home is small, fewer people should be invited, unless there is a nearby home of a friend or relative where those not immediately needed can stay.

Siblings at birth: Those who already have children may want to discuss having them present for the birth. Some things to take into account regarding the participation of siblings are:

*The age of children and their individual needs
*The timing of the birth: should a child be awakened in the middle of the night? (This will also depend upon the child.)
*Mother's comfort level; can she ask for the children to be removed if they are interfering with her concentration or crawling on her, have they previously seen her naked, etc.?

*The child's desire to be present

The children need to be informed regarding the sounds, faces, and other aspects of the hard work of labor. There needs to be an adult who is comfortable with the choice to birth at home with midwives assigned to be with each child (if possible) no matter what they choose to do. The adult needs to be committed to being with the children even if they do not wish to be in the room for the actual birth or if they need to leave the house for any reason. If necessary, have another adult on call for back-up, in case the person in charge of supervising the children must leave. These people should be comfortable with the choices the parents have made, because if they are not, the children will pick up on it and may become insecure or frightened as a result.

Ideally, anyone who is to be at the birth should come to at least one prenatal visit before you make your homevisit during the last trimester. That way both you and they can get a better sense of what they are getting themselves into and the mother has this information to use when making a decision.

PROBLEMS ASSOCIATED WITH THE SECOND TRIMESTER

As pregnancy advances, caring for women with problems becomes increasingly complex. While serious problems can occur before this point, now you have to consider a possibly viable fetus as well as the well-being of the woman. Problems which began in the first trimester and have persisted become more critical, as the mother can be debilitated from fatigue, nausea, vomiting and the like. This following section covers those problems and complications which most commonly present themselves during mid-pregnancy. When problems overlap from the first to the second trimester, most of the possible causes and differential considerations are the same except as noted below.

*Nausea and vomiting

*When fetal diagnostic tests come back positive

*False pregnancy
-Pregnancy earlier than expected
-Small for dates growth

*Miscarriage in the second trimester
-Ectopic pregnancy
-Loose cervix
-Preterm labor
-Abdominal condition unrelated to birth

*Loose cervix
-Onset of preterm labor in a woman with a normal cervix

*Abdominal pregnancy
-Abdominal condition unrelated to birth

*Sacculation of the Pregnant Uterus (very rare)
-Pregnancy earlier than expected

Nausea and Vomiting

Nausea which persists into the second trimester is a cause for concern. At this time blood volume expansion is beginning to accelerate; if this does not happen adequately, the danger of toxemia developing in the third trimester is greatly increased. Reasons for nausea at this time are much the same as for the first trimester:

*Hypoglycemia
*Low blood pressure
*Multiple gestation; this is a particularly problematic cause, since the hormone levels from multiple placentas put an extra metabolic load on the liver.
*Hydatidiform mole which has not yet been discovered (this serious cause is discussed in a separate chapter in the section on Problems Associated With the First Trimester)
*Abdominal pain which accompanies nausea may signal the late presentation of an imminent to rupture ectopic pregnancy or a serious coexisting medical complication (see separate chapter on Ectopic Pregnancy in the Problems Associated With the First Trimester section and the chapter on Abdominal Pain in the section on Problems That Can Occur at any Time).
*Headaches may accompany nausea in cases of simple hypoglycemia as well as more serious conditions (see separate Headache chapter in the section on Problems That Can Occur at any Time).

For more information on the differential diagnosis of nausea, see all of the separate chapters mentioned above. If no underlying medical condition is the cause and ectopic pregnancy has been ruled out, the remedies are the same as given in the chapter on Nausea and Vomiting in the section on Problems That Can Occur in the First Trimester.

Anti-nausea medications: If all other therapies have been exhausted, there are pharmaceuticals which can be used as a last resort. The easiest drug therapy to try is available over the counter: one 25 mg. Unisom tablet and one 25 mg. B_6 tablet is the equivalent of one dose of drug Bendectin, a product taken off the market in 1984 because many women felt their babies birth defects were related to its use during pregnancy. The company denied this connection. However, if pregnancy has advanced beyond the 12th week and nausea is still a serious concern, the risk of birth defects is low compared to the risk of ongoing nutritional compromise. Unisom contains doxylamine, an antihistamine which causes drowsiness and should be taken no more frequently than every 8 hours. Physicians regularly recommend this over-the-counter substitute for the drug which was used for years as their primary pharmaceutical line of defense against pregnancy-related nausea. (Abrams, 1990)

Bonine and Antivert are prescription drugs containing meclizine hydrochloride, an effective anti-nausea medication. They are both contraindicated for those with difficult breathing, asthma, or pulmonary disease. Either may cause drowsiness, dry mouth and rarely blurred vision. Alcohol should be avoided during treatment. One or 2 tablets of Bonine or 25 to 50 mg. of Antivert are taken every 24 hours. Dosage should be gradually reduced over the course of several days as nausea is resolved. (PDR, 1991)

Phenergan is sometimes recommended for nausea during pregnancy. Rectal suppositories are supplied in 12.5, 25 and 50 mg. doses. This drug has an antihistamine effect and is contraindicated in those known to be hypersensitive to or to have a idiosyncratic reaction to promethazine or to other phenothiazines. It causes extreme drowsiness and nervous system depression, lowers the seizure threshold in those with seizure disorders and may cause jaundice in some people. It can skew hCG pregnancy test results, causing both false negative and false positive tests. It also increases glucose levels. It is rated pregnancy category C in the Physician's Desk Reference (PDR) (see the chapter on Prescription Drugs, Well-being section, for details). Other side effects include increased or decreased blood pressure, rashes, light sensitivity, and increased nausea and vomiting; alcohol should be avoided during use. The initial dose is a 25 mg. suppository, followed by the smallest possible effective dose every 4 to 6 hours. As nausea stabilizes, the dose should be tapered off gradually over the course of several days. (PDR, 1991)

If nausea continues to be severe, hospitalization for IV nutritional therapy and IV anti-nausea medication is warranted.

Once nausea is stabilized, the woman will need to eat additional protein and calories to make up for the lack of adequate nutritional intake over the course of the previous weeks. Monitor blood volume expansion by checking the hemoglobin a couple of times over the course of the next few weeks to make sure the woman is recovering from this early pregnancy stress.

References and further reading:

Abrams, Richard, Will It Hurt the Baby?, Addison-Wesley Pub. Co., Inc., Reading, MA, 1990.
PDR (Physician's Desk Reference), 1991.

When Fetal Diagnostic Tests Come Back Positive

While the parents may have wanted fetal testing, they were hoping for reassurance that the baby was normal. When a problem is discovered, they will have to face the fact that something is wrong with their baby and what to do about it. Grief responses such as shock, anger and bargaining may surface for the parents as they grapple with this knowledge. Their options are abortion or carrying the pregnancy and preparing for a baby with special needs. In some rare instances, fetal surgery may be available, a significantly risky and expensive process for both mother and baby during which the baby will not be anesthetized; a pretty difficult way to start life. Partners may be at odds about what course to take. While fetal testing is widely recommended, the emotional implications of this technology are not well acknowledged. Nature never intended that parents would have such information, pregnancy as a time of unconditional attachment is severely disrupted by the technology available today. The anguish of this dilemma is often lost on those who have never faced it, and the parents turmoil is not acknowledged in our culture. Helping them explore their feelings, their fears and their choices in a nonjudgmental way will go a long way toward bridging this painful cultural gap.

Our culture tends to assume that women will abort in these cases, and offers little support for them to seriously consider allowing the pregnancy to continue. You can suggest that they explore what the condition might mean for their child by meeting other children with a similar condition; it is important to give them permission to consider this option. People can and do live happy family lives when one member has a disability. If they choose to continue the pregnancy, they may want to birth in the hospital if the baby will need immediate care which you cannot provide. Be aware, however that sometimes doctors recommend surgical delivery for virtually any fetal problem; often this is totally unwarranted. Your research into the nature of the fetal condition can help all of you make a decision about the appropriate place of birth. If homebirth is chosen, a pediatric visit should be arranged for the baby soon after birth.

If abortion is chosen, you can recommend whatever termination services you are aware of, although their genetics counselor will probably have recommendations for them as well. You might offer to accompany her or if she does not want you there, at least offer continuing postpartum care. There may be parent support groups in your area. Check with a local hospital or her genetic counselor.

Whatever the mother and her partner chooses, grief will be a big issue. Either the grief of losing her fantasy "perfect" baby, or the grief of terminating the pregnancy. Also see the chapter on When a Baby Dies in Early Pregnancy, in the Problems Associated With the First Trimester section, as many of the issues discussed there will be relevant for these women as well.

References and further reading:
Hershey, Laura, "Choosing Disability," Ms., July/August, 1994.

<u>False Pregnancy</u>

A false or phantom pregnancy (pseudocyesis) occurs when superficial physical changes and symptoms lead a woman to believe that she is pregnant when she is not. Sometimes this occurs because a woman is desperate to be pregnant or because she is entering menopause and is ambivalent about her changing fertility status. Sometimes it occurs due to denial about a completed miscarriage; the woman continues to believe that she is pregnant even though she has lost the baby.

The mind is a powerful thing, and a woman can cease menstruation or have only scanty or irregular periods, and may experience belly enlargement due to gas, disposition of fat or abdominal fluid. Breast changes such as enlargement, increased pigmentation and sometimes discharge may occur. probably due to hormonal imbalances. A woman may even imagine she feels fetal movement which may be due to contractions of the intestines or the abdominal wall. She may report many of the symptoms of early pregnancy such as nausea. Of course, none of this is done consciously, but is an attempt by the woman's psyche to believe that she is, indeed, pregnant.

Typically the woman comes to you early in pregnancy and is absolutely certain that she is pregnant. She does not wish to have any confirmatory tests because she is so certain. I do not rush to do tests to determine if she is pregnant, because generally speaking most women this sure of themselves are indeed pregnant. You may not discover the truth until she enters the second trimester and the positive signs of pregnancy fail to be detected. Even if you are experienced you can still be fooled, for some women raise their pulse rate to mimic fetal heart tones. Be sure to check the mother's radial pulse simultaneously as you listen for the fetal heart. First and foremost, you must not dismiss the questions which arise in your mind or your intuitions when your findings do not coincide with her certainty; if you do, you could go for months writing off your concerns.

Knowing how to deal with a woman you suspect is having a false pregnancy can be difficult, especially if she is quite sure that she is pregnant. In my practice, when I had such suspicions (it happened twice) I postponed encouraging the woman to have the situation checked out until I was quite sure by abdominal palpation that she was either much earlier in pregnancy than she thought or that she was not pregnant at all. While pelvic exam may be revealing in some cases, slight uterine enlargement is often present, especially if she has stopped menstruating. Remember that during abdominal palpation the pregnant uterus, as it enlarges, has a definite border along the top and sides; in a false pregnancy this border will not be detectable even though the abdomen is distended.

As the weeks go by it is important for you to comment on your findings as you see them. You can tell her that her uterus seems quite small, its borders are hard to find and that you cannot hear the fetal heart. Once 16 to 20 weeks or so rolls around and no definite evidence of pregnancy has made an appearance, you can encourage her to have the situation checked out with a blood test or an ultrasound exam. By now your questions regarding her pregnancy status will have eased her into the notion that it is worth looking into, and you may get the happy news that she is indeed pregnant, but much earlier than she thought. While gradually and gently breaking the news that she is not pregnant is good in some respects, it is not necessarily kind to allow a woman to go for months believing that she is pregnant. You must judge the situation on an individual basis.

If it is discovered that she is really not pregnant, remember this will be no light matter to her. She has thought and felt that she was, and may experience the same kind of grief as a woman who has had a miscarriage. This may be particularly devastating if the woman realizes she was never pregnant. She may feel that her body fooled her and that she is not in harmony with her bodily processes, especially if infertility has been a long-time burden. Encourage her to feel her emotions fully and try to come to terms with her relationship to this experience before she tries to become pregnant again.

References and further reading:

Greenhill, J., Principles and Practice of Obstetrics, W. B. Saunders, Co., Philadelphia, PA, 1951.

Miscarriage in the Second Trimester

This chapter assumes you are already familiar with the chapter covering Miscarriage in the First Trimester, since many of those suggestions and remedies apply to second trimester situations as well. After the 24th to 25th week of pregnancy, miscarriage becomes reclassified as premature labor (Gilhooley, 1995). This is the technical cutoff for fetal viability (or a fetal weight over 600 grams [about 1 lb. 5 oz.]), 50 to 60% of these babies may survive with the most intense intensive care, although long term neurologic problems are common (ACOG, 1995). Miscarriage during the second trimester is likely to be due to different factors than those which occur during the first trimester, although some problems overlap, as follows:

Ectopic pregnancy: While it is uncommon for an ectopic pregnancy to remain undetected until the second trimester, this can occur if the conceptus has implanted in an area which allows for considerable expansion before symptoms of pain and bleeding appear, such as the interstitial area of the uterine tube. If a woman has an abnormally small uterus, an intrauterine pregnancy could lead to rupture of the uterus as the pregnancy advances. Although technically this is a uterine rupture, it may mimic a late ectopic pregnancy in some respects. See the chapter on Ectopic Pregnancy in the section on the Problems Associated With the First Trimester and the chapter on Uterine Rupture in the section on Problems Associated With the Third Trimester.

Maternal blood sensitization to which the fetus is susceptible: If the mother is negative for a minor blood factor and she has been previously sensitized, it is possible for a fetus that is positive for that blood factor to be severely compromised and even miscarried in the second trimester.

Uterine or cervical damage or abnormalities (especially in DES daughters): See the chapter on Loose Cervix for more information about cervical abnormalities that precipitate early labor. If the uterus is abnormally small, labor may begin prematurely. In these rare cases, nothing can be done to correct the situation and the baby may be born before term.

Incarceration of the uterus: If a retroverted uterus becomes trapped in the pelvic cavity, cramps, pain and pressure suggestive of miscarriage may occur. If this seems to be the cause, see the chapter on Incarceration and Sacculation of the Pregnant Uterus at the end of this section.

Placental abruption: The placenta can begin to separate from the uterine wall at any time due to poor attachment with or without the additional complication of high blood pressure. Poor placental attachment is primarily due to inadequate nutrition or a congenital abnormality of the uterine wall and will be heralded by bleeding. Look for constant hardness of the uterus and extreme uterine tenderness, possibly a rising fundus in concealed abruption, and bleeding from the yoni which is too slight to explain maternal shock symptoms in a partially concealed abruption. A completely revealed abruption will present with painless bleeding from the yoni. Placental abruption is handled much the same in the second or third trimester, The fetus is usually not expected to survive a major abruption that takes place during the second trimester. (Refer to the third trimester chapter on Placental Aburption for more information.)

Hydatidiform mole: This placental abnormality may not be obvious until the second trimester. At this point some of the symptoms such as the doughy consistency to the uterus, large for dates fundal height, inability to elicit ballotment of fetal parts, and escalating secondary symptoms of toxemia may be more evident. (See chapter on Hydatidiform Mole in the Problems Associated With the First Trimester section for more details.)

Maternal infection: A multitude of maternal infections can affect the well-being of the fetus, and in some cases, lead to premature labor or fetal death. Many of these conditions are discussed at length in <u>Diagnostic Tests</u>. Maternal "flu" symptoms, foul discharge from the yoni, fever, or a recent known exposure to an infectious disease should raise suspicions. Be especially alert for the possibility of Listeriosis and Chlamydia.

Fetal malformation: Sometimes babies die due to malformations which are not lethal in the early months of gestation.

Unexplained fetal death: There are times when the destiny of a person is such that her very short life occurs entirely within her mother. These babies die for no detectable reason. Things to discuss with the parents include genetic studies, work-ups for undetected infection (especially syphilis) and autopsy to try and tell if some hidden but lethal defect is the cause. (Also see the chapter on When the Baby Dies Before Birth in the Third Trimester section for more information about how to deal with fetal demise.)

<u>**Risks peculiar to second trimester miscarriage:**</u> One of the risks of second trimester miscarriage is the possibility that the fetus will deliver but the placenta will remain attached to the uterine wall. This is most likely to happen between 12 and 16 weeks of pregnancy and occurs for two reasons. The fetus is heavier at this point than it has been and is connected by a very slender umbilical cord. The slim cord can easily break during the birth, especially if the fetus has been dead for some time. Secondly, the uterine size is still relatively small. A primary mechanism of placental detachment involves the area beneath the placenta

becoming smaller after the amniotic fluid and baby are out of the uterus, causing the placenta to peel off the uterine wall. Without much reduction in uterine size, this process may happen incompletely, causing the placenta to remain attached, or it may detach only partially and cause bleeding. If the miscarriage is occurring for a reason such as loose cervix, the site of placental attachment may be very healthy. A healthy placenta at this gestation is not ready to detach and will have more difficulty releasing. The uterine muscles cannot clamp down when the uterus is not empty, which leads to more bleeding from the exposed area beneath the partially detached placenta. In addition, the mother's blood volume is still not as expanded as it would be after 28 weeks, so she has less of a margin of blood loss before she becomes shocky. The is especially true in cases of placental abruption secondary to poor nutrition, as the blood volume will not be expanded as much as it would be at this point in a woman who is well nourished.

Presenting symptoms: If there is a problem with the pregnancy, symptoms of second trimester miscarriage will most often start out with bleeding and rhythmic backache or uterine cramps which are felt above the public bone. If a loose cervix is the cause, there will be no bleeding, cervical changes will commence, eventually resulting in contractions and sometimes rupture of the membranes. True labor is often described as a pulling sensation in the lower uterine segment, located in the area above or behind the pubic bone. As pregnancy advances, passage of the enlarging baby and placenta through the cervix will require the cervix to be increasingly more dilated. By the second trimester, the uterus needs to work hard, and lower cramps may signify that cervical dilation is occurring. Women can have second trimester uterine cramps that are not due to miscarriage. Ask if the cramps are coordinated with the uterus becoming firm. If so, this is concerning. If not, there could be other factors of concern (see list below) but she is less likely to be going into labor unless she has an abnormal cervix (as may a DES daughter). Nevertheless, any woman who suspects that she is in labor should be seen and examined right away so that the woman can correlate her symptoms with what is really taking place. The following things should be ruled out:

Does she really have a urinary tract infection? UTI symptoms can mimic false labor. With a true UTI, any backache present is continuous, not rhythmic and no distinct cervical changes are noted on internal exam. Obtain a clean catch urine specimen for culture and sensitivity. Meanwhile if a UTI seems likely, start the woman on herbal therapies to relieve urinary symptoms. (See Diagnostic Tests).

Is she dehydrated? A hot summer day, illness, being busy and not drinking, or a combination of these can cause a woman to become dehydrated. As the blood volume becomes more concentrated, contractions are triggered. Women on marginal diets are especially prone to this since their blood volume will also be marginally expanded. Have the woman drink at least a quart of plain water within a half-hour and see if contractions slow down or disappear.

Is she undernourished? Nutritional problems or even good basic nutrition which is inadequate for activity or stress levels may lead to early labor. Once protein, calories and salt are evaluated, recommend 1000 mg of calcium citrate and 500 mg of magnesium after meals daily for women at mild risk and give a double divided dose for those at high risk of otherwise uncomplicated early labor.

Has she passed any fluid from her yoni? If the woman has a loose cervix and ruptured membranes, chances are she is dilated. Typically the rather fragile bag bulges through a partly dilated cervix for a few days and then breaks. In these cases, miscarriage is much more likely. (See Chorioamnionitis chapter in Diagnostic Tests) Passage of fluid may also be due to:

> **Decidual endometritis:** The membranes may weaken and rupture secondary to a intrauterine infection with or without other symptoms. It is likely that an infection will be causing other symptoms such as fever, pain or cramping. However, this will not be so in all cases. If the fluid is bloody or yellow, rule out infection with cultures. It may be necessary to perform a sterile speculum exam to obtain a fluid sample issuing from the cervix that isn't mixed with organisms from further down in the birth passage. If a speculum exam is performed, visualize the cervix for effacement and dilation and to obtain *Beta*-strep from the lower yoni and chlamydia culture from the cervix.

> **Leakage from the space between the chorion and amnion:** During early development there is a space between the chorion and amnion. This usually disappears as the two fuse: however, this fusion is not always complete. In such cases it is possible for the chorion to break and release fluid, leaving the amnion intact and leaking a finite amount of clear fluid containing no vernix, meconium or lanugo. Labor does not follow and the chorion either reseals, remains in place with a hole in it or eventually becomes rolled up around the placental border.

> **Leakage from the amniotic cavity itself:** A rupture of both membranes would also cause fluid to issue from the yoni. In some cases, if the mother remains very still for a week or two, such a hole in the membranes can repair itself. It is likely that many cases in which midwives believe such repair to have occurred were actually a rupture of the chorion only, where the amnion remained intact. In some rare cases of complete rupture of membranes, the fetus continues to develop outside the chorionic sac. The membranes shrink and become bunched up around the base of the umbilical cord. This is

called extrachorial pregnancy or *gravidatas exochorialis*. In cases where the amnion breaks, it can become rolled into a strand as the fetus moves, wrap around the neck or limbs, and produce amputation or even death. If amniotic fluid does not surround the fetus, poor lung development may also result since the baby will have no fluid to breathe prenatally.

Obviously the second trimester is too early for the baby to be born and do well. If rupture of membranes has occurred and no evidence of infection is present, attempts should be made to forestall labor. These recommendations are the same as for preterm prelabor rupture of membranes which occurs during the third trimester: see that chapter for more information. Women choosing this option must be watched closely for evidence of infection: elevated maternal temperature or pulse, uterine tenderness, rapid fetal heart rate, or lack of fetal movement. I recommend that you do a homevisit to assess the condition of mother and baby at least once daily. The mother should notify you of any changes immediately.

As a totally benign watery discharge of unknown origin Hydrorrhea gravidarum:: Some women have small gushes of clear fluid one or more times throughout pregnancy. This is neither amniotic fluid nor urine. It may be that the uterine lining at times emits clear fluid which becomes accumulated between the uterine wall and the chorion and gradually works its way down toward the cervix where it finally breaks through the cervical mucus and is discharged. Some women have a gush of fluid with orgasm, particularly during masturbation, which may originate from the female prostate glands lining the urethra. (Sevely, 1987)

The discharge of a finite amount of clear fluid is most often nothing to be concerned about. I've seen as much as a cup of fluid come out prenatally with completely intact membranes presenting in labor.

Is there bleeding from the yoni? In most cases, bleeding is from the placenta however, small amounts can be from an inflamed cervix. Placental abruption, if minor, can sometimes be resealed with the help of oral vitamin E (2000 IU and vitamin C with bioflavinoids 1000 mg. daily for one to two weeks). Monitor carefully for shock symptoms and signs of increasing intrauterine pressure and pain, as well as increased bleeding, which would signal continued internal bleeding. (See the chapter on Abruption in the Third Trimester section.)

Is her cervix changing? Whether you do an internal exam to find this out will be partly determined by whether it seems as if the membranes are intact. If they are ruptured, doing an exam via the yoni greatly increases the likelihood of introducing infection. If they are intact, an internal exam lets you know what, if anything, these symptoms mean about the status of the cervix, useful information as to how much time you have to try to stop labor. If the cervix is not changing and there is no fluid and no bleeding, order urine tests to rule out UTI and suggest anti-miscarriage therapies as indicated to stop labor.

If the cervix is changing, determine how rapidly relative to when symptoms appeared and their severity now. If there is no external bleeding, there are no signs of internal hemorrhage, and you feel you have time, start the woman on an herbal regime of your choice. I have found 5 drops of False Unicorn Root Tincture every 5 to 15 minutes until uterine activity stops to be very effective. It can shut a cervix back down and reverse effacement back to where it should be for gestational age. (I've seen it do this with the baby low, the cervix two centimeters dilated and 90% effaced.) Once contractions have subsided, space out dosages gradually over the course of the next 5 to 7 days. (For other herbal remedies see the chapter on Miscarriage in the First Trimester). Breast stimulation (including nursing) and yoni penetration should be avoided until things have stabilized.

If the cervix is changing and you suspect loose cervix: If a woman has a history of intrauterine DES exposure or second trimester miscarriages, you must consider loose cervix as a primary probable cause. Typically, there may be slight bleeding, increased vaginal discharge or a vague feeling of pelvic pressure. Eventually these women start to feel cramps alerting them to the possibility of cervical changes only after effacement is progressing and dilation is underway. They need to get off their feet immediately and given herbs to help quiet the uterus; however herbs alone will not correct this problem if the cervix is very abnormal. Some women will be able to get by with using herbs *and* staying in bed for the duration of the pregnancy others may benefit from the placement of a cerclage. See the chapter on Loose Cervix later in this section for more details.

When to transport: Obviously, if things quiet down and the cervix seems normal, there is no need to transport. If that is not the case, whether or not you go to great lengths to transport will be determined by the gestational age of the fetus, the mother's wishes and the type of care you have access to. Consult a pediatrician, if possible, to ask about the realistic chances of the baby surviving in your area given the presumed gestational age. If the baby is 20 weeks along or more the situation is borderline. You are better off transporting, especially if your community is hostile to homebirth. The more advanced a pregnancy is when labor begins, the more you are at legal risk as a care provider for keeping a woman at home. Once a baby reaches viability you are legally bound to record the birth or death with the state and dispose of the remains in a legally acceptable manner. Most hospitals will actively strive to save babies born at 24 to 25 weeks or later, depending upon where you live. The reason why this cut-off point is not a hard and fast rule is because neonatal care is attempting to save younger and younger fetuses; as they become more successful, the survival limit is pushed earlier. (Gilhooley, 1995)

Examining what was passed: Always examine what the woman passes to try and determine if a complete miscarriage has occurred. By this time there should be a visible fetus which looks quite human and a placenta. By 15 weeks of pregnancy the placenta has a more definite shape with a less fluffy appearance. Later placental tissue will be thin, soft, and a light mottled red to pink color. Since the placenta is not very dense in early pregnancy, it will be fragile. If you discover grape-like cysts on all or part of the placenta, save the tissue in a glass container in the refrigerator and refer to the chapter on Hydatidiform Mole, in First Trimester Problems. Encourage the parents to look at the baby with you there for support. The tissue can also be sent to a lab for pathological evaluation, which may be important if the baby does not appear to be normally formed. The baby will look like a baby (unless severely macerated). Encourage the parents to plan for how they will relate to the baby's body at birth and how they want to handle burial or cremation. See the chapter on When a Baby Dies Before Birth in the section on Third Trimester Problems for more details on grieving a second trimester death.

Missed labor (dead fetus syndrome): If the baby dies after 20 weeks of pregnancy and is retained in the uterus for more than 48 hours without the onset of labor it is referred to as a missed labor. Rarely, the fetus remains within the uterus for many months or even years and becomes calcified. Signs that the baby is no longer alive include a cessation of fetal movement. As time passes, the uterus will gradually become smaller, the signs of pregnancy will diminish and finally disappear, and the woman will no longer "feel pregnant." (Danforth, 1986) If you suspect fetal demise, it is wise to get the situation documented via an ultrasound. Even with no detectable signs of life, a scan will sometimes discover a live fetus.

If the fetus has dies, some women may wish to remain at home and await the onset of labor. If the membranes are intact and there are no signs of infection, this is a reasonable choice. However, once again, you must remember that her blood volume will not be as expanded as it would be at term and therefore blood loss following the birth would be of serious concern. In addition, the risk of clotting compromise developing in the mother is increased the further along a pregnancy is when death occurs. A baseline clotting panel should be ordered at the time the fetal demise is diagnosed. Follow-up tests should be done at two week intervals or whenever evidence of clotting compromise becomes evident (such as easy bruising, excessive bleeding from injuries, etc.) See the chapter on The Clotting Mechanism and Bleeding Disorders in Diagnostic Tests for more information, including what tests to perform). Women should know that second trimester miscarriage involves laboring to birth the baby, with more cervical dilation required the further along the pregnancy. Dealing with the actual birth of a dead baby will be discussed in Volume II of this textbook. Also see the chapter on the Third Trimester section entitled When a Baby Dies Before Birth for more information.

If you transport: Medical protocols vary from place to place regarding what might be done to attempt to stop labor if the fetus is alive. To a certain extent, at what gestational age they try to stop labor has to do with the sophistication of the available neonatal intensive care unit. The woman will be evaluated for urinary tract infection, if time permits, and may be given a Ringers Lactate solution intravenously if she is felt to be dehydrated, however 5% dextrose in water or 0.25% normal saline are better choices if tocolysis is to be used as well. If the pregnancy is between 34 and 37 weeks, care is individualized and many practitioners may just let labor proceed, since babies born at 34 weeks or later have a survival rate within 1% of those born at term.

Determining if preterm labor has begun and intervention is warranted has been a precarious judgement call for many years. A new test identifies a protein called fetal fibronectin (fFN), which is present in fetal and placental tissue throughout pregnancy and in yoni secretions in early pregnancy and a week or two prior to the onset of both preterm and term labor. Currently, studies show that a woman with a negative fFN test has a 1 in 200 change of delivering within a week. Thus, those with symptoms of early labor plus a positive fFN are more likely to be truly at risk than those who have a negative test. This test will be available in labs and may also be produced in a dip-stick form which could be used at the bedside. Of course, one more test does not address the link between poor nutrition and preterm labor, but it may be useful in an emergent situation, although it is being suggested as yet another test to subject all women to in the name of prophylaxis.

If the pregnancy is not yet 34 weeks along, most hospitals will attempt to stop contractions by giving the mother a tocolytic drug such as ritodrine or terbutaline, which is intended to suppress uterine activity. Terbutaline is specifically contraindicated for tocolysis by the FDA and causes increased heart rate, transient hyperglycemia, hypokalemia, pulmonary edema, decreased blood flow to the heart and irregular heart beat in the mother and hypoglycemia and accelerated heart rate in the fetus at times, but is widely used anyway (PDR, 1991, p. 1004). An alternative drug commonly used for tocolysis is magnesium sulfate IV, which is a nervous system suppressant. Mothers should know that, "to date, no studies have convincingly demonstrated an improvement in survival or any index of long-term neonatal outcome with the use of tocolytic therapy. On the other hand, the potential damages of tocolytic therapy to the mother and newborn are well documented." Tocolysis may delay birth for a few days to one week, which allows time for the administration of corticosteroid drugs to assist in the maturation of the fetal lungs, justifying short-term prolongation of pregnancy in cases where the baby is likely to be born with immature lungs. (ACOG, 1995) Parents must weigh the use of corticosteroids for this purpose carefully, since the long term consequences of this therapy are unknown at this time, although the short term benefits of a baby that can breathe on its own at birth are certainly a compelling reason to allow their use if birth is inevitable.

Emotional issues: Talk to the woman about what was going on in her life just before the symptoms began; help her sort through her emotions and what her needs are at this time in the life in general and in this situation in particular. If transport is necessary, accompany her and stay with her in the hospital as much as possible. Some practitioners may want to perform a surgical birth if the baby is quite early. Be sure she understands the risks of surgery as well as giving her a realistic idea of what she can expect in terms of neonatal care and the chance that her baby will die, depending upon its gestational age.

If you suspect a medical problem which may mimic some symptoms of miscarriage: Read the chapter on Abdominal Pain and seek a medical consultation without delay.

References and further reading:

ACOG Technical Bulletin "Preterm Labor," No. 206, June 1995.

Danforth, D, et.al. ed. Danforth's Obstetrics and Gynecology, 5th ed., J.B. Lippincott, Phil., 1986.

Gilhooley, Joe, neonatologist, Oregon Health Sci. U., conversation regarding fetal viability, 5/95.

Garite, T, & Lockwood, C., "Fetal fibronectin (fFN): A New Immunodiagnostic Test for the Diagnosis and Prediction of Impending Preterm Delivery," in press for Contemp. OB/GYN, last quarter, 1995.

Greenhill, J., Principles and Practice of Obstetrics, W. B. Saunders, Co., Philadelphia, PA, 1951.

Sevely, J., Eve's Secrets: A New Theory of Female Sexuality, Random House, New York, 1987.

Loose Cervix

The medical model refers to a loose cervix as incompetent. Women with this condition do not feel supported by this language; therefore, this text will call this condition loose cervix. Any of the following can predispose to loose cervix:

*Malformations of the lower uterus and cervix (check DES exposure)
*Previous deep cervical tears, especially if unrepaired
*Cervical amputation from annular detachment during a previous labor (details on this complication can be found in Volume II)
*Deep conization for dysplasia (especially for someone with an anatomical weakness to begin with)
*Cervical trauma from induced abortion or other forced cervical dilation, especially with a constitutionally weak cervix; (the use of tapered cervical dilators and laminaria [a narrow stick of expansive material is inserted in the cervical passageway; the stick swells with moisture to gradually dilate the cervix]) have reduced injuries.

Some women have been told that a loose cervix precipitated a premature birth in a previous pregnancy, and have gone on to carry babies to term with no interventions other than major dietary improvement (Brewer, 1983).

Signs and symptoms: Loose cervix, whatever the cause, results in painless effacement and dilation as the weight of the conceptus increases and puts more pressure on the inner os; if there are no other complicating factors frank bleeding does not occur. This usually occurs in the second trimester, but in some cases may be delayed until the early third trimester. Vague sensations of pressure in the yoni or an increased yoni discharge may or may not accompany otherwise silent cervical changes. Frequently, significant effacement and dilation occur (often to two or more centimeters) before any noticeable uterine activity or lower back pain begins to alert the mother to a problem. At that point sometimes the membranes are bulging through the partially dilated cervix, further complicating the picture and making preterm rupture of membranes likely. Premature labor caused by an abnormal cervix will be harder to stop with natural methods than premature labor due to other causes and it is more likely that birth will occur.

What to do: The treatment of loose cervix varies depending upon the gestational age of the baby and the amount of cervical changes which have taken place prior to discovery. A cervical exam is in order, but you must introduce your fingers slowly and gently. Be alert for the possibility of a prolapsed balloon of membranes protruding through the partially open cervix; this will feel like a soft, fluctuant bubble of water and will rupture if you are not gentle. If you find such a bubble and can slide your fingers over to one side to reach higher up for the cervix, then do so, otherwise, do not risk rupture by persisting with a difficult exam. If changes are minimal, the woman can stay off her feet and take anti-miscarriage herbs as recommended in the chapter on Miscarriage in the Second Trimester. If the cervix is quite loose, the woman will have to stay off her feet, only getting up to use the toilet, for the remainder of the pregnancy. Herbs may help but will *not* be sufficient if the cervix is quite abnormal. If this route is chosen, you should perform gentle internal exams periodically to determine if cervical changes are occurring. Sometimes, once women correlate the sensations they have already experienced with the cervical changes to date, such as feelings of pressure or aching, they can monitor for cervical changes themselves and frequent internal exams will not be necessary. You can also teach the woman to check her own cervix. Sexual activity should be avoided.

If cervical changes are more advanced or proceeding to active labor, transport may be your best alternative. See the chapter on Miscarriage in the Second Trimester for general information on what might be done for preterm labor in the hospital. If the membranes are bulging through the cervix but not yet ruptured, they can be gently replaced by filling the urinary bladder which causes the membranes to recede within the cervix without being touched (Aarts, et.al., 1995). This should be accomplished in hospital. To prevent further prolapse of the membranes while awaiting transport, you can try to relieve pressure down by having the mother lie head-down on a slant board and taking herbs while you discuss what her options are and contact the collaborating physician.

Cervical cerclage: Prior to 26 weeks of pregnancy, the woman may also opt to have her collaborating physician place a cervical suture, called a cerclage, to hold the cervix closed until 37 weeks, when it would be removed. If there is a history of second trimester loss which seems related to loose cervix, a cerclage can be placed prophylactically before 18 weeks; this affords the best results in retaining the pregnancy. A spinal or general anesthetic is used. If the stitch is placed via the yoni, it can be removed by the same route and normal birth can proceed. The stitch of choice is controversial and several techniques are used; Gabbe recommends the McDonald's technique, which is a purse-string suture involving four or five bites as high on the cervix as possible. The stitch is placed with nonabsorbable suture and tied in front for ease of removal. More rarely, if the cervix is exceptionally short, a transabdominal suture is required. This is placed between the upper cervical passageway and lower uterine segment via an abdominal incision; a surgical delivery will be required to accomplish the birth. Placement of a cerclage also requires that the mother rest off her feet frequently and refrain from lifting heavy objects.

Emergency cerclage is performed in an attempt to halt early labor. It is used in women who have no other complicating factors. A cerclage becomes more risky the more dilated the cervix is at the time of placement. Most physicians will recommend antibiotics prior to and for the first 24 to 48 hours after surgery and tocolytic drugs to be taken for the duration of the pregnancy. Although there is no proof that antibiotics reduce the risk of infection after emergency cerclage, most practitioners will recommend them anyway (Aarts, et.al. 1995).

Risks of cerclage: Cervical injury is the most frequently encountered problem once a cerclage is in place. As pregnancy advances, the suture may become displaced or begin to rip out (3 to 12%). Replacing the cerclage results in a much lower success rate. Premature rupture of membranes and infection are other associated complications. Aarts et.al. believe that the suture should be left in place after PPROM if the fetus is not yet viable and there is no evidence of fetal distress or infection. The mother must be closely monitored. If cerclage is performed electively in the early second trimester, the risk of infection varies from study to study, averaging around 15%; however, if done with a dilated cervix and bulging forewaters, the risk of rupture of membranes and/or infection rises to 30 to 68%. The risk of the procedure versus the risk of the imminent birth of a very early baby must be weighed by the parents. Suture removal can prove difficult. Scar tissue which either prevents dilation or breaks during dilation may form, leading to cervical lacerations which can extend up into the uterus.

Once the suture is removed, have the mother take Evening Primrose oil, Black Currant oil or Borage oil capsules as recommended in the chapter on Prenatal Care From the 29th Week Until Birth to minimize problems due to scarring. If on exam scarring seems severe, capsules of Evening Primrose can be placed in the cervical fornices at term or at the onset of labor.

Emotional care: Women who have loose cervices are often frightened and worried. A psychological set-up which requires them to hold the baby in may leave them and their baby unprepared to allow the birth to occur when the time is right. Affirmations such as "My body gives birth at the perfect time for my baby," may help. Breech presentation may be an associated factor, especially if the woman spends most of her pregnancy lying down. Also, staying in bed for months not only gets boring, but decreases muscle strength. By the time labor rolls around, the woman may feel weak and apprehensive about the work of labor. Talk to her about all these factors and help her find ways of coping. There are some exercises, such as Kegels, which she can do to strengthen her muscles. Fortunately, her cervix should open relatively easily if no suture was placed or if scar tissues have been softened sufficiently.

References and further reading:
Aarts, et.al., "Emergency Cerclage: A Review," Ob and Gyn Survey, Vol. 50, No. 6, June 1995, p. 459-469.
Brewer, Gail, The Brewer Medical Diet, Simon & Schuster, New York, 1983.
Gabbe, S., et. al. ed. Obstetrics: Normal and Problem Pregnancies, 2nd ed., Churchill Livingstone, New York, 1991.

774

Abdominal Pregnancy

The overall incidence of abdominal pregnancy is about 1 in every 3,400 pregnancies, however with modern prenatal care and testing methods, the actual rate today is not nearly this high. (Williams, 1971). Without the use of routine ultrasound, detection of an abdominal pregnancy may not take place prior to the second trimester and may be delayed until the third. However as pregnancy advances with a viable abdominal pregnancy, the need to accurately assess the situation becomes increasingly important. It is extremely rare for an abdominal pregnancy to progress so smoothly that a woman will reach the end of the third trimester with an assumed intrauterine pregnancy which is, in fact, located outside the uterus.

A primary abdominal pregnancy occurs when the ovum is fertilized before entering the uterine tube and implants outside the uterus, usually to the peritoneum covering the posterior surface of the uterus (Moore & Persaud, 1993); this type is very rare and eliminates some of the warning signs that the pregnancy is not intrauterine. A secondary abdominal pregnancy occurs after an ectopic pregnancy in the reproductive tract ruptures and continues to develop. It is even possible to have a multiple gestation which is heterotopic (compound) where one fetus is intrauterine and another is developing in the abdomen.

Abdominal pregnancy most commonly occurs as the result of a ruptured ectopic pregnancy which continues to be viable. Usually ectopic pregnancies will present with severe symptoms prompting rapid detection and treatment. However, symptoms of ectopic pregnancy may have been mild or may have subsided without bleeding, confusing the clinical picture and allowing an abdominal pregnancy to progress undetected. If the location of the implantation site is such that the umbilical cord allows the fetus to grow in the abdominal cavity, or an ectopic pregnancy ruptures and expels the entire conceptus into the abdominal cavity, an abdominal pregnancy may continue undetected for a time. These women probably had signs and symptoms of a ruptured tubal pregnancy which was mistaken for the threatened miscarriage of a normal intrauterine pregnancy. Symptoms of an abdominal pregnancy are:

*Gastrointestinal disturbances such as diarrhea, constipation, gas, pain, nausea and vomiting
*High frequency of transverse lie
*Fetal movement becoming increasingly painful as pregnancy advances
*Small parts unusually easy to palpate
*Fetal heart tones unusually easy to hear
*Inability to stimulate a contraction of the musculature around the fetus
*The uterus felt on internal exam as a relatively small mass and fetal parts distinguished as being outside of it

*The cervix displaced from its normal central location to one side or
the other (discovered during an internal yoni exam)
*Dilation may occur up to two centimeters, but the cervix does not
efface (Varney, 1980)

Only about 25% of all extrauterine pregnancies diagnosed after the fifth month of gestation will result in living babies. About 33% of these will have major and minor anomalies, including some which are incompatible with life (Greenhill, 1951). Undetected abdominal pregnancy may end with the fetus dying and becoming surrounded with lime salts and forming a **lithopedion** or **stone fetus**. Rarely the fetus continues to grow and may even go to term. Death of the fetus can also lead to maceration and infection causing severe maternal illness and possibly death. **Mummification**, where the fetus dries up without calcification, may also occur. (Greenhill, 1951)

If you suspect that a woman is carrying an abdominal pregnancy, whether the fetus is alive or not, she should consider an ultrasound exam. Obviously, if the baby is alive, birth will require surgery. Because the placenta and membranes may be attached to a variety of tissues and organs which are not designed for their implantation and normal release, the placenta will be left in place for the system to break down on its own. The mother will have an increased possibility of postpartum infection; herbal remedies such as Echinecea tincture and supplemental vitamin C with bioflavinoids can help to minimize this. The attending physician will probably want to give a course of prophylactic antibiotics, which in this case, is not a bad idea.

References and further reading:

Greenhill, J., Principles and Practice of Obstetrics, W. B. Saunders, Co., Philadelphia, PA, 1951.
Moore, Keith, & Persaud, T., The Developing Human, 5th ed., W. B. Saunders Co., Philadelphia, PA 1993.
Varney, Helen, Nurse-Midwifery, Blackwell Scientific Pub., Boston, MA, 1980.
Williams Obstetrics, 14th ed., Appleton-Century-Crofts, pub., New York, 1971.

Incarceration and Sacculation of the Pregnant Uterus

Retroversion of the uterus occurs in 6 to 19% of all pregnancies and usually does not cause problems. However, in approximately 1 out of every 3000 pregnancies (usually multiparas), the uterus remains retroverted as pregnancy advances and becomes wedged in the pelvic cavity. Sacculation of the uterus is a very rare variation of this problem (Oxhorn mentions 38 reported cases as of 1986), defined as a ballooning of a portion of the uterine wall.

Incarceration of the retroverted uterus:

In most cases of retroverted uterus the weight of the advancing pregnancy will cause it to rise out of the pelvis, and the pregnancy will proceed normally. When this does not occur, several things can happen:

*The uterus contracts and expels its contents causing a miscarriage. This may be due to reduced blood flow to the uterus. The overall fetal loss rate may be as high as 33%.
*The uterus continues to grow until becoming incarcerated (trapped backwards) in the pelvis between 14 and 16 weeks.
-Once trapped, the uterus may spontaneously correct its position with the condition going undetected.
-The uterus may remain trapped, leading to increasing problems as the pregnancy advances.

Symptoms: If the uterus remains lodged entirely within the pelvic cavity past the 14th week of pregnancy, it is referred to as an incarcerated uterus. Symptoms can be divided into three categories:

1. Pressure-type symptoms:
   -Pelvic discomfort
   -Low abdominal or back pain
   -A sensation of pelvic fullness
2. Urinary symptoms
   -Pain on urination
   -Frequency of urination
   -Retention of urine due to elongation of the urethra by the displacement of the cervix, loss of the ureterovesical angle and pressure from the trapped uterus
   -Dribbling of urine due to pressure and an overdistended bladder
   -Urinary tract or kidney infections may develop
   -Lower abdominal tenderness and distention

       -Swelling, sloughing of the bladder wall, and rupture may
        eventually result if the problem remains undetected
  3. Gastrointestinal symptoms
     -Rectal pressure
     -Nonproductive straining to move the bowels
     -Progressive constipation

Physical exam before 20 weeks of pregnancy: Examination reveals that the abdomen appears full, fluctuant or distended due to an overdistended bladder. Upon internal exam a bulge or mass is found in the posterior fornix, the birth passage is slanted upward toward the symphysis pubis and the cervix is displaced anteriorly, often behind or against the pubic bone. The cervix may be pulled so deeply inside the yoni that it is impossible to reach. Bimanual exam finds a large, soft round mass in the cul de sac with no uterine mass felt abdominally. The extremely anterior cervical placement is the most consistent finding. If you are unable to correct the situation with the simple techniques described below, or you are unsure of your findings, an ultrasound exam may help clarify the situation.

Differential diagnosis: When incarceration or sacculation are suspected, be sure to rule out the following conditions:

    *Uncomplicated urinary tract infection
    *Miscarriage with a normally positioned uterus
    *Ovarian cyst
    *Fibroids (especially cervical)
    *Extrauterine pregnancy (tubal or abdominal)
    *A pocket of blood in the pelvis (hematocele)
    *Pelvic mass of another type
    *Accessory uterine pouch (diverticulum)
    *Other lower abdominal or pelvic conditions (infection?)

After 20 weeks of pregnancy: The symptoms listed above will worsen, with the rare case having no symptoms whatsoever. As pregnancy advances, preterm labor or early prelabor rupture of membranes may occur. Labor is not effective at resolving the misplacement, making normal delivery unlikely. If a surgical delivery is attempted, accidental incision of the elongated cervix or bladder may occur if the problem remains unrecognized.

     Physical exam findings as described above become increasingly exaggerated. The fundus is consistently small-for-dates and the fetus may appear to be lying transverse or oblique.

Getting the uterus "out of jail" before 20 weeks: Typically, the retroflexed uterus begins to come forward by the 12th week, although the fundus may remain sloped backwards for several more weeks after that. If a woman has reached 14 weeks and you are unable to palpate any part of the uterus abdominally, you can have her begin to assume a knee-chest position (shoulders on the floor, butt in the air) 6 to 8 times daily for 15 to 20 minutes each time. This will allow gravity to assist in the process of bringing the uterus forward. If that doesn't work, perform an internal exam with the woman in a knee-chest position or on her back with her bottom elevated and attempt to reposition the uterus by putting pressure up and forward with your fingers from the posterior fornix. If this doesn't work and the woman has no symptoms, have her continue postural exercises and try repositioning it yourself one week later.

If symptoms are already apparent, gentle catheterization of the bladder should be done either by you or a doctor to relieve anterior pressure, so that an attempt at manual repositioning can be made. If this fails, recommend that she see an obstetrician for surgical correction. It is likely that the doctor will first attempt to reposition the uterus with the woman under general anesthesia, since this will afford maximal muscle relaxation. If this fails, a laparoscopy incision may be made followed by another attempt at manual repositioning. This may be successful when the other attempts had failed, because the incision breaks the seal that has formed with the uterus lodged in the pelvis. If this doesn't work, the round ligaments may be grasped through the incision, and, with simultaneous manual pressure in the posterior fornix, be pulled forward using gentle, steady traction. If that fails, a larger incision is made and the same basic maneuver reattempted. Once the uterus is in the abdomen, a pessary can be placed in the yoni to support the uterus for 5 to 7 days to help it stay there. The uterus should then remain in the correct position due to its size.

After 20 weeks: If diagnosis is delayed, manual or surgical attempts to reposition the uterus may cause serious complications. Nothing should be done unless the mother is experiencing significant symptoms. Recommend that she continue to perform the knee-chest exercises as given above. Monitor closely for preterm labor or rupture of membranes and consult with a bio-technical care provider.

Sacculation of the uterus:

Rarely, when incarceration occurs, a portion of the body of the uterus remains trapped in the pelvis while the anterior wall expands into the abdomen to accommodate the growing fetus. A sac or saccule is formed by the stretched anterior uterine wall, while the pelvic mass is formed by the uterine fundus.

The saccule is a functional, transitory pouch containing all layers of the myometrium and is present only during pregnancy. It appears most frequently in multigravidas. In 50% of cases the placenta is located in the pouch; in 25% part of the fetus is in the pouch; in the remaining cases the sac turns out to be empty.

The pouch may occur in the anterior or posterior wall of the uterus. The reasons sacculation occurs are not clear. Theories include:

    *Uterine abnormalities
    *A myometrial defect causing a portion of the uterine wall to be thin.
        Pregnancy causes the thin area to bulge out. Once the birth occurs,
        the pouch collapses and disappears.
    *A nerve defect leading to ballooning.
    *Weakening of the uterine wall by the trophoblast, placenta accreta,
        or previous surgery.

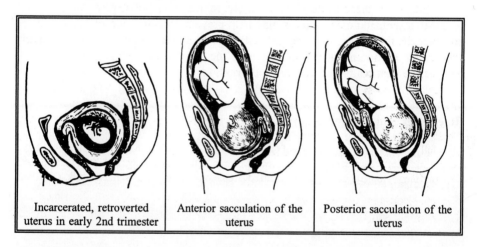

| Incarcerated, retroverted uterus in early 2nd trimester | Anterior sacculation of the uterus | Posterior sacculation of the uterus |

Signs and symptoms: Diagnosis can be very difficult and is often not clear until surgery is underway for other suspected causes such as ectopic pregnancy or stalled labor. Typically, sacculation presents as:

    *Abdominal pain
    *A sensation of heaviness in the pelvis
    *With anterior sacculation, the presenting part is felt in front of and
        above the symphysis pubis
    *On internal exam, the yoni is found to be elongated and the cervix
        high and usually anterior, squashed between the pubic bone and
        the presenting part
    *Frequent urination from pressure on the bladder
    *Painful urination, caused by stretching of the urethra and compression
        of the neck of the bladder
    *Reduced or complete inability to urinate, leading to retention of urine
        and subsequent swelling above the pubic bone

What to do: If you suspect sacculation of the uterus, an ultrasound exam can shed more light on the possibility. Refer the woman to an obstetrical specialist. Having her position herself on a slant board with her feet higher than her head or perform the knee-chest exercise several times daily may help to reduce or reverse the situation. Sacculation can impede the normal passage of urine and interfere with the normal progress of labor.

Reoccurrences:

Either of these conditions is likely to recur in subsequent pregnancies. Surgical suspension of the uterus may help prevent reoccurrence of incarceration, however if the uterus was sacculated due to a structural abnormality, early pregnancy positioning of the mother with the knee-chest position (as described) may be the best course of action for prevention.

References and further reading:

Greenhill, J., Principles and Practice of Obstetrics, W. B. Saunders, Co., Philadelphia, PA, 1951.
Lettieri, L., et.al., "Incarceration of the Gravid Uterus," OB/Gyn Survey, Vol. 49, No. 9, p. 642.
Oxhorn, Harry, Human Labor and Birth, 5th ed. Appleton-Century-Crofts, E. Norwalk, CT, 1986.

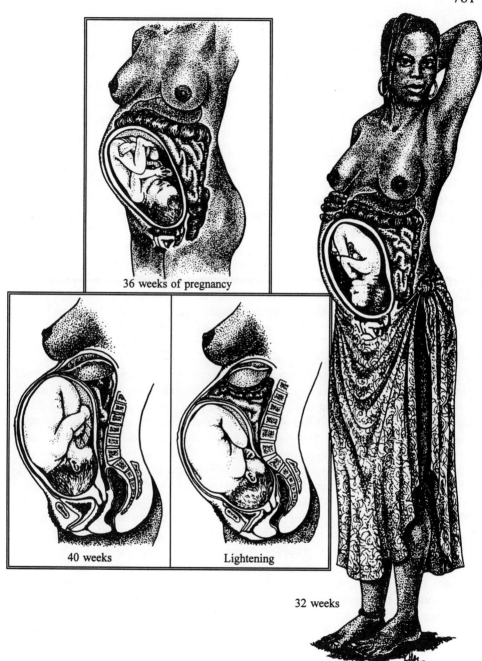

36 weeks of pregnancy

40 weeks

Lightening

32 weeks

PRENATAL CARE: The Third Trimester
(From the 29th week of pregnancy until birth)

<u>Prenatal Care From the 29th Week Until Birth</u>

<u>An overview of the third trimester</u>: During the third trimester the woman's body accelerates its preparations for birth. The baby is increasingly easy to palpate and hear. The mother looks more and more pregnant. Birth plans need to be firmed up. Problems, when they occur, become more difficult to judge and deal with because the needs of a baby that has a better and better chance of surviving if it is born early must be considered.

During the first weeks of this trimester the blood volume continues to build, peaking at approximately 30 weeks. Adequate expansion paves the way for optimal fetal growth and development during the critical last months before birth. Fetal growth accelerates over these last months, fat layers are developed and iron is stored. Babies with healthy placentas will continue to grow right up until birth.

In many first-time mothers and in some mothers with other children the baby will "drop," or settle down into the pelvis, during the last four to eight weeks of pregnancy. This process is referred to as **lightening**. First-time mothers are more likely to experience the baby dropping than women who have had babies before, due to their stronger, never-before-stretched abdominal muscles. Lightening relieves pressure on the intestines, stomach and diaphragm while producing more pressure on the rectum and bladder, so that once again the woman may feel a more frequent urge to urinate. (If a woman is urinating more often than every two hours, rule out a urinary tract infection.) Lightening usually indicates that the pelvis and the baby are a good fit and portend good pressure down and adequate pelvic capacity for labor; therefore it is a favorable indication. However, most women who do not experience lightening go on to have yoni births, so do not consider its absence a bad sign by itself. Gradual muscle and ligament softening accelerates during the last trimester in all women due to the increasingly active uterus and the rising levels of prostaglandins and other hormones. Pelvic relaxation plus more pressure down may make walking difficult as well as put pressure on pelvic nerves. Discharge from the yoni may increase and thicken. Any woman, especially those with other children, may have crampiness, groin pain and persistent lower backache. Looser bowel movements are common a day or two before labor begins. Vulval varicosities may be particularly bothersome during these last weeks as well.

Throughout the third trimester mild uterine contractions slowly work to soften the cervix, and some effacement and even dilation may begin as well. Some degree of dilation before the onset of labor is more common in multiparas than in primigravidas but can be normal in either. Cervical changes will prompt twinges, shooting pains and achiness from the cervix and the lower uterus (low down in front); some women lose bits of mucus occasionally tinged with blood, from their cervices, although labor is still a few days off. As long as toning contractions and these cervical sensations are not coordinated (occurring at the same time) they reflect normal, healthy preparation for labor. As the end of pregnancy nears, a gradual transition occurs: the toning contractions become stronger, more regular and do not stop. Painful pulling sensations above the pubic bone or in the back become coordinated with uterine contractions and cervical changes happen more rapidly. Labor has begun!

Secondary signs and symptoms of toxemia: The majority of women who are becoming toxemic will wait until the third trimester to display secondary symptoms that their blood volume is inadequately expanded. Carefully watch women whom you know to be very active, who have had questionable diets, who are under a great deal of stress or in whom fetal growth has been less than ideal. And remember that ANY woman can experience a fall in blood volume and become toxemic if her diet is not what it should be or if changing circumstances cause her nutrient needs to outstrip her intake. (See the chapter on Toxemia in the section on Problems Associated With the Third Trimester.)

Visualizing the birth: If a woman has not already begun visualizing her birth, recommend that she begin to do so during this trimester. She should focus on the experience she wants to create, rather than the form it will take. Tell her to see herself coping confidently with whatever labor brings her, the specifics of normal birth with the baby head down, facing the mother's back and flexed for delivery, the baby pink and breathing at birth, good perineal stretching and normal placental delivery with minimal bleeding, uterine contractions after the birth, and an easy postpartum and nursing experience. Remind her to use positive phrases worded as though the desired result is a current reality (instead of affirming "my uterus will not bleed after birth" she would affirm "my uterus clamps down and stops bleeding."

Frequency of visits: For the woman who is not having any unusual problems necessitating more frequent visits, the following schedule can be followed during this trimester:

*Monthly visits until 28 to 32 weeks
*Every 2 weeks until 36 weeks
*Weekly until labor begins

In recent years some midwives have started to increase the frequency of visits, to every two or three weeks beginning at the 24th week, to allow for more time to develop relationships. You will have to judge what seems appropriate for each woman as well as what you can realistically offer as a practitioner.

Prenatal care in late pregnancy:

Weeks 29 to 30: This is when the mother's blood volume peaks. An adequate diet up until now should have provided the raw materials needed to lay down this important physiologic foundation of increased circulating blood volume so that the placenta can be adequately perfused during this last period of fetal growth and nervous system development. This occurs in some women as the blood volume rapidly rises. If blood volume hasn't expanded, it is usually from this point on that you will begin to see the true secondary symptoms of classic toxemia.

   If small-for-dates fetal growth detected at a previous visit has not caught up with itself by now, review the diet again and make specific suggestions for a high protein diet and calorie loading within the mother's dietary choices. Suggest more fluids as well. If she is very active, ask her to curtail some of her exercising or other activities to spare more calories. Be empathetic! Explain the physiology of small-for-dates growth.

   This is the time to recheck her hemoglobin (if you have a hemoglobinometer) or to draw blood for a laboratory analysis. A hemoglobinometer will tell you on the spot if a woman's hemoglobin has dropped adequately to reflect a well expanded blood volume. If she is not eating enough, a drop may have occurred but may be less than you expected, given her starting point. Just a week or two of increased protein and calories can make the difference.

Weeks 31 to 33: The baby is easy to feel now and is filling up the uterus more; at the same time it is still able to move fairly freely within the amniotic fluid. If suggestions in the chapter on Ensuring Vertex Presentation at Term in this section have been followed, the baby should be vertex by the 33rd week. If it is not, try to determine why and discuss external version with the mother. The well-nourished fetus often weighs at least 4½ lbs. by 31 weeks. Small-for-dates growth should have caught up with itself by now with good dietary counseling and changes. If it has not and you suspect an underlying problem, discuss diagnostic options (ultrasound) with the mother to detect if something other than nutrition (fetal defects?) could be causing a problem.

   Sometime between now and 34 weeks you can begin having the mother keep a fetal movement chart, if you want to include this as part of your recommendations. The value of fetal movement charts is that they can be reviewed at each prenatal visit and patterns can be seen (for example the fetal movement increasing or decreasing) even though the requisite minimum number of movements have been felt for that day. This provides a baseline of movement to judge any changes the mother reports; having the mother begin to chart only after a possible problem is noted may not be as informative. Charting gives you a concrete reference tool to alert you to problems before they develop into a major emergency. On the other hand, keeping such charts may make some women feel unnecessarily nervous; I have never routinely recommended that they be kept in my practice.

Women who have other children may want to consider taking them to sibling childbirth classes. In many areas, such classes are offered by childbirth educators and are frequently tailored according to the age of the child.

These are the last months of pregnancy. Find out how (or if) a woman is dealing with her work schedule and encourage her to take time off until the baby comes. If she is a first-time mother, she may not realize that she will not have lots of private, uninterrupted time to herself or with her partner for quite a while to come. Discuss fears about labor, birth, parenting and relationship changes which may be coming up strongly now that she is approaching the threshold of labor. Also go over her sleeping hours, when she gets to bed and how well she is sleeping. Discuss the fact that if she goes to bed at 11 or 12 pm every night and then begins early labor at 1 or 2 am she will have had very little sleep. She should start now going to bed earlier and sleeping late, not skipping meals and generally prepare herself for the eventual work of labor, birth and postpartum (none of which lend themselves to long periods of uninterrupted sleep).

Remind the mother that she needs to stay hydrated! Dehydration can cause the uterus to be more active, the blood volume to marginally contract and the amniotic fluid volume to decrease. It is very important!

This is a good time to make plans for the home visit, which needs to be done in the last month of pregnancy. Make sure you have maps, directions and an appointment time which allows as many people on the birth team as possible to be present. Be sure she has ordered her birthing kit or is gathering supplies (or that she is about to do so). Waiting until the last minute means she may be caught with the vendor out of stock on certain items.

Weeks 34 and 35: The baby is steadily gaining weight and its lungs are maturing daily. Women have traditionally been told to expect fetal movements to slow down as term approaches. As the baby gets bigger, less and less room is available for large movements. Kicking, stretching and aggressive small limb movements gradually become gentle, rolling, shifting movements as intrauterine room is taken up by the enlarging fetus. When asking a woman about fetal movements, be sure to explain that the *quantity* of movement should be about the same, but the *quality* of movements will change. About the same amount of actual movement is still taking place. Once women tune into this change, they usually report that their baby's activity level is the same as it has always been, a reassuring sign. If the baby is persistently posterior, see the suggestions in the chapter on Dealing With Posterior Babies During Pregnancy in this section.

Many midwives have women begin supplementation to boost their vitamin K intake at the 34-week point. Vitamin K is a vital component of the clotting mechanism, but it is poorly transported across the placenta. The normal newborn's clotting factor levels are lower than those of adults, meaning factor deficiencies can occur more quickly than in adults. The best way to ensure that the fetus has an optimum supply of vitamin K is to supplement the mother during the last month to 6 weeks of pregnancy. Alfalfa infusion (1 to 2 cups daily) or tablets (up to 3 grams daily/2 15 grain tablets equals 1 gram) can be taken until birth. Quinone, a potent oil-based oral vitamin K_1 supplement can also be used; taken 1 to 2 drops daily during the last 6 weeks of pregnancy. Higher cord blood levels are noted in newborns whose mothers started supplementation as late as 5 days prior to birth, so women coming late can still begin supplementation. The use of Shepherd's Purse tincture is *not* recommended, however, as its potent clotting enhancing properties may actually increase the risk of abnormal clotting, especially in women with varicosities. (See <u>Diagnostic Tests</u> for details regarding vitamin K and clotting compromise.)

Right around now is when I do a pelvimetry exam. Pregnancy hormones have risen to levels which soften the tissues sufficiently to make the exam more informative. Use this exam to teach yoni stretching as well.

Cob-web cleaning session: Candice Whitridge, a nurse-midwife in California who has done births in a variety of settings, has what she calls a cob-web cleaning session around the 36th week. She tells the couple in advance that she does this with all her clients with the intention of airing concerns and clarifying roles so that labor can go as smoothly as possible. Both partners need to be present. At the interview she asks them to honestly express their expectations of each other in regard to the birth and postpartum period. Each one is asked if they believe that the woman can birth normally. What fears does each one have at this point? What other expectations or concerns do they have? What expectations do they have of the birth team? It is also a good time to discuss pain in labor. When asking these questions, it is important to allow plenty of time for discussion. Look each person straight in the eye as you address them and expect an honest response. Such sessions can be very revealing and healing, paving the way for clear relationships during the intense time of labor.

Weeks 36 to 37: If birth should occur at this point, most babies will be able to breathe on their own if the dates are accurate and the mother is truly 36 weeks along. While some earlier babies may also have mature lungs, the earlier the baby, the more likely that this will not be the case. Therefore, 37 completed weeks of pregnancy is a good cutoff point to allow early labor at home (see separate chapter on Premature Labor, this section).

Women are growing increasingly uncomfortable as the baby gets bigger, with marked downward pelvic pressure in some cases. Smaller, more frequent meals will help the mother get the foods she needs without feeling constantly bloated.

If a breech presentation is still a concern, try once again to do an external version if the mother agrees. It is time to discuss options in the event that the baby remains breech. If the baby is transverse, the woman will require a surgical delivery if all efforts to turn it fail. Have you ruled out silent placenta previa or undetected pelvic growths which may be impeding fetal rotation?

At the 36 week visit primigravidas, YBAC candidates, women with cervical scars, those who have been on any type of hormone regulating contraceptives (the Pill, progesterone-containing IUD, Depo-Provera injections or Norplant contraceptive implants) for several years prior to conception or any woman who has experienced anovulatory cycles prior to conception can begin to take three 500 mg. capsules of Evening Primrose oil daily (Borage oil Black Currant oil capsules can also be used) to provide the precursors to the prostaglandins which soften the cervix and prepare it to dilate. Consider this a dietary supplement, providing the body with the raw materials it needs to produce prostaglandins. In addition, all women can take the following homeopathic remedies to encourage an efficient labor:

-Cimicifuga 12C, 1 pellet on Monday
-Caulophyllum 12C, 1 pellet on Wednesday
-Arnica 12C, 1 pellet on Friday

Continue to take each remedy once weekly until the 40th week. (Brennan & Kramer, 1989)

If, by the 36th week, only minimal or no uterine activity is happening, start the mother on tinctures of Blue and Black Cohosh and Ginger (10 drops each) 3 to 4 times daily. This will usually encourage toning contractions. If it doesn't within a week, have the mother begin daily nipple stimulation (see recommendations for less than well-nourished mothers in the chapter on Postdatism and Postmaturity in the section on Problems Associated With the Third Trimester).
In mainstream obstetrics and in some midwifery practices it is standard of care to do a series of internal exams during the last month of pregnancy in an effort to determine how the cervix is ripening (readying itself for birth) and to ascertain when labor may begin. Routine internal exams increase the likelihood of infection as well as encouraging prelabor rupture of membranes (Lenihan, 1984). Since women can have a long, closed cervix and go into labor that day or can have a cervix dilated to 3, 4 or 5 centimeters for weeks before labor begins, routine examination of the cervix is truly unnecessary. Only if a woman has excessive scar tissue from previous cervical surgery or tears or for other reasons might have an exceptionally rigid cervix is it be wise to do a couple of exams near term to find out if the cervix is responding to attempts to soften it with prostaglandin precursors.
Give a woman instructions for what to do if labor begins (see separate chapter, this section). Advise her that you will want to talk to her directly to discuss early labor signs; she should call rather than have someone call for her whenever possible.

Weeks 38 to 39: At this point or earlier, women are becoming sick of being pregnant; they are ready to get on with the labor and get the baby out! Fetal movement and amniotic fluid volume should still be normal. If the mother is a

788

smoker or has abused other substances earlier in her pregnancy, have her start fetal movement counts at 38 weeks (or at 36 weeks).

An alternative homeopathic regime which encourages the timely onset of contractions and an efficient labor pattern calls for taking single, daily doses of 30X Cimicifuga and Caulophyllum, alternating each remedy until a total of seven daily doses are taken of both. (For example, on Monday, take 30X Caulophylum, on Tuesday take 30X Cimicifuga, etc. until a total of seven doses are taken of each remedy.) Begin at the onset of the 38th week, take them for the next 14 days, and stop. This should make labor shorter and more efficient. It is not recommended to women who have a history of rapid labors. Choose one of the homeopathic regimes I have mentioned; do not recommend both at once. (Tipton-Healy, 1994)

Uterine cramps and cervical pains will be occurring more frequently in well-nourished women. If you have suggested herbs to prompt more uterine activity, be sure to find out if the woman is taking them and if she has noticed any increase in uterine activity as a result. Labor could begin soon; be sure she knows not to skip meals and to stay hydrated, to have food in the house, to take naps if she is tired and to go to bed early. Recheck the financial agreement and be sure it is being followed. Make plans to tie up any loose money ends before labor begins.

Week 40 to 41: By now women are often dismayed that they have not had their babies yet. Those who often go overdue are resigned. Women should be reminded of the standard of care in the community regarding testing protocols for overdue pregnancies and it should be made clear how your protocols differ or to what protocols you may be bound due to state laws. Discuss what toning contractions and cervical sensations, pressure down and fetal movements are doing and emphasize that a reduction of fetal movement from now on could mean a problem is brewing; encourage her to keep her fluid intake up, drinking at least 6 to 8 glasses of clear fluids daily. Her fluid intake will directly impact amniotic fluid volume. Also explain that well-nourished women often carry to their due date and beyond and that you expect labor to begin at any time. It is also a good time to review a woman's original due date information. It is remarkable how often new data which impacts the date you set comes to light in these situations. (See separate chapter on Postdatism and Postmaturity Syndrome, this section). Now is an appropriate time to do an internal exam to assess any cervical changes which may have occurred so far. If the cervix is not very soft (ripe), 6 to 8 500 mg. Evening Primrose oil, Black Currant oil or Borage oil capsules can be inserted into the posterior fornix every day or so to help soften it.

Week 42: If a woman has gotten to her 42nd week still pregnant (after all these years) consider giving (or increasing) Blue and Black Cohosh and Ginger tinctures during the week with the goal of having the baby by the 21st day after the due date. Sometime during this week you may also recommend a Biophysical Profile (see <u>Diagnostic Tests</u>). Often, women go into labor on the eve of the scheduled biophysical. These recommendations assume that you have calculated the due date to take into account such variables as the length of the woman's menstrual cycle and family history of long gestations.

Discussing lab tests:

Aside from a hemoglobin check at 28 to 30 weeks, you will want to remind women of the standard of care in your local community concerning cultures for *Beta*-strep and genital herpes (if she has a history of herpes). Strep cultures can be done at 36 weeks or if the membranes rupture prior to labor. Herpes cultures need not be done if no lesions are visible (see Diagnostic Tests for more details). The only other reason an otherwise healthy woman may need to hear about lab work is in the event she is overdue. There are two tests that are used in this case, the non-stress test, which evaluates fetal heart rate and activity patterns, and the biophysical profile, which is the best one to use since it looks at five parameters of fetal well-being. It evaluates fetal breathing movements, heart rate, activity level, muscle tone, amniotic fluid volume and, in some areas, placental well-being. However, as midwives we also have a consistent record of fetal heart rate variability associated with movement when we count the heart rate for five second intervals. Refer to the chapter entitled Postdatism and Postmaturity Syndrome at the end of the section on Problems Associated With the Third Trimester for further information. (Methods of evaluating the fetus with and without the aid of ultrasound are also discussed in detail in Diagnostic Tests.)

Other things to discuss:

Review the discussion check list in the chapter entitled Books and Handouts in the section entitled An Overview of Prenatal Care for a review of topics to discuss.

References and further reading:

Brennan, P. & Kramer, P., Guide to Homeopathic Remedies for the Birth Bag, 7727 Sharon Hollow Rd., Manchester, MI, 48158, 1989.

Kilpatrick, Sarah, et al., "Maternal Hydration increases amniotic fluid index in women with normal amniotic fluid," OB/GYN, Vol. 81, No. 1, January 1993, pp. 49-52.

Lenihan, J., "Relationship of antepartum pelvic examination to premature rupture of the membranes," OB/GYN, Vol. 83, No. 1, Jan, 1984, p. 33-37.

Tipton-Healy, Paula, "Homeopathy for the Childbearing Year," Midwifery: the Ancient Art of Touching the Future, Helping Hands Conference, Salt Lake City, UT, July, 30, 1994.

Fetal Development in the Third Trimester

Third trimester development prepares the baby to live outside the uterus. Organs mature, particularly the brain, lungs, and nervous system. Fetal growth and weight gain is normally accelerated at this time. If a baby is having problems due to inadequate blood volume, genetics or other conditions, this will become apparent due to a lag in fetal growth during these weeks.

26 to 29 weeks: The eyes are partially opened and eyelashes are present by 26 weeks. Lanugo, a soft fine "baby fur" that covers the body, and scalp hair are well developed. In many cases, the lungs are now capable of breathing room air; however, a significant number of these babies have difficulty if born this early. The nervous system is mature enough to direct rhythmic breathing movements and control body temperature. Toenails are visible and enough subcutaneous body fat is present beneath the skin to smooth out many wrinkles. The quantity of white fat increases to about 3.5% of body weight. By the 26th week the spleen is an important site of red blood cell formation; however, this ends by 28 weeks, and the work is transferred to the bone marrow. Descent of the testes begins between 28 and 32 weeks of gestation.

30 to 34 weeks: By 30 weeks the pupils of the eyes respond to light. At the end of 34 weeks the skin is smooth and pink, and the upper and lower limbs have a chubby appearance. White fat is now 8% of body weight. Fetuses 32 weeks and older usually survive if born prematurely.

35 to 38 weeks: Babies 35 weeks along have a firm grasp and spontaneously orient to light. By 36 weeks almost all babies' lungs are sufficiently mature to breathe room air without any problems. The circumferences of the head and abdomen are about equal by 36 weeks. After that, the circumference of the abdomen may become larger than that of the head.

By 37 weeks the nervous system is sufficiently mature to carry out some integrated activities. Most fetuses are now plump. Growth slows during this time, and normal babies reach a crown-rump length of 14.4 inches (360 mm) and weigh about 7 lbs 8 ozs. (3400 grams). The baby adds 14 grams of body fat a day during these last weeks of gestation. Boys tend to be somewhat larger than girls.

By full term (38 weeks gestation and 40 weeks of pregnancy) the skin is bluish-pink. The chest is prominent and the breasts protrude slightly in both sexes. The testes are usually descended into the scrotum. The head is one of the largest areas of the fetus. "Full-term" is considered to be from 37 to 42 weeks of pregnancy. From now on, when born, babies can breathe and suck, the two most important abilities for the newborn to have in order to survive outside the uterus.

Moore, Keith, & T. Persaud, <u>The Developing Human</u>, 5th ed., W. B. Saunders Co., Phil., 1993.

Emotional and Psychological Changes of the Third Trimester

The third trimester begins the important task of maternal psychological transition from being pregnant to readiness for the baby to be born into the outside world. One can see that the whole concept of "bonding" is from a male external point of view, since birth represents increasingly separate existence for both mother and baby. In order for this separation to occur without trauma, attachment must have taken place beforehand. If attachment issues have been postponed or poorly integrated in the second trimester (due to prenatal testing, work, other children or other demands on her attention), the mother will have a more difficult time accomplishing this important psychological task.

Attachment issues begin to manifest during this trimester, as the mother and family prepare for the arrival of a new baby by preparing a physical space for the baby and gathering clothes and other baby items. In some cultures these activities are delayed until some point after the birth, and in those cases, lack of home preparation does not indicate poor attachment. These women still make important personal and emotional preparation for their upcoming birth. Such preparation is important if the mother is to let go of her fantasy child and accept her real child at birth. She may spend much time engaged in introspective thought about herself and her baby, even excluding other family members. She may be preoccupied with how the baby will look and what its sex may be.

In order to have the emotional resources to nurture her newborn the mother needs to feel supported and nurtured herself. She needs to be able to feel dependent upon those around her for support. A number of fears may surface as the woman contemplates the upcoming labor and birth, such as fears about her own or her baby's death, premature labor, postmature labor, control issues, dealing with pain and the unknown, and her ability to get the baby out. She may busy herself so that these fears stay in the background. In giving birth to new life, women often find they are face to face with their own mortality and thoughts of the baby dying or their own death in labor may be prominent in their mind. Women may only be vaguely aware of these fears or afraid to voice them. Be sure to acknowledge that these thoughts are common, and that in some ways labor is the closest she may ever be to the threshold between life and death while she is still very much alive. Surely, her life will never be the same after the birth. Encourage her to talk about her specific fears and concerns and to do whatever she must to move through them (one woman wrote out her will before she gave birth).

There is also anticipatory grief as the mother moves from complete attachment to impending separation from her baby. She grieves the loss of the attention she has gotten as a pregnant woman. While first-time mothers may not anticipate it, there is often a feeling of emptiness once the baby has been born.

As all this emotional work goes on, the physical reality of the pregnancy itself becomes increasingly obvious. The woman has more trouble moving around, and begins to have sensations indicating that her body is preparing itself for labor.

792

She becomes tired of being pregnant. She may feel ugly, fat, huge, clumsy and in need of much reassurance. These important psychological milestones prepares her to take on the rather daunting task of labor; *anything* to get the pregnancy over with. Women who do not become tired of pregnancy tend to go overdue! Many problems which may rise during labor can be traced back to unmet psychological tasks. For example, if unresolved feelings of ambivalence persist after the fourth month, uterine dystocia during labor is common (Pederson, 1981).

Emotionally and spiritually, the mother's psyche is becoming increasingly more open as pregnancy advances. Many women report that they have a harder time concentrating and feel "spaced out" much of the time. Women often become more introspective and communication with the baby should be supported. This important process opens the woman on all levels so that she can open her whole being to channel the life of the baby during labor.

Dreams: Women may dream of the baby being abnormal, of misplacing the baby, being trapped in small places, giving birth or injuring the baby. Psychologists often report that the more anxious the dreams during the last trimester are, the less problems a woman will have during labor.

Sexuality: Many women have decreased sexual desire in the third trimester due to feelings of awkwardness plus the difficult logistics of finding a comfortable position. Be sensitive to this possibility when you remind heterosexual women that semen contains prostaglandins and can therefore help ripen the cervix. Female orgasm releases oxytocin which stimulates the uterus. Talk to couples frankly about gentleness, reminding partners that sexual activity will not harm a normal pregnancy as long as the membranes are intact and good hygiene is observed, and that this is the time to try new positions all of which can help ease the situation. While no woman should feel pressured to have sex, she needs to remember (for herself as well as her partner) that she will probably have to wait at least 3 to 6 weeks after the birth to resume sexual activity. Additionally, many women do not feel inclined to be sexual for quite a while after birth due hormonal influences coupled with the constant physical contact they will have with their babies, especially if breastfeeding.

References and further reading:

Pederson, Gail, Birthing Normally, Mindbody Press, 1981.
Perez, Polly, "The Emotional Work of Labor," IJCE, Vol. 3, No. 3, Aug. 1988, pp. 30-1.
Varney, Helen, Nurse Midwifery, Blackwell Scientific Pub., Inc., Boston, MA 1980.

The Home Visit

While some midwives do every prenatal visit in the woman's home, most do not. Between the 34th and 37th week is a good time to plan to do a home visit. One reason for doing a home visit is to double check directions and make sure you know how to get there. A big advantage of doing it closer to term is that landmarks and foliage will appear much as they will when you actually have to go to the birth. A home visit will often give you more insight into the family dynamics of the client than you have been able to glean from office visits alone. Here are a few things you will want to do to prepare for the home visit:

*If you have not already done so, be sure the woman brings you accurate, written directions to her home prior to the proposed home visit date.
*Also obtain a map of her area if it is unfamiliar to you.
*Plan the visit when as many potential members of the birth team as possible can be present. If this is impossible for some, encourage your client to have them come to an office prenatal so you can meet them and answer any questions they may have.
*Be sure to inquire about the schedules of siblings and attempt to include them in the home visit as well.
*Whenever possible, plan your home visit during daylight hours so you can see landmarks and street signs more easily.

Here are a few things you may want to include in your home visit:

The birth room: Check out the proposed site of the birth itself. While plans often change during the labor, always help the parents arrange the proposed birth room to allow maximal access to the bed, the mother and the equipment. Have a dresser or vanity top cleared off to accommodate equipment, and move the bed and, if necessary, other furniture around to allow you and other birth attendants to work on both sides of the bed.

Sometimes it becomes necessary to place the mother on a firm surface for the birth; that usually winds up being the floor. If the only floor space is between the bed and the wall opposite the door to the room, this is a set up for becoming boxed in, unable to assist or reach equipment or have the mother move about easily. In this case, have them push the bed to the wall (moving any furniture necessary to accomplish this). If the room is small, remove unnecessary furniture from the room to allow more freedom of movement. Alternatively, choose another larger or less furnished room for the birth.

Check to make sure any birthing stool you may carry will fit into the room and assess how traffic will flow as a result. Assess the available lighting and help select table or floor lamps to put in the room if lighting does not seem sufficient.

As for you, carry a good flashlight and have the parents have one on hand as well.

The birth bed: Most midwives feel bed births need to take place on a firm mattress. Waterbeds cause the mother's bottom to sink down into the mattress and prevent easy and quick changes of position should they become necessary (as may be the case with a shoulder dystocia). If the mattress is not firm, have the mother get a board to place between the mattress and the box spring, or slide the mattress onto the floor. Another idea is to have a foam pad covered with blankets on the floor and forget the soft mattress altogether.

The bathroom: Check out the bathroom for hygiene as well as to assess the shower or bathing facilities. A large bathtub or jacuzzi is ideal, but most women are lucky just to have a tub. It is especially helpful to have a tub available for first time mothers. Be sure to point out if anything exceptional needs to be done to prepare for the birth, such as a major scrubbing of an old, stained tub. Running water and indoor toilet facilities are, of course, ideal. If these conveniences are not available, inspect what is. For example, if a woman is using an outhouse, you will want to know *before* you need to help her make decisions where hygiene and a clean environment are crucial, such as rupture of membranes prior to labor.

Transport route?   If a transport during labor, birth or postpartum should become necessary, how will you remove the mother from her home? Note the location of stairways, doors, 90° angles, narrow halls and passageways, etc. Make a mental note of your best route of exit. Some midwives insist that the mother give birth on a first floor to avoid difficult or impossible transports in the event that the mother cannot walk to the transport vehicle herself. Be sure that the partner or some other person who is sure to be present knows the route to the nearest hospital and to the hospital of choice (if these are not the same). Have them drive the routes to make sure they are aware of how to get there from her home. Don't assume you know the best routes from a multitude of different locations unless your community is quite small. In addition, maps and directions should be posted by the phone in case the person who knows the route cannot be there to help. (Another alternative is to have copies of the hospital directions in the chart as well.)

The birth kit: Have the mother show you her birthing supplies and where they are stored. Ask her if she has gotten everything on your list and discuss the relative necessity of and sources for those items she is still lacking. If your client has ordered a prearranged birth kit from a birthing supply vendor, you can be reasonably sure that what you want her to have is included. The vendor will include a backorder or out-of-stock list of those supplies not enclosed in the first shipment. If the mother has gathered her supplies herself, you'll want to check more closely to be sure she has understood what you had in mind when giving her the list of items. Also check to see how she is coming along with collecting any miscellaneous household items or supplies you may have requested.

Food for the mother: Find out if the mother has already purchased any electrolyte balancing fluids recommended on your list (a couple of bottles are good to have on hand). Also go over what foods are good for labor: light, easily digested proteins such as yogurt or cottage cheese, foods she likes that are nutritious, miso soup mix and other soups, juices, teas, toast, crackers, etc. Of course, a laboring woman can have any foods she desires and can keep down (I encourage intake of foods that have some nutrition, not just empty calorie junk).

After the birth it is nice to have a stocked kitchen as well as frozen dishes ready to pull out and heat in the oven. The mother can start to cook extra portions of any meals she prepares and freeze them now if freezer space is available. If not, perhaps a friend or relative can allow her to borrow freezer space or friends can organize a schedule for bringing meals over for at least the first week after birth.

Food for the midwives: Always include this on the list of things to gather so the parents will not overlook this important consideration or assume your dietary preferences. If you have done this, the woman will often ask you specifically what you would like her to have on hand. Give them a list of simple foods that are acceptable to you and easy to prepare (vegetables to steam, rice to cook, tofu or another acceptable protein, bread, butter, popcorn, etc.) If you choose not to direct the parents to the foods you prefer, good luck. If you find yourself miles from a store at a three day birth in a blizzard eating Strawberry Shortcake cereal with reconstituted coffee whitener, don't say I didn't warn you!

Oven, telephone, water, utilities, heat: While these items may be a given in many birthing situations, do not assume this to be the case in all of them. Be sure the parents have a phone and, if they are very rural, ask if calls can be placed outside the local area. I talked to a midwife who was at a birth in rural Texas; upon being paged she was appalled to learn that she could not call outside the tiny local exchange to which the client subscribed! Find out if the phone is rotary or pulse tone only, as this will hinder your ability to retrieve pager messages if your pager requires a touch tone phone to do so. If there is no phone, ideally she can run a long extension cord from a neighbor's for the labor. If not, have her locate the nearest neighbor phone or public phone and be sure you have access to it day or night. A list of pertinent phone numbers (ambulance, doctors, etc.) should be placed by every phone. This list should also include the address and directions to the client's home. If no phone is in the home, the list should be placed by every external door on the door frame or right next to it on the wall (post-it notes can be used) so it can be grabbed on the way out to the telephone. If you often work very rurally, have a wide geographic range that you cover or if a number of your clients have no phones (such as the Amish) consider getting a portable phone.

An oven can be used to heat up baby blankets, boil water, and sterilize instruments (which is an important consideration if you have several women due at once). If they do not have one (or, as I found out at one birth, they had one but it didn't work!) you will want to know this in advance.

Find out what kind of heat is used in the home and how efficient it is. Obviously this is of most concern during the winter. If wood is used to heat the home, impress upon the parents the fact that the baby will need plenty of warmth both during the birth and the weeks postpartum. They should stock up on ready-to-use wood accordingly. For a midwinter birth in a cold climate, consider recommending the use of a space heater for the birth and postpartum room.

Pets: Meet any mobile pets and get a feel for how the family interacts with their animals. Dogs, especially, can become very worried about their owner during labor and you want to be sure the dog knows you are on the birthing woman's side. Animals may have the run of the house; request that they be confined during labor to avoid such mishaps as the cat jumping onto the tray of instruments, etc.

Baby preparations: Unless cultural mandates forbid it, it is normal for the family to be preparing for the baby. You want to take a look at where the baby will sleep (even if the mother is planning to sleep with her baby, she will also usually prepare a bed elsewhere for day naps), clothing, diaper plans and so forth. If no baby plans are being made, this is a very concerning sign. Discuss why this is so and talk to the parents in more depth about their feelings regarding the coming birth.

Postpartum help: The parents will need to make provisions for such things as laundry, food, screening calls and visitors, overseeing the care of siblings, etc. for the days following birth. Sometimes the partner can take time off from work to help with some of these tasks, but should not have to bear the total burden alone. It is ideal if there are friends or relatives who can do these things for the mother so that she can attend to the baby. In fact, caring for the baby and herself should be the only tasks which the mother must do for the first two to three weeks after the birth. This fact must be made very plain to grandmothers and others who imagine that helping mom will consist of sitting and holding the baby while the new mom loads laundry and deals with the other children.

For those who want to pitch in, some midwives have a list of needed tasks such as laundry, dishwashing, taking older children to the park, and picking up a child after school for the mother to post on her front door. Ask people who offer to help to bring over dinners; assign a night per person for the first few weeks postpartum. Never refuse food, it can always be frozen!

Another option for postpartum assistance is a doula service. These provide women who come to the home to care for the mother and other children for several hours during the day for a fee. These services are becoming widely available, the local childbirth educators, health food store or community resource guides are usually good places to inquire about what may be available in the local community.

Honoring Pregnancy and Birth as a Rite of Passage

In most cultures pregnancy and birth are seen as tremendously important turning points in a woman's life. This awareness is often acknowledged by ceremonies which are associated with late pregnancy, the birth or the welcoming of the baby. In western culture, this sacred acknowledgement has been diminished. Instead we have the very mechanized but just as ritualistic and culturally influenced forms of initiation that are represented by hospital birthing routines, childbirth education classes, and on a more personal and social note, the baby shower.

A baby shower is a gift-giving party held in honor of a pregnant woman by her family, friends or work associates. Its intention is to have fun and provide the mother with most of the things she will need to care physically for her coming baby. Gifts are usually useful baby items and the focus is on the "having a baby" part of pregnancy rather than on the woman and the passage she is about to make through labor and birth into motherhood.

In the late 1960's, as homebirth became more prevalent, first world western women, sought out ways to address the spiritual components of entering into motherhood, the task of labor and the actual channeling of life on the planet as the baby emerges. Preparing the woman to undertake these momentous spiritual tasks is the goal of modern-day rituals surrounding pregnancy and birth.

Depending upon the community and the spiritual background of the women you care for, you can encourage them to have ceremonies for each other that recognize the inherent spiritual passage that birth is for the mother, the child and the partner.

The Blessingway: One such traditional ritual is found in the Navaho culture and is translated as a Blessingway. These Native Americans honored those who were entering any kind of passage or hardship with a spiritually uplifting ceremony to mark the event and prepare them for the transformation the event would bring.

Since the 1960's a variety of books have become available which describe different ceremonial poems, songs, stories and activities to symbolically honor and prepare the woman for the upcoming event. Sadly, white western culture has become quite removed from its European ritualistic heritage. White women have borrowed from other cultures, particularly the Native Americans, to try and reconstruct ceremonies which include activities that address the spiritual and emotional work which is needed to prepare for labor and motherhood. In doing so, native cultures have often felt that their rituals were being misused, misunderstood and appropriated (as whites have done with their land, their resources and other aspects of their culture).

Creating a ceremony:

The intent of birthing rituals is to gather around the pregnant woman, honoring her and celebrating her life and the transition she is about to make. A complete exploration of ceremony would be a rather substantial book in itself; here we will go over just a few of the ways a ceremony can be formulated which will give you an idea where to begin in creating meaningful rituals. It helps to have an overview of what the ceremony will entail. Below is an example of some things which many women and midwives find are powerful components of such ceremonies:

* Prior to the ceremony, prepare the home or outdoor area with flowers, pillows for participants to sit on, candles, and incense. Attractively arrange any musical instruments or other items needed during the ceremony on a small table or a cloth within easy reach.
* As women arrive, have a welcoming, introductions and explain why you are gathered today
* Cleanse and set apart the space with prayer, incense, or singing (as appropriate to the religious and philosophical beliefs of the group)
* Establish a group mood with more singing, chanting or prayer
* Have the person being honored sit in the center of the circle, make her comfortable and brush her hair, crown her with flowers, wash and massage her feet with fragrant oil.
* One by one, each participant who has brought a special offering to share comes before the honored one and reads a poem, sings a song, dances, plays music, offers a blessing, or presents a gift, explaining the meaning of the gift, if appropriate. Gifts are often objects from nature or small handmade items such as a handwritten poem.
* Various ceremonial objects placed in the circle could at some point be explained (a flower representing conception, a cooking vessel representing the womb, a shell symbolizing the watery home of the pregnant womb, an open seed pod representing birth, a gourd representing transformation).
* A gourd or other meaningful object can now be passed from person to person, giving each the opportunity to speak what is in her heart or remain silent; each person can offer a blessing to the baby and mother if a theme is desired.
* A strong, hot bittersweet tea can be brewed in advance for either the honored woman or the midwife to share with each participant. This symbolizes sharing the pain and strength of labor with each person, linking them all in the event to come.
* Pass a ball of yarn around from person to person, wrapping the

strand around each one's wrist as it goes from person to person (a symbol of connectedness).

*A pair of scissors is passed around; each woman cuts the yarn around the wrist of the woman next to her and ties a small piece to the woman's left wrist, with the honored one last of all. This symbolizes each person taking the circle with her. The yarn can be left in place until the mother and baby have safely completed the passage of birth.

*A reading can be done for the mother with cards, the I Ching or other divination method, if appropriate to her beliefs.

*More singing, chanting or prayer can be offered as the ceremony draws to a close.

As the community becomes more accustomed to the format of rituals, other features can be incorporated, such as offering the mother a full body massage (especially nice when the circle is small and composed of only close women friends), having the group form an archway for each woman to pass through, symbolizing birth, or incorporating a hot tub into the ritual. As you get more comfortable with ritual for the sake of spiritual and emotional attunement, other ideas will occur to you.

Send out invitations suggesting that those invited bring a song, poem, flower or small meaningful gift for the one to be honored, a dish for a pot-luck meal, flowers or whatever seems appropriate. Decide if it will be a women-only event or if men are welcome as well. Another option is for any men involved to be encouraged to honor the father at an all-men's ceremony.

Songs and chants: The songs and chants or prayers used during a ritual should be in harmony with the beliefs of the honored guest. There are literally hundreds of songs which have become popular over the last decades; it is fascinating to travel to different parts of the country and hear the variety of tunes put to the same words. Here is a beautiful chant which can be recited while passing the ball of yarn as suggested above:

As women has always woven, so we weave this yarn into the circle of our lives.
As women have always woven time and the fates, so let us weave this yarn into the circle of our lives.
As women have woven the seeds with the earth, so let us weave this yarn into the circle of our lives.
As women have always woven baskets and tools, so let us weave this yarn into the circle of our lives.
As women have always woven threads into clothing and shelter, so let us weave this yarn into the circle of our lives.
As women have always woven words into poetry, so let us weave this yarn into the circle

of our lives.
As women have always woven, so we weave this yarn with the Goddess who is with us.
The Goddess is always with us. May we feel her presence in our daily lives.

As the last piece of yarn is cut, the following chant may be used:

We call on the Goddess whose body we see and feel reflected in our bodies.
We call on the Goddess whose blood, like our blood, flows with the cycles of the
    universe.
We call on the Goddess whose circle is never broken, whose circle we are a part of
    wherever we go.
Today we do not break this circle but each of us carries part of it into the world.
The circle is never broken.

Numerous other chants and songs as well as additional suggestions for how
to conduct ceremonies may be found in the following books:

Women's Rituals: A Source Book, by Barbara Walker, HarperSanFrancisco, Pub.,
    New York, NY, 1990.

Celebrating Life: Rites of Passage for All Ages, by Tzipora Klein, Delphi Pres.,
    Inc., Oak Park Il, 1992.

These two books describe a variety of popular elements which can be
included in ceremonies for many occasions with specific suggestions for certain
dates (Summer Solstice, etc.).

Circle of Song by Kate Marks, Full Circle Press, Lenox, MA, 1993.

Songs of the Earth, by Anna Kealoha, Celestial Arts, Berkeley, CA, 1989. Both
    of these books offer music and songs for rituals. Circle of Song also has a
    section addressing different elements which can be included in rituals
    (dances, etc.)

Ensuring A Vertex Presentation at Term

NOTE: Review the chapter on The Art of Palpation in the Basic Skills section before reading this chapter.

Breech presentation is a common feature of early pregnancy. As pregnancy advances to term, the rate of breech presentation drops dramatically, to a fairly constant rate of 3.7% of all term births:

PREVALENCE OF BREECH PRESENTATION	
WEEKS OF PREGNANCY	% OF BREECH PRESENTATIONS
28	25
30	17
32	11
34	5
36	5
37-40	3.7

(Flamm, 1995)

Because the majority of babies will have turned on their own after 36 weeks, it has been the tendency in the medical model of care to wait until a woman is near term to attempt to influence the baby's position. However, it is my observation that the baby that has been breech all along is likely to remain so until birth. Waiting to address the issue until pregnancy is advanced lessens the chance of a successful result.

You will be able to palpate the fetal position with more certainty during the third trimester and this ability increases as term approaches. You can usually tell if the baby is breech or vertex by 26 weeks; at that point or shortly thereafter you have more information about the location of small parts and the baby's back. How do you proceed if the baby is not head down? Opinion varies within the midwifery community about the desirability of a woman giving birth to a baby in the breech position; some midwives feel it is fine and actually look forward to breech births, and others are scared or unable to deal with them, for both political as well as clinical reasons.

Our western culture, with all its fear around birth, is particularly afraid of breech births. While it is true that breech births can require skilled manipulation to accomplish the delivery, and breech babies generally have more anomalies and birth-related injuries, an easy breech birth is the easiest birth there is—the baby just falls out (from the midwife's point of view, if not the mother's)!

Of course, nothing can absolutely ensure that a baby will not be breech at term. In my practice of 12 years I have found a significant correlation between the mother's emotional state and the position of her baby *in utero*. While many techniques and opinions prevail on this controversial topic, I offer my insights and techniques to ensure a vertex presentation at term. I was able to accomplish this goal in all but .8 percent of the births I attended. (Those that made it to term were the ones I missed or whose mothers would not allow me to attempt a version.)

Preventive measures to use throughout pregnancy: Always be alert for signs that a woman is carrying breech. She may feel small movements down low in her pelvis or complain of a bruised feeling under her ribs (caused by pressure from the hard head). There may be no lower pelvic pressure or the woman may say this pregnancy feels somehow different than any previous ones. The fundal height may also seem off—either high or low for dates, depending upon how the baby is positioned. The presenting part often remains high, even in primigravidas, as pregnancy advances.

The location of the fetal heart tones is a very unreliable indication of breech presentation and should never be depended upon to cinch the diagnosis. When you are palpating a woman, ask her about her sense of fetal movement (where? what kind?) and position. Fetal movements down low (can be hands); also remember that a woman carrying a frank breech, with its feet splinted up toward the fundus, may only feel movement higher up in her uterus because no small parts are down low. Follow these pointers for palpating at all times:

*Have the mother lie on a flat, hard surface (a carpeted floor is ideal).
*Always palpate both fetal poles (a big hard butt can feel like a head, especially if the baby is in a frank breech presentation, if you don't compare it with the other end!)
*Determine head flexion. If you are unsure of what you are feeling at one pole, turn around and try the same technique at the opposite end for comparison.
*A well-flexed head with the face directed toward the back of the pelvis can feel deceivingly like a butt because it may not ballot freely.
*Keep in mind that posterior babies can fool you, because it may be difficult to get the head to ballot separately from the body.

It is very helpful to have someone else on hand to palpate with you. If you both find the fetus is "lying in a lump," that is, so tightly curled up that you can't tell one end from the other, or you suspect the head is very tucked under and therefore cannot be distinguished with ballotment, have the mother assume a hands-and-knees or knee-chest position and do pelvic rocks for a few minutes (gently rock her hips towards the floor by swaying her back, then straighten her back). This often encourages the baby to lift its head. Then have her lie down and palpate again. If the position is still in doubt, see her again in a week or two. In the meantime, have her visualize the baby head down, face toward her spine and talk to the baby about letting the midwives know where it is at the next visit. Also ask her to give more conscious attention to where she feels fetal movement.

Have the mother carefully notice fetal position between visits. If the baby makes a lot of large, turning movements (somersaults), this is a good sign, since these babies are likely to turn on their own.

Physical problems which affect the position of the baby: There are numerous physical problems which can influence the fetal position. Maternal factors include:

-Tense, tight uterine and abdominal walls which prevent the baby from turning (a mother's fear can make for tight muscles)
-Poor abdominal or uterine muscle tone
-Pelvic obstruction (tumor, cyst, fibroid)
-Pelvic injury or deformity which makes the head fit poorly in a vertex position
-Uterine abnormality (especially if a septum divides the uterine cavity)
-Placenta previa (see separate chapter)
-Poly- or oligo-hydramnios (too much or too little amniotic fluid)

Fetal factors may include:

-Multiple pregnancy
-Anencephaly
-Hydrocephaly or other abnormality preventing engagement of the head
-Very tight cord around the baby's neck or other body part
-Short cord
-Amniotic bands (fetal parts become entangled in rolls of previously ruptured amnion, thus restricting movement)
-Intrauterine fetal death

Any of these factors may be present in babies that resist all attempts at turning them or which revert to a non-vertex presentation quickly after being turned. Keep in mind, however, that no physical reason for breech presentation can be found in the majority of those which continue until term.

Visualization of the baby: One of the most important techniques for the mother to use is visualization of the baby in a head-down position at all times during pregnancy. A mother may be thinking of looking at her baby face to face or thinking of holding the baby in her arms and not in her uterus, head down. This may give the baby the message that head up is where its at. It may be necessary to provide pictures of babies *in utero* in an ideal position (head flexed, arms by

804

sides, cord floating free, baby facing mother's back) to help if she is having trouble seeing the baby inside. Family members can join in visualizing the baby head down and ready for birth.

Emotional factors: I have found that emotional factors play an essential role in other-than-vertex presentations. This is not to say that women carrying vertex babies don't have problems, but in my experience, women who carry breech or transverse for a length of time have some underlying emotional upset which is a contributing factor. Because I have found emotional factors to be a key to babies turning and staying vertex and because medically managed versions do not address this issue, I believe this is why many babies turned in medical practices return to their breech position.

Typical examples of emotional factors that influence the baby to be breech are: mothers who are preoccupied or not paying attention to the pregnancy (common around the 28th to 30th week in working mothers or those with other children); an unstable emotional environment; poor communication in the couple's relationship; or fear related to the birth, the location of the house, or any aspect of delivery. A history of breech births in the family or the fact that the mother was born breech herself can influence the mother's and baby's expectations for what birth will be like; you can counter this with strong affirmations and visual images of vertex babies which the mother can post around her home (on mirrors, etc.).

The distinct relationship between maternal distress and fetal position I observed in the practice in New England may be related to the general fear surrounding breech births in the larger society. In an insulated cultural setting where women do not fear birth, such as on the Farm in Summertown, Tennessee where the midwives are quite open and receptive to doing breech births with good medical support, the babies may at times choose to come breech without such a consistent correlation with maternal distress. In my practice we were not fearful of breeches, however, we did not work in a very favorable political environment to do breeches at home. We definitely put out a clear message to the babies we worked with that we wanted them to be head down. I think that made quite an impact on our success rate in getting babies to turn vertex.

From the baby's point of view: Breech and transverse positions symbolize comfort for the mother and baby, as the position places the head nearer the mother's heart. These positions may also be related to maternal fear of birth, or the baby's fear of birthing into a threatening environment. Women with underlying psychological issues regarding their own abilities, or those who work on life's problems by manifesting physical problems for themselves may carry in an other-than-vertex position more persistently. Babies can be breech in order to get the attention not only of their mother but also that of the care provider. Especially in cases where a physiological factor is influencing the baby's position, this is the baby's way of saying wake up and take notice!

In order for visualization, breech-turning exercises or version to work, the emotional environment must change, at least to the point where the mother acknowledges the problem and compensates by concentrating attention on the baby. If maternal attention is all that is needed, visualization is frequently effective; breech tilt exercises (described below) provide time and attention for the fetus as well. If relationship problems (such as lack of attention from the partner, or financial woes) are factors, having both partners visualize and talk to the baby may work. The main message to the baby is that whatever the external circumstances, the baby will need to come out one way or the other, and being breech or transverse won't make it any easier.

The breech tilt: If visualization alone does not lead to spontaneous version, have the mother begin the breech tilt exercises at 30 to 32 weeks. Have her prop one end of an ironing board or other long flat surface to about the height of the couch seat. She should then pad the board with a blanket and lay on it head down for 15 to 20 minutes, 6 to 8 times daily. While there, she should massage her abdomen, preferably in a face/head forward position with one hand cupped around the occiput and one cupped around the breech, moving the face forward and lifting the baby's bottom in a rotating motion. As soon as the baby turns, have her get up and walk or squat to help fix the position of the baby. Jill Breen, a Vermont midwife, has noted that if the mother performs the tilt for three days in a row and then stops the fourth day, the baby seems to turn vertex on its own in anticipation of the exercise.

Other methods that have worked: Midwives have used a variety of methods to turn babies when the tilt has failed:

*Have the mother walk on her hands in a swimming pool
*Place a transistor radio in the mother's pants and play it for 10 minutes 6 to 8 times daily.
*Move a flashlight over the belly from the fundus to the pelvis while the mother is in the tilt position. To do so, press the lighted end of the flashlight into the abdomen on the side of the baby's face and move it directly down toward the pelvis. The idea is the baby will follow the light.
*Draw a picture of a head down, face to her back (LOA) baby on the mother's belly with a washable marker if she is having trouble with visualization.
*Homeopathic Pulsatilla in 200C potency or higher, especially for babies that have had an unstable lie. Have the mother take one dose every three days while doing breech tilt exercises.
*Stimulation of the acupuncture point Bladder 67 (located on the little toe at the outer corner of the nailbed) can help turn breech or transverse babies; place a tiny cone of Moxa on the points on each

little toe and burn it for 15 minutes daily
*Recommend Webster's breech turning technique (a chiropractic technique, see the end of this chapter)

External cephalic version: A manual version can be done by the midwife if all attempts to turn the baby up until now have failed. Sometimes the situation calls for a bit more intervention and your efforts will be quickly, easily and permanently effective. Some women may be hesitant to manipulate the baby the way they need to in order to accomplish a self-version, and you will be able to project enough confidence and skill into the task to accomplish your goal.

To perform versions (manual external turning of the baby), you must be good at palpation and taking fetal heart tones. You must be as sure as possible about the fetal position; get a second opinion or an ultrasound if you are not sure! You must also feel comfortable with the procedure and the relative risk involved. The risks involved in version are cord entanglement and placental disruption, either of which may lead to fetal death. In particular, anterior placentas make version more difficult and more dangerous because of the increased possibility of placental disruption. Be especially gentle if you and the mother agree that version is warranted. However, it is my opinion (and experience has borne this out) that performing versions around the 32nd week of pregnancy, when the ratio of fetus to fluid is still such that turning is a relatively easy, gentle process, minimizes all these risks. Since the percent of babies remaining breech more or less levels off at 34 weeks, some midwives may prefer to wait until 34 weeks to do a version.

Doctor-assisted versions: The medical model views version as a highly risky procedure. Unfortunately, one study, done in 1985, using general anesthesia, cited an unacceptable perinatal mortality rate. It concluded it must be version that was dangerous and not how it was being done (Kasule, et.al, 1985). No other study to date has had any perinatal deaths or even serious morbidity attributable to version (Goer, 1995). In spite of this, the risks are addressed by giving the mother uterine muscle relaxing drugs and performing version with direct ultrasound visualization. Ultrasound is used to ascertain fetal position and monitor fetal response to the procedure. Drugs are used to minimize the chance of precipitating preterm labor as well as enhance the ability to manipulate the baby. Of course, this exposes mother and fetus to the side effects of the drugs, as well as excluding women with certain medical conditions who cannot take the drugs (Goer, 1995).

Furthermore, in my opinion, using drugs to relax the uterus removes a sensitive safety barometer from the process; one of the mother's physiological responses to the procedure. If the uterus begins contracting during version and particularly if it stays contracted it is a signal to slow down, wait until the contraction has passed, and perhaps be more gentle. To prevent the uterus from such a response seems to me to add more risk, not less!! Gentle version in a healthy mother does not start labor any more than firm, confident palpation does.

I have not found uterine contraction to occur excessively or unremittingly in the versions I have performed.

In addition, many doctors will only attempt version once, usually after the 37th week of pregnancy or later (per ACOG guidelines), feeling that the risks outweigh the benefits before that since the baby may revert to breech or may turn on its own. While this is true in part (many babies will turn vertex if left alone), it has been my observation that the baby that is breech at term is usually the one that has been breech all along. Waiting until the baby is big, the fluid is diminished and the uterus is full to the brim means that firmer pressure must be used to turn the baby. Midwives have reported that women often come back from hospital versions bruised and that doctors' arms often shake with the strain of turning the baby this late. It is easy to see how such force could increase the risks inherent in the procedure. Such a forceful procedure is not necessary if you turn the baby early! Also, having the mother in a relaxed environment helps her relax and makes version that much easier; overemphasizing the risks with drugs and machines does not assist relaxation. Of course, you should discuss the option of having a version performed in the hospital before you agree to do one yourself. Women who feel uncomfortable with any manual interference may be willing to try the Webster chiropractic technique described later in this chapter, which does not include abdominal manipulation.

Midwife-assisted version: The exam surface should be at a level which allows the midwife maximum leverage in moving the baby; a carpeted floor is ideal. I may kneel to the woman's side or between her legs (which is often preferable, particularly if I anticipate that the version may not be so easy). Before I attempt version I explain to the mother that pressure is required to turn the baby, but that she should immediately tell me if she feels any pain. It is necessary to help her differentiate pain from pressure. After asking her to empty her bladder, I help her consciously relax, positioning her with her back flat on a firm surface and using pillows under her knees and head as necessary so that her abdominal muscles are fully relaxed. The more relaxed she is and the safer she feels in allowing you to turn the baby, the less likely it is that she will interpret pressure as pain, or that her uterus will contract, or that you will do any damage. It may help to prop the mother's bottom up somewhat, especially if the baby's bottom is not above the pelvic brim.

After you have listened to the fetal heart tones and reevaluated the fetal position, you may find it necessary to have the mother do pelvic rocks in a hands-and-knees position to encourage the baby to rotate to an anterior position, lift its head and float the bottom up out of the pelvis; it really helps make version easier if the head is not fully flexed and the bottom is loosened up. After the mother has resituated herself, listen to the heart once more before you begin. Begin a combination palpation/massage of her belly, talking to her, helping her breathe deeply and fully relax. The technique for external version: (numbers refer to

808

drawings in the following chart) Study the hand positions, especially for the head.

1. Cup your hands around the baby's head and apply firm, even pressure to the occiput. Reach down and stabilize the breech, or gently scoop it out of the pelvis, if necessary. Jiggle the baby gently as you go. As the baby begins to move, place your other hand on the breech to hold it in place. (2.) If this does not get the baby moving, use both hands to cup around the occiput and walk your fingers toward the pelvis while pushing the head along in front of your hands. Once you begin to get the turn going, use one hand or have an assistant stabilize the breech, hold the baby in place, and have your assistant listen for heart tones.

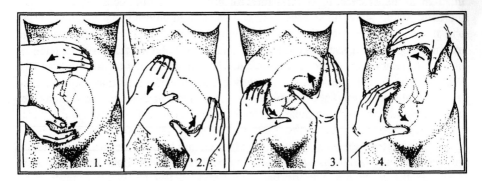

2. & 3. Getting the baby past the transverse point requires the most pressure; don't let go of the head. Listen to the fetal heart.

3. & 4. Frequently, once the head is just past the midline the baby rapidly rotates into a vertex presentation. If it does not, continue to cup your hand on the head and jiggle the baby gently, inching it toward the pelvis by pressing your fingers firmly around the contours of the head and walking your fingers toward the pelvis while simultaneously inching the breech pole up toward the fundus in the same way (Sorger, 1989).

As you do the version, talk to the mother and the baby; tell the baby what you are doing. Go slowly and sense with your hands what is going on. It is preferable to turn the baby face forward; however, move the baby in the direction it goes most easily. (When doing version earlier in pregnancy [before term] it is not critical to maintain head flexion). Gently jiggle the baby as you bring it around. This helps dislodge the baby and get it moving. (Sorger, 1989) Don't be so gentle that you are totally ineffective, as with palpation, pressure and getting a firm feel for the baby are important for success. I have not found using either oil or powder helpful in performing versions; they make my hands too slippery to get a good grip on the baby. After the version is complete, listen to the baby for a few minutes to be sure all is well. Once the baby turns, have the mother get up and squat or walk to settle the baby down into its new position.

If version is proving difficult, listen to the fetal heart tones more often. The literature reports that the FHT may drop momentarily during version. If it does, listen until it returns to normal. I have not really noticed this; it may have to do with the amount of force used and the size of the fetus being turned. <u>Human Labor & Birth</u> gives 3 minutes as a reasonable time for the fetal heart rate to normalize when it does drop. (I must say I have rarely seen it drop at all and 3 minutes to baseline seems quite long to me.) Don't force the issue, if the baby won't turn or if it reverts back to a breech position there may be a good reason; talk to the mother about an ultrasound exam to see what the problem might be.

In my experience, most versions are easily accomplished in 2 minutes or less (this is an estimate, most were accomplished quickly and relatively easily). The longest time it has taken me to do a version was 5 minutes (by the clock). The baby was transverse the mother (a first-timer) was quite tense, and the baby reverted to transverse shortly afterwards. Later, after the mother had an ultrasound assuring her that there were no problems, version was accomplished quickly and easily and the baby stayed head down. The latest version I ever did was 3 days after the due date, with the mother's bottom propped up, it was easy and quick. It is my experiences that frank breech babies are the most difficult to turn, apparently because the legs wedge the baby against the uterine wall, preventing easy rotation (maybe this is why most term breech babies are in a frank position).

<u>Larry Webster's Chiropractic Technique for Turning Breech Babies</u>: This technique was developed by Larry Webster, an Atlanta chiropractor. It is included so that you can give it to a woman's chiropractor (do not attempt to do it yourself if you have no training!). It has worked when everything else has failed to turn a baby, out of one group of 700 women carrying breech, only 18 of their babies failed to turn with this technique.

> **Step one**: Place the woman in a prone position. Flex each leg toward her buttocks; find the side of most resistance. Adjust sacrum (P-A on that side, contact point sacral notch below P.S.I.S., use light thrust due to softened ligaments of mother.) There are two possible occurrences after adjustment:
>
> 1. The most resistant leg releases to equal the least resistant leg (80%)
> 2. The least resistant leg comes back to equal the most resistant (20%).
>   You are looking for an equalization of resistance on flexion of legs on the buttocks. This equalization should take place before going on to step two. If the woman is evaluated on her side, the lower leg will automatically be 1 inch more resistant; allow for this

810

in your evaluation.

Step two: Place woman in a supine position. On the side opposite of sacral adjustment, draw a line 45° lateral and inferior from the umbilicus; draw another line from the ASIS inferior and medial 45°. Where they bisect hold an I-S contact with your thumb (3 to 6 oz. of pressure). Rotate thumb from bisect point 15° in either direction until muscle bundle is felt. Hold thumb contact for 60 to 90 seconds. You will feel the muscle drop away from your pressure. Stop at this point. Do not adjust another segment that day.

Adjust every 2 to 3 days for 2 weeks; the baby should turn. If during the second or third visit there is equal resistance on both buttocks, do not adjust. On alternate days you can adjust elsewhere along the spine. (Vallone, 1990)

<u>Transverse lie:</u> Unlike a longitudinal presentation, when the baby is lying sideways it cannot come out at all unless it comes *very* premature or dead (in some cases). Therefore, there is a big message here that something needs attention. Persistent transverse lie is much less common than breech presentation, occurring in only 1 out of 500 term pregnancies. Anything which prevents engagement of the head or the breech makes transverse presentation more likely. It is also more common in multigravidas because of the laxness of the uterine and abdominal muscles. Factors which need to be ruled out include: placenta previa, multiple pregnancy, obstructing tumor (such as ovarian cyst or uterine fibroid), fetal anomaly, polyhydramnios, pelvic contraction, and uterine abnormalities. However, cases do occur where no such associated factors are present. The diagnosis of transverse lie during abdominal examination includes these findings:

*The abdomen appears asymmetrical and wider than it is tall
*The fundal height may be small for dates
*Palpation of the fundus and the pelvic areas of the uterus reveal no
    fetal poles, which are instead found on either side
*The fetal heart is heard below the mother's navel
*Neither the head nor the breech can be felt during an internal exam

Transverse lie can be handled in the same way as for a breech presentation. If the baby refuses to turn or turns and then reverts back to a transverse position, an investigation as to any interfering factors as listed above is warranted. If everything is tried with no results, the woman should be told that a surgical delivery is necessary should the baby remain transverse. Typically, transverse presentation is associated with early rupture of membranes, since uterine contractions cause pressure changes and no fetal pole is filling the pelvis; in such cases cord prolapse is more likely. Therefore, women anticipating a surgical delivery should waste no time getting to the hospital as soon as labor begins.

Unstable lie: An unstable lie exists when the baby shifts its position from vertex to breech or transverse a number of times during the course of the pregnancy. This reflects an ambivalent emotional climate and may be a message from the baby that something really needs attention (anomalies?). These possibilities should be discussed with the mother; otherwise, recommendations are the same.

General guidelines: Here is a capsule review of what to do:

> *Palpate at every visit, regardless of how early the pregnancy may be
> *Have the woman pay close attention to fetal movements
> *Recognize the psychological, emotional and environmental factors which contribute to other-than-vertex presentations
> *Be alert to symptoms of a breech presentation
> *From 25 weeks, have all mothers consistently visualize their babies head down and pay attention to the baby
> *From 30 weeks, if the baby is not vertex, ask about psychological factors, fears, etc. and begin the breech tilt
> *Review other methods of encouraging rotation in this chapter and suggest whatever seems appropriate and acceptable to the mother
> *From 32 weeks, if baby is still breech, continue as above and discuss version; do version if the baby seems fixed in a breech position (it never responds to maternal effort to change position)
> *Discuss the pros and cons of waiting to have a version performed by a doctor using ultrasound and uterine relaxing drugs
> *Have a chiropractor perform the Webster technique as appropriate

References and further reading:

Bradley-Watson, P.J., "The decreasing value of external cephalic version in modern obstetric practice," Am. J., Ob/Gyn, 10/1/75, Vol. 123, No. 3, pp. 237-40.

Chalmer, Iain, ed., Effective Care in Pregnancy and Childbirth, Vol. 1, ed. Chapter 42, "Breech presentation and abnormal lie in late pregnancy," by G. Justus Hofmeyr.

Flamm, Bruce, "The Term Breech Fetus; Averting the Cesarean Section," workshop, Perinatal care symposium, Strategies for improving maternal and neonatal outcomes, 6/16/95.

Goer, H., Obstetric Myths Versus Research Realities, Bergin & Garvey, Westpost, CT, 1995.

Kasule, J, et.al, "Controlled trial of external cephalic version," Br J ObGyn, Vol. 92, 1985, p. 14.

Leonard, Carol, midwife, conversations regarding external cephalic version, Fall, 1987.

Oxhorn, Harry, Human Labor and Birth, 3rd, & 4th editions.

Robertson, et.al., "External cephalic version at term: Is a tocolytic necessary," Ob Gyn, Vol. 70, No. 6, 1987, pp. 896-899.

Scaling, S, External cephalic version w/out tocolysis, Am J Ob/Gyn, Vol 158, No 6 Pt 1, p. 1424.

Sorger, Leo, Breech births, workshop MANA Conference, Boston, 1989.

Vallone, Sharon, Chiropractor, Hartford CT, Webster tech. for workshop, MANA conf. KS, 1990.

<u>Anticipating a Breech Birth</u>

Generally speaking, if no interventions as outlined in the last chapter are employed, breech presentation at term will occur in about 3 to 4% of all pregnancies. Prior to 28 weeks of pregnancy the incidence is about 25%. As pregnancy advances, the incidence decreases because in most cases left to nature, the fetus will convert to a cephalic presentation by 34 weeks gestation. About 15% of all babies presenting breech at the onset of labor are preterm.

Breech presentation is a normal variation of pregnancy. Since it is a longitudinal lie, the baby can be born spontaneously. However, because it is so much less common than cephalic presentation, the care provider has less opportunity to become skilled at the manipulations which must be employed if the baby is having trouble coming out. Lack of opportunity plus the increasing safety of surgical delivery has made for a great deal of fear about spontaneous breech birth in our culture. Any woman and midwife contemplating completing the birth of a breech baby at home or in a birthing center cannot do so in a vacuum. Given the fearful climate in which we must work, all the pros and cons of out-of-hospital breech delivery must be weighed carefully before a decision is made.

Let's say you have tried everything and in spite of that the baby is remaining breech. The medical model is still strongly in favor of universal Cesarean section for breech presentations in many locales, despite the fact that studies do not support the notion that this reduces fetal risk. By the 36th week or so (maybe sooner), you should review the pros and cons of spontaneous vs. surgical breech birth and explore all locally available options for spontaneous breech birth so that the parents can make an informed decision about where and with whom to give birth.

Find out which doctors, nurse-midwives or independent midwives in your area will attend spontaneous breech births (if any) and under what circumstances. Know something about their experience (numbers of breeches attended? outcomes?). Some will only attend term, frank breeches. Others will attend anything but a footling. Some may rule out first time mothers since they don't have "proven pelvises" and their reaction to labor is an unknown. It will be helpful for the parents to know their criteria in advance and, when possible, their yoni birth success rate. What is their surgical delivery rate for breeches?

Let the parents initiate inquiry regarding if you will attend them at home. If they assume that they need to birth in hospital, let them know you might be available to attend them if desired (if that's the case), but do not try to convince them otherwise. Since breech birth is still such a political hot potato, this serves as a liability protection for you and your practice.

Discuss the risks: Matter-of-factly outline the risks of spontaneous breech birth, as follows:

*Rapid head decompression causing intracranial hemorrhage

*Head getting stuck in a partially dilated cervix
*Injuries to internal organs
*Impaired placental circulation developing during the birth
*Prolapsed cord
*Baby trying to breathe before the head is born
*Extended arms creating the breech version of shoulder dystocia
*Increased fetal morbidity and mortality
*The risks of surgical birth with breech presentations
*Mother "losing it" and being unable to cope with manipulations necessary to accomplish the birth

Many of these risks are increased if the baby is premature. And, because premature babies are more likely to be breech, the total rate of birth-related trauma is greater overall for breech babies. While risk factors need to be described to the parents, it is also important to point out that hospital breech births often occur with the assistance of fearful care providers who may not have extensive breech experience. Hospital practitioners typically do not attempt to work with women to confront their fears nor do they attempt to connect emotionally with the baby. Many techniques which midwives will use routinely, such as maternal position changes, will not be used in many hospital settings. The particular skills and techniques that you bring to the birth will vary given your background and experience; during your discussion you should include what you would do to remedy a problem whenever appropriate. (How to deal with breech births, including the midwifery remedy for some of these problems, is fully covered in Volume II of this text.)

Rapid head decompression causing intracranial hemorrhage: Premature babies have softer skull bones than those at term. Breech presentation causes the head to come through the pelvis relatively rapidly and thus produces more rapid compression and decompression of the skull without the benefit of the gradual molding that occurs in a vertex presentation. This can result in anything from no damage whatsoever to minor, undetectable bleeding to massive intracranial hemorrhaging to skull fracture. This risk is lessened in the term baby because its skull bones are firmer. However, intracranial hemorrhage is more likely even at term than in a cephalic presentation.

Head getting stuck in partially dilated cervix: The head is the largest part of the baby, regardless of gestational age. The premature baby's body is significantly smaller than its head. There is a risk that the smaller body could slip through a partially dilated cervix and the head get hung up on the cervix, which would cause it to be stuck and difficult to dislodge. If the baby is presenting small parts such as a footling or kneeling breech, this danger is increased. Because some of these risks are eliminated if the baby is of moderate size (6 to 8½ lbs.) and in a frank breech position (which minimizes the risk of the head getting stuck and of cord prolapse) the frank breech position poses the least amount of risk for the baby in this regard. In this case, the baby's butt will fill the cervix and lower pelvis; in a term baby, the butt is about as big around as the head, making it a good dilator, and thus increasing the likelihood that descent will not begin until the cervix is completely taken up. A well-fitting presenting part also minimizes the chance of cord prolapse. A related problem involves the birth of a baby with a deflexed head. If the head is fully tilted backwards, it increases the likelihood of the head getting hung up on the pelvic bones during descent. An ultrasound exam can be done near term to check to see if this is a problem; conversely, the palpation technique described for assessing fetal head flexion can be used for breech presentation just as it can for vertex presentation (see the chapter on The Art of Palpation, Skills section.) The fetal head can also be converted from a flexed to a deflexed position during the birth from improper handling or spontaneously. The one advantage of being in the hospital in this situation is that the physician can use forceps (called Piper's forceps) to deal with the deflexed head. Forceps will not be available at home and vacuum extraction cannot be used for this problem.

Injuries to internal organs: A great deal of manipulation of the baby's body may be required for the birth to be accomplished. These manipulations increase the likelihood that the baby will be injured. Such injuries include liver, kidney or adrenal gland damage from pressure on the torso, broken or damaged limbs, skull, clavicles, neck or spine and dislocated legs or arms. Injuries usually occur due to rough or improper handling and are also more likely during a premature birth.

Impaired placental circulation developing during the birth or cord prolapse: It is possible for the placenta to separate while the head is still in the yoni: placental circulation may also be disrupted if marked reduction in the size of the placental site occurs after the birth of the body.

Cord compression is inevitable during a breech birth as the head passes through the pelvis. If the baby is large, the cord will also be somewhat compressed as the body passes through the cervix. Cord prolapse may occur, especially if the baby is premature, because the presenting part is less likely to be engaged and will not fill the pelvis as well as a term baby during labor. Cord prolapse is also more likely for the same reason in any baby that is in a footling or kneeling breech position, however the soft fetal legs adjacent to the cord somewhat mitigate the risk of acute, life-threatening compression (Cruikshank, 1986). Keeping the membranes intact during the birth will also help cushion the cord.

If the baby's oxygen supply is diminished due to placental or cord problems, the baby may experience sufficient distress to cause it to attempt to breathe while the head is still inside. This can cause the baby to inhale mucus, fluid or meconium (the passage of which is normal in a breech birth) and lead to respiratory problems or infection after the birth, or it may cause the baby to die before the birth of the head.

Extended arms creating the breech version of shoulder dystocia: If the baby's arms become extended over its head or crossed behind it neck, this will delay descent during pushing and make the delivery of the arms and shoulders much more difficult. The necessary maneuvers used to free the baby's arms increase the risk of injury to the neck and the nerves of the arms (although injury is certainly not inevitable).

Increased fetal morbidity and mortality: The baby is more likely to die during a breech birth for any or all of the reasons stated above. The worst prognosis is for the premature baby. Mortality is highest for double footling presentations and lowest for frank breeches at term, however when prematurity and cord prolapse are accounted for, nonfrank breeches do no worse than frank presentations (Myers & Gleicher, 1986). Fetal anomalies are twice as frequent among breech babies compared to those presenting vertex (6.3% versus 2.4%) (Confino, 1985). Fetal disorders associated with breech birth include congenital dislocation of the hip, hydrocephaly and related spinal disorders, and some less common defects. About 15% of fetal deaths occur during labor. The remainder are divided about equally between death *in utero* before labor, congenital abnormalities incompatible with life, and neonatal death.

The danger of injury seems just as great regardless of maternal parity, with difficult births resulting in a 20% risk and easy births in a 3.5% risk. Fetal outcome is worst in surprise breech births, probably in large part because the attendant panics. While breech mortality is typically higher than for babies born vertex, surgical delivery does *not* improve neonatal survival rates (Schutte, et.al., 1985). Long term complications of breech births, regardless of birth route, include such problems as cerebral palsy, epilepsy, mental retardation, and hemiplegia. In summary, breech birth is riskier than vertex, regardless of how the baby comes out.

Risks to breech babies during surgical delivery: When considering risks, the overall risks of yoni birth vs. surgical delivery must be taken into account. The uterine incision must be large enough to prevent the head getting caught as the baby is removed from the uterus. If, at the time of surgery, the woman is not in labor or so early in labor that the lower uterine segment is not well thinned out, a low vertical incision rather than a low transverse incision may be necessary, increasing her risk for future childbearing to a small degree. Overall the maternal mortality rate is four to five times greater in cesarean section than for yoni birth and the risk of complications such as postpartum infection is higher as well.

Babies can and do become injured during extraction through the uterine incision for the same reasons that they become injured during yoni births. A Cesarean requires a total breech extraction, a complicated and risky procedure whereby the fetus is manipulated through the incision. This is inherently more dangerous than the assisted delivery anticipated in the majority of yoni births (Gimovsky & Schifrin, 1992). This is compounded by nervousness among clinicians about dealing with breeches and their lack of opportunity to gain skill at breech manipulations. Numerous studies show that Cesareans do not eliminate birth injuries common to breech presentation, including intracranial hemorrhage, skull fractures, seizures, cerebral palsy, developmental delay, mental retardation and spasticity. When birth weight and gestational age are taken into account, outcomes are similar for babies born via surgery or per yoni. (Croughan-Minihane, et.al., 1990; Green, et.al., 1982; Schutte, et.al., 1985) Studies emphasize that with proper selection of babies, with particular attention to a flexed head and average fetal weight, the presence of congenital defects and gestational age, yoni birth for a breech is a reasonable choice. In other words, merely choosing a surgical delivery does not eliminate and usually does not even reduce the risks inherent in breech birth.

Mother "losing it" and being unable to cope with necessary manipulations to accomplish the birth: Even if the parents feel comfortable with the other risks, as the midwife you must make an honest assessment regarding each woman's ability to tolerate internal manipulations (should they become necessary) and to do what she is told during the birth. She may have to breathe through an urge to push for an hour or more while waiting for the cervix to be fully taken up. She may have to put up with a significant amount of internal manipulation. A breech birth is no time for a woman to start whining about how she can't do it, can't get up, can't change position, or how you are hurting her. Such resistance and delay could cause her to tighten up, her cervix to clamp down, and her pelvic muscles to grab the baby and prevent you from getting it out. Fear can cause the same response.

You can predict such responses to a certain extent from the way a woman deals with internal exams during pregnancy. And, regardless of how non-interventive you may be, it is a good idea to plan on doing an internal exam or two during prenatals to get an idea of what you may be working with in labor. Women should be told that their cooperation is essential to a safe breech birth, but do not let their assurances that they can handle it be your sole consideration in deciding to take on a breech birth. You must also feel that she can handle whatever may be necessary, and see her clearly demonstrate this in her reactions to exams prior to birth. A multipara will at least have a history of how she responded to her previous labor to go on. A primigravida is at more risk because her response to labor is an unknown, and you don't know how big a baby she can have until she has one. Her muscles are tighter, which may make manipulations more difficult. However, they are considered statistically better candidates for breech birth because they are also more likely to have a frank breech position and better muscle tone tends to keep the baby's head well flexed. (Norwood, 1984, p. 130)

Describe your experience with breech births: Regardless of how comfortable the parents may feel with the risks of breech delivery, it is your job to make sure they understand your background, training and experience regarding attendance at breech births. As with all things, you must be scrupulously honest about this. Tell them exactly how many breech births you have attended; specify the number of these births you only observed, the ones at which you assisted someone with more experience than yourself, and the ones you actually caught. Were the births hard, requiring much manipulation to accomplish the births or did the babies fall out with no assistance from you? Were the observations at home or in the hospital? Who received the baby? What is your hands-on training? Have you practiced the difficult maneuvers with models (an acceptable training method since breech births are relatively rare)? How familiar are you with various methods of assisting the birth such as dealing with extended arms, stuck heads, etc.?

Your honesty now will help them make an intelligent decision as well as serve as a measure of protection for you should something go wrong at the birth. Your honesty will also help you make a realistic assessment of what you can take on as a midwife and help prevent you from getting in way over your head. A breech birth should not be attempted by a midwife who does not have a good feel for normal birth in general. You need the experience to be patient and at the same time to act promptly in the event of a possibly unfamiliar emergency. If in doubt about your competence, do not take on the birth yourself.

Discuss the political climate in your community and the prevailing medical attitudes about breech birth: Are all the doctors in your area still doing surgery for breeches? Are they just waiting for something to go wrong at a homebirth so they can arrest a midwife? Parents should understand what risks they are asking you to take as well as the kind of response they can expect should something come up that necessitates transport.

Assess the parent's responsibility level: Regardless of how wonderful the parents may feel about you or about the prospect of a good outcome for their birth, you must independently consider how much personal responsibility they are willing to assume for making this choice and for working with you. If they are slack about appointments, if the mother hasn't been eating right or is irresponsible in other ways, take this as a *big red flag* that you should not go out on a limb for them. If you have any doubts at all about any aspect of your relationship, decline to help them at home and offer support in a hospital setting. Don't be stupid; doing whatever people want whenever they want regardless of the circumstances is not the same thing as being a good midwife.

Clinical considerations: Apart from the mother's tolerance level, your clinical assessment of the woman should include careful pelvimetry and a developed ability to estimate fetal size. Keeping in mind that the maternal pelvis is flexible, the following findings on pelvic exam do not bode well:

818

*An interspinous diameter less than 9.0 cm.
*Forward inclination of the sacrum
*A narrow subpubic arch

Ideally, the mother is a large woman with ample pelvic room and a small to moderately sized baby. A baby that is less than 8½ lbs. is less likely to cause problems, but the fetal size must be assessed in relationship to maternal proportions. If a woman has delivered a 10 pounder before and this baby feels smaller; great! If the mother has had successful breech births before, this is a good sign as well.

Visualizing the birth: As with a vertex birth, have the mother see the baby coming out easily, with its cord floating high in the uterus, arms by its side and its chin tucked to its chest, born pink, breathing right away and nursing well after birth. She should also continue to visualize and talk to the baby about coming out vertex; the baby can still turn, even if labor has begun!!

Ongoing evaluation is essential: Continue to assess all of the above clinical considerations as well as the parents' attitudes throughout the rest of the pregnancy. If something comes up that makes you uncertain, get another opinion or make other plans.

References and further reading:

Confino, E. et.al., "The breech dilemma, A review," Ob Gyn Surv, Vol. 40, No. 6, 1985, pp. 330-337.
Croughan-Minihane, M., et.al., "Morbidity among breech infants according to method of delivery," Ob Gyn, Vol. 75, No. 5, 1990, pp. 821-825.
Cruikshank, D., "Breech presentation," Clin. Ob Gyn, Vol. 29, No. 2, 1986, pp. 255-263.
Gimovski, M, Schifrin, B., "Breech management," J. Perinatol, Vol. 12, No. 2, 1991, p. 143-51.
Green, J. et.al., "Has an increased cesarean rate for term breech delivery reduced the incidence of birth asphyxia, trauma, and death?" Am J Ob Gyn, Vol. 142, No. 6 Pt. I, 1982, pp. 643-648.
Huchcroft, S, et.al., "Late results of cesarean and vaginal delivery in cases of breech presentation," Can Med Assoc J., Vol. 125, 1981, pp. 726-730.
Myles, Margaret, Textbook for Midwives, 9th ed., Churchill Livingstone, London, 1981.
Myers, S, Gleicher, N., "Breech delivery: why the dilemma?" Am J. of Ob Gyn, Vol. 156, 1986, p. 6-10.
Norwood, Christopher, How to Avoid a Cesarean Section, Fireside Books, New York, 1984.
Oxhorn, Harry, Human Labor and Birth, 5th ed., Appleton-Century-Crofts, Norwalk, Ct, 1986.
Schutte, M., et.al., "Perinatal mortality in breech presentations as compared to vertex presentations in singleton pregnancies: an analysis based upon 57,819 computer-registered pregnancies in the Netherlands," Eur. J. Ob Gyn Reprod. Biol, Vol. 19, No. 6, p. 391-400.

Dealing With Posterior Babies During Pregnancy

One variation on the baby-position theme is the persistently posterior fetus. Although this is usually not a problem during pregnancy, a posterior labor and birth can be more problematic than most; troubleshooting early is a good idea. Valerie El Halta, an experienced midwife now practicing in Michigan, offers the following tips for picking up on posterior positioning during pregnancy:

> *The mother may comment that she feels lots of movement in front, and that the baby seems to be "all hands and feet." While this perception can be associated with multiple gestation, a posterior baby may give the same impression.
> *The mother may complain of urinary frequency even more than is usual for late pregnancy. This is due to the baby's forehead pressing against her bladder. This may even lead to a minor degree of urinary incontinence.
> *Fetal heart tones may be difficult to hear or may be faint. If you suspect posterior positioning, have the woman roll on the side and listen. If you can't hear the heart tones on one side, try the other.
> *While the breech may be easily distinguished in the fundus, it may be difficult to find the back, and the head may appear engaged.
> *Be particularly alert if you find the baby to be ROA. Babies that are ROA have a greater tendency to rotate to a posterior position than LOA babies. (El Halta, 1991)

If the baby is still posterior by the 36th week in first-time mothers or 37 weeks in multigravidas, one or more of the following suggestions (gathered from a variety of sources) may help:

> *I have often found posterior babies in women who tend to sleep on the same side every night. The baby's back is usually on the side the mother prefers for sleeping. Simply having her change sides can help. Also, having the mother prop one hip up with a pillow and bring her top leg over and up, flexing the knee, will move her pelvic joints around and help the baby to turn.
> *Have her do pelvic rocks (assume a hands-and-knees position, then arch the back slowly, flatten it out, then arch, repeat in several cycles). Pelvic rocks can be done for 10 minutes six to eight times daily until the baby turns. A variation on this exercise has the mother rock, crawl a few feet exaggerating her leg movements, then do another cycle of rocks.
> *Have the mother straddle an armless padded chair seat, so that she is facing its back. Now she should move her bottom back to the

edge of the seat, and lean forward so that her belly hangs down. She can rest her arms on the chair's back. Now, she should relax her abdominal muscles by taking deep, abdominal breaths. Recommend that she assume this position at least 4 to 6 times daily for 20 minutes. During the day, the mother should use this position to rest, rather than a reclining position.

*Have the mother lie on a slant board (as for a breech presentation) several times daily for 15 to 30 minutes at a time, as tolerated. (El Halta, 1991)

*Have the mother take warm baths and gently massage her belly and encourage her baby to "roll over." (El Halta, 1991)

*Alaskan midwives have found that babies assume a posterior position to keep their backs warm. Have the mother wrap a wool shawl around her belly to encourage the baby to turn (Marie, 1990).

*Have her visualize the baby turning face down (LOA) and talk to it about turning. (El Halta, 1991)

*Chiropractic adjustments can help correct any subtle pelvic misalignment that could be a contributing factor.

*The woman should avoid sitting with her bottom scrunched up in low-slung furniture or in bucket seats in cars with her knees flexed and higher than her hips. This constricts the pelvic inlet and discourages proper rotation as does crossing the legs. Upright, forward-leaning postures and those placing the hips higher than the knees are best as these all open the pelvic inlet. (Sutton, 1994)

*Regular exercise gets the joints of the pelvis moving and encourages anterior rotation.

*Use homeopathic Pulsatilla 30C or 200C in persistent cases or recommend the Webster chiropractic technique for rotating breech babies (see chapter on Ensuring a Vertex Presentation at Term).

If a woman has had a posterior labor or birth in the past, the baby has been posterior near term or has been persistently ROA, see the mother in early labor to determine the position of the baby. This will give you the opportunity to assist the rotation of the baby before active labor, when it can be much more difficult. (El Halta, 1991) How to deal with a posterior labor is addressed in Volume II.

References and further reading:
El Halta, V., "Posterior Labor—A Pain in the Back! Its Prevention and Cure," Special Delivery, Vol. 14, No. 3, Fall, 1991, pp. 3-4.

Marie, D., "Keep baby warm to turn babies," Midwifery Today, Nov. 16, 1990, No. 16, p. 10.

Scholles, Holly, conversation regarding posterior positioning, June 1995.

Sutton, J. Scott, P. "Optimal fetal positioning," MIDIRS, Vol. 4, No.3, Sept. 1994, p. 283-6.

The Onset of Normal Labor at Term

Usually, the first time you hear from a woman who might be in labor is by telephone. It is a good idea to instruct women to call you as soon as they think something is happening. This accomplishes two things: first, it allows you to know what may be going on, and you can plan your day accordingly. Second, it allows you the opportunity to help her figure out what may be happening, give her guidance for handling early labor, make decisions about calling people who intend to be at the birth, and so forth. What a drag it is to be out somewhere without your birth bag and suddenly get your first call from a woman in heavy labor who has been in light labor all day unbeknownst to you! The issues you must address are discussed in logical order below:

Is this really labor? Let her describe what she is feeling, then begin to ask her questions to try and figure out what might be going on. The three main signs of early labor are bloody show, contractions and rupture of membranes. True labor often begins at night, when the uterus is typically most active. Remember that prenatal toning contractions gradually build throughout pregnancy and then transform themselves into increasingly intense contractions which change the shape and dilation of the cervix and generally do not stop until the uterus returns to its pre-pregnancy size at about 6 weeks after birth. Birth is the crescendo of this process.

Typically, during the last month or so of pregnancy bouts of toning contractions come and go with intermittent sensations in the cervix and lower uterus. I detest the term "false labor" and it is, in fact, a misnomer. There is nothing false about the preparatory work of the uterus, and to call it that is a message to the woman that her body is working against her or playing tricks on her. It also lends credence to the myth that one is either in labor or not, and denies the gradual rhythmic process that is truly how the female body deals with all sexual and reproductive energies. To help you and the woman distinguish between the onset of labor and early or intense preparatory uterine activity:

PRELABOR OR PREPARATORY UTERINE ACTIVITY	LABOR WHICH WILL RESULT IN BIRTH
Uterine activity is intermittent and contractions vary in intensity.	Uterus settles into a regular, rhythmic pattern of activity which continues.
Pattern of uterine activity changes when the woman changes her activity.	Uterus keeps contracting regardless of maternal activity.
Contractions may remain regular for some time, but they do not build in intensity, and they taper off after a while.	Contractions remain regular and become increasingly stronger.

PRELABOR OR PREPARATORY UTERINE ACTIVITY	LABOR WHICH WILL RESULT IN BIRTH
Uterus feels firm or tight with contractions but not really painful (not always the case, but generally true).	Contractions and painful sensations are happening simultaneously. (The uterus may not feel hard during contractions in early labor.)
Sensations feel crampy, achy, sharp or shoot up from cervix, but are not perfectly coordinated with contractions.	With contractions, sensations feel like pulling up low down in front near pubic bone or rhythmic aching in lower back (a few women only feel labor in their lower back, hips, anus or down their thighs).
No bloody show in most cases.	Small amounts of mucus streaked with dark blood are passed, (up to 1 or 2 Tbsp.) as the contractions are changing the shape of the cervix and causing the mucus plug to release (especially true for primigravidas).
Contractions may last for several minutes at a time or may be of irregular duration.	Contractions begin to regulate; they are short at first and then gradually build in length and intensity; rarely do they exceed 60 seconds before 5 cm. dilation.
Upon internal exam, no cervical changes other than slight effacement, softening with occasional dilation of 1 to 2 cms. (sometimes more in multiparas), can be detected. *There are no detectable cervical changes when a contraction is occurring.*	Upon internal exam, the cervix can be felt responding to the contractions by becoming shorter, smoother, tighter and more dilated. It may be pulled posteriorly or anteriorly in the mother's pelvis (especially in primigravidas). If not dilated at all, tension in the cervix will still be apparent during contractions.
The amniotic membranes, if they can be reached, remain fluctuant during contractions.	The amniotic membranes, if they can be reached, become tense with contractions.
The membranes may rupture, releasing a quantity of clear or stained fluid.	The membranes remain intact.

Unless a woman has a cervical anomaly (as could happen in a DES daughter) it is uncommon for a first-time mother to have significant changes in her cervix without some fresh bloody show; that is red to dark red streaked mucus. (Brown streaked or pale pink show may be seen without significant changes.) If everything else is ambiguous, the presence or lack of fresh show in a primigravida may cinch your diagnosis. This is not necessarily so with women who have already had a baby; since their cervices will have opened before, they may have little show until later in labor or none at all.

Whenever you are trying to assess if a woman is in labor, also keep in mind that late pregnancy symptoms such as frequency of urination (from pressure on the bladder) and aches and pains in the back and lower pelvis can also be caused by a urinary tract infection as well as some other conditions. If you suspect such a problem, see the information on urinary tract infections in <u>Diagnostic Tests</u> and the separate chapter in this book on Urinary Tract Infections, as well as the chapter on Abdominal Pain in the section on Problems That Can Occur at any Time.

If you have determined that a woman is really not in labor yet and it is at night, reassure her that this is important work for her body to do to get ready for labor. Tell her to take a hot bath, even drink a glass of wine if necessary, and try to get some sleep. If it is during the day, do the same, but encourage her to do something which will distract her such as go to the movies or the zoo, take a walk or rent a video movie. It is important that she not sit around "watching her belly." Remind her that labor comes on gradually and that things could change at any time. Review the differences between preparatory uterine activity and labor. Have her call you if what is going on begins to look more like actual labor.

How strong is it? If you determine that a woman is probably in labor or if you still aren't sure, you next need to assess how active her labor is. One way to do so is to keep her on the phone during several contractions and listen to how she responds. Although she may tell you the contractions are strong, a woman in early labor will talk through them, giving little or no indication that anything is happening. More active labor will produce breathiness, halting speech or cause her to put the phone down. Notice the length of the contraction and for how long the fact that she is having one is obvious in her voice. Are there only a few seconds of breathiness in the midst of a very long contraction, or do the contractions build more quickly with the strong part lasting longer? A multipara who is responding to contractions may be in much more active labor than a primigravida responding the same way. With first time mothers you must also assess how anxious they are and whether they are overreacting to early labor. Sometimes this assessment is impossible to make on the phone, but attempt to do so.

Ask about bloody show or the passage of fluid, both of which usually indicate that active labor will begin within 24 hours. For first time mothers, remind them that this is very, very, very early labor (if it seems to be) and that they should ignore what is happening as much as possible. This will conserve psychological and physiological energy for the work that is ahead. Also remind first-timers to pace themselves for a 36 hour experience; that includes 24 hours of early labor and 12 hours of active labor. That way, if it is shorter, great, and if not, they will have conserved their energy accordingly. She should eat a high complex carbohydrate meal, drink at least 8 oz. of clear liquids every hour and get to bed early. (The process of labor will be discussed in Volume II. See the separate chapter on Rupture of Membranes Before the Onset of Labor in this section if necessary.) If the woman has given birth before, check your records to remind yourself how rapidly she had her last baby; you can usually count on a second labor to be half as long as the first, and others may be increasingly shorter. Assess when to go to her home by how long she is reporting uterine activity has been occurring; it may be time to leave! For multiparas in very early labor, it is

824

essential to remind them not to wait until the last minute to call you back, or you might miss the birth! Either way, plan on talking to the mother later in the day to note progress and decide what's next. If labor seems to be underway, you might remind the woman to start brewing the infusion for her herbal bath, if you use them in your practice. (more about the herbal bath can be found in Volume II of this text as well as Healing Passage.)

If she has a prenatal history of an ROA or posterior baby, or has a history of a previous posterior labor, you may want to pay her a visit sooner rather than later to assess the fetal position. How to deal with posterior positioning during labor is also covered in Volume II. (El Halta, 1991)

What if someone else calls for her? Occasionally a woman will have someone else call you on her behalf. Inevitably this results in a lack of adequate information on which to base your decision about what to do next or on what is happening. Always ask to speak directly to the woman so you can ask her the many specific questions you'll need to in order to make a judgement. If that is impossible (say they are calling from a pay phone or a neighbor's) have the person who called write down your questions and call you back with her response. If you know that someone will be calling for the woman, you might have a list of questions to give them at a prenatal visit to ensure that you will get the information you need.

References and further reading:

El Halta, Valerie, "Posterior Labor—A Pain in the Back! Its Prevention and Cure,"
    Special Delivery, Vol. 14, No. 3, Fall, 1991, pp. 3-4.

PROBLEMS ASSOCIATED WITH THE THIRD TRIMESTER

The problems discussed here can only occur toward the end of pregnancy or are most likely to manifest near the end; differential considerations are listed below. All others are discussed in the section on Problems That Can Occur at Any Time.

*Nausea and vomiting
-Toxemia
-Abdominal condition unrelated to pregnancy

*Toxemia
-Misinterpretation of secondary symptoms in a healthy woman
-Contracted blood volume and compromised liver function
-Medical condition superimposed upon the pregnancy

*Pendulous Abdomen

*Preterm labor
-Misinterpretation of normal uterine activity
-Loose cervix
-Infection

*Bleeding in the third trimester
-Cervical changes
-Aburption
-Placenta previa
-Uterine rupture
-Ruptured vasa previa

*Rupture of membranes before the onset of labor
-Yoni fluid not originating from the amnion
-Rupture of chorion with amnion intact
-Leakage of urine mistaken for amniotic fluid

*When the baby dies before birth

*Scar dehiscence and uterine rupture in the third trimester
-Abdominal condition unrelated to pregnancy
-Pregnancy-related bleeding and pain unrelated to scaring

*Postdatism and postmaturity syndrome
  -Inaccurate dates
  -Normal variation with a healthy fetus and mother
  -Problematic variation in an inadequately nourished mother

Nausea and Vomiting in the Third Trimester

Nausea and vomiting during the third trimester may be present as an ongoing problem from early on in pregnancy, however, third trimester complaints usually appear after a period of absence in those women who have also had these symptoms in early pregnancy. Occasionally a woman will feel nauseous from the increasing pressure a large baby puts on her digestive system. Suggest small, frequent meals, and review the remedies used for nausea in early pregnancy. Now is not the time for a woman to stop eating. Some other causes to consider include:

*The flu
*Kidney infection
*Toxemia (upper right quadrant pain may also be present; see the chapter on the Differential Diagnosis of Toxemia in <u>Diagnostic Tests</u> and the one on Toxemia in this section)
*Silent uterine rupture (see separate chapter, this section)
*Appendicitis
*Listeriosis
*Intestinal parasites (was there recent intake of possibly contaminated water, as might occur on a camping trip or missionaries in the field? Rule out Giardia)
*Food poisoning
*Abdominal pregnancy
*Cancer of the stomach or gall bladder

Toxemia

NOTE: The chapter entitled How Pregnancy Impacts Maternal Anatomy and Physiology covers why toxemia develops. This chapter covers detecting and dealing with toxemia.

The "classic symptoms" of toxemia are secondary indications only; just as everyone who has a headache doesn't have a brain tumor, every pregnant woman with high blood pressure, proteinuria and swelling doesn't have toxemia. If the diet is good and she feels great, a woman may have many signs of "pre-eclampsia" and be fine! Likewise, a woman may have a severely contracted blood volume and not have any classic "pre-eclamptic" signs except not feeling well (headaches, insomnia, nausea, etc.), a rising hemoglobin and a small fetus until she is *near death*. Remember, metabolic toxemia is a just that, a metabolic disorder resulting from liver malfunction and leading to a contracted blood volume. It is not a set of secondary symptoms alone. If a contracted blood volume is not present, she doesn't have metabolic toxemia.

Keep in mind that other disease conditions can mimic metabolic toxemia. It is easy to assume toxemia is the problem just because a woman is pregnant. This is especially true if her real condition has never been diagnosed. Lupus and various other conditions related to hypertension (see that chapter) can be causative. Seizures can be caused by other things as well. If you are unsure as to the origin of the problem refer women to a specialist for the organ system you suspect is involved for evaluation. Remember that bio-technical care providers do not acknowledge the etiology outlined here and consider all conditions producing the same secondary symptoms as pre-eclampsia, regardless of the underlying cause.

If things are going along smoothly, Betty Hosford, a CNM at the New Jersey School of Midwifery, has noted some clinical signs that suggest all is well:

*The hemoglobin at 28 weeks should be equal to what it was early in pregnancy (if it was borderline) or less than it was in early pregnancy (if it was above 12.5 gm.) It should NOT be rising unless she was very anemic at the beginning; and even with good therapeutic results, the value probably won't get above 11 to 12 grams. The hematocrit should also fall proportionately.

*A well-grown fetus equals a healthy placenta and expanded blood volume.

*Around 28 weeks (when blood volume peaks), a drop in blood pressure (as much as 12 points systolic and 10 points diastolic) may be indicative of blood volume expansion, although blood pressure is so influenced by emotional and activity-related stresses that it is not, by any means, conclusive.

*A weight gain of 5 to 10 pounds between 24 to 28 weeks is

encouraging and reflects an expanding blood volume.

*The presence of intermittent edema and distended veins suggest a well-expanding blood volume.

*Hyperreflexes may occur in any woman who is over excited, stressed or anxious during medical exams and can be a benign finding.

*Many women experience refractive visual disturbances from fluid changes brought about by an expanded blood volume, sometimes eye wear prescriptions must be changed during pregnancy to compensate.

*An absence of nausea, vomiting, upper right-quadrant pain, dizziness insomnia and headaches and a general sense of well-being characterize the well-nourished woman during pregnancy.

*Minor degrees of proteinuria (trace to +2) may occur during pregnancy and do not always indicate a problem. If readings are more than a trace in the otherwise well woman, increasing fluid intake can help dilute the urine and Nettle infusion can help strengthen the kidneys. Discharge from the yoni or urinary tract infection are other reasons protein may appear in the urine. (Read section of Protein under Urine Tests in *In Vitro* Reagent Tests.)

*A perfectly healthy woman may have excessive swelling and elevated blood pressure if she is losing salt via perspiration or needs more in her diet. Just two weeks of restricted salt intake causes a drop in blood volume. Increase salt and fluids and these symptoms will usually resolve. Leg cramps can also be symptomatic of inadequate salt intake.

The following are secondary signs of pre-eclamptic syndrome *usually* resulting from metabolic toxemia:

*Poor weight gain in a woman who was thin and underweight before pregnancy.

*Frequent headaches, black outs, feeling faint, and waking at night all indicate hypoglycemia and the need for more food.

*A rising hematocrit or hemoglobin from a normal baseline (12 to 13 grams); even if slight, this can spell trouble, as can a hemoglobin that is remaining at 13 gm. or higher, especially without intensive supplementation (unless the woman lives at a high altitude.)

*A plateau in fetal growth or a consistently small-for-dates size from 22 weeks on. Often a slightly small fetus (and correspondingly small fundal height) is your first tip that a woman is not getting enough food to meet her nutritional needs (this will be confirmed by a rising or stable hemoglobin). Dietary improvement can result in marked fetal growth and a hemoglobin drop in just 1 week.

*No change or a slight rise in blood pressure mid-pregnancy. Again, consider all possible variables that may affect blood pressure; blood pressure is a poor criteria to use alone. When significant blood pressure changes occur, they often do not present until a contracted blood volume is well established. (See chapter on Hypertension in Pregnancy, general problems section.)

*Diminished urinary output; this occurs as the lack of adequate blood volume becomes more critical and the body tries to retain fluids.

*Proteinuria; this shows up as toxemia becomes most severe, not in the early stages. The majority of proteinuria in pregnancy is related to contamination from vaginal discharge, urinary tract infection or is benign. If proteinuria does appear in toxemia, the kidneys are being severely stressed.

*No change in weight from 24 to 28 weeks with a sudden gain in the 3rd trimester. (Of course, if you stress the need for increasing dietary intake, and a woman really starts to eat, such a sudden gain may indicate that her blood volume is finally increasing.)

*Persistent edema that does not vary with time of day or activity. If edema is pathologic, the veins will not be distended because more fluid is in the tissues than the circulation. Also, the swelling may be more uniform throughout the body, not in the extremities alone.

*Serum albumin level below 3. (A value of 4 is ideal, but it may range between 3 and 4 in a woman with a well-expanded blood volume).

*Elevated liver enzymes. Some elevation of alkaline phosphatase is normal due to the fact that the placenta produces this enzyme and liver enzymes may be slightly elevated with intrahepatic cholestasis. (See chapter on The Liver and Pregnancy in Diagnostic Tests.)

*Lymphocytes below 15%

*A drop in the platelet count caused by a contracted blood volume that leads to aggregation of platelets.

*Blurred vision from blood vessel alterations usually associated with high blood pressure; a sign of severe compromise.

*Upper right-quadrant pain, nausea, vomiting and a general unwell feeling; these are secondary symptoms of severe liver compromise and an overload of placental hormones and toxic digestive byproducts which the liver is not metabolizing efficiently.

*Hyperreflexes as the nervous system becomes increasingly irritated by vasospasm; they may indicate impending convulsions.

Never draw a conclusion based on secondary symptoms alone, regardless of what they may be.

Early warning signs: I repeat, *the earliest clinical sign of a real problem is often a stable or rising hemoglobin/hematocrit (and possibly RBC count) which occurs as the blood volume begins to contract.* Early on, this will be *accompanied by a minor degree of small-for-dates fetal growth.* At this point, usually be between 22 to 29 weeks, the mother may still feel fairly well. This is one good reason to begin careful abdominal palpation from the onset of care and to become good at estimating early fetal growth with your hands. The liver is not severely compromised at this point, but it is inadequately supplied with nutrients. If you do a Liver profile now, liver enzymes will likely be normal. After a few weeks, subclinical liver compromise will often be evident in a Liver profile test; reflected in either rising enzymes levels or falling blood protein levels or both. Kidney function tests will not become abnormal until other lab work has been abnormal for a while, since kidney compromise usually commences *after* the blood volume contraction is well underway. If you have any doubt, always run a Liver profile test and check the hemoglobin. If problems are identified at this stage and diligent attention is paid to increasing protein and other nutrients, the hemoglobin will start to drop rapidly and fetal growth will improve, reflecting that the blood volume is beginning to expand. If you do not catch it at this point, symptoms will worsen, but may not necessarily include high blood pressure or proteinuria. You must be alert, keeping in mind the underlying physiology of toxemia, not just the secondary symptom picture.

Whenever you have a question about whether a woman is toxemic, check the hemoglobin. It is your earliest and most sensitive gauge of well-being. If it has dropped, the fetus is a normal size-for-dates, and the woman feels well, you can rule out toxemia with no further investigation, especially if the woman's diet is adequate. If you are still unsure about this or feel you need further documentation, order a liver profile (called a chem screen or panel or an SMA in some areas) and pay particular attention to albumin and liver enzyme levels.

When toxemia is suspected: If you suspect a problem or if a back-up practitioner suspects toxemia and you need more concrete, medically acceptable data to present in favor of health, take the following steps:

*Review the diet and make any necessary changes.
*Assess and discuss possible psychological issues that may prevent a
    mother from eating or feeling good about weight gain (for example
    not really wanting to be pregnant, or a past history of anorexia).
*Assess absorption of nutrients (are indigestion, allergies, diarrhea, or
    or other digestive upsets present?)
*Be sure calories and protein are adequate in light of the woman's
    stress and activity levels. A diet which is not adequate in both
    protein and calories leaves mother and baby severely compromised.
    Brewer has found that when a woman eats one-third less calories

than she needs for her energy output, half of the protein she eats will be burned for calories. This may leave a woman at risk for an inadequately expanded blood volume even though she makes high quality dietary choices. For example, a 1500 calorie diet with 90 grams of protein is one-third below the RDA figure of 2400 calories for pregnancy, and would only provide 45 grams of protein for building fetal tissues and for blood volume expansion.

*Encourage women to drink to a healthy thirst, (six to eight glasses of clear fluids daily) but don't overdo it. Forcing large quantities of fluids will cause diuresis and will dilute the blood stream without the benefits of the needed albumin, as well as skew lab results, thus confusing the clinical picture. Any necessary diuresis will occur naturally when the blood volume begins to normalize.

*Assist the woman in using all resources (such as WIC and food stamps,) to obtain the foods she needs.

Differentially diagnose secondary symptoms to be sure it is metabolic toxemia. (Renal or neurological problems, certain tumors, lead poisoning and, *very* rarely, autoimmune reactions or other conditions may produce similar symptoms.)

You should be seeing a drop in hemoglobin/hematocrit from the 12 week value (unless you were using herbal therapies to correct a low hemoglobin) and liver profile results for normal pregnancy (serum proteins may be slightly low/normal with good blood volume expansion—as long as everything else looks good this is okay). You may see a slight drop in the red cell count. If all lab results are negative and you still have concerning symptoms, have a specialist evaluate for the suspected problem (for example, with the kidneys, etc.).

If you feel some degree of true toxemia exists, the most important thing is to provide the system with enough fluid and nutrients to try to make up for lost time; *focus on protein, nutrient rich calories, fluids and adequate salt.* Different midwives have different approaches: lots of eggs, a whole stewed chicken with vegetables, super high-potency protein drinks; anything that appeals to the mother is fine! Have the mother eat a high protein item every waking hour. Initially recommend an increase to 150 to 250 grams of protein daily (250 to 350 grams or more with multiple gestations), with 3000 to 4000 calories and 500 mg of choline daily. Increase calcium to 1200 mg and magnesium to 400 to 600 mg daily. What you actually recommend will depend upon lab results, whether it is a multiple gestation, and the symptom picture when you detect the problem; the worse the picture, the more protein and calories you should recommend. You want to give the liver enough raw materials to make up for a long-standing lack as rapidly as possible. The placenta continues to grow throughout pregnancy, and any improvement can make a big difference in the health of mother and baby. An inadequate increase may allow the liver to maintain things so that symptoms do not worsen, but not offer sufficient amino acids to turn the situation around. (If the woman has a history of liver disorders, recommend less protein [120-150 grams for a single fetus] her liver may be overwhelmed otherwise and monitor her lab work closely for changes.) Recheck lab tests four to seven days later. Don't wait any longer, if what you are suggesting is not making a difference, you need to know. Often, women feel an immediate and profoundly increased sense of well-being. If the second lab report shows some improvement, keep up the high protein intake until all values are where they should be for her gestation. Recheck again four to six days later; if the third lab result shows no change, increase the protein. Keeping the protein intake this high for several weeks will have no adverse effects in a woman with a normal liver. Once liver enzymes and blood proteins have normalized, the hemoglobin has dropped appropriately, the fetus is an appropriate size-for-dates and secondary symptoms have subsided, the woman can cut back to 100 grams of protein daily (150 or more with multiples). At this point, she has caught up with her deficiencies and needs to maintain liver support so she doesn't get sick again. If nothing you are doing is helping, actively search for other causes, especially if symptoms are worsening.

If left untreated these women are at risk for large-scale complications. It is important that they understand the gravity of the situation, that they feel personally responsible and able to improve their condition, and that they are willing to work closely with you. Unfortunately, even if a woman is in very serious condition, standard hospital treatment is likely to aggravate the situation. Hopefully, you can get the collaborating practitioner to read Gail Brewer's book, The Brewer Medical Diet (out of print, but her new book, The Very Important Pregnancy Book, has the same information) and Tom Brewer's Metabolic Toxemia of Late Pregnancy. Call Tom Brewer to help outline a beneficial therapy in or out of the hospital at his toxemia hot line: (802) 388-0276, 50 Buttolph Dr., #201, Middlebury, VT 05753.

Caring for women living at high altitudes: The oxygen content of the air is reduced the higher up you go, so women above 5,000 feet elevation will respond to the reduction in oxygen concentration with generally higher hemoglobin levels that remain high throughout pregnancy. If the mother does not start pregnancy in an anemic state, the approximate hemoglobin changes you should see follow:

ALTITUDE	EXPECTED HEMOGLOBIN DROP BY 28 TO 30 WEEKS
Less than 5,000 feet	2 grams
5,000 to 8,000 feet	1 to 1.5 grams
Over 8,000 feet	Slight drop or none at all

The higher the altitude, the more you must rely on liver profile results, especially albumin levels and liver enzyme values, to monitor for adequate blood volume expansion. (Braun, 1994) This means you may miss a very early problem based on lab work alone. When liver enzymes start to rise, you have no time to waste in beginning dietary adjustment, but it is still not too late.

Acute blood volume contraction: A rapid reduction of a normally expanded blood volume can occur if the woman experiences a drop in dietary intake or a sudden rise in her stress and activity level. Often these factors accompany each other. It will usually take about 2 weeks until such a drop becomes severe enough to manifest symptoms; however, if the woman is carrying a multiple gestation, the drop may be very rapid and quickly lead to secondary symptoms and liver compromise.

Interpreting lab work: Laboratory testing can go a long way in helping you differentiate benign secondary symptoms which suggest toxemia from red flag secondary symptoms pointing to metabolic derangement. The variety of secondary symptoms and the timing of when they appear during the course of worsening blood volume contraction will vary among women and the same can be said for lab values. While in most cases the astute clinician can troubleshoot the problem and turn it around before full-blown secondary symptoms are evident, it will be useful for you to understand how different secondary symptoms are reflected in lab results (see following chart). Note that liver enzymes remain in a normal nonpregnant range in healthy women with the exception of Alkaline Phosphatase. This is elevated during pregnancy because it is produced by the placenta; in healthy women carrying one fetus, it may rise as much as 2 times over her nonpregnant normal range; in multiple gestation it may rise even higher. (Hellman & Pritchard, 1971) Also remember that values for an individual that are fine may fall outside "normal" ranges. While I want you to understand how toxemia may be reflected in lab values, the tests provide adjunctive information only and should never take precedence over your clinical impression of health. The mother's sense of well-being and fetal growth are the *most important* factors, regardless of what the tests may indicate. Keep in mind that women often do not realize they feel un-well until the begin to feel better, so explore how she feels carefully and in detail if lab results are questionable.

Emotional issues: There are always emotional and psychological factors related to any physical condition. Talk to the woman about her specific worries and stresses, which are as much a part of the picture as her lack of adequate dietary intake. Helping her work through her emotional issues will go along way to reducing her inner level of tension and clearing the way for the symptom picture to resolve.

This chart is designed to give you an idea of how toxemia may progress in the normal, nonanemic woman. Anemia can mask blood volume contraction; you must be alert to the normal response to supplements during pregnancy (see Diagnostic Tests).

DEGREE OF TOXEMIA	HEMOGLOBIN	LIVER ENZYMES	BLOOD PROTEINS	URINALYSIS	URIC ACID	BUN & CREATININE	FIBRINOGEN	PLATELETS	ASSOCIATED SECONDARY SIGNS & SYMPTOMS
Mild	Minimal or no change for dates	Alk. Phos. normally elev. others normal	Normal	Protein: Negative	Normal	Normal-low	Normal	Normal	Baby small-for-dates, mother basically feels well
Moderate	Slightly elevated for dates	High	Normal to slightly low	Protein: Negative	Normal	Normal-low	Normal	Normal	May have insomnia, increased swelling, poor weight gain for dates, blood pressure elevation; may feel vaguely unwell
Severe	Elevated for dates	High	Low	Protein: Negative Urine may be concentrated, output may be diminishing	Normal to slightly elevated	Normal-low	May be rising	May be low	Same plus headaches, marked swelling, increased spurts of weight gain (fluid retention), elevated blood pressure & hyperreflexia (in some), liver pain
Crisis (close to death)	Elevated for dates	Alk. Phos. ↑ 3 X normal others very high	Very low	Protein: Neg. to +3 Urine may be concentrated, Casts & cells may be found	3 X normal	Normal-low	2 X normal	May be low	Same plus visual disturbances, diminished urinary output, twitches, leading to convulsions, coma & possible death of mother & baby

A review of cases: The medical model asserts that toxemia is a disease of unknown origin.   Tom Brewer has given us the most complete understanding of the pathophysiology of toxemia to date and no other treatment plan works so consistently as his.   Even so, our knowledge of this subject is rudimentary at best, due to the lack of interest in the nutritional factor by researchers world-wide. Because it is almost impossible to find information detailing how toxemia can truly be reversed, I thought it would be helpful to present some case histories from my own files and one from the file of a midwife with whom I worked closely to demonstrate how women have been treated and gone on to have healthy pregnancies.

Case 1:   Maria was a 32 year old multipara of Mexican descent who was in the United States illegally.   She was not literate in English, so no written diet diary was submitted.   She described a history of vomiting 2 to 3 times weekly, frequent headaches, depression from being away from her home and a dietary pattern which included long periods between meals, inadequate intake and lots of processed foods throughout pregnancy.   At her first prenatal visit she was in her 37th week of pregnancy with a fundal height of 32 cm; the baby also felt small-for-dates.   Also noted was swelling in her hands and feet, +2 reflexes, and a blood pressure of 110/70.   I recommended that she eat every 2 hours and when she woke up during the night.   I encouraged her to increase her intake and to eat her traditional Mexican diet of beans, rice, meat, corn tortillas, cornbread, milk and greens.

At her next appointment 9 days later her fundal height was 37 cm; she had no swelling, headaches, dizziness or vomiting.   There was an obvious, dramatic increase in fetal size and she reported that the baby was more active.   She was eating at night, had increased her overall dietary quantity and frequency of intake, and making better food choices as recommended.   She carried to term and her newborn weighed 8 pounds, 8 ounces.   No tests were done as the situation had clearly been turned around.   No ultrasounds needed for intrauterine growth retardation, just good foods!

Case 2:   At 9 weeks of pregnancy Lynn presented the following dietary history:

Day 1	Ovo-lacto veg. Checklist
Orange juice w/nutritional yeast	Milk (4) 4*
Yogurt w/cottage cheese, **raisins** & bran	Eggs (2) 2
1 boiled potato	Protein (6) 1 1/8
2 boiled eggs	Dark greens (2) 1½
Water	Grains, starchy veg./fruits (5) 5¼ 1/3
Apple, nuts & **raisins**	Vit. C foods (3) 3½
Large salad w/lettuce, tomato & carrot	Vit. A foods (2) 0
Cottage cheese	Fats & oils (5) 0
Water	Iron rich food (5 daily) 2
Brown rice w/tomato sauce & mozzarella	

Day 2	Ovo-Lacto Veg. Checklist
Cream of wheat w/whole milk, bran, wheat germ, oats, oat bran, **honey & molasses**	Milk (4) 2½
Spinach	Eggs (2) 1
A little plain yogurt, **raisins** & rst. soybeans	Protein (6) 3 ½ 1/8
Water	Dark greens (2) 1½
Whole wheat pasta w/tomato sauce & broccoli w/mozzarella	Grains, starchy veg./fruits (5) 6½
4 oatmeal cookies	Vit. C foods (3) 2
Chicken soup w/carrots, spinach, tofu	Vit. A foods (2) ½
1 egg	Fats & oils (5) 0
1 **orange**	Iron rich foods (5 daily) ½
A little plain yogurt w/**raisins**	

*Portions needed in ( ), right-hand # is portions eaten today. Sweet foods are highlighted; and indicate the need for more protein or calorie intake.

As you can see, her food choices were basically good ones, but she needed more in almost every category, especially calories, green vegetables and protein.

At 9 weeks of pregnancy her hemoglobin was 12.5; she was walking 3 miles twice daily. Her pre-pregnancy weight was 102. She perfectly fit the description of the slim active woman with a high metabolism. This is a typical case where the care provider may dismiss diet as a problem because the diet is basically good; however Lynn's intake proved inadequate to meet her needs, as the following highlights from her prenatal care demonstrate. Note the weight gain spurt which occurred after she altered her diet and exercise level. Lynn birthed at 39 weeks of pregnancy and her baby weighed 7 pounds, 5 ounces.

Weeks of pregnancy	Fundal Height	Weight gain	Comments
17	17 cm.	110	
21	20 cm.	115	
25	23 cm.	120	
28	24 cm.	120	Hemoglobin 13 grams; baby felt small. Recommended an increase in calories & protein & to reduce walking to 1 mile daily.
32	28 cm.	128	Fetus showed significant growth. (Note weight gain spurt.)
34	30 cm.	129	Fetal growth maintaining itself, mother eating well, exercising much less.
34½	32 cm.	130	
35½	35 cm.	130	
36	34 cm.	130	

Case 3: Kathy was a multipara, 5'5" tall with a pre-pregnancy weight of 250 pounds. At her initial exam, she presented 6 days of omnivorous diet diaries from which I have extracted the following two days as representative of her intake. From the diet diaries, you will see that her protein intake was sporadic and usually inadequate. She completely neglected some food categories and has an inadequate intake of protein, greens and vitamin A rich foods. Even though she was somewhat overweight, I did not recommend that she forgo eating fats and oils completely; these foods not only provide the precursors for hormone production, but also provide calories which spare the protein intake for the needs of the pregnancy. Note on Day 2, when she ate no eggs or milk products, she ate many sweet foods instead.

1 Day diet History	Checklist
½ cup Shredded wheat w/1 T. **Maple syrup**	Milk (4) 2
1 cup Coffee	Eggs (2) 0
1 cup Milk	Protein (6) 7
1 Burrito with cheese	Dark Greens (2) 1
1 Chicken soft taco	Grains, starchy veg./fruits (5) 6
1 **Apple**	Vit. C foods (2) 0
2 16 oz. Flavored carbonated water	Vit. A foods (1) 0
1 cup water	Fats & oils (2) 1
2 Onion buns	Iron rich food (4 oz. weekly) 0
3 Fish fillets	
1 T mayonnaise 1 T catsup	
½ tsp. mustard	
½ cup Green beans	

Day 2 diet History	Checklist
6 oz. Coffee	Milk (4) 0
4 cups water	Eggs (2) 0
1 cup Polenta w/1 t. butter	Protein (6) 5 1/7
& 2 T **Maple syrup**	Dark Greens (2) 1
1 dried **fig**	Grains, starchy veg./fruits (5) 4 3/4
1 **apple**	Vit. C foods (2) 4½
1½ cups **Raspberry juice** (no sugar)	Vit. A foods (1) 0
1 Nonfat tofu dog	Fats & oils (2) 1
1 **Kiwi** fruit	Iron rich food (4 oz. weekly) 0
1 6" Whole wheat tortilla	
5 oz. Black cod fish	
2 cups Salad (Lettuce, tomato,	
cucumber, mushroom, zucchini)	
2 t. Tartar sauce	
16 oz. Perrier water	

Day 3 diet History	Checklist
2 cups shredded wheat, 2 tsp. **Maple syrup**	Milk (4) 12/3
1 cup milk	Eggs (2) 0
1 cup Oolong tea	Protein (6) 1½
2 cups Vegetable noodles	Dark Greens (2) 1
1 cup Beef broth	Grains, starchy veg./fruits (5) 5
3/4 cup Green beans	Vit. C foods (2) 0
2 T Parmesan Cheese	Vit. A foods (1) 0
3 pieces Whole wheat French toast	Fats & oils (2) 0
4 T **Maple Syrup**	Iron rich food (4 oz. weekly) 0
1 Carrot	
16 oz. Flavored carbonated water	

Kathy has two other children, the first weighed 8 lbs. 8 oz. and the second weighed 9 lb. 10 oz. at birth. Although she was told she had borderline gestational diabetes with both previous pregnancies, no dietary changes or restrictions were advised. She had no prior history of toxemia. Her fundal height measured large-for-dates with both pregnancies. She had a history of urinary tract infections and of irritable bowel syndrome, which was in remission during this pregnancy. This pregnancy was an unplanned surprise. Her recent history included Cat Scratch disease (resolved before the onset of care), during which she lost 20 pounds.

The following record summarizes pertinent findings from Kathy's prenatal records.

At 35.2 weeks the primary midwife called me for a consultation. I noted that Kathy's initial lab work showed a hemoglobin of 13.1, which only dropped two-tenths of a gram by 26 weeks; this was my first clue that her problems were likely to be related to a contracted blood volume, not kidney compromise. This, coupled with her stress level, dietary history, weight loss with a lack of any significant gain, and sporadically poor appetite; were all factors which often pointed to toxemia. Note that she didn't have a weight gain spurt between 24 and 28 weeks, which often signals the increase in blood volume which occurs at that time. Even though her fundal height measured large-for-dates, the midwife reported that the baby had recently begun to feel small to her on palpation and that fetal size had previously been hard to evaluate because of Kathy's weight. This is an important distinction to make for fundal height can be influenced by a variety of factors (see separate chapter on Measuring the Fundal Height, Skills section). Increasingly problematic right-sided back pain suggestive of kidney problems (but with no CVA tenderness and negative UA) also suggested referred pain from her liver. This midwife understood the importance of adequate nutrition, but like so many others, she missed significant clues because she thought the woman was "basically eating well." Note that the midwife had even recommended supplemental protein at the 12 week visit.

WKS PREG.	WEIGHT	BLOOD PRESSURE	URINE ANALYSIS	FUNDAL HEIGHT	COMMENTS
6.5	250	102/62	Neg.	N/A	Hemoglobin 13.1 (7 weeks), nausea w/morning sickness
12.1	245	100/62	Neg./dark	19	Occasional nausea, energy & appetite poor; rec. 15-30 gms. protein powder as a dietary supplement daily & 2 Tbsp. chlorophyll daily
15.1	245	110/62	Neg/light	19	Her father in process of dying, her home was broken into; reports she is eating well (diet diary not rechecked); fleeting FHT heard w/fetascope; taking protein powder
19.1	246	118/70	Negative	22	Father doing better, stress reduced; eating lots of small meals (diet history not rechecked); baby hard to palpate due to weight of mother; relying on fundal ht. for appropriate fetal size
22.2	245	110/70	Negative	23	Baby heard w/fetascope (previously listening w/Doppler)
26.2	246	110/68	Trace ketones	29	Freq. urination w/slight burning; Possible UTI, rec. Cranberry juice; told to eat more frequently, poor appetite; Hemo. 12.9
27.6	247				Visit to check on report that fetal movement is low, rec. kick chart, fetal heart tones show normal range & variability; no urinary problems
28.4	246	110/78	Clear Yellow Negative	30	Baby very active; slight pitting edema (rec. Red Clover tea for edema)
31.1	246	110/68	Trace glucose	32	2-hr. post-prandial GTT 112 gm.
33.1	248	110/70	Negative	35	Suspected breech presentation; appt. for ultrasound scheduled; baby easier to palpate & feels small-for-dates
34.3					Difficulty urinating, diminished output, pain in upper back on right (no CVA tenderness); diminished fluid intake; rec. increase fluids & Burdock inf.; at 34.6 weeks rec. Dr. consult (on-call Dr. ordered a Urinalysis on phone consult; he did not examine her—UA neg.)
35	247	120/80	Negative	38	Slight pitting edema, hands swelling, blood pressure 100/70 on recheck; Hemo. 12.6; difficulty urinating, symptoms as above worsening
35.1					After 24 hrs. on Burdock Rt & Echinecea tincture w/no improvement, rec. consult w/her Dr. (an internist) who did no tests & no exam & suggested her difficult urination was because the baby was low in her pelvis; he was unconcerned about her back pain
35.2			Dark yellow		Diminished urinary output continuing; ordered Chem. screen

Both consulting doctors dismissed her complaints as minor because none of these providers knew how to link-up the secondary symptoms to the laboratory evidence indicating that her blood volume was reduced. The midwife had only offered palliative relief for the edema with herbs and had advised other herbs for suspected urinary tract infection. In the presence of a truly contracted blood volume, recommending diuretic herbs may actually aggravate the fluid imbalance already underway. Her test results were as follows:

LABORATORY FINDING:	NORMAL RANGE:	WEEKS OF PREGNANCY							
		7	26	35.2	35.6	36.4	37	38.1	39
Hemoglobin	11-12 past 28 wks.	13.1	12.9	12.6	11.9	12.1	11.8*	12.5*	12.4
BUN	10 to 25 mg.			7	16	15			12
Creatinine	< 1 mg.			0.5	0.5	0.5			0.5
Uric acid	2.5 to 8.5			5.9	5.4	6.3			5.7
Albumin	3.5 to 5 gm.			3.5	3.6	3.6			3.4
Total protein	6 to 8.5 gm/dl.			6.1	6.2	6.4			5.9
SGOT	5 to 40 IU/liter			46	20	16			11
SGPT	5 to 55 IU/liter			79	58	26			7
Alkaline Phosphatase	non-preg. 22 to 99 IU/L ↑ 184 in preg.			128	123	117			128
Platelets	150-440 Th/cmm.	259	233	203	224	245			183
Urine analysis	negative	neg.	neg.	Neg.	Neg.	Neg.			Neg.

Lab results at 35.2 weeks: Kathy's test results reflect an inadequately expanded blood volume with a hemoglobin level of 12.6. Note that her urine tests are normal, indicating kidney function is not yet compromised; it is further evidence that her symptoms are related to a lack of blood volume, not a primary abnormality of the kidneys. Her liver enzymes are clearly elevated, indicating liver stress. Blood proteins are borderline, but may in fact be artificially elevated due to the blood volume contraction which exists. I recommended that she immediately begin to eat 250 grams of protein and 3000 calories daily, take 500 mg. of choline daily along with a B-complex supplement, that she increase her fluid intake and that laboratory tests be redone in a week. Her salt intake was determined to be adequate. Within 12 hours of beginning this program, Kathy began to urinate normally; in fact she started to diureses (swelling began to reduce but never completely disappeared). Her overall sense of well-being also immediately improved, with increased energy and better sleeping patterns; the midwife noted she looked better with better skin color. These deceptively minor symptoms were immediately obvious when she began to get adequate nourishment.

Wks Preg.	Weight	Blood Pressure	Urine Analysis	Fundal Height	Comments (Refer to Table of Lab Results)
35.6	254	118/70	Neg.		The diagnosis of borderline clinical toxemia was confirmed, as lab results showed a dramatic reduction in her liver enzyme levels and a fall in her hemoglobin as nutrition improved. Weight gain reflects recent blood volume expansion. Fetus felt significantly larger on palpation. Because SGPT/SGOT levels were still elevated, I rec. continuing 250 grams of protein & 3000 calories daily at this point.
36.4		105/80	Neg.		A 0.2 gram rise in her hemoglobin was not alarming (some normal variation will occur from day to day). Other results showed a continuing resolution of liver stress.
37	258	110/78	Neg.	39	A further drop in her hemoglobin prompted me to recommend reducing protein intake to 150 gm. daily
38.1	258	110/78	Neg.	38	Just ran out of protein powder (on her way to get more), edema slightly increased.
39	260				
40	262	112/72	Neg.	41	Baby feels 8-8½ lbs.

Kathy started labor spontaneously at 41.1 weeks of pregnancy. At that time she weighed 264 pounds and her fundal height was 43 cm. At the initial labor check her blood pressure was 120/80 and in active labor it was 130/90. She birthed a healthy 9 lb. 8 oz. baby.

While this is only one example, Kathy's case study is important for several reasons. First, she is not a primigravida. Secondly she had a slow build-up of secondary signs and symptoms, which were not alarming to her midwife because they were not severe and not any of the "big three" secondary symptoms of proteinuria, high blood pressure and rapid weight gain. Despite numerous indications (including negative lab tests) to the contrary, her midwife and two collaborating physicians persisted in ascribing her symptoms to kidney malfunction. Her blood pressure was essentially normal, although other physiologic adaptations were taking place to compensate for the lack of blood volume expansion she was experiencing. Problems with fetal growth were obscured by the fact that her fundal height was large-for-dates. The clue that exposed the real problem was the hemoglobin at 26.2 weeks, which did not reflect adequate expansion; with this in mind the entire symptom picture fell into place. This problem could have been caught at 26.2 weeks if it had been recognized as the start of toxemia. Only by understanding the underlying pathophysiology of blood volume contraction was this so apparent. Finally, abundant laboratory evidence corroborated not only the diagnosis but the effectiveness of treatment. Why was the midwife not concerned about toxemia during labor? Because it was clear that the toxemia had been resolved. The midwife involved says she learned a great deal from this experience. Kathy could have easily wound up in the hospital seriously ill if this had not been caught in time. Encouragingly, even with rapidly escalating oliguria, her condition began to reverse within 12 hours after the onset of therapy addressing the real problem.

A few suggestions for increasing protein and calorie intake: When large quantities of protein are necessary, protein drinks are one of the best ways to go. For example, here are just a few suggestions of what can be added to protein drinks made with prepared protein powder and milk to boost their protein and calorie content:

FOOD	CALORIES	PROTEIN
Instant non-fat dry milk powder (1/3 cup dry)	81	8 grams
Oil (1 Tbsp.)	120	none
Banana	105	1.1 grams
Whole raw egg	79	6 grams

For reference and further reading:

Braun, Jennifer, Colorado lisenced midwife, personal communication, 1994.
Brewer, Tom, Metabolic Toxemia of Late Pregnancy, Keats Pub., New Canaan, CT, 1982.
Hellman, L, & Pritchard, J. Williams Obstetrics, 14th ed., Appleton-Century-Crofts, NY, 1971.
Hosford, Betty, CNM, workshop on Nutrition during Pregnancy presented at the National MANA conference, New Orleans, LA, October, 1989.
James, Dawn, "New Thoughts About Pre-eclampsia," presentation 9/15/89, Royal College of Medicine, London Eng. President, Pre-eclamptic Toxemia Society, Ty Iago, Carmel, Caernarvon, Gwynedd, LL54 7AB, Wales, England.
Jones, Joy, "Brewer Pregnancy Diet," in Rothman, Barbara Katz, ed. Encyclopedia of Childbirth: Critical Perspectives, Oryx Press, Phoenix, AZ, 1993.
Sala, J. & Lentz, J., "Pregnant women with systemic lupus erythematosus," MCN, Nov/Dec 1986, Vol. 11, No. 6, p. 387.
Shanklin, D. & Hodin, J., Maternal Nutrition and Child Health, Charles C. Thomas, Pub., Springfield, IL, 1979.

Pendulous Abdomen

Pendulous abdomen is typically seen in women who have had several babies and whose abdominal muscles are very lax due to lack of appropriate postpartum exercise. Less common causes are:

*Defective abdominal muscles
*Contracted pelvis
*Increased forward inclination of the pelvis
*Various types of curvature of the spine (scoliosis)
*Multiple gestation
*Polyhydramnios
*Tumors

During subsequent pregnancies as the uterus enlarges and rises up out of the pelvis more and more, the abdominal muscles are not strong enough to hold it up and in place; it falls forward instead. The pendulous abdomen can pose several problems during pregnancy. It flops forward, straining the uterine ligaments, causing the abdominal muscles to undergo more stress. There may be a sense of weight and distention as well as dragging pains in the thighs, abdomen and rectum, chafing of the lower abdomen and thighs, and occasionally varicosities and edema of the vulva develop due to impeded circulation. Back pain may be severe as the uterine ligaments are pulled forward from the lower spinal area. A pendulous abdomen causes the baby's presenting part to be lifted up and over the pubic bone, eventually hampering engagement or descent, especially during labor. The risk of cord prolapse is greater upon rupture of membranes due to the fact that no fetal part is really filling the pelvis.

A pendulous abdomen is easy to spot: it looks like the equivalent of an exaggerated beer belly, with the fundus well in front of the pubic bone. It is most apparent when the woman is standing. The best remedy for this, once pregnancy is underway, is to bind the abdomen. Pregnancy corsets are one solution, and a woman with a serious problem may wish to try one on to see if that is what she wants to use. A good one should provide support from the bottom up. There are basically three items on the market which deal with this problem. For those with a small amount of abdominal prolapse Loving Lift, Action Lift and Baby Hugger provide elastic belly supports which criss-cross in the back and support from below. Others include the Reenie maternity belt by Leading Lady, (about $17.00 in 1994). These products offer good support and will meet the needs of the majority of women. A complete body suit which offers support from the shoulders is made by Mary Jane and is called Glorious ($37.50). It has the disadvantage of being difficult to use because it is one piece and requires disrobing for using the toilet. Jeunique Natal support also offers intermediate support. Finally, for the most severe situations, there is a corset made by Contour Form which runs $120.00.

It has stays and laces to provide maximum back and belly support for the grand multipara. It may be worth the investment if she plans to have more children. (Check your local phone directory for a corset shop.) Be sure to check fetal position carefully, you don't want better support to prevent a breech from turning!

An old sheet, a strip of muslin or a 6" Ace bandage can also be used to make a binder. Turn to the chapter on Cultural preferences, Contact section, and follow the directions for Japanese belly binding, wrapping it tightly. It might be a good idea to have the woman lay down and use her hands to support her belly; then she should stand, continuing to support her belly from below while another person starts to wrap her belly for her. She may even find it more comfortable to bind her belly when she sleeps. The belly binder can be worn throughout labor as well.

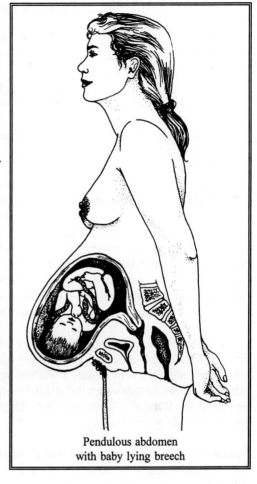

Pendulous abdomen
with baby lying breech

References and further reading:

Greenhill, J., <u>Principles and Practice of Obstetrics</u>, W. B. Saunders, Co., Philadelphia, PA, 1951.

Preterm Labor

Once a mother is past 24 to 25 weeks of pregnancy, a threatened miscarriage is redefined as preterm labor. Premature labor is the onset of uterine activity which causes cervical changes that may lead to the birth of an immature fetus; it is usually considered to be before the 36th or 37th completed week of pregnancy, depending upon who you talk to. There are two basic ways that preterm labor can present:

*The onset of symptoms suggesting that a woman is moving towards
   true labor and birth of an immature infant
*Preterm rupture of membranes

Physiological considerations: The reasons underlying the onset of preterm labor are somewhat different than those associated with miscarriage, although some factors do pertain to both complications. Chief among these reasons is inadequate maternal nutrition. Remember this means not getting enough of what's needed even if the food choices are basically good ones. Poor nutrition leads to an inadequately expanded blood volume. In turn, the mother's body may try to deal with this crisis by rejecting the pregnancy. In a woman whose blood volume is marginally expanded, dehydration can cause an acute drop in blood volume which can trigger the onset of uterine contractions. Even if the blood volume is adequate, a severe illness with loss of bodily fluids (vomiting or diarrhea) can cause an acute drop in blood volume and lead to preterm labor as well.

Poor nutrition also makes a woman more susceptible to various infections that can lead to preterm rupture of membranes, the most common complication leading to the birth of a preterm infant. Once the membranes have ruptured it is much more likely that uterine activity will accelerate and birth will occur.

Undetected or inadequately nourished multiple gestation: This is one of the chief causes of preterm labor. In undetected cases, maternal nutrition is often adequate for one baby but woefully deficient for more. Once a woman with undetected multiple gestation nears or passes the 28 week mark (the point when blood volume should have peaked), she is at great risk for the onset of preterm labor. In questionable cases it is a good idea to recommend an ultrasound exam to determine if multiple gestation is a factor in order to avoid this tragic, but usually preventable, situation.

Reproductive abnormalities: Even if a woman is well nourished and has a well expanded blood volume, uterine and cervical abnormalities can prevent her from carrying a pregnancy to term. A variety of abnormalities can occur; those most likely to precipitate early labor involve short cervices and those which have abnormal musculature. While most loose cervices will begin to dilate in the second trimester, it is possible for dilation to be postponed until the third. (See chapter on

Loose Cervix in the section on Problems Associated With the Second Trimester)
Herbs such as False Unicorn root tincture, 5 drops every few hours, can also be
recommended, but should be stopped once 37 weeks is reached.

If the uterus is abnormally small or misshapen it may not be able to
accommodate a pregnancy beyond a certain point and labor may begin. In these
rare cases, there is nothing that can be done to prevent labor.

Other complicating factors: In addition, signs and symptoms of preterm labor
may overlay other complications such as:

*Abruption (see separate chapter, Third Trimester section)
*Urinary tract infection (see <u>Diagnostic Tests</u>)
*Uterine rupture (see separate chapter, Third Trimester section)

<u>**Diagnosing preterm labor:**</u> Typically a woman will call you to say she suspects
she may be in preterm labor. It is then your job to determine if this is true and
make suggestions regarding what to do next.

*Is your uterus getting firm?
*What do your contractions feel like?
*What other symptoms are you experiencing?
*Have you lost any fluid from your yoni?
*Have you discharged any bloody mucus (show)?
*Are any cervical changes taking place?

Is your uterus getting firm? What do your contractions feel like? When the
presenting symptoms are limited to uterine activity, it is important to distinguish
exactly what is being felt. Toning contractions are normal and healthy. In well-
nourished women they increase in frequency throughout the second and third
trimesters and may occasionally be associated with spasms of the round ligaments,
shooting pains from the cervix, or crampy feelings. As long as these sensations are
not *coordinated* with the coming and going of toning contractions they are usually
no cause for alarm. Unless a woman has a cervical abnormality which results in
painless dilation (which can happen, especially in DES daughters), early dilation
generally produces some sensations that coincide with detectable uterine activity.

On the other hand, a few women will only feel contractions in their lower
back or may be confused by uterine sensations which *are* related to labor. If the
uterus is getting hard at the same time that rhythmic achiness, cramps, or pulling
sensations are occurring, or there is a sensation of increasing intrayoni pressure this
calls for an internal exam. Pulling sensations in the vicinity of the symphysis pubis
which are coming with every contraction are the most common sensation felt by
women who are actually changing their cervix. (Also review the table in the
chapter on The Onset of Labor at Term, this section, for further suggestions.)

848

Abruption can mimic early labor by creating sensations of pain and pressure. See the chapter on Bleeding in the Third Trimester for more information.

What other symptoms are you experiencing? Sometimes, a woman may mistake symptoms of a uterine infection for the onset of normal labor. She may also confuse the flu, intestinal cramps, urinary tract infection, or pain from an ovarian tumor with labor. Take into account what you already know of a woman's history, to find out what else may be going on.

Have you lost any fluid from your yoni? Preterm rupture of membranes complicates the picture considerably. Refer to the chapter on Rupture of Membranes Before the Onset of Labor, this section, if she has passed any fluid. The combination of fluid and contractions greatly increases the likelihood that labor will proceed to birth. Act accordingly, and if uterine activity is present, recommend transport if the baby is less than 36 weeks of pregnancy by good dates.

What to do if contractions are the only presenting symptom:

*   ***Get the woman off her feet**. This means that she stay horizontal, at least until contractions stop. After that she should not spend long periods of time on her feet (no more than 15 to 20 minutes) and not lift heavy things (including small children). These precautions minimize downward pressure on her cervix. However, constant bed rest is not indicated unless the woman has a cervical abnormality; otherwise its only real benefit is the conservation of calories. If there is a cervical or uterine abnormality, bed rest will minimize stress from the enlarging uterus.
*   ***Correct dehydration:** Start by asking the mother how much fluid she has had today. Tell her to drink 2 large glasses of water over the next 1 to 2 hours. Have the mother drink to a healthy thirst; at least 6 to 8 glasses of clear fluids daily.
*   ***Give herbs that will stop contractions:** A variety of herbs can be used to stop early contractions. I have personally had very good results with False Unicorn Root tincture, 5 drops every 5 to 15 minutes (depending upon the strength of the contractions) until the contractions taper off, then continue to take it, spacing out the dose to every ½ hour, then every hour, then every 3 or 4 hours, for the next several days, until she is not taking any at all. If contractions begin again, start back up on the frequent doses. False Unicorn root will actually reverse dilation and effacement and cause the presenting part to lift up out of the pelvis, returning everything to an appropriate condition for the weeks of pregnancy. I've personally seen this happen several times.

Other midwives have had good success using half a dropperful of valerian root or skullcap tincture three times daily (Loprinzi-Kassel, 1995); or equal parts of cramp bark and wild yam tinctures (Schlinger, 1995). (See the chapter entitled Miscarriage in the First Trimester for other herbal suggestions.)

Assess her diet: Discuss recent dietary patterns; a marginally contracted blood volume can precipitate early labor. Once protein, calories and salt are evaluated, recommend 1000 mg of calcium citrate and 500 mg of magnesium daily for women at mild risk and multiply this dose to two or three times daily for those at high risk.

*Stop breast (esp. nursing) or sexual stimulation until things stabilize.

Often the above recommendations will quiet things down. If more help is needed and the membranes appear to be intact:

Perform an internal exam to determine whether any evidence of labor is present by assessing the condition of the cervix during a contraction. If cervical changes are occurring, it is still possible to stop labor in many cases. However, the earlier the pregnancy and the more the cervix is effaced (thinned out) and dilated (opened), the less likely it is that you will be able to stop it. Compare how much change you are finding with how long the mother reports that uterine activity has been taking place. Remember that some cervical changes may be normal (effacement may start as early as 30 weeks in some women). If you can feel the membranes, keep your fingers in contact with them during a contraction to see if they tighten up; if they do, this is a good indication that they are affecting the cervix. Assess the consistency of the cervix during a contraction in the same way. Also, note if there is any bloody show. Be gentle with the cervix as you don't want to stimulate it unnecessarily. An internal exam can help determine how much time you have to try low-tech interventions to turn things around.

If cervical changes are occurring in a woman with a known cervical anomaly, it is unlikely that the cervix will return to its previous condition regardless of what you do. Again, these women *can* benefit from bed rest, as it decreases the pressure on the cervix as the baby gets bigger. A cerclage can be placed early in the third trimester if bed rest and herbal therapies are not arresting cervical changes by themselves. Perform an internal exam several hours to several days after the first, depending upon the situation, to determine whether cervical changes have stopped.

Rule out urinary tract infection: Because of the high correlation preterm contractions and cramps with urinary tract infection, it is a good idea to rule this out with a clean catch culture of the urine (for more details see <u>Diagnostic Tests</u>).

Emotional issues: Once you have begun work on the physical situation, talk to the mother about her emotional and mental status. Preterm labor is often a cry for help from the mother. Typical psychological factors which may play a part include anxiety about going to term and experiencing full term labor, concerns about getting a full term baby out, lack of support at home, fears and concerns about parenting issues or her baby's safety (abusive partner?), concerns about the baby's well-being (unconscious desire to get the baby out where she can see it and it can be safe), unconscious integration of cultural messages that the uterus is a dangerous place for the baby. Asking the mom what she needs right now on other levels can open up this discussion. Once she is clear on her emotional issues, have her talk to her baby and her uterus about waiting until term to give birth.

If nothing you do works and labor seems to be progressing (do another internal exam to assess if cervical changes are reversing themselves or proceeding) transport is in order if the baby is younger than 36 weeks gestation. Accompany the mother to the hospital, if you can, to offer further support. Assisting at a preterm birth is covered in Volume II.

<u>What to do if contractions are not the only symptom or sign</u>: You must consider other pathological conditions which have nothing to do with labor, such as urinary tract infection. Bloody show is a good sign that the cervix is changing and must be taken to mean just that until an internal exam proves otherwise. It is important to distinguish "heavy bloody show" from bleeding due to placenta previa or abruption (see separate chapter, this section). Rupture of membranes complicates the picture. Do not perform an internal exam if you suspect the membranes have ruptured (read the chapter on Rupture of Membranes Before the Onset of Labor, this section, for more details). Transport is your best alternative if the woman is truly preterm and labor is progressing. Not doing an exam will spare the woman one invasive procedure, as they will probably want to do a sterile speculum exam at the hospital.

Until about 34 weeks, treatment options which will be offered will be similar to those offered for women at risk to give birth during the second trimester; see the end of the chapter on Miscarriage in the Second Trimester for those details. After 34 weeks, babies born with access to neonatal care usually do quite well and no attempt is made to curtail labor unless the fetal lungs are found to be immature.

<u>References and further reading</u>:
Loprenzi-Kassel, Clarabeth, midwife, Veneta, OR, editing comments, 5/95.
Oxhorn, Harry, <u>Human Labor and Birth</u>, 5th ed., Appleton-Century-Crofts, Norwalk, Ct, 1986.
Schlinger, Hilary, midwife, Ithica, NY, editing comments, 5/95.

Bleeding in the Third Trimester

By far, the most common cause of minimal third trimester bleeding is normal cervical change. In addition to passage of the mucus plug, a woman's cervix may bleed slightly due to softening and women commonly have some spotting after yoni penetration. Be sure to rule out infection if the cervix is the source of bleeding.

There are a number of uncommon or rare causes of bleeding in the third trimester; however, about half of the non-cervical bleeding you see will be due to either placental abruption or placenta previa. In the other half of cases, the cause is often less clear and often no cause is ever determined. (Enkin, 1995) The most serious threats to the pregnancy are life-threatening hemorrhage and preterm birth.

Placental abruption: Whenever a portion of the placenta's surface separates from the uterine wall after the 20th week of pregnancy but before the actual birth of the baby, the placenta is said to be abrupting. Hemorrhage into the decidua basalis causes it to divide, leading to separation of the part of the placenta adjacent to the split. A hematoma (contained blood clot) forms between the placenta and the uterus. Abruption is directly related to poor nutrition and frequently accompanies hypertension. Associated factors include:

*Toxemia
*Malnutrition combined with hypertension
*Over-distention of the uterus from polyhydramnios or multiple pregnancy
*Short umbilical cord
*External trauma

Malnutrition or substance abuse (notably cocaine) is a prerequisite for placental separation except in cases of maternal trauma or an abnormality of the uterine wall or placental surface. Healthy placental attachment depends upon a good maternal diet. A poor diet leading to poor attachment combined with high blood pressure is a set-up for abruption because the higher pressure of maternal blood perfusing the placenta literally pushes the poorly attached placenta off the uterine wall. If the mother is well-nourished, high blood pressure by itself doesn't increase the incidence of abruption. (Boyd & Scott, 1985)

Placental separation always causes bleeding, but distinguishing it from other causes of bleeding can sometimes be tricky. Abruption may present as follows:

External or apparent abruption: In this case the edge of the placenta lifts up and bleeding begins. The blood works its way down between the uterine wall and the membranes and appears as bleeding from the yoni. It may be dark and clotted (because it took a while to work its way down to the cervix) or bright (because the abruption is nearer the cervical os and blood is coming out before it begins to turn dark). Since there is little or no build-up of blood, this type of abruption is not painful or only mildly so. The degree of anemia and shock is roughly equivalent to the amount of bleeding observed.

Mixed or combined abruption: Here some of the bleeding appears as discharge from the yoni and some of it is remaining behind the placenta or trapped high in the uterus. In this case there might or might not be some pain related to pressure into the uterine wall caused by the build up of blood. However, even if the amount of bleeding is not sufficient to cause pain, there could still be more bleeding than is apparent because pressure is being released by blood passing from the yoni.

Classic, internal or concealed abruption: The type of abruption most commonly described has the classic symptom picture of sudden, increasing uterine pain from blood building rapidly behind a partially or completely detached placenta. This build-up irritates the uterus and often, though not always, precipitates the onset of contractions. The woman may mistake this pain for the onset of a rapidly accelerating labor. Her uterus remains hard between contractions because of the trapped blood. The woman's vital signs soon begin to show evidence of shock (rapid pulse, a temporary rise then fall in blood pressure followed by feeling faint) even though there is no obvious cause for this. At some point she may have some bleeding from the yoni, but it will not be enough to account for her degree of shockiness. The fetal heart tones may be weak or absent and the mother may report violent fetal movements prior to a cessation of all movement.

The build-up of blood behind the placenta will prevent the uterus from effectively closing off the bleeding vessels opened by the placenta's release; therefore bleeding continues and increases. At times the hemorrhage will cause the fundal height to increase. If you are unsure what is going on, mark the fundal height with a felt tipped pen when you first suspect a problem; a rising fundus will give you an idea of how much bleeding is occurring inside the uterus.

This is a life threatening situation for both mother and baby, if it is still alive. Transport immediately!

The slow leak concealed abruption: A small abruption can take place which does not threaten the life of either mother or baby. A small portion of the placenta separates and bleeds, and the blood coagulates. A firm, adherent clot is formed beneath the abrupted area. Neither you or the mother will be aware of this until the clot is found during the placental exam after the birth. In other cases, a significant portion of the placental surface is damaged, causing a reduction in nutrient transport and leading to intrauterine growth retardation of the fetus.

A variation on this type is the concealed abruption which causes a rupture of the membranes near the site of bleeding. Blood then enters the uterine cavity, and mixes with amniotic fluid. This leakage releases pressure and thus this abruption may be painless. When the membranes rupture, a port wine stained fluid is released, indicating that bleeding is occurring somewhere.

Painless atypical abruption: If a posteriorly implanted placenta abrupts, you may find only bleeding from the yoni with an accompanying backache, even though the abruption is severe enough to cause fetal death. The uterus is not tender, relaxes between contractions if the woman is in labor, and allows for easy palpation and auscultation of the fetal heart.

Regardless of how it manifests, there are four grades of abruption:

GRADE	BLEEDING	MATERNAL/FETAL CONDITION
0	Apparent only after birth, a small retroplacental clot is found when inspecting the placenta	Mother and fetus asymptomatic at all times
1	Mild, with some but not excessive bleeding	Mother not in shock, fetal heart tones heard
2	Moderate	Mother in shock, fetal heart tone heard
3	Severe; uterus tender & may be hard to the touch; fetal parts may be hard to find, because palpation obscured due to accumulated blood	Mother in shock, no fetal heart tones

<u>Placenta Previa:</u> Placenta previa occurs when the placenta is implanted partially or completely over the internal os of the cervix. The incidence is 1 out of every 200 births. If enough of the cervical opening is obstructed, cervical changes such as softening, effacement and dilation will cause the placenta to separate or tear around the margins of the internal os with accompanying rupture of underlying blood vessels and bleeding. While placenta previa can become symptomatic in the late first or during the second trimester, it is most common for this to occur after the seventh month of pregnancy (28 weeks and on) as this is when significant cervical changes most commonly begin. Predisposing factors include:

*Women over 35 are three times more likely to have a placenta previa
*A large, thin placenta. These are more likely to cover the cervix simply because they take up more of the uterine surface
*Multiparity. (Theory is that the trophoblast seeks out a new area to implant during each pregnancy; if several pregnancies preceded this one, there will be less such areas in the uterine lining.)
*If the lining of the upper uterine segment is deficient, the placenta may spread out over more of the uterine wall in an effort to maintain an adequate blood supply.
*Endometritis following a previous pregnancy
*Uterine scars. In one study, the rate of previa in an unscarred uterus was 0.26%; 0.65% after 1 CS, 1.8% with 2 CS scars, 3% with 3,

and 10% with 4 or more, a 38-fold increase. The risk of placenta accreta in conjunction with previa rose from 5% in an unscarred uterus, to 24% with 1 scar, 47% with 2, 40% with 3, and 60% with 4 or more CS scars. (Clark, et.al., 1985) Also, having had five or more D & C's increases the risk of previa.

*Repeated pregnancies with short intervals in between. There may not be sufficient time for the previous placental site to heal, thus reducing the available space for a new placenta to implant

*A history of previa. Women with a history of previa are 12 times more likely to have a recurrence

*Multiple gestation (due to the large placental implantation site[s])

*Any disturbance of the healthy formation of the uterine lining. This may cause the embryo to implant lower in the uterus than is usually the case.

Placentae previae are classified as follows:

DEGREE	DEFINITION
1. Total or central	Placenta completely covers cervix at all times
2. Partial	Placenta partially covers cervix at full dilation
3. Marginal	Placental edge reaches the margin of the os at full dilation.

Symptoms of a placenta previa include:

Painless "warning hemorrhage" after 7 months (rarely earlier): Typically the mother has a sudden, painless, bright red discharge of blood from her yoni. This may be precipitated by penetration of the yoni (as the finger or penis causes trauma to the placenta through the cervix) or it may happen with no such stimulation. Frequently women call saying they woke up in a pool of blood or had a sudden discharge of blood at the toilet. Often such a hemorrhage will stop spontaneously and the woman can resume normal activity for a time before another warning hemorrhage occurs. Other times a slight continuous trickle of blood continues which can lead to anemia and possible depletion of clotting factors.

These are called warning bleeds because they alert you to a problem before torrential hemorrhaging which does not stop and is life threatening begins. Rarely no such warning hemorrhages occur, and the first sign of previa will be continuous hemorrhaging as the cervix begins to change at the onset of or at some point during labor.

Uterine tone is normal: In a previa, uterine tone is always normal because blood is not building up between the uterine wall and the placenta.

Blood is bright red: Because the placenta is near the cervix, the bleeding will usually be fluid and bright red. Sometimes soft, bright red clots will form if blood has pooled in the yoni prior to discharge (as may occur during the night).

The fetal presenting part is high and often breech or transverse: Because the placenta is obstructing the lower uterine segment, the baby often most comfortably lies either breech or transverse.

The maternal condition is equal to the degree of blood lost: Shock equals blood loss because the bleeding from a previa is revealed.

Congenital fetal anomalies: Fetal defects may be accompanied by a placenta which seeks an inappropriately low implantation site.

If placenta previa is present you are likely to find:

      *The woman feels no uterine pain unless labor has begun
      *The uterus is soft and not tender
      *The presenting part is high
      *The fetal heart is usually heard
      *Shock is rare, because bleeding is noted before symptoms of shock begin.

    While any condition can present atypically and confuse the clinical picture, this chart comparing previa and abruption will assist with differential diagnosis:

FINDING	PREVIA	ABRUPTION
Onset	Quiet & sneaky	Sudden & stormy
Bleeding	External	External &/or concealed
Color of blood	Bright red	Dark venous
Anemia	= Blood loss	> Apparent blood loss
Shock	= Blood loss	> Apparent blood loss
Toxemia	Absent	May be present
Pain	Only contractions	Severe & steady
Uterine tenderness	Absent	Present
Uterine tone	Soft & relaxed	Firm to stony hard
Uterine contour	Normal	May enlarge & change shape
Fetal heart tones	Usually present	Present or absent
Engagement	Absent	May be present
Presentation	May be abnormal	No relationship

(Oxhorn, 1986)

Uncommon causes of bleeding: Bleeding and other symptoms may come from a variety of sources. The most typical include:

Yoni or cervical lesions: These are far less common causes of third trimester bleeding. Growths such as cervical polyps or cancer can lead to tissue breakdown and bleeding. Cervical or yoni infection can also cause bleeding but not to the extent that is likely to be caused by either abruption or previa.

Vasa previa: Rarely, a cord vessel will traverse the fetal membranes before inserting into the placenta. If such a portion of the bag overlies the cervix and ruptures, the vessel can be torn in the process and fetal bleeding will result. If the cervix is dilated you may be able to feel or see the vessel as a long rounded object in the membranes. An APT test can be done to determine if the blood is of fetal origin (see Diagnostic Tests). Poor fetal heart tones would also be an indication of fetal compromise. If you suspect a ruptured vasa previa, transport without delay.

Uterine rupture: Bleeding from the yoni may occur in a silent rupture. See the separate chapter on this topic for more information.

What to do if abruption is suspected: See the mother immediately and assess the situation yourself (if she is bleeding profusely, advise her to have someone else drive her to the hospital and meet her there). Palpate the uterus and listen to the fetal heart rate. Evaluate the mother's pulse, blood pressure and color for signs of shock. If mother and fetus appear stable and you suspect a small abruption has occurred, review the diet and make necessary changes, ask again about substance abuse and recommend 3000 IU of Vitamin E and 5000 mg. of Vitamin C with bioflavinoids daily for 2 weeks. This should assist the placenta in maintaining and strengthening the rest of its implantation site. If the mother notes more pain or bleeding she is to call at once, or get someone to drive her to the hospital if you are, for any reason, unavailable. If you are unclear about the cause of bleeding, an ultrasound should be done to locate the placenta.

If a major abruption has occurred or you are unclear about how much blood was lost or if bleeding is continuing, transport. A slow bleed may not be immediately life threatening, but it can lead to a depletion of maternal clotting factors which may result in DIC (disseminated intravascular coagulation). A clotting lab study should be done to evaluate clotting status prior to any surgery.

What to do if previa is suspected: Generally speaking you should never do an internal exam (per yoni or rectum) if you suspect placenta previa because your examining fingers could further traumatize placental tissue and initiate a torrential hemorrhage. Even in the hospital, an internal exam is not done unless the woman is in surgery ready for a surgical delivery in case previa is discovered.

If bleeding occurs and then stops, the safest option is to send the woman in for an ultrasound exam to determine the placental location. Since more ultrasounds are being done early in pregnancy, it has been discovered that often placentas which are situated in the lower part of the uterus early in pregnancy are later found in a normal fundal location. As pregnancy advances, the placenta moves up the uterine wall. This is in part due to the enlargement of the uterus, with the attached placenta being brought along, and is also apparently due to the fact that the placenta itself can, at least to a certain extent, migrate up the uterine wall. Any woman who has been told she has a low lying placenta can visualize it moving up to a more ideal location as the pregnancy advances. Preterm birth is the major problem accompanying placenta previa. When previa is found, women may return home to await 37 weeks and a surgical birth, with recommendations to avoid heavy lifting, rest frequently and call at once if bleeding resumes.

Whenever bleeding occurs: Maternal well-being should be monitored with assessment of vital signs as soon as possible and a hemoglobin check 36 hours after bleeding has ceased. Anemia should be treated. Fetal movement and heart rate should be assessed as well. Rh negative women should have blood drawn for a Kleihauer-Betke test to determine if fetal blood has entered her system and an antibody screen, followed by a prophylactic injection of Rho(D) immunoglobulin if the screen is negative. Prolonged bleeding from a previa (or for any reason) can lead to a reduction in clotting factors and make a clotting crisis more likely. A clotting panel can be done to determine if normal clotting status is being maintained (see Diagnostic Tests for more details. When it occurs, preterm birth is most likely to take place within the 7 to 10 days after a bleeding episode.

References and further reading:

Boyd, P. & Scott, A., "Quantitative structural studies of human placentas associated with pre-eclampsia, essential hypertension and intrauterine growth retardation," Br. J. of OB/GYN, Vol. 92, July 1985, pp. 714-715.

Chattopodnyay, Sisir, et.al. "Placenta Previa and Accreta After Previous Cesarean Section," Eur. J. of Ob Gyn Repor. Bio., Vol. 52, 1993, pp. 151-156.

Clark, et.al., "Placenta previa/accreta and prior cesarean section," Ob Gyn, Vol. 66, No. 1, 1985, pp. 89-92.

Enkin, M., et.al., A Guide to Effective Care in Pregnancy and Birth, 2nd ed., Oxford U. Press, NY, 1995.

Oxhorn, Harry, Human Labor and Birth, 5th ed., Appleton-Century-Crofts, Norwalk, Ct, 1986.

Rupture of Membranes Before the Onset of Labor

The placental membranes form a protective barrier between the sterile world of the fetus and the outside. They contain the fluid in which the fetus grows and which protects it from injury. By far, one of the most nerve racking and aggravating experiences of pregnancy is the rupture of membranes without the onset of labor shortly thereafter. For our purposes PROM will stand for prelabor rupture of membranes at term and PPROM preterm prelabor ROM. How this situation is handled greatly depends upon whether the rupture occurs before or after the baby reaches full term, 36 weeks of pregnancy by excellent dates and 37 weeks if the dates are at all in doubt or maternal nutrition has not been what it should be.

Risk factors: Prelabor rupture of membranes occurs in about 10% of term and up to 30% of all preterm pregnancies. In spite of efforts to determine exactly why this occurs, the cause remains unexplained in most cases. The most common known risk factors are:

*Poor maternal nutrition leading to inherently weak membranes (and making the mother more prone to infections)
*Trauma to the membranes from pelvic examination or penetration of the yoni during sexual activity
*Loose (incompetent) cervix
*Preexisting chorioamnionitis from a variety of organisms (gardnerella, chlamydia, gonorrhea, listeria, mycoplasmas, etc.)
*Polyhydramnios

Once rupture of membranes occurs, the primary maternal and fetal risk is intrauterine infection with or without generalized sepsis. At term, there is a direct correlation between the length of time from rupture to the onset of labor (the latent period) and the development of maternal infection. For pregnancies less than 37 weeks, the risk of maternal infection is not significantly greater if the latent period is prolonged. Maternal risk of infection is related to the mode of birth, with those having oxytocin induction at increased risk (probably due to the adjunct digital exams and internal electronic fetal monitoring which often accompanies induction) and those having surgical deliveries most at risk. (Goer, 1995; Morales & Lazar, 1986) However, in all cases, the risk of infection is increased if internal exams are performed during the latent period.

Fetal risks include:

-Prematurity (poor fat reserves, weak suck, not ready to be born, immature immune system)
-Respiratory distress syndrome (RDS) in babies born before their lungs have matured. Lungs are almost always mature at 36 weeks, and

virtually always mature at 37 completed weeks of gestation. The major cause of neonatal death is RDS (not infection) in babies born before 34 weeks.

-After 35 weeks, when the majority of babies have mature lungs, sepsis takes over as the main cause of death and injury. As in the mother, a prolonged latent period before 37 weeks does not significantly increase the risk of fetal infection as long as internal exams are not performed.

-Cord prolapse occurs when the umbilical cord falls out of the cervix before the birth. The smaller and earlier the baby, the more likely this becomes, because the baby has not settled down in the pelvis and fluid can flow down through the hole in the bag, past the high presenting part, carrying the cord with it through the cervix or beside the presenting part, creating an occult prolapse (detectable in fetal heart tone variations; see Volume II for more information.)

-Breech presentation is more common, because many babies are breech earlier in pregnancy and will rotate to vertex as term approaches. Up to 30% of all preterm babies are breech.

In summary, how the fetus will fare depends upon its maturity and the presence of intrauterine infection. However, when and if an internal exam is done significantly impacts neonatal infection rates as well. One study (Shutte, et.al., 1983) of 321 women who had PROM for more than 24 hours before birth showed that two factors influenced the onset of clinical symptoms of fetal and neonatal infection: gestational age and an interval of more than 24 hours between the first internal exam and birth. The relationship between infection and the time interval between rupture of membranes and birth disappeared if no internal exams were performed.

When to expect the onset of labor: Somewhere between 50 to 70% of all women who break their waters early will go into labor within 48 hours. The time this takes is influenced by several factors:

*Gestational age
 -80% to 90% of those near term will begin labor within 24 hours
 -35% to 50% of those before 36 weeks will begin labor by 24 hours.
 -Only 10% of those before 36 weeks will take more than 14 days to begin labor.
*This latent period is shorter when the fetus is more mature.
*First-time mothers tend to have longer latent periods than multiparas.
*Intrauterine infection decreases the length of the latent period.

860

*Those who rupture their membranes at night are much more likely to begin spontaneous labor within a day or so than those who do not. Women who rupture membranes due to the presence of infection or who do not begin labor within 48 hours do not show a correlation in this regard. (Cooperstock, et.al., 1987)

Diagnosing rupture of membranes: Typically you will receive a call from the woman announcing that she thinks her waters have broken. If the woman is early, she may be quite upset or afraid. It is now up to you to find out if the bag is broken and advise the mother accordingly. You have these things to determine:

*If the fluid is from the membranes.
*If so, is it coming from the rupture of both the amnion and chorion (a frank or complete rupture) or a rupture of only the chorion, leaving the amnion still intact.
*If the membranes are the source of the fluid, is the fluid coming from a hole near the cervix or is it coming from a leak high in the bag?
*The well-being of the baby.

Try to find out how much fluid she may have lost. This process is similar to discovering how much blood a woman may have lost; however, since clear fluid will be less alarming to most women than blood (especially if they are close to term), you may get a more objective estimate in some cases (although she may be just as terrified if she is preterm). Did she recently have intercourse? (Fluid could merely be semen.) Did she soak a pad? Did it penetrate her clothing?, underwear?, outerwear? Is she still leaking or gushing? Is she soaking washcloths or towels? How big a puddle did she make on the bed? Once you have an idea of how much she lost, ask such questions as "Do you think it might be urine?" "Have you been leaking urine at all with stress, laughing, sneezing, or coughing?" Most of the time it isn't urine.

The passage of a small amount of clear or translucent milky fluid which does not continue is most likely to be something other than a frank rupture. If possible, have the woman catch some fluid in a clean container so that it can be examined for ferning (which indicates amniotic fluid, although urine will also fern sometimes) and for fetal lung maturity.

It is also possible that fluid could be coming from a leak high in the bag, closer to the fundus than the cervix. This could occur if an abruption is putting pressure on the junction of the bag and placenta or if some other factor is causing the bag to be weakened higher up. It is usually impossible to determine this without an internal exam, which is not recommended. Those leaks which are typically termed "high" that reseal are usually due to the chorion breaking while the amnion remains intact.

Is the fluid clear, and if not, what color is it? Colored fluid increases the likelihood that a frank (complete) rupture of both chorion and amnion has occurred. Meconium stained fluid will be greenish or brownish tinged. However, it is possible for meconium to seep through an intact bag and stain yoni mucus or the fluid which is sometimes trapped between chorion and amnion (an ominous sign because it indicates long-standing and severe staining).

Port wine stained fluid indicates placental bleeding from higher up in the uterus which is leaking into a hole in the bag and becoming homogenized with clear fluid before it passes through the cervix. Such an abruption may be otherwise asymptomatic or produce seemingly normal uterine contractions. (see APT Test in Diagnostic Tests). Rarely, a fetal cord vessel will traverse the membranes and may overlie the cervix and rupture, causing bleeding (a velamentous insertion of the cord with accompanying vasa previa). This is more likely in a multiple gestation. An APT test can be done to determine if the blood is of fetal origin (see Diagnostic Tests). Poor fetal heart tones would also be an indication of fetal compromise. If you suspect a ruptured vasa previa, transport without delay.

Ask the mother to save anything she has soaked with fluid so that you can examine it for amount and color as well as vernix: This is most important when the fluid is stained or you are in doubt whether the bag is ruptured or not. Ask her to catch at least some of it on a white towel, tissue or pad so you can tell what the color really is.

How does she feel? Ask specifically about fever, abdominal pain or tenderness, persistently elevated maternal heart rate or foul smelling yoni discharge prior to the passage of fluid. You are looking for signs of infection. Keep in mind that the bag can break in the presence of subclinical yoni or intrauterine infection.

How is the baby moving? Normal fetal movement is a good indication that the baby is okay and the cord is not prolapsed. If the baby is quiet at the moment ask the mother if the baby has been moving, and ask her to palpate the baby now to see if she can stimulate movement. If little or no movement is detected and she has a fetascope, she or someone else can check for the fetal heart rate right then.

If the mother reports wild or rapid fetal movements which suddenly ceased, this is an ominous sign. A baby may have convulsive movements before dying if its oxygen supply has been cut off. Cord prolapse is especially likely the earlier the baby is and anytime the presenting part is not filling the pelvis prior to rupture of membranes (of particular concern in preterm situations or with multiparas).

If you suspect cord prolapse and the mother lives close by, go over right away to check; if she lives farther away, discuss how she feels intuitively about the baby's welfare. Suggest that she go straight to the hospital, where you can meet her, if she has concerns for the baby's well-being. If she doesn't feel there is a problem and doesn't want to go straight to the hospital, go over to check immediately.

Babies may also slow their movements in response to systemic compromise due to infection. This is usually reflected in a gradual decline in activity over the course of several hours or even days. Careful attention to fetal movement patterns becomes critically important once the bag is broken.

Clinical means of confirming rupture of membranes: Once your questions have determined that rupture of the membranes is likely, there are certain things that can be done to more definitively diagnose if this has occurred. If indicated, one or more of these techniques may be used. Nitrazine and Fern testing are discussed in Diagnostic Tests as well as later in this chapter. Additional methods are:

*Have the mother lie down and see if more fluid comes out. Now palpate the baby's presenting part by balloting it back and forth (to move it, but not to dislodge it if it is down in the pelvis). Next have her roll over. If any of these cause fluid to come out, the probability of ruptured membranes is almost certain. In many cases you can stop at this point if you feel rupture of membranes has been clearly demonstrated. Nitrazine and Fern testing could also be performed on fluid released during this exam.

*Sterile speculum exam: using scrupulous sterile technique, a speculum is inserted so you can see if fluid is issuing from the cervix. If not, try pressing gently on the abdomen and moving the fetal presenting part to see if this causes fluid to be released. A speculum exam, although sterile, is still intrusive. If you do one, take this opportunity to obtain a swab culture for *Beta*-strep from the upper yoni by rolling the swab firmly around the outer surface of the cervix, in the fornix (do not insert the swab in or near the cervical passageway). Only one sterile speculum exam should be performed. The concept of a sterile exam is rather inaccurate since the yoni cannot be rendered sterile.

*pH testing; amniotic fluid is alkaline, semen is neutral to alkaline (7.2 to 8). The pH of fluid that bathes the yoni walls may be altered by the pH of the yoni. During a speculum exam, you can either use a sterile hemostat or sponge forceps to transport a small piece of nitrazine paper to fluid pooling in the posterior fornix. Or, you can use a long-handled nitrazine swab to dip directly in pooled fluid. If the fluid is clearly acid, the membranes are probably intact. If the fluid tests alkaline, the membranes are probably ruptured. Blood, urine and infected yoni secretions can also cause an alkaline reading; therefore, a positive reading should be confirmed with a Fern test whenever possible.

*A properly prepared slide of amniotic fluid will show a characteristic ferning pattern under a microscope. Be careful to obtain fluid from the posterior fornix for this test, as samples from the internal cervical os can appear to fern normally. (see <u>Diagnostic Tests</u>). If you don't have access to a microscope, The Lens, a fertility device for checking saliva, can also be used to check for ferning in amniotic fluid. (order from Around the Moon, P.O. Box 3325, Applegate, OR, 97530 800-797-FERN) For most accurate results, the sample should be completely dry prior to examination; do not use a hair dryer for this purpose.

*A drop of dried yoni fluid can also be stained with Nile blue. If orange cells from fetal skin are seen under the microscope, the membranes are ruptured.

*An ultrasound can be done to look for fluid; if little or none is seen, this is highly suggestive of rupture of membranes, but not an absolute indication.

Diagnostic procedures are not 100% reliable, however. Short of seeing fluid actually pouring from the cervical os on sterile speculum exam, all tests must be considered equivocal. When fluid is not seen draining from the cervix multiple tests may show either false positive results (meaning it says the waters are broken when they are actually intact) or false negative results (i.e. it says the bag is intact when it is actually broken). By 24 hours post rupture the rate of false-negative results for tests of pH, ferning and nile blue reaches 50%. Therefore, any tests deemed necessary should be done as soon as possible after rupture is suspected and multiple tests should be performed whenever possible. (Gorondeski, et.al., 1982) Another study suggests that either fluid should be seen actively pouring from the cervix *or* both nitrazine testing and ferning should be positive before PROM is confirmed. If only one test is positive and no fluid is seen issuing from the cervix, diagnosis must be considered equivocal. (Davidson, 1991)

Do not perform a manual yoni exam unless you suspect cord prolapse; if possible perform a sterile speculum exam to see if cord prolapse has occurred. Digital exams increase the incidence of infection in mother and baby and should be postponed until the mother is well into active labor. Some midwives try to avoid exams completely in these cases.

<u>**General precautionary advice**</u>: If the woman is at term, absolute diagnosis is not so critical unless there is a history of positive *Beta*-strep cultures, since labor will likely follow in short order anyway. Once rupture of membranes has been determined, advise the woman of the following precautionary measures:

*Insert nothing in the yoni (fingers, penises, or tampons) unless she

864

suspects the cord may have prolapsed, (which is possible, especially if the baby is early). If she thinks cord prolapse may have occurred she should lie down or get in a hands-and-knees position and insert her fingers into the yoni to feel for cord. Whenever possible, she should have someone else do this who can wash their hands thoroughly beforehand. (Iodine scrub and sterile gloves may be in the birth kit, which is another good reason to include gloves in your birth kit supply list.)

*No oral sex.

*Take her temperature first thing in the morning before rising (basal) and every 4 hours during the day and record it. A temperature over 100.4°F (38°C) is cause for concern. She should also watch for other signs of infection such as elevated pulse, foul yoni discharge, and uterine tenderness. She should call immediately if any of these are noted. Transport is advisable if you suspect established infection.

*Drink plenty of clear fluids and keep her salt intake up. Dehydration can cause her temperature to rise, and liquids help replenish the amniotic fluid.

*Continue to eat well, labor could start at any time.

*Scrupulous hygiene should be observed when using the toilet. White unperfumed toilet paper should be used to wipe from front to back only. Many midwives advise showering after each bowel movement as well. Public rest rooms should not be used. The household toilet facilities should be cleaned frequently, preferably by someone other than the woman. If she has more than one bathroom, the woman should reserve one toilet in the house for her exclusive use.

*A squirt-bottle filled with diluted Provodine iodine or Rosemary infusion can be used to rinse the vulva from front to back after using the toilet, but care should be taken that the solution does not enter the yoni. (Cultures should be taken before any kind of rinse is used; see below.)

*No sit-down baths or hot tubs; showers only until labor is well underway.

*She should avoid wearing a pad or underwear whenever possible. If necessary, change pads each time she uses the toilet. Prolonged wearing of the same pad may foster the overgrowth of pathological organisms and is therefore not recommended. Use plain old fashioned sanitary pads (not super absorbent chemical pads) or clean cotton diapers. This will help the woman pay attention to changing her pad frequently and give a better idea of how much fluid is coming out.

*Chart fetal movements on a daily basis (see <u>Diagnostic Tests</u>).
*Elicit a fluid thrill in several areas of the uterus to assess fluid volume. (See chapter on Assessing the Volume of Amniotic Fluid in Skills section.) A significant lack of fluid could cause cord compression, even though no frank cord prolapse has occurred.

Dealing with the issue of infection: You have two choices when confronted with rupture membranes: wait for labor or induce. If you choose to deal with prelabor rupture of membranes by waiting until labor begins, the risk of infection is a major complicating factor. In cases of preterm rupture of membranes, the possibility that the fetus will have underdeveloped lungs is more likely and makes the wait worthwhile. If the woman is at term and breaks her bag at night, labor will usually begin within 48 hours. Whenever the situation is handled by waiting for the spontaneous onset of labor, the following additional steps can be taken to monitor for the onset of infection:

*White blood counts with differentials. These can be done daily or every other day if labor is taking days to start. If suspicious symptoms develop, do a white count immediately and order a STAT result. (A STAT request means the lab will do the work as soon as possible.) Watch for rises in the polys or bands, either of which may indicate an infection. Lymphocytes may be normally elevated if the mother is taking prophylactic echinacea.
*A *Beta*-strep culture can be done. This should be a regular culture which requires 24 hours for the first reading, as quick tests are too inaccurate. A sterile speculum exam is not necessary. A culture can be taken by swabbing inside the lower third of the yoni. According to the CDC, another culture should be taken from the anorectum as well. Be sure no antibacterial perineal rinses have been used at the toilet before this test is done. More details on current CDC protocols for strep can be found in <u>Diagnostic Tests</u>.
*Monitor fetal heart tones and record at least once daily. Persistent fetal heart rate elevations over 180 beats per minute suggest the presence of infection in the baby. Hot showers and maternal dehydration may also cause the fetal heart rate to go up temporarily; wait 45 minutes to one hour after showers or fluid intake to check. Be sure to take these factors into account when you (or the parents) listen.
*Have the mother take echinacea tincture (½ dropperful four times daily) plus 5000 mg vitamin C with bioflavonoids and a good prenatal multivitamin daily.
*The mother should continue to eat well, with extra servings of

complex carbohydrates daily to fuel up for labor.

Pharmaceutical antibiotics should not be given prophylactically. They have not been proven of benefit if the mother is not infected and may mask infection in the newborn. If *Beta*-strep is detected in the culture, it is probably best to stimulate labor, even if the baby is preterm; if you transport, antibiotics will be given in the presence of a positive strep culture. A preterm baby is less resistant to developing an active infection in the presence of pathological organisms. Keep in mind that while infection, when it occurs, is a serious complication, many cases of prelabor rupture of membranes occur without infection, even when the waters are broken for several days or even weeks.

Suggestions for dealing with PPROM before 37 weeks:

With preterm PROM, waiting with its incumbent risk of infection must be weighed against the risk of fetal lung immaturity (read more in Diagnostic Tests). When no infection is present, waiting is in the best interests of the baby, since rupture of membranes for at least 24 hours stimulates increased surfactant production. In these cases the following additional recommendations can be followed:

*Reassess due date, review records, and carefully palpate for fetal size. Use all available data to reassess probable maturity of baby.
*Note that vernix (white, creamy flakes) in the fluid is a good indication that the fetal lungs are mature.
*Have the mother begin taking Evening Primrose oil (three 500 mg. capsules daily) or Borage oil to ripen the cervix for an early birth. (These should be taken orally, *not* inserted into the yoni.)
*Once 37 weeks rolls around, go ahead and try to induce labor.

Suggestions for dealing with term PROM:

It is possible for the membranes to rupture as the first sign of labor. When this occurs labor usually follows rather quickly, within hours or by the next day. Women should observe all the precautions as listed above. As a prudent anticipatory move on your part, you can opt to go ahead and do a standard *Beta*-strep culture by swabbing at the introitus, just in case this woman is in the minority who will not start labor before 24 hours is up. Initial results will be available after 24 hours. In addition:

*Question her as outlined above and advise her about the risk of infection, fetal movement considerations and precautions. Then, if it is at night (as it often is) ask her if she is having any contractions. If she is not or they are mild, tell her to go back to sleep. She needs her rest for the work ahead (and so do you). Have her call you upon arising the next morning for further discussion. Tell her that it is likely that she will be in labor by the next morning.

*The next day, if labor has not begun, review the results of the *Beta*-strep culture and discuss the situation with the parents. If the culture is negative, you are in good shape for waiting for labor to begin. Other options include attempting to induce labor at home, or transporting for hospital induction. Home inductions do work, but are more difficult to get going if the mother has never given birth before. (See Volume II for how to induce labor).

When fluid has been passed but its origin is uncertain: A finite amount of clear fluid may be from the yoni but is often not from the amnion and usually no cause for concern. If your investigations do not turn up evidence of ruptured membranes, the baby seems fine, the mother is unconcerned, there is no evidence of infection and the fluid has stopped coming out, relax. It certainly won't hurt for the mother to watch her hygiene as recommended, but the chances of a frank rupture having occurred in such cases is very slim.

References and further reading:

Cooperstock, M., et.al., "Circadian incidence of premature rupture of membranes in term and preterm births," Ob/Gyn, Vol. 69, No. 6, 1987, pp. 936-941.

Davidson, K., "Detection of premature rupture of the membranes," Clin. Ob Gyn, Vol. 34, No. 4, 1991, pp. 715-721.

Goer, Henci, Obstetric Myths Versus Research Realities, Bergin & Garvey, Westport, CT, 1995.

Gorodeski, I., et.al., "Reevaluation of the pH, ferning, and nile blue sulphate staining methods in pregnant women with premature rupture of the fetal membranes," J. Perinat Med, Vol 10, 1982, pp. 286-291.

Morales, W, Lazar A., "Expectant management of rupture of membranes at term," South Med J, Vol. 79, No. 8, pp. 955-958.

Oxhorn, Harry, Human Labor and Birth, 5th ed., Appleton-Century-Crofts, Norwalk, Ct, 1986.

Schutte, M., et.al., "Management of premature rupture of membranes: the risk of vaginal examination to the infant." Am. J. Ob Gyn, Vol. 146, No. 4, 1983, pp. 395-400.

When the Baby Dies Before Birth

A baby may die while still *in utero* at any time during pregnancy. This tragic event is usually first discovered by the mother, who has noted that fetal movements have ceased and calls you, alarmed or at least worried about the baby's well-being. When women have been encouraged to tune into their baby's movements throughout pregnancy, they seem to notice lack of movement within hours, not days, of their baby's demise. At times these babies are really fine; the mother may have simply lost track of fetal motion due to changes in the character of movement that take place in late pregnancy, but such a report should always be evaluated further.

When you get such a call, it is wise to see the mother without delay. If the parents have a fetascope or stethoscope and can hear the baby themselves, that will at least assure you that the baby is alive. However, a slow fetal heart rate must be compared to the maternal pulse; it is possible for anyone, especially a nervous parent, to mistake the maternal pulse for the baby's. Even if they can hear the baby, see them immediately to make an assessment yourself.

Keeping in mind that fetuses do sleep, a lack of fetal movement, even with a heartbeat, may mean that the baby is conserving energy in a compromised state and could be in danger. Talk to the baby about making its condition clear to you and the mother (the mom can do the same thing before you see her). Listen for the rate, variability and reactivity of the fetal heart. Perform the fetal reactivity test using abdominal stimulation as described in <u>Diagnostic Tests</u>. Attempt to stimulate the baby with abdominal palpation, and see if you get a response in the heart rate. Listen for at least several minutes. Next, discuss tests which assess fetal well-being such as the Biophysical Profile (BPP). The BPP takes into account five parameters of fetal well-being (respiratory movements, muscle tone, fetal movements, heart rate, volume of fluid, and in some areas the condition of the placenta). It is therefore a better assessment tool than a single test, such as a Non-Stress Test, by itself (see <u>Diagnostic Tests</u>).

If no heart beat can be detected with a fetascope, use a doppler if one is available. Typically, there is a uniform, ominous silence and stillness over the uterus. If no heartbeat can be heard, arrange for an ultrasound exam to determine the condition of the baby without delay. It is possible to have a live fetus with an inaudible heartbeat. Accompany the parents for the exam if you possibly can, so you will be there to comfort them in the event that the baby is dead. Other clinical signs and symptoms suggesting that the baby is not alive include:

* The mother reports a feeling of weight, or of a body lying heavily in the abdomen.
* The disappearance (either sudden or gradual) of other symptoms of pregnancy such as breast changes.
* Cessation or reduction of uterine growth with the uterus feeling

smaller, firmer and evenly resistant over its surface

*After a week to 10 days, the skull becomes characteristically softened, with the bones freely movable and the scalp hanging over them like a loose sac. This may be felt during an internal exam or more rarely during palpation. The rest of the baby's body loses its characteristic feel on palpation. (Greenhill, 1951)

While the above signs are important to know, the advent of ultrasound has rendered these signs less relevant to modern practice. In addition, an alert mother will sense trouble much more quickly than the time it would take for these symptoms to manifest. An ultrasound exam will give a definitive answer in most cases. Having documentation of a prelabor fetal death will make it easier for you legally to offer to assist the birth at home if the parents so desire.

If the baby is not dead, information from the tests will determine the choices presented to the parents by mainstream care providers. Anything may be recommended from going home and waiting for term labor to daily or weekly retesting to immediate surgical delivery, depending upon the situation.

If the baby has died, the parents will be in shock and disbelief. Unless other complicating factors are present, such as bleeding from the yoni, the parents have time to go home and decide what they want to do. Their options are:

Check into the hospital for immediate induction: This usually entails inserting prostaglandin gel near the woman's cervix to ripen it. This will take about 24 hours. (8 500 mg. Evening Primrose oil or 3 1500 mg. Borage oil capsules can also be inserted at home for the same purpose.) Once the cervix is ripe, the woman will go back to the hospital for oxytocin induction. Since she may be reluctant to admit that the baby is dead (it will all feel like a nightmare to her at this point), induction can take some time to get going.

Obstetricians may use prostaglandin suppositories to soften the cervix and initiate contractions. This can be dangerous, especially past 28 weeks; uterine rupture has been reported. Treatment often produces severe nausea, vomiting, diarrhea, elevated blood pressure, bronchial constriction, rapid heart rate, seizures and fever. Prostaglandin gel is safer, can be used near term, and does not produce such severe side effects. Laminaria inserts can also be used to begin to open the cervix and carry none of these pharmaceutical risks, although there is some chance that the insert could rupture the membranes.

Stay home and wait for normal labor to begin, then go to the hospital for the birth: Many hospital based practitioners will feel uncomfortable with this option and the mother must be clear with them that she is making her own decision, not being pressured into anything by her midwife.

Wait for labor and then birth at home: Of course, this means you will be attending the birth and you must decide if you feel up to the job in relationship to your clinical skills, the political climate, and emotionally. About 80% of women retaining a dead fetus will go into spontaneous labor within 3 weeks. How to assist at the birth of a dead baby is covered in Volume II.

Watching and waiting: Whenever the parents decide to wait for labor to begin, there are certain precautions to take:

Monitor maternal clotting status: The mother's clotting status can be compromised due to absorbed thromboplastic substances (which cause the acceleration of clot formation) from the placenta or fetus which can lead to a gradual depletion in maternal fibrinogen levels. Fibrinogen is one of the many clotting related agents in the blood. Disseminated intravascular coagulation (DIC) gradually develops in about 25% of women who retain a dead fetus for more than 4 weeks, but rarely occurs sooner than that.

Various clotting values can vacillate from day to day, ranging from normal to very low. More typically, fibrinogen falls from normal pregnant levels back to a nonpregnant range. In some cases it continues to drop as low as 100 mg./dl. or less. The platelet count may also drop, but severe thrombocytopenia does not usually develop. The onset of easy bruising or bleeding (as from the gums or nose) suggests dangerously low platelet levels. Spontaneous correction to normal levels occurs after delivery, but often the recovery is slow. Liver-supporting herbs, especially Yellow Dock and Dandelion root tinctures, may help speed this process.

Clotting studies should be done after the fetal death is confirmed to get a baseline, then repeated 2 weeks later and every week thereafter until birth, or as indicated. Liver supporting herbs will help boost factor production. (See chapter on the Liver and Pregnancy in Diagnostic Tests for tips.) If abnormal values or suspicious symptoms present themselves, the plan to wait for spontaneous labor should be abandoned and the birth should take place in the hospital. Clotting factors should be restored to normal levels before induction is attempted (see Diagnostic Tests for more information about which tests to run).

Preparing for labor: If the fetus dies before term, it may take two to three weeks for labor to begin, because the woman's body is not ready to go into labor and because she may need time to psychologically integrate what has happened. Uterine stimulant herbs, nipple stimulation, and Evening Primrose oil capsules (500 mg., three times daily) may be used during this time to help stimulate the uterus and soften the cervix. The mother can also take homeopathic remedies as recommended in the first chapter in the third trimester section, Prenatal Care from the 29th week until Birth. Have the mother take her temperature 3 to 4 times daily and insert nothing into her yoni. Internal yoni exams should be withheld until labor is well underway. If membranes rupture and labor does not begin immediately, transport to the hospital for an induction, as the risk of infection is greatly increased.

Six to eight intact 500 mg. Evening Primrose oil capsules can be placed in the posterior fornix (behind the cervix) and allowed to dissolve. This can be repeated every 8 to 12 hours. Evening Primrose provides the raw materials the cervix needs to make more of its own prostaglandins and therefore side-steps the dangers of adding hormone directly. It can ripen a cervix remarkably in 24 to 36 hours. This should be done only if is seems necessary and only after other things have been done to prepare the body for labor, since introducing something into the yoni slightly increases the risk of rupture of membranes and infection.

Have the mother visualize a normal birth, normal placental delivery, and minimal bleeding. Speak to her specifically about not manifesting her grief through a birth complication. Explain in advance that it would be a good idea to set the baby aside until the placenta is out and all bleeding is under control, before she says hello and goodbye. This will allow her to give as much attention as she can to the process of completing the birth without problems. Suggest that she select clothes for the baby and think of other ways she may want to relate to the baby's body once born (anointing the baby with fragrant oils, bathing the baby, etc.) The spirit of the baby is often very much present during the birth.

If labor is delayed, the parents should be told that the baby may look dark or bruised, that the body will be very limp and filled with fluid, and that the skin may be peeling. In some cases, the fluid and baby may have a foul odor at the time of birth (watch the mother carefully for infection). The parents should know these things ahead of time since they will be imagining what it may be like to see the baby. Addressing their fears out loud may help them prepare for the birth. Also, ask them what they need from you every time you see them, as you may not always be able to anticipate their needs and should not try to. They may need things explained to them several times, since denial, shock and grief may make it hard to take information in the first time it is presented. Support them to share the reality of the situation with other siblings, as they will have their own feelings to work through regarding the death.

Remember that a woman who has carried a dead fetus for a week or two has had a gradual drop in blood volume over that period of time. This factor must be taken into account when assessing blood loss at any time during the birth.

How to deal with the actual birth will be covered in Volume II; postpartum grieving considerations will be covered in Volume III.

References and further reading:

Greenhill, J., Principles and Practice of Obstetrics, W. B. Saunders, Co., Philadelphia, PA, 1951.

Scar Dehiscence and Uterine Rupture in The Third Trimester

Spontaneous uterine rupture during pregnancy in a woman who has an unscarred, normal uterus and no history of invasive procedures (such as dilation and curettage) is virtually unheard of. In women who have had uterine incisions from surgery, damage from invasive intrauterine procedures, or uterine abnormalities, rupture during pregnancy is rare but does occasionally occur. While the uterus may rupture at any time during the course of pregnancy, it is most likely to happen closer to term, since uterine enlargement will increase the chances that the scar will give way. The rather ominous term "rupture" is often used to describe all types of uterine disruption. Many scar problems which do occur are relatively benign and may go completely undetected, even though they may get lumped in with statistics of more traumatic rupture events. When rupture occurs during labor, it usually happens in women who have had previous surgery, many babies or when a woman is unusually sensitive to the effects of oxytocic drugs.

In a review of the literature, Clark (1988) noted that scar separation after a low transverse Cesarean incision, the most common variety, is rare. Ranges from 0.5% to 2% are reported (Clark, 1988: Haq, 1988) and most cases were benign. Classical or T incisions pose a greater risk of traumatic rupture, with many occurring preterm; one study cited a 4% risk with classical incisions (Haq, 1988).

Predisposing factors: Uterine rupture may be precipitated by any of the following underlying causes:

* *Thinness or other defect in the uterine wall due to congenital anomalies
* *Implantation of the placenta within anomalous areas of the uterus such as a rudimentary horn
* *Sites of uterine puncture or other injury which were never repaired such as those which may occur during an induced abortion
* *Previously repaired surgical incisions in the uterus
* *Sites where a portion of the uterine wall was removed and then repaired, such as a fibroid which had grown within the uterine wall
* *Concealed prenatal hemorrhage from the placenta (a rare cause)
* *Placenta percreta (placenta has grown into and through the uterine wall and may invade adjacent organs; creates a weak area in the uterine wall)
* *Previous extensive cervical laceration which weakens the lower uterine segment
* *Endometritis and myometritis (inflammation of the endometrium or the uterine muscle)
* *Hydatidiform mole

*Cornual resection for ectopic pregnancy
*Hysterotomy
*Amniocentesis during pregnancy can lead to a weakened area in the myometrium (extremely rare) (Oxhorn, 1986)

Types of rupture:

***Silent, bloodless, benign dehiscence** of a previous cesarean scar
***Incomplete:** includes only the myometrial layer of the uterus; the peritoneum covering that portion of the uterus remains intact.
***Separation of uterine layers:** the serosa and part of the external myometrium are torn, but the tear does not extend into the uterine cavity. A severe intraperitoneal hemorrhage may occur which eludes diagnosis.
***Complete:** all the layers of the uterus are involved and there is direct communication between the uterine and abdominal cavities.

Clinical presentation: How a uterine rupture presents during pregnancy depends upon a number of factors:

*Cause of rupture
*Degree of rupture (complete or incomplete)
*Position or location of rupture
*Extent of rupture
*Amount of bleeding into the intraperitoneal space
*Size of blood vessels involved and amount of bleeding
*Extent of extrusion of the fetus and/or placenta from the uterus
*Degree of retraction of the myometrium
*General condition of the woman

Rupture related to previous surgery: The most common type of prenatal rupture is related to separation of a uterine scar. (See the chapter on Types of Uterine Surgeries in the section on Special Circumstances regarding the different types of incisions.) Keep in mind that VBAC women may experience sensations of pulling, aching, soreness, pains and twinges, throughout pregnancy and labor which are all within normal limits as long as they do not persist and increase. Many women notice pain in the layer of tissue between the skin and the uterus overlying the Cesarean scar which is due to adhesions in the tissue being broken as the uterus enlarges. Many scar separations are not accompanied by pain or tenderness (Clark, 1988).

874

Most complete scar separations (ruptures) are extensions of an existing window which developed prior to the onset of labor, usually before the 37th week. Any scar that has made it to the threshold of labor intact is likely to stay that way throughout the birth unless the injudicious use of oxytocin or intrauterine manipulations provide sufficient stress to cause a rupture.

Atraumatic "window": This usually occurs during the healing process and is defined as a hole along the line of the incision. This window is healed all around its edges and is really an opening along the line of the scar where the edges did not heal to each other but did heal separately. A woman may have such a window in her scar and proceed to carry her pregnancy and give birth normally. If the window is large enough, membranes and even fetal parts can protrude through it, causing the edges of the window to spread (a traumatic extension of the window). This, however, is very rare.

Windows in the scar usually cause no problems by themselves and, unless another surgery is performed or a uterine exploration is done postpartum, often go undetected.

Traumatic extension of a window: A window in the scar may be widened by the pressure from the enlarging pregnancy, causing an increasingly painful, tearing sensation. The onset of pain may be very gradual, becoming constant, and may be mistaken for an abruption of the placenta. This may not occur before labor contractions have begun. The woman's pulse may rise and bleeding from the yoni may or may not occur. Once the scar has given way as much as it is going to, a bubble of intact membranes may prolapse into the abdominal cavity followed by some or all of the fetus. This release of pressure will often cause the pain to vanish and may result in a delayed or missed diagnosis. One woman reported a bubbling sensation as amniotic fluid was released into her peritoneum (Schlinger, 1995)

Atraumatic dehiscence: A dehiscence refers to an area along the line of an incision in which some, but not all, of the layers of the uterus have healed together. It also appears to be a result of healing rather than a result of labor stress. This does not pose a dangerous situation for either mother or baby.

Traumatic opening of a uterine scar (rupture of most of or the entire incision): Typically, when a low transverse scar truly ruptures, it separates along the line of the incision, opening gently and neatly like a seam or zipper. This process is often asymptomatic and benign. Symptoms of trauma are most likely to occur when the scar is nearer the uterine fundus and may present in a variety of ways. Some cases may mimic other abdominal conditions or urinary tract infection. There may or may not be bleeding which produces swelling over the lower uterine segment. Some women have a fever; in others, the uterus may feel as hard as a board.

How a traumatic rupture will appear can be divided into four basic presentations:

1. Silent or quiet rupture: Silent rupture begins without the usual signs and symptoms. Diagnosis is difficult and may be delayed since nothing dramatic happens. A rising pulse rate, pallor, and perhaps slight bleeding from the yoni may occur. The woman may complain of some pain and may feel she is having contractions but no cervical changes are found on exam. This presentation is most often seen when a previous Cesarean scar has a traumatic separation.

2. Typical: Symptoms develop over a period of a few hours and include abdominal pain, vomiting, faintness, bleeding from the yoni, rapid pulse rate, pallor, tenderness of the uterus on palpation and absence of the fetal heart sounds. If this goes unrecognized, hypotension and shock develop.

3. Violent rupture: This is the example used when scare tactics are employed to talk women out of attempting a yoni birth after a Cesarean. The woman may think she is suddenly in heavy labor. A violent pain is followed by a sensation of something having given way and of sharp pain in the lower abdomen. After this the contractions cease, the character of the pain changes, and the woman may become anxious. The fetus is expelled from the uterine cavity and can be easily palpated; it feels close to the examining fingers. Sometimes the uterus and fetus can be palpated in different areas of the abdomen (the uterus, once empty, may contract down, becoming quite small). The presenting part moves freely. Fetal movements may cease and no fetal heart sounds can be found. Signs of maternal shock follow and complete collapse may occur.

4. Rupture with delayed diagnosis: Gradual deterioration of the woman's condition makes it apparent that a serious underlying problem exists. She may demonstrate unexplainable and unresponsive anemia. Investigation discovers a palpable hematoma along a broad ligament of the uterus and signs of peritoneal irritation such as cramping and contracting of the ligament develop. The woman may gradually slip into shock due to blood loss, or suddenly become shocky if the hematoma ruptures.

What to do: If the woman is symptomatic and you suspect uterine rupture, transport without delay. If the woman is completely asymptomatic but seems to have fetal parts protruding through an opening in her uterus, send her in to be evaluated by a hospital-based care provider.

Spontaneous rupture of the normal uterus: This rare complication usually occurs during labor. It is discussed in Volume II.

876

References and further reading:

Clark, S., "Rupture of the Scarred Uterus," <u>Ob Gyn Clin North Am</u>, Vol. 15, No. 4, 1988, pp. 737-744.
Haq, C., "Vaginal Birth after cesarean delivery," <u>Am Fam Physician</u>, Vol. 37, No. 6, 1988, pp. 167-171.
Oxhorn, Harry, <u>Human Labor and Birth</u>, Appleton-Century-Crofts, Norwalk, Ct, 1986.
Schlinger, Hilary, midwife, Ithica, NY, editing comments, 5/30/95

Postdatism and Postmaturity Syndrome

Postdates pregnancy is defined by a pregnancy which exceeds the 42nd week. In many obstetrical practices, being postdates is a high risk category and increases the barrage of interventions that the medical model will force upon a woman until she gives birth. This is because a few babies from postdate pregnancies will exhibit postmaturity syndrome; a compromised baby suspected to result from the extended length of pregnancy. This chapter assumes you have taken into account such variables as family history of length of gestation, parity, and length of the menstrual cycle in arriving at an individualized due date and now have a woman who is approaching 40 weeks or more.

Is the due date correct? In order to find out if a problem truly exists, the first thing to do is reexamine the due date. (Refer to the chapter on Calculating the Due Date in the Basic Skills section for a full discussion.)

Postdatism vs. postmaturity syndrome: In a well-nourished woman who salts to taste and drinks to thirst pregnancy usually proceeds to term and often 1 to 2 weeks past the 40 week mark. In fact, 42 weeks may be the normal gestation for humans. When a well expanded blood volume has stimulated a well grown and well nourished placenta, neither baby nor placenta will suffer before birth occurs. Fetal growth continues, fetal movement and heart rate variability maintain themselves normally, the volume of amniotic fluid is adequate, blood volume remains appropriately expanded providing optimal placental profusion and everything is fine.

Such a pregnancy may be postdates by the classic definition of the term, but it is NOT postmature. Most women assumed to be postdates have been misclassified based on an inaccurate due date. Their babies are quite healthy. In fact, congenital anomalies, infection and intrauterine growth retardation account for much of the perinatal mortality generally lumped into the postmature category. About 10% of babies are postdates, of which only 5% to 26% exhibit postmaturity syndrome. (Nichols, 1985a) One study of 7005 infants, which excluded babies from mothers with conditions known to affect fetal size, found the mean birth weight increased as pregnancy advanced and no babies less than 2500 gms. were born after 42 weeks. No evidence of weight loss or lower weight for length was found. The study concluded that there is a lack of convincing evidence that the postterm baby of a healthy mother is at increased risk of distress or nutritional deprivation. (McLean, et.al., 1991)

While physicians are talking about dysmaturity on the one hand, they don't want pregnancy to go beyond 42 weeks because of the fear that the baby will grow too big!! Obviously, a large healthy baby of a well-nourished mother is not suffering from intrauterine starvation. Furthermore, performing Cesareans for "macrosomia" (defined as any baby larger than 4000 gm. or 8 lb. 13 oz.!) does not decrease the rate of asphyxia or injury. (Boyd, et.al., 1983)

When is there cause for concern? In any of the following cases, you may have to be more concerned about the possibility of inadequate blood flow to the placenta, the real culprit in creating a compromised baby, regardless of gestational age:

*Women who have been poorly nourished for reasons such as vomiting, nausea, poverty, etc., for more than a week during the pregnancy; however, the placenta grows throughout pregnancy so any improvement in diet can be beneficial.
*Any woman who smokes or takes excessive amounts of poorly assimilated calcium supplements or antacids containing calcium during her pregnancy *and* has a marginal diet.
*Women who have had placental bleeding unrelated to previa, as this may indicate a poorly adhered placenta. Dietary improvement and vitamin E (up to 2000 IU. at the time of bleeding) can help strengthen the placental bed.
*Women experiencing no uterine activity (i.e. toning contractions) by the 34th week of pregnancy or no cervical twinges or low menstrual-like sensations by 37 weeks. This can represent inadequate hormonal activity. Equinox Botanicals Prenatal Uterine Tonic, started at 34 weeks, can help to balance this out.
*Women who have had pituitary or hypothyroid disorders. Sometimes these problems are not evident until labor doesn't ever begin. Watch for appropriate breast changes during pregnancy and adequate toning contractions without herbal assistance. (If there is a history of hypoactivity, glandular supplements may help; if hyperactivity has been a problem, homeopathic preparation of either pituitary or thyroid (3X potency) can be alternated every other day during the entire pregnancy to gently support the gland without overstimulation. Which you use will depend upon the gland involved. Consultation with a naturopath is recommended.)

Anything which causes poor placental implantation, interferes with circulation to the placental surface or otherwise leads to improper fetal nourishment can lead to a situation that does not support a healthy pregnancy until birth and, therefore, what is termed postmaturity syndrome or dysmaturity in the newborn. In these cases you may get any of the following problems, depending upon the degree of severity: meconium staining; a baby with loose skin, appearing to have lost weight; little or no skull molding due to calcification of the bones; or a placenta inadequately supplied with blood to compensate for the lower oxygen supplied to the uterus during contractions. These newborn problems were first described in a small study of 37 infants ranging between 285 to 325 days of gestation (41 to 46.4

weeks). Clifford described three grades of severity, but the ages of the infants widely overlapped within each grade; no control infants were examined and no evidence that problems related to placental insufficiency was presented (Clifford, 1954). In fact, postmaturity syndrome is not exclusively related to postdates babies nor do its signs have clinical importance (Shearer & Estes, 1985) other than to demonstrate malnourishment of the fetus *in utero*. Those symptoms ascribed to postmaturity may simply be due to a baby with a degree of intrauterine growth retardation who has gone past term. The postdates babies at highest risk are those weighing less than 2500 gm (5 lb. 8 oz.), not surprising if poor maternal nutrition is the real problem. The most frequent cause of death in these cases is congenital malformation. (Sims & Walther, 1989)

Placental factors: A placenta compromised by inadequate blood flow from a poorly expanded blood volume or vasoconstriction of the uterine arteries (as might be the case in a smoker) results in a poorly nourished baby (Fox, 1991). While postmaturity has been commonly blamed on placental insufficiency, and felt to be the result of infarcts (dead spaces) and calcifications, these problems *by themselves* are not such a problem if blood flow to the placenta is adequate. The fact that the villous surface of the placenta expands right up until birth means that the placenta does not "get old" in the way it has been thought (Fox, 1991) and that any improvements the mother makes which increase blood flow to the placenta (improving her diet, quitting smoking, etc.) will benefit the pregnancy right up until the end.

Many mainstream practitioners encourage women to take antacids (especially Tums) to relieve heartburn, feeling that they will get an "added benefit" because these products contain calcium. However, this calcium is not well assimilated, as is frequently apparent from looking at the placenta after birth. If an excessive amount has been taken, the placenta may be full of calcifications. Poorly assimilated supplements, hard (mineralized) drinking water or smoking can also cause excessive placental calcifications. The combination of many calcifications and a marginally expanded blood volume are a set-up for trouble. Furthermore, a calcified placenta is more fragile and more likely to break up during detachment after the birth. If a woman comes to you with such a history, you must take these factors into account. Bio-technical providers are also recommending aspirin for high blood pressure (See the chapter on Hypertension in Pregnancy, general Problems section, for the reasons). Since aspirin and other salicylates interfere with prostaglandin production, this may increase the chances of a prolonged pregnancy as well.

Dealing with postdatism in a well-nourished woman: First, recheck the due date and previous pregnancy history of the client and her mother (i.e. what was her mother's length of gestation?). Recurrent postdates pregnancies may be normal for a particular woman and are often seen among women in the same family. Check

880

uterine size and fetal growth, contraction activity, cervical sensations, heart rate variability and reactivity, and amount of amniotic fluid at each prenatal. Have the mother keep a daily fetal movement chart (see Diagnostic Tests). See her weekly until birth. Make sure she continues to eat well *and to drink plenty of clear fluids—six to eight glasses daily* or more if she is more thirsty or lives in an extremely dry climate. I suspect that some women unconsciously reduce their fluid intake at the end of pregnancy, because the increasing pressure from the presenting part results in more frequent urination. In the normal situation, amniotic fluid volume is directly related to maternal fluid intake; it is therefore important that women know how vital it is to keep drinking. (Kilpatrick, et al., 1993) If all signs look good, relax and wait for labor to start. In my experience, some women who are fairly well-nourished have reduced amniotic fluid volume when they carry to 43 weeks, but no other symptoms; attention to daily fluid intake should lessen this possibility. Less fluid or the suspicion of it calls for discussion of a biophysical profile test and diligent fetal heart monitoring in labor. Oligohydramnios correlates with fetal distress, probably due to cord compression. However, the amount of amniotic fluid does not correlate with outcome, and it is unclear to what extent reduced fluid is characteristic of prolonged pregnancy or when intervention solely for this factor is warranted. (Shearer & Estes, 1985)

Dealing with postdatism in a less-than-well-nourished woman: In situations that you feel either from history, clinical signs, or intuition on your part or the mother's may develop into true postmaturity syndrome, monitor at each prenatal as described above. Depending on your findings and the individual situation, you may also want to employ any of the following:

* *Beginning at 36 weeks have the mother record fetal activity daily and review this chart at every visit.
* *Assess the fetal heart rate for good variability and accelerations with fetal movement at every prenatal. (See chapters on Fetal Activity Test and Assessment of Fetal Movement in Diagnostic Tests.)
* *Give Equinox Botanicals Uterine Tonic for the 6 weeks before term.
* *If, in spite of therapies, no uterine activity is present, have the mother do nipple stimulation starting at 38 weeks. This can be done by rolling the nipple end between the fingers or by applying gentle suction with a breast pump. If stimulation causes contractions longer than 1 minute in duration, stop that session at that point.
* *To ripen the cervix, have the mother take three 500 mg doses of evening primrose, borage or black currant oil daily beginning at 36 weeks and continuing until birth.
* *Starting at 36 to 37 weeks, three tablets daily of glandular pituitary extract may help to prime the pituitary gland to produce adequate oxytocin. (Do not use this if there is a history of hyperactive

pituitary function; instead use a homeopathic preparation of pituitary (3X) one dose every other day throughout pregnancy).
*Heterosexual intercourse provides prostaglandins in the form of semen. If the mother has a male partner and is so inclined, frequent sex will help ripen the cervix.
*At 36 weeks, begin the following homeopathic remedies:
-Cimicifuga 12C, 1 pellet on Monday
-Caulophyllum 12C, 1 pellet on Wednesday
-Arnica 12C, 1 pellet on Friday
Continue to take each remedy once weekly as suggested until birth. This will help prime the uterus for the timely onset of effective labor and minimize physical trauma to mother and baby.

If clinical evaluation suggests a problem or if the woman is past 42 weeks of pregnancy, do not hesitate to discuss a biophysical profile to assess fetal well-being. While prenatal testing is not, by any means, 100% reliable as to the condition of the baby, at least this test offers five variables from which to judge well-being and also is fairly reliable if severe distress is discovered (see Diagnostic Tests). If you feel it is advisable to attempt labor induction in a woman who has reached or passed term, see Volume II or the postmaturity chapter in Diagnostic Tests for suggestions.

Psychological factors and postdatism: For a variety of reasons, conscious or unconscious, a woman may be holding off her labor. She may be afraid she can't do it, waiting for a friend or relative to arrive (or leave!), ambivalent about her birth choices, or uncertain about her ability to mother or her relationship with her partner. In the midst of evaluating physical signs, be sure you are sensitive to emotional symptoms as well. In addition, there is the cultural stress around going beyond her due date. This fact cannot be dealt with in a vacuum, and your relatively gentle interventions to encourage physiological readiness for labor will serve to insulate women, to a certain extent, from the medical hysteria in the larger society. A woman's feelings about these factors should be discussed as well. A solid relationship throughout pregnancy will provide the framework through which conflicts and problems can be expressed and released.

Helping the mother deal with being overdue: Inevitably, families and friends are anxious and excited when a woman nears her due date. When she carries beyond it, they can be real pests! Typically, people call on a daily basis, questioning the mother about any symptoms of labor and asking what the midwife has said or recommended. The best thing she can do is have an answering machine screen her calls or, if she can afford it, use the new device that lets her know the number of who is calling before she picks up the phone. In this way she can avoid

882

some of this aggravation. With all the cultural hysteria over postmaturity, the last thing a woman needs is family and friends adding to the stress.

Labor induction: If necessary, inducing labor with herbs is one alternative to going to the hospital for induction with oxytocin. Herbal induction stimulates a physiologic labor and is much easier on both mother and baby than oxytocin induction. This will be discussed in Volume II.

References and further reading:

Boyd, M., et al., "Fetal macrosomia: prediction, risks, proposed management," Ob Gyn, Vol. 61, No. 16, 1983, pp. 715-722.

Clifford, S., "Postmaturity—with placental dysfunction," J. Pediatrics, Vol. 44, No. 1, 1954, pp. 1-13.

Fox, H., "A contemporary view of the human placenta," Midwifery, Vol. 7, No. 1, March, 1991, pp. 31-39.

Kilpatrick, Sarah, et al., "Maternal Hydration increases amniotic fluid index in women with normal amniotic fluid," OB/GYN, Vol. 81, No. 1, January 1993, pp. 49-52.

McLean F, et al.: Posterm infants: too big or too small? Am J of Ob Gyn, 164(2), 1991, p. 619.

Nichols, C., "Postdate pregnancy. Part I: A literature review," J. Nurse-Midwifery, 1985a, Vol. 30, No. 4, pp. 222-239.

Shearer M., Estes, M., "A critical review of the recent literature on post-term pregnancy and a look at women's experiences," Birth, Vol. 12, No. 2, 1985, pp. 95-111.

Sims, M., Walther, E., "Neonatal morbidity and mortality and long-term outcome of postdate infants," Clin Ob Gyn, Vol. 32, No. 2, 1989, pp. 285-293.

SPECIAL CIRCUMSTANCES

Information in this section should be used as an adjunct to the general information discussed in the sections addressing each trimester of pregnancy.

884

Working With Women Who Want Labor Support for a Hospital Birth

As your reputation as an experienced midwife grows, you may begin to hear from women who are planning a hospital birth but wish to have a midwife provide them with labor support at home and then accompany them to the hospital. These calls typically come from first-time mothers or from women who have no contraindicating medical conditions but nevertheless perceive that they should not choose a homebirth based on their "risk status." This self-screening could be due to previous birth-related complications, the mother's age, or the number of babies she has already had. Other women will seek you out as a compromise measure, perhaps wanting a homebirth themselves but unable to talk their partner into it. At any rate, you will be faced with how to handle such requests.

To the uninitiated, this request appears benign enough, and you may think, "Why not?" There are several points to consider. First of all, you are a midwife, not merely a labor support person. While you can certainly provide labor support, your skill level and expertise in dealing with the variations of normal pregnancy and labor as well as your ability to detect problems will be far more highly developed than a woman who only offers labor support; after all, you are in a more responsible position. Because you bring your skill level and perspective as a primary attendant, it can be very hard to simply provide labor support. Chances are, the woman hopes this is the case, or she would be hiring someone who only offers labor support instead. In other words, she may want your expertise but may not trust the process of birth enough to stay home, which really means she doesn't trust herself.

The expectation that you can use your skills but function in a limited role, especially after the woman enters the hospital, needs to be carefully considered. My motto is "once a midwife, always a midwife." It is almost impossible, and perhaps even unethical, not to apply skills that you have developed. Therefore, don't think you are in a less responsible role just because you are calling yourself a labor support person; until the woman is in the hospital, you are just as responsible as ever. Furthermore, you may bend over backward working with such women during pregnancy and labor, but you then must take them to the hospital and turn over care to their primary provider. Sometimes this works out fine, but often you will have to mutely watch all your careful support go down the tubes as the woman's head is filled with frightening possibilities, her confidence in her body is undermined and she winds up with a highly interfered with birth. Of course, these choices are hers to make, but they can be a big heartache for you as well. In addition, being a primary caregiver hired to provide labor support fosters further fragmentation of care; something which you may or may not wish to support.

Finally, being the primary midwife bringing a woman from a planned homebirth to the hospital for a specific, presumably necessary intervention is very different than assuming a role which requires to you advocate for her and support her to *avoid* unnecessary interventions instead. In this process, you can't help but wonder "what are we doing here, anyway?" (oh yes, you remind yourself, the mother *chooses* to be here). Role-switching may not sit well with collaborating physicians either; doctors who are normally happy to help you with a transport may not be so happy for you to be advising a woman to deviate from their normal management of labor, thus disrupting your relationship for future transports. Some of the concerns addressed here are somewhat mitigated if the woman has a physical condition which truly contraindicates homebirth, but many of them apply in all cases.

Consultation visit: Offer a consultation visit to discuss all the usual issues, including their thoughts about homebirth and midwifery care. What exactly do they expect from you as a labor support person? Be specific; do they want yoni exams?, fetal heart tone checks? Give them a clear idea of your expectations regarding their clarity of choice, the need for prenatal visits and good nutrition and the type of relationship you hope to build with them prior to birth.

Be aware that some women will seek a midwife for labor support with the intention of staying at home for the birth if things are going well. I highly discourage you from leaving such an option open. Fence-sitters are refraining from stepping into responsibility by making a clear choice. If everything looks great during labor, you might be tempted to allow them to make such a last minute decision. Then, if an unexpected complication occurs, you could be in a very compromised position because of their unwillingness to commit in the first place. This is especially true if the woman has manipulated the situation around the unwillingness of her partner. If a homebirth is desired, they should make this decision prenatally; be clear that changing their mind in labor is not an option and stick to this.

Prenatal care: As a homebirth midwife, it is likely that your way of caring for women will be very different from that of the primary care provider a woman has engaged. You will need to be assured of normal parameters of well-being for the woman and her baby, just as you would for any woman you are expecting to assist during labor. Therefore, I strongly urge you to consider offering this woman full, or at least some, prenatal care. Doing so will help you establish a relationship and will also help you gauge just how much "alternative" care she is interested in. Offering prenatal visits is, however, a double edged sword. You may frequently find yourself at odds with recommendations that she has been given by her primary care provider. In such cases, sit back and hear what she has been told, give your opinion if requested, and then remain unattached to what she chooses to do.

It sometimes happens that women very much want to trust the natural process of birth, but they do not. Therefore, they choose a physician for primary care and come to a midwife for support. You may not realize this at first, but be aware that such women can project their desire to trust birth onto you and their distrust of birth onto their doctor. You can get caught in the middle, with the woman's dualistic persona requiring the doctor to recommend lots of interventions and then requiring you to fix them. See the chapter on Dealing With Emotional Issues with Clients in the section on Sustaining Health and Well-being for ideas about how to help women reintegrate this split within themselves.

Fees: Because you will be spending the same amount of time with this woman as you would with any woman you attend, I encourage you to charge a full fee for your services. If she only wants labor support, let her hire a labor support person. If you take her on, she will be taking up a slot in your monthly schedule of births and she will be getting more expert care. You should be compensated accordingly.

Caring for Women-of-Size

Our culture has a tremendous loathing of large, especially fat, women. While being overweight certainly can take its toll on the physical self, living in a culture that ridicules women-of-size does not help matters, and leads instead to high levels of stress. Women who are overweight actually have some points in their favor when it comes to pregnancy. First of all, they have ample stored energy to withstand the occasional cold or bout of flu, and can compensate for the nausea and vomiting of early pregnancy more easily because of the extra calories they have on hand.

Prenatal exams: The more tissue there is between your palpating hands and the baby within the uterus, the harder it will be to feel small parts adequately to determine fetal position, the harder it will be to hear the fetal heart and the harder it will be to assess the volume of amniotic fluid. Version will be harder to perform as well. Expect to begin to be able to feel fetal parts and hear heart tones even with a Doppler later in pregnancy than usual. Fundal height measurements will be harder to obtain and will often be more than anticipated based on the weeks of pregnancy indicate they should be. Many large women have an "apron" of abdominal skin that hangs down; lifting this tissue, or having the mother pull up on her belly to render the skin taunt can help during all necessary abdominal exams. The woman-of-size may have difficulty moving around as pregnancy advances, and may even have difficulty maintaining perineal hygiene.

Weight gain issues: The woman who is carrying extra pounds may be particularly concerned about gaining more weight during pregnancy. Advise her to cut out all junk foods and refined carbohydrates (such as white bread, pasta and sugars) to concentrate her diet on high quality proteins, vegetables and whole grain products (as you would advise any woman to do) and to walk or swim daily. If she improves her diet, she may not gain weight. In some cases weight may actually be lost during pregnancy. Most of the time, however, such women gain modest amounts of weight. Any of these are fine as long as a woman is not trying to diet and as long as she does not restrict her food intake. Likewise, neither weight nor dietary restrictions should be imposed in a misguided attempt to control the size of the baby. Eating well, eliminated empty-calories foods and exercising will help with this and will not be harmful.

Medical complications: Obesity may bring with it some associated medical complications, such as essential high blood pressure, and because of the difficulty in palpating the uterus these women may be more prone to certain birth complications such as undetected other-than-vertex presentations or surprise multiple gestation!

As far as the woman-of-size being at higher risk for birth, much of this is

888

related to nutritional choices and lack of exercise which may have contributed to the obesity in the first place. Keep in mind that some people have a genetic predisposition to obesity as well. When women improve their diets and begin to be more active, some of their obstetrical risk is reduced, as is true for any woman.

Cultural attitudes: Certainly the biggest problem for women-of-size is not so much their size but the white western views regarding them. To say that such women have been treated unfairly, with little respect and often outright mistreated is an understatement. Remember too, that excess weight gain sometimes begins in a childhood during which abuse, either physical, sexual, or both, are the norm. That "apron" of belly may afford protection for the genitals and obesity in general counters our cultural norms about what is attractive, serving to insulate a woman from unwanted sexual advances.

Multiple Gestation

While in some preliterate cultures the birth of twins has been considered a blessing, modern obstetrics has made pregnancy and birth with multiple gestations almost a curse. The level of fear, technology, and general anxiety that the woman carrying multiples is subjected to is very high. Medical management of multiple gestations leads to a high toxemia rate with twins and an even higher rate with triplets due to their disregard for the protective effects of good nutrition. Even though I do not think this level of fear is warranted or helpful, undoubtedly pregnancy and birth with multiples carries with it some unique risks.

Embryology: The conception of multiple pregnancy has become more common in women being treated for infertility than in the general population. The primary methods which cause more multiple gestations involve the use of hormones to stimulate the release of several ova during a cycle, *in vitro* fertilization (IVF) and embryo transfer. In fact, *in vitro* fertilization produces multiple gestations in up to 22% of cases. The embryology of multiple gestation differs from that of a singleton gestation in some respects. First and foremost is the way two or more babies are conceived instead of one. There are two ways this can occur.

Dizygotic twins (DZ): Twins may originate from two zygotes (two fertilized eggs). This occurs in 66% to 75% of all twin pregnancies. These are also called fraternal twins; they are no more genetically similar than any two siblings with the same biological parents. Mixed sex dizygotic twins may occur. The frequency of DZ twins varies from race to race and increases with maternal age. The incidence is about 1 in 500 Asians, 1 in 125 Caucasians and as high as 1 in 20 in some African populations. These babies have two separate placentas, even though they usually fuse together along one edge. The tendency to conceive DZ twins is carried by the mother; a maternal family history of DZ twins makes additional twin gestation three times more likely than in the general population. If a multiple birth has occurred in the firstborn babies of a mother, she is five times more likely to conceive multiples in a subsequent pregnancy. Maternal age also plays a part; women under 20 birth DZ twins once in every 1000 births, the rate rises to 14 per 1000 between ages 35 to 40; past age 40 the rate once again declines. All twins conceived as a result of IVF and embryo transfer will be dizygotic.

Monozygotic twins (MZ): Identical twins, when one fertilized egg splits into two zygotes, account for 25% to 33% of all twins. About 35% of the time, MZ twins occur during the time starting with the two-cell (blastomere) stage through the morula stage (the first 3 days after conception). The split produces two identical blastocysts. Each embryo then develops its own amniotic and chorionic sacs. The placentas may be separate or fused. The fact that some MZ twins have separate placentas is why they may be easily misdiagnosed as DZ twins. In 65% of the cases, the splitting occurs by division of the inner cell mass (embryoblast) of the blastocyst at the end of the first week of development.

Fetal-to-fetal connection between the blood vessels in the placentas is called **anastomosis.** It occurs to some degree in virtually all MZ multiples. These connections may be artery-to-artery, vein-to-vein, artery-to-vein or a combination of these. A sufficient artery-to-vein link between placentas can produce a potentially serious complication called Twin-to-Twin Transfusion Syndrome (discussed later in this chapter). Twins at risk for this problem typically have separate amnions, a single chorionic sac and a common placenta. When two chorions are present, clinical problems from the presence of anastomoses are rare.

Late division of pre-embryonic cells (during the second week) results in MZ twins that share one set of membranes (amnion and chorion). The umbilical cords of such twins often become so entangled that they are rarely born alive.

TYPES OF MONOZYGOTIC TWINS	
DAY AFTER FERTILIZATION WHEN ZYGOTE SPLITS	**MODE OF TWINNING**
Less than 4 days	Dichorionic, diamniotic
4 to 8 days	Monochorionic, diamniotic (75%)
8 to 13 days	Monochorionic, monoamniotic
More than 13 days	Conjoined twins

ZYGOSITY	SEPARATE CHORION & AMNION	SINGLE CHORION		TWO CHORIONS	
		SINGLE AMNION	TWO AMNIONS	FUSED PLACENTAS	TWO PLACENTAS
Monozygotic	35%	Uncommon (4%)	65%-75%	25%	10%
Dizygotic	100%	---	---	40%	60%

Conception of higher order multiple gestations: Triplets may be conceived when one zygote divides into two identical zygotes and one of these zygotes again divides, producing identical triplets. One zygote may divide, producing identical twins with an additional fertilized ovum producing a genetically different sibling. Superovulation (either the natural, or more commonly, the pharmaceutically-stimulated release of more than one ovum) results in different zygotes which can be of the same sex or of different sexes but are no more genetically related than any other siblings. Similar combinations occur in higher order multiples.

Superfecundation: the fertilization of two or more ova during the same cycle by sperm from two different men. This can be confirmed by testing for genetic markers.

Superfetation: occurs when a second ovum is fertilized within a uterus that already contains a developing conceptus fertilized in a previous cycle. In these rare pregnancies the babies are of different gestational ages.

Twin blood types: Anastomosis (communication) of fused placentas occasionally occurs in DZ twins and results in erythrocyte mosaicism. This results in a mixed blood type called blood group chimera; these babies have blood cells of two different genotypes that are from different zygotes.

(Section based on Moore & Persaud, 1993)

Prenatal care considerations:

Diagnosing multiple gestation: Identification of multiple gestation is not always straightforward, but these signs and symptoms should alert you to investigate:

   *Woman became pregnant using *in vitro* fertilization or ovulation-
      inducing drugs
   *Family history (dizygotic twins only; the incidence of monozygotic
      twinning is the same regardless of race or family history)
   *Ravenous appetite
   *Large-for-dates uterine growth, especially if the size indicates you
      should be able to hear the fetal heart or find fetal small parts, but
      you cannot, particularly after 20 weeks. Also consider:
      -Polyhydramnios with a single fetus
      -Large single baby
   *Unexplained anemia develops
   *Polyhydramnios develops
   *Rapid and more than usual weight gain
      -May be a normal weight gain spurt for some women
   *Woman reports feeling fetal motion everywhere
   *Feeling three large parts on palpation
      -Rule out fibroids or other growths
   *Hearing two distinct fetal heartbeats, the difference between them
      being at least 8 beats per minute with a region of less intensity
      between the two areas of greatest intensity
   *A crease felt in the fundus, down the front or elsewhere on the uterus
      (this distinguishes the line along which the twin membranes are
      lying and implies that two bags are present)
      -May also occur in a distorted uterine contour with one baby or an
         abnormal uterus, and may be absent in twins

892

Ultrasound to confirm multiples: Once suspected, multiple gestation can be confirmed with an ultrasound exam. While this exposes the babies to an unproven technology, it also confirms your suspicions, and dietary adjustments can be made so the babies will be carried to term. Detecting multiples with palpation alone is not always easy; in fact it is frequently quite tricky, especially if you do not have lots of experience with multiples or if the mother is a first-timer.

Early on, a quick ultrasound exam can be done to determine if more than one fetus is present. A later ultrasound can be done at about 36 weeks. Frequent routine ultrasounds are not any more necessary for multiples than they are for singleton births. Here is a summary of things to look for whenever an ultrasound is done after 20 weeks during a multiple gestation:

> *Fetal gender (if different, indicates dizygotic twins and therefore eliminates the possibility of Twin-to-Twin Transfusion Syndrome)
> *Membrane separating the sacs and number of layers (two layers indicate the babies share a chorion; 4 layers indicate two chorions, two amnions and separate placental systems; no line of separation indicates monoamniotic twins at high risk for cord entanglements)
> *Number and location of placentas
> *Circulatory connection between placentas (some labs can do this)
> *Fetal size-for-dates and fetal size in relationship to each other
> *Signs of fetal defects
> *Amniotic fluid volume in each sac and relative to each other

When ultrasound is done early on, it is possible to note the presence of two or more babies and then have one baby die and be reabsorbed in the first trimester. With the advent of ultrasound, it has been recognized that this happens much more frequently than anyone previously thought. Some threatened miscarriages which go on to term with one baby are undoubtedly the miscarriage of a twin. If you should encounter a woman who has had this experience or who has it while under your care, be sure and talk to her about her grieving process and give her space to feel sad about the loss of one baby. Emotional issues may be complex in these situations. There may be feelings of relief that she isn't having twins, guilt and grief over the loss, plus happiness about the remaining pregnancy. Helping her come to terms with the normalcy of this emotional milieu will help her resolve her feelings.

Fetal positioning: Since twins are the most common multiple gestation, their positioning is discussed most often in textbooks. Obviously more babies mean a more complicated combination of presentations to deal with; for example, triplets have 12 possible combinations (which includes babies lying oblique). The combinations of possible positioning for twins are illustrated below. It is always best for the first baby to be vertex, as this minimizes problems with locked babies at birth and ensures that a well fitting presenting part and a good cervical dilator are present for the initial opening of the cervix during labor. Estimates of the frequency of each presentation combination vary, but an average is given with each (combinations involving oblique lie are not illustrated).

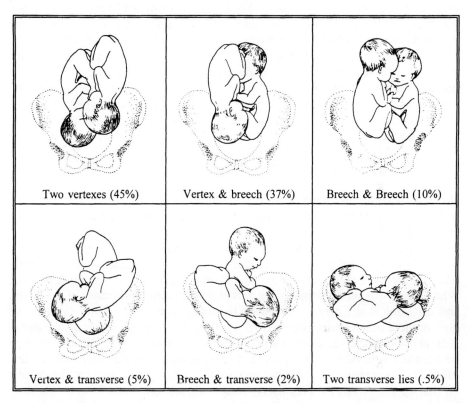

| Two vertexes (45%) | Vertex & breech (37%) | Breech & Breech (10%) |
| Vertex & transverse (5%) | Breech & transverse (2%) | Two transverse lies (.5%) |

Prenatal care: For the healthy, well-nourished woman, prenatal care with a multiple gestation is similar to any other prenatal care. The signs and symptoms of pregnancy may be aggravated for her, nausea may be worse due to the hormonal input from two (or more) placentas, cramps, back aches, "bigness," poor balance and fluid retention may all occur more readily and are all normal variations. In some women, blood pressure may normally be higher during pregnancy since there is more blood for the heart to pump.

Women who are seeing mainstream care providers may be told to expect their babies to come a month before their due date, at 36 weeks of pregnancy. This is how the medical model adjusts for the fact that they haven't figured out how to keep babies in there until term. Not only does this make the mother anxious about prematurity and set her up to expect it, but the doctors tend to get anxious if the mother goes past this point to term or overdue. Tell women to expect to carry to term and explain to them why their back-up providers have told them not to expect this and why you do!

Emotional issues: The prospective parents of more than one baby often feel overwhelmed at the task before them. Feelings of ambivalence about the pregnancy and questions about whether more than one baby is really wanted may plague the mother and cause her to feel more guilty than other women during early pregnancy. Especially if infertility has been a problem, these feelings will be particularly hard to resolve or even discuss. As the midwife, create an opening for both parents to speak about their feelings by pointing out the heightened feelings of joy, ambivalence, guilt and the questions regarding the ability to parent which inevitably occur to most parents expecting a multiple birth. Fears about finances and her living situation may be part of the emotional picture as well. It is also important to directly address her medically-related fears and concerns, especially if she has already seen medical model providers who have frightened her about her risk status.

Nutritional concerns: One of the most significant features of multiple gestation is the presence of two or more placentas and the need to nourish two or more babies. Each fetus requires a 40 to 50% increase in the mother's total non-pregnant blood volume (one baby, a total of 150%; for twins 200%!!) This means that nutrition is of critical importance to the health of the pregnancy. It is directly related to how big the babies will be and whether the mother carries them to term. While this is true for all pregnancies, it is especially obvious in cases of multiples; undernutrition is the major reason why the toxemia and prematurity rates are so high in these pregnancies. *Each extra fetus requires the equivalent of 1 quart of milk in protein and calories daily (30 grams of protein and 500 calories) in addition to the basic diet*: that amounts to 4 additional portions from the Milk and Milk substitutes table or 2 more portions from a Protein table found in the chapter on Dietary Counseling for Pregnancy, Well-being section. In addition to this basic intake, more calories or protein may be needed to compensate for individual stress or activity levels. Extra salt may be needed as well. Eating small frequent meals almost constantly may be the only way a woman can keep up with her needs, especially if she is carrying more than two babies. As pregnancy advances, high protein drinks made with protein powder can play a significant role in keeping intake adequate. Be sensitive to the needs of the individual woman; do not hesitate to recommend an increased protein intake if for any reason it seems necessary.

Admittedly, the more babies a woman is carrying, the more difficult it will be for her to meet her nutritional needs. Some women have found it helpful to substitute skim milk or skim soy milk for clear fluids in order to pack in the protein. Curtailing activities which utilize many calories may be advisable as the pregnancy advances, fetal growth accelerates and the room in the maternal digestive system is encroached upon by her ever enlarging uterus. Large quantities of high bulk foods should be abandoned for protein and calorie-packed foods which provide maximum nutrition and require minimum room for digestion; this means no empty calorie foods!!

Unfortunately, one of the biggest drawbacks of undetected multiple gestation is that the woman doesn't eat what she needs early on. She then goes into premature labor right around the time when the blood volume should peak, which is often when the body can't support the extra burden of more than one baby any longer without the additional blood volume. The risk of premature multiples rises rapidly after 26 weeks, with blood volume peak expected around 28 weeks.

Vitamin and Mineral Supplementation: Multiple gestations requires extraordinary amounts of all nutrients and women should be encouraged to take a natural brand multi-vitamin and mineral supplement daily. A woman may want to take twice or even three times the recommended daily dose, depending upon how many babies she is carrying. In addition, she can take extra Vitamin C with bioflavinoids, calcium (be sure it is easily assimilable) and iron. Anemia is of special concern in a multiple pregnancy, because more babies are relying on maternal iron stores to build their own stores during the last three months. A general program of supplementation with particular emphasis on adequate iron intake is important. Check the hemoglobin frequently to monitor anemia and to make sure that the blood volume is expanding adequately.

Lab work to monitor the pregnancy: Since pregnancy with multiples carries with it such increased demands on the mother, it is wise to get a baseline Liver Profile (Chem screen, SMA-12) at the onset of care in all cases. Repeat the screen, along with a hemoglobin and hematocrit, at 26 weeks; do all tests again at 28 weeks and at 32 weeks and from 36 weeks test every week or two until birth. While this may seem like a lot of tests (you're right, it is), it is an excellent way to monitor for subclinical evidence of liver stress and will allow you to act before it turns into a big problem. (Refer to Diagnostic Tests for review of how to interpret these tests. Refer to the chapter on Toxemia in the Problems Associated With the Third Trimester section if the test results are abnormal.)

Fetal size: If both placentas are functioning normally, and maternal nutrition is adequate, babies from multiple gestations can potentially be as large as singleton babies and follow normal fetal growth curves. Some medical-model care providers expect a slowdown in fetal growth rates after 30 to 32 weeks with twins, even sooner with higher order multiples (Gabbe, et.al., 1991). This slowdown exactly correlates with when maternal blood volume should have peaked, and reflects the inadequate diets of many women carrying multiples. However, this correlation is not seen universally and some studies indicate that fetal size should equal the size of a singleton fetus throughout gestation.

Generally speaking, the babies should be roughly the same size; however, a difference in the weights of newborns of as much as 1 pound has been noted in otherwise normal babies. There can be a disparity of growth rates for a number of reasons, including normal variation, intrauterine growth retardation of only one baby, Twin-to-Twin Transfusion Syndrome (TTTS), or fetal anomalies. Monozygotic twins have the highest incidence of size discordance. If the growth rate of the babies seems significantly unequal, the possible cause should be sought.

Amniotic fluid volume: In most situations, amniotic fluid dynamics in multiples occur as for singleton births. However, it is possible for one or more fetuses to develop an abnormal quantity of fluid due to various underlying complications, although sometimes no apparent reason is found.

Polyhydramnios may occur in the bag of the larger twin in chronic Twin-to Twin Transfusion Syndrome, with oligohydramnios in the sac of the smaller twin. Polyhydramnios may also accompany certain fetal abnormalities, maternal diabetes and some cases of toxemia. Oligohydramnios in the bag of one twin is also referred to as "stuck twin" and occurs most often in the presence of uteroplacental dysfunction. It is also seen in certain types of fetal malformations of genetic origin or in cases of congenital infection. These causes are no different than in singleton pregnancies. (See the chapter on Amniotic Fluid Volume Abnormalities later in this section for more information.)

Acute hydramnios refers to the very rapid accumulation of excess fluid over the course of a few days to two weeks. This condition is almost always associated with monoamniotic pregnancy. The woman may experience varying degrees of upper abdominal discomfort, difficulty breathing, and marked edema of the abdomen, vulva and legs. This usually occurs between 21 and 28 weeks of pregnancy and may lead to premature rupture of membranes or preterm labor. The babies are often normal, but may be too premature to survive. In some cases, drainage of fluid via transabdominal amniocentesis can help to prolong the pregnancy, but the risks of precipitating labor are great, given that drainage must be performed repeatedly. (Danforth, 1986) Try finding an appropriate homeopathic remedy to balance the fluid volume; this will have to be prescribed for the individual woman's symptom picture.

What about bed rest? Premature labor is a primary complication of multiple gestations. Medical care providers often recommend bed rest beginning around 26 to 32 weeks as a deterrent to premature labor. While this may help in cases of loose (incompetent) cervix, it is not the most common reason why bed rest is recommended. The stated reason usually has to do with the overdistention of the uterus which results from multiple gestation. Bed rest keeps the mother off her feet, thereby reducing downward pressure and theoretically preventing premature labor. While the rapid onset of polyhydramnios certainly produces overdistention, and higher order multiples might reasonably be considered to distend the uterus beyond its normal capacity, the carriage of twins and sometimes triplets to the point when women often go into premature labor (between 26 and 36 weeks) is not so extremely different than carriage of one large baby. Keep in mind that women who go into premature labor supposedly because their uterus is overdistended, frequently deliver two or three babies that together barely weigh what one large term baby would weigh. Those women who carry healthy pregnancies to term may have two or even three 7 to 8 pound babies. Something is not quite right about the "overdistention theory of premature twin labor." There must be more to it than this, and the "more" is maternal nutrition!

Bed rest certainly spares calories. Care providers seldom make the connection between blood volume expansion, carrying to term, caloric intake and bed rest. If a woman starts early getting the foods she needs, in the majority of cases bed rest will not be necessary; it depresses the appetite and makes the woman feel like she has a serious disease, not a pregnancy. If premature labor threatens, having a woman go on bed rest and eat, eat, eat, can be used as a temporary measure to help her catch up with her nutritional needs. (Note that no randomized studies demonstrate that bed rest results in prolonging gestation in multiple pregnancies [ACOG, 1995]. Some doctors may recommend a cerclage suture to prevent prematurity in women with normal cervices, but this doesn't work either [Dor, et.al., 1982].)

Visualization: Having more babies means that it is more likely that one or more of them will not present head down. Therefore, encourage the mother to visualize all babies head down from early on, since they will tend to settle into one position and stay there sooner than one baby because they have less room to maneuver.

Palpation: Palpation of multiples can be difficult since one baby can be on top of another or partially obscure the parts of the other from your palpating fingers. The area of placental attachment is also larger, which means if it is covering the anterior portion of the uterine wall, it may be even more difficult to feel or hear the babies until the pregnancy is advanced. The more babies there are, the smaller they will tend to be due to the difficultly in providing adequate nourishment. However in twin and triplet pregnancies with proper maternal diet it is entirely possible to have normal sized infants weighing at least 7 pounds. It is most desirable that the first baby be head down; this minimizes the likelihood of the babies getting caught on each other during the birth.

Version during multiple gestations: When indicated, it is both safe and desirable for women to practice the breech turning techniques offered in the chapter on Ensuring Vertex Presentation at Term. It is also possible for a highly experienced practitioner to perform external versions during a twin pregnancy. However, this is more difficult to do at best; it is not a good idea to do so without experienced guidance until you feel competent with versions in singleton pregnancies and with palpation in multiple pregnancies.

898

Where the birth should take place:

As is the case with breech presentations, women carrying multiple gestations should be allowed to initiate the discussion of birth of their babies outside a hospital. In well-nourished mothers, homebirth with multiple gestation is not so much a medical as a political risk, since many of the problems which place multiple gestation at high risk are due to an inadequate diet to support more babies and placentas; however, there are a few problems intrinsic to multiple births which need to be carefully spelled out. In order to consider birth at home with multiples the following criteria may be employed:

*Both parents must freely seek to birth at home
*Both parents must understand and feel comfortable with the potential risks particular to multiple birth (as discussed below)
*Fetuses must appear to be normally sized, of similar size relative to each other, and in good positions (ideally the first one is vertex)
*The mother must be healthy and willing to eat adequately for multiples
*Midwives and parents must both feel intuitively positive about proceeding with an out-of-hospital birth as pregnancy progresses
*A one-step-at-a-time approach is useful when dealing with any out of the ordinary situation
*The issues regarding breech presentation must also be addressed, since one or more babies may present breech (see the chapter on Anticipating a Breech Birth in the section on the Third Trimester)

If, for any reason, the hospital is decided upon as the appropriate place of birth, clients may continue to be followed prenatally and accompanied to the hospital with care continuing postpartum as they so desire.

Discussing risk factors with parents: There are several risks unique to multiple pregnancy and birth. The most common of these involve nutritionally reducible risks such as abruption of the placenta, premature labor, small-for-dates infants, and postpartum maternal hemorrhage. While the risk of postpartum hemorrhage is partly due to the larger placental site in multiples, all these risks are most likely to occur in women who have not been eating enough to support a multiple gestation, or who may only begin to eat enough late in their pregnancy. Other risks of multiple gestation include:

*Cervical or uterine abnormalities, which increase the risk of miscarriage or premature labor regardless of her nutrition.
*The risks inherent in a breech or transverse presentation exist if a baby is not head down.

*A transverse baby cannot be born unless rotated to a longitudinal lie. Rotation may be difficult or impossible and carries the risk of arm or cord prolapse or uterine rupture if attempted during labor.

*Two or more babies positioning themselves so that one baby gets caught on the other during descent into the pelvis. The most common and most deadly of all locked presentations occurs when the first baby is breech and the second is vertex. In this case the heads can become locked under the chins and prevent the birth of either baby. This complication is rare, occurring in one in every 1000 twins births; when the first baby is breech, the incidence rises to one in 100 cases. (Oxhorn, 1986)

*Polyhydramnios: this is more frequent in multiple gestations, increasing the likelihood of nonvertex presentation.

*Fetal anomalies, which are found more frequently in multiple gestation.

*A seven times greater incidence of velamentous insertion of the cord (fetal umbilical vessel(s) run through a portion of the amniotic sac before reaching the cord proper). The risk of a vessel tearing when the membranes rupture or otherwise becoming damaged during the birth are high.

*Cord prolapse: the risk is higher with multiples, especially those that are premature or not vertex.

*Entanglement of the cords if both babies are in the same amniotic sac (rare): this can cause fetal death of one or both during pregnancy or labor.

*Twin-to-twin transfusion syndrome, which may occur in monozygotic multiples (see discussion below).

While fetal mortality with twins is higher than in singleton births, the main reasons for this are fetal defects and prematurity. Gross mortality varies from 9 to 14%. Special risks exist for the second or subsequent babies after the first one is born:

*Reduction of uterine capacity after the birth of the first baby may cause the placental blood flow to be altered and result in fetal hypoxia.

*The placenta can also be prompted to separate before the next baby is born due to the reduction in size of the uterine cavity, causing bleeding and depriving the unborn baby(ies) of oxygen. I believe that this is less likely when the mother is well-nourished, because the placenta will be more firmly attached.

*The second fetus may get hung up in the actively contracting upper uterine segment, preventing descent.

*Rarely, the placenta will partially separate and cover the internal os, thus producing an acute case of placenta previa and preventing the birth of the second twin. This will cause bleeding and jeopardize the unborn baby.

-There is an increased incidence of other-than-vertex presentation in second and subsequent babies.

Complications of multiple gestation:

Birth defects: There is a general agreement that anomalies occur more frequently in multiple gestations, but the degree of difference is debated. Various studies show a rate of 1.4% for singletons, 2.71% for twins and 6.1% for triplets. Both twins are affected in 14.8% of these cases (Onyskowova, et.al., 1971). Dizygotic twins may experience birth defects as might any other siblings in a family. Monozygotic twins may be discordant for a variety of birth defects and genetic disorders; that means only one twin will be affected even though they are from the same zygote. In addition to environmental differences and chance variation, the following reasons for such discordance are recognized:

*The mechanism of embryological development may produce defects such as vascular abnormalities.

*Postzygotic changes, such as somatic mutation leading to discordance for cancer or somatic rearrangement of immunoglobulin or T-cell receptor genes may occur.

*Chromosome aberrations can originate in one blastocyst after the twinning event

*Uneven X chromosome inactivation between female MZ twins can result in one twin expressing the maternal X and the other the paternal X.

Anomalies unique to multiple gestation include acardia and conjoining. Acardia occurs in one of monozygotic twins, triplets, or even quintuplets about 1 in every 30,000 births. These babies either have no heart or a very malformed one as well as multiple other defects. Such twins share one chorion and have vascular anastomoses which support the life of the baby with defects. Chromosomal abnormalities may at times be involved. Monozygotic babies are also more prone to a defect called symmelia which involves fusion of the lower limbs, as well as midline spinal defects and exstrophy of the cloaca, a type of urinary tract defect.

If the embryoblast or embryonic disc does not divide completely about 13 to 15 days post ovulation, various types of conjoined twins may occur. Conjoined (Siamese) twins are identical (MZ) twins that do not completely separate. It is estimated that the overall incidence is 1 in every 50,000 births and 1 in every 600 twin births. Conjoined twins may or may not share vital organs through the joined area. They are named according to the anatomic regions which are attached and the majority are female pairs; the ratio of female to male pairs ranges from 2 to 1 to 3 to 1. Major congenital anomalies of one or both babies are not uncommon and most are prematurely stillborn. Today, diagnosis can be made by ultrasound.

In cases where the babies are viable, or even if they have died, surgical delivery is the best option for both mother and babies except in cases where the joined area will allow them to be born naturally one after the other (as is the case if the tops of the heads are joined). When the danger exists that both babies will be born parallel, the possibility of them getting stuck during yoni birth and the subsequent trauma to both mother and babies makes surgical birth the safest alternative for all concerned. Whether or not such babies can be surgically separated after birth depends upon what organs they share, if there are anomalies in one or both babies, and if they have separate hearts.

Most known chromosomal abnormalities occur in multiple gestations. DZ and MA twins are usually discordant for these anomalies. Discordance means that one twin is normal while the other is affected. Such MZ twins are known as heterokatotypes. It is assumed that an abnormal distribution of genetic maternal occurred at about the same time as the twinning (postzygotic nondisjunction). The incidence of Down syndrome is no more common than in singleton pregnancies.

Abortion of a baby with anomalies: For a discussion of how to counsel women regarding fetal testing, refer to the appropriate chapters in Diagnostic Tests. Women who choose to have fetal diagnostic testing with multiples may be faced with the fact that one baby is normal while the other has a genetic defect. Choices are to carry both babies to term, abort both babies, or abort the baby with defects, leaving the other baby to be carried to term. (See the chapter When Fetal Tests Come Back Positive in the Second Trimester section for counseling suggestions.)

Both abortion options are problematic. One normal baby will be lost if the entire pregnancy is terminated. If only one fetus is to be selectively aborted, the unsavory options for this second-trimester procedure include cardiac puncture with exsanguination, removal of the baby by hysterotomy (a mini-Cesarean), injection of calcium glyconate or potassium chloride into the heart, or induction of air embolism through a fetal cord vessel. Potassium chloride injection may be the safest of these options. This process is fraught with risks such as selection of the wrong fetus, technical inability to accomplish the procedure, premature rupture of membranes, infection or loss of the entire pregnancy, plus the emotional impact on the surviving baby.

Identification of the appropriate twin depends somewhat upon how the defect can be identified. If the defect is genetic it may or may not be visible on ultrasound exam. If the twins are different sexes or the affected fetus has a visible defect, identification is much easier. If there are no visible signs, reliance on previous diagnostic testing (often done elsewhere, several days or weeks prior to the decision to terminate one baby) is not adequate. Fetal blood sampling and rapid karyotype testing should be performed to reidentify the affected twin. A sample of fetal tissue should be obtained after the procedure to confirm that the correct twin was terminated.

If the twins are monozygotic and share a chorion, selective termination of one twin poses additional risks. If vascular connections exist between the babies, a lethal agent injected into one twin may enter the circulation of the normal sibling and result in death or permanent damage. Even if the procedure is successful, the remaining twin could bleed to death into the collapsed circulatory system of the dead twin. Except in rare cases, attempted termination of one such twin has lead to the death of the surviving baby within a short time. Three successful cases involved hysterotomy and one involved injecting normal saline solution into the pericardium (bag) around the heart of the twin with defects. (Gabbe, et.al. 1991)

Fetal reduction: With the advent of so many means of helping infertile women become pregnant there has been a corresponding rise in the number of higher order multiple pregnancies that are conceived. Since good nutrition is not on the modern medical "plate," so to speak, one solution to the increased risks of toxemia, premature labor and associated complications with multiples has been to selectively abort some of the babies to give the rest a better change of survival. Obviously the moral, ethical and emotional crisis that such a choice presents to the parents is formidable, not to mention the impact on the surviving babies. Given the option of aborting some of her healthy babies versus attempting to eat well, my guess is that most women will choose to eat better. Unfortunately, the medical model has not yet come to this solution.

When the woman does want to reduce the number of babes she is carrying, a small dose of potassium chloride is injected into the fetal thorax under real-time ultrasound guidance during the first trimester using either a transabdominal or transyoni approach. The risks to the surviving babies are the same as for the selective abortion of a fetus with defects.

Twin-to-Twin Transfusion: A particularly dangerous and hard to diagnose problem known as Twin-to-Twin Transfusion Syndrome (TTTS) occurs with some monozygotic twins. This results in a transfer of blood from one baby to the other. Vascular anastomoses of the placentas (blood vessel communications between babies) are present in virtually all monochorionic twin gestations. They may be between arteries, between veins, between arteries and veins, or a combination. Although such vessels are often seen passing through the dividing membranes, the most clinically important anastomoses may be within placental cotyledons. The type, size and extent of the vascular connections determines the severity of TTTS.

In TTTS the arterial circulation of one twin is connected to the venous circulation of the other. This results in a one-way donor/transfuser link between the two circulatory systems. Such shunts are not always open and are subject to alterations in fetal cardiac output, regional blood flow or pressure brought on by differences in fetal growth rates or a mechanical event affecting only one baby such as transient incomplete cord compression; this may account for variations in the severity of TTTS.

Acute TTTS from the first twin to the second twin usually occurs at birth. Therefore it is important to emphasize to the parents that the cord must be clamped immediately upon the birth of each baby to minimize this problem, since it cannot be detected ahead of time. After all babies are out, the cord of the last baby can be left unclamped if desired.

Chronic TTTS typically presents in the mid-second trimester with clinical findings ranging from a size difference between twins to size discrepancies plus acute polyhydramnios in one sac and oligohydramnios in the other (if the net transfer of blood is large).

Clinical diagnosis of chronic TTTS is difficult. Frequently the first sign will be rapidly developing polyhydramnios (excess amniotic fluid), which may be described as developing "before the woman's eyes." Medical management includes amniocentesis to draw off fluid from the uterus, which facilitates performing further tests and can give an idea of how fast fluid is building up. (Little or no reaccumulation of fluid is inconsistent with the acute hydramnios associated with chronic TTTS.) An ultrasound is then done to determine if any of the following clues are present:

*Same sex twins with a single placenta
*Thin (two layer) separating membrane between the sacs
*Significant difference in fetal size (not always present)
*Polyhydramnios in one sac with oligohydramnios in the other
*Evidence of hydrops or cardiac failure in 1 twin, (usually the largest)

These signs together provide an almost certain diagnosis. The bladder of the small twin may be invisible while the large twin may have a full bladder that does not completely empty and a normal but enlarged heart. Identification of two chorions pretty much rules out TTTS. The absence of other findings besides infection does not rule out TTTS 100%, but does suggest that any TTTS present is minor, is not likely to account for a size discordance before 25 weeks and is therefore unworthy of further study. Doppler velocimetry has not proven useful in diagnosing chronic TTTS. (Keith, et. al., 1993)

The mortality rate for twins with chronic TTTS manifesting before 25 weeks exceeds 80%. In chronic TTTS, the over-transfused (recipient) twin is usually larger, while the under-transfused (donor) twin smaller. The recipient twin may suffer hypertension, hyperviscosity (thick blood) and heart failure, while the donor twin typically has hypotension and poor circulatory profusion.

Death of one twin *in utero*: Sometimes one twin will die before birth. This is estimated to occur in 2.2 to 6% of twin pregnancies, depending upon the study.

904

Often this results in the dead twin being transformed into a *fetus papyraceous*. In such cases the fluid from the dead twin is reabsorbed by the mother's body and pressure from the live twin results in the dead baby becoming dehydrated and compressed. This can occur regardless of the relationship of the two placentas and occasionally is the end result of TTTS.

Whenever a dead fetus remains *in utero*, it is important to keep careful watch on the mother's clotting status. Release of thromboplastic materials from the dead baby can result in alterations in the mother's clotting mechanism which make her prone to disseminated intravascular coagulation (DIC). Draw a baseline clotting panel when the death is discovered and do a follow-up in two weeks, then weekly after that. If symptoms of clotting problems become evident, transport immediately. (See the chapter on Clotting Disorders in Pregnancy in Diagnostic Tests, for more information.)

If the twins are monozygotic, additional complications are more likely for the surviving twin. It is possible for thromboplastic material to pass through the vascular connection in the placenta to the living twin, resulting in a liveborn baby with DIC or structural abnormalities. This occurs in 17% of MZ twins which suffer the death of one baby. These complications are quite unlikely in twins that have separate chorions.

Aside from these problems, the surviving twin may also experience growth retardation, fetal distress in labor, abnormal heart rate patterns and elevated bilirubin levels. Psychologically, the surviving twin will carry the burden of having lived while its sibling died. When parents are open to the possibility, talk to them about how the child might respond to this and encourage them to discuss the loss with the child early on; this will make it more likely that the child will process through the experience emotionally. S/he may also be able to remember events while *in utero* which the parents can record for the child to review when older. The parents will have a complicated emotional process to face as well, grieving the loss of one baby while celebrating the survival of the other.

References and further reading:
ACOG Technical Bulletin "Preterm Labor," No. 206, June 1995.
Danforth, D. et.al., ed. Danforth's Obstetrics and Gynecology, 5th ed., J.B. Lippincott, Phil, 1986.
Dor, J. et.al., "Elective cervical suture of twin pregnancies diagnosed ultrasonically in the first trimester following induced ovulation," Gyn Ob Invest, Vol. 13, 1982, pp. 55-60.
Gabbe, S., Obstetrics: Normal and Problem Pregnancies, 2nd ed. Churchill-Livingstone, NY 1991.
Keith, L., et.al., "Triplet and higher order pregnancies," Contemp. OB/GYN, Vol. 38, No. 6, June, 1993, p. 36.
Moore, Keith, & T. Persaud, The Developing Human, 5th ed., W. B. Saunders, Co., Phil., 1993.
Onyskowava, A., et.al., "The frequency and the character of malformations in multiple birth (a preliminary report)," Teratology, 4:496, 1971.
Oxhorn, Harry, Human Labor and Birth, 5th ed., Appleton-Century-Crofts, Norwalk, CT, 1986.
Weiner, Carl, "Challenge of twin-twin transfusion syndrome," Contemp. OB/GYN, Vol. 37, No. 5, May, 1992, p. 83.

Caring for Women Who Have Disabilities

The special needs of people who have disabilities have not been addressed adequately in our culture. This is particularly true in regard to reproductive issues. Often, women with disabilities have not been offered sex education while growing up. They may have trouble getting birth control due to our culture's tendency to asexualize those who are disabled. Conversely, others have been forced to use birth control or sterilized without their knowledge or consent. Abortion may be either forced upon a woman or denied to her under the assumption that she is not competent to make such a choice.

In the United States, financial benefits such as social security or Medicaid may be reduced or cut off entirely should a disabled person marry. When a disabled woman does have children, the state sometimes tries to remove the child from its mother's care based on her disability alone. Adoption has also been an option closed to those with disabilities, although this is slowly beginning to change. (For example, Adoption Resource Associates in Watertown, MA states that they do not discriminate on the basis of disability.) While this book will not be able to address each disability in depth, this chapter will offer an overview of issues to consider when caring for a woman with a disability. More information may be found on a number of disabling conditions in the section covering Medical Conditions and Disabilities Which May Preexist Pregnancy.

Accessibility: When you are looking for office space or remodeling existing space, consider its accessibility for women with disabilities. At least one parking area should be wheelchair accessible, that is, large enough for a van with additional room on the side for exiting the vehicle in a wheelchair. For a building to be wheelchair accessible doorways need to be at least 32" wide. Ramps need to be in place in each area where steps would be required; they should be no steeper than 1:12 (12 inches of ramp for every one inch of height); they should be properly railed so as not to pose a danger to a blind person. Bathrooms should be large enough for a wheelchair to pull up beside the toilet, with grab bars on the other side of and behind the toilet. Bathtubs should have a grab bar on the opposite wall, and a bench seat and anti-slip mat should be provided, and transfer boards or stools should be available. Showers should be wheelchair accessible. Toilet paper holders, door latches and hooks should be accessible from a wheelchair, and the chair should be able to roll up to and preferably under a sink. An elevated toilet seat adapter should be provided as well. Exam surfaces should be low enough for easy transfer from a wheelchair. Doorhandles are preferably lever-type. Consider installing a TTY, a device which makes telephone communication accessible to those who are hearing impaired. Braille signs will help blind women be more independent. Your usual handouts can be tape-recorded for women who are visually impaired. Find out where to go for sign language interpreters before they are needed. Also be aware that some people have environmental sensitivities, meaning the use of incense, air freshener, chemicals in carpets (especially a problem in new wall-to-wall carpet), potent cleansers, perfumes, fancy soaps and the like should be avoided.

Being conscious: If you are able-bodied, being in the presence of a woman with disabilities who wants to mother will bring up any prejudices and fears which you may have. Remember that most people with physical disabilities are of normal intelligence. Ask whether a woman needs assistance, rather than assuming. The woman is the best expert on her abilities, her needs, and what assistance she may require. Find out as much as you can about the disability itself before meeting the woman, this will allow for maximum sensitivity in how you discuss her situation with her and also relieves her of being your teacher in this regard. You should be able to offer general information pertinent to her condition without being asked while being open to hearing how she copes with her situation. Be honest with her about your previous experience serving women with disabilities. Speak directly to her, eye-to-eye, in a matter-of-fact way, just as you would any other woman. Don't try to pretend that the disability doesn't exist, and don't make a fuss over her *because of her disability*; make a fuss over her because she is pregnant and beautiful and full of all the hopes and fears and joys of motherhood, the same as any client. If several midwives will be caring for the same woman, be sure chart review takes place consistently, that everyone takes responsibility for learning about the disability and that the disability is labeled prominently but discreetly in her records as a reminder. At the home visit, look over any adaptive equipment she may have and do some "dry-runs" for positioning and wheelchair transfers so the birth team can get a feel for what will be necessary during the birth.

Visual impairment: If the woman is blind, take the time to orient her to the unfamiliar environment. A guide dog is a working animal; do not interact with the dog without first asking permission. Discuss getting to know the dog during pregnancy so s/he understands who you are before labor, when dogs often feel the need to protect their owners. Always go around the room and name those present and announce when a person is coming or going; converse as you would if you were on the phone with the person. Allow her to feel any equipment or teaching aids. Handouts which you normally offer should be given to her as well; a partner or assistant can read them to her or ask if she would prefer to have them on tape. Partially sighted women may be able to see handouts if the print is large. Ask!

Hearing impairment: Find out the extent of hearing loss and if the woman prefers to communicate through lip reading, writing or sign-language with an interpreter before your first visit. If she prefers an interpreter, find out if there are community resources that will provide one. Or, you might learn sign-language yourself (a good idea if you want to work with other women with hearing impairment in your community.) When speaking, always look at the woman, facing her directly and making eye contact, even if she chooses an interpreter. If she prefers to lip read, speak normally and check in frequently to be sure that what you are saying is getting across, (even good lip readers only catch about 25% of the conversation). If the woman speaks, she may be hard to understand; listen carefully and do not hesitate to ask her to repeat herself, if necessary. Your ear will soon accustom itself to her voice.

Mobility impairment: Women often see their wheelchair or crutches as physical extensions of themselves. Do not move any supportive equipment without asking first. Do not lean on a wheelchair or rest your hands on it. When speaking, arrange yourself so that you are at eye level with the woman by being seated or kneeling beside her chair if no seat is available. As pregnancy advances, a wider chair may afford more comfort as the woman gains weight and her center of gravity shifts. If a woman has a personal care assistant, you should ignore the attendant and speak directly to the woman.

Those with cerebral palsy may not speak clearly; they are probably used to repeating themselves when not understood, so don't hesitate to ask. Careful attention to a woman's speech patterns will quickly train your ear so that she can be understood. Anyone with a neuromuscular impairment may have trouble with fine motor skills; you or her attendant may need to assist with such things as obtaining a urine specimen.

Plan exams at a time that doesn't interfere with a woman's normal bowel and bladder routine. Ask the woman what position will be most comfortable for exams and offer to do as much of an exam as possible with her in her wheelchair. If a spasm occurs, support the limb or area in spasm and wait until it is gone before proceeding. Women with spinal injuries should receive pelvic exams in a semi-sitting position to minimize the chances of triggering a hyperreflexive reaction (see specifics in the chapter on Disorders Related to the Nervous System.) Pelvic exams can be done in a variety of positions; knee-chest, supine with feet together and knees spread, side-lying or some variation, work with the woman to find the position most comfortable for her. A woman with mobility impairment may need extra time allotted during visits for self-catheterization, removing a brace or transfer to and from a wheelchair. As she gains weight, be sure to check for circulatory problems and the development of pressure sores. Have the woman bring an assistant for transfers or allot enough time for you to become acquainted with the best ways to perform transfers if you will be assisting her.

The usual aches and pains of pregnancy may be particularly problematic for women who have back injuries, joint problems or whose mobility is impaired. Having a regular massage or chiropractic adjustments throughout pregnancy will help; many of the usual remedies for these complaints may offer relief as well.

Preconception counseling:

How will the woman integrate parenting with her disability? Find out what resources are available in your community for women with disabilities. Is there peer counseling that could review the issues outlined here with her? If no such resources are available, you will need to fill that gap. Women with disabilities who are seeking to parent may be afraid to ask questions for fear they will be perceived as unfit to parent; they may feel (not without cause) that they have been prejudged as poor candidates for motherhood. Discuss the following questions, many of which are faced by all parents and some of which will be particularly relevant to her situation.

> *How well adjusted are you to your disability? (This may be more relevant for those whose disability is more recent.)
> *If you will require daily help in caring for a child, is this help available? (Check with state funding regulations on assistant care, if relevant)
> *Is the natural course of your condition likely to lead to a reduction of your ability to parent in the future? If so, is your partner able and prepared to take on the responsibility of being increasingly responsible for the child(ren)?
> *Do you have a network of friends or relatives nearby whom you can call on for physical and emotional support?
> *Have you looked after other people's children in your current state of ability?
> *What adaptions does you home need to allow you to parent? Do you have the resources to make these changes or are you willing to move?
> *If you will be relying on public financial assistance, have you researched how that might be impacted if you have a child?
> *Do you feel you would be a burden to your children? Is this a real possibility or due to guilt?
> *How do you and your partner relate around your disability? If you are planning to be a single parent, how do you foresee that working?
> *Do you feel confident in your own ability to face the challenges of parenting a growing child?

Obviously there is no right or wrong answer to any of the above questions, but they can provide a starting point for a discussion of the complex considerations that need to be taken into account. They can be utilized even if a woman comes to you already pregnant, since there are likely to be some points that she has not yet considered.

According to mothers with disabilities, the conditions which hamper them the most include lack of balance, involuntary movements, anxiety, inexperience, lack of access from a wheelchair, inability to hear the baby cry or see the baby while s/he is active (if hearing visually impaired), problems with lifting the baby, and worrying about the baby's safety, as well as isolation from other mothers. If any of these are relevant to the woman, help her explore how she will cope with them (for example, a device which flashes a light can be used to alert a deaf mother to a baby's cry). If she would like, an appointment with an occupational therapist can be arranged to perform baby-care activities with dolls to access what types of adaptive aides may be most helpful, especially if it is her first child.

Emotional issues: It is important to ask open-ended questions about a woman's fears and concerns, helping her explore their origins as you would with any woman. While some women may have a prolonged sense of ambivalence regarding the pregnancy, others will welcome it as something their body can do normally. Many women may worry that parenting may be unfair to their child. Delve into the origin of this fear, while assuring her that what really matters is the quality of time she spends with the child, not what they do together. While there may be frustrations on both sides when the mother cannot engage in certain activities with her child or when certain phases of growing up are difficult, this is inevitable in all parent/child relationships. If the mother and her associates accept her disability, the child will learn to do so as well. Able-bodied people aren't all perfect parents; far from it. As long as a woman has a healthy attitude of self-responsibility regarding her disability, her child is unlikely to feel burdened.

Self-consciousness and fear of public disapproval of pregnancy may also be an issue, especially if the woman's disability is quite visible. Your encouragement, reminding her how well she is doing and how good she looks, will help build her self esteem during this emotionally vulnerable time.

Prenatal testing: If a woman's (or her partner's) disability is inheritable, this issue may be emotionally charged. Genetic counseling, the various tests available and the fact that abortion of the baby is the only "treatment" the medical model will offer must all be addressed. Some parents may choose testing in order to prepare for the birth of a baby with special needs. Complex feelings of valuing one's own life, guilt over not wanting to knowingly impose a disability on a future child, questions such as "what if my parents had had access to genetic testing and had aborted me?," "would I be able to parent a child with the same disability I have?," feelings about abortion, and possible differences of opinion between a woman and her partner on this issue will make the whole topic of prenatal testing a loaded one. Remember that for recessive traits the biological father must also carry the gene for them to manifest in the baby; for some conditions his status can be determined. As with all parents, the risks and benefits of the various kinds of tests available should be explored as well their relevance to their situation. Emphasize that these tests are only options, not requirements. Real reproductive choice includes the option to bear a child with disabilities; and is not quality control of the perfect baby "product."

Physical considerations: The woman will know her disability better than anyone else, but she may not have a clear idea of how pregnancy, labor and birth will interact with her overall physical condition. Each disability is unique and the degree to which an individual is affected will vary; therefore, together with the woman, prepare a list of questions that she can discuss with her primary care provider or with one specializing in her particular condition. These should cover the safety of pregnancy and labor for the mother, whether, s/he considers yoni birth advisable, and whether the woman's body can support the pregnancy sufficiently to birth a healthy baby. Daily medication is frequently a part of life for those with disabilities; the possible effects of any drugs on the pregnancy, the baby and the contractibility of the uterus should be explored. Do these drugs preclude breastfeeding? If there are pregnancy-related concerns, can other drugs be substituted? If infertility has been a problem, the possibility that drugs may be causative should be explored. The risk of pregnancy to the baby and mother will depend on her health prior to conception and the disability in question.

When referring women for a medical opinion, try to find out what preconceived notions the provider may have about parenting with disabilities. If you cannot locate a supportive practitioner in your area, call one of the following community centers to see if they have someone on staff knowledgeable about the disability in question on staff or if they know of someone to contact in your area:

> Through the Looking Glass, 801 Peralta Ave., Berkeley, CA 94707, (510) 848-1112.
> The Project on Women and Disability, One Asburton Pl., Rm 1305, Boston, MA 02108, (617) 722-7440
> The Health Resource Center for Women with Disabilities, Chicago Rehabilitation Institute and the Prentice Women's Hospital, Chicago, IL.

The mother may require additional support systems during pregnancy; this should also be explored. For example, the additional weight gained during pregnancy may further impair a woman's mobility. If the woman's current assistants cannot meet her needs during pregnancy or will require additional help, it will be important to know this and make provision for it in advance.

Home or hospital birth? A woman with a lifelong disability may have had many painful or frightening hospital experiences; for many the idea of homebirth may carry special appeal. However, women who need major medical support or intervention to safely give birth or whose babies will need such support (either because of a known disability or due to the effect of maternal drugs) are best off birthing in a compassionate hospital setting. (For example, women who have cerebral palsy or spinal injuries may require drugs to relax their muscles to make yoni birth possible.) If the situation is borderline, get more than one opinion.

If homebirth is planned, ideally you will be able to arrange specific collaborative care with a hospital based practitioner if transport is required. The hospital staff should know of the woman's plans to birth at home and what her particular needs are regarding her disability should transport be necessary.

Prenatal care: Women who have disabilities will need the same kind of support, information and encouragement as other women in your care. Some women may appreciate home visits for prenatals, affording them maximal accessibility and comfort for exams, etc.. If a woman is paralyzed below her chest she may not feel uterine sensations; it will be important to point out how her uterus looks when a toning contraction is occurring. If she has use of her arms, she can learn to feel for both contractions and fetal movement with her hands. Similar adaptations will need to be worked out with the mother so she can experience her pregnancy as fully as possible.

References community resources and further reading:

Basen, G, et.al. eds. Misconceptions: The Social Construction of Choice and the New Reproductive and Genetic Technologies, Voyager Pub., Quebec, 1993.

Campion, M., The Baby Challenge: A Handbook of Pregnancy for Women with Physical Disability, Tavisstock/Routledge, New York, 1990.

Carty, E, et.al., "Guidelines for serving disabled women," Midwifery Today, No. 27, Autumn 1993, p. 29.

op.cit., "Childbearing and parenting with a disability or chronic illness," Midwifery Today, No. 28, Winter, 1993, p. 17.

Disability Rag Resource, Journal, special issue in parenting, Avocado Press, Louisville, KY

Finger, A., Past Due: A Story of Pregnancy, Disability and Birth, Seal Press, Seattle, WA 1990.

Haseltine, F, et.al., Reproductive Issues for Persons with Physical Disabilities, Paul H. Brooks, Pub., Co., Baltimore, 1993.

Martin, D "A Call for Reform: Disability Health and Benefits Programs that Penalize Recipients," Mainstream Magazine, Feb. 1994.

Mathews, J., A Mother's Touch, Henry Holt, New York, 1992.

Saxton, M., "Women Disability and Reproduction," Sexuality and Disability Journal, Summer, 1994.

op.cit., "Reproductive Rights: A Disability Rights Issue," Sojourner, Vol. 20, No. 11, July 1995, pp. 8-9.

Lesbian Mothers

More and more lesbian women are choosing to have biological children either by themselves or with a partner. In most cases, a biological child is easier to come by than an adopted one for a lesbian mother. Biological children are also harder for the state to remove from the mother's custody. Lesbian mothers and couples face special challenges in choosing to parent, largely due to the lack of acceptance of gays and lesbians in North American society. Some of the issues specific to childbearing include:

Obtaining the sperm and getting pregnant: Obtaining sperm is easier than it used to be for lesbians. Some sperm banks will ship sperm directly to women anywhere in the United States. Alternately, fresh semen may be available from a male friend or relative who has had his medical history examined and has been tested for hepatitis, syphilis and HIV.

The woman to carry the baby should keep track of her fertility cycles so she can inseminate at an optimum time. A Turkey baster can be used to introduce the sperm, followed by the insertion of a diaphragm to keep the semen in place. The woman can lie with her hips elevated for 30 minutes to encourage the sperm to travel up into her cervix.

Often, lesbians become so caught up in the process of becoming pregnant that they do not seriously consider what it will be like to parent a baby, a toddler, a teenager. It is important to help them explore these issues.

The pregnancy and birth: Ironically, lesbians are often quite willing to jump into the most mainstream of care settings without much thought as to the environment of birth and how it will be to actually give birth. This may be because lesbians have often made such conscious efforts to resist cultural pressures to be a certain way that they have given little consideration to the emotional and spiritual side of giving birth. Pay special attention to informing them and helping them get in touch with their feelings about the pregnancy and birth.

A boy or a girl? Most of the time, lesbians seeking to conceive have decided that they are not attached to the sex of the baby. Nevertheless, they are women who have chosen not to make men a primary focus in their lives. It is important to discuss how they feel about the sex of the baby and help them to resolve any issues related to this before the birth. Some lesbians may try to increase their odds of having a female infant. A group of women in Amherst Massachusetts found that keeping fresh semen in a baby food jar under their clothes next to their bodies for 12 hours and then introducing it into the yoni greatly increased the percentage of female babies. This is worth a try if a girl is desired. Frozen sperm produces a high percentage of boys. Discuss how they will feel if the baby is of a gender they would not have chosen, and how they will resolve raising a boy in a predominately women-only community.

The non-biological mother: The non-biological mother may feel left out of the process of pregnancy and birth and may be more sensitive to having another woman take care of her partner than some men might be. How she feels and how she views her role as the non-biological parent should be discussed. Some women will want to try and lactate so they can co-breastfeed the baby. This will be easier if the woman has breastfed in the past. A lact-aide can also be used to supplement the baby while she nurses from the non-biological mother. In some cases, the non-biological mother can formally adopt the child, thereby becoming a legal guardian. Their plans in this regard should be discussed as well.

Just like any other birthing family: While there are unique aspects to the lesbian parenting situation, in most respects these families are like any others, with the same hopes and concerns, as well as the same emotional issues to address.

Resources and further information:

The Family Next Door, P.O. Box 21580, Oakland, CA, 94620, (510) 482-5778 (newsletter for lesbian and gay parents)

Momazons, P.O. Box 02069, Columbus, OH, 43202, (614) 267-0193 (newsletter for lesbian parents)

Gay and Lesbian Parents Coalition International, P.O. Box 50360, Washington, DC, 20091 (202) 583-8029 (newsletter, annual conference)

Fenway Community Health Center, Lesbian/Gay Family and Parenting Services, 7 Haviland St., Boston, MA, 02115, (617) 267-0900 ext. 282, (independent fertilization program, services and support groups)

Chicago Women's Health Center, 3435 N. Sheffield, Chicago, IL 60657, (312) 935-6126 (office fertilization and prenatal care, one year waiting list)

Feminist Women's Health Center, 580 14th St., N.W., Atlanta, GA, 30318, (404) 874-7551 (office fertilizations, fertility awareness classes)

Pacific Reproductive Services, 444 Deharo, Suite 222, San Francisco, CA 94107 (415) 861-3558 (lesbian owned sperm bank, on-site health screening, most donors can be made known to the child when they reach age 18, will ship throughout the country)

The Sperm Bank of California, 2115 Milvia St., Berkeley, CA 94704 (510) 841-1858 (offers identity release and anonymous donors, will ship to home or provider's office; lesbian friendly)

Xytex, 1100 Emmett St., Augusta, GA 30904 (800) 277-3210 (ships sperm to provider's office or direct to homes, donor files and sometimes photos are available for review, contact David Towles for more information)

National Center for Lesbian Rights 870 Market St., Suite 570, San Francisco, CA 94102 (415) 392-6257 (legal advocacy group)

Lavender Families Resources Network, P.O. Box 21567, Seattle, WA, 98111, (206) 325-2643 (legal support for custody issues, etc.)

Martin, April Lesbian and Gay Parenting Handbook, HarperCollins, 1993.

Pies, Cheri, Considering Parenthood: A Workbook for Lesbians, Spinster, 1985.

914

Prenatal Care of Rh- Mothers

NOTE: For complete information read the chapter on Blood Types and Incompatibilities in <u>Diagnostic Tests</u>. This chapter summarizes the main concerns during the prenatal period.

Rh- women should be assessed as to their Rh antibody status at the onset of care, at 28 to 30 weeks and at 36 to 38 weeks, or as indicated. Should an antibody titer develop, further tests should be done on a weekly basis, or more often if necessary. A titer of 1:16 or below which develops late in pregnancy is considered to be clinically insignificant with respect to fetal risk.

The use of Rho(D) Immunoglobulin (Rhogam) (FDA category C) is currently being given prophylactically to women at 28 weeks gestation in an attempt to eliminate rare instances of sensitization during the latter part of pregnancy. The dose used varies among locales and is either the prenatal dose of 50 µg or a standard 300 µg dose, which is also the dose used postpartum. The rationale for prenatal prophylaxis is to prevent sensitization due to any blood mixing which may occur during the last trimester. The effect on the fetus of such prophylaxis has not been well explored and there is speculation that it can have adverse fetal effects, including death. The only Rho(D) immunoglobulin products currently produced in the United States are preserved with thimerosal, which could be one source of problems. (Thimerosal is a mercury derivative and an allergen for some people. WinRho SD, a Canadian thimerosal-free product, is now distributed in the United States by Univax Biologics, Inc., Rockville, Maryland, 20852.)

The affect of Rho(D) immunoglobulin administration on the fetal blood is also not understood. Babies have been born with minor sensitization resulting from prenatal Rho(D) immunoglobulin; this occurs because the immunoglobulin is introducing Rh antibodies into the mother's system. Due to these unknown factors, Rho(D) immunoglobulin administration during pregnancy is controversial. This should be explained to women so that they can make their own decision as to whether to receive Rh immunoglobulin at 28 weeks.

If invasive prenatal testing such as amniocentesis or chorionic villi sampling is done, Rho(D) immunoglobulin is recommended. Should a condition involving uterine bleeding occur, tests can be ordered (Antibody screen, Rosette, type and factor and, if results indicate, a Kleihauer-Betke) and the need for Rho(D) immunoglobulin discussed.

Should the father of the baby prove to be Rh-, precautions are not necessary, as the baby will also be Rh- except in very rare cases of genetic mutation (this occurs in about 1 out of every 100,000 cases).

Women with religious or other objections to receiving Rho(D) immunoglobulin need not be refused care as long as antibody screens are negative or below 1:16 (as noted above). After the birth, cord blood can be taken regardless of the anticipated choice to ensure an informed decision.

Yoni Birth After Cesarean (YBAC)

NOTE: Also read the next two chapters on Previous Uterine
Surgeries and Working with Women Who Have Had Difficult
Yoni Births

Working with a woman who has previously given birth via surgery presents
a unique and challenging set of circumstances for the midwife. There are a number
of physiological and psychological factors which come into play which may make
this pregnancy and birth more difficult; at the same time, it is very rewarding when
she finally, this time, gives birth via the yoni. The aspects of care that are unique
to the YBAC mother shall be reviewed in this chapter.

Risks of YBAC: While much has been made about YBAC risks among North
American obstetricians, YBACs have been standard of care in Europe for many
decades. Some common myths are that the scar is highly likely to rupture, that
multiple Cesareans increases this likelihood and that multiple gestations and breech
presentations also increase these risks. While the risk of disruption of uterine
integrity certainly exists, it remains small, even for those who have had multiple
Cesareans or Classical incisions. Neither multiple gestation nor breech birth
appears to increase the risk of scar separation. (Davies & Spencer, 1988) In fact,
rupture of the unscarred uterus occurs more often and does more harm than rupture
of the scarred uterus (Martin, et.al., 1988). In addition, the scar which has
remained intact up to the threshold of labor is very likely to remain intact through
the birth (Macafee, 1958). In her literature review, Henci Goer (1995, p.42) found
reference to only 46 ruptures during 15,154 labors, a rate of 0.3% (benign scar
separations are a more common occurrence). The possibility of other unforeseen
events occurring which may necessitate transport such as intrapartum hemorrhage,
fetal distress, or cord prolapse is about 2.7%, roughly 10 times the rate of rupture
during labor (Enkin, 1989). So, while a risk is present, it must be considered in
context with the overall risks inherent in birth. When viewed in this light and
compared to the greater, multiple risks inherent in Cesarean surgery, yoni birth after
a Cesarean becomes the only sane standard of care. Therefore, as a midwife, the
question is whether or not to attend a woman at home; in most cases, the
advisability of yoni birth is a given.

The consultation visit: Ask the woman to bring her previous medical records
from both the hospital and her care providers. Make sure she asks for her complete
chart, including a surgical report; not merely a summary of the case. This will
allow you both to review the chart with an eye to dispelling any misunderstandings
regarding what occurred. She should bring her file to the initial visit if she does
not have it at the consultation visit. At this point, an overview of the circumstances
surrounding the decision to do surgery, the type of scar on the uterus and any

attendant complications are what you need to know. The type of scar on the abdomen may be different than the one on the uterus; if in doubt, check the surgical report. It is important to address any questions she has about risks of birth with a scarred uterus in general and her risk factors in particular. Then, move on to the other topics relevant to the consultation interview; it is important that a woman feel that her whole situation is being addressed, not that she is merely a "walking scar," as so many medical model providers project.

The initial history: It is important to review the previous birth experiences from the mother's point of view as well as to go over the hospital records. Review, in detail, the physical and emotional climate of her previous pregnancy and birth. Elicit her perceptions about such things as the strength of her labor, when procedures were performed and what her understandings were at that time about why these things were being done. Her perceptions will impact her current feelings about her pregnancy and upcoming labor and birth. Get the partner's perceptions, if s/he was present for that birth, about why things were being done and what s/he felt about how things happened. Try to let the mother explain what she felt and understood to be happening before you launch into your own interpretation of what you are hearing and what you see written in the chart. It helps everyone to have a clear clinical picture of what went on in what time frames, and of progress in terms of dilation, effacement and station of the presenting part. Frequently it will be found that what the parents were told does not coincide with medical records. In fact, the records themselves will often contradict each other! Reviewing the case and describing how you might have handled the situation can give women some perspective on how you can help them have a different experience for this birth.

The type of uterine scar, any complications from surgery, etc.: The types of uterine incisions are discussed in the next chapter. You want to know if there was any infection following the birth, how her scar healed (did it open and drain? were tubes put in to facilitate this?) What has her nutrition like after the surgery? While having had an infection may make a woman more afraid about her scar's integrity, it can, in fact, make the site of the infection that much stronger, as more scar tissue may build up in response to the disruption. It could also cause one or more of the tissue layers to heal apart (a dehiscence) which is not, in itself, usually a problem (Wainer-Cohen, 1994). Endometritis may, however, leave the scarred area more susceptible to the development of placenta accreta. Good nutrition and an easily assimilated multi vitamin and mineral supplement will help to optimize the situation as much as possible now. Make sure her diet remains excellent!

A few doctors may still be attempting to test the integrity of the scar. Two tests may be suggested. Hysterography uses radiopaque dye and x-ray to visualize the scar prior to conception. Amniography is done during pregnancy to detect dehiscence and involves amniocentesis and x-rays. Neither of these tests are predictive of the strength or integrity of the scar, since dehiscence and or defects may be present in scars which maintain their integrity throughout pregnancy and birth. The thickness or thinness of a scar does not predict its likelihood to rupture. Fortunately, as YBAC has become more accepted, these dangerous and unnecessary tests have fallen by the way-side in most areas.

Is another surgical birth necessary and is homebirth advisable? Regardless of the reason for the previous surgery, in almost every case a woman can give birth naturally with a subsequent baby. Yoni birth is ill advised only in those cases where a physical deformity prevented birth or in which so much scarring is present on the uterus that carrying a pregnancy to term would put the mother at great risk for uterine rupture. Other reasons such as failure to progress, no urge to push, cord prolapse, placenta previa, placental abruption, breech or posterior presentation, cephalopelvic disproportion (CPD) and twins are not necessarily repeating complications and some reasons, (such as breech, posterior presentation or twins) were often no reason in the first place. Studies confirm that YBAC with twins, breeches or a history of CPD are not contraindications. (Ophir, et.al., 1989)

As far as the type of incision goes, the mother who has a low transverse uterine incision is at the lowest risk for scar-related problems such as dehiscence and rupture. Those with classical or T-shaped incisions are at more risk for rupture, which tends to be more traumatic than the usually benign scar disruptions which occurs in women with low transverse incisions. While some types of incisions pose more risk, the highest risk is still probably around 5% (some scars are more rare and limited data is available, from looking at the existing data, 5% seems to me a generous estimate of risk for all types of Cesarean scars, with the order of risk as follows: low transverse [0.5% Haq, 1988; to 2% Clark, 1988], low vertical [1.3% Enkin, 1989], Classical and inverted T [probably about the same for both; 2.2% to 4%, depending on the study] upright T and J-incision [probably somewhat higher, but no specific data is available]). Women with upright T, J-shaped or classical incisions or those who have experienced a previous uterine rupture may want to birth in the hospital, although finding a practitioner that will assist them to have a YBAC will be more difficult. However, in these cases scar disruption is *most likely* to occur during pregnancy with accompanying fetal distress and possible death or not at all. The mother must weigh the risk of rupture with a YBAC with the risks of major surgery and multiple Cesareans. As the midwife, you must assess whether you are up to dealing with the increased risk at home, especially since rupture of these incisions tends to be more traumatic than scar disruption in a low transverse incision. Studies indicate that a history of multiple surgical births does not increase the risk of rupture (Farmakides, 1987; Porreco & Meier, 1983; Roberts, 1991).

Multiple surgical births do significantly increase the risk of placental problems. In one study, the rate of previa in an unscarred uterus was 0.26%; 0.65% after 1 CS, 1.8% with 2 CS scars, 3% with 3, and 10% with 4 or more, a 38-fold increase. The risk of placenta accreta occurring in conjunction with previa rose from 5% in an unscarred uterus to 24% with 1 scar, 47% with 2, 40% with 3, and 60% with 4 or more CS scars. (Clark, et.al., 1985)

In the midwifery community there has been question as to whether fetal distress is a repeating complication. The baby and mother are in a symbiotic relationship during pregnancy. Fetal distress can be the baby's way of protecting the mother from difficult emotional or physical issues (for example, labor has to be interrupted due to fetal distress before painful maternal memories are triggered). Of course, in every pregnancy there are two destinies involved, the baby's and the mother's. The outcome of birth "works" in some way for the baby as it does the mother; however the mother's ability to change her relationship to the process and her larger life patterns can change the way the baby responds as well.

The emotional climate of birth and the YBAC mother: It is important for the woman to understand that nothing happens by accident. Regardless of how blatantly unnecessary the surgery may have appeared on reviewing the chart, the woman, nevertheless, allowed the surgery to be done. This does not mean that she is "to blame" and this should not be inferred in your discussion; you should, however, invite her to notice the connection between events. Unconsciously she (as we all do) set herself up for the outcome of the birth and needs to look at how such events supported her in her life at that time. For example, if a first time mother unconsciously knew that the way her mother always took care of her best as a child was when she was unable to care for herself, i.e. when she was sick, she could have unconsciously set up the Cesarean (by choice of doctor, allowing the staff the give her drugs at a critical point in labor, etc.) to be sure she had the mothering she needed from her own mother so she could, in turn, nurture her newborn.

Often, too, the woman who winds up with a Cesarean has been sexually abused. Remembered or not, the abuse may make the stretching of the pelvic tissues and the passage of the baby a very unsafe and frightening experience. Giving over control in labor may recapitulate the feeling of lack of control over the abuser. Some women responded to sexual abuse by "freezing;" in labor this can lead to failure to progress. The variety of nuances this can take are infinite, and they are very hard for some women to look at. However, taking responsibility for the underlying psychological strategies involved in the process and outcome of birth can be the key to making a difference for a woman in a new situation.

Regardless of the circumstances, the drama and intensity of birth highlights a woman's psychological and emotional patterns. She cannot birth apart from how she lives the rest of her life. Therefore birth is an opportunity to see these patterns in high relief and, hopefully, become more conscious of them as a result. Support women to view their birth as a growing experience.

Affirming a new and different birth: Most of the time a woman who has experienced a surgical birth has felt completely disempowered. Not infrequently, she has undergone numerous ultrasound exams, internal exams, fetal monitor tracings, blood tests and a multitude of other interventions, all of which serves to externalize her sense of control and safety. Subtle and not-so-subtle remarks may have left her feeling completely powerless, as if they could do nothing to affect the course of events she found herself trapped in. Often, she arrives at the threshold of surgical birth feeling like her baby is being rescued from her body or that she is being saved from an endless, ineffective labor.

How different it is for such a woman to be told, quite categorically, that she and she alone can make a difference in her birth; that the MOST IMPORTANT things that need to be done are what she ALONE can do: that she, in fact, has central and almost complete control over how her pregnancy and birth goes!; And that taking care of herself by eating well and avoiding drugs, cigarette and alcohol eliminates the need for all those tests and interventions.

Emotionally, women have had a dramatic event that magnifies some pattern in their life which they now wish to change. An array of issues come to mind: passivity in the face of (male) authority, being a "good girl" and following instructions, control issues, fear of success, attention getting, poor body image . . . the list goes on. Just making the effort to seek a care provider that will encourage them to believe in themselves is for many women a major breakthrough. Affirmations and visualizations of yoni birth done on a daily basis, with specific emphasis on seeing themselves moving past the point where they had surgery before, will help to contradict their negative belief patterns. Counteract negative messages with affirming statements such as:

*My body knows how to labor and give birth.
*My uterus has strong, powerful contractions in labor which bring my
 baby down and out.
*My placenta separates and births easily and my uterus clamps down
 after birth.
*It is safe to let the baby come out.
*I am strong and capable of birthing my baby.
*I deal with whatever labor brings me.
*Birth heals and cleanses my pelvis.
*Contractions caress and massage the baby and prepare it for birth.
*My baby is head down, facing my back and has its chin on its chest.
*My uterus is healed and whole.

You and the woman can make up additional affirmations which apply to her individual situation.

Detecting a split in beliefs during pregnancy: Sometimes women who have had difficult births in the past are split within themselves about who or what to trust. Part of them wants to trust their intuitive sense that birth works and that they are okay. The part that is afraid gives an open ear to the voices of doctors, tests and technology which assert that birth is dangerous and needs highly skilled assistance just in case something goes wrong. It may happen that you, the midwife, become caught in the middle of this split, so beware. If you feel this is happening, point it out to the parents by discussing their feelings of trust in birth versus technology.

Benign symptoms related to the uterine scar: Many women have reported feeling twinges, aches, pains and sometimes pulling sensations in and over their uterine scars as pregnancy advances, and sometimes right through labor. As long as such symptoms do not persist and increase, they are usually only the benign discomforts that occur with any scar that is being thinned and stretched. This is not to say that pregnancy causes unusual thinning of the scar itself but that the normal, overall thinning of the uterine wall which accompanies uterine enlargement naturally includes the area where the scar is located (be sure to be clear about this when you explain this to the woman). Reassure her that many YBAC mothers have reported such sensations during normal pregnancies that ended in normal yoni birth. (See the chapter on Uterine Dehiscence and Rupture for serious symptoms and what to do in the section on the Third Trimester.)

Nutrition and the YBAC mother: When a woman has had the disappointment of experiencing a surgical birth for a previous baby, good nutrition can help her feel empowered as well as significantly increasing the chances she will have a yoni birth this time around.

Many problems which lead to surgical solutions for childbirth are essentially preventable with the adequate intake of a whole foods diet as outlined in the nutrition chapters. A few of these problems include abruption, toxemia, prematurity, and some complications of multiple births. Many other problems, such as unexplained stillbirth, infections, poor healing, anemia, coagulation problems, weak contractions, poor hormonal response and others may be related to poor nutrition as well. Their recurrence can be minimized with a good diet.

Encouragement about getting bigger and having a vigorous baby will support a woman to continue to eat well. It is vital that she focus on what she eats, not what she gains, so her baby will have all it needs. It is particularly important to address any messages the woman may have gotten about limiting weight gain to limit the size of the baby, emphasizing that this is *dangerous advice!!*

Where is the placenta? Because of an overall increased risk of placenta previa and accreta in the presence of uterine scars, listening low down in front above the pubic bone for placental sounds is an especially important part of prenatal care for all YBAC women. If a low lying anterior placenta is discovered, you might want to discuss the increased risk with the woman so you can both decide if proceeding with homebirth is wise. (See chapter on Bleeding in the Third Trimester in the section on Problems Associated With the Third Trimester for more information.)

Preparing the YBAC mother for labor: The previous surgery has created a powerful message that she can't do it; her body doesn't work. Often the most difficult point in labor will be getting past where she had surgery the first time. Once she is beyond that point, the rest is an unknown for her. Your most important contribution to the YBAC mother is your belief in birth, your faith that she has the strength and where-with-all to have this baby naturally, and your patience.

A mother may ask you not to tell her when she was at the same dilation as when she had her surgery for the previous birth. When a woman is close to the same dilation, telling her that she is one centimeter past that point is often the best strategy. Of course, you must decide about such things on an individual basis.

Often women have had surgery before they were even in active labor, at anywhere from one to four centimeters of dilation. While this can occur due to an extremely rigid cervix resisting strong contractions, most often it occurs because the first-time mother does not understand how strong labor must get to birth the baby. Women often perceive early labor contractions, which are, after all, the strongest they have ever felt, as overwhelming. It is up to you to clarify that early labor is not active labor and, regardless of how badly it hurt during their last labor, it needed to get stronger. Working with these women on issues of fear of pain, of birth and of losing control is important.

If the surgery was done for some kind of unexpected emergency and, in fact, appears to have been necessary, the woman may be appropriately relieved that she was in a setting which allowed for this intervention to occur. She will need help believing that birth can be normal for her. Again, getting past the point when the emergency occurred in the next labor will be a major hurtle.

Some women may have had a surgical delivery prior to even beginning labor. For these women the entire specter of birth is an unknown. Although this is true for a first-time mother as well, having gone through the mechanical process of having surgery to have a baby may make the impending labor and birth that much more frightening. In these cases, remind the woman that she does not know how her body will respond to labor, and that she never failed at labor because she never got a chance to experience it.

Women may have problems with the passive part of labor (having contractions and dilating) or the active pushing phase of labor. Rarely, some women may have problems with both. Encourage women to think about how they deal with other passive and active elements of their lives as they consider how they will deal with labor this time around.

The mother who has birthed surgically is far removed from the birth of the placenta. Remember, as you must with all mothers, to emphasize the importance of this last part of the birth and review with her the mechanism of the delivery of the placenta.

References and further reading:

Clark, et.al., "Placenta previa/accreta and prior cesarean section," Ob Gyn, Vol. 66, No. 1, 1985, pp. 89-92.

Farmakides, G. et.al., "Vaginal birth after two or more previous cesarean sections," Am J Ob Gyn, Vol. 156, No. 3, 1987, pp. 565-6.

Davies, J., Spencer, J., "Trial of scar," Br J of Hosp Med, Vol. 40, No. 5, 1988, pp. 379-381.

Enkin, M, et.al., Effective Care During Pregnancy and Birth, Oxford U. Press, New York, 1989.

Goer, H., Obstetric Myths versus Research Realities, Bergin & Garvey, Boston, MA 1995.

Macafee, C., Irish J. of Med Science, Vol. 38, 1958, p. 81.

Martin, et.al., "Vaginal birth after cesarean section: the demise of routine repeat abdominal delivery," Ob Gyn Clin North Am, Vol. 15, No. 4, 1988, pp. 719-736.

Ophir, E, et.al., "Trial of labor following cesarean section: dilemma," Ob Gyn Sur., Vol. 44, No. 1, 1989, pp. 19-24.

Oxhorn, Harry, Human Labor and Birth, 5th ed., Appleton-Century-Crofts, Norwalk, CT, 1986.

Roberts, L. "Elective section after two sections—where's the evidence?" Br J Ob Gyn, Vol. 98, No. 12, 1991, pp. 1199-1202.

Wainer-Cohen, Nancy, YBAC expert & co-author of Silent Knife, phone conversation, 4/23/94.

op. cit. Estner, L., Silent Knife, Bergin & Garvey, Boston, MA, 1983.

Previous Uterine Surgeries

When you are working with women wishing to have a yoni birth after a previous uterine surgery, it is useful to know exactly what kind of incision she had and the stated indications for both the surgery and that particular style of incision. If the woman was never told or is unsure, this information can usually be found in her medical records. In most cases, this will apply to women who have undergone previous Cesarean surgery as well as other procedures. Knowing the type of incision will help you assess the woman's risk of scar disruption during the pregnancy or birth and will also assist in your analysis of why the surgery was done and what problems the physician thought s/he was likely to encounter during the operation, as different incisions are performed in different circumstances.

The vast majority of women having surgical births will be given a low transverse uterine incision. Note that the location and direction of the incision in the abdominal skin does not always correlate with the uterine incision that was used and should not be assumed to indicate the type of uterine cut that was made. Preterm Cesareans are usually done with low vertical or classical incisions because the lower uterine segment is not thin enough to allow a low transverse incision, as would be the case if the surgery was done after labor had been ongoing for a while.

Types of incisions: The types of uterine incisions used for surgical births are illustrated below and described in the table on the following pages.

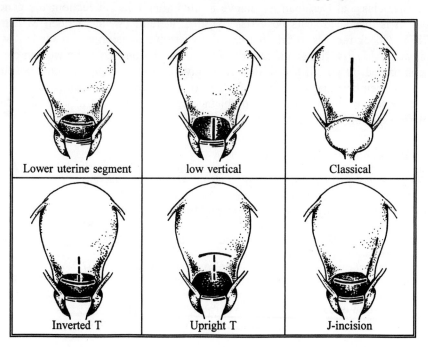

Risk factors: The primary risk factor involves separation of the scar with or without associated complications such as fetal distress, maternal hemorrhage or fetal death. Generally speaking, the higher up a vertical uterine incision extends, the greater the risk of subsequent, relatively benign scar separation (dehiscence) or scar rupture (traumatic tearing open of the scar, which may cause pain or bleeding, but most consistently causes fetal distress). Classical and T- or J-shaped incisions pose significantly more risk of rupture than does a low transverse incision (4% or more versus 2% or less). These incisions are more likely to give way during pregnancy as well. However, when you consider that the overall maternal mortality for Cesarean section has been reported to be at least four times higher (Petitti, 1982) to as much as 26 times higher (Evrard & Gold, 1977) than for yoni birth, the relatively small risk of uterine scar separation is put into perspective. Dehiscence and uterine rupture are covered in a separate chapter in the Third Trimester section.

Other uterine surgeries: Other than Cesarean section, the primary reason surgery is performed on the uterus is for tumor removal. Usually this applies to fibroids. In most cases the removal of small fibroids does not impact any future pregnancies. However, if the fibroid was large and embedded in the uterine wall, and especially if a portion of the wall was taken out when the fibroid was removed, uterine integrity could be compromised. Another less common reason involves surgical correction of uterine anomalies. When surgery is done outside of pregnancy, the uterus is less active, thus healing is less complicated. Hysterotomy is a second trimester classical Cesarean to remove a fetus after failed induction; the general opinion is that such scars pose less risk than at term (Wainer-Cohen & Estner, 1983). Check records to find out exactly where the incision was made and what was done. Ideally, if a significant risk of scar separation exists, the woman can be accompanied by you, if she so desires, to give birth in a compassionate hospital.

Remember that a history of other types of abdominal surgeries such as appendectomies are not usually a problem. Be aware, however, that as the uterus enlarges, pulling pains may occur due to scar tissue adhesions.

Reference and further reading:

Clark, S, "Rupture of the Scarred Uterus," Ob Gyn Clin No Am, Vol. 15, No. 4, 1988, p. 737-44.
Donald, Ian, Practical Obstetric Problems, Lloyd-Luke, Ltd., London, Eng. 1979.
Douglas, C., "Rupture of the uterus," Nursing Times, Feb. 17, 1977.
Evrard, John & Gold E., "Cesarean Section and Maternal Mortality in Rhode Island: Incidence and Risk Factors, 1965-1975," Ob Gyn., Vol. 50, Nov. 1977, No. 5.
Gabbe, Steven, et al., Obstetrics: Normal and Problem Pregnancies, 2nd ed. Churchill-Livingstone, New York 1991.
Hag, C, "Vaginal Birth after cesarean delivery," Am Fam Physician, Vol. 37, No. 6, 1988, p. 167.
Oxhorn, Harry, Human Labor and Birth, Appleton-Century-Crofts, E. Norwalk, CT, 1986.
Petitti, D., et al., "In-hospital maternal mortality in the United States: Time trends and relation to method of delivery," Ob Gyn, Vol. 59, 1982, pp. 6-11.
Wainer-Cohen, N., Estner, L., Silent Knife, Bergin & Garvey, Boston, MA, 1983.

Type	Location	Advantages	Disadvantages
SKIN INCISIONS:			
Vertical	Midline, vertical, hypogastric incision; extends from symphysis pubis to navel and above the navel if necessary	Excellent exposure of the uterus, rapid entry into abdominal cavity; often used in cases of acute fetal distress	Weakens abdominal muscles, scar is very visible
Pfannenstiel transverse suprasymphyseal Popularly called the "Bikini cut"	Semilunar incision just above the public hairline, with the angles inclined slightly upwards toward the anterior-superior iliac crests	Good cosmetic results; abdominal wall is stronger and post operative pain is less than with vertical cut; dehiscence is rare	Exposure is not as good; takes more time to perform, not good in true emergencies
UTERINE INCISIONS FOR SURGICAL DELIVERY:			
Lower segment transverse incision	The fold of peritoneum attached to the bladder is dissected away and pushed downward; a small transverse incision is made in the lower uterine segment; the incision is widened with the fingers, stopping before reaching the uterine vessels. To avoid injuring the fetus, the cut can be made with the scalpel handle.	Low in the uterus; splitting muscle laterally leads to less bleeding; cutting the placenta is rare except w/previa; the head is usually beneath the incision and extracted easily; the thin lower segment is easy to sew back up and blood loss is less; the repair is covered by the bladder flap; incidence of rupture in subsequent pregnancies is low, rarely occurring before term; if rupture occurs it is usually not traumatic.	A uterine vessel may be torn if the cut is made too far laterally or the baby is big, causing hemorrhage; contraindicated in abnormalities of the lower uterine segment (fibroids, varicosities); previous scars may prevent easy access; if the lower segment is still thick (i.e. it is early in labor), the operation is difficult; often cannot be used in placenta previa; takes longer due to bladder involvement; a true emergency may preclude its use.
J-shape	Surgery begins with a lower transverse incision which is extended as a vertical cut to one side of the uterus	Allows access to baby in cases where the lower uterine segment is narrow or a large baby cannot be brought out through the original incision	Greatly weakens the uterus; produces extensive scarring; increases the likelihood of rupture in subsequent pregnancies

TYPE	LOCATION	ADVANTAGES	DISADVANTAGES
Inverted T-shape	Same as above except vertical extension is in the center of the uterus	Same as for J-shaped incision	Same as for J-shaped incision
Lower segment vertical incision	The bladder flap is removed as for a regular transverse incision; a vertical incision is made with a scalpel and is enlarged with blunt scissors to avoid injury to the baby.	Can be carried upward when necessary; good for large babies or when lower segment is poorly formed, for transverse lie, or in fetal anomalies such as conjoined twins; may be done for placenta previa.	Muscle is cut, leading to more bleeding; may accidently extend into the upper segment
Classical upper segment	A longitudinal midline incision is made into the anterior wall of the uterus, then enlarged upward and downward with blunt scissors.	Used where there is difficulty in exposing the lower segment (large blood vessel, high or adherent bladder, fibroid), impacted transverse lie, anterior placenta previa, or uterine malformation; in some areas (esp. the North East US) it is used for delivery of premature babies because it is felt to be less traumatic for them.	Thick myometrium is cut & bleeding is profuse; baby is born breech, often with more aspiration of fluid; if the placenta is anterior, cutting it will cause profuse fetal hemorrhage; incision faces peritoneal cavity with more chance of seepage from infected uterine contents; higher incidence of abdominal contents adhering to the uterus; higher incidence of uterine rupture in subsequent pregnancies
Upright T	Classical incision is extended laterally across the upper uterine segment.	Used rarely when reaching the baby or the location of the placenta makes it seem necessary.	Maximally weakens the integrity of the uterus for future childbearing
Extraperitoneal	the lower uterine segment is incised without entering the peritoneal cavity.	Devised in preantibiotic era to prevent the use of hysterectomy in grossly infected cases; prevents spillage of infected amniotic fluid into peritoneal cavity.	Difficult to perform; accidental entry into the peritoneum does occur; increased injury to the bladder; rarely used in 1st world countries today but is still used on women in other areas of the world

Working with Women Who Have Had Difficult Yoni Births or Suffered a Previous Fetal Death or Early Infant Loss

A woman who has had a previous yoni birth, can still come to her next pregnancy scarred from interventions or emotional trauma during the previous experience. Women who have been categorized as high risk due to high blood pressure, toxemia, small-for-dates fetal growth, or other problems, or who have been given pain medications during labor, had a forceps delivery or have suffered with a large, painful or poorly healed clitorotomy have all had traumatic experiences. This can contribute to fears and concerns as they move through another pregnancy, labor and birth. Many of the suggestions that apply to women who have had surgical births apply here, so read that chapter as well as this one.

Discuss the specific events of the previous labor, and encourage the mother to get in touch with her feelings regarding the experience. Any woman who has had a traumatic birth can benefit from writing letters to her previous care providers expressing her feelings about what took place. She does not have to send such letters and can view them as a way of working out her many complex feelings about the situation. She can talk to her baby and visualize how she wishes the birth had gone. Affirmations specific to her circumstances can also help her to counteract the fears she brings with her to this pregnancy.

As the pregnancy advances, be aware of the timing of any problems that occurred during the previous pregnancy. These landmarks may be especially anxiety ridden for the woman, especially if she had a baby die or almost die before. However, once those critical periods have come and gone, women are typically more relaxed. Be aware of any underlying fears and keep encouraging women to ask questions and express their feelings as care progresses.

Previous infant loss: If a woman has experienced an early infant loss, either through death, abortion, or separation (such as placing the baby for adoption), a new wave of grieving will accompany the joy she feels in anticipating the birth to this baby. She may still harbor guilt that she was somehow responsible for the other loss and may fear that she does not deserve a healthy baby now. Even without added guilt, she may fear for the infant's health or safety. Help her move through her feelings by providing frequent opportunities for her to express her feelings about the coming baby during prenatal visits. How she accomplishes this will depend upon how fully she dealt with her initial grief at the time of the previous loss. If she remained shut down or was placed on tranquilizers or mood altering drugs, her process is likely to be much more difficult. Counseling will prove helpful in such cases. Her feelings will probably not be fully dealt with until the new baby has passed the point when the last baby was lost. It is important to support her to feel her feelings fully, so that she can eventually move beyond her acute emotional response and fully relate to her new baby in the present.

Working with Women Who Have a History of Infertility

Women who have had a history of infertility, including those who have gone to great technological lengths to get pregnant, will occasionally choose, once pregnant, to forego all additional high-tech care and come to you! Since they often know of their pregnancy sooner than other women, such clients may seek care quite early on. Fertility specialists do not usually provide prenatal care; once a woman has conceived, she is expected to transfer her care to another provider.

Find out what drugs, technologies and techniques the woman may have utilized to achieve conception and if any side effects or repercussions are predicted by those who provided her care. Specifically, you want know the diagnosed reason for the infertility (was it secondary scarring from IUD use or pelvic inflammatory disease, has the scar tissue been removed?) How long have they been dealing with infertility issues? Do they have other children (sometimes secondary infertility occurs in previously fertile couples; this can happen with a history of Cesarean section).

Clomid (clomiphene citrate) is a widely used drug which stimulates ovulation. It may be used in women who are not ovulating or to encourage the ovary to ripen and release more than one egg if *in vitro* fertilization is to be used. Pregnyl (chorionic gonadotropin) is also used for this purpose. Multiple eggs means more eggs to fertilize and introduce into the mother, thus increasing her chances of conceiving. This procedure also increases her chances for multiple gestation, since several fertilized eggs are introduced in the hope that at least one will implant. Typically it is recommended to the mother to have daily progesterone injections during the first weeks of pregnancy to ensure that the body can support it; many women take progesterone for the entire first trimester. New drugs can be looked up in a Physician's Desk Reference.

While infertility is primarily physiological, women who have had trouble conceiving have accompanying emotional and psychological issues which arise. Regardless of which partner is deemed infertile by the medical system, never assume it is just one partner's "problem." People functioning in a couple dynamic will often bounce issues back and forth as they unconsciously work to achieve equilibrium. Discuss with both partners their mental and emotional processes in considering pregnancy. Encourage discussion of ambivalence, how infertility affected their relationship, and their fears and concerns now that the woman is pregnant. Next, help her choose affirming statements to use daily to help reestablish trust in her body's ability to take on the tasks of pregnancy, labor and birth. Stay alert to clues that emotional issues may still be unresolved or unacknowledged. Do not assume that a history of infertility is "no big deal" or that it will not impact how labor will go. The same emotional issues which were associated with an inability to conceive may resurface in some form late in pregnancy or during labor. It is your best bet to establish as honest and open a relationship as possible now so that any issues which arise later can be resolved.

Independent Fertilization

Independent fertilization (IF), known under the medical model as donor insemination (DI), may be used whenever a woman or her male partner is experiencing certain types of infertility. In addition, more and more single women and single or coupled lesbian women are choosing independent fertilization as a way to conceive without the involvement of a male parent.

General considerations: Find out if any medical history is available on the sperm donor. Was the donation arranged by the parents with or through a friend or relative? If a known donor was used, is there a written agreement outlining his desire for involvement (or lack thereof) in the child's life. While this might clarify the relationship, the mother should know that a known father cannot sign away his legal rights as a parent. Will he seek custody in the future? Will his parents be involved as grandparents? These questions are especially pertinent to single women.

Was a sperm bank used? Some banks are set up to reveal the donor to the child when the child turns 18. Have the parents explored this option? A discussion of when they plan to tell the child, what they plan to say and what provisions they have planned, if any, for the child to contact their biological father are appropriate. If there is no provision for the child to ever know their biological father, discuss how they came to that decision and what they plan to tell the child.

There are several different profiles of people who use independent fertilization. They are:

Couples in which the man is sterile: These men may want their fertility status to remain secret and are most likely to be prone to feelings of inadequacy. Often they are acutely aware that they are not the real father of the child, and the mother may have extra power and privilege in the relationship dynamic. When the circumstances surrounding conception are kept a guarded secret they become an underlying family bomb, waiting to go off. Many times this situation is aggravated by care providers who encourage men to see IF as an immediate and easy solution to their fertility problem with comments like—"No one has to know they aren't your kids." This sets up a pattern of denial and secret-keeping which may go on for years. In this situation the man never really comes to grips with his infertility, and never grieves the loss of his genetic children so that he can clear the emotional slate to relate to the children he does have. This scenario presents the most emotionally complex dynamic. Be aware that some couples may not even tell you the real status of the conception.

Couples in which the man had a previous vasectomy: Perhaps the man had children with a previous partner and then decided he didn't want any more, or has a genetically inheritable health problem he does not wish to pass on to his children. Either way, this man has chosen his inability to have genetic offspring and therefore may not feel as insecure about the situation as the sterile man described above. He may regret his choice, but can see IF as a solution and does not necessarily feel there is a terrible secret to keep.

In some cases the man may have thought ahead and frozen some sperm just in case he ever changed his mind about wanting a family. When the sperm used is from the man who will also parent the child, the situation is pretty clear cut; the child knows s/he has a father and who that father is.

Couples where the man has an undesirable genetic trait he does not wish to pass on to offspring: This situation is usually far easier psychologically, does not lend itself to "secrets" and makes for a clearer emotional reaction to the decision. Here, the man is choosing the IF option. While there may be emotional difficulties with this decision, they are less likely to be as problematic as in the case of male infertility.

Single mothers: If a woman does not wish to marry or has not found the right partner but wants to start a family, she may choose IF as an alternative. These women are typically up front about their decision and willing to share this with their children. Single women will ideally have a network of family members and friends who can support her during the postpartum period. Even though she is single, a heterosexual mother will usually not encounter legal difficulties in keeping her children, however single lesbians who are out in their community may in some areas. You should discuss her feelings about single parenthood, her concept of a family, any concerns she may have about having or raising a son, how her family feels about her choice, and how she plans to balance work and parenting.

Lesbian couples: Many lesbians are starting families these days and IF is one solution to obtaining sperm. The dynamics within such couples about how or if they will let the child know who the father is (if known to them) or what they will tell the child about his origins are often not very clearly thought out. Discussing this with them will be helpful.

Encourage any parent who has received IF to carefully consider their emotional needs now and the emotional needs of their children in the future regarding their heritage and roots. Recommend that they read Lethal Secrets: The Psychology of Donor Insemination by Annette Baran and Reuben Pannor, which outlines the psychological concerns in detail.

Teen Pregnancy

Teenagers and younger girls can and do become pregnant. High rates of unprotected intercourse result in over 1 million adolescent pregnancies each year. Most of these are unintended and unwanted, and over 50% end in induced abortions. The United States has more teen pregnancies than any other developed nation. This is in part due to misguided attitudes on the part of some parents who feel that sex education is offering teens a license for sexual promiscuity; therefore, lack of sex education is felt to be ideal. Some religious and political attitudes subscribe to the idea that sex education is a private matter to be handled in the home, however, many parents feel ill-prepared to talk to their teens and therefore the issue may go poorly addressed. Teen pregnancy cuts across all class and racial lines but is most prevalent in poor and black communities.

A very high percentage of these girls have a history of sexual abuse either by a parent or another relative. A higher percentage of pregnant teens are battered than is true of their adult counterparts. Be alert to these possibilities throughout your caregiving relationship. Often, these girls have not had any sexual education and may have some strange ideas about sexual activity and its relationship to becoming pregnant.

Deciding to carry the pregnancy and keep the baby: The question of whether to carry the pregnancy or have an abortion is an important one. Parents or the boyfriend involved may pressure the girl one way or the other, to the point that she feels powerless to examine the issue and make a choice for herself. Often, teens feel both guilty about abortion and overwhelmed at the prospect of parenting. Other teenagers seem to have no concept of what parenting means and may have a very childish attitude, not grasping the responsibility involved. The loss of the balance of her own childhood is another consideration, and those who decide to keep the pregnancy should be referred to teen educational programs that accept pregnant girls. Talk in detail about what it means to parent. Adoption alternatives should be discussed as well (see the next chapter).

Conducting prenatal care: Teens can be treated like other pregnant women. However, they are also children who may be in denial and disbelief that they are in the midst of an unplanned pregnancy. This may cause her to seek care late in her pregnancy. They need to feel nurturing attention, while not feeling as though all the adults are making their decisions for them. A young teen may not have the maturity to express her feelings and make her needs known. Private, lengthy appointments, going slow with physical exams, and seeing her by herself at some visits will help to build trust and hopefully open the lines of communication. Remember to ask her what she needs rather than make any assumptions. Often, teens will be accompanied to prenatal visits by a mother or sister. This may prevent some girls from feeling comfortable about revealing problems in her home life, her desires about the pregnancy, birth, or baby and any questions she may have about sexuality. Realizing this, it may be appropriate to tell support people that you need to talk with her in private. This medical model tactic can be used to your advantage in such situations. Be tactful, if the girl is a minor, parents or guardians have the legal right to be present.

Discuss the teen's financial situation. Although young teens may still need to live with their parents, older girls may be able to obtain state or federal financial aid such as welfare and food stamps.

You should make every effort to meet the father of the baby. If he is much older than she is, problems such as abuse may be present. Be alert for this possibility. Discuss what his role will be in parenting the baby: if he will not be involved, discuss legal issues related to custody.

When explaining pregnancy physiology and warning signs to teens, be sure that you use simple language and define your terms. Encourage the girl to ask questions and give her handouts and books to take home and read. Do not assume that she is disinterested because she is shy about asking questions. Explore what childbirth classes might be especially useful to her. Some communities have teen-oriented classes. Talk to her about breastfeeding, recognizing that it brings up a great deal of embarrassment for many teens, but can also present an opportunity to make her feel capable and powerful in her mothering role.

Adjustment issues: Once the decision to keep a pregnancy is made, encourage teens to be proud of their role as mothers. Often, self-esteem is low in pregnant teens, many of whom come from abusive backgrounds. Teens may get pregnant out of an unconscious desire to have someone to love them, to cement a relationship, or to get away from a bad home situation. Now, having made the choice to continue the pregnancy, they need positive reinforcement around their new responsibilities. Teen mothers can be strong birthers, with their young bodies dealing well with labor and birth. If they eat right and eliminate substance abuse they are not at higher risk for prematurity or toxemia, but young girls (less than 15) may have problems birthing a full term baby of average size because their bone structure has not fully matured. This does not mean, however, that weight gain or dietary limitations should be suggested, as this will only increase the likelihood of other complications.

Nutrition: Nutrition for the pregnant teen is a challenging topic: she should be encouraged to eat as well as any other pregnant woman. She needs support and a good basic understanding of why nutrition is important and how directly her dietary habits, as well as other ways she can care for herself, can impact the health of the pregnancy. Focusing on what she can do will go far in helping her feel more in control of her life and her situation.

Young teens have bodies that are still growing and need additional protein and calories to compensate. Also encourage exercise, especially if the girl is worried about getting fat. Eating disorders are rampant among teens; this coupled with embarrassment about the pregnancy, and its advertisement of her sexual activity, may compound her feelings about getting bigger. Constantly praise and reassure her about her size as the pregnancy advances.

Substance abuse: Drug, alcohol and cigarette use should be reviewed carefully, with the recognition that teens may not grasp the importance of telling you the truth. It is up to you to make clear why these things are important to avoid, once again emphasizing how much control she has over the health of her baby.

Sexually transmitted diseases: Teens need this topic specifically addressed with details regarding what constitutes sexual contact so that they understand the behaviors which place them at risk. Start with a basic overview of sexual anatomy. If possible discuss these issues in private with the girl and then readdress them later when the partner is present as well. Use active listening, having her repeat what you have told her, to be sure she understands what you are saying.

References and further reading: (books available through Cascade birth supply's Imprints catalogue).

Altendorf, J, Klepacki, L., "Childbirth education for adolescents," NAACOG's Clinical Issues, Vol. 2, No. 2, 1991.
Arthur, Shirley, Surviving Teen Pregnancy, explains options to teens.
Barr & Monserrat, Working with Pregnant and Parenting Teens, a teacher's manual for teen pregnancy.
op. cit., Teenage Pregnancy Set includes three books on pregnancy, exercise and breastfeeding for teens.
Lindsay, Jeanne, Teen Dads, discusses responsibility and parenting issues for teen fathers
op. cit., Parents, Pregnant Teens and the Adoption Option, for the parents of the pregnant teen.
op. cit., Pregnant Too Soon: Adoption is an Option, for teens, with personal stories.
Loprenzi-Kassel, ClareBeth, midwife, Veneta, OR, editing comments, 2/95.

934

Adoption Issues

A woman contemplating her options for dealing with an unwanted pregnancy has three basic choices: carry the pregnancy and either keep the baby or put it up for adoption, or abortion. Since the relinquishing mother will require ongoing prenatal care, we will discuss adoption here.

What to do? You should examine your own feelings and prejudices regarding the "type" of women who choose adoption. If you feel teenagers shouldn't be mothers, that older women have no business placing a baby for adoption, or that adoption is a woman's only alternative to parenting, your opinions will color how you discuss the matter with the woman and not allow her a clear space for her decision. The choice to continue the pregnancy, as is true of the choice to abort, must be the mother's choice. While we can explain the various health and emotional factors to the best of our ability, we have no right to impose our idea of the "correct" choice on the mother. Her three options may all carry tremendous burdens for her; but she needs to examine each one so that her decision is right for her. Neither adoption nor abortion is an easy choice. The element of choice involved does not diminish the pain which accompanies either decision. To carry a child and then place it for adoption requires tremendous love on the part of the mother; adoption is not abandonment. The choice to abort carries emotional issues similar to those which arise for women experiencing an early pregnancy loss; see When a Baby Dies in Early Pregnancy for how to help women who choose to abort. Other abortion-related issues will be addressed as an interconceptional matter in volume III.

If the biological father is also part of the picture, try to interview them both; fathers, being biologically distant from the process of pregnancy, may be in even less in touch with their feelings and grief around the baby. Fathers can and do sometimes put up a big fight around both abortion and adoption decisions. Helping the birthparents discuss the pros and cons of their decision and helping the father feel involved in the decision can help smooth the legal issues. This is especially true if the biological father will be required to sign the consent papers. Making a free choice without coercion will lay a foundation for the healing which will need to follow. Also, keep in mind that as the pregnancy progresses, the mother will naturally rethink her decision at every point and must be allowed to reexplore the option to parent. Vacillation is common as term approaches; just listen to her and support her to examine her alternatives in any way she must, no legally binding decision is made until the papers are signed.

Resources and support: Find out what resources are available for emotional support for birthparents. Concerned United Birth Parents is a national group offering such support. (800) 822-2777. Call local social service agencies for more contacts in your area. Suggest that both birthparents and grandparents read Suzanne Arms excellent book <u>Adoption: A Handful of Hope</u>, which should provide rich topics for further discussion.

Basic adoption procedures: Adoption is the legal process whereby the guardianship of a child is permanently transferred from the biological parents to adoptive parents. Each jurisdiction has its own adoption laws which vary in the number of days after birth the consents may be signed; consents are never signed prior to the birth. Time periods for withdrawal of consent also vary. Be sure to consult legal counsel and understand each paper before it is signed. Once the papers are signed, there is a probationary period before the adoption is finalized. The average time is about 6 months, although this period may vary as well. The birthmother's consent is always required for the adoption to proceed, no one can sign on her behalf, even if she is a minor. In some places the biological father is also asked for consent when he is available. The birthparents retain all rights until the adoption is final, after that, all rights are transferred to the adoptive parents. There are a number of ways that legal adoption may be orchestrated:

Traditional closed adoption: This refers to total confidentiality with no identifying information exchanged, although nonidentifying information is provided to both parties. The birthmother should ask for this information in writing so that she can refer to it in the future. The opportunity to exchange letters, photos, etc. before as well as after the birth may be offered, but there is no guarantee that this will occur. In many places the birthmother can sign a waiver of confidentiality at the time of adoption which would allow her child to seek information about its birthparents upon reaching the age of majority.

Open adoption: This usually refers to the exchange of identifying information between the birthparents and the adoptive parents, and to the possibility of face-to-face contact between the parties involved. The extent of openness may include meeting each other, having adoptive parents at the birth, handing the child into the hands of the adoptive parents, continuing exchange of information after placement (letters and photos), or continuing contact with the child. Having the adoptive parents at the birth may be too much contact for some birthmothers, and may interfere with their time with the baby, to be alone and to say goodbye. How much contact is appropriate for her needs, both during the pregnancy and the birth must be thought through carefully.

Agency adoption: This refers to social agencies lisenced and regulated by the jurisdiction to facilitate adoption; some have a religious affiliation. Counselors meet with prospective adoptive parents and assess their living situation with a home study. They will also help the birthmother weigh decisions and provide emotional support. Agencies vary in their degrees of openness in the adoption process. One advantage to the birth mother may be the lack of connection with a specific adoptive family. In the United States, locate an agency by contacting the local social services department, the Child Welfare League of America, or the Family Service Association. In Canada, contact you provincial ministry of social services or Children's Aid Society.

Private or independent adoption: These adoptions take place as a result of collaboration between the birthparents and a private intermediary such as a lawyer, physician, or independent adoption facilitator. These persons are often working for the adoptive parents, and therefore are not there to assist the birthmother in her decision-making. Private or independent adoptions are not legal in all areas. Adoptive parents may be paying a substantial fee for the services of the intermediary, although it is illegal to give or receive money for the procurement of a child. Adoptive parents may offer to pay for medical expense and other costs incurred during the pregnancy. They may or may not offer some degree of openness. The birthmother should engage her own lawyer to represent her in the process, who should do a background check on the intermediary, since adoptive parents going this route may be desperate for a baby and there may not be any study of their suitability for adoption.

The pregnancy: Deciding to keep the pregnancy and place the baby for adoption will cast a shroud of ambivalent feelings over the entire experience. Many women may present themselves for care quite late in pregnancy as a result. Even during the pregnancy, women will be looking foreword to the inevitable loss of parting with their baby and begin an anticipatory grieving process. This grieving process is complicated, however, by the fact that the baby will be alive, allowing the mother space to fantasize about her baby's life with its adoptive parents and thus diverting her away from dealing with her loss and grief. Her grief may also leave her feeling overwhelmed and as though she has made the wrong decision; this is not necessarily the case and the more prepared she is for the grief to follow, the better she will deal with the decision once made. In order to let go, attachment must first take place. Since the pregnancy and the immediate postpartum period will be the only time the mother will have to be with her newborn, she can use this time to get to know her baby, take good care of it with good eating habits and generally appreciating this special time which she alone can share. She can think of a name for the baby during pregnancy. Naming her baby, even though the adoptive parents will likely give the baby another name, is an important step for the birthmother in claiming her experience, in recognizing the individuality and the relationship she has with this baby and in letting go. She can also plan how she wants to handle the time she will send with the baby prior to adoption. For some women, a ceremony, ritual or religious activities such as a christening or baptism may serve as a way to formally say goodbye. Remind her that before any papers are signed it is her baby; she can see and breastfeed or bottlefeed her baby, spend time with and care for her baby in any way she wishes. Seeing the baby will make the baby and the loss more real, although it may be hard to imagine at the time of birth, contact with the baby will make the grieving process more complete. *Attempting to avoid pain does not make it go away, it merely means that the pain will resurface at a later time and must be dealt with then.* However, while explaining this and encouraging women to see and relate to their baby, their wishes must, of course, be respected. Whatever the woman can do the grieve this loss will help her in dealing with pregnancy and mothering in the future.

Legal aspects: The legal representatives for both sets of parents may have little understanding of what homebirth or midwifery care is all about. They may insist, or try to insist, that tests and technology be used which the birthmother would rather avoid. It is therefore important to be clear about your practice parameters and find out if the birthmother's legal representative is open to advocating for her in these situations. Hopefully you will be able develop a resource file of agencies, lawyers and other support services that understand why a woman might choose midwifery care.

The midwife's role: Even though a healthy baby is anticipated, this birth is very like a birth that will end in a neonatal death from the point of view of the birthmother. Your job is to provide a sympathetic, open ear to her emotional needs. After the birth you can take some photographs, snip a lock of hair, take hand and footprints, and save a baby shirt or blanket from the time of birth and mementos of the birth. Talk to the mother about this and ask if there are any special requests she has along these lines. If transport is necessary, developing a birth plan (including confidentiality issues, visitor stipulations, time with the baby after birth, the status of the birthfather, her attorney and any labor and birth specifics) which can be given to the attending nurse may help smooth out some of the awkwardness that this situation may produce.

The adoptive parents: If this is an open adoption situation and the parents have been asked to be present at the birth (this should be the birthmother's decision), you should meet privately with the adoptive parents, perhaps at a home visit, to discuss homebirth and your role as midwife. You should ask them directly what their expectations are in being at the birth and speak to them about how important it will be for the birthmother to have time to say goodbye to her baby. As is true with any birth, the birthmother's needs must come first and if the adoptive parents are asked to leave, they should understand that staying is not an option. There is a strong feeling that birthmothers know how long they need to say goodbye to their babies and this can vary greatly from woman to woman. Tell the adoptive parents this in advance. Hopefully this will minimize their anxiety while they are waiting for the birth mother to come to terms with her decision and take the next step. Will they want you to continue to provide postpartum newborn care?

938

The birth grandparents: Especially if the mother is young, the birth grandparents will probably be integrally involved in the decision to place the baby for adoption. Out of their own feelings of guilt over their imagined deficiencies as parents and an overwhelming feeling of being out of control, they may try to impose their opinions on their daughter. While they may not want the girl to "give away their grandchild," they may offer not support for helping her to parent. Encourage them to seek counseling if you have the opportunity and warn them that their feelings of grief and loss may be intense.

Women who have previously placed a baby for adoption:

Especially if this is her next pregnancy, she will relive that experience through this one and may feel a variety of emotions which she should be encouraged to express; ask her how she is feeling frequently throughout her care. She may question whether she deserves to have a child now or that she will lose the child once it is born. If her previous adoption was forced upon her or she was totally numb to the grief of her loss, she may have gotten pregnant again quickly in an unconscious attempt to resolve those complex feelings. If unresolved grief surfaces, assist her to visualize how she would have liked to deal with the time after birth, or how she would do it differently now, may help. Writing a letter to the adoptive parents may help, if that is possible. Your willingness to take the time to hear her feelings and concerns will go a long way in helping her to come to this birth clear enough to receive this baby with joy.

References, resources and further reading:

American Adoption Congress, 1 (800) 274-6736
Arms, Suzanne, Adoption: A Handful of Hope, Celestial Arts, Berkeley, CA, 1990.
Panuthos, C & Romero, C., Ended Beginnings, Bergin & Garvey, MA., 1984.

Pregnancy and Biological Fathering After 35

There is no data that supports the myth that healthy women with no preexisting medical conditions who are over the age of 35 are at greater physiological risk for bearing children than younger women. The risk of conceiving a child with a trisomy genetic defect is greater after age 35 and increases as the woman becomes older. Since the risk of such defects (primarily Down syndrome) at age 35 equals the risks of the tests to determine if the fetus has Down syndrome, 35 is the age when routine genetic screening is first recommended by mainstream medicine.

Women over the age of 35 having their first baby may have unique psychological issues. These women typically have made a conscious choice not to have children during their twenties and many of them will have pursued careers and otherwise will have a good handle on their life and how they want it to be. Often, long standing relationships that have been "just the two of us" are faced with the prospect of permanent disruption by the addition of a new family member. In short, her life has probably been in control and under her control for some time. Being pregnant brings up any unconscious control issues big time! Regardless of how wanted the child may be, these changes can be unsettling as the woman and her partner make room in every aspect of their life for another person. A baby can be a real wrench in the works and can require considerable adjustment. Not every midwife finds this true with women over 35. I practiced on the East and West coasts and have found this to be true; however, if you live in an area where the attitude about life and "getting ahead" are quite relaxed, such parents may simply bring maturity and centeredness to the pregnancy without so much extra baggage.

How the couple will handle these changes will, of course, vary with individuals and how much support they have from their larger community. As the midwife, it is up to you to help them discuss the real and imagined changes they will face and how they can cope with them.

Older Fathers: Men over 55 are more likely to father infants with Down syndrome by a small margin. Achondroplasia, myositis ossification, Marfan's syndrome and acrocephalosyndactyly each have a highly probable paternal age specific new mutation expression. The number of mutants per million gametes has been calculated to range from 3 to 13 for these four disorders, the risk to men age 45 and older is increased 4 to 5 fold in comparison to men aged 20 to 25. Other autosomal dominant disorders with similar mutation rates have not shown such a correlation.

Three autosomal dominant disorders appear to have slight paternal age effect. These are retinoblastoma, neurofibromatosis and tuberous sclerosis. Tumors are associated with all three. Thus, children who inherit the germ cell mutation carry an increased risk for somatic cells to transform into tumor cells.

In X-linked recessive mutations age effect relates to the maternal grandfather since potential fathers either don't reproduce or have unaffected children (daughters will be carriers and sons will get the normal Y, not the abnormal X from affected fathers). Hemophilia A, Lesch-Nylan syndrome and Duchenne muscular dystrophy all show a higher mutation rate in male germ cells.

Males aged 40 or older have a 20% greater risk of fathering a child with some kind of birth defect compared with males under 40 years of age, including ventricular septal defect and atrial septal defect at a slightly higher rate. This makes the risk 4 to 6 per 1000 live births.

References and further reading:

Brassil, M., et.al., "Obstetric outcomes in first-time mothers aged 40 years and older," Eur J of Gyn & Repro Bio, Vol. 25, 1987, p. 115-120.

Holz, K., et.al., "Outcomes of mature primiparas in out-of-hospital birth center," J of Nurse-Mid, July/Aug. Vol. 34, No. 4, 1989 p. 185-189.

Mansfield, P., McCool, W., "Toward a better understanding of the advanced maternal age factor," Health Care Women Int, Vol. 10, No. 4, 1989, pp. 395-415.

Meagher, Kirsten, genetics counselor, Kaiser Sunnyside, Clackamas, OR, phone conversation re: genetic risks in older fathers 6/23/95.

Third Baby Syndrome

I first heard this term from an experienced nurse-midwife. I was describing some of the issues coming up for one of my clients and she asked which baby this was (it was her third). The midwife then went on to explain what she called third baby syndrome. This occurs in women who have had two healthy pregnancies. Usually the first birth was the longer one. During the second pregnancy, the woman felt much more confident, because she recognized the sensations from the first pregnancy and knew that things turned out fine before. The second labor is usually only half as long as the first, and the woman was relieved it was so much easier, relatively speaking.

Now, having had those two experiences, pregnant with her third child, she doesn't quite know what to expect. Psychologically she feels that she has been lucky; after all, look at all the problems everyone else she knows has had. She not only knows more about what can happen during pregnancy, she often feels her "number is up" for a problem. She worries about everything. Every little symptom of pregnancy, which she is aware of now more than ever due to past experience, becomes a "real" problem. She calls and asks more questions and frets over things which she would have ignored in the past. Part of the reason for this is that women often experience their pregnancy with a third baby differently than their first two. It becomes easier for them to fear something is wrong because things feel so different. This often carries through right into labor, with the course of labor, pushing and birth going differently than it did with previous babies. Of course this psychological picture can occur with a second baby or a fourth or fifth baby, but typically it occurs with the third.

As the midwife, you can reassure a woman when symptoms are clearly within normal limits. When they are not, you can ask her point blank if she really feels there is a problem. Does she have an intellectual conversation in her head going on about this issue or is this a gut level, intuitive warning that something is amiss? Usually, when asked like that, most women can discriminate the two and will let you know which it really is. Having this distinction articulated can also help women calm their fears.

Bottom line, your job is to reassure women when things are normal but not to lean so heavily in that direction that you ignore a real warning sign of a problem. When in doubt, get the opinion of another experienced midwife. If that is a dead end, start with the least invasive means of getting more information and work your way through all the medical tests available until the mother says she has sufficient information or you know what the problem really is.

Grand Multiparity

A grand multipara is a woman who has given birth to several babies. How many babies varies, depending upon the reference. Remember that parity is defined by the birth of babies, alive or dead, weighing 500 gm. or more or carried to an estimated length of pregnancy beyond 20 weeks. Taber's Medical Dictionary (1985) and Hughes (1972) say it is a woman who has given birth seven or more times. As more women have chosen to limit the size of their families, some sources have changed the definition in response. Myles (1981) uses five births as the cutoff point and Oxhorn (1986) states a parity of 6. In recent years, there has been talk of reducing the defining number of births even more, but nothing official has been decided at this time.

Certain subcultures within North America typically have as large a family as they can. These include the Amish, Mennonites, Muslims, Orthodox Jews and some branches of Christianity. Often when women have their "last" baby at home with midwives, they opt to have one or two more because the experience was so transformative. Therefore, just because modern textbooks do not often discuss it, grand multiparity is hardly a thing of the past.

The woman who is having her seventh pregnancy or higher faces some potentially greater risk factors than women who have less children. However, whether many of these risks will manifest depends upon her overall health, muscle tone, nutrition, the amount of time that has elapsed between pregnancies (2 years is ideal) and her living situation (i.e. how supported does she feel in her family and community). Prenatal care is the same, whether a woman is pregnant for the first time or the 20th, although there are some things to be aware of that may impact the grand multipara more than women of lesser parity. She is at more risk for:

*Lax abdominal muscles and lax uterine tone, increasing her risk for:
   -Other-than-vertex presentations
   -Pendulous abdomen
   -Inefficient labor pattern
   -Spontaneous uterine rupture (especially if oxytocin is used)
   -Uterine inversion
*Anemia
*Diabetes
*Varicose veins and hemorrhoids
*Severe afterbirth pains

With a watchful attitude and attention to excellent nutrition and physical exercise, the essentially healthy grand multiparous mother receiving adequate prenatal care to troubleshoot for problematic developments does not face excessive risk in childbirth and can be cared for by midwives at home.

References and further reading:

Hughes, Edward, ed., Obstetric and Gynecologic Terminology, F.A. Davis Co., Phil. PA 1972.
Hughes, P., Morrison J., "Grandmultiparity—Not to be feared? An analysis of grandmultiparous women receiving modern antenatal care," Int. J. Gyn Ob, Vol. 44, No. 3, 1994, p. 211-17.
Myles, Margaret, Textbook for Midwives, 9th ed., Churchill-Livingstone, New York, 1981.
Oxhorn, Harry, Human Labor and Birth, 5th ed., Appleton-Century-Crofts, Norwalk, CT, 1986.

944

NOTES:

PROBLEMS THAT CAN OCCUR AT ANY TIME

Obviously, a lot of problems can occur at any time. The ones most likely to occur in a given trimester are mentioned in those sections. This section is a catch-all for those problems and symptoms which rarely occur as well as more common problems that are not clearly associated with any particular trimester. Disorders and infections which are covered in <u>Diagnostic Tests</u> are not reiterated here in detail and may not be mentioned in this section at all. <u>Healing Passage</u> has details regarding prolapses of the yoni wall and uterus. Please check <u>Diagnostic Tests</u> and <u>Healing Passage</u> if you do not find the problem you are looking for discussed in this section or elsewhere in this text.

Abdominal Pain

This chapter assumes that you have already ruled out the most common pregnancy-related causes of abdominal pain, such as:

*Round ligament stretching (see chapter Aches and Pains, this section)
*Threatened miscarriage (see chapter in First Trimester section)
*Urinary tract infection (see separate chapter in this section)
*Ectopic pregnancy (see separate chapter, First Trimester section)
*Fibroids (red degeneration, torsion [twisting], see chapter, this section)
*Labor
*Abruption (see separate chapter in Third Trimester section)
*Illness, food poisoning or another type of poisoning (See Poisoning
    chapter in this section)
*Uterine rupture (see separate chapter in Third Trimester section)
*Abdominal pregnancy (see chapter in Second trimester section)
*Torsion of the pregnant uterus (see separate chapter in this section)
*Sacculation of the uterus (see chapter in Second Trimester section)
*Hematoma of the rectus sheath (see Aches and Pains chapter)
*Acute hydronephrosis or hydroureter (see Aches and Pains chapter)

Described below are several other relatively common non-obstetrical causes of abdominal pain which can occur during an otherwise normal pregnancy:

Pelvic inflammatory disease or chorioamnionitis: Any pathological organism within the reproductive tract can cause active infection either in the mother, placenta, membranes or fetus with accompanying lower abdominal pain, tenderness, fever, malaise, and at times purulent discharge from the yoni. This represents a serious threat to both mother and baby. Get a medical evaluation right away!

Appendicitis: The incidence of appendicitis during pregnancy varies from 0.38 to 1.41 per 1,000 pregnancies. The overall fetal death rate is 8.5%; this rises markedly to between 35% and 70% when the appendix has ruptured.

In the nonpregnant woman the appendix is located in the right lower quadrant (65%), the pelvis (30%), or behind the cecum (5%) in a horizontal position. Uterine enlargement during pregnancy displaces the appendix. After the 12th week the appendix begins to move upward and to rotate at the base. These changes continue until the 8th month, when 93% of women in one study were found to have their appendixes above the iliac crest, and in 80% the appendix was rotated in a upwards direction from the base. Because of this displacement, the symptoms and complications of appendicitis can differ from those in the nonpregnant woman. With infection, the appendiceal channel becomes obstructed, abdominal pain is felt around the navel or epigastric area, regardless of the position of the appendix. If the appendix ruptures, contact of the inflamed appendix with the parietal peritoneum alters the point of maximal tenderness, causing pain to be felt in the lower right quadrant at or above the iliac crest or in the right flank. Some women may not feel pain at all if the appendix does not touch the parietal peritoneum; this is one reason for the higher incidence of gangrene and rupture during the late second and third trimester. Pain is localized as follows:

*1st trimester: lower right quadrant (100%)
*2nd trimester: lower right quadrant (80%)
*3rd trimester: upper right quadrant (20%)

If pain is localized in the right lower quadrant when the woman lies down and shifts when she lies on her left side, the pain is most likely within the uterus or ovaries. If it remains in the lower quadrant, appendicitis should be ruled out. General signs and symptoms other than pain include:

*Loss of appetite (not a consistent symptom during pregnancy)
*Nausea and vomiting
*Increased frequency of urination (also normal in pregnancy)
*Rebound tenderness (75%) (Ask the woman to cough and to show you where the cough produced pain; then palpate gently with one finger to map the area of pain. If necessary press the flats of your fingers into the painful area firmly and slowly, then quickly withdraw them. Ask her to compare which hurt more, the pressure or the withdrawal. Have her show you exactly where it hurt. Pain induced or increased by quick withdrawal is rebound tenderness, indicating an inflamed peritoneum.)
*Instinctively guarding the area with her hands (60%)
*Fever over 100.2°F (37.9°C) (18%)
*Pus in the urine, if the inflamed appendix touches the kidney (typically no bacteriuria is found)
*An elevated white blood count (some elevation is normal during late pregnancy; therefore unless the count is over 15,000 the WBC is not very useful in diagnosis).
*Rigid abdomen (but it is difficult to elicit rectus muscle spasm and rigidity due to uterine enlargement).

Appendicitis can be confused with kidney infection (acute pyelonephritis). The upward movement of the appendix often produces pain along the side of the body between the ribs and the ilium (flank) or the costovertebral angle. To differentiate the two, do a urinalysis with culture. If pus is present with bacteria suspect kidney infection, if not, suspect appendicitis. If you suspect appendicitis, transport without delay before rupture occurs. Surgery should be anticipated.

Other less common reasons for pain mimicking appendicitis include:

*Twisted ovarian cyst
*Degenerating myoma (fibroid)
*Ruptured corpus luteum of pregnancy
*Ruptured dermoid cyst
*Infarction of a normal ovary
*Pneumonia
*Endometriosis of the appendix with decidual reaction

Cholecystitis (inflammation of the gallbladder): This is associated with gallstones in 85% to 95% of all cases. Women of childbearing age are twice as likely as men to develop gallstones. Oral contraceptives increase the risk of stone formation, and stones more frequently occur in multiparas as well. Cholesterol dissolves in bile, but if the equilibrium of the gallbladder is altered by an increase in cholesterol, the bile can no longer dissolve it adequately and cholesterol stones form. Stone formation may be accelerated in pregnancy due to hormonal changes, a normal rise of cholesterol in the blood and bile, increased gallbladder volume with decreased emptying, and a decrease in bile salts or malabsorption of bile juices. Gallstones may be asymptomatic or produce pain due to blockage of the gall bladder ducts. Symptoms are the same whether a woman is pregnant or not and include:

*Nausea, vomiting and complete loss of appetite, sometimes with fever
*Tenderness and sometimes muscular rigidity in the upper right quadrant
*Midepigastric pain that radiates to the upper right quadrant, around
     the side to the back, or directly to the right shoulder blade
*Pain that occurs suddenly and may be described as excruciating,
     lancing, a deep ache or cramping and colicky, building to peak
     intensity in 15 to 60 minutes and subsiding over several hours
*Distention of the gallbladder
*Distention of the right colon
*Aggravation of symptoms from eating greasy foods
*Light colored or gray stools may occur if gall ducts are obstructed
*Generalized rebound tenderness (see appendicitis for technique) in
     cases of rupture

Other things to consider are:

*Severe acute viral hepatitis (see Diagnostic Tests)
*Alcoholic hepatitis
*Penetration or perforation of a duodenal ulcer
*Appendicitis

*Kidney infection
*Myocardial infarction (heart attack)

Physical assessment of the gallbladder includes palpating the liver (see chapter on the Physical Exam, Skills section) and the gallbladder for tenderness. To palpate the gallbladder, have the woman lie down on a firm surface. Hook your left thumb or the fingers of your right hand under the ascending bone margin along the inner edge of the rib cage about two-thirds of the way down from the xiphoid process on the woman's right side (i.e. at the point where the outer edge of the rectus abdominous muscle and the lower margin of the rib cage intersect). A sharp increase in localized tenderness which causes the woman to catch her breath is a sign of a problem. This maneuver is called Murphy's Sign. Tenderness may also be elicited in the normal liver with this maneuver but it will be vague and less localized. (Bates, 1991)

The lab tests that are the most helpful in differentiating gallbladder obstruction from other conditions with similar symptoms test for 5'-nucleotidase and the amylase:creatinine clearance ratio values. Ultrasound can also be used to spot gallstones 95% of the time.

TEST	FINDING	SIGNIFICANCE:
Amylase excretion/ Creatinine (2 hour urine test)	70-775 Somogyi units/hr. or 13-15 u./hr. 1500-6000 Somogyi units/24 hr. or 277-1110 u./24 hr.	Amylase is an enzyme which changes starch to sugar; indicative of pancreas function
	Elevated	Acute pancreatitis, peptic ulcer, choledocholithiasis, values increase about five points per unit in pancreatitis, in the other conditions, less than 5%
5'-Nucleotidase	10.6-17.5 U/liter	Widely distributed enzyme which appears in the serum in liver diseases
	Increased	Cholecystitis caused by chlorpromazine, extrahepatic obstruction, liver cancer, biliary cirrhosis

Once you have it narrowed down to gallbladder difficulties, if the symptoms are mild to moderate you can have the woman try any of the following home remedies to help the gallbladder pass stones and prevent further problems. Pain with no fever or swelling may respond well if the mother takes olive oil and uses castor oil packs. Any time pain and fever, nausea or vomiting appear together, bio-technical diagnosis should be sought without delay.

*If gallstones are the problem, have the mother take 3 tablespoons of the greenest, darkest olive oil she can find mixed with the juice of 1 to 2 lemons or 1 grapefruit before going to bed and again upon rising. This great natural remedy lubricates the bile ducts and in some cases will actually help the gallstones pass into the intestine. Passage may be painful but will relieve the symptoms.

Additionally, this remedy is not harmful.

*The application of castor oil-soaked flannel covered with plastic, with a heating pad applied on top can also help to heal the area. Once the acute attack has subsided, have the woman continue to take olive oil with lemon every day to lubricate and encourage gallbladder health.

*The pure juice of apples, pears and beets can be drunk daily to cleanse the liver. (Pregnant women should never fast!)

*Foods such as apples, applesauce and shredded raw beets are also cleansing to the liver. Olive oil and lemon juice can be used in food preparation and as a salad dressing.

*Women should eat small amounts frequently throughout the day rather than large meals

*Sugar, animal fats, fried foods, spices, margarine or other hydrogenated oils, soft drinks, commercial oils, coffee, chocolate and refined carbohydrates should be eliminated from the diet.

Bio-technical care includes giving chemicals to dissolve the stones and surgical removal. Surgery should be delayed if symptoms arise in the last trimester. None of the newer forms of bio-technical therapies are appropriate in pregnancy.

Acute pancreatitis: Pancreatitis occurs less during pregnancy (0.01% to 0.1%) than in nonpregnant women, however, when it does, the death rate is much higher. Acute pancreatitis is most often associated with gallstones, chronic ingestion of alcohol, surgery, trauma, metabolic disorders, genetic predisposition, infection, drugs, connective tissue disease, penetrating duodenal ulcer or obstruction of the pancreatic ducts. However, pancreatitis which appears during pregnancy is most often without obvious cause.

Inflammation develops when enzymes from cells within the pancreas are released and begin to digest other cells in and around the pancreas. This releases more pancreatic enzymes, which accelerate the process. Necrosis (tissue death) develops; this either heals itself spontaneously and/or with medical support or continues leading to systemic deterioration, including circulatory collapse, hypocalcemia, and kidney or respiratory failure or both. Clinical symptoms include nausea and vomiting, abdominal pain, fever and shock.

Serum amylase and lipase may be elevated in pancreatitis as well as in other diseases of the gastrointestinal system. Elevation of one or both can occur with intestinal obstruction, liver trauma, acute salpingitis (pelvic inflammatory disease), ruptured ectopic pregnancy, peptic ulcer disease and common duct stones. Interpretation of the serum amylase assay is further confused during pregnancy, as it may increase, decrease or remain unchanged during normal gestation.

The amylase:creatinine ratio (Cam/Ccr%) is easy to calculate; it requires simultaneously collected urine and blood samples. The ratio is elevated in pancreatitis. The normal nonpregnant ratio is between 1% and 4% (averaging 3.0 to 3.7%). Pancreatitis causes elevations that vary from 6.6% to 14.5% in the nonpregnant. During pregnancy the ratio is normally lower between the 12th to the 28th gestational week. Therefore, a value that would be normal outside of pregnancy is abnormally elevated in pregnancy. Elevation also occurs in cases of toxemia, severe burns, diabetic ketoacidosis, ruptured duodenal ulcer or cardiac surgery. In hyperemesis gravidarum, serial Cam/Ccr% values can help rule out pancreatitis as the real cause. The following table gives examples of normal pregnancy CAM/Ccr% values derived from a graph in a study done by DeVore, et.al. in 1980. Actual values may vary depending upon the type of test used.

12 WKS	16 WKS	20 WKS	24 WKS	28 WKS	32 WKS	36 WKS	40 WKS
2.3-2.7	2.25-2.6	2.15-2.55	2.35-2.45	2.25-2.5	3-4.4	2.75-3.4	2.5-3

Other things which may produce similar symptoms are:

*Perforated ulcer (especially peptic [stomach]—see below)
*Acute cholecystitis and biliary colic
*Dissecting aortic aneurysm
*Connective tissue disorders with blood vessel inflammation
*Pneumonia (see chapter on Colds, Flus and Pneumonia, this section)
*Diabetic ketoacidosis (check urine for glucose and ketones)

If you suspect pancreatitis or any of the above conditions, transport immediately!

Peptic ulcer disease: Peptic ulcer is occasionally seen in childbearing women. Previous disease often becomes asymptomatic during pregnancy. Pregnancy appears to reduce the gastric acid output, and placental hormones deactivate histamine, both of which play a role in aggravating this condition. In some cases, ulcers may worsen or show no improvement in symptoms. Peptic ulcer is precipitated by an increase in the secretion of hydrochloric acid and pepsin, causing irritation to the stomach lining. Eventually an open sore develops in the lining.

Symptoms include mild to severe midepigastric pain, described as burning, cramping, pressing or boring. The pain lasts 15 to 60 minutes, is relieved by food or an antacid, and is made worse by drinking coffee, taking aspirin or ingesting alcoholic beverages. The pain may occur intermittently throughout the day as well as in the early morning. Women rarely vomit unless the ulcers are the result of a stomach or duodenal tumor. Vomiting of blood or blood in the stools (making them sticky and black) is caused by the erosion of blood vessels around the ulcer. Bleeding may leave the woman fatigued and anemic. Keep in mind that black stools can also be caused by poor assimilation of supplemental iron. Physical examination reveals only occasional tenderness in the midepigastric area. Serum electrolytes and liver function tests are usually normal. Women with gastro-intestinal ulcers need to avoid spicy foods and take plenty of vitamin E (at least 1000 IU daily) and eat lots of high quality, dark green olive oil. Also rule out:

*Simple heartburn (see Bowel and Digestive Upsets, this section)
*Chronic cholecystitis
*Acute pancreatitis
*Acute appendicitis
*Other bowel disease

Bowel abscess: The presence of a bowel abscess may confuse your ability to distinguish the problem when abdominal pain presents. If you suspect a bowel tumor or abscess, check for occult blood in the stool (keeping in mind that hemorrhoids can cause blood to appear in the stool; however, this blood is usually visible during wiping at the toilet). Test kits are readily available in drug stores. If occult blood is found, refer the woman to a specialist for further diagnosis.

Bowel obstruction: Especially in women who have previously had abdominal surgery, scar tissue adhesions may lead to intestinal obstruction presenting with crampy abdominal pain, distention, vomiting and eventually an inability to pass gas or defecate. Seek a medical evaluation without delay. (Gleicher, 1985 p. 821)

Liver rupture: Rupture may occur as the result of severe toxemia or trauma. It presents with sudden upper right quadrant or epigastric pain, nausea and vomiting and in some cases shock, hypotension and hemoperitoneum. Transport!

References and further reading:

Bates, B, A Guide to Physical Examination and History Taking, 5th ed., Lippincott, Phil, 1991.
DeVore, Gregory, "Non-obstetric abdominal pain in pregnancy: What's the cause?," Contemp. OB/GYN, Vol. 22, #1, July, 1983, pp. 65-86.
Gleicher, Norbert, ed. Principles of Medical Therapy in Pregnancy, Plenum Pub., NY, 1985.
op. cit., et.al., "The amylase/creatinine clearance ratio in normal pregnancy and pregnancies complicated by pancreatitis, hyperemesis gravidarum, and toxemia," Am. J. of Ob/Gyn, Vol. 136, 1980, p. 747.
Niewiarowski, Tomasz, Fisher, R., "Effects of upper GI dysmotility in pregnancy," Contemp. Ob Gyn, Vol. 38, No. 2, p. 67-81.

<u>Aches and Pains of the Bones, Muscles, Ligaments and Pelvis</u>

Most women experience various sensations in the area between the lower abdomen and the upper thighs throughout pregnancy. These are caused by pressure from the enlarging uterus, fetal movement, and circulatory changes.

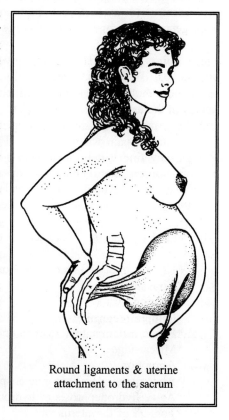

Round ligaments & uterine attachment to the sacrum

<u>Round ligament pain</u>: By far the most common soft tissue complaints during pregnancy are aches, pains, spasms or stitches in the round ligaments. As the uterus enlarges in early pregnancy and as toning contractions accelerate in late pregnancy, the round ligaments can occasionally become cramped, producing mild to severe discomfort such as sticking or pulling pains on either side of the symphysis pubis, along one or both sides of the uterus and up to the level of the navel. Sometimes these sensations are felt in the groin instead of or in addition to the sensations described above. As pregnancy advances, toning contractions may cause the round ligaments to become uncomfortable more often.

*For an acute spasm, have the mother bend toward the point of pain to allow the muscle to relax. She should breathe deeply during the spasm and, if possible, lie down on her side until it has passed.
*St. John's Wort tincture can be used to relieve all kinds of spasms (5 to 20 drops per dose, taken with symptoms).
*Massage the area with caster oil or apply a caster oil pack. (Soak flannel in castor oil and apply to the area, cover with plastic, then apply a heating pad. Leave in place for 30 minutes.)
*A hot water bottle can be applied to the painful area
*Have women avoid sudden movements involving outward movements of the legs, such as when rising from bed or exiting a car.

<u>Increased pelvic blood flow</u>: Vulval and venous engorgement within the yoni due to the expanded blood volume of pregnancy is heightened by less-than-prompt blood return due to pressure from the enlarged uterus. If a woman has varicose

veins in her vulva or yoni, this sensation of pressure may be more dramatic and may increase as pregnancy advances. One of the best remedies for this sensation is orgasm, and in fact, the engorgement of pregnancy (which mimics the engorgement of sexual excitement) is sexually stimulating to some women.

Pelvic joint pains: The joints between the pelvic bones are relaxed as term approaches. While this increases pelvic dimensions during labor, it makes all the joints more mobile, gives rise to difficulty with walking and may put pressure on nerves in the area, causing discomfort. Up to one centimeter of separation of the symphysis pubis is considered normal; however, at times it may be more, giving rise to extreme pain when walking. The best remedy for this is bed rest. Some women may find it helpful to wrap a tight binding around their hips to provide support. Joint relaxation may also cause the coccyx to become painful, a condition referred to as coccyalgia or coccydynia. This can also be handled with rest, and by sitting on a hemorrhoid pillow to relieve pressure symptoms.

Differential diagnosis: More serious causes of pelvic pain are as follows:

>   *Urinary tract or kidney infection
>   *Appendicitis
>   *Ovarian cyst
>   *Ectopic pregnancy
>   *Pelvic inflammatory disease or intrauterine infection
>   *Miscarriage
>   *Abruption
>   *Abdominal conditions (see chapter on Abdominal Pain, this section)
>   *Acute hydronephrosis or hydroureter (see below)
>   *Torsion of the uterus
>   *Incarceration or sacculation of the uterus

Rule these out before you assume pelvic pain is due to a benign condition. Simple joint pain may be relieved with St. John's wort tincture, up to 20 drops with symptoms, homeopathic remedies and regular chiropractic care.

Acute hydronephrosis or hydroureter: This is a very occasional problem of pregnancy and occurs due to the relaxation and kinking of the ureters which commonly takes place as pregnancy advances. Obstruction of a ureter may occur at varying levels at or above the pelvic brim with recurrent episodes of loin or lower abdominal pain radiating to the groin. Repeat midstream urine specimens are sterile. Diagnosis is by excretory urography or ultrasound and urethral catheterization. Positioning the woman on the unaffected side may relieve the pain. If it does not, ureteral catheterization or nephrectomy (removal of the kidney) may be required. Catheterization immediately relieves the pain.

Uterine tenderness: Sometimes women have tenderness in certain spots on their uterus. This may be due to a history of endometriosis prior to pregnancy, fibroids, or for unidentifiable reasons. If the pain only occurs during palpation and no other symptoms are present, simply take care when palpating and listening to fetal heart tones during examination. Tenderness or pulling sensations along old surgical delivery scars are common symptoms among YBAC mothers; unless these persist and increase they are not cause for alarm. A homeopathic remedy often works for unusual, otherwise undiagnosable, complaints. The sudden onset of tenderness may indicate an intrauterine infection and warrants further investigation.

Leg cramps: Adequate sodium, calcium, magnesium and potassium intake will help to prevent leg cramps. Very often, cramps are due to inadequate salt intake as well. It is felt by some natural health care providers that carbonated drinks (including water), can interfere with the body's calcium balance and should be avoided. Foods such as bananas, grapefruit, oranges, cottage cheese, yogurt, salmon, sardines, dark greens, seaweeds, soybeans, almonds, and sesame seeds will all help provide the nutrients needed to avoid leg cramps. Sometimes excess calcium can cause leg cramps. A "funny, achy or restlessness" in the lower legs at night may also point to anemia. If cramps do occur, recommend the following:

*While sleeping or sitting, elevate the legs higher than the heart
*Do not stand in one place for too long. Shift your weight from one
    leg to the other
*Do not point toes outward; point them upward to relieve cramps
*Walk a mile daily to help with leg circulation
*When experiencing a cramp, apply a hot water bottle or heating pad
    to the cramping area and apply manual pressure until it subsides

Keep in mind that what may feel like a cramp to some women may actually be clots in varicose veins deep in the legs. If varicose veins are present or suspected the woman should not massage the area to relieve pain until a clot is ruled out. (Read the chapter on Vascular Problems for more information.)

Soreness under the ribs or xiphoid process: This is usually caused by the baby's position; it frequently accompanies a breech presentation, with the hard head pushing up into the soft tissues under the rib cage. If the baby rotates to vertex or the baby "drops" in a first time mother during the last weeks of pregnancy this pressure is often relieved. Point out that this sometimes means the baby is lying breech so the mother will know to alert you to this during her visit. If so, you will want to discuss options for changing the baby's position to vertex (see separate chapter on Ensuring Vertex Presentation at Term in the section on the Third Trimester) Have the mother change positions often to minimize the discomfort. Also be sure to rule out liver or gall bladder tenderness (see Abdominal Pain, this section and Toxemia chapter in section on Third Trimester Problems) or gas, as well as baby kicking, which can lead to a sore diaphragm. Homeopathic Arnica in 30C doses 3 to 4 times daily can help with any sore, bruised feeling.

Backache: As the mother's weight and posture shift to accommodate a changing center of gravity (due to the enlarging uterus) backaches often occur. The enlarging uterus stresses the ligaments which attach the uterus to the sacrum. Spinal pain may be aggravated by the fetal position, so be sure to look for posterior positioning of the fetus if back pain is a problem. See the chapter on Dealing Posterior Babies in Pregnancy in the Third Trimester section for more information.

One of the best preventive measures to avoid backaches is to wear flat shoes and visit a chiropractor regularly. Not standing in one position for long periods of time, and avoiding forward bending and strong upward stretching may also help, although stretching that isn't too abrupt or extreme may be beneficial. Lifting should be done by squatting and pushing up with the knees, not by bending from the waist. Carrying a toddler on the hips can aggravate back pain as well. Encourage women to try sleeping with a pillow between their legs, and suggest they support their bellies if pendulous abdomen is a factor. Many women may find a back support in their car seat helpful, as cars were not designed with pregnant women in mind. Even if a woman does not have a pendulous abdomen, a belly support may help relieve back aches as pregnancy advances. Loving Lift and Action Lift and Baby Hugger provide elastic belly slings which crisscross in the back and support from below (see Appendix for ordering information).

A castor oil pack can be made by soaking a piece of flannel in castor oil and placing it on the painful area, covering it with plastic and then applying a heating pad for 30 minutes. Soaking a small towel in apple cider vinegar, squeezing out any excess and applying it to the painful area for 15 to 20 minutes may also help.

Be sure to distinguish simple back pain from causes such as kidney infection (check for CVA tenderness) or referred pain from the liver or urinary tract (which will not produce CVA tenderness on exam). Women from Pakistan, Northern India, Iran and Bedouin tribes or elsewhere where women are not exposed to much sunlight may have osteomalacia, the adult form of low-calcium rickets, which may lead to a variety of aches and pains in the bones. (See the chapter on Skeletal and Joint Disorders in Medical Conditions section for more information).

Yoni and uterine herniations: Mild to moderate degrees of herniation (cystocele, rectocele, etc.) may cause dragging pains in the lower back and abdomen during pregnancy. This may make walking very uncomfortable. Pelvic floor exercises may be done daily throughout pregnancy, but since everything is relaxed by the pregnancy hormones, no dramatic improvement should be expected.

Conception is rare when the uterus is totally prolapsed, and when it does occur, progress to term is unlikely. However, partial degrees of uterine prolapse are frequently associated with pregnancy. Early on, this may cause the cervix to protrude from the vaginal opening. As pregnancy advances it may actually improve the situation because the enlargement of the uterus often draws the prolapsed portion of the lower uterine segment and cervix back into the vagina.

Incarceration (entrapment of an extremely retroflexed uterus in the abdominal cavity) may occur as the uterus enlarges, and can lead to abortion. If this does not occur, progress to term can be expected. Assuming a knee-chest position for 20 minutes several times daily during the first 6 months of pregnancy will help to prevent this problem. If incarceration does not occur, the pregnancy usually proceeds without problems. Weak ligaments and muscles make a woman more likely to sustain additional damage during birth, and a prolapsed uterus may invert (turn inside out) more easily during placental delivery.

Osteoporosis: Osteoporosis results from demineralization of the bones and is rare in women in their childbearing years, rarer still in pregnant women. Severe back or hip pain, a decrease in height and increasing difficulty with weight bearing are characteristic symptoms which appear in late pregnancy or postpartum. Diagnosis is by radiologically proven fractures or bone mineral density assessments. Pregnancy may be a stress that unmasks a defective maternal skeleton (likely since a higher number of affected women have a history of bone fractures). Decreased absorption or utilization of calcium may play a part. Calcium supplementation does not seem to prevent this disorder. However, bone remineralization may occur in some cases if the mother drinks Oatstraw or Horsetail tea daily, 1 cup steeped only 5 minutes. If hypersensitivity to touch should develop, the intake should be reduced until this side-effect subsides. Women with fractures due to minor to moderate trauma, or back or hip pain which persists postpartum may want to be evaluated for bone density.

Hematoma of the rectus sheath: This very rare condition usually occurs in multiparas as a result of coughing or sudden expulsive effort. Muscle fibers and branches of the deep epigastric veins are torn leading to acute abdominal pain, signs of shock mimicking peritoneal infection and a vague abdominal swelling. If this occurs above the navel a localized hemorrhage generally results, if below the navel the hemorrhage is more generalized. A consult should be sought without delay. Small areas of localized bleeding are usually left to reabsorb, however surgery to evacuate the clot and ligate bleeding vessels is often necessary. Homeopathic Arnica, 30C or 200C can be given as soon as this condition is suspected to minimize trauma and further bleeding.

References and further reading:
Balch, J, & P. Balch, Prescription for Nutritional Healing, Avery Pub., Garden City, NY 1990.
Dunne, F., et.al., "Pregnancy-Associated Osteoporosis," Clin. Endocrinol, Vol. 39, 1993, p. 487.
Garrey, M. et.al., Obstetrics Illustrated, Churchill-Livingstone, London, Eng., 1980.
Miller, A & Callander, R, Obstetrics Illustrated, 4th ed., Churchill-Livingstone, NY, 1989.

Amniotic Fluid Volume Abnormalities

This chapter will address the implications of abnormal quantities of fluid. The chapter entitled Assessing Amniotic Fluid Volume in the Basic Skills section discusses how to determine the volume of fluid and distinguish a normal amount from too much or too little. If an abnormal quantity of fluid is suspected, assess the situation over the course of several prenatal visits; fetal growth spurts and lags as well as fluid volume are not always consistent from week to week in normal pregnancy. If the fluid volume is extremely abnormal, more prompt evaluation is appropriate.

Polyhydramnios (polly-hi-DRAM-nee-os) or hydramnios (too much fluid):
Normally the volume of amniotic fluid at term does not exceed 1000 ml. Hydramnios refers to the accumulation of excessive amounts of amniotic fluid; it is generally considered to be 2000 ml. or more, with amounts as high as 15 liters on record. The composition of the fluid is the same as in normal pregnancies. The most commonly associated conditions are maternal diabetes (5 to 25%), Rh incompatibility (11%), multiple pregnancy (8%), and congenital malformations (18 to 39% depending upon the study). Associated fetal anomalies include gastrointestinal, cardiac, urinary tract and central nervous system defects. However, the cause is never found in 60% of cases. The more severe the hydramnios, the more likely it is associated with a fetal abnormality. The cause for hydramnios is not completely known; abnormalities in fetal voiding or swallowing seem to be related, however, hydramnios may exist in the absence of these factors. Hydramnios predisposes a woman to other-than-vertex presentation, preterm labor, dysfunctional labor, postpartum hemorrhage and cord prolapse upon rupture of the membranes.

Minor degrees of hydramnios (2 to 3 liters) occur once in every 150 to 280 pregnancies and are not usually a problem. Amounts over 3000 ml. (3 to 4 liters) occur rarely (1 in every 3000 pregnancies) and lead to maternal symptoms such as abdominal discomfort, difficulty breathing, gastrointestinal reflux, restriction of movement, and pressure which causes the abdominal wall and extremities to swell. Severe cases may cause nausea and vomiting. Overdistention of the uterine wall may lead to generalized pain in the uterine muscle itself. Bed rest, salt restriction and diuretics do not help and should not be recommended; however, in severe cases women will be extremely uncomfortable and should be advised to quit working and allow ample time for resting. An abdominal binder will help support the overdistended belly. A homeopathic remedy specifically prescribed for the woman may help to balance the system. Acupuncture may also provide some relief.

Chronic hydramnios is usually first suspected after the 28th week of pregnancy, when large-for-dates growth, a tense uterine wall, and difficulty hearing fetal heart sounds and palpating small parts become obvious. At this point the parents should be informed that the amount of fluid seems excessive and that this can sometimes be associated with multiple gestation or problems with the baby. A stage-I ultrasound scan can confirm the diagnosis, however, if you feel certain that too much fluid exists you may want to talk to the parents about foregoing a stage-I scan and immediately having a stage-II scan performed, which will give more information about the condition of the baby while minimizing ultrasound exposure. Magnetic resonance scanning can also be helpful in providing details about the baby's condition. Because of the frequent association with diabetes, glucose testing should be discussed if no other cause is found. A Coomb's test will also rule out blood incompatibilities as the source of the problem.

If symptoms become extreme, fluid can be drained via amniocentesis. Fluid is removed at the rate of about 500 ml. an hour to minimize the chances of changes in uterine size causing placental separation or initiation of contractions. The fluid may collect again rapidly, and the procedure must then be repeated. The prostaglandin inhibiting drug Indomethacin is also being used instead to reduce fluid volume by decreasing fetal urine production. This drug poses a number of serious risks for both mother and fetus. Fetal effects include a variety of heart problems. It is contraindicated in babies who have severe intrauterine growth retardation or certain heart defects such as critical aortic stenosis. Constriction of the ductus arteriosus may occur in the normal fetus and can lead to an overprofusion of the fetal lungs resulting in further problems after birth which vary depending upon the gestational age of the newborn. Babies with esophageal atresia, neuromuscular dysfunction, hydrocephalus or other conditions which may be associated with poor swallowing activity may show only a limited response. This drug suppresses maternal fever and can therefore mask infection, amniocentesis is recommended prior to administration to rule out infection if fluid removal has already been performed. It also depresses maternal platelet function and urine production, may cause headache, vertigo and jaundice and should not be used if the woman is hypertensive or carrying a multiple gestation. Use of this drug requires weekly fetal echocardiograms to look for severe ductal constriction in the fetus and amniotic fluid volume assays are needed every 3 to 4 days to be sure *oligohydramnios* is not developing! Fortunately, fluid regulation is rarely needed.

Acute hydramnios occurs in 2% of cases, with the rapid accumulation of huge amounts of fluid over the course of a few days to two weeks. This is usually associated with monoamniotic twin pregnancy. (See the chapter on Multiple Gestation for more information.)

Oligohydramnios (o-lih-go-hi-DRAM-nee-os) (too little fluid): It is very rare for true oligohydramnios, defined as less than 400 ml. of fluid, to develop. Varying degrees of fluid reduction can occur, with volume occasionally reduced to only a few milliliters of thick fluid. Fetal renal agenesis and other obstructions of the urinary tract lead to severe oligohydramnios, since the fetus is unable to urinate. When oligohydramnios occurs early in pregnancy, it presents a serious situation for the fetus. Adhesions between the amnion and parts of the baby may form, leading

960

to severe deformities, including amputation of fetal parts. Without fluid to breathe, underdevelopment of the lungs often results, leading to irresolvable respiratory distress at birth. Since the baby is being subjected to an abnormal degree of pressure from all sides, it may look peculiar at birth, minor deformities such as club foot may develop and the skin may be thick and leathery. Other causes include prune belly and Turner's syndromes, trisomy 18 and 22, and fetal death. Intrauterine growth retardation is often found in conjunction with fetal abnormalities. An ultrasound will help determine whether anomalies or IUGR are factors. Severe oligohydramnios (amniotic fluid volume <1 cm on ultrasound) is associated with a 40-fold rise in perinatal mortality, a 14-fold increase in major anomalies and nearly an 8-fold increase in IUGR. (Skovgaard, 1993)

Acute oligohydramnios may develop in the second or third trimester if the mother is undernourished or dehydrated. In this case, fluid volume is reduced but not completely eliminated. Minor degrees of oligohydramnios may lead to cord compression during labor. However, oligohydramnios detected with ultrasound in unselected populations is a poor predictor of perinatal outcome. If dehydration is the cause, hydration should normalize the fluid volume in a day or so; nutritional status should also be reviewed. Fluid will also diminish in the third trimester if the fetus is experiencing acute or chronic hypoxia for any reason, such as complicated maternal hypertension, toxemia or drug use, often with accompanying asymmetrical IUGR. A process called "brain sparing" directs oxygen to the brain while decreasing blood flow to other organs including the kidneys, thus reducing urinary output, the primary component of amniotic fluid in late pregnancy. (Gregor, 1991) Increased hydration probably won't increase fluid volume in complicated cases, reflecting compromised fetal status. Careful monitoring, nutritional improvement, fetal movement counts, and labor induction upon fetal maturity are warranted.

Also, a study of 53 women has found a correlation between oligohydramnios (AFV <5 cm) and an increased likelihood of finding pathologic microbes in the amniotic fluid in cases of term prelabor rupture of membranes. The correlation of AFV of <5 and infection had a sensitivity of 71%, a specificity of 89%, a positive predictive value of 75% and a negative predictive value of 87%. Although a small study, it is a factor to consider when dealing with PROM at term. (Romero, 1994)

Danforth, D. ed. Danforth's Obstetrics and Gynecology, 5th ed., J.B. Lippincott, Phil., PA, 1986.

Gregor, C., et al., "Antepartum Fetal Assessment: A Nurse-Midwifery Perspective," J Nurse-Midwifery, Vol. 36, No. 3, May-June, 1991, pp. 153-167.

Kilpatrick, S., et al., "Maternal hydration increases amniotic fluid volume in women with normal amniotic fluid," Ob Gyn, Vol. 81, No. 1, Jan 1993, pp. 49-52.

Moise, K "Indomethacin as treatment for symptomatic polyhydramnios," Contp ObGyn, 5/95, 53.

Moore, Keith, Persaud, T., The Developing Human, 5th ed., W. B. Saunders Co., Phil., 1993.

Oxhorn, Harry, Human Labor and Birth, 5th ed. Appleton-Century-Crofts, E. Norwalk, CT, 1986.

Romero, R., et al., "Is oligohydramnios a risk factor for infection in term premature rupture of membranes?," Ultrasound Ob/Gyn, Vol. 4, 1994, pp. 95-100.

Skovgaard, R, Silvonek, A, "Oligohydramnios," J Nurse-Midwifery, Vol. 38, No. 4, 1993, p. 208

Bowel and Digestive Upsets

Constipation: The normal peristaltic action of the gastrointestinal tract is slowed during pregnancy due to the influence of muscle relaxing hormones. This serves to enhance the absorption of nutrients, but also encourages the production of additional metabolic wastes (providing more work for the liver) and increases water absorption from the stool, potentially leading to constipation.

Contrary to popular belief, however, it is not normal for women to be constipated during pregnancy. If women are drinking the proper amount of fluids and eating a whole foods diet, the factors listed above are not sufficient to produce constipation. In part, the belief that women are chronically constipated has been fostered by the tendency among North American practitioners to prescribe poorly assimilated iron supplements such as ferrous sulfate. It is true that constipation can be brought on more easily in women who have a tendency toward sluggish bowels when they are not pregnant or if women eat constipating foods such as refined carbohydrates during pregnancy.

If a woman says she is constipated, first find out exactly what she means by this term. True constipation is the difficult passage of hard, dry stools at less frequent intervals than is normal for that individual. Many people used to a low fiber "typical American diet" are chronically constipated to a certain extent. In addition, past events that were emotionally traumatic such as forced enemas or sexual abuse can lead to chronic constipation in adults (the bowels represent one thing the child can control).

General recommendations to avoid or remedy constipation are:

*Stop taking all vitamin supplements (particular vitamin and iron supplements may not be utilized well by individual women. In order to monitor the progress of other corrective measures, remove this possible source of the problem first.)
*Stop taking antacid preparations (if heartburn is a problem, see recommendations in Bowel and Digestive Upsets in this section)
*Drink plenty of clear fluids (not more than 8 glasses a day unless she wants more)
*Eat unrefined carbohydrate foods
*Drink prune juice or black cherry juice regularly
*Avoid foods known to be constipating to the individual
*Eat plenty of vegetables to provide more fiber in the diet
*Get moderate exercise every day
*Tune into when the bowels move and set aside a regular time to have a movement; the feet and legs should be elevated on a small stool in order to help the rectal muscles relax. Whenever the urge to defecate occurs, respond as soon as possible, don't put it off.
*Drink a hot liquid immediately followed by a cold liquid; this is an

old trick for stimulating the peristaltic action of the colon to bring on a bowel movement.

Usually these suggestions will quickly turn the situation around. If you recommend more fiber (as in bran added to breads and cereals or eating dried fruit), remember that dry foods must draw fluid from the system in order to be digested; too much of a good thing can hinder rather than help the problem. It is best to derive bran from the whole grains in breads and pastas and to use whole grain rice. Dried fruit can be soaked in water before eating.

If the woman is in acute discomfort from constipation, the quickest, most benign remedy is the use of one or two glycerin suppositories inserted into the rectum. The glycerin will help lubricate the lower rectum and dried fecal matter, as well as mildly stimulate the bowels to move without producing so much intestinal activity that the uterus will be stimulated unduly. This will make the movement easier to pass and should provide relief within a few hours. However, no form of laxative should be used regularly to assist in moving the bowels, as this will encourage dehydration. Additionally, oil-based laxatives can interfere with the absorption of vitamins A, D, and K. Products mixed with water which are designed to increase dietary bulk can be used as a last resort if women find that they cannot stay regular with the recommendations listed above.

Another by-product of constipation is the production of excessive metabolic toxins which are normally produced during the process of digestion. These toxins are broken down by the liver. Therefore, constipation stresses the liver by giving it even more work to do. Yellow dock root is a mild liver stimulant and an alterative (system balancing) herb which has mild laxative effects and provides a source of iron. This can be recommended to those women who have a chronic problem with constipation.

Once the constipation is under control, reintroduce vitamins and mineral supplements one at a time. If they seem to be aggravating the problem, switch to a different brand. Extra magnesium may actually help relieve constipation for many women. A poorly assimilated iron source may be the problem, even in a multi-vitamin. Vitamin C and chelation can aid iron absorption. Be sure not to over-supplement iron. If the stools are black, iron is not being assimilated properly and is being discharged via the bowels (assuming no abdominal symptoms suggest internal bleeding, which can also leave the stools black).

If constipation does not clear up with simple measures such as these, consider an underlying problem such as fibroids in the lower uterine segment putting pressure on the lower bowel (see separate chapter on Fibroids, this section.)

Diarrhea: Diarrhea occurs less frequently than constipation during pregnancy. If it does occur, however, it can become serious. It usually accompanies an illness, such as the flu or mild food poisoning. When diarrhea occurs, first suggest the recommendations given below:

*Stop taking all vitamin supplements (for the same reasons outlined above)

*Stop taking antacid preparations (if heartburn is a problem, see Bowel and Digestive Upsets, this section)

*If food poisoning is suspected, take 2 Tbsp. of apple cider vinegar in water with a tablespoon of honey; this helps change the pH of the stomach and discourages the growth of harmful bacteria, however, this may not be sufficient to arrest the process if the poisoning is already symptomatic.

*Drink plenty of water or electrolyte balancing fluids such as Third Wind if diarrhea is severe

*Eat unrefined carbohydrate foods

*Avoid foods known to be undigestible to the individual or those to which she is allergic

*Eat plenty of cooked vegetables to provide more fiber in the diet, avoid raw vegetables and fruits until the diarrhea has resolved

*Get moderate exercise every day

Diarrhea can quickly lead to dehydration, electrolyte imbalance and malnutrition. One of the best and most benign remedies is to eat basmati rice and live culture yogurt. The yogurt will help to repopulate the colon with beneficial bacteria and the rice will provide bulk. An exception to the no fruit rule is green bananas, which will also assist in correcting mild to moderate diarrhea as will mashed bananas mixed with roasted carob powder. Whole Slippery Elm bark can be brewed in water or chewed to release its soothing qualities. Powdered slippery elm bark dissolved in water with honey added can be fed to women who are very weak, as it is very nourishing and soothing to mucus membranes. Homeopathic remedies can work well if the proper remedy is selected. An over-the counter Bio-technical diarrhea medication can be taken, if necessary, to curb the acute symptoms; select a brand that does not contain aluminum.

For women with severe diarrhea who also have small children in day care or who have recently been drinking from possibly contaminated waters (foreign travel? camping trip?) the possibility of an amebic form of diarrhea should be ruled out (see Giardia, Amebiasis and Shigella chapters in Diagnostic Tests). Also inquire about recent dietary intake to determine if food poisoning is likely.

Flatulence (gas): Women who dramatically change their diet from refined junk and processed foods to more whole grains and fresh vegetables may find that they have more gas as a result. This is often because the body is not used to digesting these more complex foods. Primary offenders are bran, cabbage family vegetables (such as cabbage, broccoli, cauliflower, kale, and collards), excessive sugar intake and milk products. Women should keep track of what they are eating to determine what causes the most gas. Eating four or five small meals rather than three large ones may also help. Chewing the food thoroughly before swallowing mixes it with saliva and helps to break it down better before it enters the system. Suggest cooking foods quickly in a perforated steamer instead of boiling food for long periods. Walking daily will aid digestion, and setting up a regular time for a bowel movement may help as well.

Beans are one of the most problematic foods when it comes to gas. Bean-O is a product which provides enzymes to help with digestion; it must be taken before any beans are consumed. To reduce the gas-producing sulfur compounds in beans, bring one cup of beans to a boil in five cups of water for one minute. Drain and add five cups of fresh water. Bring to a boil again and cook according to directions. Adding raw garlic to the cooking water will also help reduce gas.

Food allergies can also cause the production of gas. Eliminating suspect foods from the diet for a week or two should help track down the offenders. If this simple step does not produce results, a naturopath can help with allergy diagnosis. Snoring, which may be enhanced by nasal congestion, nausea and swallowing air may lead to more belching and gas as well.

Heartburn (esophagitis): When the more delicate esophageal lining makes contact with acid or alkaline gastric contents, a burning sensation is produced. Heartburn is increased during pregnancy, because the hormones which relax the soft tissues in preparation for birth cause the muscle that normally closes off the esophagus from the stomach to relax as well. This, in conjunction with the upward pressure from the enlarging uterus, can cause gastric contents to slosh up into the lower esophageal canal, where a burning sensation is produced. Spicy foods aggravate heartburn even more. Women may suffer from heartburn at various points in their pregnancy and to varying degrees. Palliative measures can help relieve or at least minimize heartburn. These include:

*Avoiding spicy foods as well as those a woman knows to be hard to
digest or which produce gas and indigestion outside of pregnancy
*Walking (not lying down) after meals to get digestion going
*Not eating large meals late at night (or, eating only bland foods)
*Drinking milk before, during and after meals
*Taking any of the following supplements may help enhance digestion
and/or neutralize heartburn:
*NF formula's liquid calcium/magnesium supplement, 1 tsp. to 1 Tbsp.
as needed
*Tablets of comfrey with pepsin
*Papaya enzymes (also eating raw papaya or drinking papaya
juice may help)
*Digestive enzyme tablets
*Slippery elm bark powder in capsules, as needed
*Plain baked potatoes

*Thoroughly chewed raw almonds, cashews or filberts
*A tablespoon of cream or milk may help by coating the stomach.
*Avoiding eating and drinking at the same time.

Commercial antacids such as Tums or Mylanta should be taken *only as a last resort* and be used in strict moderation. Alka-Seltzer, which contains aspirin, should never be used. The use of baking soda can lead to the formation of stones in the urinary tract and should be avoided as well.

Antacids neutralize stomach acids, thus arresting digestion. Neutralized acids later rebound, producing even more stomach acid. Interference with digestion can lead to constipation and diarrhea. Excessive use of antacids which contain magnesium can lead to lethargy, circulatory collapse, respiratory paralysis and coma if taken to excess. Poorly assimilated calcium from these products deposits in the placenta and leads to placental calcifications later in pregnancy. Antacids are not a good source of calcium!

Chest Pain

It is common for pregnant women to experience various kinds of upper torso pain during pregnancy. Pressure from the enlarging uterus frequently causes shortness of breath, particularly on exertion. The diaphragm may become sore as the baby presses its little head or bottom up under the mother's ribs. In fact, a distinct soreness up under the ribs is a tip off that the baby may be lying breech. With these normal nuisances in mind, the next most common reason is a lung infection. Below are other more severe conditions which also cause chest pain:

Heart attack: Mid-sternum chest pain with sensations such as pressing, squeezing, tightness, heaviness or occasionally burning is the primary symptom. Other symptoms include sweating, nausea, shortness of breath, pain radiating down the left or sometimes both arms, and fever. Stabbing, momentary twinges of pain are usually not signals of heart attack. Some women experience benign heart palpitations (temporary rapid heart rate), which should be further evaluated if it persists or increases or if associated with other accompanying symptoms.

Viral pericardium: Upper respiratory symptoms and low-grade fever may precede sharp or dull chest pain behind or to the left of the sternum which is aggravated by lying down, coughing, breathing deeply and swallowing and relieved by sitting up and leaning forward. This turn of events may indicate a viral infection of the bag which encases the heart. This rare complication requires immediate follow-up.

Pregnancy cardiomyopathy: Women with cardiomyopathy have heart failure, usually right sided, either at the end of pregnancy or most commonly postpartum. They are usually multiparous, black, older and poor, with a history of hypertension.
Cardiomyopathy in pregnancy may take an obstructive form. The heart enlarges and the muscle action becomes disorganized. Women present with chest pain, fatigue, fainting, edema, arrhythmias and symptoms of heart failure. Jugular venous pressure is elevated and the heart is enlarged. A third heart sound gallop is usually present, frequently accompanied by regurgitation murmurs. Hypovolemia must be strictly avoided. Epidural anesthesia is contraindicated. Pulmonary, peripheral and cerebral embolisms are possible complications. Possible causes are thought to be immunological or infective conditions.

Pulmonary embolism: Embolism occurs when a foreign substance, typically a blood clot, finds its way into the circulatory system of the lungs. The primary presenting symptoms are chest pain, difficult, rapid breathing and lack of oxygen. Be alert to this possibility in women who have large varicose veins.

Pneumothorax: This is a puncture of the lung tissue which allows air to become trapped between the outer lung surface and the chest cavity. It may occur in susceptible women during pushing. These women complain of the sudden onset of chest pain and breathlessness. The diagnosis is confirmed by chest x-ray. Cyanosis and hypotension may also accompany pneumothorax. The area should be aspirated if the lung is more than 25% collapsed.

What to do: If you suspect a any of these serious problems, get a consultation from a bio-technical care provider without delay. If the woman is in acute distress, administer 5 to 6 liters of oxygen by mask and be prepared to offer CPR if necessary.

References and further reading:

Gleicher, N., ed. Principles of Medical Therapy in Pregnancy, Plenum Pub., New York, 1985.

Colds, Flus and Pneumonia

When common colds occur in pregnancy, the best treatment is bed rest, fluids, extra vitamin C and the use of properly prescribed homeopathic remedies. Difficult breathing may be due to simple congestion secondary to a cold, pneumonia or bronchitis. Keep in mind that poisoning and heart problems may also be less common but serious reasons why a woman would develop difficult breathing. (See the chapters on Chest Pain and Fever for more information.)

Pneumonia: Pregnant women are somewhat more susceptible to developing pneumonia than the general population. Pneumonia is defined as an inflammation in which the lungs fill with fluid. It produces dullness over the obstructed lung area on percussion and crackling sounds during auscultation. Pneumonia in the pregnant woman should be taken very seriously, since it can lead to death if not treated. Bed rest and full scale care is recommended so that the condition does not worsen. Be sure to differentiate pneumonia from kidney infection (see chapter on Urinary Tract Infections, this section).

Bronchitis: Bronchitis is an inflammation of the bronchial tubes, leaving the lungs clear. It produces normal breath sounds and resonance on chest percussion. The woman presents with fever, cough, purulent sputum or chest pain. The majority of infections are bacterial in origin and should be treated promptly with antibiotics. Flu viruses are also a common cause which will not respond to antibiotics. In these cases bed rest and cold care as described above are recommended. (See Diagnostic Tests for details regarding specific cold and pneumonia producing conditions.)

Dental and Gum Problems

It used to be said that a woman would lose a tooth for every baby. This adage grew from the belief that the fetus draws calcium from the mother's bones and teeth. In fact, the increase in dental caries that may be seen during pregnancy has been traced to elevated levels of acidophilic organisms in the mouth due to the hormones of pregnancy. However, dental problems are usually a tip-off that oral hygiene and dietary intake are inadequate. The teeth are often the first part of the body to show the effects of general ill health. In order to maintain good dental health at any time during life, remind women to:

*Find out what kind of dental history "runs in the family." If a woman's siblings and parents have lost teeth or had gum disease this means her teeth and gums may be constitutionally weak, placing her at higher risk for problems if she does not take care of her teeth.
*Understand the link between diet and dental health (sugar promotes cavities, as do sticky foods and sodas)
*Brush 2 to 3 times daily with a medium to soft bristled toothbrush, being sure to work the bristles down into the gum margin and between the teeth, as well as the tops and sides. The type of toothbrush really does make a difference; encourage women to spend money on a good brush designed to get at plaque.
*Use a non-fluoride toothpaste that has gum-strengthening additives such as Blood Root, Myrrh Gum or Propolis.
*Floss at least once daily, preferably before bed (pooled saliva works with bacteria in food particles to inflame gum tissues); also encourage women to carry toothpicks or floss with her during the day in case of sticky food problems that need attention.
*Brush the tongue during regular brushing; this also helps reduce bacteria and plaque in the mouth.

Bleeding gums: While mainstream practitioners generally consider bleeding gums a normal variation of pregnancy, it most certainly is not! Although the hormones of pregnancy may make the gums slightly softer than those of nonpregnant women, this does not mean that a woman in optimal health should expect bleeding gums. Low vitamin C levels contribute to bleeding gums. A vitamin C supplement with bioflavinoids can help alleviate this problem.

Bleeding gums usually reflect a need for increased vigilance with dental hygiene as well. Suggest that the woman make a paste with hydrogen peroxide and baking soda and brush her teeth with this twice daily. She can also use this paste or moistened Myrrh Gum powder to massage into the gums twice daily. Lastly, she can dip her dental floss into Myrrh tincture or hydrogen peroxide before using it. These things in combination should clear up minor gum problems quickly.

Hypertrophy of the gums: Some women develop a puffy, soft gum line which tends to enlarge in spots during pregnancy. This is a benign response to the extra blood volume and hormonal changes from pregnancy and should be cared for as above.

Epulis of pregnancy: A painless, very vascular, friable red tumor sometimes appears along the anterior maxillary region. It is usually in response to calculus deposits, poor oral hygiene, denture irritation or other trauma, although it has been known to develop without preexisting gingival disease. Epulis commonly appears at the end of the first trimester and disappears spontaneously shortly after birth. While usually appearing only on one side, bilateral tumors have been reported. The tumor is composed of a collection of acute and chronic inflammatory cells and multiple vascular channels in a lose edematous network. There may be areas of local bleeding or ulceration; they are most often painless and rarely grow large enough to necessitate surgical removal. (Gleicher, 1985, Hellman & Pritchard, 1971)

Tooth decay: Occasionally a woman will have a tooth problem flare up during pregnancy and will want to know the relative risks of X-rays and dental anesthesia. First, be sure to rule out a sinus infection, which can cause smelly mucus and pain which may mimic a dental abscess. An x-ray may even be fooled! Therefore, always check the suspect tooth for signs of a problem (although tooth problems are not always visible on inspection) and determine if a sinus infection is a factor before sending her off to the dentist (Hartley, 1994). If tooth decay is suspected, the dentist will probably want to do an X-ray. Of course, X-rays are always risky. Women should avoid X-rays whenever possible (especially during the first three months) and insist on being shielded if they cannot be avoided. (See chapter on X-rays in <u>Diagnostic Tests</u> for more information.) If X-rays are necessary, after exposure the woman should take a bath in hot water with ½ pound of sea salt and ¼ pound of baking soda added. It is also helpful to eat extra miso, sodium alginate rich seaweeds, kelp, buckwheat grass, and take niacin supplements for several weeks. Sodium alginate attracts radioactive materials and carries them out of the body. Homeopathic X-ray in a potency of 30C or 200C can also help minimize the harmful effects.

If anesthesia becomes necessary, a local injection should be used rather than a general anesthetic.

Replacing fillings: If a deteriorated filling must be replaced during pregnancy, the woman may choose to have a dental composite filling, which does not contain mercury, a toxic metal. However, systematic replacement of mercury fillings with alternative materials should be postponed until after the pregnancy, because this procedure can cause systemic upsets in mercury-sensitive individuals.

Professional cleaning: Routine dental prophylaxis without X-rays or fluoride treatments can be performed with no problem during pregnancy. If a woman needs extensive ultrasonic deep gum cleaning, it would be ideal to have this done prior to pregnancy and for her to get her gums in a healthier state before she conceives. However, if this is done during pregnancy, remind the woman of the unknown effects of ultrasound. It may also be possible for an extensive cleaning to be done with conventional instruments over the course of several appointments; have her discuss this possibility with the dentist and hygienist. Be sure to suggest that she get a second opinion regarding the need for ultrasonic cleaning.

References and further reading:

Cassidy-Brinn, Ginny, Woman-Centered Pregnancy and Birth, Cleis Press, San Francisco, CA 1984.

Gleicher, Norbert, ed. Principles of Medical Therapy in Pregnancy, Plenum Pub., New York, 1985.

Hansen, Lori, et.al., "Otolaryngologic Manifestations of Pregnancy," J of Family Practice, Vol. 23, No. 2, 1986, pp. 151-55.

Hartley, Carla, midwife & educator, founder of Ancient Arts Midwifery Institute, P.O. Box 788, Claremore, OK, 74018, editing comments, December, 1994.

Russell-Manning, Betsy, ed., Home Remedies for Candida, Greensward Press, San Francisco, CA, 1988.

Hellman, L, & J. Pritchard, Williams Obstetrics, 14th ed., Appleton-Century-Crofts, New York, 1971.

Dizziness

Dizziness (vertigo) refers to a sensation of motion, lightheadedness, unsteadiness and faintness. It can be caused by a variety of relatively benign problems. It usually results from a lack of oxygen to the brain and may precede fainting (syncope). In pregnancy and in women taking oral contraceptives, or in those who are premenstrual or menstruating, dizziness sometimes apparently occurs due to hormonal fluctuations, although a correlation has not been clinically proven. It is postulated that such dizzy spells may be due to slight changes in blood flow to the ear secondary to tiny clots. Dizziness may also be related to inner ear or genetic hearing problems and when the two occur together infection, Meniere's disease, fluid in the ear or more rarely otosclerosis need to be ruled out (see chapter on Hearing Impairment and Loss, this section).

Hypoglycemia: One of the main reasons pregnant women become dizzy is hypoglycemia. For some women, just postponing a meal in pregnancy can cause them to experience severe symptoms of low blood sugar, including spilling ketones in the urine. The remedy, of course, is to eat immediately! Protein and unrefined carbohydrates will gradually stabilize the blood sugar. Fruit or fruit juice can be used to bring the blood sugar level up more quickly if a woman is at the point of passing out. Follow this with protein or unrefined carbohydrates, since concentrated sweets by themselves can create a yo-yo effect, with the blood sugar dropping again quickly.
Dizziness may accompany morning sickness. Have the woman lie back down with a very cold cloth across her eyes and breathe evenly and deeply until the dizziness passes. Darkening the room may also help. (El Halta, 1989)

Anemia: Since the hemoglobin is what carries oxygen to the brain, dizziness can be brought on by anemia. The anemic woman would easily become dizzy on exertion or upon rising, when blood is channeled from the brain to other parts of the body. The remedy is to correct the anemia.

Blood pressure fluctuations: Low blood pressure can be brought on by hypoglycemia or may be normal for an individual woman. Hypotensive women usually become dizzy on rising or during quick temperature changes such as exiting the shower or hot tub and should change positions slowly.

Blood loss or concealed hemorrhage: Dizziness is an early sign of shock and may tip you off that a woman is bleeding internally or that any visible blood loss is having an adverse effect. If you suspect blood loss, have the woman lie down quietly with her feet higher than her head, keep her warm and check vital signs (pulse, blood pressure, respirations, degree of awareness). Have an assistant keep her conscious by maintaining eye contact and talking with her while you look for and rule out possible causes of bleeding (see chapters on Miscarriage, Ectopic Pregnancy in the First Trimester section, and Bleeding in the Third Trimester in the Third Trimester section). If bleeding is suspected or discovered, transport immediately.

Toxemia: Dizziness can be a secondary symptom of nervous system compromise and may become apparent as toxemia advances. See the separate chapter on Toxemia in Third Trimester section for complete information.

Meniere's disease: Meniere's disease can be aggravated by pregnancy. The diagnosis is based on four criteria:

* *Abrupt onset of whirling vertigo, associated with nausea and vomiting, lasting hours, with complete freedom from vertigo between attacks.
* *A frequently fluctuating, low-frequency hearing loss, often one-sided, accompanying the vertigo
* *Ringing in the ears accompanying the vertigo that is low pitched and persistent between attacks
* *A sensation of fullness in the ear

The cause is not certain, but seems to be related to fluid retention with the predominant feature being dilation of all endolymph-containing structures. The natural course of the disease is fluctuating and unpredictable. While surgery and drugs (particularly diuretics and low-salt diets) are often used in treatment, these should be avoided during pregnancy. Homeopathic remedies and acupuncture are good possibilities for treatment.

References and further reading:

Gleicher, Norbert, ed. Principles of Medical Therapy in Pregnancy, Plenum Pub., New York, 1985.

El Halta, Valerie, Moving Midwifery Forward, Garden of Life, Pub., Aug. 1989.

Hansen, Lori, et.al., "Otolaryngologic Manifestations of Pregnancy," J of Family Practice, Vol. 23, No. 2, 1986, pp. 151-55.

Ear Problems and Hearing Impairment

Hearing impairment may appear for the first time during pregnancy. There are several reasons why this might occur:

Ear stuffiness: A sensation of fullness, deafness or fluid in the ear may be occasionally described by pregnant women. Hormonal changes may be involved, but this relationship is supported only by the clinical association of the two events. In some cases, fluid may be seen behind the tympanic membrane on otoscopic exam. Hearing tests usually find mild hearing loss if fluid is present. A complete examination by a head and neck specialist should be done to rule out tumors as a causative factor, particularly in cases where only one ear is affected or when fluid is present. A head cold or other congestion may be related, and should be cleared up with herbs or drugs. In the uncomplicated case these symptoms resolve after the birth. In the meantime, holding the breath and pushing may equalize the pressure in the Eustachian tubes, providing temporary relief. Acupuncture may alleviate simple hearing loss due to fluid imbalances.

Patulous eustachian tube: Normally the eustachian tube is closed at rest and opens in response to yawning, talking and swallowing. The abnormally open tube either remains open constantly (patulous) or has a reduced resistance to airflow (semipatulous). Outside of pregnancy, this condition is usually secondary to recent and rapid weight loss, abnormal tubal structure or altered nerve supply to the controlling muscle. It is a poorly understood problem that is more common in pregnancy with onset of symptoms appearing most often during the last trimester. Symptoms only occur on the affected side and include hearing a hollow-sounding resonance while speaking and breathing (called autophony); a blocked sensation or popping sounds and amplification of environmental sounds. Hearing tests are usually normal, although the tympanic membrane may appear thin and bulge with expiration and retract with inspiration, leading to a sense of motion within the ear. Tinnitus, a sensation of noises within the ear, varies and may be increased by forced expiration. Symptoms are often aggravated by systemic or topical decongestants because they shrink the mucous membranes and thus enlarge the eustachian tube even more. Symptoms may worsen when the woman is sitting or standing and improve when she lies down. Alternations in humidity, barometric pressure and altitude may result in changes in the symptom picture. Improvement is often noted during upper respiratory tract infection with mucus congestion, whereas exertion, fatigue, and anxiety seem to aggravate symptoms. Fortunately, the condition usually resolves after birth. Increasing the environmental humidity in the home or work-place may help (discuss using a non-ultrasound humidifier). Inhaling sharply through the nose with the mouth closed and nostrils pinched several times daily may also provide relief in some cases (this is called the Müller maneuver). A homeopathic remedy or acupuncture may also be of great benefit.

Sudden sensorineural hearing loss: This is an uncommon problem of pregnancy which has often been associated with toxemia or hypertensive disorders. It may be due to obstruction of the circulation in the cochlea and 8th cranial nerve from tiny clots or emboli, which is supported by the fact that this problem is frequently seen in conjunction with an increase in platelet numbers and adhesiveness. In uncomplicated pregnancies, such hearing loss may be due to the elevated estrogen levels which result in increased coagulability. A hearing evaluation will help to rule out other possible causes such as viral infection, tumor, a fistula between membranes in the ear, and Meniere's disease (see Dizziness, this section).

Otosclerosis: Hearing loss may be due to otosclerosis, a genetic disorder with an autosomal dominant inheritance pattern. Its effects on family members are similar, but there is a difference in the extent to which the gene causes hearing loss from family to family. About half of those who carry this gene will manifest loss of at least some of their hearing ability. Stapedial otosclerosis occurs in about four of every 1,000 Caucasian adults, but is rarely found in Oriental or Black peoples. Cochlear otosclerosis is more serious and is also more rare, occurring in about 4 out of every 10,000 people. Otosclerosis makes itself known in those between ages 15 to 45 with the peak decade of incidence in 30 to 40 year olds.

In otosclerosis the bone within the temporal portion of the skull surrounding the internal ear is metabolically disturbed. Normal bone is destroyed and replaced with disorganized bone which is thicker and more vascular than normal bone. The tympanic membrane looks normal to slightly pink. Otosclerosis results in progressive hearing loss which can appear or worsen during pregnancy. One study has shown that subsequent pregnancies may increase the impairment, but others have not found this correlation. Hearing is not necessarily affected in all pregnancies or to the same degree in each pregnancy when loss does occur. Occasionally a woman's hearing normalizes after she gives birth, but for most the effects are not reversible. It is not known why pregnancy triggers this condition, although patterns of otosclerosis changes show episodes of impairment during lactation and menopause, so high estrogen levels may play a part. Oral contraceptives, some of which have high estrogen levels, do not seem to have any effect.

A primary clue to recognizing the possibility of otosclerosis lies in a family history of hearing loss; 50 to 70% of women with this condition report other cases in the family. Hearing loss that improves in the presence of background noise is also associated with sound conduction defects. These women may be soft-spoken, since the voice is transmitted through bone. They may have a buzzing or ringing in their ears. Intermittent dizziness usually lasts only a few minutes, although it may last as long as several hours in 5% of cases.

Types of hearing loss: **Conduction deafness** occurs when the ear's normal amplification system is diseased or bypassed, as when the ear canal contains a foreign body. If the tympanic membrane or the ossicles are fixed and cannot

976

vibrate, the person hears by sound transmission through the skull. Usually this means they hear sounds over 50 dB; normal speaking is in the 40 to 50 dB range. Amplification from a hearing aid can help in this case.

Sensorineural deafness occurs due to problems with sound reception. The defect is within the cochlea, the auditory nerve or the hearing centers in the brain.

Evaluation: First, examine the ears with an otoscope to look for any obvious abnormalities. If a foreign body is discovered and you can visualize it sufficiently, you might try to remove it gently with a pair of fine-nosed tweezers, taking care not to push it in further. If you cannot retrieve the object, send the woman to an eye, ear, nose and throat specialist for removal. If no obvious inflammation or other problems are discovered, testing the hearing with tuning forks provides the most valuable information. The best tuning fork to use is either the 256 or 512 Hz.

Weber test for lateralization of sound: Strike the tuning fork on the heel of your hand so that it is vibrating smoothly. Place the handle on top of the woman's head or the middle of her forehead. Ask where she hears the sound. Normally she hears it equally in both ears.

Rinne's test to compare air and bone conduction: Strike the tuning fork on the heel of your hand so that it vibrates smoothly. Place the handle on the mastoid prominence behind the ear, then hold it in front of the ear canal. Ask her in which position the sound is loudest. Normally it should be loudest in the second position, demonstrating that air conduction is louder than bone conduction.

TEST	STAPEDIAL OTOSCLEROSIS (CONDUCTION DEAFNESS)	COCHLEAR OTOSCLEROSIS (NEUROSENSORY DEAFNESS)
Rinne's test	Bone conduction is greater than air conduction in the affected ear	Air conduction is greater than bone conduction in the affected ear but there is decreased hearing in both
Weber test	Lateralization of sound to affected ear. No external noises distracting the perception of sound through bone	Lateralization of sound to the unaffected ear where the healthy nerves are working best

After making a preliminary evaluation, refer these women to a hearing specialist to discuss options for treatment which may include hearing aids (in some cases) and surgery in others.

References and further reading:
Gleicher, N., ed. Principles of Medical Therapy in Pregnancy, Plenum Pub., New York, 1985.
Gussman, Debra, "Otosclerosis and Pregnancy," MCN, Vol. 5, Nov/Dec, 1980, pp. 408-411.
Hansen, Lori, et.al., "Otolaryngologic Manifestations of Pregnancy," J Family Prac., Vol. 23, No. 2, 1986, pp. 151-55.

Edema (Swelling)

Physiologic edema of pregnancy: A normal increase in interstitial tissue fluids occurs due to the hormonal changes as well as the increased blood volume of pregnancy. This may increase as pregnancy advances; even pitting edema can be normal. In fact, it is now recognized among mainstream practitioners that healthy women usually have some swelling. This reflects a well expanded blood volume. Physiologic swelling fluctuates with the woman's activity level throughout the day and may be more pronounced in those women who report noticeable swelling prior to their menses. The presence of distended blood vessels with edema is evidence that the blood volume is well expanded. In most cases of physiologic swelling more edema will be seen below the waist than above. Typically women do not awake with physiologic swelling, it develops throughout the day (although a few women will wake up somewhat puffy from the waist down, with quick resolution when they become active). It can also be alleviated by changing position, resting, or walking. Standing in one position for too long or going without movement (such as sitting in a car) can encourage the development of edema in the lower limbs.

Swelling related to acute salt depletion (sweating): Normal swelling can increase when a woman is pregnant during the summer months or whenever she is naturally perspiring more freely. This swelling is an acute reaction to a short-term imbalance in the protein/sodium ratio in the bloodstream due to the loss of sodium through perspiring. If corrected, it will not become a pathological condition. The simple solution to this is to drink more fluids and eat more salt. While a woman need not make her food unpalatable, adding slightly more salt than she ordinarily would will usually reverse this trend. If this alone does not resolve the edema, slightly increase the protein in her diet as well.

Pathological swelling of pregnancy: Pathological swelling progressively increases, does not tend to fluctuate throughout the day and tends to be generalized (from head to toe) rather than primarily in the lower body. Pathological swelling results when circulatory fluids seep into the spaces between the cells surrounding the blood vessels. Blood vessels are not distended and may even be less noticeable due to swelling. In the otherwise normal woman with normal kidneys, pathological swelling occurs because the protein/sodium ratio in the blood stream is out of balance and therefore incapable of retaining the fluid in the circulating blood volume where it needs to be. As fluid becomes trapped in the interstitial spaces, the hemoglobin rises, reflecting a contracted blood volume. The point at which a marginally contracted blood volume will begin to cause pathological swelling varies among individuals. Therefore lack of excessive swelling cannot be taken as "proof" that the blood volume is adequate.

Since pathological swelling's ultimate cause is dietary inadequacy, it is reasonable to assume that a woman is already suffering from an inadequately expanded blood volume before swelling becomes apparent. This protein/sodium imbalance represents insufficient dietary intake which can be corrected by reviewing the diet and adding more salt, protein and nutrient rich calories as necessary. If this imbalance is not corrected, pathological swelling can persist and increase, draining more and more fluid from the circulation into the surrounding tissues. The end result can be a hypovolemic crisis which precipitates premature labor, placental abruption or stillbirth depending upon how acute the problem and how inadequate the diet was to begin with. Even if the dietary intake has been good, just two weeks of inadequate salt intake can begin to cause a reduction in the circulating blood volume due to fluid being shifted into the intercellular spaces outside the blood vessels. (See chapter on Toxemia, Third Trimester section, for more information.)

Medical conditions which cause swelling: The primary underlying medical conditions which cause swelling are kidney disorders and heart failure. In most cases these conditions will already be diagnosed and the woman under treatment prior to conception. If you suspect an underlying condition, get a consultation without delay.

Electrical Injuries and Shocks

The majority of deaths related to electrical accidents are from occupational hazards, but lightening and in-home hazards can also result in significant injury as well. The extent of injury depends upon such variables as current, resistance, voltage and duration of contact. Alternating current presents the greatest hazard because of its effects on the muscles. The intensity of the current will produce heat and thus influence the extent of the injury. Flow of the current requires the completion of a circuit through two contact points. The amount of flow is related to voltage and resistance; the higher the voltage and the lower the resistance the greater the flow. In human anatomy, bone is the most resistant and nerve tissue the least. Moisture decreases skin resistance to electrical currents. Contact points help define the possible extent of damage with the head and chest being the most dangerous. Persons exposed to high voltages usually show the most injuries but fatal heart effects may be produced by less than 1000 volts of exposure.

Three types of injuries are noted: localized burns at contact areas which produce charring and necrosis; flash burns, which look like second and third degree thermal burns, result from external electrical arching to the ground; and flame-type thermal burns due to ignition of nearby articles such as clothing. When such burns occur disorientation may be present. Tissue destruction, clot formation, shock, convulsions, coma and kidney failure may sometimes occur as well.

Fetal effects are poorly defined, but theoretically the amniotic fluid should be an excellent conductor of electricity to the fetus. However, 11 cases of *in utero* exposure to lightning resulted in 6 live births without obvious effects.

What to do: Maternal treatment does not differ from that of the nonpregnant population. First, remove the source of the electricity. Ideally you will turn the electricity off at the source, such as the breaker or fuse box. If you can't, unplug the item or push it out of the way with a nonconductive item such as a completely dry wooden-handled item. Wet objects will act as conductors and their use will cause the rescuer to be electrocuted. If moving the source of electricity is impossible, try to manipulate the victim away from the source with a dry wooden-handled item. Do not attempt to separate the source and the victim with your hands or any conductive object and do not touch the victim until she is separated from the source of the current. Check for breathing and pulse; administer cardiopulmonary resuscitation if necessary. Once the woman's vitals are stable check for injuries such as burns. If available, apply water gel pads to burned areas; run cold water over them if not. Give homeopathic Urtica Urns in 30C or 200C potency to minimize the severity of the burns. Have the woman receive a medical evaluation as soon as possible.

References and further reading:
Gleicher, N., ed. Principles of Medical Therapy in Pregnancy, Plenum Pub., New York, 1985.

Eye Problems and Visual Disturbances

Pregnancy-induced changes in the eyes will reverse themselves after the birth. Visual disturbances may be due to:

*Fluid retention in pregnancy (the most common cause; this can be a normal variation of pregnancy)
*Vascular pressure secondary to high blood pressure or other vascular disturbances
*Underlying organic disease unrelated to pregnancy, such as glaucoma

Visual disturbances:

Refractive errors: If a woman reports blurred vision, a simple screening measure can be used to determine if she is experiencing a refractive error or organic disease. Have the woman look through a pinhole in a piece of cardboard or stiff paper. This will at least partially correct a significant refractive error. Large alterations in refraction are unusual during pregnancy, but may occasionally occur. Difficulty with reading or near vision may occur as well as blurred vision for distance in those who are farsighted. Thickening of the cornea may also cause refractive errors. Such visual disturbances will resolve after birth.

Organic disease: Nonrefractive visual errors may be caused by a number of underlying conditions unrelated to pregnancy such as opacities or irregularities in the normally clear ocular media, and disease of the retina, optic nerve, or intracerebral visual pathways. Reports of visual problems accompanied by such symptoms as unilateral visual impairment, irregularity of pupil response, pain, pressure, or other problems need to be evaluated by an ophthalmologist without delay.

Contact lenses and pregnancy: The normal pregnant woman experiences changes in her tear volume as pregnancy advances. These normal changes may make the wearing of contact lens uncomfortable or impossible. Those wearing hard lenses will have the most difficulty. Protein and mucus tends to accumulate on the lenses more easily during pregnancy, and frequent cleansing is recommended. The cornea is also less sensitive to irritants during pregnancy; so contact lens wearers need to be especially mindful of protecting their eyes from irritants and keeping their lenses clean. Some women may find they cannot wear their lenses at all during late pregnancy, when these changes are most pronounced. Women should also be made aware that standard contact lens solutions often contain thimerosal, a mercury-based preservative. Solutions designed for use in "sensitive eyes" do not and should be used instead.

Glasses and pregnancy: Those who wear glasses may notice changes in their vision, with a tendency to be more myopic (nearsighted) during pregnancy. In some women, this may produce eye strain and, if the changes are very severe, may even necessitate a change in prescription

Pathological symptoms: Visual disturbances which involve consistently seeing little clear or silvery spots before the eyes (floaters), especially when accompanied by high blood pressure or headaches, may indicate a serious underlying condition. First, rule out toxemia. To do so, assess the size of the fetus, the fundal height, the mother's overall sense of well-being, and draw blood to perform a liver profile (chem panel) and a hemoglobin check. If the chem panel looks good (normal liver enzymes and albumin levels, and a hemoglobin that has responded appropriately to blood volume expansion), then address any high blood pressure as simple hypertension unless you suspect a more serious cause. If the liver profile is not normal, increase protein intake dramatically in an attempt to remedy this situation, which reflects a contracted blood volume (see separate chapters on Hypertension in this section and Toxemia, Third Trimester section, for more information). Worsening visual disturbances should be evaluated to rule out underlying disease.

Eyelid disorders:

Droopy eyelids (ptosis): For unknown reasons some pregnant women develop droopy eyelids; this problem usually resolves after birth. There is no accompanying abnormality of pupil dilation or weakness of other eye muscles which would be present if a tumor on the third cranial nerve were the cause. If the condition does not improve after birth, surgery can be performed. A homeopathic remedy is probably your best bet for resolving this problem during pregnancy.

Pigmented eyelids: The "mask of pregnancy" may extend to the eyelids. This is evidence of a folic acid deficiency.

Inflammation: Acute or chronic diffuse inflammation of the edges of the eyelids is common during pregnancy. This may manifest as a flaky or ulcerative condition usually caused by *staphylococcus*. Symptoms include itching, burning, redness and irritation of the eyelids. Some women may lose eyelashes. If suppurative, oozing lesions may be found at the base of the lashes. Rinsing the eyes several times daily with Calendula, Chamomile or Eye Bright infusion with a pinch of Golden Seal added per cup should clear this problem promptly. Dietary assessment and supplementation with extra vitamin C, bioflavinoids, and zinc will help strengthen all membranes. Women who wear contact lenses should switch to glasses until the condition has completely cleared.

Sty (hordeolum): This localized eyelid inflammation of the glands at the base of the eyelashes is usually caused by staph infection. It presents as a painful, red, localized swelling of the lid margin. The application of hot chamomile compresses every few hours for several days will usually cause it to drain. Antibiotics are rarely needed.

Chalazion (chronic granuloma): These swellings are located in the meibomian glands which are found high up on the inner surface of the eyelid. They may present as acute painful lumps or a firm, nontender, gradually enlarging swelling. Hot compresses tend to relieve these swellings as well. When asymptomatic these lesions disappear over several weeks or months.

Conjunctiva disorders:

Subconjunctival hemorrhage: Eye hemorrhages may result from any kind of intraocular stress. This may be produced by severe vomiting, straining (especially during labor), trauma or, rarely, blood disorders. An asymptomatic, flat, red, sharply delineated area appears under the bulbar conjunctiva that fades within 2 weeks. Homeopathic Arnica (30C or 200C) can be given 3 times daily to help resolve it.

Conjunctivitis: Inflammation of the normally transparent conjunctiva covering the globe of the eyeball and the inner surface of the eyelids is a common problem. It often presents with diffusely dilated blood vessels. Vision may be temporarily blurred from tearing or mucus and a mild gritty feeling may be present, especially during blinking. Toxic fumes, chemicals, pollen allergies, or microorganisms may be causative. If inflammation is due to an irritating substance, cool compresses, rinsing the eyes with normal saline (contact lenses solution) and removal of the offending substance will usually resolve symptoms.

Inflammation caused by infection can be due to viral, bacterial or chlamydial organisms. There may be copious mucousy, pus-filled discharge. If there is extremely profuse discharge, rule out gonorrhea. Immediate Gram stain and culture of the discharge is called for, as gonorrhea can lead to infection and perforation of the cornea. Antibiotic treatment should be begun promptly after a specimen is collected. Cultures should also be obtained from oral and genital swabs of the woman and her partner.

Herpes may produce inflammation, but viral infection is most commonly produced by adenovirus. This extremely contagious infection can be passed by hand-to-eye contact. Swollen lymph nodes in the neck, swollen eyelids and a watery or mucoid discharge are frequently seen. Conjunctival follicles may be visible on slit-lamp examination by an ophthalmologist. This condition will resolve on its own, with the acute phase lasting a few days to 2 to 3 weeks. Vision may be mildly affected.

Chlamydial conjunctivitis is often clinically indistinguishable from viral conjunctivitis and should be ruled out in any follicular conjunctivitis lasting more than 2 weeks or occurring in any pregnant woman near term. About 90% of those with an ocular infection will also have a genital chlamydial infection, which can lead to eye infection or chlamydial pneumonia in the newborn.

Cornea changes: A woman's cornea may become thicker during pregnancy due to fluid changes. Changes in the cornea may affect visual acuity; however, normal pregnancy usually has little clinical effect on the vision. A decrease in corneal sensitivity may occur after the 31st week of pregnancy, returning to normal 6 to 8 weeks postpartum. Kruchenberg's spindles, a melanin pigmentation of the posterior cornea seen on slit lamp examination and usually associated with secondary glaucoma, may be seen in normal women during pregnancy. They have no effect on vision.

References and further reading:

Gleicher, Norbert, ed. Principles of Medical Therapy in Pregnancy, Plenum Pub., New York, 1985.
Imafidon, Chris, & J. Imafidon, "Commentaries: Contact Lenses in Pregnancy," Brit. J. of Ob/Gyn, Nov. 1992, Vol. 99, pp. 865-868.

Fatigue

Fatigue is a hallmark of early pregnancy. In those women who are unduly stressed (including emotionally or psychologically), it may persist throughout pregnancy. The best remedy is to nap during the day. Be sure the woman is getting enough nourishment to meet her individual energy requirements, since hypoglycemia can cause chronic fatigue. Eliminate underlying problems such as anemia, subclinical infections, dental problems (which can lead to overall debility) and rule out heart complications. Emotional issues can also cause a person to feel fatigued; do not hesitate to discuss possible emotional factors if the fatigue seems excessive or prolonged. Note that multiple gestation may be accompanied by excessive fatigue beyond the first trimester, especially if it goes undetected and nutrition is inadequate. Yellow Dock root tincture has an energy-balancing effect and can be given to increase vitality, even if a woman is not anemic.

Acute fatigue can be a sign of impending illness and indicates a need to rest and build up resistance by supporting the immune system. Question the woman carefully for other symptoms which may point to a more serious problem; fatigue can indicate heart problems, cancer, or immune compromise such as AIDS (read chapters on HIV and Syphilis in Diagnostic Tests).

Fainting

The most common cause of fainting (syncope) in pregnancy is hypoglycemia. Usually the blood sugar is low, the blood pressure drops, and hot weather, slight dehydration, standing too long and/or lack of oxygen (as might occur when standing in a crowded room) combine to cause a woman to faint. Such fainting may be accompanied by a wave of nausea. While this may be alarming to those around her, particularly in a public setting, usually all that is needed is to apply cool cloths to her head, sit her up slowly, and lead her to the nearest place where she can sit down, eat, drink, and recover her equilibrium. Such incidents are usually isolated events.

Recurrent fainting or near-fainting spells require careful evaluation and may necessitate consultation. Causes of fainting in pregnancy other than hypoglycemia may be more serious, and require further investigation or referral:

*Anemia
*Blood loss
*Electrolyte disturbances (dehydration?)
*Oxygen deprivation which may be caused by:
  -Anemia
  -Hypothermia
  -Fever
  -Heart problems
  -Poisoning
  -Liver or kidney failure
  -Diabetes
*Intracranial lesions resulting in coma (woman passes out and will not come to) which may be due to:
  -Infection
  -Trauma
  -Vascular rupture or other vascular disorder
  -Tumor
  -Pulmonary embolism (accompanied by respiratory distress)
*Toxemic coma

Intracranial disorders: Ischemic (deficiency of blood) disorders of the brain may be caused by arterial obstruction which may be due to plaque formation on the sides of the vessels, clots on the left side of the heart, or venous channels that gain entrance to the arteries through a patent formane ovale. The incidence may be higher in women who smoke and in those who have been on oral contraceptives prior to pregnancy, and may be associated with mitral valve prolapse in women with no other problems or symptoms. Venous thrombosis of large intracranial veins is being reported in younger women, but the incidence is low in the United

States. Symptoms vary dramatically but mild ones such as weakness, headache, slight fever, malaise and nausea are common.

Angiography, a test which can confirm ischemic cerebral vascular disease, involves the injection of radiopaque dye followed by x-ray study to determine where it circulates. Sometimes a CAT scan is done as well. Adequate shielding should be provided for all areas of the body not to be examined. If X-rays are necessary, the woman can take a bath in hot water with ½ pound of sea salt and ¼ pound of baking soda added after exposure. It is also helpful to eat extra miso, sodium alginate rich seaweeds, kelp, buckwheat grass, and take niacin supplements for several weeks. Sodium alginate attracts radioactive materials and carries them out of the body. Homeopathic X-ray in a potency of 30C or 200C can also help minimize the harmful effects.

Intracranial hemorrhage may, in some cases, be directly related to long-standing hypertension, which has led to arteriovenous malformations and aneurysms (dilated portion of blood vessels). However, hypertension is not an associated factor in a significant percentage of cases.

Bleeding from aneurysms is most often into the subarachnoid space but bleeding from an arteriovenous malformation may be subarachnoid or into the brain itself. Symptoms include headaches, neck pain, and coma. Subarachnoid bleeding does not change the reflex response or muscle tone; intracranial bleeding may lessen both.   Diagnosis includes a spinal tap except in cases of increased intracranial pressure, displacement of the pineal gland (indicating a mass) or when the skin at the proposed puncture site is infected. CT scan and angiography may also be useful. (Also see the chapter on Vascular Problems in this section).

Toxemic coma: Although rare, it is possible for a woman who is severely ill with toxemia to pass right into coma without first experiencing convulsions. Symptoms such as headache, visual disturbances, nausea, vomiting, epigastric pain and *low* blood pressure, fever and slight jaundice are present prior to the onset of coma. This form of severe toxemia is frequently fatal. (Greenhill, 1951)

What to do: Any woman who has symptoms associated with fainting other than dizziness, who passes out and will not come to, or who has additional symptoms which raise suspicions of a serious underlying cause, such as acute, severe headache or signs suggesting cardiac compromise, should see a bio-technical medical care provider for evaluation without delay! If she will not come to, have her taken to the nearest hospital that provides obstetrical care and then contact her collaborating medical care provider.

References and further reading:
Gibbs, Charles, "Sudden sensorium derangement during pregnancy," Contemp. Ob/Gyn, Vol. 20, #1, July 1982, pp. 55-64.
Greenhill, J., Principles and Practice of Obstetrics, 10th ed., W. B. Saunders, Co., Phil., 1951.

Fetal Heart Rate Abnormalities

For a description of normal parameters and terms such as baseline, variability and reactivity, see the chapter on Fetal Heart Rate Assessment in the section on Basic Skills. This chapter discusses variations from normal and what they might mean.

Baseline abnormalities: Some fetuses who demonstrate consistent bradycardia have no apparent problems and experience a healthy labor and birth. In such cases, the heart rate is rarely below 100 bpm, which may simply indicate that a normal baby has a lower baseline than most. I have personally seen this in several babies who were fine. Listening carefully throughout pregnancy will help you differentiate such a normal, albeit uncommon, variation from a true problem.

Severe, persistent bradycardia ranging between 20 to 80 bpm. (but usually falling within 50 to 70 bpm) can be due to a heart abnormality referred to as fetal heart block, with complete disassociation between the electrical impulses controlling the auricles and ventricles in almost every case. The incidence of congenital heart disease, especially ventricular septal defect, is as high as 40% in these babies, warranting a discussion with the parents regarding the use of an ultrasound exam to detect heart abnormalities. Fetuses that have heart block but no heart abnormalities usually do well, however some may experience heart failure or hydrops. Maternal collagen disease can cause congenital heart block, and should be ruled out whenever heart block is found.

Arrhythmias of the heart rate can sometimes be heard. Most are transient and not clinically important (Gabbe, 1991, p. 469). If you detect an arrhythmia, continue to listen for several minutes, stimulate the baby to move and see if and how often the irregularity repeats, if it continues or if it has a regular rhythm. Chart your findings and discuss them with the mother. If an arrhythmia is persistent over the course of several visits or you detect other fetal heart abnormalities along with it, discuss having the fetal heart evaluated with ultrasound.

A rare but significant finding is a sinusoidal pattern, which ranges between 120 to 160 bpm. However, it has a smooth, undulating wave-like pattern of uniform long-term variability ranging between 5 to 20 bpm. No short term variability is noted. The pattern is continuous; short-term or intermittent changes do not qualify and are usually benign. True sinusoidal patterns typically reflect severe fetal anemia, as in Rh isoimmunization, or hypoxia.

Bradycardia: When the FHR falls below 100 bpm, oxygen deprivation may be an associated complication. Beat-to-beat variability will also be reduced or absent. This type of bradycardia often precedes imminent fetal death and is an indication for immediate birth.

Maternal drug intake may also cause a reduction in the fetal heart rate. Any drugs which cause maternal bradycardia will also cause fetal bradycardia. *Beta-*

988

blockers used to control maternal hypertension are the drugs most frequently responsible. Maternal hypothermia is another rare cause of fetal bradycardia.

Sporadic periods of prolonged deceleration may occur in pregnancy during which the heart rate drops for a period of 1 to 10 minutes and then quickly returns to normal. Very short episodes may be associated with such factors as the baby momentarily becoming entangled in or "tripping over" its umbilical cord, or maternal position (especially supine). It is thought that this is associated with fetal hypoxia. Watch for evidence of abnormal heart rate patterns during labor in these babies. Whenever you hear the FHR drop, change the mother's position and continue to listen; this may correct the bradycardia if maternal positioning was causing the baby to put pressure on its umbilical cord. If a deceleration should occur during a procedure such as external version, stop at once and listen for when and if the heart rate returns to normal. Listen constantly if further attempts at version are made, but only after a discussion of the situation with the parents.

Tachycardia: Tachycardia occurs when the fetal heart exceeds 160 bpm. Periods of tachycardia may be precipitated by a variety of maternal factors such as dehydration, overheating (hot baths or exercise), oxygen deprivation, fever, infection or hyperthyroidism. Precipitating fetal factors include anemia, blood loss, side effects of drugs administered to the fetus. Drugs used to inhibit labor such as parasympatholytics characterized by atropine and the beta sympathetic drugs, also result in fetal tachycardia. Fetal hypoxia is the most serious cause. The degree of oxygen deprivation is usually mild and the heart rate seldom exceeds 180 bpm, however, the fetus can still be considerably compromised. Tachycardia which lasts less than 10 minutes is most accurately described as acceleration.

Maternal overheating from bathing, exercise or saunas is the most frequent cause of fetal tachycardia. Hot baths in mild saline solution or waiting for 30 to 45 minutes after a bath to check the heart rate may help to eliminate this temporary factor. The next most frequent cause is maternal dehydration, easily remedied by having the mother drink 10 ounces of fluid in a 30 to 45 minute period and then reassessing the heart rate. Next comes maternal infection. When the infection is not in the uterus, fetal tachycardia is due to maternal fever. Intrauterine infection may lead to fetal heart rate elevation before maternal fever begins.

Supraventricular tachycardia is characterized by a heart rate exceeding 180 bpm which may be continuous or intermittent. If continuous, the fetus is at risk for congestive heart failure, necessitating delivery if near term or careful monitoring for signs of heart failure using real-time ultrasounds if premature.

Variability: If the fetal nervous system is normal, a variety of factors may influence fetal heart rate variability. The fetal state is the factor that most frequently affects changes in the heart rate variability, as explained in the chapter on Fetal Heart Rate Assessment. Since changes in adult respiration, blood pressure and temperature effect variability in the adult, we have reason to believe that similar changes will occur in the fetus. This includes whether the fetus is awake, asleep, or active, as well as its movement, temperature, oxygenation and exposure to drugs.

Maternal drug ingestion may significantly affect fetal heart rate variability. Those drugs used most frequently which have an impact are narcotics, sedatives, tranquilizers, and *beta*-blockers, all of which decrease variability to varying degrees depending upon the maternal dosage.

Oxygenation also has an effect. Acute and moderate fetal hypoxia increases variability. Variability greater than 25 bpm may represent shifting oxygen and carbon dioxide levels, however in the absence of repetitive decelerations, there is usually no change in fetal oxygenation. Increased variability that is followed by loss of beat-to-beat variability can be ominous. Only after prolonged hypoxia is the variability likely to be reduced. Of note is the sleeping fetus, who may temporarily show a marked reduction in variability; however, this should return to a more active pattern in a maximum of 80 minutes. Sleeping babies usually show minor variability, whereas the severely hypoxic fetus may have none.

Reactivity problems: Remember that young healthy fetuses may not show a reactive heart rate until their nervous system is more mature. If the baby is older than 32 weeks gestation, a lack of reactivity could indicate that the baby is sleeping. If the baby is moving and no reactivity is detected, it indicates that the baby's cardiovascular system is not responding appropriately to normal stress.

What to do: If worrisome patterns in the FHR are irresolvable with the simple measures outlined here, you must consider that significant fetal compromise may be taking place. Often a random or transient abnormality is benign; assess both your own and the mother's intuitive sense of fetal well-being as well as other options such as monitoring fetal movement, ultrasound exam, and consultation with the collaborating physician. If heart problems are found, often the choice is the birth of a preterm baby that may not do well or waiting until term, when the condition of the fetus may be such that it does not survive late pregnancy or will die when the additional stress of labor is imposed.

References and further reading:

Gabbe, Steven, et. al. ed. Obstetrics: Normal and Problem Pregnancies, 2nd ed., Churchill Livingstone, New York, 1991.
Pauerstein, Carl, ed., Clinical Obstetrics, John Wiley & Sons, New York, 1987.

Fetal Size/Dates Discrepancies

This chapter assumes you have already reviewed and compensated as appropriate for all the considerations set forth in the chapter on Overall Assessment of Fetal Size and Growth and are now convinced that there is, indeed, an abnormality.

If small-for-dates: There are two varieties of small infants:

*Small (light) for gestational age (SGA): those that are normally or constitutionally small due to genetic variations
*Intrauterine growth retardation (IUGR): a baby that is normally proportioned but fails to achieve the size expected for their gestational age due to impaired growth

The primary reason babies are small-for-dates is either incorrect dates or inadequate nutrition. If dates seem correct and you have advised dietary improvement, the mother has actually improved her diet and fetal growth is still small-for-dates, assess ways to lower her stress level and reevaluate. Even in a small woman who might be expected to have a small normal baby, in most cases some fetal growth will occur if dietary changes are made; you will see growth from visit to visit, normal fetal activity and a normal, reactive heart rate.

If no significant improvement is obvious after the mother has faithfully followed your instructions, you may be dealing with a baby that is truly suffering from intrauterine growth retardation. This problems affects 3 to 7% of all pregnancies. These figures cover all cases of IUGR, however, and include many cases which would have been corrected if adequate nutritional counseling had been implemented in a timely fashion; therefore the rate of unavoidable IUGR is actually lower. IUGR is a serious problem, regardless of why the baby is small. About 20% of stillborn babies are IUGR, and perinatal mortality for growth-retarded infants may be 6 to 10 times higher than for those of normal size. Most IUGR stillbirths occur after the 36th week of pregnancy and before labor begins. There are a number of factors which are associated with true IUGR:

Serial ultrasound exposure?! See the medical management comments below for a description of the study which found one-third more IUGR in babies exposed to intensive serial ultrasound exams during pregnancy.

Fetal infection: Infections, particularly involving herpes, cytomegalovirus, rubella and toxoplasmosis, can cause fetal damage which makes it impossible for the fetus to utilize nutrients. Herpes gestationes, while not truly an infection, is also associated with growth retardation. Infections may also produce cellular or organ damage leading to poor growth patterns.

Toxic exposures: Maternal poisoning from ingestion of potentially lethal doses of certain drugs as well as concentrated exposure to chemicals such as certain pesticides or heavy metals (notably cadmium) may lead to growth retarded babies.

Congenital malformation: Various genetic and congenital anomalies lead to IUGR because poor growth is part of the genetic picture. Abnormalities of cell replication and reduced cell numbers produce early onset of impaired growth that is symmetrical. Organ defects such as heart malformations may lead to a poorly perfused and therefore poorly grown baby.

Placental problems: Many placental problems are due to poor nutrition; however, damage can occur if the mother is exposed to certain toxins, is traumatically injured, or if the placenta is malformed for unidentifiable reasons. Some of the specific problems include decreased placental mass, accreta, abruption, prolonged gestation in the presence of an abnormal placenta, and inadequately nourished multiple gestation. Obviously a small placenta or one left partially nonfunctional from an abruption will deliver less nutrients to the fetus. Since placental growth is stimulated by the amount of blood perfusing the placenta and since placental villi continue to develop past term the importance of nutrition as a major corrective measure to promote adequate transfer of nutrients cannot be overemphasized.

Intrinsic placental abnormality or disease: A poor implantation site which does not afford the placenta adequate contact with the maternal circulation, a single umbilical artery or other cord malformation, or vascular disease which interferes with nutrient transfer may all cause problems with fetal growth.

Decreased placental blood flow: This problem may be caused by maternal vascular disease, hypertension due to underlying disease, postural hypotension or hyperviscosity of the blood (thick blood, which is most often due to a contracted blood volume correctable with adequate dietary improvements). Toxemia leads to asymmetric IUGR with normal head growth but a reduction in the size of the fetal heart, thymus, spleen, pancreas and adrenal glands.

Maternal digestive conditions: Ileojejunal bypass surgery removes a large portion of the maternal intestine and deceases its ability to absorb nutrients, regardless of the woman's dietary intake. Disease conditions such as ulcerative colitis or Crohn's disease may also lead to IUGR.

Decreased oxygen availability: If the mother lives at a high altitude, she has a hereditary disorder of hemoglobin, suffers from a lung disorder or cyanotic heart disease, or smokes, oxygen delivery to the fetus will be reduced. However, again, in many cases, good nutrition will compensate for these factors.

Drug ingestion: Various recreational drugs (such as cocaine and alcohol) and prescription drugs (especially Hydantoin and Coumarin) are associated with the birth of IUGR infants.

Prior history of IUGR infant: While studies clearly correlate prior history as a factor, habitual maternal dietary patterns and stress levels are most likely causative in women who do not have medical conditions, genetic factors or toxic exposures which place them at higher risk for a growth retarded baby.

Ask yourself these questions when a baby is small-for-dates:

*Is this a normal variation given the size of the parents?
*Is the fetus abnormal?
*Is there a problem with placental transfer of nutrients?
*Is there a problem with maternal transfer of nutrients?

In true IUGR, not much can really be done. If every effort to relieve stress, remove the intake of offending substances and optimize nutrition do not cause the fetus to catch up with its growth, discuss various options for further fetal evaluation, including ultrasound examination to detect fetal defects. Knowledge that the fetus may be suffering from a congenital anomaly may help the parents make an informed decision about the location of birth and postpartum pediatric care. If asymmetrical growth is noted, this increases the likelihood that a contracted blood volume is the cause and warrants investigation as to why the mother may not be assimilating nutrients.

Medical management: Bio-technical medical care providers manage IUGR with serial ultrasounds to determine the extent of the problem and with properly timed delivery based on the results of amniocentesis to determine fetal lung maturity. While ultrasounds may be able to identify causative factors such as anomalies, it should be emphasized to parents that no difference in perinatal outcome can be demonstrated when serial ultrasounds are used and that ultrasound is notoriously inaccurate at assessing fetal size, especially as pregnancy advances (this is one reason why serial exams are preferred). There is no bio-technical solution to IUGR, ultrasounds merely document the situation. The primary value of a single evaluation to midwifery clients is that additional knowledge regarding the baby's condition allows them to make an informed choice to birth in the hospital or to stay home. Staying home may be a reasonable choice, if, for example, the baby is discovered to have a defect incompatible with life or to be small but otherwise normal.

In addition, a large study utilizing imaging ultrasounds and continuous wave doppler flow studies at 18, 24, 28, 34 and 38 weeks in one group and a single imaging ultrasound at 18 weeks in the control group found that *there were one-*

third more IUGR babies in the intensive group. (Newnham, et.al., 1993, p. 890) This sobering finding should be made known to parents, who may not want their already compromised infant to be compromised further by multiple tests which will do nothing of benefit and may make the situation worse.

If large-for-dates: As with small-for-dates babies, the most common reason for a baby to appear "large-for-dates" is a wrong expected date of delivery. Women who eat well often carry babies that are larger than "average," keeping in mind that a large term baby is defined as any baby weighing over 8 lb. 5 oz. in some areas. If women are short or short-waisted, they may appear to have a large baby when in fact this is not the case. If all factors have been taken into account, including the possibility of polyhydramnios and multiple gestation, the most likely reason for a truly large-for-dates infant is undiagnosed maternal diabetes.

Maternal diabetes: Review the history for evidence of diabetes in the family and ask the woman about the classic symptoms of diabetes such as excessive thirst, ravenous appetite with weight loss or failure to gain, and slow healing of wounds. A family history of large babies born early or stillbirths may indicate undetected diabetes. If a suspicious history is revealed, have the woman tested for diabetes (see the chapter later in this section on Gestational Diabetes and the chapter on Diabetes and Pregnancy in <u>Diagnostic Tests</u> for more information). Babies of truly diabetic mothers exhibit asymmetric growth patterns including enlarged organs and increased fat and muscle mass resulting in a disproportionate increase in the abdomen and shoulder girdle. Head growth is not usually altered so brain growth is normal. These features constitute true macrosomia. Such babies may die in the last 6 weeks of pregnancy, often deliver prematurely and have a variety of problems including certain birth defects and hypoglycemia after birth.

In other cases, large babies will be found to "run in the family" with no history of diabetes. A woman on an excellent diet may have a 10 to 11 pound healthy baby at term. These large babies exhibit symmetrical increases in both head and abdominal circumferences.

Fetal hypothyroidism: If the fetus is suffering from thyroid problems, large-for-dates growth may be a factor, but is not always present.

What to do: An ultrasound exam can be done to try and determine the size of the baby and whether growth appears symmetrical or asymmetrical. After 30 to 33 weeks of gestation, the presence of an abdominal circumference greater than the 90th percentile for fetal growth is a fairly reliable indicator that the baby is large-for-dates, although generally speaking the later in pregnancy an ultrasound is done the less reliable an indicator it is of fetal size.

If a woman is found to be diabetic, her blood sugar must be regulated to give the baby the best chance for survival. Unfortunately, conception in an uncontrolled diabetic state will often cause severe congenital anomalies. If a woman is a diagnosed diabetic, her blood sugar will ideally be well controlled prior to conception.

The primary risk factor with the birth of a large infant is shoulder dystocia with accompanying trauma and asphyxia. However, every large baby does not have shoulder dystocia. If there is no evidence of diabetes, and the baby seems exceptionally large you should discuss the possibility of shoulder problems with the mother, review the mechanism of shoulder delivery so that she can visualize it clearly and discuss how you would handle this emergency, including your views on the best delivery positions to avoid a problem.

References and further reading:

Gabbe, Steven, et.al., ed., Obstetrics: Normal and Problem Pregnancies, 2nd ed. Churchill-Livingstone, New York 1991.
Newnham, et.al., "Effects of frequent ultrasound during pregnancy: a randomized controlled trial," Lancet, Vol. 342, pp. 887-891.

Fever

Normal body temperature is generally considered to be 98.6°F (37°C). Fever is defined as an elevation above an individual's normal range. As long as the maternal oral temperature does not exceed 104°F (40°C) the fetus is not at risk from maternal overheating. (Also see the chapter on Hyperthermia in the section on Sustaining Health and Well-being.) A number of conditions may cause a temperature elevation; some of these are serious, while others are temporary or easily treated.

*Maternal overheating, as from a hot shower or hot tub soak
*Strenuous exercise
*Dehydration
*Illness (usually colds and flus but also be alert for Listeriosis or chorioamnionitis)
*Life-threatening, poorly managed toxemia
*Infective endocarditis

Many infectious diseases which may cause fever are discussed in detail in Diagnostic Tests. Ask the woman about any of the common reasons for temperature elevation. If those have been ruled out, ask about recent exposures to others who are ill. Barring common illnesses, rule out intrauterine infection, severe toxemia (there will be plenty of other signs before fever sets in) and finally, infective endocarditis.

Infectious endocarditis: Infection of the heart muscle may follow episodes of bacteremia, in which the bloodstream is showered with bacteria during invasive procedures. It presents with fever, heart murmur and anemia, and may be accompanied by headache, malaise, fatigue, musculoskeletal pain and the development of small blood vessel ruptures or petechiae. Be alert for this possibility in women with congenital heart conditions such as mitral valve prolapse. When it occurs it is usually associated with an invasive or traumatic event such as dental work or labor. If the woman is at risk and you can find no other cause for her condition, send her in for a cardiac evaluation without delay.

Treatment of fever: If you suspect a serious condition such as endocarditis, have the woman see a medical practitioner without delay. Simple fevers can be treated by giving the mother the following (this regime can also be used in conjunction with whatever prescription medications are being taken):

*1000-2000 mg. Vitamin C every 4 hours
*250,000 IU Beta-carotene daily, divided into 50,000 IU doses

996

　　*Echinacea tincture 2 droppersful
　　*4 Garlic capsules

　　Rotate doses every waking hour; i.e., have her take the vitamin C the first hour, Beta-carotene the second hour, Echinacea the third and Garlic the fourth. Continue until all symptoms are gone, then cut the doses in half and continue for one more week. (Bitterman, 1995) If symptoms do not improve rapidly, seek consultation with a medical practitioner.

　　Elder flower infusion is also a fever regulator. It can be mixed with equal parts of Peppermint to relieve cold symptoms and regulate the temperature. It is very safe.

References and further reading:

Bitterman, Connie, "Herbs for pregnancy and birth," ATM conf. workshop, Dallas, TX, 5/95.
Gleicher, Norbert, ed. Principles of Medical Therapy in Pregnancy, Plenum Pub., New York, 1985.

Fibroids

"Fibroid" is the popular name for benign tumors or growths which occur within the uterine cavity; they are attached to the uterus or grow within the layers of the uterine wall. Since the tumors are derived from muscle tissue, they are more accurately referred to as myomata or leiomyomata. It is estimated that 10% of white women and 30% of African American women in the United States will have a fibroid by age 30. They tend to be more common once a woman has passed her childbearing years.

Although it is possible for a woman to know of the existence of her fibroids prior to becoming pregnant, this is not always the case since the majority of fibroids tend to be asymptomatic. This is why fibroids are included here rather than in the section on preexisting medical conditions. It is estimated that only 20% to 50% of all fibroids cause symptoms. Submucous and interstitial fibroids are most likely to cause abnormally heavy menstrual bleeding when symptoms do occur. Other symptoms associated with fibroids include abnormal bleeding, pain and pressure. Fibroids are implicated in some forms of infertility, but their exact role is not clear.

Examining for fibroids: Palpation reveals one or more smooth rounded swellings which may be growing within the uterine wall. It is also possible for the tumor to be suspended within the uterine cavity on a thin stem (pediculated), if it is large enough, it can be mistaken for the fetal head or that of a suspected twin. Fibroids do not usually complicate pregnancy, however their presence may cause some women to have an increased incidence of miscarriage. If the fibroid is attached to the posterior wall of the uterus and is large enough it may become trapped within the lower pelvis as the pregnancy advances.

Types of fibroids: The location of a fibroid has some bearing on how it may impact the pregnancy and labor and upon what complications it may produce. Keep in mind that fibroids are usually asymptomatic. What follows are the different varieties of fibroids and their possible impact on pregnancy:

Cervical: located in the wall of the cervical passageway, these may produce:

> *Frequency, urgency, and urinary retention due to occlusion of the junction of the urethra and bladder
> *Pain with yoni penetration due to pressure on the fornices and shortening of the birth passageway
> *If near the lower bowel, rectal pressure or constipation
> *Obstruction of labor

Intramural (interstitial): Located in the myometrium or uterine muscle wall, these fibroids stay put as they grow and are the most common. They have a rounded shape since there is equal pressure on them from all sides. Uterine contractions can cause the tumor to be squeezed either inward or outward from its central location in the uterine muscle layer. Those pushed in toward the uterine cavity are called submucosal, those that move toward the surface of the uterus are called subserosal. Migration can cause a fibroid to become irregularly shaped and cause the point where it is attached to become long and thin, resulting in a pediculated tumor. Some interstitial fibroids may become flattened against the uterine wall so that the baby can be born. Intramural fibroids are associated with the following problems:

*If extensive, interference with contractility of the uterus in labor (and possible postpartal hemorrhage)
*Migration into subserosal or submucosal locations with related complications
*Moderate association with miscarriage

Subserosal: bulges from the uterine wall just beneath the peritoneum on the outside of the uterus. This type of interstitial fibroid may lead to:

*Torsion (twisting) of the stem, leading to tissue death & decay within the fibroid
*Adhesions to other pelvic structures
*Red degeneration (necrosis and edema) in pregnancy, which may lead to bleeding from the yoni

Miscarriage is least likely with this type of fibroid, but if a subserosal fibroid interferes with labor, it is the most problematic, as it has the least likelihood of being drawn up and out of the way by uterine contractions.

Submucosal: located beneath the endometrium and projecting into the uterine cavity, this type constitutes only 5% of all fibroids. Associated problems include:

*Torsion of the pedicle, tissue death and decay
*Severe menstrual bleeding leading to anemia
*Infection and discharge from the fibroid due to necrosis and sloughing of overlying endometrium
*Red degeneration (necrosis and edema) in pregnancy which may lead to bleeding from the yoni

Miscarriage is highest with this type of fibroid. Submucosal fibroids seem to disrupt endometrial vascularization and may distort the uterine cavity, thus impeding implantation.

Intraligamentous: a fibroid pushed into the broad ligament may develop an entirely new blood supply.

Pediculated: any fibroid which has developed a thin stem attaching it to the uterus.

Parasitic: a fibroid which has been completely extruded from the uterus and has developed an accessory blood supply.

Common problems and risk factors: Women with fibroids often complain of uterine pain during pregnancy; this may simply be due to sensitivity or it may indicate degeneration (see below). If a fibroid is located in the lower segment of the uterus or the cervix it may become situated beneath the presenting part and prevent labor from progressing. In this case fetal descent would not occur. Intrauterine fibroids can also interfere with the uterus clamping down after birth or during miscarriage, and therefore may predispose a woman to hemorrhage. Likewise, if the placenta attaches entirely or partly to a fibroid, normal placental detachment would not be likely to occur. Whether you provide care for a woman with a fibroid that has caused problems in other pregnancies will depend upon your skill and experience levels as well as the particulars of her previous problems. Asymptomatic fibroids, a normal pregnancy and normal progress during labor mean a normal outcome is more likely; however, an asymptomatic prenatal course does not rule out the possibility of placental detachment problems or postpartum hemorrhage. Women should be aware of the possible complications associated with fibroids so that they can make an informed decision regarding location of birth and choice of care provider.

Degeneration of a fibroid: Red degeneration (less commonly cystic degeneration) of larger fibroids with necrosis (tissue decay) and bleeding into the tumor, which becomes red and soft. A fibroid may undergo rapid growth due to the hormones of pregnancy. As it outgrows its available blood supply, circulatory impairment results in infarction (tissue death), irritating the uterus and leading to pain, miscarriage or premature labor. This usually occurs during the second half of pregnancy or during the postpartum period. It can cause considerable pain, local tenderness and discomfort which usually disappears within a few days. If it does not disappear or pain increases and persists during the days following its onset, the woman should be referred for a consultation with an obstetrical care provider. Surgery is rarely necessary. Degeneration is characterized by the onset of abdominal pain of all degrees of severity. Vomiting often accompanies such pain, and the temperature and pulse may be elevated. The tongue is often coated and the woman looks ill. Usually the tenderness is over the actual site of the fibroid.

Differential diagnosis: Rule out other causes of abdominal pain or enlargement (see separate chapter, this section) such as:

*Appendicitis
*Multiple gestation
*Ovarian tumor
*Double uterus
*Fibroma of the abdominal wall
*Fat
*Hematoma
*Abdominal hernia

At times it may be difficult to distinguish whether a fibroid alone is present, whether there is both a fibroid and a pregnancy or if there is just a normal pregnancy. The following points may help in your evaluation:

FIBROID	PREGNANCY
1. Normal pregnancy symptoms are absent.	1. Symptoms appear at expected times.
2. Menses are present.	2. Menses cease.
3. The fibroid is usually asymmetric or nodular.	3. The uterus is usually symmetric or characteristically shaped.
4. The fibroid is usually hard.	4. The uterus is soft.
5. Contractions of the fibroid are rare.	5. Contractions of the uterus are usual and involve the entire organ.
6. The cervix is retracted, high in the pelvis, is hard, and feels like an appendix to the fibroid.	6. The cervix is low in the pelvis, large, soft, and is part of the uterine wall.
7. Fetal heart tones are not heard.	7. In most cases fetal heart tones are audible at the usual times, unless the fibroid is obstructing auscultation.
8. Ultrasound confirms a fibroid without an accompanying pregnancy.	8. Ultrasound finds a pregnancy, with or without an accompanying fibroid.
9. All pregnancy tests are negative.	9. Pregnancy tests are positive.

Once you are sure it is a fibroid, treatment includes rest, hydration and pain relief, if necessary. Lobelia, Skullcap or Valerian tinctures may help, or Tylenol with codeine can be used if the pain is severe.

References and further reading:
Greenhill, J., Principles and Practice of Obstetrics, 10th ed., W. B. Saunders, Co., Phil., 1951.
Kolder, Veronika, editing comments, 7/95.
Lichtman, Papera Gynecology: Well-Woman Care, Appleton & Lange, East Norwalk, CT, 1990.

Foot Problems

Several factors work together to causes changes in the feet during pregnancy. Normal fluid retention plus weight gain cause the feet to widen and enlarge slightly. The hormones which soften all the tissues cause the joints in the feet to spread. Even though the swelling and weight gain will gradually be reduced after the birth and the joints will return to their approximate preconception position, this process will not always completely restore the feet to their original pre-pregnancy size and shape. Pregnancy often renders a woman's feet permanently larger by a half to a whole shoe size.

During pregnancy it is not uncommon for women to discover that their shoes are uncomfortably tight and their feet ache; standing for periods of time only makes these symptoms worse. Symptoms are compounded by wearing high heels, especially those higher than 2 inches. High heels will also make a woman's balance more precarious, as her center of gravity changes with advancing pregnancy. Therefore, recommend that women purchase shoes which have relatively flat heels and good arch support early in pregnancy to minimize such discomforts. A good pair of cloth or leather walking shoes or Birkenstock type shoes is ideal. Shoes should be tried on at the time of day when the feet are most swollen to give a better idea of correct fit. For some women, more shoes of a larger size will have to be purchased later in pregnancy.

Soaking achy feet in bath salts such as Bath Therapy brand will also help considerably in easing acute foot discomfort. Hot foot baths of celery seed infusion (a few tablespoons of seeds to 2 quarts of boiling water, steeped half an hour; this can be refrigerated, reheated and reused) is also reported to be helpful (Hartley, 1994). Following the bath, the woman should prop her feet up for 20 minutes. Propping her feet can also be done at work during breaks or at lunch time.

Orthotic inserts are also available. These special supports are inserted into the shoes to reduce foot, back and leg pain. They are available in two different sizes, one for the first six months of pregnancy and a second to be used during the last trimester. Check for them at a local surgical supply store.

Loose house shoes or slippers which are worn while at home may also reduce foot fatigue for some women. In most cases, wearing the correct shoes along with avoiding standing for long periods of time will solve or at least minimize foot problems.

"Nervous feet": Fidgety extremities may be due to anemia or mineral deficiencies. Investigate this further. (Scholles, 1995)

References and further reading:
Hartley, Carla, midwife & educator, founder of Ancient Arts Midwifery Institute, P.O. Box 788, Claremore, OK, 74018, editing comments, December, 1994.
Scholles, Holly, licensed midwife, Portland, OR, editing comments, 1/95.

Gestational Diabetes

Gestational diabetes is a term used for decreased glucose tolerance during pregnancy. It became a clinical entity in 1979. Prior to that time pregnant women were evaluated for diabetes according to standards set for the non-pregnant population. After 1979 a special range of glucose levels began to be used during pregnancy. The creation of this scale and of the category known as gestational diabetes is very controversial because the research it is based on used oral glucose tolerance tests (OGTT) with no dietary histories taken into account. In addition, study populations included such confounding variables as women with previous poor pregnancy outcomes or risk factors in their current pregnancy as well as mixing in women known to be diabetics and then comparing their outcomes with the general population, thus thoroughly obscuring the true risk of various glucose levels in pregnancy (Goer, 1995). It was determined that women in certain blood sugar ranges had an increased risk of developing diabetes later in life, but careful comparison of the data has found that the baby is at no greater risk (Chalmers, 1989). In fact, the only fetal variable of any significance is that the baby may be 8 lb. 13 oz. or larger, however race, age, parity and maternal weight have far more impact on fetal weight than does "gestational diabetes" (Keen, 1991; Green et.al., 1991; Farmer et.al., 1988) Furthermore, the test used for screening in pregnancy is a random oral glucose tolerance test after a 50 g. glucose load. If positive, a 3 hour OGTT is done which not only requires fasting, but is notoriously inaccurate (Chalmers, 1989).

If gestational diabetes is diagnosed, the medical profession will view a woman as high risk. A huge epidemiological research project which culminated in the publication of Effective Care During Pregnancy and Birth concluded that routine blood glucose screening using OGTTs in pregnancy should be abandoned; random glucose readings on clients is the only recommended action (no glucose load, no fasting). The only correlate of significance is that women diagnosed with gestational diabetes are at higher risk for developing overt diabetes later in life. Limiting refined sugar and other refined carbohydrate intake, as midwives advise anyway, is a prudent step in reducing her risk. However, this protocol has not filtered down to the average bio-technical clinician.

The pros and cons should be explained to each client so that she can make her own decision regarding testing. If she decides in favor of testing, discuss the screening procedure outlined in the chapter on Urine Tests Results under Glucosuria as a possible alternative to screening with an OGTT.

If glucose screening is desired for any reason, first test a first-morning blood sugar after an overnight fast (not an extended fast) without any special dietary adjustments. This is the most accurate way to screen for a true problem; a finger-prick test should be less than 120. If this value is high or borderline, next perform a two hour postprandial test:

*Three days of carbohydrate loading with complex carbohydrates, to
    equal a total of 150 grams daily (no sugar or white flour)
*Fast 8 to 12 hours
*Obtain fasting blood sugar (finger prick should be less than 120 mg/dl)
*Eat a large breakfast of foods normally ingested
*Engage in 45 minutes of exercise such as walking between tests
*Obtain another sample at 2 hours (should be less than 140 mg/dl)

Giving a woman a concentrated refined sugar load before testing is not recommended; she can have a physiological reaction to the glucose overload which can mimic diabetes (called starvation diabetes). This is a shock reaction, not true diabetes. When the pancreas is presented with an unusually high glucose load, insulin is not produced fast enough to compensate. A temporary pseudodiabetes results, causing test results to be abnormally high. When the pancreas catches up and an insulin surge brings the blood glucose level down, this rebound effect actually demonstrates hypoglycemia. The time it takes for this to occur varies, but a 1 to 3 hour OGTT may not be long enough to detect a delayed rebound effect. This is the reason 5 to 6 hour OGTTs have been used to diagnose hypoglycemia.

Other factors that can skew results include infections, lack of exercise, poor diet, smoking, caffeine intake and fear or anxiety. Some people have abnormal results in the morning, but are normal if retested in the afternoon. All interfering factors should be removed or cleared up at least three days prior to testing. See Diagnostic Tests for a full discussion of diabetes and pregnancy.

Pregnant women who do show glucose intolerance are often those with a family history of diabetes and a genetic tendency for their estrogen to bond to insulin in the presence of B$_6$ deficiency. These women often respond dramatically to 100 mg doses of B$_6$ three times daily which uncouples the estrogen and allows the insulin to be utilized. Because of the deficiency, this regime can be safely continued throughout pregnancy. (Wright, 1995)

References and further reading:

Brewer G: The Brewer Medical Diet for Normal and High Risk Pregnancies, Simon & Schuster, New York, 1983.

Chalmers I, et al: Effective Care in Pregnancy and Birth, Oxford U. Press, 1989.

Farmer, G. et al: The influence of maternal glucose metabolism on fetal growth, development and morbidity in 917 singleton pregnancies to nondiabetic women; Diabetologia, Vol. 31 1988, pp. 134-141.

Goer H: Obstetric Myths versus Research Realities, Bergin & Garvey, Boston, MA 1995.

Green J; et al: Influence of maternal body habits and glucose tolerance on birth weight, Ob Gyn, Vol. 78, No. 2, 1991, pp. 235-240.

Keen H: Gestational diabetes, Can epidemiology help? Diabetes, 40:s2:3, 1991.

Wright, J: Lecture on clinical nutrition, Conf. Amer. Assoc. Naturopathic Physicians, Snowmass, CO, with ref. to Adele Davis, 1995.

Headaches

Headaches can be divided into three major categories.

- ***Vascular headaches** occur from persistent vasodilation of the intracranial vessels due to disturbed vascular tone. Migraines are the most common type of vascular headache, and are discussed in the section on Medical Conditions Which May Preexist Pregnancy.
- ***Muscle contraction headaches** or tension headaches commonly manifest cranial sensations of a tight band or neck pain.
- ***Traction and inflammatory headaches** arise from disorders that involve pain-sensitive intracranial structures such as the meninges, blood vessels and the periosteum of the skull. This type should be suspected in those who have persistent headaches which are not relieved by analgesics. If fever, elevated white count and neck stiffness are noted, assume meningitis and advise a cerebral spinal fluid examination without delay. Those with neurologic signs or convulsions associated with headaches may have a tumor or bleeding from an arteriovenous malformation in the brain and should be evaluated accordingly. Mental confusion or coma may accompany these headaches.

Common causes of headache in pregnancy: Two primary causes of headache in pregnancy are hypoglycemia and dehydration. These can be easily remedied by eating small amounts of food frequently throughout the day and drinking a glass of water every two to three hours. If the headache is currently occurring, recommend eating, drinking and sleeping it off. Simultaneously soaking the hands and feet in hot lemon water may help (Hartley, 1994). Anemia may also cause headaches, since less oxygen is getting to the brain. Headaches associated with visual disturbances may be due to eye strain, especially in cases where the vision is altered due to normal fluid retention from the pregnancy. Headaches are often the result of exposure to toxins (insecticides, pollution), smoking or dietary intake of coffee, chocolate, or sugar. Exposure as well as withdrawal from offending substances can cause headaches. Recent onset of headaches, especially those in the front of the head or those which recur regularly, are more concerning, as these kinds of headaches are often related to toxemia.

Here are some questions to ask concerning headache symptoms:

Have you ever had headaches like these before? This is, by far, the best gauge of whether this symptom is a relatively benign aggravation or a new manifestation which you need to be worried about. Headaches which do not differ in their character, frequency or duration from before pregnancy and which were present for some time prior to pregnancy are not "fine," but are probably not symptomatic of serious underlying problems. Make notes of how the headache feels, frequency, etc. to get a baseline (if not already obtained during the initial exam). Be sure bowel movements are regular, and discuss possible allergens (dietary and environmental), stress levels and emotional concerns (headaches represent energy blockages and are often emotionally related). If the headaches are just the same as they have always been and the woman is not concerned about them, provide support, suggest rest and other palliative remedies as described above, but do not worry about them. Homeopathic remedies and delving into the emotional factors which surround the onset of such headaches may help to get to the bottom of the pattern and alleviate them entirely.

If the headaches have appeared for the first time during pregnancy, ask the following questions as well:

What does the headache feel like, where is the pain? The sudden onset of an uncharacteristic, severe headache may be a warning sign of a severe underlying problem. Follow the woman closely for accompanying symptoms. If the headache and other symptoms (especially neurological), become progressively worse, get a medical evaluation without delay. Throbbing headaches could be due to tension, but may more rarely be due to the imminent rupture of an intracranial blood vessel, especially if the throbbing becomes increasingly severe.

How frequent are the headaches? Headaches which have appeared for the first time during pregnancy and which are getting worse or closer together may mean there is an underlying problem. Get it checked out! Women with persistent headaches of recent onset after the 24th week must be evaluated for toxemia.

Are there associated symptoms? Nasal congestion, emotional stress, eye strain, fatigue, unexpressed anger and the need to have more time and space to herself can all precipitate headaches. Vomiting, edema of the optic nerve and hypertension may accompany pseudotumor cerebri (see chapter on Hypertension, this section, for more details).

References and further reading:

Bates, Barbara, A Guide to Physical Examination, 5th ed., J.B. Lippincott Co., Philadelphia, PA, 1991.

Donald, Ian, Practical Obstetric Problems, Lloyd-Luke, Ltd., London, Eng., 1979.

Gleicher, Norbert, ed. Principles of Medical Therapy in Pregnancy, Plenum Pub., New York, 1985.

Hartley, Carla, midwife educator, Ancient Arts Midwifery Institute, P.O. Box 788, Claremore, OK, 74018, editing comments, December, 1994.

HEADACHE	LOCATION	SEVERITY	ONSET	ASSOCIATED SYMPTOMS	AGGRAVATING FACTORS	RELIEVING FACTORS
Tension	Usually bilateral, may be all over or in the back of the head & upper neck or the frontotemporal area	Mild & aching or nonpainful tightness & pressure	Gradual	Anxiety, tension, depression	Sustained muscular tension, emotional stress	Variable
Migraine	Frontal, temporal, occipital or generalized, often one-sided	Throbbing or aching, variable severity	Rapid, peaking in 1-2 hrs.	Nausea & vomiting; may be preceded by visual or neurologic disturbances	Alcohol, some foods, tension, noise & bright light	Quiet, dark room, sleep
Eye strain (more rarely Glaucoma)	Around & over eyes; may radiate from occipital area	Steady, aching	Gradual	Eye fatigue, sandy feeling in eyes, redness	Prolonged use of eyes, esp. for close work; computer monitors that flicker; visual alterations	Rest of the eyes; have vision assessed
Sinus	Above the eye	Aching, throbbing variable	Variable	Local tenderness, nasal congestion, discharge & fever	Coughing, sneezing, jarring the head	Nasal decon- gestants
Toxemia	Usually generalized but may be isolated in the occipital or occasionally the frontal area	Often severe	Persistent	Contracted blood volume, dehydration; caused by poor diet!		Increase protein, salt, calories & fluids now!

Hemoglobin Variations

A full discussion of the varieties of anemia, testing and interpretation of results can be found in <u>Diagnostic Tests</u>. This chapter provides an overview of how one might approach anemia in the clinical setting.

A hemoglobin of 12.5 or higher is considered normal in the first trimester. A drop of at least 2 grams is expected by the 28th to 30th week of pregnancy, reflecting adequate blood volume expansion. A greater drop may be seen with multiple pregnancies.

Low hemoglobin: A hemoglobin of 12 or less before 20 weeks necessitates evaluation and therapy. Evaluation may include:

>   *Review of the diet
>   *Physical exam and questions regarding signs and symptoms of
>   problems
>   *Lab analysis, as indicated which may include:
>   -Hemoglobin, hematocrit
>   -Reticulocyte count
>   -Peripheral blood smear
>   -Red blood cell indices
>   -Serum iron, TIBC, % saturation
>   -PRBC folate, serum folate
>   -Quantitative electrophoresis
>   -B_{12} levels

In general therapy may include:

>   *Nettle leaf infusion dark green vegetables, prunes, grape juice,
>   organic iron supplements, Yellow Dock tincture

In cases of a low reading, a slight rise or stabilization of the count may indicate improvement due to hemodilution and fetal storage. You may see a dramatic rise in the TIBC and serum iron levels before the hemoglobin starts to rise. However, when supplementation is being well absorbed basic lab work will show a response in 5 to 7 days, therefore, following the hemoglobin and hematocrit will be sufficient in most cases. Anemia appearing to be non-nutritional in origin should be evaluated and treated, as appropriate.

High or rising hemoglobin: A rising hemoglobin in the absence of intensive nutritional therapy for diagnosed anemia should be considered an ominous sign reflecting hemoconcentration until this is ruled out. The following steps should be taken, as indicated:

*Review dietary intake and make changes as necessary
*Assess fetal growth
*Perform SMA-12 (liver profile) as indicated
*Review fluid intake and adjust as appropriate
*See the chapter on Toxemia in the section on problems that can occur
    in the Third Trimester for more information.

Caring for women living at high altitudes: Since the oxygen content of the air is reduced the higher up you go, women who live above approximately 5,000 feet elevation will respond to the reduction in oxygen concentration with generally higher hemoglobin levels that remain high throughout pregnancy. The approximate changes you should see mid-pregnancy are described below:

ALTITUDE	EXPECTED HEMOGLOBIN DROP BY 28 TO 30 WEEKS
Less than 5,000 feet	2 grams
5,000 to 8,000 feet	1 to 1.5 grams
Over 8,000 feet	Slight drop or none at all

The higher the altitude, the less of a drop you are likely to see. Therefore, rely on liver profile results, especially albumin levels and liver enzyme values, to monitor for adequate blood volume expansion in these women. (Braun, 1994)

References and further reading:

Braun, Jennifer, CDEM, Colorado Midwive's Assoc. meeting and workshop, April 1994.

Laryngeal Disorders

Hoarseness: Hoarseness (laryngopathica gravidarum) may be noted during pregnancy.   Temporary changes in the laryngeal mucosa consisting of edema, mucosal drying and sometimes crusting may be caused by fluid retention.   Such changes or the vocal changes described below may also predispose a woman to coughing.

More seriously, laryngeal edema may cause airway restriction.   In the very few cases on record, some had to be relieved with tracheotomies.   If hoarseness is progressive with increasing airway restriction, the possibility of this crisis needs to be anticipated.   Homeopathic remedies should be used to balance the situation before crisis occurs.

Voice alterations: Changes in voice quality (dysphonia) include breathiness, deepening of the voice, difficulty with high notes, cracking of tones, vocal weakness, and the rapid sequential production of at least two sounds resulting from vibration of the false vocal cords which produces rough, grunting, or groaning sounds.   Examination of the throat reveals red and swollen vocal cords with vascular dilation and small submucosal hemorrhages.   Singers frequently experience such changes during their menstrual cycles and in pregnancy.   Advise women to avoid straining their voices to prevent permanent damage.   Barring underlying disease, these changes are temporary and the voice should return to normal after the birth.   Women should be advised to have the condition evaluated if it has never been noted in relation to their menstrual cycles.   A homeopathic remedy prescribed for the woman's individual symptoms should provide some relief.

Airway distress: Difficult breathing commonly occurs during pregnancy as pressure from the uterus restricts movement of the diaphragm.   Singers may need to compensate by altering their breath control accordingly.

References and further reading:

Gleicher, Norbert, ed. Principles of Medical Therapy in Pregnancy, Plenum Pub., New York, 1985.

Hypertension in Pregnancy

The definition of hypertension in pregnancy:

Before 1972 the definition of hypertension in pregnancy was a pressure of 140/90 or higher on at least two occasions, six hours apart. In 1972 the definition was changed to any rise in the baseline systolic pressure of 30 points or more and/or a rise in the baseline diastolic pressure of 15 points or more on two occasions at least 6 hours apart. (The two readings stipulation has been ignored in many practices). The redefinition of hypertension in pregnancy placed many healthy women into a new high risk category. The 18th edition (1989) of William's Obstetrics reports that the "30/15" criteria mentioned above "is vague and clinically useless." It recommends returning to 140/90 as the cutoff for diagnosing hypertension in pregnancy. Since I always felt the 30/15 definition was contrived anyway, I recommend the 140/90 cutoff point as well.

Interpreting blood pressure readings:

It is normal for the blood pressure to vary widely (de Sweit, 1984). Start prenatal care as soon as possible to get a relative baseline of vital signs. Take the blood pressure after the woman has relaxed from her trip to the appointment, waiting at least 15 to 20 minutes into the visit. Keep in mind that normal people often have wide variations in their blood pressure; readings taken just a few minutes apart can be very different.

Dr. Kevin Dalton's research at the University of Cambridge, England, (1989) showed that this variability occurs during normal pregnancy as well. He attached portable blood pressure monitors to normal, healthy women. Blood pressure was assessed at one-minute intervals throughout the day. He found that the systolic pressure fluctuated up to 40 points and that diastolic readings fluctuated as much as 22 points. This range might be seen in a 10 minute period even when the woman was asleep! He found an average fluctuation between 20 to 30 mmHg. within a ten minute period. This supports the research done by Madalene Sawyer (1981), which showed variability of 20 to 40 mmHg. systolic and 15 to 30 mmHg. diastolic within a 15 minute period in normotensive, hypertensive, *and* toxemic women.

Low blood pressure: Low readings such as 90/60 are often seen in young women, vegetarians, and women who exercise regularly. Adequate blood volume expansion may be reflected by a slight drop beginning about 16 weeks; this is a good sign! Sometimes very low blood pressure presents a problem. Symptoms include nausea, dizziness on rising, fainting, visual disturbances, and breathlessness with exertion.

Anemia may be an underlying cause. Exercise, rising slowly, and correcting hypoglycemia or anemia will all help if the problem is low blood pressure.

High blood pressure: Benign blood pressure elevations in a well-nourished woman may be due to any of the following:

*Anxiety, or simply a harried trip to the appointment. Stress factors and ways to alleviate them should be discussed.

*Multiple gestation and the accompanying extra blood volume.

*Technical errors: review the instructions in the chapter on The Physical Examination (Skills section) and recheck later in the visit.

*Lack of salt in an otherwise well-nourished woman. This can cause edema as well as high blood pressure. Be sure she is salting to taste and using more if she is perspiring (i.e. in hot weather). Just two weeks of less-than-adequate salt intake causes the blood volume to begin to fall, even if all other dietary intake is adequate.

*Inadequate calcium, magnesium or B_6 intake. (Loprenzi-Kassel, 1995)

*Inadequate dietary or fluid intake; review the diet carefully and make necessary adjustments.

*Obesity is often associated with high readings due to an inaccurately sized cuff. However, if the properly sized cuff shows that a higher reading is correct and the diet is good, this alone is no cause for concern.

*Lack of exercise may also be a factor, particularly in women-of-size. (Schlinger, 1995)

If you get a high reading with the women upright, have her lie on her left side for the second reading (use her right arm to check the blood pressure). Many practitioners feel that a reading taken with the woman lying on her left side is the most accurate gauge of the blood pressure in pregnancy (if this reading is within normal limits, relax!). (Luce, 1990) Also remember that the fifth phase reading (very last sound) is the most significant diastolic pressure (unless the fifth phase reading goes down to zero, in that case the fourth phase reading is more significant). Be sure to take this into account when judging your findings.

The systolic reading is especially sensitive to a woman's stress level. Often the systolic pressure is elevated but the diastolic pressure is roughly within the usual range when a woman's stress level is high. This is a perfectly normal variation and nothing to be concerned about.

If you detect a high reading at one visit and *don't make a big deal of it*, it will usually be back down in a visit or two. Sometimes this elevation may extend over the course of several visits, then, just as suddenly, drop back down; I have often seen this in practice. Or you may see a fluctuating blood pressure from visit to visit, which reflects a labile state. I have also seen women spike a blood

1012

pressure and keep it high, seemingly more in response to her caregiver's distress over the reading than due to any problem of her own. Women are frequently risked-out of homebirth over what amounts to a completely benign finding.

Labile blood pressure: Some women have labile (rapidly changing) blood pressure. Readings rise significantly with stress or anxiety. Sometimes this manifests during medical examinations ("white coat hypertension"), during an exceptionally busy day, or even with the excitement surrounding the onset of labor. Wait until late in the visit to check the blood pressure, after the woman has had a chance to relax. If it is high, recheck it a bit later with the client lying on her left side. You will usually see a drop; if you do then you can be sure all is well if she is otherwise fine. If it remains high, you can either not worry about it, secure in the knowledge that her diet is good, or you can have someone check her blood pressure at home. This will often reveal a lower reading than you see at visits.

Essential hypertension: Essential hypertension results from no known cause and commonly appears with age. However, it is also particularly common among young African American women. The definition of hypertension is an artificial cut-off point and what is defined as "high blood pressure" may not be a problem in an individual. The threshold for diagnosing hypertension in pregnancy is a reading of 140/90 during the first half of pregnancy; this identifies less than 2% of all women. In the second half of pregnancy 21.6% will exceed this limit at least once. Essential hypertension may be diagnosed before pregnancy or reveal itself during pregnancy. After all, when, other than in pregnancy, is a woman having her blood pressure checked all the time?

The lower limit of 140/90 defines mild hypertension and 170/110 or greater defines severe hypertension. Hypertension of 170/110 reflects a mean arterial pressure of 130 mmHg, the level at which acute vascular damage may occur. The risk of hemorrhagic stroke exists when the blood pressure exceeds the range of vascular autoregulation. (de Sweit, 1984)

Hypertension need not be treated unless it rises to 170/110 or more. The purpose of treating mid-range hypertension (140 to 170 systolic and 90 to 110 diastolic) is to prevent long term complications which are not relevant for the short term of pregnancy. However, mainstream practitioners often do recommend treatment of hypertension reaching 160/110 or higher. Their management includes antihypertensive drugs and, in pregnancy, often low salt, low calorie diets and diuretics. Such management has, predictably created higher risk pregnancies with accompanying poor outcomes. Drugs should be avoided whenever possible. Methyldopa, a widely used drug in the United States, reduces uterine contractibility as well as contributing to platelet malfunction and other problems (see HELLP syndrome in the chapter on The Clotting Mechanism in Diagnostic Tests). *Beta*-blockers, which slow heart rate, also affect the lungs by causing bronchiole constriction.

Many medical practitioners now advocate no pharmaceutical treatment unless the diastolic pressure exceeds 110 mmHg. Electrocardiogram and optic fundus (retinal) exam will help determine if organ damage has begun. Proteinuria and impaired creatinine clearance point to renal damage which may underlie hypertension. Sporadic episodes of hypertension may call for checking catecholamine levels to exclude pheochromocytoma (a rare adrenal gland tumor which can produce dangerous hypertension in pregnancy). (de Sweit, 1984)

The impact of hypertension on pregnancy: About 85% of women with essential hypertension have normal pregnancies with successful outcomes. They show the normal 5 to 10 mmHg (or sometimes more) reduction in diastolic pressure by the 16th week of gestation followed by a steady rise toward pre-pregnancy values by the end of the third trimester. Women whose blood pressure fails to fall in early pregnancy do less well; this appears to correlate with longstanding hypertension. Complications such as intrauterine growth retardation are also more likely in those with chronic hypertension and those with organ damage related to longstanding hypertension or when hypertension is a secondary sign of toxemia.

Maternal hypertension is commonly blamed for low-birth-weight infants. British studies (Boyd, 1985) show that hypertensive women with no complicating factors who are undrugged and on unrestricted diets grow big, healthy placentas and babies! The report saw such a beneficial difference in these pregnancies that they labeled them a "favored population!" These women do not become high risk when they maintain an adequate diet. To declare hypertension benign, you must make certain that the woman has been eating and salting sufficiently with adequate absorption, that she is drinking to thirst and that no underlying medical conditions exist. If so, you can usually relax. The following remedies can help when hypertension results from a benign cause:

*Relaxation techniques can be used several times daily and the lifestyle modified as much as possible to reduce stress and anxiety.
*Strong spices: especially mustard, black and white pepper, ginger, and nutmeg should be avoided.
*A number of foods and herbs help to reduce simple hypertension:
-Watermelon and buckwheat
-Raw garlic, parsley and onions in large quantities. Garlic oil capsules, 2 to 10 daily, have worked for some women.
-Cucumber — 1/2 cup of fresh juice or a whole fresh one daily. Overripe, yellowish cucumbers are the most effective.
-Juice of half of a fresh lemon or lime plus 2 tsp. cream of tarter in half a cup of water, once daily for 3 days. This can be repeated once after a rest of 2 days.
-Hops tea (1 tsp. to 1 cup boiling water steeped 20 min.) can be safely and effectively used nightly during the last 4

months of pregnancy. (Hormonal precursors contraindicate
its use during the first 5 months.)
-Passion flower (2 to 4 capsules daily, or 15 drops of tincture 3
times daily; must be taken for several weeks to obtain the best
result.)
-Skullcap infusion (1 oz. to 1 qt. boiling water; cover and
steep 4 to 6 hours) 1 to 2 cups daily; builds and strengthens
the nervous system.
-Hawthorn berries work cumulatively to strengthen the heart
and is said to help ameliorate and prevent congenital heart
defects. (1 oz. crushed dry berries in 2 cups cold water
steeped overnight, brought quickly to a boil, strained and
sipped, 1 cup daily. Tincture dosage is 15 drops 2 to 3
times daily.)
-Fenugreek seed infusion (1 oz. to 1 pint boiling water, steep
½ hour). Start with ½ cup daily.
*Vitamin supplements containing magnesium, calcium, and potassium
in a balanced formula.
*Moderate exercise can be very beneficial. Apart from providing
relaxation and sparing calories, bed rest is useless, although widely
recommended!
*As always, be sure fluid intake is adequate throughout the day;
recommend an 8 oz. glass of clear fluid every 2 to 3 hours or so.

Serious causes of hypertension:

Other medical conditions causing high blood pressure may make their
appearance prior to or at any time during pregnancy. Such conditions include:

Benign intracranial hypertension (pseudotumor cerebri): This self-limited
condition of pregnancy occurs in women in their 20s and 30s and is often seen with
obesity. It usually presents between the second and fifth month of pregnancy and
often disappears after birth. It presents with headache, vomiting and edema of the
optic nerve. Overproduction or underabsorption of cerebrospinal fluid is the
pathophysiologic abnormality; the cause is unknown. If edema and visual
compromise are severe, hospitalization with steroids, bed rest and diuretics will be
recommended by mainstream providers but care must be taken not to compromise
the blood volume in doing so. Homeopathic remedies offer a safer option for
dealing with symptoms but must be prescribed on an individual basis.

Metabolic toxemia is the most serious pregnancy-induced cause of hypertension,
and it is preventable with a good diet. No drop or a slight rise in blood pressure

around the 28th week may be a tip off to problems (but do not use this as your only criteria!). Hypertension is not necessarily an early sign of true toxemia. Once toxemia is established, high blood pressure may appear, but other problems such as the mother feeling unwell, a rising hemoglobin, and poor fetal growth will already be apparent.

The pathophysiology of toxemic hypertension is simple: the body is trying to nourish an entire extra organ (the placenta with fetus attached) without sufficient blood volume to do so. Inadequate expansion or a drop in blood volume causes the body to respond as if a hemorrhage has occurred. The kidneys secrete renin, which triggers blood vessel constriction. In a true hemorrhage, renin temporarily raises the blood pressure to provide sufficient blood flow to sustain vital organs. In toxemia, the blood pressure may remain high because the blood volume does not normalize. The kidneys also attempt to increase the blood volume by reabsorbing water and salt and returning it to the circulation; as reabsorption increases, urine excretion falls off. However, since there isn't enough intake of albumin and salt to hold the fluid in the circulating blood volume, it leaks into the tissues, producing pathological edema. The kidneys step up water reabsorption, fluid keeps filtering out into tissues and renin production increases, pushing the blood pressure up even more. Pathological weight gain occurs as more and more fluid is retained. (based on Jones, 1989)

An individual woman may compensate for her contracted blood volume for a long time before her blood pressure rises. Some women may be severely toxemic and never manifest high blood pressure until immediately before or even after the onset of convulsions. This is the danger of trying to make any single secondary symptom the criteria for diagnosis.

If hypertension is due to toxemia, the diet needs immediate attention (see chapter on Toxemia, Third Trimester section). Increase her protein, salt, calories, and be sure she is drinking to thirst. A more thorough evaluation is in order: Is she having digestive or assimilation problems such as nausea, vomiting, diarrhea, or preexisting colon or stomach trouble? Is there unrecognized liver weakness from previous disease? Is she under unusual stress that increases her nutrient needs? These things need correction so that she can maintain a healthy pregnancy.

High blood pressure readings due to toxemia will tend to fluctuate throughout the day. In true toxemic hypertension the high blood pressure itself causes arterial wall damage. A concentrated blood volume promotes abnormal platelet aggravation in the vessels, thus narrowing the channels and increasing the blood pressure even more.

Headaches and blurred vision may occur with or without hypertension. These are symptoms of pressure and vessel constriction in the brain and often precede convulsions. Placental abruption may occur as high blood pressure pushes a poorly attached placenta with clotted blood pooled beneath it away from the uterine wall. True toxemia-induced hypertension is very dangerous and needs to be ruled out! An SMA-12, (also called a Chem screen or Liver profile) a hemoglobin value, evaluation of fetal growth and a careful dietary and stress history will assist in differential diagnosis.

Some bio-technical practitioners are recommending aspirin for toxemia-related hypertension out of the recognition that platelet aggregation (clumping) occurs in some toxemic women. This abnormal clotting is enhanced by a contracted blood volume. (An unexamined possibility is that severe clotting malfunction may actually be precipitated by the increased stress from drugs prescribed for hypertension prior to the onset of clotting compromise.) The cure is not in artificially thinning the blood, but in adequate volume expansion through dietary improvement. (For further information refer to Thrombocytopenia and toxemia in the chapter on The Clotting Mechanism and Bleeding Disorders and the section on HELLP syndrome in the chapter on The Liver and Pregnancy in Diagnostic Tests.)

Conn's syndrome (primary hyperaldosteronism): This is a rare cause of hypertension and is diagnosed on the basis of hypokalemia (potassium deficiency) combined with hypertension. Successful pregnancies have been reported with and without treatment.

Kidney disease, cysts, and tumors can cause elevated blood pressure readings, with values that remain consistent throughout the day. If a woman has a history of kidney problems, she should be checked by a renal specialist before becoming pregnant. Kidney compromise may cause proteinuria. If renal disease is suspected during pregnancy, be sure an accurate differential diagnosis is made, since kidney disease can have serious consequences. In the past, toxemia has been considered a kidney malfunction because symptoms are superficially similar. (See chapter on Toxemia later in this section and the chapter on The Liver Profile Test in Diagnostic Tests for details.)

If an asymptomatic kidney infection is discovered, an infusion of Uva Ursi leaf can be taken daily for 10 days (seek antibiotic treatment if symptoms appear). Non-sugar cranberry juice and increased vitamin C will also help clear infections. To strengthen damaged kidneys, Nettle leaf infusion can be taken 2 cups daily or as desired, throughout pregnancy.

Heart problems that limit physical activity make a woman higher risk due to the extra stress placed on the heart by blood volume expansion. If a woman reaches the 30th week without severe symptoms (after blood volume peaks), she will probably make it to term without problems. Rarely, a heart condition causes the blood volume to be abnormally expanded outside of pregnancy. This is one occasion when a low salt diet and diuretics may be needed during pregnancy as well. Even so, careful monitoring is important to maintain adequate blood volume for pregnancy. Such a woman usually cannot birth at home; evaluate based upon the actual problem. Hawthorn berry infusion (as mentioned above) can help with any heart problem.

Pheochromocytoma is a rare, benign adrenal gland tumor. This is, however, very dangerous in pregnancy, causing extreme, unstable hypertension, sweating, facial flushing, apprehension, nausea and vomiting, palpitations, proteinuria and toxemic symptoms such as headaches. Fetal and maternal death rates are reported to be as high as 50%. If you suspect this rare and serious disorder seek medical consultation immediately. Treatment with *alpha*-adrenergic blockade drugs can help improve maternal survival. (For more information see the chapter on Adrenal Function in Diagnostic Tests.)

Lupus erythematosus: Lupus can mimic toxemia; its symptoms can be so subtle that it often goes undiagnosed for quite a while. Edema, hypertension, proteinuria and seizures are all symptoms of Lupus. In addition, mental manifestations may resemble postpartum psychosis. Autoantibody tests will help to clarify the situation. (For more information see the chapter on Lupus in Diagnostic Tests.) Other connective tissue disorders such as polyarteritis nodosa and scleroderma, may produce hypertension as well.

Cerebral and other vascular disturbances can be life threatening and are rarely asymptomatic. Elevated blood pressure can cause a vessel to rupture in the brain or can dislodge a clot. Sudden, severe or throbbing headaches, visual or neurological disturbances need immediate assessment. High blood pressure in combination with varicose veins is especially concerning. Heavy support stockings are worth the investment to ensure that the veins receive adequate support. This minimizes venous blood pooling and consequent clotting during pregnancy, in labor, and after birth.

Hyperthyroidism needs regulation before and during pregnancy, when the thyroid is stimulated to even greater activity. If holistic treatment is desired, an experienced naturopath can help monitor levels and help them remain normal throughout the prenatal period. (See chapter on Thyroid Function in Diagnostic Tests for more details.)

Central nervous system disorders such as brain tumor, epilepsy, or stroke can cause high blood pressure. Epileptics may want to change anti-seizure medication prior to pregnancy, while all have side effects, some are strongly contraindicated due to teratogenic effects. Some epileptics may choose to stop taking anti-seizure medications before pregnancy, replacing them with dietary and herbal means to regulate and strengthen their nervous system. Skullcap or Passion flower infusion can be especially helpful, as well as a macrobiotic diet. An experienced naturopath can be used as a consultant both prior to and during pregnancy.

1018

Hydatidiform mole is a placental malformation that can cause toxemic symptoms, high blood pressure, uterine growth that is large-for-dates, bleeding, and vomiting. An exceedingly high level of the placental hormone human Chorionic Gonadotropin (hCG), will be present in the blood and urine. (See chapter on Hydatidiform or Vesicular Mole in the section on Problems Associated With the First Trimester.)

Malignant hypertension is extreme, fulminating high blood pressure that is often deadly and of undetermined cause. Herbs, as mentioned, probably won't hurt, but medical supervision is definitely indicated.

Liver disease unrelated to toxemia is sometimes associated with high blood pressure. Even if the liver is supplied with adequate nutrients, if function is compromised it may not be able to meet the increased demands of pregnancy. The liver needs as much support before and during pregnancy as possible to minimize problems. Spring Dandelion Root tincture (half a dropperful 4 times daily) can be used to strengthen the liver. If this seems too strong (which may be indicated by liver tenderness), switching to Yellow Dock root tincture is a good second choice. Choline (500 mg. daily) along with a B-complex supplement will also help support and heal the liver.

As you can see from the above list, high blood pressure is often a secondary symptom of an underlying problem for which the vascular system is trying to compensate. Attending to the root problem will usually result in a normalization of the blood pressure. If a woman is eating and absorbing her food well, you can rule out toxemia and continue to look for the real cause of her distress. Don't hesitate to seek medical help as necessary.

References and further reading:

Boyd, Patricia & Scott, A., "Quantitative Structural Studies on Human Placentas Associated with Pre-eclampsia, Essential Hypertension, and Intrauterine Growth Retardation," British J of Ob & Gyn, Vol. 92, July, 1985 pp. 714-721.

Dalton, Kevin, J., MD, "Home telemetry: a need for reassessment of PET," report presented at the Royal College of Medicine, London, UK Sept. 15, 1989.

Jones, J, "The Brewer Pregnancy Diet," handout published by Perinatal Support Services, 715 Monroe St., Evanston, IL 60202, single copy 50 cents, 1989.

Loprenzi-Kassel, ClareBeth, midwife, Veneta, OR, editing comments, 2/95.

deSweit, Micheal, edl. Cptr 6: Hypertension in Pregnancy, Medical disorders in Obstetric Practice, by C. Redman, Blackwell Scientific Pub., Oxford, Eng., 1984

Sawyer, Madaline, et.al., "Diurnal & Short Term Variation of Blood Pressure: Comparison of Preeclamptic, Chronic Hypertensive & Normotensive Patients," Obstetrics & Gynecology, 58:3, Sept. 1981, pp. 291-6.

Injuries During Pregnancy

The most common causes of serious maternal injury during pregnancy are car accidents, falls and physical abuse. Serious accidents cause the death of the fetus far more often than the death of the mother; medical evaluation and treatment can be vital to the well-being of both.

The effects on the fetus: The effect of maternal trauma on the fetus depends upon the type and severity of the trauma, the gestational age of the fetus and the extent of disruption of normal uterine and fetal physiology. During the first week after fertilization the conceptus has not implanted in the uterine wall and is relatively resistant to traumatic stimuli. Once implanted, traumatic disruption of the placental villi can cause placental abruption and the death of the fetus. The uterus is relatively protected in its position behind the pubic bone before the 12th week of pregnancy. As the pregnancy advances, the symphysis pubis, sacral promontory and spinal column can strike the enlarging uterus during trauma.

Fetal survival depends on adequate profusion of the placenta with oxygen and is directly related to the mother's systemic blood pressure. If the mother goes into hypovolemic shock, vasoconstriction further compromises uterine perfusion. In a normal pregnancy, the fetus has considerable reserve to tolerate a certain amount of variation in uterine blood flow and oxygenation. However, if the mother experiences full cardiac arrest prior to 24 weeks, the chances that the fetus will survive are very slight.

Trauma to the uterus can also injure the myometrium, leading to chemical changes which may produce uterine contractions. Fetal membranes may rupture leading to labor or infection. Rupture of the membranes prior to 24 weeks of gestation may result in poor fetal lung development or bone deformities if the volume of amniotic fluid does not return to normal. Injury to the placenta may lead to fetal anemia, hypovolemia or both. Poor oxygenation of the fetus may cause abnormal fetal heart rate variations and may serve as the first indication of a disruption of fetal well-being.

Physiological effects on the mother: Maternal clotting factors are increased during pregnancy. Trauma can cause the release of clotting factors, as would occur with abruption of the placenta, which can quickly lead to disseminated intravascular coagulation (See Clotting Disorders in <u>Diagnostic Tests</u>). Decreased gastric mobility and emptying time predispose pregnant women to aspiration of gastric contents into the lungs. Signs of intra-abdominal injury such as rebound tenderness and abdominal guarding may be diminished, presumably because the gradual stretching of the peritoneum and abdominal musculature by the gravid uterus makes the area less sensitive. The urinary bladder is displaced upward and forward; it becomes an abdominal organ around the 12th week of gestation and is thus more prone to injury. The larger the uterus, the greater the risk of its injury. The increased blood flow to the uterus predisposes the mother to massive blood loss if the uterine vasculature is injured.

Types of injuries: Head injury and hemorrhage account for most injury-related deaths during pregnancy. No data suggests that serious injuries result in higher mortality when compared to nonpregnant women. However, increased risks from rupture of the spleen and retroperitoneal hemorrhage due to blunt abdominal trauma have been reported. On the other hand, bowel injury is less frequent when a woman is pregnant.

Uterine rupture due to blunt trauma is unique to pregnancy and occurs only about 0.6% of the time. It tends to occur during the most severe accidents involving direct abdominal trauma. Fetal morality approaches 100%, but maternal mortality is less than 10%. Most maternal deaths involving uterine rupture are due to accompanying injuries. The more severe the maternal injury, the greater the likelihood the baby will die; however, minor injuries can result in fetal death as well. Except for maternal death, the most common cause of fetal death is abruption of the placenta. Fetal deaths due to direct injury or uterine rupture have also been described, but are much less common.

Abruption complicates about 1 to 5% of all minor maternal injuries and 20 to 50% of all major maternal injuries. In these cases, abruption occurs because the uterine wall beneath the placenta becomes deformed from the trauma, causing placental separation. The simultaneous increase in pressure beneath the placenta from the accumulated blood causes it to separate more, leading to fetal hypoxia and death.

Direct fetal injury is uncommon since the maternal soft tissues protect the fetus quite well, absorbing impacts and diminishing their force. Cranial injuries are the most frequently reported fetal injury. Most of these occur in the third trimester when the engaged fetal head is injured during maternal pelvic fractures.

Immediate care of the seriously injured pregnant woman: Stabilization of the mother's vital signs is the top priority in dealing with severe maternal trauma. If you have any natural remedies on hand, give 200C to 1M Arnica orally every 15 to 30 minutes and Rescue Remedy (a Bach flower combination remedy). Place one pellet or one drop of the remedy inside her lower lip. Tell the woman what has happened and what injuries she has. Have someone talk to her constantly and maintain eye-to-eye contact if she is conscious. Initial resuscitation measures include clearing the airway, maintaining ventilation of the lungs, blood replacement and assisting venous return by displacing the uterus from the inferior vena cava. Oxygen should be given routinely in such cases, even if the woman is breathing on her own. Because the uteroplacental circulation is dependent on maternal blood volume, replacing lost blood is critical to maintaining adequate transfer of oxygen to the fetus. If the pregnancy is past the 20th week, the volume of fluid replacement via IV should be increased 50% over what would be given a nonpregnant woman of the same weight because of the increased plasma volume of pregnancy. Blood replacement should be used if IV fluids such as Ringer's Lactate do not produce adequate stabilization. If an emergency transfusion is necessary before the mother's blood type can be determined, group O Rh- blood should be used.

The woman should be placed in the left lateral position, especially if she is past the 20th week of pregnancy. However, if injuries are severe the spine could be involved and the head and spine should be kept in line. If side-positioning seems unwise, her right hip should be slightly elevated with a hand or wedge. If that cannot be accomplished, have someone push the uterus to the left with their hands as the mother lies supine. These measures will prevent compression of the inferior vena cava by the uterus and facilitate blood flow to the fetus. If blood loss is severe or the woman's condition quite unstable, military antishock inflatable trousers (MAST pants) can be used to relocate blood from the lower extremities upwards to supply the vital organs. This will improve circulation in the upper body, control pelvic and abdominal hemorrhage and raise the blood pressure. However, it is possible for these trousers to compress the uterus against the inferior vena cava and thereby decrease blood flow to the uterus. They should only be used if the mother is in extremely critical condition due to external blood loss, the uterus is below the pubic bone or the baby is known to be dead.

An assistant should also push the uterus to the left to reduce pressure on the inferior vena cava if the mother goes into cardiac arrest. If there is no response within minutes to advanced cardiopulmonary resuscitation, surgery (called thoracotomy) to allow for open chest massage of the heart should be considered, with emergency surgical delivery of the fetus, if it is still alive. While open chest massage has not proven very useful in cases of blunt chest trauma in nonpregnant persons, it can improve cardiac output. Cesarean section can improve maternal venous return when the mother is near death; it has been reported to aid maternal resuscitation. The fetus is most likely to survive if a Cesarean is performed within five minutes of losing maternal vital signs, but is justified if there are any signs that the baby is alive.

In less severe situations, after the mother has been stabilized, the fetal heart rate should be assessed. For pregnancies past the 20th week, fetal heart monitoring should be initiated and the mother should be observed for at least 4 hours, even if the injury was relatively minor. Continued observation beyond the four hour minimum is warranted if there is bleeding from the yoni, uterine tenderness, uterine contractions, rupture of the amniotic membranes, poor or questionable fetal heart rate patterns, or fetal death.

Anticipating abruption of the placenta: In virtually all cases beyond 20 weeks of pregnancy, injured women who develop abruption of the placenta have frequent uterine activity—more than 8 contractions per hour—during the first four hours after the trauma. In women who have at least 3 contractions in a 20-minute period, 25%

1022

will go into premature labor or develop aburption. Abruption usually becomes obvious shortly after the injury, but it has been known to take up to several days to develop.

In hospital, cardiotocographic monitoring (doppler measurement of fetal heart activity and measurement of uterine activity) can be performed for the four hours immediately following severe trauma to monitor for uterine contractions and fetal heart rate changes which indicate compromise. Women who do not develop signs of problems in the first four hours will most likely proceed with a normal pregnancy to term.

Ultrasonography is not as effective in evaluating possible abruption, but can be used to estimate amniotic fluid volume and fetal gestational age and well-being if the fetus is thought to be injured or dead or if monitoring presents unclear evidence of fetal compromise.

Evaluation of serious maternal injuries: Mainstream practitioners recommend the use of x-rays to evaluate severe injuries, regardless of whether the fetus will be exposed in the process. The fetus receives the highest dose if it is the direct path of the beam; otherwise scatter and leakage are the chief sources of exposure. The fetal risk depends on the amount of radiation exposure and the gestational age at the time. After 20 weeks of gestation, radiation is unlikely to cause fetal abnormalities. Adverse effects are not expected with exposure up to 1 cGy (1 rad) or less during pregnancy, and doses of 2 cGy (2 rads) or less have not been associated with an increased risk of childhood cancer. Concerns are greater if the fetus is exposed to 5 to 10 rads or more. Maternal cervical spine and chest films with shielding of the abdomen produce negligible exposure of the fetus. A single pelvic film delivers well under 1 rad to the fetus.

Beyond plain old x-rays, there is the CT SCAN (computerized tomography of the body using x-ray), which can be used to assess extraperitoneal and retroperitoneal organs and the genitourinary tract with three-dimensional images. The exposure of the fetus will vary with the size of the mother, the fetal position, type of machine, method of shielding and the number of pictures obtained. If the fetus is in the direct path of the beam, exposure generally ranges between 5 to 10 rads. The choice to use a CT SCAN must be made based on the mother's condition and balanced between the benefit to the mother and potential risk to the fetus. (See chapter on X-Rays in Diagnostic Tests for more details about x-ray exposure.) Ultrasound is of limited value in assessing maternal trauma. Diagnostic peritoneal lavage (washing of the peritoneal cavity to determine if bleeding exists) has been successfully used in all trimesters. An incision is made above the mother's navel to insert the instruments under direct visualization in order to avoid damaging the pregnant uterus.

The lab tests which may be ordered are geared to the clinical circumstances. At minimum in most cases a Compete Blood Count, screening for blood type and antibodies, and the Kleihauer-Betke test (which detects fetal blood cells in the maternal circulation) are needed. If the woman is not obviously pregnant or does not know her pregnancy status, a *Beta*-pregnancy test should be done as well. If a woman has had several organ systems injured, additional tests may be done, including blood type and crossmatch as well as other tests such as Prothrombin Time, Partial-thromboplastin Time, Platelet Count, and levels of Fibrinogen and the products of fibrinogen degradation. If the mother is Rh-, Kleihauer-Betkie test results can be used to determine how much $Rh_o(D)$ immunoglobulin should be administered. (See various chapters in Diagnostic Tests for details about these tests.)

Fetomaternal hemorrhage: Maternal trauma increases the risk that fetal blood will cross the placenta into the maternal circulation. This occurs more commonly with anterior placental attachment or when the mother reports uterine tenderness after trauma. Complications include blood factor sensitization of the mother (mainly with the Rh factor), newborn anemia, arrhythmic heart beat in the fetus and fetal death due to blood loss. When internal uterine bleeding is suspected, a Kleihauer-Betke test of maternal blood can be used to detect the presence of fetal blood, and further tests can be performed sequentially to monitor the amount of blood being lost by the baby. If the mother is Rh-, Rho(D) immunoglobulin should be given in adequate doses to prevent maternal sensitization.

Evaluation for fetal injuries: Electronic fetal monitoring (EFM), imaging ultrasound and Biophysical profile tests (BPP) are used to determine the well-being of the fetus. However, EFM and BPP tests rely on physical responses primarily mediated by an intact brain stem. They may remain normal in the presence of other brain injuries which do not affect the brain stem, such as intracranial bleeding into a cerebral hemisphere. Imaging ultrasound examination may not detect injuries obscured due to fetal positioning. However, in most cases when the protocols outlined in this chapter are followed and the fetus appears well during the first four hours after maternal trauma, the fetus is unharmed. Fortunately there are only two cases on modern record where an apparently well fetus was found to have severe neurologic injuries after birth. In cases of severe maternal injury where the usual fetal studies are normal, discuss with the parents and collaborating physician whether further evaluation of fetal well-being using a transyoni ultrasound probe or an MRI is desirable.

Supporting the mother: Once the initial physical crisis is under control, talk to the mother about how she is feeling (scared, tired, worried) and encourage her to visualize the baby and placenta as well-oxygenated and healthy. If she has already lost the baby, help her to deal with her grief, shock and general distress. It will all feel like a nightmare to her. If the baby's situation is relatively stable, turn your conversation to the events of the accident. Talking about what happened will help her discharge emotions and will allow you to find out if what happened was related to domestic abuse or other issues which need to be addressed. Review her chart for evidence of past abuse and, if indicated, ask her directly if someone was violent with her; remember that abusive behavior often escalates when a woman is pregnant. If the woman is hospitalized, a social worker should be available on staff to help the woman work through her feelings. If she has a private therapist, that person should be notified of the accident if the mother so desires.

If x-rays were necessary, the woman should take a bath in hot water with ½ pound of sea salt and ¼ pound of baking soda added. It is also helpful to eat extra miso, sodium alginate rich seaweeds, kelp, buckwheat grass, and to take niacin supplements for several weeks. Sodium alginate attracts radioactive materials and carries them out of the body. Homeopathic X-ray in a potency of 30C or 200C can also help minimize the harmful effects.

References and further reading:

Anquist, K. Warren, et.al., "An unexpected fetal outcome following a severe maternal motor vehicle accident," Ob & Gyn. Vol. 84, No. 4, Part 2, Oct. 1994, p. 656.

Parker, Barbara, & J. McFarlane, "Identifying and Helping Battered Pregnant Women," MCN, May/June, Vol. 16, 1991, pp. 164.

Pearlman, Mark et.al., "Blunt Trauma During Pregnancy," NEJM, Vol. 323, No. 23, 12/6/90 pp. 1609-1613.

Insomnia

Many women report that they wake at night and sometimes cannot go back to sleep or that they cannot initially fall asleep very easily. Some sleeplessness may be due to positioning problems as the uterus gets larger, preoccupation with emotional issues or an underlying hesitation (as going to bed might mean having to deal with a partner who wants certain intimacies that a woman does not feel up to providing). Very often, however, a major component of this problem is hypoglycemia. Typically a woman wakes at night, feeling that she has to urinate. She does so and returns to bed only to find herself unable to sleep. She may not even recognize that she is hungry; however, 7 to 10 hours is a long time to go without nourishment and not something she is doing during the day. Recommend eating before bed time and keeping a high protein snack nearby; a glass of milk, nuts, crackers and cheese, or a yogurt. In the vast majority of cases eating at night will remedy this annoying problem! B vitamin deficiency is also associated with sleep disorders, so be sure B intake is adequate, especially in women who are unusually stressed. Old textbooks report that insomnia is a secondary symptom of toxemia, no doubt due to the chronic undernourishment involved.

Exercise shortly before bed time elevates lactic acid levels in the blood which can cause the baby to become temporarily more active, thus interfering with maternal rest. Advise women to reduce their evening activity level. (Hartley, 1994)

Emotional or psychological issues may cause a woman to sleep poorly. Ask what she thinks about when she lies awake. If she is very intellectually oriented and has trouble turning her mind off so that she can relax, she can use Skullcap tincture as a sedative (1 to 10 drops in hot water or directly under the tongue). More can be taken if necessary as Skullcap is nonnarcotic and very safe for use in pregnancy. After the fifth month Hops tincture or infusion can be drunk before retiring. A glass of warm milk and a hot bath or a cup of Chamomile or Catnip infusion (steeped for half an hour) can also be used. Hypnotherapy may also help.

As pregnancy advances, getting comfortable becomes increasingly difficult, which often leads to problems with sleeping. Some women find that they are most comfortable sleeping alone during the last weeks. Supporting the belly with pillows, sleeping propped up, and changing positions often may also help, but will probably not cause the woman to sleep as though she were not pregnant. Frequent urination starts up again in the third trimester and is normal. If a woman is urinating more often than every two hours, rule out a urinary tract infection. Remind the woman that sleeping more lightly and waking frequently during late pregnancy is Nature's way of preparing her for the frequent feedings and for being tuned into the newborn every night for the first year or two of motherhood.

References and further reading:
Balch, J, & P. Balch, Prescription for Nutritional Healing, Avery Pub., Garden City, NY 1990.
Hartley, C., midwife, Ancient Arts Midwifery Inst., Claremore, OK, editing comments, 12/94.

Jaundice

Jaundice, (the skin turning yellow), may appear for a variety of reasons:

Viral Hepatitis: See <u>Diagnostic Tests</u> for full information.

Hyperemesis gravidarum: Profound vomiting, dehydration and ketosis may be accompanied by occasional jaundice and hepatic dysfunction. (See chapter on Nausea and Vomiting in the section on First Trimester Problems for more details.)

Intrahepatic cholestasis of pregnancy (ICP) and its milder form, pruritus gravidarum, are the most common forms of jaundice in pregnancy. ICP begins anytime after the 12th week of pregnancy and clears within 48 hours after birth. Women who have taken high estrogen oral contraceptives are at more risk. Although not hazardous to the mother, according to some studies the rate of prematurity and fetal distress is increased. Bio-technical physicians may prescribe cholestyramine, 12 to 16 grams per day, to control itching, tapering the dose to 8 to 10 g daily as symptoms subside. This may cause malabsorption of fat soluble vitamins and a prolonged prothrombin time; which can be monitored and treated with vitamin K to prevent hemorrhage. ICP may recur in successive pregnancies. (See remedies in The Liver and Pregnancy chapter in <u>Diagnostic Tests</u>.)

Extrahepatic cholestasis: Non-liver related cholestasis may be due to large bile duct obstruction from gallstones, carcinoma of the bile ducts or certain drugs. Gall bladder problems are discussed in the chapter on Abdominal Pain in this section.

Acute fatty liver: Acute fatty liver is often associated with overt toxemia. Some studies have shown its incidence to be associated three times more frequently with male fetuses than female. Predisposing factors include exposure to toxins, viruses, toxemia, protein and vitamin malnutrition and depression of protein synthesis by tetracyclines. (See <u>Diagnostic Tests</u> for further information.)

Severe toxemia: Jaundice may occur but is not associated with actual liver failure.

Liver failure may be caused by a drug reaction (anesthesia with halothane), Wilson's disease, viral hepatitis, or chronic liver disease. Restlessness, confusion, hallucinations, drowsiness, convulsions, and vomiting rapidly progress to stupor, coma and death. Jaundice may already be present or follow within a few days. Disseminated intravascular coagulation occurs; sometimes renal failure does as well.

Extrahepatic bile duct cancer: A very rare cause of rapidly developing jaundice accompanied by weight loss and abdominal pain. (Gleicher, 1985, p. 1078)

Gleicher, N., <u>Principles of Medical Therapy in Pregnancy</u>, Plenum Pub., NY, 1985.

Nerve Pain and Pressure Symptoms

Normal physiological relationships are altered during pregnancy due to weight gain, edema, increased pressure from the enlarging uterus and hormonal influences which soften tissues in preparation for birth. This can lead to a variety of aggravating symptoms caused by pressure on various nerves. Keep in mind that acupuncture, chiropractic adjustments or homeopathic remedies may be able to minimize or relieve the symptoms from any of these problems, as they are all very effective in treating neurological conditions.

Bell's Palsy is a unilateral facial paralysis of sudden onset related to the seventh nerve, and is most common in the 30 to 50 age group. It occurs in nonpregnant women at a rate of 17 per 100,000 yearly; the incidence rises to 57 per 100,000 among pregnant women. Bell's Palsy may appear at any time but is seen most frequently in the third trimester or the first 2 weeks postpartum. The facial nerve passes through a long bony canal as it leaves the skull; the normal fluid retention which occurs may be responsible for the increased incidence of this problem in pregnancy. Toxemia seems to increase its occurrence.

Onset is typically sudden and painless; symptoms vary according to the location of the compressed area of the nerve. Most severely, compression of the geniculate ganglion results in the loss of ipsilateral tearing, heightened sensitivity to sound, paralysis of the facial muscles including the muscles of the eye, mouth and forehead, and loss of taste in the anterior two-thirds of the tongue. If the lesion is farther from this area, tearing may remain functional but the rest of the symptoms are likely to be present. Lesions located still further from the geniculate ganglion toward the surface of the skull may leave hearing unaffected but will involve taste and muscle functions. Lesions at the styloid foramen will produce weakness of the facial muscles only.

Bells' Palsy does not affect the course of pregnancy. Recovery of functions is related to the extent of the initial impairment with partial palsies recovering better than complete initial palsies. Loss of taste is associated with an overall less favorable prognosis. Bio-technical providers may recommend 40 to 60 mg. of oral prednisone daily, which increases the chances of recovery if begun within a week of onset. Surgical decompression provides no benefits. If functional loss is minimal, no therapies are recommended since the chances of recovery are good. The one mild case of Bell's Palsy I have seen responded well to oral intake of Skullcap and St. John's Wort tinctures and topical applications of Skullcap poultices on the side of the face in front of the ear several times daily; this cleared a Palsy that appeared in early pregnancy within two weeks with no reoccurrence. This woman had a history of a difficult forceps delivery when she was born that resulted in some injury to the side of her face where the palsy appeared.

Sciatic pain: The sciatic nerve is the largest nerve in the body. It arises from the sacral plexus, leaves the pelvis through the greater sciatic foramen, runs through the hip joint and down the back of the thigh. Irritation of this nerve is common during pregnancy as pelvic joints move due to hormonal influences and as the weight of the uterus increases. Many women find that chiropractic adjustments relieve such pain. In addition, St. John's Wort tincture, between 5 to 20 drops per dose when symptoms occur, can seemingly work magic on some women's sciatic pain; however, it does not work for everyone.

Foot drop: Foot drop is caused by injury to the lumbosacral cord, which contains nerve fibers from the 4th and 5th lumbar spinal segments, and presents as weakness of movement at the ankle joint and an outward turning of the foot. There is also loss of sensitivity along the lateral aspect of the leg and the sole of the foot. These symptoms resolve after birth. A chiropractor experienced in dealing with pregnant women can help keep the pelvis properly aligned. Getting off the feet, taking a hot bath, massage and slow range-of-motion movements on the affected side may also relieve acute pain.

Brachial plexus pain: The brachial plexus area is found below the clavicle near the shoulder joint. Fluid retention and postural changes may cause sensations of tingling and numbness in the shoulder and arm. Sometimes there is a familial neuropathy of this nerve; an additional symptom suggesting this is muscular wasting on the affected side. Other spinal and cranial nerves may be affected as well. Rest will help with the symptoms, as well as St. John's Wort tincture (5 to 20 drops with symptoms).

Intercostal neuralgia: Some women may experience an intermittent nerve pain that comes around one side from the back into the intercostal space between two ribs. Using a straight backed chair, a hard mattress and lateral flexion of the spine toward the painful side may relieve this to a certain extent. A chiropractic adjustment will also be helpful.

Other pregnancy-related palsies: Various peripheral nerves can be compressed by maternal positioning or pressure from the presenting part of the fetus. They may be dealt with as described above.

"Nervous feet": Fidgety feet may be a sign of anemia or of mineral imbalance.

Carpal Tunnel Syndrome The median nerve passes from the forearm to the hand behind the flexor retinaculum muscle. During pregnancy, weight gain and edema reduce the narrow passage for this nerve, which may lead to tingling, pain and stiffness in the thumb, index, middle and radial half of the ring finger on the affected side. These symptoms often appear or worsen at night and may cause wakefulness. Less commonly, weakness may also occur leading to clumsiness of manual function. Carpal tunnel syndrome is precipitated and aggravated by repetitive hand and wrist motion which may occur in jobs that require keyboard use (typing or computer entry). When a significant degree of carpal tunnel syndrome is present, percussion over the medial nerve at the center of the wrist can cause a tingling sensation along the region supplied by the median nerve (referred to as Tinel's sign).

Drinking skullcap infusion can help to heal damaged nerves. Vitamin B_6 has also been shown to relieve some cases of carpal tunnel syndrome. Have the woman try 25 mg daily along with a B complex supplement while implementing wrist stabilization (described below). Regular exercise helps mobilize fluid and is very beneficial. Acupuncture may also be helpful.

Stabilizing the wrist in a straight position at night will help minimize this problem. Advise women not to sleep with their heads resting on their hands or wrists. If carpal tunnel syndrome is severe, the woman should wear wrist supports at night and when working at a keyboard. Alternatively, an ergonomic keyboard can be purchased to minimize further damage, especially if the problem was present prior to pregnancy. (The Kinesis Ergonomic Keyboard is one of the best [22232 17th Ave. SE, Bothwell, WA 98021-7425, (425) 402-8100]). If carpal tunnel syndrome is only being caused by pregnancy-related changes, the condition will resolve after birth in most cases.

Numb thigh (meralgia paresthetica): The lateral femoral cutaneous nerve (L2, L3) of the thigh passes through the inguinal ligament. The weight gain of pregnancy may lead to pressure anywhere along this nerve, causing prickling, tingling, heightened sensitivity and numbness of the anterolateral aspect of one or both thighs, usually beginning around the 30th week of pregnancy. There is no relation to age or parity of the mothers affected. This condition typically resolves within three months after birth. If the thigh is painful, a skullcap compress can be placed in the inguinal area on the affected side. Drinking a cup of skullcap infusion daily or taking St. John's wort tincture (five to 20 drops with symptoms) may also be helpful.

Chorea gravidarum: This extremely rare condition often begins in the first (50%) or second (33%) trimester, but may start at any point in pregnancy. It produces involuntary, irregular, nonrepetitive movements mainly of the extremities and facial muscles. It can range from minimal involvement to marked, persistent movement resulting in exhaustion. It is associated with generalized muscle weakness and poor muscle tone, emotional lability and fatigue. All movements cease during sleep. Its appearance is strongly linked to a history of rheumatic fever; at least 35% of those affected have a positive history. Its probable cause is a reactivation of subclinical damage to nerves as a result of rheumatic encephalopathy. Evaluation includes a cardiologic exam to rule out current rheumatic fever with carditis and other tests such as an electrocardiogram, antistreptolysin titer, and throat culture to

1030

other tests such as an electrocardiogram, antistreptolysin titer, and throat culture to assess other possible strep infections. Wilson's disease, lupus, thyrotoxicosis, and polycythemia should also be considered in the differential diagnosis; if other family members had chorea, Huntington's chorea must be considered as well. A homeopathic remedy may be useful in relieving symptoms. Rest, quiet and sometimes sedation may help. The disease undergoes spontaneous remission before birth in 30% of cases, the rest usually resolve by 6 weeks postpartum. Twenty percent will have a recurrence in a subsequent pregnancy.

Gestational neuropathy: Women may exhibit short-term memory loss, confusion with alertness and loss of control of the muscles around the eyes due to severe nutritional deficiencies, which may result from excessive vomiting. Aggressive nutritional improvement and supplementation, with special emphasis of the B vitamins (especially B_1, B_2, and B_{12}) will remedy this problem, but prevention is obviously the best remedy.

References and further reading:

Garrey, M. et.al., Obstetrics Illustrated, Churchill-Livingstone, London, Eng., 1980.
Gleicher, Norbert, ed. Principles of Medical Therapy in Pregnancy, Plenum Pub., New York, 1985.

Nasal Congestion and Other Nasal Problems

Congestion: Nasal congestion is common during pregnancy, occurring most often after the third month. Pregnancy hormones stimulate the nasal mucosa as well as increase vascular congestion. The mucus secreting glands throughout the body are more active. Often allergic responses are heightened due to hypersensitivity to placental hormones, fetal proteins, or antigens within the body. In some women allergic reactions may be caused by estrogen deficiency. Snoring may be a problem. Not much can be done except to avoid those foods which the woman knows to cause excessive mucus production in her body. Freeze-dried Nettles in capsules has helped some women with this problem; take with symptoms, starting with 4 capsules and adjusting dosage as relief occurs.

Snoring: Less commonly, women may start to snore in the third trimester as a result of sleep apnea (apnea is a temporary cessation in breathing). If sleep apnea is causative, changes the normal pattern of blood flow and oxygenation in the body may lead to cardiovascular problems with accompanying diminished blood flow to the placenta. If snoring appears and is accompanied by difficulties with sleeping in general which are not remedied by such things as going to bed and arising at consistent times and the other suggestions in the insomnia chapter in this section, a sleep disorders center can evaluate the woman for sleep apnea. (Doghramji)

Nosebleeds (epistaxis): The increased blood volume of pregnancy plus the softening effects of higher hormone levels can make the small capillaries in the nose more likely to rupture, causing a nosebleed. While nosebleeds are more common for women during pregnancy, this does not mean that they are necessarily a normal response. An adequate diet, with special attention to getting enough vitamin C with bioflavinoids and calcium can help prevent nosebleeds, just like it can with bleeding gums. Hypertension, the use of certain drugs (notably aspirin), clotting disorders, pressure changes within the nose (nose blowing, sneezing or dependent head positions) and atherosclerosis may be predisposing factors.

Dry heat, whether in the winter from artificial heat sources or from dry air in the summer, can greatly contribute to the tendency for the nose to become irritated and begin to bleed. The woman can use a non-ultrasound humidifier or vaporizer in her home, especially at night, to prevent over drying of the nasal passages. She can also use a nasal atomizer filled with plain warm water with a pinch of salt added to spray into her nose to relieve dryness.

Should a nosebleed occur, the woman should be advised to apply firm pressure and tilt her head back while sitting down, if possible. These measures are usually effective in stopping the flow when the bleeding originates from the anterior portion of the nasal passage. When the bleeding originates from higher up

1032

in the nose, it may become profuse since there is no way to apply direct pressure. If severe, hospitalization for cauterization of the bleeding site may be necessary. For this type of bleeding, cayenne pepper taken as a teaspoon in a glass of water or in capsules may be effective. A homeopathic remedy may also be helpful (Homeopathic Belladonna is for sudden, hot, bright red bleeding which is worse with any motion. It may be a good first remedy to try, if the symptoms fit the remedy picture).

Granuloma gravidarum (hemangioma or telangiectatic polyp): This is a painless, very vascular, friable red tumor of the nasal mucus membrane which usually appears during the first trimester of pregnancy and disappears spontaneously shortly after birth. While usually appearing only on one side, bilateral tumors have been reported. It is composed of a collection of acute and chronic inflammatory cells and multiple vascular channels in a lose edematous network. There may be areas of local bleeding or ulceration. It may be attached directly to the nasal passage or suspended on a tiny stem (pendeculated) and measure up to 3 to 4 cm. in diameter. Polyps frequently occur on the mucosa of the nasal septum near the opening of the nostril. Nasal obstruction and nosebleeds are common symptoms. If removed, they have a tendency to recur. They also have a tendency to recur during subsequent pregnancies. The best course of action is to avoid surgery, utilizing homeopathy in an attempt to resolve the tumor.

References and further reading:

Balch, J, & P. Balch, Prescription for Nutritional Healing, Avery Pub., Garden City, NY 1990.
Gleicher, Norbert, ed. Principles of Medical Therapy in Pregnancy, Plenum Pub., New York, 1985.
Doghramji, Karl, director, Sleep Disorders Center, Dept. of Ob Gyn at Thomas Jefferson U., Philadelphia, PA.

Poisoning During Pregnancy

Poisoning refers to a variety of illnesses caused by the absorption of toxic chemical agents. Poisonings may be acute, subacute or chronic and result from accidental or intentional exposure via ingestion, injection, inhalation or direct skin contact. Most physical effects of poisons simulate other illnesses, therefore poisoning must be considered in cases of coma, seizures, psychosis, acute hepatic failure, acute renal failure, and bone marrow depression. More subtle manifestations are less likely to be recognized as the result of poisons. The woman may be reluctant to admit intentional poisoning; the accurate diagnosis of poisoning requires the midwife to be alert for this possibility.

Maternal physiology, poisoning and immediate first aid: Placing a woman on her left side may aid in the excretion of poisons via the kidneys due to the cardiovascular changes of pregnancy. Pulmonary blood gas alterations necessitate close monitoring for the development of acidosis. The increased plasma volume may cause poisons to be more diluted in the system, which may be beneficial. Pregnant women have an increased sensitivity to vomiting, which may help eliminate poisons; however, the relaxation of the pyloric value of the stomach may cause caustic agents to be more damaging than in nonpregnant persons. Reduced motility in the intestines may enhance absorption of agents in the gastrointestinal tract.

Identifying the poison: Try to identify the poisoning agent whenever possible by contacting pharmacists, discussing the circumstances with all possibly knowledgeable parties, obtaining samples from the woman's mouth or clothing, and looking for empty containers in her home or where she is found. Contact a local Poison Control Center for assistance (check your phone book or call 911 for the number of a center near you). Don't overlook the possibility of environmental exposure from crop spraying, work related exposure, chemical agents in the home such as termite control agents, or a defective furnace producing carbon monoxide fumes.

Some poisons have clearly associated symptoms; for example carbon monoxide produces cherry-red discoloration of the mucus membranes, belladonna may produce neurological depression and cyanide causes a bitter almond odor. However, most poisons produce nonspecific symptoms. Toxicologic assays are usually available to rule out alcohol, barbiturates, salicylates, cocaine, and heroin, but more sophisticated tests for other poisons may not be readily available. Therefore, specimens of all body fluids should be preserved for future analysis.

Initial maternal therapy: Want of a diagnosis must not delay therapy, which should be directed at preserving vital functions. The severity of the poisoning is best judged by a clinical evaluation. Place the woman on her left side, if possible.

1034

Avoid placing the woman flat on her back or have an assistant support the uterus to one side to prevent supine hypotension. Obtain baseline and then periodic assessments of vital signs and neurologic function. Maintain an open airway and begin artificial respiration as indicated. Keep the woman warm with blankets. The level of consciousness can quickly be assessed by her response to painful stimuli. Pupil reactivity and limb reflexes are not reliable indications in cases of poisoning. Press a knuckle into the sternum, to make the following assessment:

GRADE	RESPONSE
I	Woman is drowsy or asleep but will respond to vocal commands
II	Woman is unconscious but responds to minimally painful stimuli
III	Woman is unconscious & responds only to maximally painful stimuli
IV	Woman is unconscious & shows no response to painful stimuli

Once the woman is transported, heart function should be monitored with an echocardiogram and IV hydration be given if needed. Shock may ensue due to depression of nervous system function, heart arrhythmia, or as the primary effect of some poisons. Possible reasons for shock must be evaluated and corrected. Poisoning often results in metabolic abnormalities due to diarrhea or vomiting, and electrolyte-balancing fluids may be necessary. Careful regulation of fluids is important because it is easy to induce pulmonary edema in the pregnant woman. Specific therapy is usually not necessary to counteract the central nervous system effects of poisons; generally anticonvulsants should be used along with correction of metabolic imbalances. Cerebral edema may be relieved by high-dose steroids and mannitol diuresis when increased intracranial pressure is present.

Many poisonings result in coma, which usually resolves on its own; supportive care is the most important treatment. If blood tests show that coma is due to hypoglycemia or insulin overdose, 50% dextrose at 1 ml/kg up to 50 ml. may provide immediate correction.

Preventing absorption: Since many poisons are ingested, prompt interference with digestion may prevent further absorption. Water or milk may be initially utilized to dilute the stomach contents. Vomiting should be induced unless specifically contraindicated due to the poison involved. Although gastric emptying is most effective if done immediately, since some poisons depress gastric emptying and peristalsis, significant amounts of ingested poisons are often recovered several hours after ingestion.

Vomiting often follows poisoning. If it does not, putting an index finger in the back of the throat to stimulate a gag reflex may assist in emptying the stomach and is the safest means of inducing vomiting during pregnancy. Ipecac syrup can cause cardiac arrhythmias and central nervous system effects and should not be used during pregnancy. Apomorphine, 0.06 mg. by intramuscular or 0.01 mg. by intravenous administration usually produces vomiting. However, vomiting may occasionally be prolonged after intramuscular injection, and there is also a question about its safety for the fetus. Do not induce vomiting if the woman is convulsing or in a coma because of the danger of pulmonary aspiration. Vomiting is contraindicated after poisoning with strong caustics (it increases the risk of gastrointestinal perforation) or liquid petroleum products (due to the increased risk of lung irritation).

Gastric lavage (pumping the stomach) is not more effective than vomiting but can produce immediate results and may be used if the central nervous system is compromised. It cannot be used if strong caustics have been ingested. The woman is placed on her side with her head and shoulders lowered. A mouth gag is used to maintain an open throat. An endotracheal tube prevents aspiration; gastric contents are emptied with gentle suction, followed by lavage with 200 ml. of warm water or normal saline until the solution runs clear. Fluid and electrolyte balance should be closely monitored during saline catharsis.

Interfering with absorption: Many poisons may be absorbed by 30 to 50 g. activated charcoal mixed with 100 to 200 ml. of plain water taken orally. In conjunction with this, 250 mg/kg of magnesium or sodium sulfate (taken orally to a maximum total dose of 30 g.) or magnesium citrate (up to 300 ml. of a 25% solution), is frequently used in those with normal kidney and heart function.

Poisons contaminating skin or eyes should be removed by copiously flushing the area with clear water. Ventilation with fresh air assists in eliminating inhaled poisons. An ice pack or tourniquet can be used to slow the absorption of injected poisons. However, incision and suction is only used for venomous snake bites.

Eliminating absorbed poison: Preventing absorption is more effective at lowering peak blood levels than using methods to eliminate absorbed poisons. A large number of agents are eliminated via the kidneys. Circulatory support is the main way to stimulate urinary secretion. Agents such as organochlorine, pesticides, organic acids, and some drugs are excreted in the bile. Cholestramine is a drug used to decrease absorption of toxins from the bile as it passes through the digestive system. Its safe use in pregnancy has not been established; however, its use is warranted in cases of ingestion of such poisons as chlordecone (Kepone). Hemodialysis may aid in eliminating some poisons such as boric acid, barbiturates, chlorate, ethanol, glycols, methanol, salicylate, sulfonamides, theophylline, thiocyanate or any agent with small molecules, low lipid solubility and low protein binding. No effective means of speeding the elimination of most poisons is known.

Antidotes: There are specific antidotes for a few poisons; accurate identification of the toxic agent is necessary for their use.

Fetal effects of maternal poisoning: Fetal heart monitoring should begin as soon as possible after maternal poisoning is identified. The fetal effects depend on the maternal response to the agent in question, its ability to be transferred across the placenta, the gestational age, maturity of the fetal metabolism, length of time the poison is in the mother's system, maternal metabolic effects, and the relationship of the episode to the time of birth. Some poisons may have minimal maternal effects yet produce significant long-term effects in the fetus since the fetus concentrates some poisons in its system.

Non-ionized, lipid-soluble drugs of low molecular weight such as barbiturates and narcotics transport rapidly across the placenta. Other factors affecting placental transport are the concentration of the agent across the placenta, protein binding, and the fetal and maternal blood flow. Early first trimester poisonings may either produce miscarriage or no apparent effects. Fetal damage may be apparent in other first trimester situations. Neurologic defects or growth retardation are the most likely problems from acute or chronic second and third trimester exposures. Even small doses of many drugs can produce side effects in the infant after birth if the mother takes them close to the time of labor or delivery because the fetal liver is immature.

Heavy metal exposure: The most common source of exposure to toxic metals is the industrial work-place. However, environmental exposure from contaminated water, soil, air and food is increasing. **Lead** is most commonly inhaled from contaminated dust; old plumping pipes are a significant source as well. (Lead toxicity is covered in Diagnostic Tests).

Cadmium is a widely distributed mineral. Processes such as refining lead and zinc ore, combustion of oil and coal, waste disposal, and scrap metal recovery are significant sources of contamination. Food is the main source for those not directly involved in industry. Toxic symptoms include labored breathing, coughing and wheezing, eventually progressing to emphysema. Nausea, vomiting, abdominal pain and diarrhea occur after acute exposure. Kidney damage eventually results, with accompanying proteinuria. Fetal growth retardation, severe newborn anemia and possible malformations may result from maternal exposure. Cadmium has a particular affinity for the placenta and may interfere with nutrient absorption. Minimal maternal exposure may therefore interfere with growth and blood formation in the fetus.

Mercury is used in the production of lamps, lights, batteries, electrical equipment and pesticides and is found in contaminated water and fish. Microorganisms convert various mercurial compounds into the most toxic form of mercury, methylmercury, which is readily absorbed by the gastrointestinal tract and can cross the blood-brain barrier. Adverse effects include kidney and brain damage. Mercury concentrates in the fetal blood and brain tissue. Even if the mother appears unaffected, delayed onset of severe neurologic damage including instability of the neck, convulsions, poor growth, and deformity of the limbs may present in children exposed *in utero*. The studies available do not clearly demonstrate if the risk is similar in all trimesters, but do indicate fetal sensitivity during the last 3 months of pregnancy. Breastmilk must also be considered a major source of contamination. Decreased fertility in adults is another possible consequence. Mercury dental fillings may also release mercury into the system, especially when the are removed. Women who desire to have their mercury fillings replaced with composites should be advised to wait until after they give birth to do so (Schlinger, 1995).

Nickel is used in metal alloys, nickel plating, and is found in coal and petroleum products. Nickel carbonyl is the most toxic form; inhalation may lead to immediate headache, nausea, vomiting and substernal pain, followed by fever, chills, labored breathing and a cough. In severe cases convulsions and death may result. The only evidence for fetal effects from nickel carbonyl exposure are from animal studies. A transient 15 minute maternal exposure to 0.3 ml. per liter in the air was associated with malformations, especially of the eye, in 28% of the fetuses tested. While the cause and effect relationship of these defects to nickel exposure remains unclear (a hormonal imbalance is a possible contributing factor) it seems prudent to remove pregnant women from all exposure to nickel during pregnancy.

References and further reading:

Gleicher, Norbert, ed. Principles of Medical Therapy in Pregnancy, Plenum Pub., New York, 1985.
Schlinger, Hilary, midwife, editing comments, 1995.

 1038

Radiation Injury

This chapter will cover accidental exposure to radiation from various sources. For a discussion of exposure from medical X-rays, please see <u>Diagnostic Tests</u>.

General pathophysiology: Three things must be considered when trying to determine possible effects of radiation exposure: the type of radiation, (i.e., α or β particles, neutrons or X or y-ray photons); the amount of ionizing radiation, measured in roentgens, and the duration of exposure, measured in rads. Matter exposed to ionizing radiation causes ion pairs to form, dislodging the target atoms's orbital electron, resulting in a low linear energy transfer. The absorbed dose is the number of ion pairs absorbed within a volume of tissue; if tissue absorbs 100 ergs of ionizing radiation in 1 g of matter, this equals 1 rad (radiation absorbed dose), which also equals one rem (a rad equivalent in humans or animals).

Maternal pathology: Effects can be divided into threshold and non-threshold categories. Acute radiation syndrome includes skin changes, weight loss, suppression of the bone marrow, gastrointestinal inflammation and death; all are examples of threshold effects. Survival at doses of about 200 rem is common, although sickness, hemorrhage and death follow in 10 to 30% of cases in 30 days. Doses over 100 rem. result in a 60 to 95% fatality rate in 30 days with acute illness and early deaths. Radiation sickness does not usually occur in doses less than 25 rem. Doses of about 50 rem. result in temporary male sterility; doses over 300 rem produce permanent sterility in women.

Genetic mutation and cancer are the two major non-threshold effects. Genetic mutation effects are difficult to evaluate. Cancer occurrences vary with the type or amount of exposure, but no linear correlations can be drawn between type of cancer and the radiation exposure. Onset of detectable disease is usually delayed for a latency period lasting 2 to 15 years.

Medical exposures from diagnostic techniques produce no known maternal effects (although I have personally noted spaciness after even dental x-rays!). Larger exposures are hard to qualify; however, genetic effects on the inhabitants of Hiroshima and Nagasaki indicate that stillbirth, major congenital defects, death during the first week of life, death of liveborn children, and frequency of sex chromosome anomaly is seen more often with approximately 156 rem of maternal exposure. Children may also be born with chromosomal changes directly linked to the maternal exposure.

Fetal pathology: It appears that the risk of miscarriage rises to 23% in women exposed to extremely high levels of radiation based on studies done on women living near the sites of the bomb dropped on Hiroshima and Nagasaki. A quarter of their infants died in the first year of life and 29% surviving the first year were microcephalic. Studies also show that women receiving less radiation had occurrences of about 5% in each listed category. Adverse effects were noted in children of mothers who received as little as 10 to 19 rads of exposure; more than 50 rads of whole body maternal exposure produced a small head circumference rate of 50% which was the most prominent abnormality noted. Mental retardation was often an associated complication. These risks increased as maternal exposure doses increased.

What to do: A woman should consult radiation physicists to help her determine the amount of exposure if she is exposed to radioactive substances during her pregnancy. Exposure at or above 10 rads may be considered a threshold at which fetal effects might be seen. The parents should be advised of the possible affects of the radiation exposure and options explored. After exposure the woman should take a bath in hot water with ½ pound of sea salt and ¼ pound of baking soda added. It is also helpful to eat extra miso, sodium alginate-rich seaweeds, kelp, buckwheat grass, and take niacin supplements for several weeks. Sodium alginate attracts radioactive materials and carries them out of the body. Homeopathic X-ray in a potency of 30C or 200C can also help minimize the harmful effects.

References and further reading:

Gleicher, Norbert, ed. Principles of Medical Therapy in Pregnancy, Plenum Pub., New York, 1985.

1040

Salivation

Excessive salivation (ptyalism or sialorrhea) occasionally occurs during pregnancy. It usually starts quickly and is characterized by the production of excessive saliva, sometimes more than 1,900 ml per day. It is often associated with pregnancy-related nausea and found in women who may have difficulty swallowing their saliva as a result; it is therefore postulated that there is no true increase in the amount of saliva, but an inability to swallow the saliva normally secreted. Ptyalism usually begins at two to three weeks of gestation and may continue or even increase in amount until after the birth.

Women may report thin, watery oral secretions which leave a bitter taste in their mouth. Secretion may diminish during sleep, but some women report that excessive salivation at night wakes them up. Women may have distended cheek pouches and excessive expectoration and may have to wipe their mouths frequently when talking. Speech difficulties may arise from swollen salivary glands and because the tongue is enlarged, red and coated. Ptyalism seems to run in some families and many of these women will show identical symptoms during each pregnancy, with the salivary flow increasing in volume each time and returning to apparently normal levels postpartum. Women may feel fatigued and depressed because of the considerable discomfort, inconvenience and embarrassment caused by this condition.

*Various dietary adjustments have been suggested, such as increasing carbohydrates, decreasing fluids and limiting fats. Some women have had limited success by eating small balanced frequent meals instead of three large meals, chewing gum and using oral lozenges.

*It has been suggested that a causative factor may be ingestion of large quantities of starch (pica), so a review of the nutritional status is warranted.

*Dehydration is not necessarily associated with this condition, but could happen if vomiting is excessive, women should be aware that natural food brands of electrolyte balancing fluids, such as Third Wind, can help alleviate any dehydration that occurs.

*Bio-technical medicine has nothing to offer in the way of corrective pharmacological agents, homeopathic remedies and Chinese medicine are two likely candidates for effective treatment.

*Cinnamon flavored gum or cinnamon bark tea may help (El Halta, 1989). Fresh cinnamon bark tea should be brewed for only a few minutes and should not be used in the first trimester as it is a uterine contractant.

Dinter, Maureen, "Ptyalism in Pregnant Women," JOGNN, Vol. 20, No. 3, 1991, pp. 206-9.
El Halta, V., Moving Midwifery Forward, Garden of Life, Pub., Dearborn MI, 1989.

Seizures

The most likely cause of pregnancy related seizures is undetected toxemia in the otherwise normal woman. However, a well-nourished woman, receiving adequate nutrition for her activity and stress levels can be suffering from other conditions which may be aggravated to the point of seizure activity due to pregnancy. There are varying degrees of seizure activity. Absence or petit mal seizures are characterized by a 10 to 30 second loss of consciousness, with eye or muscle fluttering and may occur several times daily. They pose no particular danger unless the person happens to be driving, operating dangerous machinery, otherwise engaged in an activity which requires their full attention when the seizure occurs. They are genetically determined and do not begin after the age of 20. Gross brain damage is not a feature of this disorder and drugs are usually not prescribed. Partial or focal seizures present with localized neurological symptoms such as twitching, numbness or tingling, mouth movements, hallucination of smell and vision and automatic mannerisms. Brain lesions may be causative and should be investigated. Tonic-clonic (grand-mal) seizures are much more serious and may lead to hypoxia and brain damage. Seizures which result from toxemia are tonic-clonic and are described below.

What to do: If a woman should start to seize for any reason, have someone call 911. In the meantime, certain emergency measures will minimize the chances of injury to the woman and her baby:

*Do not restrain her movements; allow her to drop to the floor while attempting to guide her so as to prevent head injury
*Move away any objects that might lead to injury
*Loosen clothing near the neck
*Maintain an airway
*Cradle her head in your lap
*Remove dentures as quickly as is safe
*Observe seizure activity
*Turn her on her side so fluid and vomitus can drain freely after movements subside
*Give mouth-to-mouth resuscitation if breathing does not resume following the seizure
*Administer blow-by oxygen by holding the tubing close to her nose Once the seizure is over, give oxygen by mask (5 to 6 liters per minute)
*Allow the woman to rest undisturbed; she may be confused, disoriented and very tired
*Record seizure activity
*Stay with the woman while medical assistance is summoned

1042

*Be prepared for another seizure (Hegner & Caldwell, 1992)

You will note that the use of a bite stick is not mentioned. Traditionally something was placed into the mouth of a seizing person to prevent them from biting their tongue or lips. This practice has fallen into disfavor because it was found that more damage to structures within the mouth occurs when a bite stick is used.

Seizures due to severe metabolic toxemia: Toxemic seizure activity is a severe consequence of an extremely contracted blood volume during pregnancy. Before toxemic seizures begin, there has usually been a period of poor dietary intake coupled with symptoms such as headache, epigastric pain, nausea and vomiting, hyperreflexia and visual disturbances, frequently accompanied by hypertension, swelling and proteinuria. However, blood pressure within a normal range does not preclude the imminent onset of seizures in the malnourished woman; blood pressure may not rise until seizures have begun or it may not rise at all.

Convulsions may occur at any time, even while the woman is asleep. Toxemic seizures are tonic-clonic and associated with loss of consciousness. She may report that she "feels funny" with a sinking or rising feeling in her stomach. The woman falls to the ground unconscious; there are a few seconds of quiet and some twitching of the facial muscles. The pupils dilate, the eyes and the head are turned to one side, the woman opens her mouth and the jaw is pulled to the side. A cry or sigh may be emitted. Her whole body becomes rigid, features become distorted, arms flex, hands clench, feet invert, toes flex and the whole body is drawn to one side in a tonic spasm. This lasts a few seconds, then the jaws and eyelids open and close violently and twitching begins in the face, then in one arm, next in the leg and finally the whole body. This violent clonic convulsion may even throw the woman out of bed. The tongue protrudes, blood-tinged foam may come from the mouth, respiration stops and the chest is rigid. The pulse is rapid (up to 120) and strong, later growing weaker, but may be difficult to assess due to the convulsion. Rarely the pulse is weak throughout. The eyes become blood-shot and protrude, the face is swollen, cyanosis is extreme and the lips are purple. Gradually convulsive movements cease, a few twitches or jerks take place, the woman lies quiet and the heart pumps violently. For a few seconds the woman may appear to be dying, but then there is a long sigh, irregular breathing begins and coma sets in. Respiration soon quiets and the woman wakes after a short time disoriented and sore in all muscles. A few minutes to an hour later another convulsion begins. Fetal and maternal mortality are high.

When convulsions recur the intervals between them become shorter and the woman remains in a deep coma. A fever of 102°F (39°C) often develops. Untreated, seizures may occur as often as every 30 to 40 minutes. Pulmonary edema and cessation of urinary output with hemoglobinuria are possible complications. As death approaches convulsions increase in frequency and intensity, temperature rises (sometimes to 107°F [41.7°C]) or drops rapidly, and the pulse rate increases over 120, becoming weak and thready. Respirations rise above 40 per minute. Peripheral circulatory collapse or shock may occur as well. Acute toxemia may also occur with severe secondary symptoms but no convulsions. The woman sinks into a coma, which is almost always fatal. (Greenhill, 1951)

There is no reason why any woman's health should deteriorate to the point of convulsions, coma and death. For full details regarding the prevention and reversal of toxemia, see the Toxemia chapter in the section on Problems Associated With the Third Trimester.

Previously well-controlled epilepsy: A woman on anti-convulsive medication whose epilepsy has been well controlled before conception may have a convulsion during early pregnancy because nausea and vomiting and more rapid clearance of anti-epileptic drugs may reduce their effectiveness.

Gestational epilepsy: About 13% of all women who have a seizure disorder have their first onset during gestation. Of those about 40% have no seizures when they are not pregnant.

Differential diagnosis: Other conditions to consider include:

> *Drug abuse (either ingestion or withdrawal)
> *Poisoning or other toxic exposure
> *Brain tumors
> *Arteriovenous malformation
> *Cerebrovascular disease
> *Hypertension
> *Intracranial trauma
> *Infection (meningitis)

References and further reading:

Gibbs, Charles, "Sudden sensorium derangement during pregnancy," Contemp. Ob/Gyn, Vol. 20, #1, July 1982, pp. 55-64.

Greenhill, J., Principles and Practice of Obstetrics, 10th ed., W. B. Saunders, Co., Philadelphia, PA, 1951.

Hegner, Barbara & E. Caldwell, Nursing Assistant, 6th ed., Delmar Pub., Albany, NY, 1992.

1044

Skin and Hair Changes

A number of benign skin changes occur during pregnancy. The causes of some changes are not well understood, but are apparently due to hormonal, metabolic, and vascular volume alterations. A few changes warrant further evaluation by a dermatologist. Homeopathic remedies, correctly prescribed for the presenting symptoms may be highly effective for many skin conditions. Numerous herbal salves are on the market to deal with skin conditions and many are quite effective. If nothing else is working, suggest Cort Sym, a fabulous homeopathic topical gel which simulates the effect of cortisone cream without the drugs. Black gel is indicated for crusting, ulcerating or hardening of the skin. Order from Energique, Inc.

Common pigment and skin changes:

Stretch marks (*striae gravidarum*): Perhaps the most universal skin change noted during pregnancy is stretch marks, reddish to purplish streaks that appear in 90% of women during pregnancy at tension points in the skin surfaces that receive the most stretching. They typically appear on the breasts, abdomen and thighs as the deeper layers of the skin tear and will eventually become jagged silvery whitish lines that fade with time but never disappear. A genetic predisposition will make for more stretch marks, but who gets them and how much seems to depend, in part, on a woman's skin quality. Poor nutrition, especially a lack of fat soluble vitamins such as vitamin E, can contribute to stretch marks that are even more pronounced. Some other things women can try are:

  *Massaging cocoa butter and other natural oils into the skin; this may
      help but will not eliminate stretch marks.
  *Mix ½ cup virgin olive oil, ¼ cup aloe vera gel, 6 opened capsules
      vitamin E oil (400 IU or more) and 4 capsules vitamin A oil in a
      blender. Store in the refrigerator and apply daily.
  *Creams containing elastin.
  *Taking extra Vitamin E, vitamin C, bioflavonoids and zinc will help
      optimize the stretchability of the skin
  *Rejuvederm (also by Energique) is a homeopathic cream for stretch
      marks

At the same time, you should let women know that their bodies will be permanently changed by childbirth. They can see their stretch marks as symbols of their passage into motherhood, a new stage of womanhood; and something to be proud of. (Loprenzi-Kassel, 1995)

Itching (generalized pruritus of pregnancy): Itching of the skin may occur during pregnancy because the skin is being stretched; this is accentuated if the skin is dry. Contributory factors, aside from the enlargement of the uterus and breasts, include weight gain and hormonal changes. Dry skin will often itch more than skin which tends to be oily, and winter may aggravate the problem, especially if the woman has a central heating system that produces dry heat. Be sure to ask about recent changes in soaps or laundry products, which could also be causative. Some things which may help are:

> *Add unrefined olive oil to the diet
> *Apply castor oil to the skin nightly
> *Avoid mineral oil based skin products (which most of them are!)
> *Increase intake of vitamin A & D rich foods
> *Take Oatmeal baths (put oatmeal flakes in a piece of cloth and allow
>   the water to filter through it as it fills the tub)
> *Massage yogurt into the skin

Pruritus gravidarum: This type of itching is unique to pregnancy and is the result of the elevated estrogen and progesterone levels which are thought to interfere with the liver's excretion of bile salts. The reported incidence is 0.02% to 2.4%. Liver supporting herbs such as Dandelion root or Yellow Dock root can help the liver do its job. Onset is usually in the third trimester with severe generalized itching. There are no lesions but the skin may be abraded due to scratching. In the most severe cases jaundice will be noted. Lab tests of liver function are usually normal or mildly elevated. Other more common conditions need to be ruled out. (For more information see the chapter on The Liver and Pregnancy in Diagnostic Tests.)

Acne: Sebaceous gland secretions increase in late pregnancy. While some women's skin will clear for the first time during pregnancy, others will get a crop of pimples to rival what they had in high school. This is because the oil glands become more active and the hormones of pregnancy promote the formation of pimples in some women. Just as in high school, about all the woman can do is eliminate those foods she knows to cause problems and keep the face, neck and back particularly clean. She should avoid wearing heavy make-up, as this will just clog the pores. The use of Accutane (isotretinoin), tetracycline and corticosteroids to control outbreaks are all contraindicated during pregnancy; topical acne preparations should be avoided whenever possible.

Candida: A fungal skin infection may occur in pregnant women, especially in hot weather and in women-of-size. Typically, a rash appears in skin folds and under the arms and breasts. Lesions appear as round, blotchy areas of redness with itching or burning and, if the rash is very established, may peel revealing bright red shiny tissue. Pinhead-sized papules are seen around the edges; it resembles a typical candida diaper rash. The area should be kept clean and dry, cotton clothing will help the skin breathe; brief periods of exposure to sunlight will also help to dry and heal the area, if it is not sunny, a hair dryer set on low and held at a distance can be used to ensure that the area is dry after baths. To avoid spread, towels, clothing and hands which touch the rash should be washed before touching other body parts, particularly the genitals, mouth and breasts. Sexual contact is best avoided until the rash has cleared. The mother should be advised not to scratch, since this will imbed the fungus deeper into the skin and make it harder to eliminate. Energique makes a Diaper Rash gel specifically for candida rashes and other homeopathic or over-the-counter bio-technical yoni salves can be applied, but ointments which have a heavy greasy base (such as A & D) should not be used, as they will form a seal over the rash and thus an ideal incubator for it to persist. Rinsing the area in dilute lemon juice or white vinegar will help clear infection by supporting the skin's acid mantle.

Generalized hyperpigmentation: This diffuse darkening of the skin occurs in about 90% of pregnant women. It varies from generalized darkening of the skin to well-circumscribed macules (discolored spots), particularly of the face and other sun-exposed areas. The areolae of the nipples, genital skin, and *linea alba* are all areas which darken in many women. Freckles, other pigmented skin lesions and new scars may darken as well. Old scars remain unchanged. Avoiding excessive sun exposure and being sure folic acid intake is adequate will help minimize this.

Mask of pregnancy (chloasma or melasma): A woman who is deficient in folic acid may develop pigmented blotches over her cheeks, eyelids and nose. Increasing the intake of fresh dark green vegetables and supplementing with folic acid should eliminate this symptom.

Moles: Refer the woman to a dermatologist for diagnosis and removal of moles with any of the following features:

> *New moles appearing during pregnancy
> *Moles which change color or enlarge
> *Moles associated with ulceration, bleeding, or pain
> *Moles that are smooth and blue-black or dark brown
> *Moles located where they are subject to irritation (such as at the belt or panty line)
> *Moles on the genitals or feet (where they are more likely to undergo malignant changes)

Skin tags: Women sometimes note the appearance of small pinhead to pea sized pediculated skin tags called *molluscum fibrosum gravidarum*. These appear as little flesh colored to pale growths attached by a small stem that are commonly found on the neck, chest, breasts, and underarms. They appear during the latter part of pregnancy as the result of hormonal changes, and will usually decrease in size or disappear completely after the birth.

Miscellaneous skin tumors: A variety of skin tumors may appear or grow more quickly during pregnancy. Any unusual skin condition should be evaluated by a dermatologist.

Palmar erythema (red palms): Reddening of the palms from venous and capillary engorgement may occur during pregnancy; it may also be related to increased levels of estrogen in the bloodstream. It is noted in up to 66% of Caucasian women. Palmer erythema is also seen in lupus, hyperthyroidism, and liver disorders. If the liver is not metabolizing hormones normally, red palms can also indicate liver stress; rule this out by performing a Liver Profile test. If the liver profile is normal, this condition is considered benign by bio-technical providers, as it will resolve after birth. If a woman is seeing a Chinese doctor, this symptom will be seen as significant and treated accordingly.

Vascular changes: High levels of estrogen may be the cause of the growth of blood vessels and congestion that is commonly seen in pregnancy. Vasomotor instability may also produce pallor, flushing and mottling of the skin. In otherwise normal women these changes are not a concern.

Spider veins (nevi araneus): These lesions are found in 66% of Caucasian women and 11% of African-American women. They present as a centrally dilated arteriole surrounded by fine, tentacle-like blood vessels, often with a surrounding area of redness. They blanch completely when a glass microscope slide is pressed over them or when a pencil point is pressed directly in the center. They usually disappear completely by the 3rd month postpartum. No therapy is indicated.

Sweating: The sweat glands increase their activity due to the influences of the hormones of pregnancy, a woman's body odor becomes stronger and may take on an odor that is unique to her. One solution is to bathe regularly. Most women report that they are warmer than usual during pregnancy and they may perspire more as well. This is due to the increased metabolism of pregnancy. Sweating is one way the body cools itself off; in hot weather women may perspire quite a bit. Wearing loose comfortable clothing, preferably of a breathable absorbent material such as cotton, can help. Taking liquid chlorophyll daily (1 to 2 Tbsp.) may help minimize odor and is a good source of nutrients. Zinc intake should also be checked (the naturopathic motto goes "if you stink, you need zinc!"). Strong deodorants and antiperspirants containing aluminum should be avoided, since the chemicals they contain get absorbed into the underarm lymph nodes and the breast tissue. "Health food brand" deodorants that do not contain aluminum should be used instead.

Increased sweat gland activity may also lead to the development of milaria, tiny epidermal entrapments of sweat. Hand or foot eczema or clammy skin may also be a problem during pregnancy.

Capillary hemangiomas: These variations on a birthmark may arise during pregnancy, appearing on the gum line, tongue, eyelid and upper lip. They usually regress postpartum, but do not always disappear completely. Large lesion may be associated with heart problems. Preexisting hemangiomas may increase in size during pregnancy. Nothing should be done during pregnancy; after birth, laser therapy, steroids and surgery are the treatments available from bio-technical practitioners.

Nail changes: Transverse grooving of the fingernails, called Beau's lines, may be noted during pregnancy; this can occur as a result of decreased nail synthesis. Brittleness, and distal separation of the nail plate from the nail bed has been reported. Any woman experiencing nail changes such as these is probably nutritionally deficient and should have a thorough dietary and supplement review.

Hair and scalp problems:

Hair growth or loss: Both diffuse scalp hair growth and increased hair growth in locations other than the scalp (hirsutism) are seen during pregnancy. An increased percentage of scalp hairs are growing during pregnancy, with decreased hair loss. Hair loss may indicate the need for more protein and calcium in the diet. Remember that hair loss is seen in secondary syphilis; be sure to review the history for this possibility.

Dark hairs may appear on the upper lip, chin, around the nipples, and elsewhere especially during the third trimester, these will usually disappear after birth. If severe or if accompanied by other signs such as clitoral enlargement, deep voice and severe acne, a full endocrinologic evaluation is indicated. A few women may notice the development of fine downy hair on their face and chest; this is a response to the increased hormone levels in pregnancy and is not a concern.

Scalp itching: Itching of the scalp may be caused by the retention of bile salts secondary to the increased estrogen levels of pregnancy. If the woman reports itching, crawling sensations or other unusual scalp symptoms, examine her scalp for the possibility of head lice (*pediculus humanus capitis*). Look for tiny red bumps or bite marks on the scalp, eyebrows, behind the ears and on the neck. If you are suspicious of an infestation, part the hair behind the ear with a pair of tissue forceps. Shine a bright light on the area and immediately look for the lice with a magnifying glass, as they will run away quickly from the bright light. Also check for nits, or eggs, which will cling to the hair shaft. The tiny egg cases will reflect the light, they are most often found at the nape of the neck or behind the ears, and do not slide easily off the hair. To inspect a specimen under the microscope, grab one with the forceps and tape it to a slide with clear tape. Set the microscope on low power. Adult lice are neutral gray or rust colored and have a long, tapered body, three pairs of legs with delicate hooks on the end and are 2 to 3 mm. long. Nits appear as whitish translucent eggs.

Pediculicide agents should be used exactly as directed on the package. Start with over-the-counter agents such as RID or A-200. Lindane lotions such as Kwell or Scabene are not generally recommended for use during pregnancy since about 10% of the application will be absorbed systemically and may rarely cause central nervous system toxicity or convulsions. Shampoo should only be applied for 4 minutes and then rinsed out. In addition, brushes and combs should be boiled, and all washable fabrics should be washed in hot water, double rinsed and then ironed with a steam iron; nonwashables should be dry cleaned and stored in sealed plastic for 10 days. Headrests should be vacuumed and sealed in plastic for 10 days. Since head lice are frequently the result of a school-wide epidemic, the children and partners of affected women should be examined as well.

Pubic lice: Another type of lice (*phthirus pubis*) may infest pubic hair, perianal hair and sometimes the hair of the armpits, trunk, thighs and eyelashes. They are mainly transmitted by sexual contact and occasionally are transmitted by contact with infested bedding, clothes, toilet seats or other articles. The woman will complain of itching, which may be accompanied by tiny bluish to slate colored flat lesions and scratch marks; these may become infected.

Using a magnifying glass, look for oval, whitish translucent nits (eggs) attached to one side of the hair shaft and for lice at the base of hairs. Adults look like tiny yellowish-gray to rust colored crabs 1 to 2 mm. in length. If the woman bathes often, mature lice will be hard to find. Snip any hair with a nit, tape it to a slide and examine it under a microscope, using a low-power objective. You may be able to see an immature louse moving inside the egg.

Pediculicide agents should be applied carefully so as to avoid mucous membranes; gel may be the easiest to use in the genital area. Instructions should be followed exactly as the package indicates. All sexual partners and family members should be examined and treated, if necessary. In addition to the delousing suggestions given for head lice, toilets and toilet seats should be scoured, rinsed and dried. Be sure she cleans up under the bowl lip. Mattresses should be vacuumed and then sealed in plastic for ten days.

While various herbal washes and oils can be used to try and eliminate both types of lice, the quantities necessary, the length of treatment, and the topical use of oils (especially Pennyroyal) make herbs a poor choice during pregnancy.

1050

Rare skin conditions of pregnancy: Rare skin conditions are frequently controlled with steroid medications and antihistamines. If a woman would like to try other forms of treatment, homeopathic remedies are an excellent modality; since these conditions produce distinct symptom pictures. While some of these conditions cause no problems, any generalized skin eruption should be differentially diagnosed before being dismissed as benign. Consider viral, syphilitic, and other possible causes. Get a consultation and run tests as necessary to track down any not-so-benign causes (see specific topics in Diagnostic Tests).

Toxemic rash of pregnancy: A rash consisting of red, elevated itching hives appears on the skin of the abdomen. It has no relationship to metabolic toxemia; no pathologic data are available.

Papular dermatitis of pregnancy: This rare rash consists of an eruption of highly itchy hives over the entire skin surface, with the appearance of 3 to 8 new lesions daily. Lesions are 3 to 5 mm. in diameter, consisting of a central raised area covered with a bloody crust 1 to 2 mm. in diameter; they do not occur in clusters and may appear anywhere on the body. Healing takes 7 to 10 days and may leave some residual hyperpigmentation. The rash may appear at any time during gestation and almost always vanishes after the birth, but may recur in subsequent pregnancies. All women with this condition have been found to have elevated urinary Chorionic Gonadotropin, (from 25,000 to 500,000 units). A 27% fetal mortality is reported, although no reason for these deaths is given. In women treated with corticosteroids, no fetal deaths occurred. (Gabbe, et.al., 1991)

***Pruritic urticarial papules* and plaques of pregnancy (PUPPP):** Rarely (14 cases were on record as of 1985), late in the first pregnancy, a woman gets an itchy pimply skin eruption presenting with edema and redness on her abdomen and in her stretch marks. These lesions can also enlarge to include the thighs, buttocks and upper arms. No laboratory test abnormalities are noted. They are not harmful and will disappear postpartum. The newborn may also have these lesions, but they are presumably benign.

Impetigo herpetiformis: This skin condition usually appears in the third trimester in conjunction with malaise, fever, diarrhea, swollen lymph nodes, delirium, tetany from hypocalcemia, dehydration or convulsions. Red patches ringed with pustules begin to appear in skin folds (usually the groin and inner thighs) and may spread to cover the entire body, enlarging around their borders. The mucus membranes are frequently affected, with painful, grayish white plaques in the mouth. The skin overlaying the pustules ruptures, leaving a central denuded area and a ring of adherent scale. Lesions beneath the nail beds may cause the nails to separate from the underlying tissue. The name of this condition is misleading, because in the 300 cases on record as of 1985, no bacterial or viral infection was found. Cultures done on the pustules are negative. Both syphilis and ringworm must be considered in your differential diagnosis. Darkfield microscopy of lesion specimens, and non-treponemal and treponeme specific tests should be done to rule out atypical syphilis. There is a high incidence of stillbirths but no known cutaneous involvement in the fetus. This condition usually disappears postpartum, but may recur with subsequent pregnancies.

Herpes Gestationes: These blistering lesions occur in about 1 in every 3,000 to 5,000 pregnancies. Lesions may appear at any time during pregnancy or immediately postpartum. Onset is signaled by fever, hot and cold sensations, malaise, nausea, headache and itching. The lesions begin as a red rash and typically make their first appearance on the abdomen; the buttocks, back, forearms, and genitalia are sometimes involved. Mucous membrane involvement is rare. Most affected women show a circulating herpes gestationes factor, a complement-fixing IgG antibody detectable only by complement immunofluorescent testing. Lesions usually disappear by 6 months after birth. More severe episodes may occur in subsequent pregnancies. Medication containing estrogen and progesterone are contraindicated at any time for women with such a history, as they aggravate the condition. While herpes gestationes is not truly a herpes infection, it may respond well to remedies for viral herpes. Syphilis should also be ruled out. Herpes gestationes is associated with a somewhat increased rate of growth retardation, fetal mortality, miscarriage and prematurity rate. High levels of circulating antibasement antibody and peripheral eosinophilia may account for this increased risk. Sometimes skin lesions appear in infants due to passive transfer of maternal antibodies; these generally require no therapy and will resolve on their own. (See the chapters on Herpes and Syphilis in Diagnostic Tests for more information). (Gabbe, et.al, 1991)

Pruigo gestationis: These benign lesions appear as raw, itchy, non-blistering papules that are limited to the extensor surfaces of the arms and legs. They usually appear during the second half of pregnancy. They are small, 1 to 2 mm. papules that are distributed symmetrically. Lesions appearing between 25 and 29 weeks are more itchy than those appearing later. Calamine lotion usually relieves the symptoms.

References and further reading:

Gabbe, Steven, et.al., eds. Obstetrics: Normal and Problem Pregnancies, 2nd ed., Churchill Livingstone, New York, 1991.
Gleicher, Norbert, ed., Principles of Medical Therapy in Pregnancy, Plenum Pub., New York, 1985.
Loprenzi-Kassel, ClareBeth, midwife, Veneta, OR, editing comments, 2/95.

Torsion of the Pregnant Uterus

Most of the time the uterus develops a slight degree of rotation, to the right in 80% and to the left in 20% of all pregnancies. Uterine torsion, or twisting, is defined as the lengthwise rotation of the uterus by more than 45°. In most abnormal situations the degree of rotation has become extreme and is usually 180° or more. The cause of this exceedingly rare complication of pregnancy is not really understood, but it is often found in the presence of some kind of uterine malformation or tumor. In 20% of all cases the following factors have accompanied this complication:

*Malpresentation of the baby, especially transverse lie
*Uterine myomas (fibroids)
*Abnormalities of the uterus
*Pelvic adhesions (from scar tissue)
*Ovarian cyst
*History of uterine suspension (surgery using the round ligaments to
      correct uterine retroversion or prolapse)
*Abnormal pelvis
*Placenta previa

Signs and symptoms: The woman will appear to be having an acute abdominal condition which includes pain, shock and bleeding, and may appear to be in hard, obstructed labor. Symptoms may mimic those of an intestinal or severe urinary tract condition. Sudden or extreme degrees of torsion result in impaired uterine circulation. The maternal mortality rate is as high as 13%, and increases as term approaches. Mortality is directly related to the degree of torsion. The perinatal mortality rate is about 30% and is also related to the severity of the torsion.

What to do: If you suspect this condition. support the mother and monitor for symptoms of shock (monitor vital signs, keep her warm, give oxygen by mask at a flow rate of 6 liters per minute) and transport without delay!!

Treatment: If the woman is close to term and she is not in acute distress she can visualize the uterus rotating back to a normal position. If acute, a surgical delivery will be performed. If the fetus is too premature for birth a laparotomy may be done in order to rotate the uterus to its normal position and allow the pregnancy to continue to term.

References and further reading:

Oxhorn, Harry, <u>Human Labor and Birth</u>, 5th ed. Appleton-Century-Crofts, E. Norwalk, CT, 1986.

Urine Test Results

Why positive urine tests occur is reviewed extensively in <u>Diagnostic Tests</u>, This chapter is designed to augment that information with details on how to deal with these issues in the clinical setting. Some of this information will overlap. (For those findings not discussed here, please see <u>Diagnostic Tests</u>.) The following protocols address dealing with positive urine test results during pregnancy. You might also want to discuss the recommendations offered with other midwives. Consult with another care provider if you are unsure about the underlying problem or if these suggestions do not result in a satisfactory resolution.

Proteinuria: Proteinuria may appear in the urine for a variety of reasons; most of them are relatively benign.

> *A trace of protein is within a normal range
> *Concentration of urine can cause proteinuria: assess adequacy of fluid intake and increase as indicated
> *Assess possibility of urinary tract infection and treat as appropriate
> *Assess possibility of contamination from the yoni or yoni infection; get a clean catch specimen if proteinuria is significant
> *Recommend at least 1 cup daily of Nettles infusion to strengthen kidneys, as indicated
> *If other signs of metabolic toxemia of late pregnancy are present, evaluate for toxemia

It is recognized that proteinuria is a late secondary sign of toxemia: all other possibilities should first be ruled out unless toxemia is otherwise clinically apparent.

Ketonuria: In the absence of complicating signs and symptoms, ketones in the urine indicate inadequate food intake. Advise increasing the amount of food eaten and eating more frequently throughout the day. If ketones are positive, especially in the presence of significant glucosuria and alkaline urinary pH, diabetes screening should be carried out.

Glucosuria: Glucosuria is a common occurrence during pregnancy and usually does not indicate a problem. Upon the first positive finding:

> *Assess recent dietary intake and recommend eliminating all sugars (white, brown, honey, maple syrup, etc.), juices, fruits and refined carbohydrates, as appropriate in relation to level of glucosuria presenting
> *Assess and encourage regular exercise

*Review current or previous history of personal and familial diabetes or kidney problems
*Assess normal limits for the individual—has this happened with previous, otherwise normal, pregnancies?
*Recommend nettle infusion or freeze dried capsules to strengthen kidneys if more than a trace of glucosuria is found

If glucosuria exceeds a trace on more than one occasion instruct client to:

*Recheck urine using the second voided morning specimen
*Return to recheck urine a few days after dietary changes have been made if the woman lives nearby
*Monitor her glucose levels at home and keep records of her diet and test results including time of day the urine was checked and the time in relationship to her last food intake (2 hours after breakfast, for example) if the woman lives farther away.
*Use a finger-stick test to compare urinary glucose readings with blood levels. A normal blood test will help distinguish benign glucosuria from a problem.

After glucosuria clears, reintroduce one or two whole fresh fruits daily and continue to check. If glucosuria does not resolve, especially if her levels during other pregnancies and earlier in this pregnancy have been normal, assume this is due to a higher renal filtration rate and continue to follow with dipstick testing, unless other diabetic symptoms develop. Recommend at least one cup of nettles infusion daily to strengthen the kidneys.

If this is a first pregnancy with unresolved significant glucosuria, especially if ketosis or other diabetic symptoms are present with frequent meals, recommend a 2-hour postprandial glucose test. Diabetic symptoms include ravenous appetite with weight loss or failure to gain, continuous thirst, and slow healing of wounds. (See the chapter in this section entitled Gestational Diabetes and the chapter on Diabetes and Pregnancy in Diagnostic Tests for more details.)

*If the two hour postprandial is positive, recommend 100 mg of B_6 three times daily and recheck in a week.
*If a postprandial is still positive, recommend a one hour oral glucose tolerance Test (OGTT).
*If the OGTT is positive, adjust diet to pregnancy diabetic diet (high calorie and complex carbohydrate plus one gram protein per pound of body weight daily) and recommend regular exercise; recheck.
*If still positive, consult a specialist for recommendations.

Blood in the urine: Blood may appear in the urine in two forms (which are distinguished on most urine test strips that include reagents for blood). When any blood is found in the urine:

> *Check to be sure test strips look normal/are stored correctly/are not out of date
> *If you have questions about the sticks, use a new bottle
> *Retest using a fresh stick and a clean catch
> *If urine is dark or specific gravity reading on dip-stick is high, have the woman drink 10 oz. of water and retest at the next urination
> *Recommend Nettles infusion to strengthen and heal the kidneys

Hemoglobinuria (free hemoglobin from broken down RBCs) may appear due to conditions outside the urinary tract such as severe burns, injuries, transfusion reaction, chemical agents (aspirin), hemolysis (especially from anemia; this can be due to lead poisoning), or alkaline urine. If hemoglobinuria is present:

> *Rule out alkaline urine, chemical agents & lead poisoning
> *Order a lab urine analysis (explain the reason to the woman)
> *Use a clean catch specimen

Hematuria (intact red cells) can be caused by bleeding within the urinary tract, a lower UTI or contamination of the sample with discharge from the yoni. Kidney stones or other kidney problems such as congenital anomalies of the urinary tract, cancer, tuberculosis, heavy smoking and hypertension may cause a positive result. In rare cases, spontaneous traumatic rupture of the kidney can occur. Hematuria may be secondary to a variety of problems such as tumors, calculi, fungal disease, endometriosis, inflammatory bowel lesions, amyloidosis and granulomas which may involve the urinary tract. Blood will often cause a positive protein reading as well. Protein or a high specific gravity may reduce the sensitivity of some tests. Benign gestational hematuria does occur and may be related to engorgement of blood vessels in the kidneys (Donald, 1979). If hematuria is present:

> *Order a bacterial culture & sensitivity to rule out urinary tract infection
> *Have the lab check for blood as well
> *If there are no symptoms and other lab tests are negative, continue to monitor and retest at the 6 week visit, if still present, suggest a consultation with a kidney specialist.

References and further reading:
Donald, Ian, Practical Obstetric Problems, Lloyd-Luke, Ltd., London, Eng., 1979.

Urinary Tract Infections

Pregnant women are more susceptible to urinary tract infections (UTI) than those who are not pregnant due to the generalized relaxation of muscles in the body (which affects the ureters) and the pressure from the enlarging uterus. Bacteria can grow in kinks in the ureters, because they are not flushed out as efficiently. Constipation is thought by some to encourage urinary tract infections, because the impacted lower bowel may put pressure on the ureters and the retention of feces may encourage bacteria to penetrate the rectal wall (Ajayi, 1988). Women should be reminded not to perform pelvic floor exercises while urinating as this will encourage infection, although an occasional contraction to assess muscle tone will not generally cause a problem. Signs of UTI include sub- or suprapubic aching or pain, burning on urination, cramps, fever and general fatigue (if the infection is well established) and lower backache (which may indicate kidney involvement).

More information about how to proceed with diagnosis and treatment is outlined in Diagnostic Tests. Once diagnosed, Uva Ursi-Plus TM (from Scientific Botanicals) can be used as an initial treatment (two capsules four times daily for three to five days and recheck). It contains mannose (the main sugar in cranberries) which attaches to bacteria and prevents it from adhering to the lining of the urinary tract.

Note that the following conditions may mimic urinary tract infection:

*Early signs of ectopic pregnancy
*Premature labor (see separate chapter, Third Trimester section)
*Torsion of the pregnant uterus (extremely rare, see chapter in this
    section)
*Incarceration or sacculation of the uterus (also rare, see the section
    of Second Trimester Problems)

Acute pyelonephritis: This is the most common renal complication of pregnancy. Symptoms are the same as for UTI, but more severe, with fever as high as 104°F (40°C). It must be distinguished from referred liver pain (in toxemia) or pneumonia on the affected side (pay attention to respiration rate and physical chest signs). Differentiating it from acute appendicitis may also be difficult, especially in late pregnancy, but usually at the onset of appendicitis, pain is referred to the center of the abdomen, vomiting is not a marked feature, the fever is not so high as in pyelonephritis, and rigors do not occur. Kidney infection should be treated without delay. IV antibiotics in the hospital may be recommended for two to three weeks, after which urine cultures should be checked at each prenatal until birth.

References and further reading:

Ajayi, V., A Textbook of Midwifery, McMillian Pub., New York, 1988.

Vascular Problems

Varicose veins: Varicose veins are enlarged blood vessels that have weakened valves. Varicosities are most commonly found in the legs, vulva, or yoni. However they may more rarely develop on the torso or breasts as well as elsewhere on or within the body. They are by far the most common vascular disorder that occurs during pregnancy. The valves normally help in directing blood flow; if they weaken, pooling of blood and subsequent enlargement of the vessels can occur. Pregnancy accentuates this problem due to the expansion of the blood volume in combination with the indiscriminate hormonal relaxation of muscles. Additionally, as pregnancy advances, the weight of the uterus impedes blood flow from the lower extremities. These factors increase venous distention, which is further aggravated if veins are not given proper support.

As pooling increases, clots may form, causing firm lumps and heat in the area. If they persist, redness, tenderness and swelling may occur. Blood stasis may lead to infection or thrombophlebitis (blood clots). Moist hot packs may be applied to problem areas, but under no circumstances should vessels be massaged. This could break up clots and cause an embolism. Exercise such as walking and swimming will keep the blood moving and minimize clot formation. Women need to engage in light activity after birth to prevent blood pooling in the veins. Women who are prone to clots should know that airline travel encourages their formation. Shepherd's Purse tincture should not be used in these women; it may lead to such an increase in coagulation ability that clots form more easily.

Vulval and yoni varicosities may only be apparent during pregnancies. Large vulval varicosities can be supported by wearing a sanitary pad with a sanitary belt; this will provide counterpressure and reduce discomfort. Trauma to vulval and yoni varicosities may occur during birth. If one ruptures, a hematoma will be the likely result; if there are lacerations, sewing around a varicosity can be tricky.

Some therapies that may minimize varicosities, regardless of location, are:

> *Nettle infusion (1 to 2 cups daily) or freeze dried Nettles in capsules (start with 3 daily). Nettles heals the vascular and renal systems and is a nutritive herb. There are no contraindications to its use.
> *Collinsonia Root tincture or tablets (available through Standard Process Labs) can be used. Start with 1 tablet 3 times daily and see if the veins improve. Increase up to 6 tablets a day, if needed. (Contraindicated in women with a history of kidney problems.)
> *An abdominal support may help prevent further damage and minimize discomfort (see Pendulous Abdomen chapter in Third Trimester Problems)
> *Vitamin C with bioflavinoids (at least 500 mg. and up to 3 grams daily); Rutin (a bioflavonoid), 50 mg.
> *Vitamin E, 400 to 1000 IU daily

*Hawthorne Berry extract (¼ tsp. 2 to 3 times daily)
*Moist towels applied daily (five minutes with hot towels alternating with 1 minute of cold towels)
*Avoiding heavy lifting.
*Avoiding constipation with plenty of fluids and fiber in the diet.
*Avoidance of restrictive pants or stockings which go part way up the leg.
*Witch Hazel bark infusion (1 oz. herb to 1 pint boiling water, steeped for 10 hours) can be used on cloths to apply to the veins.
*If a vein is an open sore, soaking the area in an combination of comfrey and plantain infusion twice daily and following the vitamin recommendations above. The woman should also have it checked by another practitioner.
*Support hose; these should be worn from early pregnancy on if any veins are visible, and especially if swelling, heat, or pain is present in a vein. A little cornstarch powder on the legs and dishwashing-style latex gloves may help in putting them on. Open toed, porous stockings which supply at least 30 mmHg. and up to 60 mmHg. of graduated pressure are good for severe vein conditions. They can be worn during labor and continued postpartum until the veins have reduced to their prepregnant size and blood volume has reduced to non-pregnant levels. Those which are fitted to the individual woman are the most effective, but in some states they are only available by prescription.
*Elevating the legs above the level of the heart, or lying on one side several times a day for 15 to 20 minutes.
*If a woman must stand during the day for extended lengths of time, elevating her legs during breaks and going up on her toes periodically throughout the day to increase venous circulation.
*Vulval varicosities can be supported with old-fashioned sanitary napkins worn securely against them and held in place with a sanitary belt.

Clots can form in deep veins as well, which may result in edema on the affected side. To further evaluate this possibility, have the woman lie down, then grasp her foot and sharply flex her ankle. Calf pain indicates the presence of a deep venous clot. (This is called Homan's Sign.) (Varney, 1980) If such a clot is discovered or suspected, give homeopathic Arnica in 30C doses several times daily and get a bio-technical evaluation and a naturopathic evaluation (if available) so that options for treatment can be explored.

Hemorrhoids: Hemorrhoids commonly appear or become aggravated during pregnancy. They arise from highly vascular submucosal cushions of the anal canal which differ from the rest of the GI tract. Rather than forming a continuous ring, this mucosa is present in only three areas: two o'clock on the posterior anal canal, five o'clock on the anterior aspect and nine o'clock on the left lateral anal wall. Hemorrhoids are the abnormal dilation of veins in one or more of these cushions. The following factors are thought to be contributory: erect posture, lack of venous valves, intrinsic weakness of anal blood vessels, back-flow into the cushions (with increased abdominal pressure or defecation), defects of venous drainage due to a tense anal sphincter during defecation and back pressure on the vessels by a pregnant uterus. Constipation and its accompanying pressure changes also play an important role. Straining and passage of hard stool leads to blood vessel engorgement; repeated straining causes dilation of the veins in the anal cushions. Dilated vessels stretch the supporting tissues and allow the hemorrhoid to prolapse into the anal canal, leading to distention during defecation.

Internal hemorrhoids originate above the edge of the internal anal sphincter (the dentate or pectinate line) and may eventually be pulled down through the anal opening. Closure of the sphincter then strangulates the prolapsed hemorrhoid, occasionally leading to thrombosis. If hemorrhoids arise below this point, they present at the anal opening as external swellings where they more commonly undergo thrombosis. An external skin tag can form from an old skin fold that was once a thrombosed hemorrhoid. Trauma, irritation, jobs requiring prolonged sitting and straining during defecation increase the risk of thrombosis.

DEGREE	SYMPTOMS OF INTERNAL HEMORRHOIDS
First	Painless, bright red bleeding during or after defecation
Second	Painless bleeding with prolapse producing the sensation of a perianal mass that reduces spontaneously
Third	Prolapse that is manually reduced by the woman
Fourth	Nonreducable prolapse

Uncomplicated external hemorrhoids are often asymptomatic unless thrombosed, although they may present with painless bleeding, irritation or itching, the sensation of a perianal mass and constipation. Thrombosed hemorrhoids swell up and appear as purple, grape-like protrusions from the anal opening, usually accompanied by dramatic and sudden moderate to severe pain. Only severely thrombosed, ulcerated or ruptured hemorrhoids may require surgery, rubber band ligation or, alternatively, Keesey (electrical destruction) treatments, if natural remedies do not promote a resolution of symptoms. Neither surgery nor electrical treatments can be done during pregnancy.

External hemorrhoids are usually obvious on visual inspection or during a digital exam; palpate at 2, 5 and 9 o'clock as described above. Ask the woman to bear down during the exam, which will help to make internal hemorrhoids more obvious. Without thrombosis, painful anal bleeding is most likely due to an anal

1060

fissure (a split in the anal mucosa; insert 400 IU or higher vitamin E capsules at night to help such fissures heal). However, it could also be caused by other types of lesions (cancer) and a visit to a proctologist is warranted if hemorrhoids are not obvious on exam or symptoms persist for more than 6 weeks in spite of treatment.

If a woman has a history of hemorrhoids, the first 12 suggestions given above for varicose veins may be helpful. In addition, make the following recommendations:

*Use a stool or other object to elevate feet at the toilet. This will put the muscles in better alignment and produce less rectal strain
*Yellow Dock root tincture (½ dropperful taken orally 3 times daily) gently supports the liver; hemorrhoids are related to liver
*Prolapsed hemorrhoids can be gently lubricated with olive oil or water-based lubricant and replaced inside. The woman can purchase a box of inexpensive gloves or finger cots at a surgical supply house for this purpose. Replacement will help minimize strangulation and prevent thrombosis.congestion.
*Vitamin E capsules (400 IU or more) can be introduced into the anal canal at night before retiring to help heal the tissues.

Do not recommend over-the-counter remedies such as Preparation H. Preparation H, in particular, contains mercury. The less questionable chemicals in the mother and baby's systems, the better. There are several topical homeopathic hemorrhoid products on the market, any of which can be safely used during pregnancy. Energique markets one such gel. Tucks pads are soaked with distilled Witch Hazel and can be used, although full strength infusion, as suggested above, is much more effective. (Schussman & Lutz, 1986)

Bruising easily: In most cases, bruises occur because capillaries and sometimes larger vessels are ruptured due to injury. Spontaneous bruising may also result from an abnormal clotting situation involving platelets. Bruising easily may be a long standing problem or one which presents as a new problem during pregnancy. In most cases it is related to the need for more B complex vitamins and vitamin C with bioflavinoids; these are nutrients which strengthen membranes and capillary beds. Vitamin K is also essential to clotting and is found in dark greens, dairy products, egg yolks, black strap molasses, safflower oils, fish-liver oils and other unsaturated oils. It can also be supplemented with 8 to 10 15-grain Alfalfa tablets daily (see Diagnostic Tests for additional sources). Homeopathic Arnica in 30C doses can be taken shortly after any obvious injuries, this results in a remarkable reduction or elimination of subsequent bruising.

If bruises begin to occur suddenly and are severe, there may be a clotting abnormality. Clotting problems from low platelets may produce petechiae, which are small patches of ruptured blood vessels producing bluish-purple spider-like subcutaneous lesions. (See the chapter on Clotting Disorders in <u>Diagnostic Tests</u> for more information.)

Cerebrovascular disorders: Intracranial bleeding is much more rare and more serious. Nonhemmorhagic stroke occurs 3 to 4 times more frequently among pregnant women than in the general population of young women. It is currently believed that arterial occlusions, rather the venous blockages, account for most strokes occurring during pregnancy. Venous blocks are more likely to occur after birth.

Arterial occlusion: A blockage may occur in any one of several arteries, although the majority involve the carotid arteries. Symptoms may be varied but include one-sided paralysis (arm may be worse than leg), one-sided changes in the senses (taste, smell, hearing, vision), blindness for half of the field of vision in the eye on the side of the lesion, temporary loss of vision in one eye due to insufficient blood flow (may last up to 10 minutes), and various types of aphasia related to the dominant hemisphere of the brain involved, such as speech impairment, memory loss and inability to understand words.

Treatment is aimed at establishing the cause of the blockage and preventing its recurrence. Damage to the neural tube does not ordinarily repair itself, so bio-technical medicine hopes rehabilitation will compensate for any lost functions. Homeopathic remedies as well as taking Skullcap infusion and applying Skullcap poultices to the affected area whenever possible can all help restore neurological function. A careful neurologic exam should be performed; this will help establish the possible location of the damage. Causative factors such as increased clotting ability and clots from the heart or peripheral vessels should be ruled out: a CT scan with adequate shielding may be needed to rule out brain tumors, subdural hematomas or other bleeding. A base-line EEG (brain wave evaluation) should also be obtained. If systemic causes are ruled out, it is assumed the stroke was caused by simple vessel occlusion, for which treatment is supportive and rehabilitative; anticoagulants are not recommended if the symptoms are stable. However, if they are progressing, heparin may be prescribed. During the balance of the pregnancy, blood pressure and glucose levels need to be maintained with minimal fluctuation.

References and further reading:
Ellis, Harold, <u>Varicose Veins</u>, Arco, Pub., Co., New York, NY, 1982.
Gleicher, N, ed. <u>Principles of Medical Therapy in Pregnancy</u>, Plenum Pub., New York, 1985.
Kassel, Joe, ND, L.Ac., conversation concerning hemorrhoids, 6/27/95.
Loprenzi-Kassel, ClareBeth, licensed midwife, Veneta, OR, editing comments, 2/95.
Schussman, L., Lutz, L., "Outpatient Management of hemorrhoids," <u>Primary Care: Office Surgery</u>, Vol. 13, No. 3, Sept. 1986, pp. 527-41.
Varney, Helen, <u>Nurse Midwifery</u>, Blackwell Pub. Co., Boston, MA, 1980.

1062

<u>Venoms, Bites and Stings</u>

While venomous bites from a variety of animals can occur, the most common include snakes, lizards, insects and spiders. Pregnancy does not alter the pathophysiology or treatment of these illnesses; the main goals are to maintain maternal vital functions and fetal well-being.

Snakes: Approximately one-tenth of all snakes are poisonous. Coral snakes are found across the southern states from Florida to Arizona. They are usually marked with alternating red and black bands separated by narrow yellow rings. They are not aggressive and tend to be nocturnal and reclusive. Their short fangs are permanently erect. Venom is ejected with multiple chewing movements. Bites result in ascending neurotoxic effects beginning about 15 minutes after the bite. Symptoms include poor muscular coordination, droopy eyelids, dilated pupils and progressive central nervous system and respiratory depression. Most deaths that occur take place within 6 to 72 hours. Recovery may be complicated by tissue damage, infection, shock, homolysis or clotting breakdown.

Pit vipers such as rattlesnakes, cottonmouths and copperheads are the other type of poisonous snake native to the United States. Several species of rattlesnakes are found across the country. The cottonmouth (or water moccasin), and copperhead (or highland moccasin) are found in swampy regions of the southern and gulf states. These snakes have a triangularly shaped head with pit-like heat sensors between the eyes and nostrils. The fangs are hinged and become erect during a strike. Venom is ejected through the hollow fangs, exiting through holes located proximal to the tips of the fangs. These snakes are aggressive and tend to strike when disturbed. Bites cause painful local swelling with edema, bruising, and blistering. Local tissue necrosis and gangrene may occur. Vascular compromise may lead to amputation of an affected extremity. Fever, nausea, vomiting, hemolysis, clotting collapse, heart failure and central nervous system excitation or depression are frequent accompanying symptoms.

The severity of the reaction to a bite is dependent on the person's age, health, the location and depth of the bite, the amount of envenomization, the size and anger of the snake, which bacteria are present on the skin surface and in the snake's mouth, and the amount of exercise or exertion following the bite as well as the initial treatment. The emotional response of the victim may confuse the clinical picture.

What to do: All types of snakes bites are handled in the same way. About 20% of those bitten will not have symptoms because no significant envenomization has occurred. This may be due to a shallow bite, condition of the snake's fangs, or fullness of the venom sacs. If no fang marks are found or if the woman does not show local or systemic symptoms within 20 minutes after the bite, significant envenomization is unlikely.

First aid should begin within 30 minutes of the attack to be most effective if a bite is found. Apply a loose tourniquet proximal to the bite; you should be able to insert your finger beneath it. This will serve to diminish lymphatic and superficial venous return while not impeding flow in deeper vessels. It should be moved closer to the body as local edema develops and removed when antivenom is administered.

After placing the tourniquet, the fang marks should be incised with linear cuts about 0.5 cm. long to the depth of penetration with a sterile implement. Suction with a bulb should be continued for one hour, during which up to 50% of the venom may be removed. Do not attempt to incise and suction the advancing edge of edema, as this is ineffective. The affected limb should be loosely immobilized in a functional position for transport to the nearest medical facility. Cooling may provide symptomatic relief but will not inactivate venom. Do not apply ice as this may encourage tissue necrosis. If you know homeopathic prescribing well, give a remedy for the symptom picture, if not, give oral Arnica, 30C doses at 15 to 30 minute intervals.

Treatment: At the hospital, neutralization of the venom with antivenom and prevention of tissue loss or the need to amputate will be the primary goals of care. Women should be tested for hypersensitivity to horse serum, the base for antivenom polyvalent medications. Sensitive individuals will be premedicated with epinephrine, antihistamines and corticosteroids to reduce allergic reaction. Antivenom is most effective when promptly administered; it is of little value after 24 hours have passed following the bite.

Poisonous lizards: There are two species of poisonous lizards, the Gila monster (found in the southwest United States), and the Mexican beaded lizard. Gila Monsters are shy, biting only if directly provoked. Venom is secreted into the oral cavity from glands in the floor of the mouth. Envenomization occurs by contamination of the wounds from the teeth. Bites produce neurotoxic and necrotic effects such as tissue destruction, pain, edema, and bruising. Other symptoms such as nausea, vomiting, ascending prickling or tingling sensations, blurred vision, labored breathing, and weakness may last for several days. Fatality is rare. No antiserum is available. Treat as for snake bite and consider antibiotic and homeopathic therapy.

Bees, wasps, hornets and fire ants: The majority of these bites are merely painful. Symptoms include local pain, heat, edema, and bruising; they may be treated with homeopathic Apis Melllifica (bee venom) as quickly as possible following the sting. However, close to 1% of the North American population is at risk for a severe, systemic allergic reaction to such bites. Immediate allergic reactions cause most fatalities, although delayed reactions can also occur.

A severe reaction presents as shock, with bronchospasm, itchy hives, patches of edematous skin, abdominal pain, nausea, vomiting, labored breathing, cyanosis, low blood pressure, coma and death. Acute renal failure may also occur. Allergic individuals should avoid areas where there is a high risk of receiving a sting and should carry an emergency kit for allergic reactions, as well as high potency Apis.

What to do: Remove the stinger if one can be found. Gently cool the area and give Apis Mel in 30C or 200C doses every 15 to 30 minutes. If a severe reaction occurs, give higher potency Apis (up to 1M) every 30 minutes until the person is stable. Epinephrine, 0.3 to 0.5 ml. of aqueous 1:1000 solution is given subcutaneously and repeated every 5 to 20 minutes as needed. Place a tourniquet proximal to the sting if it is located on an extremity. Oxygen, artificial respiration and bronchodilator drugs may sometimes have to be employed.

Spider bites: Although irritating, most spider bites are not potentially serious. In the United States only the Black Widow and Brown Recluse spiders are associated with significant morbidity and mortality.

Black Widow spiders (*Latrodectus mactans*) are found throughout the United States. The fangs of the male spider are too small to penetrate human skin; however the larger female is the leading cause of death from spider bites. A red hourglass marking is seen on her shiny black abdomen. These spiders are most active during warm months and build nests in dry, dark locations. They are not usually aggressive unless the web is disturbed or they are feeding. Bites produce a momentary localized sharp pain. Over the next 15 minutes to an hour, an intense cramping pain spreads from the site of the bite, becomes generalized and lasts for the next 12 to 48 hours. The victim's abdomen may become rigid but is not tender on palpation. Fever, sweating, nausea, vomiting, urinary retention and twitching may occur. Without treatment 5% to 10% will die of heart and respiratory failure. Elevated white count, blood and protein in the urine are frequently associated laboratory findings.

What to do: Give a homeopathic remedy appropriate to symptoms, if possible, and transport for black widow antiserum immediately. After treatment, a hot bath will help relieve muscle cramps, and calcium gluconate or magnesium sulfate will give prompt temporary relief.

All species of *Loxosceles* are venomous; *Loxoscelos reclusa*, the Brown Recluse, is most widely distributed through the southern and midwestern United States. It is brown with short, fuzzy hair and a dark pear shape on its underside. The spider is nocturnal and shy, often nesting in unused clothing; bites often occur when clothing is brought from storage and worn without cleaning or shaking first. Venom produces local tissue destruction and hemolysis. Local reactions are most common; bruising, and central pustules form at the site of the bite. Extensive necrosis with ulceration can occur which may necessitate skin grafting.

Occasionally severe systemic reactions such as fever chills hemolysis, clotting failure, hematuria and kidney failure occur. No antivenom is available. Supportive therapy such as pain relief and medical evaluation is appropriate. Homeopathic Ledum in 30C or 200C doses or another specifically chosen remedy will help speed recovery.

Scorpion bites: Scorpions have a long segmented abdomen with a bulb-shaped end segment containing poisonous glands and a stinger. Scorpions are shy, preferring moist, cool, shaded places. Most United States species are harmless, except for *Centruoides sculpturatus*, which is found in the southwest. Their bites account for only 2% of deaths attributable to venomous animals in the United States. Stings produce immediate local reactions with pain and bruising; they only rarely progress to systemic reactions such as generalized heightened sensitivity to touch, high blood pressure, sweating, dilated pupils, nausea, vomiting, tearing, convulsions and heart failure.

What to do: Antiserum is available. A tourniquet should be applied proximal to the sting for 15 to 20 minutes to slow absorption of the toxin. Cooling will produce local pain relief. Mild analgesics may be used except for morphine, meperidine, and paraldehyde which may combine with the venom to produce lethal effects. A poultice of clay or Plantain may be placed on the bite to help draw out the venom, and Arnica may be given to relieve bruising and swelling.

Tick paralysis: Some ticks produce a toxin which leads to ascending flaccid paralysis. This will reverse once the tick and all mouth parts are removed from the host. (See Diagnostic Tests for information regarding Lyme Disease, which is carried by Deer ticks.)

Animal bites: Rabies and infection of the wound are the main danger from bites inflicted by warm blooded animals. (See the chapter on Rabies in Diagnostic Tests for more information.)

Additional remedies for any bites or stings: Rescue Remedy (for emotional balancing in any crisis), may be given in one drop doses as frequently as necessary to calm the woman down. Once the acute crisis is over, a poultice can be applied to the sting or bite to help draw out more toxins. A paste of green clay, tofu mixed with whole wheat flour, grated potato, or fresh macerated Plantain leaves may be used for this purpose. Apply directly to the area, cover with plastic, wrap lightly with gauze or a strip of cloth to secure and leave in place for 30 minutes. Repeat with fresh poultice material several times daily.

Gleicher, Norbert, ed. Principles of Medical Therapy in Pregnancy, Plenum Pub., New York, 1985.

Yoni Discharge

It is normal for the yoni discharge to gradually increase as pregnancy advances, although this is notable more in some women than in others. A pregnant woman is more prone to the development of yeast infections (candida) in the yoni because of the influence of pregnancy hormones. Women can reduce the chances of having any yoni infections by taking the following precautions:

*Bathe regularly with a mild, non-irritating soap
*Wear only cotton underwear and cotton crotch panty hose
*Avoid perfumes, bubble baths, bath oil, bath salts and feminine
    hygiene products.
*Use only unscented non-deodorant sanitary products
*Use only unscented white toilet tissue

If symptoms such as burning, itching, swelling, redness, pain, or other irritation appear, the cause needs investigating. Ask about possible sources of irritation such as soaps, detergents, sanitary pads, perfumed toilet paper, and feminine hygiene products. Rule out the following:

*Chemical or allergic reaction
*Yeast
*Chlamydia
*Trichomonas
*Bacterial infection
*Warts in the yoni
*Gonorrhea
*Weeping lesions within the yoni or on the cervix

Each of the above mentioned infections is discussed in Diagnostic Tests. A lesion found within the yoni or on the labia, may be caused by:

*Syphilis
*Chancroid
*Herpes
*Venereal warts (*condylomata acuminata* or Syphilis)
*Granuloma inguinale

Each of these conditions is also discussed at length in Diagnostic Tests.

MEDICAL CONDITIONS AND DISABILITIES
WHICH MAY PREEXIST PREGNANCY

Preexisting Medical Conditions or Disabilities and Midwifery Care

Deciding whether or not an individual woman is a good candidate for a homebirth or midwifery care is not the black and white issue it may appear to be at first glance. The evaluation of a preexisting medical condition or disability is an art which can only really be developed through experience with normal, healthy women during regular full scope midwifery care.

Midwifery organizations and most midwifery textbooks list physical conditions which contraindicate homebirth or midwifery care, but rarely does one get any information regarding the specifics of why this is so. It is far more helpful to evaluate a medical condition in light of the additional risks it may pose to the mother or baby. In this way, midwives hone their clinical judgement skills becoming more competent, more independent and better able to establish a midwifery based definition of well-being. These abilities are vital to both the individual practitioner and to the continued growth and survival of midwifery.

With this in mind, this book will not merely say, "don't do this" or offer a list of conditions which are contraindicated for the provision of midwifery care. Instead, an evaluation process regarding medical conditions in general will be presented.

Chances are you have turned to this chapter because you have discovered that a woman seeking your care has some preexisting condition that you know little or nothing about. As you discuss her birthing options, there are several points to keep in mind:

*How will the medical condition affect the pregnancy? Will it compromise blood or oxygen exchange for the fetus or lead to fetal defects? Will it cause undue physical stress for the mother to carry a pregnancy given the condition in question? Unfortunately, the interaction between many conditions and pregnancy is poorly understood, and the decision regarding how to proceed may be vague in some situations.

*What impact will the pregnancy have on the condition? Generally speaking, most conditions are aggravated by pregnancy, but some actually improve or temporarily disappear during gestation.

*Medical conditions are harder to diagnose and monitor during pregnancy due to the wide range of pregnancy-related symptoms which are clearly abnormal outside of pregnancy, as well as the bio-chemical and hemodynamic changes which cause lab results to vary from nonpregnant normals. (Gleicher, 1985, p. 3-5)

*Treatment of medical conditions during pregnancy may vary from that used outside of pregnancy because of the possible adverse effects of many pharmaceutical agents on the fetus.

Keeping these thoughts in mind, ask the following questions during the first conversation you have with the woman:

*What is the exact medical name of your condition?
*Have you ever spoken to a specialist regarding its possible impact on your fertility, a pregnancy or birth? On the fetus and newborn?
*Is this condition hereditary (genetic)? If so, have any other women in your family had it, and how have their pregnancies and births gone?
*Did this condition complicate a previous pregnancy? If so, how?
*What type of bio-technical or other therapies have you used in the past for this condition?
*What are you currently using to control this condition (drugs, etc.)?
*Have you recently noticed a change in your symptoms for better or worse?

What is the exact medical name of your condition? This is a very important piece of information. The exact bio-technical name for the condition allows you to look it up. It also allows you to discuss the condition intelligently with other care providers. General information about specific disorders can be found in the Merek Manual, an encyclopedia of disorders. However, only rarely will any such a compendium have any details about pregnancy. Large obstetrics textbooks such as William's Obstetrics and Obstetrics: Normal and Problem Pregnancies, by Steven Gabbe are among several which cover a variety of medical conditions. There are other texts devoted entirely to this topic. You should have at least one current textbook of this type in your library for reference. You will find that opinions differ from text to text regarding the same condition.

Have you ever spoken to a specialist regarding its possible impact on your fertility, a pregnancy or birth? On the fetus and newborn? I have never met a women with a preexisting disorder that had not asked someone what its impact might be on a future pregnancy. In some cases, this information will be your best resource regarding what the disorder is and what its effect may be. This is particularly true of very rare disorders or physical defects. If the woman has never asked anyone about her condition, she can either call the care provider that originally helped her (if it has been some time since the condition was a problem) or she can see another care provider and get their opinion. In most cases, I have found that non-obstetric medical specialists are not hostile to a woman seeking birthing alternatives and will give an honest evaluation of the condition in question without a lot of unwelcome commentary on her choices for care or birth place. At the same time, obtain copies of any existing medical records so that you can review her care, lab work performed, and any other pertinent information.

Is this condition hereditary (genetic)? If a woman has a genetic condition, her fetus may be at some additional risk for having the condition as well. Genetic testing as well as research done to determine what affect the condition may have on an affected newborn can be discussed.

If so, have any other women in your family had it and how have their pregnancies and births gone? Naturally, the most important thing is the health of the woman seeking care. However, this additional historical information can be helpful, especially if the woman is a first time mother. Perhaps family members are aware of specialists with whom you can consult. In addition, be aware that the woman may expect certain problems in her pregnancy if other family members have experienced complications. Explore her feelings regarding her condition and the problems that arose for other women in her family.

Did this condition complicate a previous pregnancy of yours and if so how? A mild condition which leaves a woman more or less functionally normal and which did not complicate a previous pregnancy indicates that this pregnancy will also go well in most cases, if the woman's overall state of health and her health relevant to the specific condition has not worsened in the meantime.

What type of bio-technical or other therapies have you used in the past for this condition? Long term use of certain drugs can cause damage or undue stress to the kidneys or liver. Previous radiation therapy can expose the ova to high levels of x-rays which may lead to fertility problems or an increased risk of genetic problems in babies. Steroid drugs, in particular, are very debilitating. Knowledge of what therapies have been used can help you assess the mother's overall well-being as she seeks to conceive or make it through early pregnancy.

If non-bio-technical therapies have been used, the woman's body is probably in better shape. The use of other therapies is often accompanied by dietary and lifestyle changes which improve the overall state of health. The successful control of a medical condition without drugs or surgery is a good indication that a woman will be able to tolerate pregnancy better than someone whose disorder can only be controlled with heavy doses of drugs and other conventional therapies.

What are you currently using to control this condition (drugs, etc.)? Some women will have had a condition which was a problem in the past but is not currently being treated. Generally speaking, the longer the condition has been stable without specific therapy, the better are her chances of having an uncomplicated pregnancy. If she is currently taking drugs, find out whether they have been categorized for pregnancy and any associated side effects. Sometimes the dosage of medication must be changed during pregnancy; is the woman planning on continuing to consult with her physicians throughout the pregnancy? Some drugs are contraindicated in pregnancy and she should begin alternative therapy prior to conception.

Have you noticed a change in your symptoms for better or worse? A woman's current sense of well-being is also an important indication of her regenerative abilities. If you are seeing a woman for a preconception visit, take the opportunity to direct her to non-bio-technical therapies and care providers (such as chiropractors or naturopaths) that may help her with any current symptoms she may be experiencing. She can also consult an obstetrician or even a maternal-fetal medical specialist to hear their recommendations regarding her situation. If she is already pregnant radical dietary changes or beginning a specific type of therapy must be carefully evaluated for its possible impact on the pregnancy.

Once you have explored the above questions with the woman, there are some other questions you need to ask in order to decide if it is appropriate for you to work with a woman with her condition if this is not already clear:

*What is my current level of experience as a midwife?
*What did the specialist say regarding her condition?
*What organ systems are involved and what stress does pregnancy place on these systems?
*What is her general state of health now, and what is the state of health of any organs affected by the condition in question?
*What risks are present for the fetus and newborn?
*What do medical references say regarding this condition?
*How motivated is this woman to do whatever she needs to do to ensure a healthy pregnancy, birth and baby?
*Will this woman will be honest with me regarding her symptoms and self-care?
*What kind of medical back-up does this woman need and can we get it?
*How likely is this condition to require hospitalization or other care which I cannot provide in my practice setting? How frequently or likely does it appear that this will be the case?

What is my current level of experience as a midwife? This is vitally important. Whenever you are dealing with a woman who has a condition with which you are not familiar, you need to be able to fall back on a solid foundation of understanding what is normal in pregnancy. This can only be gained through actual midwifery experience, not through books and not through using other midwives as resources. This is not to say that doing research is a bad idea or that asking the opinion of our sister midwives is unwise. However, in the day-to-day work of dealing with a woman with a particular disorder, especially when you have no prior experience with that disorder, you need a broad enough base of midwifery experience to be able to distinguish what is truly a problem from what is truly a normal variation of the pregnancy itself. In some cases this can be difficult, even with a great deal of experience. You need to know how to monitor dietary intake and how to interpret laboratory results, taking into account both the pregnancy and the condition in question.

This is especially true for independent, home birth based midwives who do not have a broad-based working relationship with the rest of the mainstream medical community. They put themselves out on a limb whenever they take on an unusual case. Don't go out there with the big saw of inexperience.

A fledgling midwife is prudent to refuse to care for women who have preexisting medical conditions which are likely to compromise a pregnancy. In fact, the less experience you have, the more you can refer to those laundry lists of disorders that contraindicate prenatal care and birth with a midwife. I would still encourage you to do the research and go thorough the thought process outlined here, even if you know that you shouldn't work with a particular woman at this point in your career.

There are some conditions which absolutely contraindicate primary midwifery care and home birth regardless of your experience level. This is usually due to the nature of the condition and the compromise it poses for vital organ systems which are further strained by pregnancy and birth; it may also be due to the dangerous drugs used to control the condition or the dangers the condition poses to the fetus and newborn. Even so, women can gain much from a relationship with a midwife. You might offer to provide simultaneous prenatal care and accompany such women to the hospital as a supportive guide to the birth experience.

What did the specialist say regarding her condition? Very often you can get a definitive "everything's fine and you should have no problems" from such a specialist (be sure they understand that she is contemplating a homebirth!). This is, of course, a big relief and usually means that everything will go fine. However, it is still wise to familiarize yourself with the condition enough so that you will recognize signs of a problem should they appear and make sure that the specialist wasn't glossing over potential problems in the name of keeping the woman calm.

What organ systems are involved and what stress does pregnancy place on these systems? Pregnancy places demands on every part of a woman's body. However, the liver, the kidneys, and the heart are three organs that are particularly stressed during gestation.

The liver seems to have the best ability to bounce back from previous problems and not buckle under during pregnancy; this is probably due to its amazing ability to regenerate itself. The kidneys can be in a borderline state and be pushed over the edge into overt and dangerous symptoms by the increased blood volume of pregnancy. This is also true of the heart. However, if a woman is free of symptoms and able to function normally with her heart condition outside of pregnancy, there is a good possibility she will tolerate pregnancy well.

Another important question is: "How does this condition or the drugs used to control it affect smooth muscle?" In other words, will it impair the uterus's ability to contract during labor or thereafter? Everything else may look good, but if a massive hemorrhage is likely postpartum, the woman is a poor choice for an out-of-hospital birth. In addition, does this condition or the drugs used to control it affect the blood's ability to clot? Either insufficient or excessive clotting are both problematic during pregnancy.

What is her general state of health now, and what is the state of health of any organs affected by the condition in question? This is an especially important evaluation. Just because a woman is basically functional does not means she is in the best possible condition. Whenever indicated, run the appropriate laboratory tests to determine her current biochemical state. In this way you have a baseline of what is normal for her from which to judge during the rest of her pregnancy.

What risks are present for the fetus and newborn? The mother's condition may be within acceptable parameters for your care; however, if her condition or the drugs she is taking pose a significant risk to the newborn, you must take this into account when deciding upon appropriate care and place of birth.

What do medical references say regarding this condition? While I encourage you to look up specific conditions in medical textbooks and journals, the information in them must be evaluated with the understanding that it comes from a purely bio-technical point of view. This means that the discussion is based on pregnancies that have been managed with drugs or other therapies which do not focus on holistic healing and often do not generally benefit the overall state of health. Bio-technical therapies generally seek to control, suppress or cut out (via surgery) the symptoms or problem, not to cure. In most cases there has been little or no regard for maternal nutrition except as it may directly affect the condition in question (such as diabetic dietary recommendations). The question of what the outcome might be if alternative therapies are used and if maternal nutrition is a top priority is left wide open (how can we separate the problem and its impact on pregnancy from the therapy?). In most cases, and particularly with serious, life threatening conditions, this is almost impossible to know.

A woman who depends on regular bio-technical care and drug therapy is usually not a good candidate for independent midwifery care, simply because the therapies themselves complicate the picture, as well as contributing health depleting side effects of their own. On the other hand, a woman who has been able to control or heal her condition with other means *may* show compromise during pregnancy, but this should be much more obvious than when symptoms are masked or altered by intensive bio-technical treatments.

How motivated is this woman to do whatever she needs to do to ensure a healthy pregnancy, birth and baby? Every woman needs to be willing to eat well and eliminate smoking, drinking and recreational drugs. However, a woman with a serous medical condition may have to be even more careful. This can be difficult for women who are desperately trying to live with a physical problem which it has already imposed itself on their lives. Dietary and lifestyle changes which may be necessary in order to have a healthy pregnancy may be perceived as an additional burden. On the other hand, there may be many things such women can do to improve their condition; this is what you should emphasize: a woman's power to create an optimal pregnancy and birth. Included in this will be exploring what the condition means in the woman's life, how having it works for her and what ways she might help herself to deal with it that have not been explored (other forms of medical treatment such as homeopathy, herbs, dietary adjustments, stress reduction, etc.)

Unfortunately, pregnancy is not the best time to start radically different therapies or dietary habits. Ideally, a woman who has a serious condition will approach you before conceiving to find out what she can do to bring herself to her pregnancy in the best possible health. This is a good time to involve other bio-technical care providers in your community who have more expertise in dealing with medical conditions outside of pregnancy.

Do you think this woman will be honest with you regarding her symptoms?
The vast majority of women, whatever their health status may be, will be scrupulously honest with you about their physical condition. This is not always true in an institutional setting, especially if women fear that minor problems will be blown up into major ones by medical model care providers, but it should be true for the most part in a noninstitutional home care setting.

However, there are always exceptions to this rule. Some women are so desperate for an uninterfered-with birth that they will lie about their condition by claiming to be in perfect health or will minimize or deny dangerous symptoms if they arise during pregnancy. It is important that you make clear from the onset of your relationship that you need to know a woman's complete medical history.

If a woman is in denial about the seriousness of her condition, she may not have explored what implications her health status may have for pregnancy in advance. The woman may first have sought out regular medical care only to be bombarded with information about her risk status. She may be trying to seek refuge in midwifery care, feeling that midwives focus on normal births and therefore will not have the same opinion or will be more relaxed about her condition; in some cases this will be true. However, a woman may minimize the nature of her condition or simply never mention her condition to the midwife. (This can be particularly true of women who have a condition that does not leave them that debilitated, such as diabetes with no other organ compromise.) One of two things can happen at this point.

The midwife may take the woman's word for it and do no further research on the condition herself. This is a big mistake. First of all, she may find out too late the true impact the condition has on pregnancy, realizing after a problem has occurred that she should never have taken on this woman in the first place.

Or the midwife may investigate further and discover the true potential for problems with this condition and refuse to give the woman primary care. Of course, a full explanation of the reasons and the condition in question should accompany such a refusal. As much as possible, information should be related to the individual health status of the woman so that she understands that it is not a *carte blanche* refusal but that her *personal* risk is significant enough to warrant a refusal of care.

If you are refusing a woman for care because you feel you are not yet skilled enough to take her on, refer her to more experienced midwives for their opinion. Always call them ahead and let them (and the woman) know you will be referring a woman with this medical condition to them for a consultation. Always notify the other midwives in your community of a situation such as this. If you are attending an organizational meeting, you may, without disclosing the woman's name, describe the circumstances of your discussions and inform the other midwives why you refused her care. This way, the others will be alert to the possibility of such a woman contacting them. You must do this because a woman in serious denial about her condition may then seek other midwifery care and not tell them of her condition at all.

What kind of medical back-up does this woman need and can we get it? Sometimes you will interview an extremely motivated woman who is in basically good health but who has an unusual medical condition. You want to help her, and feel comfortable doing so, but you know that the medical community may frown on this because of her medical condition. In such a case, it is important to secure a good back-up situation in which the care provider knows you, knows the woman and her unique circumstances, and is willing to offer back-up services and, if needed, hospital attention.

How likely is this condition to require hospitalization or other care which I cannot provide in my practice setting? How frequently does it appear that this will be the case? In addition, how much medical attention is a woman likely to require? The potential need for frequent visits to receive medical interventions make home birth and midwifery care poor primary care choices. For example, a woman who has Sickle Cell anemia may have frequent pain crises due to blood cells backing up in her circulatory system. This requires intensive hospital management. Choosing to care for a woman, perhaps without good back-up, and sending her into the emergency room for such critical care is not good midwifery. It robs her of the kind of continuous care she needs and jeopardizes the life of both her and baby.

Some case histories:

The following telling examples illustrate the positive and negative points on the issue of risk screening. First, a positive story: June (not her real name) came to my practice at 25 weeks of pregnancy very disenchanted with her nurse-midwife. June had been previously diagnosed with Hodgkin's disease and Lupus. After two chemotherapy treatments for the Hodgkin's disease, she abandoned bio-technical therapy completely and began a macrobiotic diet and healing program. Both her Lupus (which was very mild with no kidney involvement) and her Hodgkin's went into remission. June was a second time mother who had had a normal birth prior to these diagnoses. At the time she came to me, June was generally quite healthy and very aware of her physical condition and what made it better or worse.

Her nurse-midwife had plenty of homebirth experience and had assured her that she would not be treated as "high risk." However, upon reading more about Lupus in pregnancy, the midwife started pushing June to receive serial ultrasounds as she felt the baby was small for gestational age. June reported that the midwife seemed much more anxious as time went on. June did not have any desire to be treated as high risk if, in fact, things were going normally. Her nurse-midwife provider cautioned her not to seek my care and that a homebirth would be too dangerous for her.

I found June to be generally well informed about her conditions in general but not very knowledgeable about their impact on pregnancy, which she readily admitted. She was open to finding out more. She was exhibiting no signs of any problems with the pregnancy itself, and contrary to the nurse-midwife's concerns, I found the baby to be growing nicely. I reviewed her most recent lab work, which did show ANA antibodies, but her kidney function and white counts were both well within normal limits.

Not knowing much about either of her conditions, I went to research them at the medical library. While the possible problems associated with Lupus certainly were concerning, this woman was not on bio-technical drugs and had no kidney damage, with fetal heart tones in a normal range (lowering the possibility of heart block in the fetus). I felt that I could take her on as long as she understood the risks involved and agreed to get lab work to monitor her condition. I gave her the chapter on Lupus from the most thorough text I could find and asked her to read it. Her Hodgkins' had been in remission for some time and did not pose a concern to me or to her nurse-midwife provider.

A lab panel done in the 36th week confirmed that her clotting factors and other results were fine. During one visit the baby seemed a little bit small for dates. This quickly corrected itself with specific dietary counseling: thereafter the baby's growth rate was fine. At term June gave birth to a very healthy, 9 lb. 12 oz. baby. (She said she was thankful the baby was "small for dates"!)

In this case I looked at the woman first: her general condition and how it was affecting the baby. Then I researched the literature to discover what hidden problems I might be faced with, and explained them to her. A mutual decision was made to begin care and continue as long as everything went well. She was motivated, had managed her own recovery to a great extent with non-bio-technical means, had been in remission for some time and demonstrated her body's ability to withstand pregnancy by growing a healthy baby.

A number of years ago, a very rural midwife without much experience reported that she had seen five stillbirths in her practice. With some further questioning it was revealed that all five of the mothers of these infants had been insulin-dependent diabetics who were under her care alone. In light of the possible problems associated with diabetes and the baby, this is no surprise. It was, however, news to the midwife, as she had no idea that there was a connection. There is no excuse for this kind of ignorance. If a woman has an unusual condition, regardless of how benign it may appear, you must research it to discover what risks it may carry.

A woman was seeing midwives for her first prenatal visit. When they checked her urine they were shocked to find that her glucose and ketones were off the scale on the dip stick. The midwife immediately ordered glucose tolerance tests and discovered that this woman was a full-blown diabetic, although her condition was not longstanding. The woman was started on insulin and told that her fetus was in great jeopardy of having anomalies, since she had entered pregnancy with her diabetes uncontrolled. The women then went from practice to practice, both home and hospital, in a desperate attempt to find someone who would help her without any intervention at all. She was sporadic about her insulin dosage and generally in shock and denial about her situation. Although a very caring practice of nurse-midwives offered to help her in the hospital with a minimal amount of intervention she continued to look for less interventive care at home and was refused at every turn. Finally, without much prenatal care, she arrived at a practice who found her to be small for dates and discovered that her fetus did, indeed, have multiple anomalies. She choose to give birth in the hospital and donate whatever organs may be useful from her baby to others.

This situation is heart wrenching; you might be tempted to attend such a woman at home out of a misguided attempt to heal her pain around the entire situation. This would be a big mistake for you and for her, since an unmonitored insulin-dependent diabetic requires constant attention to her glucose levels in labor; her baby is at great risk for stillbirth as well. The best thing to do is to stand firm in your opinion about where she will be safest and to offer to accompany her to the hospital as a labor support person if she would like.

In another case a woman approached me for care, but since she lived quite near another midwife, I referred her there. I didn't hear from her again until her 8th month of pregnancy. The woman's mother called me. She asked if I remembered her daughter, I said I did recall the conversation we had. She called to ask what her daughter should do about the fact that her membranes seemed to be ruptured. I then asked if she had seen the other midwife for prenatal care. Yes, she had. Then why was she not calling her own midwife with these questions, I asked. I was then told she had tried, but the midwife wasn't home, and they didn't have her beeper number. I asked again, "she's been seeing her for regular prenatal care and doesn't have her beeper number?" "Yes," I was told. "So," I said, "I'll give you her beeper number," and did so. At this point the mother pressed me to give her information about her daughter's condition, and said the situation with the other midwife was complicated and problematic. I said that the best thing for her to do would be to call her daughter and give her her midwife's number so that she could talk with her directly. I assured the mother that I would let the midwife know she would be calling. I then called and left a message with the midwife.

A little while later the midwife called me. Apparently this woman had come to see her for an initial visit. After taking her history (which revealed nothing problematic) the midwife asked the woman to collect a urine sample. The woman asked suspiciously why this was necessary. The midwife explained that this was a routine part of her prenatal care. When she checked the urine, the glucose was off the scale. At this point the midwife asked the woman if she was diabetic; the woman admitted that she was, but that she wanted an uninterfered-with birth. The midwife told her she could not care for her at home, suggested a medical practice she could see and offered to accompany her to the hospital for her birth, which the woman refused. The woman did not return to that midwife for further care. Upon receiving the call from the mother about her daughter, she told them that they needed to seek care in a hospital.

This woman tried to side-step two midwives in a very dishonest fashion to get what she wanted. Dishonesty like this breeds dangerous situations for all concerned. You never know how someone you haven't had a stable relationship with may react. Do not be trapped into believing that you are a hard hearted midwife for being clear enough to know and define your limits!!

A woman who was on medication for schizophrenia came to me for care. She took her medication only sporadically and was attempting to stabilize her condition with diet and vitamin therapy. These efforts had helped to a certain extent, but she would swing from being off her medication completely to taking high doses to moderate doses to vitamins again. She got pregnant during a 6 month hitchhiking jaunt during which she did not take her medication and could not remember anything about the father of the baby. She wanted a homebirth and was afraid of the hospital. At the point when I interviewed her she was back on her prescribed medication, after having taken very high dosages as soon as she realized she was pregnant to reestablish her emotional equilibrium. I checked the Physician's Desk Reference (PDR) and noted that her medication caused respiratory distress in the newborn and possible fetal distress in labor. Given the fact that she could not guarantee that she would remain on her medication or maintain the proper dosage, along with its possible effects on the baby, I recommended that she see a practice that had a very supportive CNM on staff. After consulting with them she made her own decision to birth in the hospital.

These cases illustrate how careful midwives must be to assess each woman on an individual basis so that mother and baby receive optimal, appropriate care and they are not taken advantage of in their roles as care providers.

About the descriptions that follow:

The medical conditions and diseases listed in this section cover a wide variety of problems, but they are by no means complete. Most of the information has been compiled from several medical textbooks and is presented here in abbreviated form for your convenience. Each entry briefly reviews the bio-technical opinion about the condition. Quite a few of these conditions can be positively impacted with non-bio-technical healing modalities. However, in this section I have focused on the drugs and other bio-technical treatments which the woman is likely to have used in the past or will need to consider using during her care, as these pose the most risk. In addition, there are no alternative reference materials available on many of the less common conditions. Many of these conditions are quite rare; you will probably never encounter most of them in potential clients. Looking up a condition in this section may help you to decide that it is way out of your league, or it may prompt you to look further into the individual woman's case. This section does not present an exhaustive thesis on each topic, but a starting reference point so that you may:

*Have a general definition of the condition
*Have some idea of its effects both within and outside of pregnancy
*Understand what kind of drugs a woman may have been taking and their implications for her health in general and her pregnancy in particular
*Have some idea where to look for further information
*Have a reference point from which to question the woman regarding the particulars of her situation
*Have information available to guide the woman in what to ask other care providers about her condition or in helping refer her for more appropriate care

If you do plan to care for a woman who has a medical condition, always go through the steps outlined in this chapter. *Do not rely solely on the information in this section to make your decision.* Also be sure to check in <u>Diagnostic Tests</u> to see if a particular condition is mentioned there as well. When exploring the particulars of a medical condition, keep the following points in mind:

*How the condition is affected by pregnancy.
*How the condition will affect the pregnancy.
*That diagnosis and following the progress of a medical problem is often more difficult during pregnancy, because many normal variations of pregnancy are abnormal in the nonpregnant state (such as nausea and vomiting and certain heart murmurs).
*That in many instances treatment of medical conditions during pregnancy varies from treatment in the nonpregnant state either due to the negative impact of the therapeutic agent on the baby or the interaction between the agent and pregnancy physiology.

References are listed at the end of the entire section rather than at the end of each chapter. Material is synopsized from de Sweit unless otherwise noted.

Taking on a woman with a special medical condition:

Taking into consideration any special needs she may have, care for her as you would any other woman, attending to her diet, the growth pattern of the baby, etc. Be sure to keep an eye out for problems which may be specifically related to her condition (such as the kidney and clotting problems I looked for in the woman who had Lupus). Try to remember to evaluate the woman and not the condition alone. This will help you differentiate a true problem from a personal concern due to what you know about her condition from your reading. Do not hesitate to send her to another care provider for a second opinion or for primary care if you feel unsure about her or her baby's condition.

Autoimmune Disorders

Whenever the immune tolerance of self is disrupted, autoimmunity exists. There are a large variety of autoimmune disorders. Their pathophysiology is still incompletely understood. Genetic, infectious and environmental factors may all play a part. A directly detrimental effect of pregnancy on these disorders has not been proven and, in the majority of cases, autoimmunity will not be affected by pregnancy. In fact, some of these conditions may improve during pregnancy. However, other conditions often become worse, usually during the latter part of pregnancy or postpartum. The association of potential fetal risk with the particular maternal disorder is a primary determinant of treatment in women with autoimmune disease, keeping in mind that only IgG antibodies can cross the placenta. Depending upon the disease in question, placental transfer of IgG antibodies to the fetus may cause transient fetal levels or produce outright fetal harm, depending upon which antibodies are involved. Autoimmunity may appear or be discovered for the first time during pregnancy. Cases of women near term experiencing sudden single- or multi-organ failure with hemolysis and low platelet counts have occurred. Treatment typically involves the use of corticosteroids such as hydrocortisone or prednisone.

Sjögren's Syndrome: This rare autoimmune disorder is characterized by dry mucus membranes. It is frequently associated with rheumatic disorders, sharing certain autoimmune characteristics secondary to an inflammatory lymphocytic invasion into affected tissues. Those with this condition have a variety of autoantibodies, including some types of antinuclear antibodies. The presence of Anti-Ro antibodies has been associated with congenital heart block in the infants of these mothers.

Systemic Lupus Erythematosus (SLE): Lupus is the most common autoimmune disorder of young women. Numerous lab tests are used in its diagnosis and management; it is covered in detail in Diagnostic Tests.

Lupus nephritis: In addition to the risks associated with SLE itself, lupus complicated by kidney damage poses three additional risks:

1) Acute fatty degeneration of arterial walls in the placenta can cause fetal death in mid- or late pregnancy. Symptoms mimic toxemia, with hypertension and proteinuria that resolve postpartum.
2) Exacerbation of the lupus, especially a flare-up of the nephritis, may occur during pregnancy or in the puerperium with the possibility of acute renal failure postpartum.
3) Preexisting renal insufficiency, hypertension, and nephrotic syndrome have inherent risks regardless of the cause (as discussed

in the chapter On Kidney Disease)

The possibility of problems is more likely when a flare-up of renal or nonrenal lupus symptoms has occurred during the six months prior to conception. This is true even with biopsy evidence of severe glomerulonephritis. Renal compromise results in a fetal loss rate of 30%, compared to less than 10% if the lupus has been in remission. In women with established systemic lupus erythematosus, pregnancy-induced relapse or exacerbation of lupus occurs in 60% of those with clinical activity at conception and in only 7% of those in remission.

Note that toxic by-products produced by the breakdown of aspartame (Nutrasweet) can lead to side-effects which mimic lupus and multiple sclerosis. Aspartame should be avoided whether or not a woman is pregnant.

Gastrointestinal Disorders

Ileostomy, Ileoproctostomy, colostomy: An ostomy is a surgically formed artificial opening which serves as the exit site for connections from the bowel to the outside. Ostomy operations do not seem to impair fertility and complications such a prolapse of the stoma (ostomy opening) and change of appliance fit will resolve after birth. Occasional obstruction of the ileal segment traversing the peritoneum and abdominal wall has been reported, but this is rare.

Newer procedures for ileoproctostomy with an ileal reservoir do not interfere with pregnancy. Difficult defecation has been reported during the third trimester in about 10% of cases. Continence is the same as before pregnancy. Total parenteral nutrition (TPN) may help a woman with poor absorption to carry her pregnancy to term or even to conceive. This should be considered when large portions of the small intestines have been removed leading to severe diarrhea. TPN carries certain risks (such as sepsis from the IV site), and is very costly ($5,000 monthly).

Malabsorption of fats, fat soluble vitamins, and B vitamins, ester and electrolyte imbalance, oxalates appearing in the urine, and gall stones may occur. During labor, there may be an impaired ability to push due to scar tissue obstruction or the location of the surgery.

The hormonal changes of pregnancy can affect the skin and cause poor adhesion of ostomy appliances or the need for more frequent changing. Skin wafers and extra adhesive can help with this problem. Preparations designed to provide a protective film over the skin will help the skin stay healthy and also aide appliance adhesion. The stoma will change from circular to more oval, may become shorter or longer and will become more lateral as the uterus enlarges. The stoma can be damaged if the appliance fits poorly. If the stoma retracts below the flange of the appliance, more leaks result, especially when the woman is lying down; a softer, more moldable flange may help. Lying down also changes the position of the stoma, making leaks more likely; positioning with pillows should help. As pregnancy advances the woman may require a full-length mirror to see how to apply the appliance. Labor presents few problems for the woman with an ostomy.

Jejunal-Ileal bypass: This surgery is used to help reduce weight in those who are extremely overweight. It removes a portion of the small intestines and joins the proximal 35 cm. of jejunum to the terminal 10 cm. of ileum. Complications include diarrhea, vitamin deficiency, electrolyte loss, hypocalcemia, hypomagnesemia, oxalate stones, polyarthritis and liver problems. Premature birth is increased due to nutritional compromise. Pregnancy-related problems occur most often post surgery, which is the period of most rapid weight loss. It is therefore recommended to postpone pregnancy until 1 to 2 years after surgery. Gastric bypass has not been subject to the same complications and is now the procedure of choice for obesity when this surgery is chosen. (Gleicher, 1985)

Miscellaneous Disorders of the Digestive Tract:

Celiac sprue: This is a gluten sensitivity of the small intestinal mucosa caused by ingesting gluten. The intestinal villi may be atrophied. Withdrawal of gluten causes a marked improvement. Other causes of a "flat" jejunal biopsy include Crohn's disease, cow's milk protein intolerance, soy protein intolerance, and tropical sprue. Celiac sprue classically causes diarrhea, anorexia, and weight loss with evidence of malabsorption. However, these symptoms are not always present and probably only occur in a minority of older patients. In young women, there may be an increased risk of infertility. Megaloblastic or iron deficiency anemia may accompany pregnancy. Bone pain, rarely tetany or other complications may occur due to malabsorption of vitamin D and calcium. Skin and mucus membrane changes may also occur. Supplements of B_{12}, folic acid, iron, and trace metals such as zinc are recommended along with a strictly gluten-free diet. Failure to respond should prompt investigation into possible dietary lapses, infection, use of gluten-containing preparations (drugs) or associated disease. Relapse usually occurs within 7 weeks of reintroduction of gluten to the diet.

Colon disorders: Ulcerative colitis is similar to Crohn's disease, both cause inflammation of the bowel wall, with Crohn's disease producing the more serious symptoms. Recurrences of active disease are no more likely to occur during gestation than outside of pregnancy. Some investigators have noted a high recurrence rate during the puerperium but others have not. Inactive ulcerative colitis at conception poses no risks to mother or fetus. Recurrences tend to be mild and easily managed. Treatment is the same as in the non-pregnant and stress reduction is an important consideration in keeping both conditions under control.

One study has shown a worsening of symptoms with active colitis (although others didn't confirm this). However, waiting for it to be inactive for 1 year prior to conception may be a good idea. Adrenal corticosteroids are the best groups of medications for these conditions; they do not, however, prevent relapse once the acute condition is over. Supplementation with B_{12}, folic acid (5-10 mg/daily), vitamin D, trace metals and iron may all be called for. Diarrhea generally lessens in pregnancy and constipation should be avoided with plenty of fluids; some recommend a high fiber diet (although opinions vary). If surgery is needed during pregnancy, the risk is high for both mother and fetus.

Inflammatory bowel disease may affect liver function, although this is not always clinically obvious. Severe complications such as sclerosing cholangitis and bile duct carcinoma occur somewhat more frequently in ulcerative colitis than in Crohn's disease. Liver involvement in small bowel Crohn's disease is unusual. (Also see Diagnostic Tests for more details regarding colon disorders, especially risks of Crohn's disease for the fetus.)

Esophageal problems: Increased intraabdominal pressure in late pregnancy and circulating levels of estrogen and progesterone reduce lower esophageal sphincter competence and aggravate symptoms of preexisting esophageal reflux. Even women without such symptoms before pregnancy commonly develop heartburn and other symptoms of reflux, especially in the last trimester. Aside from this problem, pregnancy does not aggravate any esophageal disease and esophageal disorders not interfere with pregnancy as long as good nutrition can be maintained.

Gastric and colon cancers: These cancers typically cause protracted vomiting, abdominal pain, constipation and rectal bleeding. Pregnancy seems to have no adverse effect on the cancer or vice versa. However, maternal prognosis is very poor.

Hiatus hernia: The stomach protrudes upward through the opening where the esophagus passes through the diaphragm. It is common in women and may be related to reflux due to the pressure of the enlarged uterus, but otherwise pose no problem during pregnancy.

Stomach disorders: Diseases of the stomach do not adversely affect pregnancy nor does pregnancy aggravate them, provided adequate nutrition can be maintained.

Stomach ulcers: Gastric or duodenal ulcer activity is not affected during pregnancy. Existing ulcers may actually improve only to erupt suddenly postpartum. Management is similar regardless of pregnancy.

The drug ranitidine is the ulcer treatment of choice in pregnancy (150 mg at bedtime or twice daily). It should only be used with frequent recurring ulcers or a history of gastrointestinal hemorrhage. Climetidine is another drug which is relatively safe for use in pregnancy, although liver dysfunction may be seen in babies who are exposed *in utero*.

Women who have had vagotomy (severing of the vagus nerve) and drainage, or have had partial gastrectomy (surgical removal of some or all of the stomach) for their ulcer disease should have no problem with pregnancy provided their nutritional status is monitored. Mild anemia is common due to iron, folic acid and B_{12} deficiencies. Bone weakening may occur due to poor absorption of calcium and vitamin D. Problems can be avoided by suggesting iron, calcium and vitamin D supplements.

Aphthous stomatitis ulceration may be due to an underlying deficiency of vitamin B_{12}, iron or folic acid. It may also herald the onset of another disease. Management consists of determining if an underlying disease process is present and whether nutritional deficiencies exist. If not, therapy seeks to relieve the symptoms.

1086

Small intestinal disorders: No small bowel disease has been shown to affect pregnancy adversely. Crohn's disease tends to relapse after birth, but has otherwise been shown to be unaffected by pregnancy in most studies. Total parenteral nutrition is a better option than immunosuppressant drugs if symptoms are severe and treatment is mandatory. Steroids may be used for inflammation if absolutely indicated.

Liver Disease:

The anatomical location of the liver is not altered until the second trimester. In the third trimester it may occupy a more posterior-superior position with displacement to the right and a subsequent reduction in dullness to percussion. Therefore, a palpable liver suggests underlying disease. (For how to examine the liver, see the chapter on The Physical Examination in the Basic Skills section.)

Budd-Chiari syndrome: In this disorder an obstruction of the venous outflow tract of the liver extends from the sublobular veins to where the inferior vena cava enters the right atrium. It is seen more frequently in those who use oral contraceptives. It causes clotting factors to increase in, but not outside of, pregnancy. Clinical symptoms include acute abdominal pain caused by a rapidly developing accumulation of fluid in the peritoneal cavity that leads to abdominal distention. It is seldom reversible and prognosis is poor, although in a few recorded cases there has been spontaneous recovery with no evidence of disease. Pregnancy is probably safe if the condition is asymptomatic.

Cirrhosis: Cirrhosis is a chronic liver disease in which dense connective tissue is formed in the body of the liver, accompanied by liver cell degeneration. It results in loss of liver function and poor blood flow; irregular menses are common as well. Cirrhosis increases the risk of spontaneous abortion. If hepatic function is well compensated without portal hypertension and liver histology is biliary, postnecrotic in type or consistent with Wilson's disease (see below) the prognosis for the mother is good. It is suggested that women with cirrhosis have their hepatic wedge pressure measured and have esophagoscopy performed to look for varicosities prior to conception. If wedge pressure is over 12 mmHg and varices are large (>5 mm in diameter), and especially if topped by dark vascular reticulum (network), the woman may want to undergo sclerotherapy before she attempts a pregnancy.

In compensated cirrhosis without jaundice or previously impaired liver function, the pregnancy should be allowed to proceed to term with attendance to rest, vitamin supplements and diet (high carbohydrate [to ensure enough calories] with no excess protein in advanced cirrhosis).

Excessive straining should be minimized during pushing to avoid a rise in portal hypertension. Excess blood loss should be anticipated, including bleeding from esophageal varices. Problems are less severe in those who have had porto-systemic shunt surgery prior to pregnancy.

Primary biliary cirrhosis: The risks of primary biliary cirrhosis to the baby are similar to those in chronic hepatitis.

Dubin-Johnson syndrome: Dubin-Johnson syndrome is a rare autosomal recessive genetic disorder. It causes mild, asymptomatic jaundice from conjugated bilirubin, and bile appears in the urine. It may be exacerbated or appear for the first time in pregnancy due to high estrogen levels. It can be distinguished by measuring the 5'-nucleotidase levels or serum bile acid levels, which are not elevated in Dubin-Johnson syndrome. Dubin-Johnson syndrome causes a high serum conjugated bilirubin when the woman is not pregnant, an abnormal BSP (bromsulfophthalein) clearance (a test done with dye), and a nonfilling gallbladder. Biopsy is the only way to make a definitive diagnosis and is usually not done. The main symptom is itching. Relative fetal risk is not known.

Hepatitis: Chronic persistent hepatitis in the mother is no threat to pregnancy; only chronic active hepatitis influences the course and outcome of pregnancy. Varices and accumulations of peritoneal fluid as well as other complications usually occur only when there is structural damage associated with cirrhosis.

Women who have chronic active hepatitis without cirrhosis may have trouble conceiving, especially when the disease is active. An increased rate of prematurity and perinatal mortality will be seen in relationship to the activity of the disease. The major complications of cirrhosis are esophageal varices, accumulations of peritoneal fluid (ascites) and the occurrence of hepatic encephalopathy (brain dysfunction caused by liver disease). Whether the woman is pregnant or not, these problems increase mortality. (See Cirrhosis in this chapter for a discussion of possible complications.)

Liver transplantation: Normal pregnancy is possible in women who have undergone liver transplant. They must take prednisolone and azathioprine.

Liver tumors (hepatic adenomas): Hepatic adenomas (tumors) may be induced by the administration of estrogen such as in oral contraceptives. Reports suggest that the possibility of rupture of the adenoma may be increased during pregnancy. Such tumors may enlarge and become symptomatic during pregnancy, and for this reason some advise against pregnancy. (Gleicher, 1985)

Heart and Circulatory Disorders

Hypertension:

Pheochromocytoma: This is a rare but dangerous disease caused by an adrenal gland tumor. It leads to extreme, unstable hypertension, proteinuria and toxemic symptoms such as headaches. Treatment with α-adrenergic blockade drugs can help improve maternal survival.

Severe pulmonary hypertension: This disorder is characterized by increased pressure within the lungs and carries a poor prognosis even outside of pregnancy. It is severe, but somewhat less so than systemic pulmonary hypertension. Vascular resistance may occur in chronic pulmonary embolism. Pregnancy mortality is 50%. Management is as for Eisenmenger syndrome (described later in this chapter).

Note: Methyldopa is a *Beta*-blocker drug which is used widely for hypertension both in and outside of pregnancy. One side effect of this centrally acting antihypertensive is the reduction of uterine contractibility. *Beta*-blockers slow the heart rate in an effort to reduce blood pressure; bronchiole constriction is an undesirable side effect as well. These drugs are classified as category D and their use should be discontinued prior to conception. Diuretics may also be prescribed for certain heart and circulatory conditions and they are also contraindicated in pregnancy.

Cerebrovascular Disease:

Arteriovenous malformations: These blood vessel defects lead to bleeding in 87% of cases with rebleeding in 27%. The greatest risk for a bleeding accident is between 16 to 24 weeks, as well as before labor or during pushing. Many recommend surgical delivery to minimize such complications.

Brain tumors: The symptoms associated with malignant brain tumors worsen during pregnancy because the pituitary gland increases in size and fluid balance changes. Edema of the brain can be controlled with drugs. Surgical decompression can be carried out during pregnancy. A brain tumor which appears for the first time during pregnancy may improve postpartum.

Embolism: Women with a history of deep venous thrombosis during a previous pregnancy are at risk for stroke with the next pregnancy. Mitral valve prolapse may rarely cause cerebral embolism (1 in 6,000) in the general population, but risk is not increased during pregnancy.

Meningiomas: Meningiomas are usually benign tumors of the meninges which may grow rapidly during pregnancy. Most improve after birth but may reappear during another pregnancy.

Neuromas: These are lesions of the cells of the intracranial nerves which may involve the auditory nerve, causing tinnitus, deafness, facial weakness, signs of increased intracranial pressure and cerebellar dysfunction secondary to local compression. The tumors may undergo rapid growth in pregnancy; they are treated with steroids and surgical removal postpartum.

Vasculopathy: Women who are known to have had an intracerebral aneurysm or arteriovenous malformation in the past and for those with Marfan's syndrome are at higher risk for pregnancy-associated cerebral hemorrhage. Women who have had prior incidents of problems may have also had surgery to remove the vascular lesion. In inoperable lesions there is a greater risk of hemorrhage during late pregnancy or pushing. Surgical delivery is advised, with an epidural and forceps or vacuum extraction as second choices.

Heart Disease:

General considerations: The increased blood volume of pregnancy increases cardiac output by about 40% as well as increasing the heart rate. These normal changes may exacerbate symptoms of a heart disorder. The normal heart is not permanently damaged by pregnancy. In most heart disorders, surgical delivery is more dangerous than yoni birth. The effects of most recently applied drugs in heart disease are unknown in regard to pregnancy.

    If the heart condition in question can be surgically corrected, treatment should be completed before pregnancy. Such conditions include the secundum type of atrial septal defect, patent ductus arteriosus and some cases of coarctation. An exception to this is valvular disease, which may necessitate a prosthetic valve. In most cases, these women should birth prior to treatment to avoid anticoagulant risks. If valve replacement has been done, Heparin is the anticoagulant of choice since it is one of the few drugs which cannot cross the placenta (Gabbe, 1991, p. 1061)

    In other cases a heart condition may have been ameliorated but not permanently corrected. These conditions include mitral stenosis and regurgitation, aortic stenosis, teratology of fallot, ventricular septal defect with moderate pulmonary hypertension, pulmonary stenosis, and a variety of other congenital malformations and acquired conditions. A year or so should elapse between treatment and conception.

    The babies of women who have a congenital heart defect are at risk for intrauterine death based on their mother's degree of functionality and cyanosis.

1090

Additionally, their babies are at risk for having a heart defect themselves, although the degree of risk varies according to the defect involved.

Infectious endocarditis is a serious risk with any heart disorder. To avoid this, dental health should be attended to and other infections dealt with promptly to avoid this. Many recommend the use of prophylactic antibiotics for any dental work and during labor, delivery and postpartum, specifically:

EVENT	RECOMMENDED PROPHYLAXIS
Labor and birth	Ampicillin, 2.0 g. IM; or IV plus gentamicin 1.5 mg.kg IM; or IV given in active labor, one follow-up dose may be given 8 hours later & postpartum
Minor or repetitive procedures in low risk women	Amoxicillin 3.0 g. orally 1 hour before procedure & 1.5 g. 6 hours later
Penicillin-allergic women	Vancomycin 1.0 g. IV slowly over 1 hour, plus gentamicin 1.5 mg/kg IM or IV given 1 hour before procedure; may be repeated once 8 to 12 hours later

(Gabbe, 1991, p. 1062)

General notes on labor: Women with heart problems typically have rapid, uncomplicated labors. Specific recommendations for assisting a woman in labor differ according to the nature and severity of the problem. Induction should not be undertaken routinely. IVs may overexpand the blood volume and put undue stress on the heart leading to pulmonary edema. Supine hypotensive syndrome is especially predicative of maternal and fetal distress in these women. Pain and anxiety in first stage should be minimized; however, inhalation anesthetics should be avoided. Spinal anesthesia causes hypotension and hemodynamic compromise and is also best avoided.

Severe heart conditions indicate the need for an epidural and forceps to minimize stress during the pushing phase of labor. Pitocin is the best drug to use in the event of bleeding. Some recommend prophylactic antibiotics only for those with an artificial heart valve. Maternal mortality is most likely in those conditions which impair pulmonary blood flow.

Classification of heart diseases is based on the following criteria:

Class 1—no resulting limitation of physical activity. Ordinary physical activity does not cause undue fatigue, palpitation, dyspnea (painful breathing) or anginal (heart muscle) pain.

Class 2—slight limitation of physical activity although comfortable at rest, ordinary physical activity results in fatigue, palpitation, dyspnea and anginal pain.

Class 3—marked limitation of physical activity. Comfortable at rest. Less than ordinary activity causes fatigue, palpitation, dyspnea or anginal pain.

Class 4—inability to carry on any physical activity without discomfort. Symptoms of cardiac insufficiency or of the anginal syndrome may be present even at rest. If any physical activity is undertaken, discomfort increases.

These classes are most relevant outside of pregnancy. The changes of pregnancy can significantly worsen preexisting symptoms in individual women.

Congenital heart disease: Left to right shunt (cyanotic heart diseases)

Aortic stenosis: Bicuspid valve stenosis is a common congenital malformation. Lesions are usually not severe, but when they are they can cause severe left ventricular hypertrophy and limit the ability of the heart to respond to increased demands with an increase in cardiac output. Symptoms are dyspnea, chest pain, and syncope, but asymptomatic lesions may also occur.
Critical aortic stenosis is usually treated by aortic valve replacement and occasionally with repair. If severe, maternal mortality is 17%. Valve replacement necessitates anticoagulant therapy and makes pregnancy even more dangerous. If the problem is only moderately severe, the woman should have her baby before heart surgery.
Limits on physical exertion and bed rest may be required during pregnancy. Ventricular failure may appear and necessitate the use of diuretics and digitalis. Vasodilator drugs are dangerous in this disorder and should not be used. Prophylactic antibiotics should be given during labor (Gabbe, 1991, p. 1064)

Atrial septal defect and coarctation of the aorta: These problems may be discovered in childbearing women because symptoms are often absent and physical findings are not blatant.

Patent ductus arteriosus: This loud murmur is usually detected in childhood, although a few women reach pregnancy without being diagnosed. If the left to right shunt is large, the circulation is hyperdynamic. This means there is a wide arterial pulse pressure, low arterial diastolic pressure, hyperactive precordium, and warm skin, perhaps with capillary pulsation. The heart may be somewhat enlarged. These signs are exaggerated by pregnancy and may lead to maternal death. However, if the defèct is small and the woman is young, her chances of tolerating pregnancy well are very good and prophylactic antibiotics are the only medical necessity (Gabbe, 1991, p. 1066)

Division of the ductus should be accomplished surgically before pregnancy is undertaken. Pregnancy without surgery is generally able to be managed safely if the left-to-right shunt is uncomplicated. Endocarditis is a risk in women with a patent ductus arteriosus. This is another reason for preconceptual surgical closure of the duct. Embolic complications are usually in the lungs. Fever and respiratory problems are signs of such an infection.

Pulmonary stenosis: This loud, long murmur is usually detected in early childhood and should be corrected before childbearing. Mild to moderate disease is well tolerated so that neither pregnancy nor labor pose a significant threat. Antibiotic prophylaxis against endocarditis is necessary. More severe cases require treatment by simple valvotomy, which is ideally performed before pregnancy. In pregnancy this operation poses considerable risk to the fetus.

Eisenmenger's syndrome: Either a large ventricular septal defect or a patent ductus arteriosus may cause this extreme form of pulmonary vascular resistance with pulmonary hypertension and right ventricular hypertrophy. Eisenmenger's syndrome represents a high risk in pregnancy. Its management is similar to the complications of ventricular septal defect (described below).

This defect consists of a right to left or bidirectional shunting at either the atrial or ventricular level combined with elevated pulmonary vascular resistance (Gabbe, 1991, p. 1042). The most common underlying defect is a large ventricular septal defect. The next most common cause is a large patent ductus arteriosus. Rarely is it associated with atrial septal defect or other less common defects. When increased pulmonary vascular resistance is detected, the defect must be closed as soon as possible because Eisenmenger's syndrome makes repair impossible and is itself irreversible. The clues to its development are diminution or disappearance of the shunt sound and appearance of pulmonary hypertension. When pulmonary vascular resistance is significantly higher than systemic right-to-left shunt it causes cyanosis, clubbing of the fingers and toes, and increased hematocrit in those affected. Attempts at surgical correction usually cause death. Many die from heart failure, pulmonary hypertension or pulmonary hemorrhage. Pregnancy poses a 50% risk of death for mother and fetus, and abortion is recommended. If pregnancy does occur, no physical activity is advised, and the mother should live at or near sea level. If the hematocrit rises above 60, phlebotomy should be performed. Great caution is required in lowering pulmonary vascular resistance with drugs. Surgical delivery and sterilization are recommended.

Secundum atrial septal defect: This straightforward defect can usually be corrected and surgery is recommended prior to conception. If the mother refuses surgery, the lesion is unlikely to complicate labor, birth or postpartum. The vasodilation of pregnancy, if anything, seems to reduce the left to right shunt. Atrial septal defect in young women does not cause heart failure. A small number of those affected will have atrial flutter, which is usually paroxysmal. Surgical closure does not prevent arrhythmia. Rarely, labor leads to paradoxical systemic embolus due to preferential flow from the inferior vena cava to the left atrium.

If a woman is over 35, atrial fibrillation may be due to an established arrhythmia and right heart failure will be incipient or present. Pulmonary vascular disease or pulmonary hypertension may also be complicating factors. If so, pregnancy is ill advised and will necessitate bed rest and vigorous treatment of heart failure. Maternal and fetal risks are very much increased.

Ventricular septal defects: This problem may be so mild that it has no effect on pregnancy or it may be so severe as to pose a risk of death to mother and fetus. Ventricular septal defects which are associated with a considerable increase in pulmonary vascular resistance reflect occlusive disease of the small pulmonary arteries and arterioles. This usually develops in childhood; if uncorrected, significant pulmonary vascular resistance occurs. These women are at high risk for death of mother or baby during pregnancy or labor. They require intensive care with strict bed rest and no physical exercise. The combination of no activity, pulmonary hypertension and vascular disease mean that anticoagulant therapy with heparin would be wise. Some advise preterm birth by surgery and sterilization.

Defects which persist as small left-to-right shunts may show an audible murmur but normal electrocardiograms and radiographs except for prominence of the main pulmonary artery. This is called **maladie de Roger**. Prophylactic antibiotics may be used to prevent infectious endocarditis; otherwise there is no increased risk during pregnancy.

If the defect is in the membranous septum, the left-to-right shunt is larger and the spontaneous closure that frequently occurs in childhood with other ventricular septal defects is rare. If there is no significant pulmonary vascular disease the same systolic murmur and thrill that characterizes maladie de Roger is found. Due to the larger shunt, excess circulation to the lungs causes pulmonary hypertension from increased cardiac output. Pulmonary vascular resistance is normal.

Those with relatively large uncomplicated left-to-right shunts through a-ventricular septal defect tolerate pregnancy well and can be compared to those with atrial septal defect, except that infectious endocarditis may occur and they are less prone to arrhythmias.

Right-to-left shunt without pulmonary hypertension produces right ventricular overflow obstruction.

Coarctation of the aorta: This defect occurs when there is a congenital narrowing

1094

of the aorta where the ligamentum and the left subclavian artery insert. It may be simple or complex and may be associated with patency of the ductus arteriosus or other defects. It may also be associated with Turner XO syndrome. It is usually detected and repaired in childhood, but some women enter pregnancy undiagnosed.

Typical features are upper extremity hypertension with lower extremity hypotension, visible and palpable collateral arteries in the scapular area, late systolic murmur, femoral pulses that lag behind the carotid pulses and are usually weaker in amplitude and notching of the inferior rib borders (seen on chest x-ray).

Surgical correction can usually reduce upper extremity hypertension, but blood pressure does not always return to normal and hypertension may occur later in life. The surgery should be performed before pregnancy; otherwise, maternal mortality is 3%. In cases without surgery, blood pressure can be controlled with α-adrenegis stimulating and blocking agents given by IV, eliminating the need for surgical birth. Coarctation of the aorta is associated with congenital berry aneurysm of the cerebellum (Circle of Willis). Hypertension during pushing may cause such lesions to rupture, resulting in cerebral hemorrhage.

Tetralogy of Fallot: This consists of a large defect in the ventricular septum, accompanied by pulmonary stenosis. There is a loud murmur; the woman is usually cyanotic, with significant clubbing of the fingers and toes. Most such defects are treated surgically during infancy or childhood. The palliative Blalock and Taussig surgical technique has improved exercise capacity but left the circulation far from normal. However, many women who have had this surgery have had successful pregnancies. Most of the surgical techniques in current use involve closing the defect. Pulmonary stenosis is relieved, constituting virtual total repair and rendering women safe to undertake pregnancy, birth and motherhood.

If a woman with this defect should request counseling, advise her to wait to conceive until after surgical repair. In most unrepaired cases maternal risk of heart failure is increased and fetal risk is proportional to the severity of maternal cyanosis. This risk includes a small fetus or stillbirth due to profound hypoxia.

Other congenital heart malformations: These include defects such as **left-to-right or right-to-left shunts, transposition of the great vessels, truncus arteriosus, single ventricle, double outlet ventricle** and a variety of **obstructive lesions**. Survival depends upon at least partial correction either by surgery or as part of the malformation. Most of these defects contraindicate pregnancy.

Mitral valve stenosis and other disorders:

Mitral Valve prolapse: This is by far the most common heart condition encountered by midwives. Authorities differ as to whether mitral valve prolapse is abnormal since the condition is so prevalent. It occurs because one or more portions of the mitral valve apparatus is too large for the heart; as a result the leaflets balloon into the left atrium during systole. The leaflets may separate, causing variable degrees of mitral regurgitation. More severe forms are caused by leaflet degeneration or redundant chordae. These may be isolated to the mitral valve or associated with Marfan's syndrome, which is a genetic disorder. Mitral valve prolapse may be associated with other congenital heart problems, notably atrial septal defect.

In a few cases, autonomic nervous system dysfunction is an associated factor, leading to excessive lability of the heart rate, tachycardia and postural hypotension. Dysautonomia (an associated hereditary syndrome characterized by mental retardation, convulsions, motor incoordination, vomiting and frequent infections) is aggravated during pregnancy. Anxiety is an associated feature and may be due to abnormal catecholamine metabolism and altered function of the sympathetic nervous system; other psychological problems may appear. Women may also complain of chest pain.

Simple mitral valve prolapse: Pregnancy is generally safe and unaffected, but standing blood pressure and heart rate during exercise should be watched. When the only sign of prolapse is a click, the need for antibiotic prophylaxis is controversial; with regurgitation it is considered more important.

Mitral prolapse with significant regurgitation: In such cases the murmur is louder, longer and more consistent. Even with modest left ventricular impairment pregnancy may precipitate heart failure. If the defect is successfully repaired, pregnancy is usually well tolerated. Severe regurgitation greatly enlarges the left atrium and ventricle and eventually leads to left ventricular failure and pulmonary hypertension, although the latter is less severe than with mitral stenosis.

Symptomatic mitral valve prolapse: When chest pain, palpitation, tachycardia, dysrhythmia, anxiety and panic attacks are present, they are best managed by blockage of the ß-adrenergic receptors with an bio-technical agent such as propranolol. With severe symptoms, thyroid levels and plasma catecholamines should be tested.

During pregnancy the enlarged uterus and vasodilation may add to postural hypotension. This may cause lightheadedness, dizziness or fainting during prolonged standing.

Significant mitral stenosis without heart failure: Most sources advise surgery with full recovery before conception. If no surgery is performed, long rest periods, no strenuous activity, salt restriction and diuretics are advised. When affected women are followed correctly, maternal mortality is low.

Atrial fibrillation would signal the need for digitalis, a ß-adrenergic blocking agent, or a calcium channel blocking agent to maintain a normal heart rate. Atrial fibrillation with significant mitral stenosis requires anticoagulant treatment. If the valve can be treated by valvotomy and does not require replacement, the operation may be carried out safely for the mother but the fetus may not survive. If valve replacement is needed, it should usually be postponed until after birth.

These women may spend many weeks in bed and should be hospitalized prior to delivery. During labor and birth the mother should be on her left side. The lithotomy position invites pulmonary edema, which may appear regardless. If so, sedation to drop the heart rate and promote cardiac filling and the administration of diuretics must be followed by surgical delivery if the fetus is viable. If not, emergency mitral operation is called for. Recently, balloon valvuloplasty has been used as a nonsurgical means to dilate mitral stenosis. It should be postponed until after the first trimester.

Mitral stenosis and heart failure: Once right heart failure and pulmonary stenosis have developed, pregnancy is ill advised. If the woman does concieve, she must be prepared for prolonged rest, much dyspnea, fatigue and swelling, and episodes of acute decompensation as well as increased risk of stroke or pulmonary embolism. Maternal and fetal death rates are high.

Mitral regurgitation not caused by prolapse: Most of the advised parameters for prolapse applies in these cases as well. In addition, the mitral valve is more apt to be calcified; therefore it is less likely to be repairable and must instead be repaired.

Those with severe left ventricular dysfunction or failure who have mitral valve regurgitation are advised that pregnancy is dangerous, it would require bed rest, and be punctuated by episodes of uncompensated congestive heart failure. The risk of death for the fetus exceeds 50%.

Miscellaneous heart problems:

Aortic valve disease: Aortic stenosis is commonly caused by tissue degeneration, often of a congenital bicuspid valve. Frequently the valve is calcified. Heart failure often develops and sudden death may occur. This and syncope or previous cardiac arrest are contraindications to pregnancy in women with uncorrected aortic stenosis. If the valve is replaced, treatment with anticoagulants and close supervision may bring women to term with relatively low maternal risk. Tight aortic stenosis may be relieved by the aortic balloon technique, if necessary.

Aortic regurgitation: This volume load is usually well tolerated in pregnancy and labor. A prolonged course without heart failure is usual, but once heart failure occurs the condition rapidly deteriorates. Usually nothing is done until symptoms of heart failure, such as difficulty breathing with exertion, make their appearance or evidence of left ventricular dysfunction can be detected by pulmonary congestion or abnormal lab tests. These symptoms indicate the need for valve replacement or repair. Pregnancy is not advised. Increased diastolic volume of the left ventricle is a result of its overload and does not necessarily indicate heart failure.

When left ventricular dysfunction and heart failure are absent, carefully supervised pregnancy is in order. Women should be encouraged to complete childbearing before heart failure and the need to consider valve replacement arises.

In many cases the causes of aortic regurgitation will not be obvious during surgery. Special care must be taken to rule out aortic aneurysm or dissection. This is especially true in Marfan's syndrome since this condition may lead to aortic rupture and is a reason to avoid pregnancy. All valvular disease of the heart necessitates antibiotic prophylaxis for infectious endocarditis.

Heart failure: When the heart cannot meet the body's metabolic requirements, heart failure may occur. Primary myocardial causes include: disorders of the myocardium such as myocarditis, various cardiomyopathies, ischemic heart disease, specific myocardial disorders such as amyloidosis, and metabolic abnormalities such as myxedema. Secondary myocardial causes include chronic pressure overload leading to cardiac enlargement and volume overload causing dilation. Contractile power is eventually diminished, decreasing pump function. Conditions which lead to these problems include valve disease, systemic and pulmonary hypertension, and congenital malformations.

In addition, extra-cardiac causes may lead to heart failure. Conditions such as severe thyroid disease, profound anemia, renal disease, and prolonged high fever may all lead to heart failure. These conditions may also provoke failure in previously compensated heart disease.

The principal signs of heart failure are caused by increased left and right ventricular diastolic pressure, engendering pulmonary and systemic congestion and reduced cardiac output. In severe cases symptoms occur even during rest. In less severe cases, symptoms appear during exercise. The combined effects of heart congestion and inadequate output are dyspnea, fatigue, and edema. These changes lead to progressive dysfunction of vital organs, especially of the liver and kidneys as heart failure progresses. The prognosis for death in severe and uncorrectable cases is 50% by five years.

Clinical features that enable physicians to diagnose and follow the course of heart failure are changes in body weight, jugular venous pressure, the third heart sound, cardiac size, radiologic evidence of pulmonary congestion, lung crepitations (crackly sounds in the lungs) and peripheral edema.

Heart failure limits physical activity and requires continuous treatment with diuretics and other drugs. Pregnancy imposes a powerful, often intolerable, load on the failing heart. Pregnancy is contraindicated and will worsen a woman's symptoms; it often results in premature birth, fetal malformation and stillbirth.

Chronic heart failure represents sustained irreversible damage to a large portion of the ventricular myocardium. The chief symptoms of heart failure are dyspnea and fatigue. These are exaggerated by pregnancy which often produces edema, breathing difficulty in any other but a sitting or standing position, difficult breathing at night and pulmonary edema. Pregnancy is an intensive care emergency in these women.

Heart transplantation: Pregnancy is not encouraged because of the immunosuppressive drugs and other therapies required and the uncertain prognosis. However, successful pregnancies have occurred. Women seeking to become pregnant should be evaluated individually prior to conception. (Kolder, 1995)

Artificial heart valves: Women with artificial heart valves may have near normal cardiac function. The need for anticoagulation agents is the major risk factor in pregnancy and should be accomplished with heparin.

Myocardial infarction (heart attack): Heart attacks are rare in pregnancy and in young women in general. They are most likely to occur in pregnancy in smokers, diabetics and women over age 35. The advisability of a woman becoming pregnant who has a history of myocardial infarction is unclear, and opinions vary. Sine MI is usually precipitated by underlying vascular disease, (primary atherosclerosis), it is usually progressive, since it is often associated with hypertension, pregnancy may be contraindicated. Prior to conception, a full cardiac evaluation with a coronary angiography is advised. (Williams Obstetrics, 17th ed., 1985, p. 594)

Rheumatic heart disease: Rheumatic fever seldom occurs for the first time in young adults; it is usually a relapse from childhood. It is relatively uncommon in the United States, England and Western Europe but is still prevalent in less developed countries. Women with a history of rheumatic fever, especially those with rheumatic heart disease, should take penicillin or (if allergic) its equivalent at regular intervals prior to conception and throughout pregnancy to prevent a recurrence. The American Heart Association recommends monthly injections of 1.2 million units of benzathine penicillin G or daily oral doses of penicillin or erythromycin (Gabbe, 1991, p. 1061).

Symptoms of acute rheumatic fever include fever, anemia, malaise and, sometimes, joint pains. Acute fever or acute streptococcal infection call for a full dose of antibiotics for ten days. Pericarditis, heart failure, cardiac murmurs and enlargement of the heart call for prompt suppression with prednisone and bed rest.

Rheumatic heart disease usually produces mitral valve stenosis with or without aortic regurgitation (which may lead to pulmonary edema). Mitral stenosis causes enlargement of the left atrium and right ventricle, a diastolic murmur, and pulmonary hypertension. A fast heart rate can impede ventricular filling, further elevating atrial pressure. Atrial fibrillation eventually supervenes causing a fall in cardiac output and escalation of left atrial hypertension especially if the ventricular rate cannot be easily controlled. This increases the chances of thrombus in the left atrial appendage and the threat of an embolic stroke.

Pregnancy drastically stresses the circulation with severe pulmonary congestion that may be manifest by progressive, exceptionally difficult breathing (dyspnea) or orthopnea (uncomfortable breathing) and progress to sudden attacks of difficult breathing during the night and pulmonary edema. Women who have not had care often come in with pulmonary edema. Long standing cases develop severe right heart failure and infectious endocarditis, pulmonary embolism and massive hemoptysis may also occur.

Ventricular extrasystole and atrial fibrillation: These problems are more frequent and more symptomatic in women of childbearing age. Ventricular tachycardia or fibrillation occurs in a small minority and has in a small percentage of cases resulted in sudden death. Stroke may also occur and is thought to be due to platelet occlusion or embolism but not thrombus unless regurgitation is severe. Platelet function is abnormal in some women with associated mitral valve prolapse.

Diagnosis is based on a systolic click occurring between the first and second heart sounds which may or may not be followed by a mid or late systolic murmur. This symptom may vary with posture and from time to time.

Left ventricular dysfunction: Pregnancy may transform this problem into clinical heart failure. Lesser degrees of left ventricular dysfunction with ejection fractions in the range of 40% are compatible with safe pregnancy and birth provided care by specialists is excellent throughout pregnancy.

Hypertensive heart disease: Hypertensive heart disease is associated with left ventricular hypertrophy, which lessens stress of the heart wall.

Hypertensive left ventricular failure: Overt clinical ventricular failure may develop as a result of hypertension, and may appear to be heart failure. The failing ventricle frequently cannot pump hard enough to generate arterial hypertension; frequently by the time left ventricular failure develops, hypertension is no longer present. Hypertension is the problem in pregnancy, not the heart condition. The thinner and taller a woman is, the less significance the heart condition has.

First determine if the heart shows evidence of disease or dysfunction aside from severe concentric hypertrophy. If the case is uncomplicated, blood pressure must be controlled before pregnancy. Cardiac evaluation before conception is recommended, as left ventricular failure would contraindicate pregnancy.

Disturbances of cardiac rate and rhythm: Superventricular and ventricular extrasystole are heart murmurs which require no treatment. Arrhythmia in the absence of disease is usually benign. Even with organic heart disease, arrhythmia that is not sustained does not require treatment. If it is sustained it must be treated. If the mother has a pacemaker to treat arrhythmia, the pacemaker itself does not pose a risk to the pregnancy or the baby.

Prenatal diagnosis of heart disease in the fetus: The babies of mothers with congenital heart defects are at somewhat more risk for manifesting a heart defect themselves. Fetal heart failure and arrhythmias are treated with a variety of medications depending upon the condition. Many fetal heart defects can be detected via ultrasound and fetal electrocardiography.

Marfan's syndrome: This autosomal dominant genetic trait involves a congenital deficiency of elastic tissue causing severe heart degeneration leading to aneurysms of the aorta and great vessels and severe aortal and mitral regurgitation resulting in heart failure. Surgical treatment is only temporary as the tissues do not hold sutures well. Pregnancy is poorly tolerated and labor may lead to heart failure.

<u>Cardiomyopathy</u>: defined as any disease of the myocardium (the heart muscle).

Coronary artery disease (CAD): Coronary artery disease may be precipitated by conditions such as lupus (especially when treated with steroids). Coronary atherosclerosis is the most common form of CAD and appears in a high percentage of those who have cardiac transplants or those with familial lipid disorders.
Angina pectoris which occurs with moderate effort may require drug treatment, but successful pregnancy is possible. If a woman has had a myocardial infarction (heart attack) but has recovered without heart failure, significant left ventricular dysfunction or unstable angina pectoris, she may be advised that her pregnancy and labor should not differ significantly from those without heart disease. The major indications that problems will occur are previous heart failure, significant heart enlargement, dysfunction of the left ventricle and ischemia (lack of tissue oxygenation) provoked by slight effort (Williams Obstetrics, 17th ed., 1985, p. 594) (Also see the entry for myocardial infarction, this chapter.)

Dilated cardiomyopathy: In this condition the cardiac chambers are dilated and are not thin walled. Cardiac output falls and filling pressure increases, both of which cause progressive dyspnea, edema and fatigue. In the majority of cases, serious ventricular arrhythmia develops. The five year prognosis period for survival is less than 50%, and heart failure becomes progressively unresponsive to treatment during that time. A few cases improve or return to normal, but there are no indications regarding who will have such a remission. This condition may be due to an autoimmune response to myocardial injury such as viral myocarditis. In some cases, alcohol abuse is a major aggravating factor. The pregnancy risk is high, with maternal mortality being greatly increased and survival afterwards decreased.

Hypertrophic cardiomyopathy: This is a severe concentric hypertrophy of ventricular myocardium in which the ventricular cavities are very small and the walls thick, elevating ventricular diastolic pressure. In many the problem is detected in childhood or infancy. Drugs and surgery may be used in an attempt to correct this condition. A variation is termed asymmetrical hypertrophy; the left ventricular outflow tract is narrowed by the hypertrophied septum and the abnormally anterior position of the anterior leaflet of the mitral valve. Major symptoms are angina, syncope, and dyspnea but this condition may be asymptomatic.

Sudden death, possibly due to arrhythmia, characterizes a small but significant subset of these patients. About half the cases are inherited. Except when severely symptomatic, these patients tolerate pregnancy, labor and drug therapy well. Severely symptomatic women who do not respond well to drugs should have surgery before conception, but the risk of sudden death is not eliminated. Familial disorders will affect the baby 30% of the time.

Severe ischemia: Ischemia (is-KEM-me-ah) is a lack of blood flow to an area due to circulatory obstruction. Symptoms include angina (chest pain) which occurs at rest or with minimal exertion and usually follows a period of classical angina pectoris (pain and oppression around the heart). Unstable angina is a reliable symptom of severe, extensive myocardial ischemia. This is a clear warning of imminent major ischemic events such as acute myocardial infarction or a fatal ventricular arrhythmia. Pregnancy is ill advised.

With less advanced conditions a treadmill test will provoke either angina pectoris or a fall in blood pressure, indicating a high risk for a severe ischemic event. Pregnancy should not be undertaken unless the cause is found and treated. Bypass surgery is recommended, after which the woman may more safely concieve.

Acute pericarditis: Whether viral or idiopathic, this condition is usually self limiting and characterized by fever, chest pain, and certain heart changes. It usually responds to simple antinflammatory treatment. It may indicate underlying myocarditis. It occasionally relapses and is resistant to simple drug therapy but will respond to steroids. Due to the adverse effect of steroids on pregnancy, women should wait to conceive until the disease process ends or is in prolonged remission.

Cardiac tamponade: Cardiac tamponade is caused by high pressure cardiac effusion (defined as an escape of fluid into the membrane which encases the heart). It is indicated by circulatory distress, high venous pressure and, usually, pulsus paradoxus. Treatment must be carried out regardless of whether a woman is pregnant or not and consists of removal of pericardial fluid. In pregnancy, open drainage through a small incision is preferred.

Constrictive pericarditis: Tight pericardial fibrosis, thickening and sometimes calcification characterize this condition. It usually involves the entire pericardium and causes loss or disappearance of pericardial compliance, which severely limits venous return and ventricular diastolic filling. Heart chamber size is reduced but filling pressures are greatly increased. Pulmonary and systemic venous pressures rise with resulting congestion, cardiac output falls, and tachycardia develops as partial compensation for the reduction in stroke volume.

Women with severe, untreated constrictive pericarditis should not undertake pregnancy, as this condition is equivalent to congestive heart failure. They can look forward to normal pregnancy, labor and delivery and normal babies a year or more after a successful pericardiectomy.

Mild constrictive pericarditis can be managed with prolonged rest, avoidance of excessive diuresis and by refraining from drugs that drastically reduce tachycardia. Excessive tachycardia associated with atrial fibrillation, however, should be controlled with digitalis.

Congenital heart block: A heart block is a portion of the heart tissue in which the spread of cardiac electrical impulses are slowed or interrupted in their normal pathway. This usually poses no problems in pregnancy. In general those with a pacemaker in place fare better than those without.

<u>**Migraine (vascular) Headache**</u>: Seventy percent of those who suffer from migraine headaches are women of childbearing age. These headaches are worse with menses, oral contraceptives and pregnancy. Some women experience the worst headaches they have ever had during the first trimester of pregnancy. As pregnancy progresses headaches diminish in some, but not all, women. There is no evidence of harm to the pregnancy or the fetus. Migraines may be triggered by stress, alcohol, caffeine, dietary items (such as strong cheese, MSG and nitrates), and lowered glucose levels. Dietary adjustment may help, as will eating frequently to avoid hypoglycemia. Eliminating alcohol (esp. red wine), strong cheeses and chocolate are especially important.

At the first sign of headache warm baths can help divert circulating blood to the extremities. Ice packs and pressure on the painful area, an upright rather than a reclining position and avoiding exercise and visual or auditory stimuli may also help to offset a headache. Noting what happens emotionally around the time of onset is important part of understanding the non-physical factors which may be related.

Fetal risk from drugs is highest during the first 8 weeks. The commonly used drug ergotamine tartrate is not recommended during pregnancy. Tylenol or Tylenol3 with 30 mg. codeine (1 to 2 tablets every 4 to 6 hours as needed) can be used if necessary. While drugs may help the headache symptoms, most drugs have not been tested extensively in pregnancy and should be avoided whenever possible.

Immunologic Disorders

Hypogammaglobulinemia:

This large and diverse group of B-cell immunodeficiencies results in a deficiency of immunoglobulins of all or some classes. The two discussed below are the most common.

Common variable immunodeficiency: This condition usually appears during the second or third decade of life; symptoms include a tendency to bacterial infections, markedly decreased serum immunoglobulins, and impaired antibody responses. IgG levels are usually below 500mg/dl, and IgM and IgA are often undetectable. Cellular immunity is usually normal. Commonly recurrent sinus and lung infections eventually become chronic. Physical exam reveals a lack of lymphoid tissue, although the liver and spleen may be enlarged. Gastrointestinal findings include malabsorption of folic acid and B_{12}, lactose intolerance, protein-losing defects and abnormal villus structure. Giardia is frequently found in the small intestine.

The outcome of pregnancy is related to the types of infections occurring during gestation. Severe infections in the mother often lead to miscarriage or fetal demise. Treatment includes giving y-globulin as an IV infusion of 4 ml/kg (200mg/kg.) of body weight every 21 to 28 days. Anaphylactic reactions may occur, so infusion should not exceed a rate of 25 ml per hour, and anaphylactic medications should be readily available. In the third trimester, increased transfer of IgG antibodies to the fetus leaves the mother with reduced levels. Because of this, IV infusions or intramuscular injections of 0.6 ml./kg. y-globulin should be given weekly with the goal of raising maternal IgG levels above 200 mg/dl. If thrombocytopenia develops, the mother should be given y-globulin intravenously. Newborns on record have not shown manifestations of maternal disease. (Gleicher, 1985, p. 949)

Selective IgA deficiency: This is the most common immune disorder with a prevalence of 1:400 to 1:800. IgA levels are usually below 5mg/dl. Women with this deficiency have many allergies and often have asthma and pernicious anemia. The body treats IgA received from any source as a foreign substance. Gastrointestinal problems such as ulcerative colitis or regional ileitis and autoimmune disease such as lupus may occur. When pregnant, these women do not experience any additional problems. Their babies may have low serum IgA, but serum IgA does not reach adult levels until 10 to 12 years of age. (Gleicher, 1985, p. 950)

Chronic mucocutaneous candidiasis:
A cellular immunodeficiency causes a chronic yeast infection of the skin and mucus membranes. Endocrine disorders are

1104

sometimes associated. If a woman does not have severe endocrine involvement, she is likely to experience a normal pregnancy. Naturopathic care should be sought to outline a diet and natural therapeutic approach to minimize symptoms. There are pharmaceutical means of treatment which should be investigated as well. (Gleicher, 1985, p. 951)

Acrodermatitis enteropathica: This rare autosomal disease is characterized by failure to thrive, skin lesions, hair loss, diarrhea and malabsorption, impaired immunity, infections and behavioral disturbances. The hair becomes reddish; skin lesions similar to eczema appear around the mouth and genital areas as well as on the cheeks, knees and elbows. Immunoglobulin deficiencies have been described, although levels are usually normal. This condition is thought to be caused by a zinc deficiency. During pregnancy, supplemental zinc should be given in doses of 300 mg daily (68 mg of elemental zinc), increased to 400 mg. daily in the last month. The goal is to maintain a maternal plasma level of 72 to 137 mg/dl of zinc. None of the women treated with zinc in this fashion have had babies with defects (which occurs in untreated women); zinc therapy also significantly improves maternal immune function. (Gleicher, 1985, p. 951-2)

Red cell aplasia: This rare disorder involves a depression in the production of red cell precursors in the bone marrow. It is also associated with low levels of immunoglobulins, white blood cells and thymus cells.   There may be immunodeficiency with susceptibility to infections, particularly those of the respiratory tract. Autoimmune disorders may also be present. Anemia may recur during pregnancy in women who have received treatment, or aplasia may develop during pregnancy. Rapid remission tends to occur after the birth. Newborns have been normal in recorded cases. Management includes treating anemia with blood transfusions. Autoimmune disorders should be treated with steroids only if blood transfusion does not help. (Gleicher, 1985, p. 952)

Myasthenia Gravis: This disorder is frequently found in women of childbearing age and involves weakness of the voluntary muscles following repetitive activity and a marked tendency to regain motor function after rest. White blood cells infiltrate skeletal muscles in 50% of those affected. (This occurs in many autoimmune disorders.) A tumor may appear on the thymus gland. Remission may be achieved by surgical removal of the thymus gland. Relapse frequently occurs during pregnancy and medication requirements may increase. (Gleicher, 1985, p. 956)

Kidney Disease

General considerations: The demand on kidney function increases considerably during pregnancy due to the increase in maternal blood volume. The kidney enlarges and the calyces, renal pelvis and ureters dilate markedly. The clinical implications of these changes follow:

1. Dilation of the urinary tract may lead to collection errors in tests based on timed urine volume (*e.g.* 24 hour tests of output of various chemicals and hormones).
2. Stasis within the ureters may predispose pregnant women with asymptomatic bacteriuria to develop acute pyelonephritis.

Acceptable norms of kidney size should be increased by 1 cm during pregnancy and the immediate postpartum since dilation of the ureters persists after birth. Elective radiological exam should be postponed until 16 weeks postpartum.

Glomerular filtration rate (GFR) and effective renal plasma flow (ERPF) increase about 50% in normal pregnancy; these changes begin shortly after conception and peak levels are present by the second trimester. The GFR reduces by about 15% during the third trimester (measured as 24 hour creatinine clearance). These changes must be taken into account, especially when assessing the course of pregnancy in a woman with known renal disease.

General tips when caring for women with renal disease in pregnancy are:

1. Carefully monitor the blood pressure. Detection of hypertension and assessment of its severity and long-term effects are important in preventing further kidney damage and eclampsia.
2. Assess renal function by performing 24 hour creatinine clearance and protein excretion tests at regular intervals. Monitor the nutritional status in heavily proteinuric women to be sure they are getting adequate calories and adequate but not excessive amounts of protein. Excess protein puts additional stress on weak kidneys.
3. Carefully assess fetal well-being and appropriate growth.
4. Detect and treat urinary tract infection promptly.
5. Provide prenatal visits every two weeks until 32 weeks, then every week thereafter. Kidney problems can reach a crisis point and become serious very quickly.

Complications requiring hospital admission:

1. Deterioration of renal function indicated by a 20% decrease in creatinine clearance, the onset of proteinuria, or marked increases in proteinuria which persist. Poor renal function leads to maternal

1106

metabolic acidosis.
2. Development of moderate hypertension; i.e. blood pressure greater than 140/90 on two more occasions at least 6 hours apart.
3. Signs of intrauterine growth retardation or placental dysfunction.
4. Change in weight gain, either cessation or excess.
5. Symptoms of impending convulsions.

Diagnosing renal disease which appears for the first time in pregnancy should take into account the following:

1. The type of chronic kidney disease, if known
2. General health considerations
3. Effect of pregnancy on blood pressure
4. Effect of pregnancy on renal function and plasma biochemistry (via lab tests)
5. Past obstetric history
6. Use of drug therapy
7. Renal failure (due to sepsis from induced abortion, chorioamnionitis, etc.)

Assessing renal function: Laboratory tests to determine creatinine clearance and 24-hour urinary protein loss will help to assess renal function. Some doctors advise against pregnancy if the creatinine level exceeds 2.0 mg/dL. This is high; a decade ago the upper limit was 1.5 mg/dl. Serum levels above 3.0 mg/dL are very dangerous to both mother and baby, and pregnancy is not recommended. At creatinine levels of 1.5 to 3.0 pregnancy should not be undertaken lightly. When the creatinine levels are high, miscarriage is common and therapeutic abortion is frequently indicated, especially in the presence of fulminating hypertension. Twenty percent of those infants that reach viability are small for dates, and fetal distress is common in the third trimester. In 70 to 75% of these women kidney deterioration continues at about the same rate that it would outside of pregnancy, but for 25 to 30% it accelerates considerably.

Mild renal impairment: Milder renal impairment is less risky. If the glomerular filtration rate (GFR) and the blood pressure are both normal before conception, pregnancy will usually be uncomplicated and maternal disease will not get worse. However, the perinatal mortality rate remains elevated for such women.

Mild renal insufficiency: Creatinine levels less than 1.5 mg/dl represent only mild problems unless accompanied by serious hypertension. Fetal risks are still significant, with higher mortality and prematurity than normal. Proteinuria and high blood pressure requiring treatment may develop in 50% of these women.

Advanced renal failure: The ability to conceive is also greatly impaired.

Pregnancy may aggravate hypertension as well as worsen maternal kidney disease. Renal failure often leads to premature labor and a poor fetal outcome due to problems such as a baby small for gestational age.

Hypertension and renal disease: Hypertension that accompanies renal disease complicates the picture considerably. Conception should not be attempted if the blood pressure cannot be kept below a diastolic level of 90 mm.Hg. with drugs that can be taken during pregnancy. Uncontrolled hypertension coupled with renal disease causes approximately 100% fetal mortality.

Glomerulonephritic Disease: Chronic renal disease is hard to evaluate during pregnancy. Acute disease is rare but does occur. In the absence of hypertension there is usually no adverse effect from the condition during pregnancy. Glomerulonephritis may be adversely affected by the coagulation changes which normally occur in pregnancy. Urinary tract infections occur more frequently as well.

Minimal change nephrotic syndrome: This disorder is characterized by the development of a sclerosing lesion and excessive proteinuria possibly due to chronic injury from immune processes associated with infectious hepatitis, syphilis or malaria, rather than actual glomerular disease. It has a relapsing and remitting course, but responds to steroids and only rarely causes renal impairment or hypertension. Pregnancy is well tolerated in those who have received prednisone only. Most childhood cases remit in adulthood, and pregnancy does not increase the risk of relapse. Although premature labor and small for dates babies are somewhat more common, fetal survival is good. Those subject to frequent relapses may prefer to remain on prednisone throughout pregnancy.

Focal glomerulosclerosis (FGS): Hardening of the glomerular filtration system leads to marked nephrotic syndrome. It is steroid resistant, often associated with hypertension, and progresses to renal failure over several years. Premature and small for dates infants have been reported, with perinatal loss rates of 20 to 30%. Increased proteinuria and hypertension are frequently seen but usually reversible. FGS may accelerate with pregnancy, but this is minimized if kidney function is close to normal at conception. If serum creatinine levels exceed 1.5 mg/dl and hypertension is present, pregnancy may be ill advised.

Diffuse proliferative glomerulonephritis (DPGN): This generalized inflammation develops in those with prolonged proteinuria. Hypertension and proteinuria worsen during pregnancy but there is no evidence of increased kidney damage. Preterm labor is more likely and fetal loss compares with those conditions described above.

Membranoproliferative glomerulonephritis (MPGN)/mesangiocapillary GN:

This causes persistent low serum compliment levels and a renal syndrome of proteinuria (often in the nephrotic range), persistent microcytic hematuria, frequent hypertension and usually progression to renal failure over a period of several years.

When maternal preconceptual creatinine levels are below 1.5 mg/dl, fetal loss is about 35%; it rises to as high as 50% with a greater degree of renal impairment. Reversible increases are seen in 50% of pregnancies. Hypertension arising during pregnancy usually persists afterwards. Some with this disorder have a circulating "C3 nephritic factor" antibody which can cross the placenta and cause transient neonatal hypocomplementemia (low complement levels). These women should avoid pregnancy unless they have normal blood pressure, no clinically overt nephrotic symptoms and renal function that is normal and stable for many months without specific therapy. Type I may be treated with dipyridamole and aspirin, but there is no consensus that any therapy is beneficial in adults (Stein's, 1994)

Nephropathy of various kinds:

Nephrotic Syndrome: This occurs when urinary protein excretion is so heavy (>3.5 g/24 hours) that blood levels of albumin fall and edema develops. Only those renal diseases in which damage is directed at the glomeruli cause this condition. It is often treated with diuretics; their use further complicates pregnancy, since women with nephrotic syndrome are already hypovolemic. This syndrome appears to double the risk of fetal loss and perinatal death. High protein diets may accelerate the loss of protein and aggravate the underlying renal disease. However, if renal function is adequate and hypertension absent, there should be few problems; in these cases a high protein diet (3 g/kg/day) is important.

Membranous glomerular nephropathy (MGN): This condition causes adult nephrotic syndrome although blood pressure and renal function remain otherwise normal for a long period of time after onset. Short courses of prednisone and chlorambucil are sometimes used to stabilize the condition. Such treatment should be completed prior to conception. The outlook for pregnancy is favorable and gestation does not damage the underlying renal lesion. If complicated by hypertension or full blown nephrotic syndrome the outcome is not as favorable, with miscarriage occurring frequently.

Mesangial IGA nephropathy: This is a common renal disorder with recurrent hematuria and persistent proteinuria which may lead to hypertension and occasional renal failure. There is no specific treatment. Fetal loss is about 15%, perinatal mortality 3 to 10% and preterm birth 10 to 15%. Marked preconception hypertension increases the fetal loss to about 50%. The risk of developing hypertension during pregnancy is somewhat increased. A serum creatinine over 1.5 worsens the fetal loss rate. Almost all affected women show progressive renal failure postpartum. After birth the babies seem to do well. In some cases this problem may be genetic.

Familial nephritis: Women with hereditary nephritis do not appear to have any special risk other than those dictated by blood pressure and renal function parameters. If creatinine is below 1.5 mg/d and blood pressure is normal, they can be expected do well in pregnancy.

Polyarteritis nodosa and Wegener's granulomatosis: Women with either of these conditions do poorly and pregnancy is contraindicated unless the disease is inactive and renal involvement minimal.

Chronic tubulointerstitial nephritis: Chronic inflammation of the renal tubules and interstitium is usually seen with persistent or modest proteinuria (.3 to 1.5 g/24 hrs). If creatinine is below 1.5 mg/d and blood pressure is normal or well controlled, pregnancy is usually well tolerated by the mother with only a moderately increased risk of perinatal death and preterm delivery. In cases complicated by high creatinine levels and hypertension, perinatal death is increased and accelerated maternal renal damage often occurs.

History of pyelonephritis: This is an inflammation of the body and pelvis of the kidneys due to infection. In women with such a history, bacteriuria may lead to kidney infection more easily than in those who have no such history.

Persistent bacteriuria despite treatment may be a clue to underlying urinary tract abnormality (usually vesicoureteral reflux). Women with recurrent urinary tract infections, hypertension and proteinuria may have an underlying kidney disorder. Check creatinine clearance and proteinuria in a non-infected 24-hour specimen. If results are abnormal, a postpartum intravenous pyelogram can determine any chronic damage and a voiding cystogram can check for vesicoureteral reflux. Normal preconceptual results of a pyelogram reassure that pregnancy will not be subject to unusual problems except the need to monitor for and treat urinary tract infections. Prognosis is most favorable in women who have normal blood pressure and adequate renal function.

Reflux nephropathy: In childhood the growing kidneys can be damaged from reflux (backwashing of urine) during voiding which causes recurrent bacterial infection. The renal scarring which can result may lead to hypertension and even renal failure in adulthood. In the later phases of disease, secondary glomerulosclerosis with proteinuria can occur.

Although opinions vary, most agree that pregnancy is associated with only moderate increases of prematurity, fetal loss, and toxemia unless renal insufficiency or hypertension already exist. High creatinine levels (above 2.3 mg/dL) may cause rapid progression to kidney failure even with well controlled blood pressure.

Recurrent urinary tract infections are common in pregnancy, but do not contribute appreciably to fetal loss. Complications are less common in those who have had their reflux surgically corrected. The majority of fetal deaths occur in those who have experienced complications from reflux nephropathy prior to conception.

Analgesic nephropathy: This disorder is caused by the chronic abuse of analgesics. It is not usually apparent until women are beyond reproductive years, and is seen infrequently in the United States. Advanced cases carry all the risks of renal insufficiency. Continued analgesic abuse can lead to infertility. Those who do conceive risk postmaturity and congenital defects.

Wilm's tumor survivors (nephroblastoma): Women face a 30% risk of fetal or perinatal death, perhaps due to the effects of therapeutic radiation on the uterus.

Polycystic Kidney Disease:

The adult form of polycystic kidney disease is caused by an autosomal dominant genetic trait. Renal ultrasound can identify about 65% of cases by age 15 and 85% by age 25. Symptoms include hematuria, hypertension, renal pain and sometimes urinary tract stones and infections. Impairment progresses over years or decades, ending in renal failure. Fifty percent of the offspring of those affected will inherit this disease. Ultrasound does not often detect this problem in the fetus.

Polycystic kidney disease does not affect fertility, and pregnancy brings no an increased rate of spontaneous abortion, stillbirth or urinary tract infection. Hypertension is more common (32%). Perinatal mortality may be higher if hypertension preexists pregnancy. When renal insufficiency is severe or associated with uncontrolled hypertension, fetal survival is rare and maternal death may occur. When functional impairment is minimal and hypertension absent, pregnancy is generally uncomplicated.

Kidney Stones and Other Renal Obstructions:

Urolithiasis: Renal calculi may cause severe abdominal or flank pain and should be treated with hydration and analgesics. Too much bed rest can lead to thrombosis in the legs.

Stones and other disorders: There is no increase in the rate of stone formation during pregnancy. In addition the presence of stones do not pose an increased obstetric risk, but urinary tract infections are more common. Renal colic is a relatively common non-obstetric cause of serious abdominal pain in pregnancy.

Urinary diversion surgery: Women with temporary obstructive urinary diversions and permanent diversions can be reassured that there are usually no problems during pregnancy except an increased incidence of urinary tract infection. Those with urostomies are more prone to urinary tract infections. An uncontaminated urine sample should be checked periodically to detect asymptomatic bacteria. To obtain a specimen, remove the appliance, cleanse the surrounding skin and allow urine to spurt into a sterile container. Catheterization of the stoma is another option. Obstruction of the ureter may occur (usually in the left) as the growing uterus compresses the ureter which crosses the vertebral column to reach the ileal conduit. (See the chapter on Gastrointestinal Disorders for additional tips on managing an ostomy during pregnancy.)

Kidney Removal and Congenital Malpositioning:

Pelvic kidneys: A pelvic kidney is one which is placed below its normal location in or near the pelvic area. It does not compromise gestation but may cause dystocia during labor, necessitating a surgical delivery. Women with this condition are vulnerable to infection, probably due to associated urinary tract abnormalities.

Solitary kidney: Women may have only one kidney either as a congenital disorder or as the result of surgical removal. These women seem to tolerate pregnancy well.

Dialysis:

Dialysis: Dialysis is a mechanical method of filtering toxins from the blood used when the kidneys are no longer functioning. Women on dialysis are usually amenorrheic or anovulatory. Those that do menstruate have irregular periods which often delays the diagnosis of pregnancy. Early miscarriage is a common problem.

Most pregnancies occur in women with some renal function or in those who started dialysis after pregnancy commenced. Pregnancy-related hypertension and toxemia are common and anemia worsens, necessitating transfusions. Ideally dialysis should be performed five times weekly to reduce intrauterine azotemia (excessive nitrogen levels) with special attention to avoiding large blood volume shifts during dialysis and meticulous control of the blood pressure. Fetal monitoring should be done throughout dialysis sessions in late pregnancy. Drug and supplement use should be carefully monitored. Nutrition is very important. (Gabbe, 1991, p. 1090) Ideally, kidney transplant occurs before conception.

Kidney Transplantation:

Prepregnancy assessment: Recipients of kidney transplants usually regain near-normal fertility, but should delay pregnancy for at least two to five years after surgery. Recipients of live grafts may do better in pregnancy than recipients of kidneys recovered from cadavers. Immediate graft function after transplant correlates with better gestational success. Maternal survival rates are not below the usual rates for transplant patients in general; however, transplant recipients may be at higher risk for ectopic pregnancy due to surgical scar adhesions. Pregnancy must be carefully monitored for kidney rejection.

The following are general guidelines for transplant recipients wishing to conceive. The absence of some of these guidelines (1, 2 and 6 below) present only relative contraindications to pregnancy:

1. Good general health for at least two years after transplantation
2. Bone structure compatible with good obstetric outcome
3. No proteinuria
4. No significant hypertension
5. No evidence of graft rejection
6. No evidence of pelvicalyceal distention on recent excretory urogram
7. Plasma creatinine of 2 mg/dL (180 μmol/I) or less
8. No evidence of hydronephrosis (obstructed flow of urine from the kidney) on intravenous pyelography
9. Drug therapy: prednisone or prednisolone 15 mg/day or less and Imuran (azathioprine) 2 mg/kg/day or less and dosages stabilized.

Prenatal visits should take place every two weeks until 32 weeks then every week thereafter. Each visit should include the following:

*Complete blood count with platelets
*Urea and electrolyte assays
*24-hour creatinine clearance and protein excretion
*Collection of a midstream urine specimen for culture and sensitivity
*In addition, plasma protein, calcium and phosphate levels, CMV and herpes hominis virus titers should be checked every 5 weeks.

Kidney grafts seem to have a filtration rate and pattern similar to a normal kidney. Fifteen percent of all pregnant graft recipients develop significant impairment of function which may persist following delivery. Women should also know that 9% of those carrying into the third trimester may have serious rejection episodes, however there is no greater incidence than in nonpregnant recipients. Symptoms include fever, oliguria, deteriorating renal function with enlargement and tenderness. When considering other tests to monitor the pregnancy itself, keep in mind that transplanted kidneys do not filter estriol normally, however human placental lactogen levels are normal in these women.

Drug use and pregnancy: Immunosuppressive drugs should be continued during gestation. Women taking Imuran have lower creatinine levels than those on cyclosporine (Sandimmune), but the latter have better graft acceptance.

Results of pregnancies in women treated with azathioprine have been extensively documented. It has been found that 16% of those women will miscarry, which is considered within normal limits. Among the fetuses that survive the first trimester, 92% will survive to infancy. An increase in toxemia (30%), preterm birth (50%), and intrauterine growth retardation (20%) has been noted.

The safety of cyclosporine is not established in pregnancy but acute rejection of the kidney may occur if a switch is made. This drug produces better immunosuppression and presumably better acceptance of the graft than some others. Liver impairment and lymphoma development have been reported.

Urinary tract infection must be treated however, all existing antibiotics pose some special problems for the transplant recipient. Nitrofurantoin (Macrodantin) is not recommended when the GFR is >50 ml/min. due to side effects. Ampicillin predisposes women to the development of resistant organisms and may not be effective long term. Trimethoprim combinations (Septra, Bactrim) are widely used in non-pregnant azathioprine patients but in pregnancy may cause synergistic nephrotoxicity. Sulfonamides and, in some cases Gantrisin, may be helpful.

The use of immunosuppressive therapy means that such women are 35 times more likely to develop malignancies. In theory, the infant which was exposed *in utero* to immunosuppressive drugs as well as azathioprine should be able to tolerate them via breastfeeding, but more information is needed.

Labor and birth: Steroids such as hydrocortisone, 100 mg intramuscularly every 6 hours, are necessary during labor. Yoni delivery should be the aim, and induction may be used if needed. These women are prone to premature rupture of membranes and it is postulated that long term steroid therapy may weaken connective tissues. Careful management of fluid balance, cardiovascular status and temperature are essential. Asepsis is mandatory and prophylactic antibiotics are recommended. Pain relief protocols are no different than for other women.

Cesarean section may be needed if there is pelvic osteodystrophy (defective bone development) related to the previous renal failure or prolonged steroid therapy. An ultrasound exam at 36 weeks gestation may be recommended to rule out kidney compression from the enlarged uterus. If a surgical delivery is needed, lower segment incision may be hindered by scarring from previous surgeries.

Newborns: Risks to live-born infants include preterm birth, respiratory distress syndrome, depressed hematopoiesis (formation of blood cells), septicemia, lymphoid hypoplasia (defective development), adrenal insufficiency, cytomegalovirus (CMV) infection and congenital abnormalities. Mothers may transmit HBsAg carrier status to their newborns. Newborn immune suppression due to maternal immunosuppressive drugs, leukopenia, and thrombocytopenia may also occur. In spite of these problems, most babies recover well.

Metabolic and Glandular Disorders

Adrenal Diseases:

General considerations: Most women with adrenal disease are diagnosed before they concieve and many have experienced infertility. In active adrenal problems, replacement hormonal therapy is continued throughout gestation. When monitoring hormone levels, normal pregnancy elevations should be taken into account.

Addison's disease (Adrenocortical insufficiency): This is brought on by atrophy of the adrenal cortex and lack of glucocorticoid and mineralocorticoid activity. Symptoms include vomiting, hypotension, mental lethargy, weight loss, dehydration, muscular weakness and hyperpigmentation due to excess ACTH secretion.

During pregnancy untreated women are at risk for death; this risk is increased in labor, since extra natural steroid production is not possible. Adrenal steroid replacement therapy may be at no increased risk. For most women this consists of oral cortisone acetate 25 mg. each morning and 12.5 mg each evening. Some may need an additional medication with the salt-retaining hormone 9-α-flurohydro-cortisone (Florinef) as well, .05 to .1 mg daily. During the first trimester nausea and vomiting may worsen adrenal insufficiency and may necessitate adjustments in drug dosages. Minor or major infections, emotional stress, or other events may also require higher doses of replacement therapy.

Primary diagnosis during pregnancy is uncommon because fetal adrenal hormones can help regulate maternal levels as well, but those with persistent nausea and vomiting beyond 20 weeks gestation should prompt concern that this condition may be causative. If suspected, tests should be done to determine if Addison's disease is present. Replacement therapy can be started immediately with no increase in miscarriage, prematurity or fetal death rates.

Acute adrenal crisis is rare, but can be life-threatening in pregnant women. It may occur if a woman discontinues her medication due to problematic symptoms such as nausea. Acute cardiovascular collapse during the stress of labor and delivery may be the first sign of adrenal hypofunction, with abdominal pain, nausea, vomiting and shock. Blood should be drawn immediately for a ACTH assay so therapy can begin as soon as possible.

Most women with **mild adrenocortical insufficiency** tolerate pregnancy well unless they experience infections or an unexpected complication. They are at increased risk for acute adrenal insufficiency during labor, delivery and the immediate postpartum period. Lab values which denote adrenocortical insufficiency during pregnancy are:

TEST	SIGNIFICANT RESULTS:
Serum Na	Normal or low
Serum K	Elevated
BUN	Low
Creatinine ACTH stimulation test	Low response of plasma cortisol
Plasma ACTH	Above normal pregnancy level
24 hour urinary free cortisol	Below normal pregnancy values
Plasma cortisol	Below normal pregnancy level (normally elevated during pregnancy)

Hypercortisolism (Cushing's syndrome): Eighty percent of these cases involve primary pathology of the pituitary. A pituitary adenoma secretes excess ACTH which inappropriately stimulates the adrenal glands to produce glucocorticoids. Symptoms include bruising, myopathy, hypertension, plethora, edema, hirsutism, red stretch marks, menstrual irregularity, obesity, headaches, acne and impaired glucose tolerance. Outside of pregnancy, overgrowth of facial hair and acne may be the earliest clues to increased adrenal hormone secretion.

Pregnancy usually doesn't occur in untreated women due to excessive androgen production and anovulatory cycles. When it does, fetal loss and preterm labor frequently occur. Diagnosis during pregnancy is difficult since abdominal enlargement, fatigue, emotional lability, mild hypotension and glucose intolerance are symptoms common to both pregnancy and Cushing's syndrome. With Cushing's syndrome, stretch marks tend to be wide and deep purple.

Treatment depends upon the cause. If necessary, surgical removal of tumors is most successful in the second trimester. Treatment with cyproheptadine has also resulted in successful pregnancies. Diagnostic studies in pregnant women include:

TEST	FINDINGS IN CUSHING'S SYNDROME IN PREGNANCY:
Plasma ACTH	Elevated or high normal suggests abnormal elevation of ACTH secretion
24-hr profile of plasma cortisol	Loss of normal diurnal pattern
Ultrasound or CT scan of adrenal glands	Adenoma, carcinoma or bilateral enlargement
CT scan or MRI of the sella turcica	Look for microadenomas of the pituitary gland

Note that normal pregnancy produces cortisol levels similar to those found with Cushing's syndrome, making diagnosis during pregnancy extremely difficult; however, there is a lack of normal diurnal variation in Cushing's syndrome. Cortisol levels in normal pregnancy follow.

Test	Time of Day	Nonpregnant	2nd Trimester	3rd Trimester
Total cortisol nmol/l	9 am midnight	324 ± 100	No data	1029 ± 200
Free cortisol nmol/l	9 am midnight	18 ± 9 6 ± 4	No data	38 ± 12 17 ± 5
Urinary free cortisol nmol/l	N/A	103 (13 to 256)	No data	229 to 680
ACTH ng/ml	15 to 70	15 to 70	20 to 70	20 to 120

Primary Aldosteronism: This condition is characterized by abnormally high levels of the adrenal hormone aldosterone, causing retention of sodium, urinary loss of potassium, and alkalosis. Although rare, primary aldosteronism should be suspected whenever hypertension along with hypokalemia and metabolic alkalosis are found in young women. If found, adrenal gland removal is indicated.

Acromegaly (Acromegalia): Growth hormone secretion from the anterior pituitary is increased, leading to elongation and enlargement of the bones in the limbs and the head (especially the frontal bones and the jaw). In addition the nose and lips become enlarged and the soft facial tissues thicken. Most of those with the active condition are infertile due to suppressed ovulation. If treated prior to pregnancy, the course of this disorder should be unaffected, although hyperglycemia may present a problem; blood glucose levels should be checked at 12 weeks.

Hypopituitarism (Sheehan's syndrome): The anterior pituitary is sensitive to blood loss after birth; hypopituitarism may follow severe hemorrhage associated with hypotension, leading to lack of lactation. Affected women rapidly become apathetic and are often thought to be depressed in the postpartum period. Persistent amenorrhea with loss of axillary and pubic hair accompanied by the signs and symptoms of hyperthyroidism and adrenocortical insufficiency should lead you to suspect this problem. Low levels of thyroxine, plasma cortisol, TSH, ACTH, FSH, LH and growth hormone that do not rise on stimulation are usually seen. Women with a positive history should be followed up for 1 year.

If Sheehan's syndrome is treated prior to conception of the next pregnancy, outcome is good. Hydrocortisone in doses up to 30 pg. per day is used for anterior pituitary deficiency and may be needed during labor. If untreated, maternal mortality, abortion and stillbirth are major risks.

Acute adrenal failure: Acute adrenal failure is rare and may result from thrombosis or hemorrhage in the adrenal glands, usually following eclampsia or postpartum hemorrhage. Symptoms include rigors, abdominal pain, circulatory collapse and vomiting. This condition is almost always fatal.

Congenital adrenal hyperplasia: This group of inborn errors of metabolism affects adrenal hormones.   It may cause ambiguous genitalia in a female infant. Fertility is reduced as well; however, if defects are corrected, pregnancy may occur in some women.   Steroids are given throughout gestation.

Hypothalamic-pituitary disturbances:

Hyperprolactinemia (macro and microadenomas):   Most women with these types of pituitary tumors remain asymptomatic during pregnancy, almost never developing a problem which results in perinatal damage or serious maternal complications.   During prenatal care, pay particular attention to the development of visual symptoms and headaches.   Formal visual assessment of the sella turcica (shallow bony depression where the pituitary gland is found) need not be done unless such symptoms develop.

Bromocriptine, the drug most often used for this condition, has not been shown to adversely affect the fetus or the pregnancy.   Both galactorrhea (excess milk production) and hyperprolactenemia may resolve spontaneously after pregnancy for reasons not yet discovered.

Women who have had ovulation induced with total pituitary hormone replacement to treat other hypothalamic-pituitary disturbances typically do well during pregnancy; but breastfeeding may be impaired if prolactin secretion has been eliminated by therapy.   Women with idiopathic hypopituitarism can often breast feed following birth.

Thyroid Disease: (See Diagnostic Tests for more details on thyroid disorders.)

Thyroid enlargement in pregnancy may be directly related to a slightly inadequate iodine intake.   There is a reduction in the renal tubular absorption of iodine before 12 weeks gestation.   The urinary excretion of iodine doubles, the plasma levels fall, and the thyroid gland is therefore forced to triple its uptake of iodine from the blood.   In partial deficiencies, the gland enlarges in order to produce sufficient amounts of thyroid hormone to meet the demands of pregnancy. Placental estrogen causes an increase in the synthesis of thyroxine binding globulin (TBG) by the liver.   By the 12th week TBG production has doubled.   Thyroid function in mother and fetus are almost entirely separate.

The fetus depends on the mother for proper iodine supplementation.   Iodine deficiency in the first 12 weeks leads to fetal neurological cretinism.   Although these babies have normal thyroid function, they have mental retardation, deafness and spasticity.   Maternal hypothyroidism in the second and third trimesters leads to true hypothyroidism and cretinism in the newborn.   There is no treatment for cretinism.

1118

Sporadic goiter: In countries where most goiter is eradicated, some may still occur due to iodine deficiency, ingested goitrogens or a defect in enzymes which help to form thyroid hormones. Thyroid antibodies may also cause a goiter to develop; two-thirds of young girls presenting with goiter have a titer. Preexisting goiters tend to enlarge in pregnancy. In simple goiter (due to iodine deficiency), iodine supplements (700 μg. daily) or iodized table salt is recommended.

Thyroid nodules: These small tumors may be cancerous. If there is a history of radiation therapy of the throat during childhood, assume such nodules are cancerous, regardless of the stage of pregnancy. Voice change, a hard fixed lump, lymph gland enlargement, or Horner's syndrome (contraction of the pupil, drooping of the eyelid, recession of the eye into its orbit and loss of the ability to sweat on the affected side of the face) demand immediate thyroid surgery. Solitary nodules with none of these associated signs may not require surgery. Tests should be done to determine total thyroxine and triiodothyronine levels to exclude a toxic adenoma.

Ultrasound is the best way to investigate if the lesion is solid, cystic or mixed. Questionable nodules can be biopsied with a fine needle. If surgery is performed, the woman should have replacement thyroxine immediately.

Parathyroid Disease: (Also see Diagnostic Tests for more details on parathyroid disorders.)

The parathyroid regulates the use of calcium in the body. Affected women are fertile and require monitoring of their condition throughout pregnancy; without this fetal and neonatal mortality rates are high.

Treatment of maternal hypoparathyroidism prevents fetal hyperparathyroidism. Vitamin D requirements may vary during pregnancy due to enhanced absorption of calcium. Treatment consists of vitamin D (50,000 to 150,000 IU per day) in the form of 25-hydroxycholecalciferol (25D) or 1,25-hydroxycholecalciferol [1,25-$(OH)_2$D; calcitrol] along with calcium supplements. Vitamin D intoxication can cause nausea, constipation, fatigue, headaches, vomiting and dehydration. If these symptoms occur or serum calcium is elevated, vitamin D supplements should be decreased or stopped and IV fluids given. Serum calcium and phosphorus levels should be checked at regular intervals to monitor for hypo- or hyperparathyroidism.

Postpartum, mothers should be observed for and be aware of signs pointing to hypercalcemia such as constipation, nausea, vomiting, loss of appetite, abdominal pain, and in more severe cases, labile emotions, confusion, delirium, psychosis, stupor and coma. Frequent urination, the need to urinate at night and excessive thirst may also occur. Hypercalcemia may occur without a change in calcium or vitamin D intake and mild cases may be asymptomatic. High supplemental levels of vitamin D may contraindicate breastfeeding.

Infants of mothers being treated for hypoparathyroidism are usually normal at birth. They are generally not at risk for developing hypoparathyroidism, except if the mother has sporadic hypoparathyroidism; the infant is at risk for the inherited disorder and should be followed to determine whether treatment will be required.

Infants born to women with hyperparathyroidism are at risk for hypoparathyroidism and tetany. Frequently a problem is not suspected in the mother until her infant presents with hypocalcemia. Fetal loss, prematurity and perinatal death are high when maternal hyperparathyroidism has been long-standing and is accompanied by kidney or bone complications. Babies may have prolonged suppression of parathyroid function, but most of them will recover spontaneously.

Diabetes Mellitus:

General considerations: Insulin dependent diabetes requires careful monitoring throughout pregnancy and gestation. Considerable fetal risk is involved; it is therefore an inappropriate choice to care for such women at home. Classical signs of diabetes are increased thirst, ravenous appetite with weight loss, and excessive urination. Urine samples show high levels of glucose, ketones and perhaps protein. **Eye damage** is often associated with diabetes severe enough to require insulin dependence. Studies conflict, but eye damage may worsen with pregnancy, especially in those who have had diabetes for more than two years.

Renal damage (nephropathy) peaks after about 16 years of diabetes, eventually afflicting 30% to 50% of those who are insulin dependent. Severe renal disease may impair fetal growth and lead to stillbirth. Significant renal damage is often accompanied by hypertension. **Protein in the urine** is a cardinal indication of such damage. Persistent proteinuria greater that .5 g per 24 hours is the accepted hallmark of overt nephropathy in diabetics, although subclinical involvement is detectable as microproteinuria. This can be measured by radioimmunoassay and may be present for 14 to 17 years before overt disease develops. Most diabetic women with nephropathy start pregnancy with proteinuria less than 2 g/24 hrs and progress to >6 g/24 hrs in the third trimester

Once established, renal impairment progresses rapidly. Hypertensive therapy cuts this rate of progression in half, thus normalizing blood pressure and decreasing the strain on and further damage to the glomeruli. Kidney disease makes large babies and polyhydramnios less likely. Hypertension is present in 30% of insulin dependent diabetic women at conception and 70% at term. Some of this may be related to toxemia, which is more common in diabetics. Perinatal mortality is about 11.5% in those women with renal impairment compared to about 3% in those with diabetes with good glycemic control.

Autonomic neuropathy (nerve damage) may also be present. This can cause a woman to be insensitive to the signs and symptoms of hypoglycemia. It can also cause paralysis of the stomach, diarrhea, postural hypotension and cardiovascular reflex abnormalities. During a physical exam, signs suggestive of neuropathy include tachycardia, postural hypotension and failure of the pupil to dilate normally in the dark. Cardiovascular reflexes can be evaluated by noting heart rate responses to the valsalva maneuver (holding the breath and pushing), standing up and deep breathing, blood pressure changes which occur from a sitting to a standing position, and whether or not a handgrip can be sustained.

Cardiovascular complications are rarely encountered in pregnant women whether they are insulin dependent or not. However, pregnant women with insulin-dependent diabetes have less than the normal pregnancy-related increase in left ventricular size and stroke volume, as well as less cardiac output. Reduced output may play a part in contributing to decreases in fetal oxygen supply. Strenuous exercise may divert even more blood from the placenta; a woman's exercise program needs review with this in mind. Myocardial infarction may occur before, during, or up to 4 weeks after birth. Maternal and fetal mortality is high.

CONGENITAL DEFECTS IN INFANTS OF DIABETIC MOTHERS	
FETAL ORGAN SYSTEM INVOLVED:	**DEFECTS NOTED:**
Cardiovascular	Complex transposition of great vessels Single ventricle Hypoplastic left heart Tricuspid atresia Ventricular septal defect Atrial septal defect
Renal	Agenesis Cystic kidney Ureteral duplication
Gastrointestinal	Small left colon syndrome Situs inversus Anal or rectal atresia
Neurologic	Anencephalus Central Nervous System defects Postnatal effects of severe maternal ketosis or hypoglycemia
Skeletal and spinal	Caudal regression syndrome

Diabetic women need careful glucose control beginning prior to conception and continuing throughout pregnancy to minimize these risks to the fetus. Hemoglobin A_{1C} levels, which reflect glucose control in the previous 6 weeks, should be monitored, they should be normal before conception to reduce the risk of anomalies. If the mother is diabetic, the baby's risk for diabetes is only slightly higher than the general population; if both parents are, the risk to the baby is 1 in 10. (Campion, 1991)

Ectopic hormone production:

The primary source of abnormally high levels of hormones is cancerous tumors. Hormone studies are not typically done and normal hormone levels change during pregnancy, making detection of such abnormalities more difficult. If lab findings indicate hormonal levels in excess of pregnancy norms, further investigation for a cancerous tumor especially of the cervix, breast, ovary, or rectum, or a lymphoma is indicated. (Gleicher, 1985)

Clinical syndromes of disorders of nucleic acid metabolism:

Gout: Gout refers to a disorder of purine metabolism and is the most common nucleic acid disorder of pregnancy. It manifests with high serum levels of uric acid, recurrent attacks of acute arthritis and, in some cases, sandy mineral deposits in joints. Gout may be either the result of an inborn error of metabolism (primary gout) or secondary to disorders such as leukemia that cause either increased metabolism or deceased renal clearance of nucleic acid precursors. The knowledge of the effects of gout on pregnancy are somewhat vague. Through 1967, Talbott reported at least 28 pregnant women with gout who had healthy full term babies. Of course, the impact of any associated disease or kidney impairment must be taken into account when assessing risk. The drugs Probenecid and colchicine as well as a high fluid intake are recommended for the treatment of gout in pregnancy. (Gleicher, 1985, p. 292)

Xanthinuria: This rare disorder of purine metabolism is associated with reduced activity of *xanthine oxidase*, an enzyme found in colostrum and liver and intestinal mucosa, resulting in low levels of serum uric acid and high levels of xanthine and hypoxanthine. Xanthine is less soluble at a pH of 5 to 7 than uric acid, therefore there is an increased tendency to stone formation in the urinary tract. Crystal deposits may also occur in skeletal muscles. High fluid intake, reduction of dietary purines, alkalinization of the urine and administration of allopurinol have been suggested as measures to minimize stone formation during pregnancy. There are few such pregnancies on record, one of which resulted in a normal baby. This may be an autosomal recessive genetic trait. (Gleicher, 1985, p. 293)

Xerodermia pigmentosum: This autosomal recessive disorder of DNA repair manifests in a variety of neurologic disorders. It often leads to an increased incidence of sunlight-induced skin cancers, extreme photosensitivity, hyperpigmentation and malignant skin legions. There are at least eight different genetic variants; the nonneurolitic forms are C, E, F and variant. The neurologic forms include groups A, B, D, and G. The most common form is group C. The most problematic complication for such women involves the stimulation of skin cancer growth during pregnancy; pregnancy may also increase the likelihood of melanoma development. (Gleicher, 1985, p. 293)

Other disorders of purine metabolism are rare and information on their effect during pregnancy is therefore scarce. (Gleicher, 1985, p. 294)

The porphyrias: This group of six related disorders is characterized by excessive production and excretion of porphyrin, porphyrin precursors, or both.

Congenital erythropoietic porphyria produces marked cutaneous photosensitivity, scarring, infections, and ulcerations of skin lesions; progressive disfigurement and mutilation having been reported. Excess hair growth in the affected areas is common. Mild hemolytic anemia and enlargement of the spleen may also occur. Treatment involves avoiding sunlight and prompt treatment of lesions. Splenectomy may improve the anemia. Few cases of pregnancy are on record, but liver disease and an increased risk of infection in those who have had splenectomy are anticipated complications. (Gleicher, 1985, p. 298)

Protoporphyria: This relatively common autosomal dominant disorder usually begin in childhood with moderate cutaneous photosensitivity, sunlight causes a burning or prickling sensation in exposed skin, followed by edema and redness. Symptoms usually disappear within a few hours; however, repeated exposures may lead to skin thickening. Although generally considered benign, associated abnormalities of the gall bladder and liver have been found; an increased incidence of gall bladder and liver disease and fatal cirrhosis have been reported. Therapy consists of avoiding sunlight and taking 120-180 mg. of *Beta*-carotene daily, which increases tolerance to sunlight. Liver function tests should be performed periodically throughout pregnancy. A marked decrease in the appearance of skin lesions has been noted during pregnancy, and there are no reports of this disorder negatively impacting pregnancy. (Gleicher, 1985, p. 298)

Porphyria cutanea tarda: This most common form is an autosomal dominant genetic trait. It usually presents in adulthood; the use of estrogen therapy, alcohol, excessive iron seem to cause it to manifest. The skin is fragile and vesicular lesions appear; milia are common on the hands and face, and excessive hair growth occurs in affected areas. Symptoms may be aggravated during the first trimester with improvement as pregnancy advances. Therapy consists of avoiding alcohol and sunlight, removing excess iron via phlebotomy and avoiding unnecessary iron supplementation. No fetal effects have been reported. (Gleicher, 1985, p. 298)

Acute intermittent porphyria: This more rare form of porphyria occurs in 1 to 2 per 100,000 overall and in 7.7 per 100,000 in Sweden. Onset occurs after puberty with recurrent episodes of abdominal, neurological and psychiatric symptoms. Crampy, colicky abdominal pain is the most common symptom and is often accompanied by constipation and vomiting. Neurologic symptoms vary and may include foot drop, wrist drop, areas of numbness and tingling in the arms and legs, and impaired respiratory function. Tachycardia may occur during acute episodes. Mental symptoms include anxiety, confusion, hallucinations and schizophrenic behavior. Photosensitivity does not occur. Treatment involves avoidance of precipitating substances (alcohol, barbiturates, ergot derivatives, estrogens, methyldopa, progesterone and sulfonamides them). Correction of acute symptoms may occur after giving a large glucose load (at least 300 g in 24 hours) either orally or by IV. Hematin (given IV in a dose of 4 mg/kg of body weight at 12 to 24 hour intervals) or sodium benzoate are alternative therapies. Pregnancy appears to be well tolerated; the condition is exacerbated in 54% of women, but of these only 24% have significant symptoms. Morphine and meperidine are safe to use for analgesia; local anesthesia and epidural anesthesia are well tolerated. A high incidence of prematurity has been noted; in mothers who experience an acute attack in pregnancy, low birth weight infants may result. The effects of Hematin on the fetus are unknown. (Gleicher, 1985, p. 299)

Variegate porphyria: This rare autosomal dominant form is most often found among the white population of South Africa. It usually presents at 20 to 30 years of age with neurologic symptoms. Treatment and impact on pregnancy are similar to intermittent porphyria. Skin lesions are characteristic of other forms of porphyria. (Gleicher, 1985, p. 299-300)

Hereditary coproporphyria: This rare autosomal dominant form has clinical symptoms similar to those of acute intermittent porphyria, with 30% manifesting cutaneous lesions as well. Maternal and fetal effects are similar as well. The use of chlorpromazine should be avoided during pregnancy. (Gleicher, 1985, p. 300)

Wilson's disease: This disease is characterized by an excessive accumulation of copper in various organ systems. It primarily manifests as a liver disorder; symptoms include degeneration of the body of the liver, muscle distortion, difficulty with speech and swallowing, and a highly emotional state. It may lead to subfertility, miscarriages and amenorrhoea. Vascular malformation, amoebic abscess or tumors may be causative. Treatment with C-penicillamine throughout pregnancy is recommended to promote copper excretion. (Gleicher, 1985, p. 296)

Galactosemia: Classic galactosemia frequently leads to death in infancy. **Galactokinase deficiency** causes cataracts. Normal infants were born in five pregnancies of women who were treated for galactosemia. In one case of an untreated mother, the baby was not born with cataracts. (Gleicher, 1985, p. 301)

Glycogen storage diseases: Conditions causing the abnormal storage of glycogen appear in about 1 in every 60,000 individuals; in most cases as an autosomal recessive trait. There are a number of different forms; those relevant to pregnancy are listed below:

Type 1: Glucose-6-phosphate deficiency causes liver and kidney enlargement, fat accumulation, flabby musculature, elevated serum uric acid and lipid levels, soft flat growths, gout, and impaired platelet function. Pregnant women may have a variety of complications including renal disease and toxemia. Hypoglycemic conclusions may also affect fetal well-being. (Gleicher, 1985, p. 302)

Type IIb: Acid Maltase deficiency results in survival to adulthood. (Type IIa is fatal during the first year of life; those with one affected child have a 25% chance of having another.) Two pregnancies of women with Type IIb resulted in normal labors and births with normal babies. (Gleicher, 1985, p. 302)

Type V: This recessive syndrome presents with muscle fatigue, cramps during exercise and occasional myoglobin in the urine. Successful pregnancies have been reported; these were uncomplicated, and spontaneous labor occurred at term. Babies were all normal. (Gleicher, 1985, p. 302)

Glycolytic pathway defects: These problems are characterized by enzymatic defects associated with hemolytic anemias. They may range from mild to moderate. The only reported cases involving pregnancy were in women with pyruvate kinase deficiency, by far the most common form associated with chronic hemolysis, which is preventable by splenectomy. Pregnancy may precipitate a hemolytic crisis. (Gleicher, 1985, p. 302)

Hexose-monophosphate-shunt defects: Glucose-6-phosphate dehydrogenase (G-6-PD) is the most common form and is discussed in the Anemia chapter in Diagnostic Tests.

Disorders of lipid metabolism: Hyperlipoproteinemia may be recognized for the first time during pregnancy. Small soft growths on the skin, abdominal pain, or elevated cholesterol and triglyceride levels may be presenting symptoms. The use of the drug clofibrate to control cholesterol levels is contraindicated in pregnancy. High lipids levels may accompany other problems such as pancreatitis. (Gleicher, 1985, p. 303-4)

Muscular and Connective Tissue Disorders

Mixed Connective Tissue Disease: This is usually a mild, lupus-like syndrome with sclerodermatous evolution (thickening and hardening of the skin accompanied by inflammation). Cases associated with antibodies to soluble nuclear antigens such as ribonucleoprotein seem to carry risks similar to systemic Lupus.

Ehlers-Danlos syndrome: This heritable disorder presents with skin and joint hyperelasticity, fragile tissue, and poor wound healing. Spontaneous rupture of arterial or intestinal tissue may rarely occur. There are eight variants, all of which carry risk for pregnancy. Pregnant women may experience an increase in bruising, relaxation of ligaments leading to scoliosis, backache and a high incidence of varicosities and hernias. During birth perineal tears or cuts may extend and severe postpartum hemorrhage may occur. However, labor is usually short and easy. Operative procedures such as the use of forceps may prove particularly damaging to the mother. Uterine scars may not sustain their integrity through pregnancy. Postpartum complications include slow healing, uterine prolapse and pubic discomfort. (Gleicher, 1985, p. 308)

Marfan's syndrome: This genetic connective tissue disorder manifests in the bones, eye and heart. The extremities may be elongated or there may be scoliosis and chest deformity. During pregnancy, dissecting aneurysm of the aorta is the most serious complication; it may occur any time during pregnancy, birth or the first few weeks postpartum. The majority of cases have occurred during the third trimester. There is no contraindication to yoni birth. Those who want to conceive should be encouraged to do so at an early age, before heart complications are severe.

Myotonic Muscular Dystrophy (Steiner's disease): Affected children born to affected mothers are more likely to have severe, profound hypotonia and mental retardation than those born to affected fathers.

Myotonic dystrophy (Dystrophia myotonia): Symptoms include muscular weakness and myotonia (repetitive contractions of muscle fibers in response to a single neural stimulus). Problems result in delayed reaction of the muscles, frontal loss of hair, opacities of the lenses of the eyes and testicular atrophy in males as well as below average intelligence. Fertility may be decreased. Symptoms may increase during pregnancy. There is an increased rate of fetal loss, prematurity and neonatal death from congenital myotonic dystrophy. Prematurity may be related to uterine myotonia or to polyhydramnios, which is frequently seen. Labor abnormalities include uterine inertia (responsive to oxytocin) and precipitous birth. Maternal weakness may prolong pushing and hemorrhage may occur due to uterine atony.

Myotonia congenita (Thomsen's disease): In this variety of myotonia weakness may become worse during the second half of pregnancy. (Gleicher, 1985, p. 935)

Myositis ossificans: Osseous structures are deposited along the facial planes of muscles. The three varieties of this disorder are not related to any problems during pregnancy. (Gleicher, 1985, p. 937)

Carnitine deficiency: Carnitine is a chemical that appears to be essential in the transport of long-chain fatty acids into mitochondria. A deficiency may produce profound muscular weakness during pregnancy or in the immediate postpartum period. An oral supplement can reverse the process. (Gleicher, 1985)

Scleroderma (Systemic sclerosis): This uncommon connective tissue disorder affects the skin, gastrointestinal tract (esophagus), kidneys and lungs. It evokes a vaso-spastic-inflammatory process in the small arterioles, especially those in the skin. The clinical features vary from calcinosis (deposits of lime salts in tissues), Raynaud's phenomenon (blood vessel spasms of the extremities, especially with exposure to cold), esophageal hypomotility, sclerodactyly (hardening of the skin of the fingers) and telangiectases (dilation of capillaries which produces a small overgrowth of blood vessels on the skin) to an intense and fulminant generalized vasoplastic syndrome with malignant hypertension and renal failure.

Women may experience fertility problems. Pregnancy does not affect the course of scleroderma unless renal involvement is present which worsens the maternal and fetal prognosis. This condition may be fatal in pregnancy. If it has been present for more than 5 years with no kidney or hypertension problems it is less dangerous but still hazardous. All affected women are at risk for hypertension and fetal distress.

Polymyositis (also called Dermatomyositis when rash is present): This is an acute, subacute or chronic inflammatory disease involving muscle and skin, often presenting with a skin rash on the face, eyelids, and over the extensor surfaces of the extremities. Arthritis, skin vasculitis, fibrous growth of tissue in the lungs, intermittent cyanosis followed by redness in the fingers, and heart problems may also occur. This condition rarely occurs among women of childbearing age. When it does, its effects are inconsistent; in pregnancy the condition may improve or get substantially worse. Fetal mortality is high; corticosteroids are the treatment of choice in pregnancy. (Gleicher, 1985, p. 934)

Vasculitic syndromes: These uncommon disorders are associated with inflammation of a variety of blood vessels. **Polyarteritis nodosa** involves medium sized muscular arteries. Swelling and inflammation may lead to vessel blockage resulting in damage to the organs fed by that vessel due to lack of blood flow. Presenting problems include gangrenous skin lesions, kidney disease and hypertension. During pregnancy, this condition can be confused with toxemia. Treatment involves the use of corticosteroids and cyclophosphamide if serious maternal compromise occurs. There is no advantage to therapeutic abortion in these women.

Wegener's granulomatosis is a rare vasculitic disorder with necrosis of the respiratory tract and kidneys and inflammation of small blood vessels. Fever, upper airway inflammation, sinus and ear infections, and abnormal urinalysis are common findings. There is little information about its effects during pregnancy. Treatment is with cyclophosphamide. (Gleicher, 1985, p. 1018-9)

Takayasu's arteritis is a rare disease of young women involving inflammation and stenosis of large and medium sized arteries with frequent involvement of the aortic arch and its branches. Renal artery stenosis and hypertension may also occur. Maternal outcome is usually excellent, but hypertension causes a high degree of intrauterine growth retardation.

Disorders Related to the Nervous System

Friedreich's ataxia: This autosomal recessive nervous system disorder occurs once in every 5,000 persons. It is characterized by degenerative changes in the spinal cord, cerebellum, and brain stem, peripheral nerves and other portions of the nervous system. Onset is often in adolescence. Eight to 10% of those affected also have diabetes; 60% to 90% have electrocardiographic abnormalities. Reproductive abilities are typically good without undue problems. One child in every 200 will be affected when born to women with the disease but no other family history.

Cerebral palsy: This vague term applies to nongenetic brain damage which results in functional and sometimes intellectual impairment. There are two major manifestations. Muscle spasticity and athetosis, or movements which eventually reach their goal but tend to overshoot the mark and deviate from their fixed course. These problems may impair motor skills, walking, bowel and bladder function, sight, speech or intelligence. The condition does not worsen with age. During pregnancy, bladder infections and constipation may be more of a problem in those whose eliminative functions are impaired. Painful muscle spasms may increase and require medication. Yoni birth is possible unless the pelvis is deformed or spasticity of the soft tissues prevents delivery. (Campion, 1991)

Huntington's disease: This is a rare autosomal dominant disorder in which the major gene expression occurs in the central nervous system. Age of onset varies and may occur from birth to age 70 or older, with most onset occurring between 35 and 43 years. Onset is influenced by genetic modifiers, environmental threshold, disturbed tolerance immunity and maternal protection. In most cases, duration is about 17 years. Clinical signs are depression, erratic behavior, progressive involuntary twitching of the facial and limb muscles and dementia. It results from a loss of cells in the brain and related nerve pathways. Genetic testing is complicated; other family members and people who are normal now may be given information that they can anticipate inevitable nerve degeneration and death in later life.

Neurofibromatosis (Von Recklinghausen's disease): This autosomal dominant disorder occurs in approximately one out of every 3,000 births. It is characterized by pigment changes such as cafe au lait spots, axillary freckling, and, usually, peripheral neurofibromas. Although there are numerous related problems, pigment changes are the most common and can be readily identified during physical exam. Women who have no family history and a mild condition may have never been diagnosed before. Brain tumors, including meningiomas, may occur in several members of a family. Pregnancy may aggravate neurofibroma formation and pigment changes. For more information contact the National Neurofibromatosis Foundation, National Office, 120 Wall St., New York, NY 10005.

Multiple sclerosis: MS causes central nervous system demyelination that predominantly affects myelinated nerve tissue. Women are affected twice as often as men and are diagnosed between the ages of 20 and 40 at the rate of 1 per 1000. Their children have a 3% lifetime risk of developing MS as well. The average patient lives 25 to 30 years after diagnosis. MS does not decrease fertility.

MS causes acute flare-ups and remissions, but pregnancy does not increase this tendency. Many studies show 20% to 40% risk of flare-ups postpartum. There are no bio-technical therapies that decrease this risk. Fatigue, weakness, fine motor impairment, bowel and bladder control problems and gait disturbances are the main features of MS and may limit a mother's ability to care for her baby. When MS presents during pregnancy, there is less disability overall than in those who start out pregnancy with MS. The toxins in aspartame (Nutrasweet) can cause symptoms which mimic multiple sclerosis; these reverse when ingestion is discontinued.

Prenatal care is not different for women with MS, but drugs and megavitamins need to be reviewed for possible adverse fetal effects. Those that are problematic need to be gradually discontinued before gestation. MS is associated with increased urinary tract infections, and this risk is even higher when a neurogenic bladder is present. Although some practitioners recommend antibiotic prophylaxis with cephalosporins or ampicillin to protect against urinary tract infections, others prefer to treat infections as they occur. In those with an uninhibited hyperreflexia of the bladder, 15 to 30 mg of Pro-Banthine or 5 mg of Ditropan may be given three times daily. The enlarging uterus may aggravate genitourinary problems or constipation.

Women with spinal cord involvement above T10 are at risk for premature or precipitous delivery. Otherwise, the conduct of labor is normal. If autonomic hyperreflexia causes spastic contractions of the pelvic floor, an epidural may help relieve this problem and allow yoni birth. Women who have received more than 10 to 20 mg of prednisone for more than two weeks prior to birth will need their drug therapy continued during the labor and birth.

There are no contraindications to breastfeeding per se; however, women on drugs such as corticosteroids, immunosuppressives, or diazepam are advised against breastfeeding because of possible adverse effects on the baby.

Myasthenia gravis (MG): This rare disease of neuromuscular transmission is characterized by muscle weakness and fatigability after the repeated use of voluntary muscles. The site of the abnormality is the neuromuscular junction which is associated with a depletion of acetylcholine receptors, probably secondary to an autoimmune response. Unlike most other neurologic problems, MG poses significant mortality risks for both mother and infant.

Fertility is not decreased in this condition and the effect of pregnancy on the disease is unpredictable. In one study almost 41% had aggravations during pregnancy, with a 3.4% maternal death rate, an 8.2% perinatal death rate and a 19.1% incidence of neonatal myasthenia. Maternal deaths are related to a crisis flare-up of the disease or its drug-related treatment.

The prenatal course includes an increase in respiratory infections because of pressure from the enlarging uterus, decreased diaphragmatic movement and hypoventilation. Urinary tract infections are frequent and require prompt diagnosis and treatment. Nausea and vomiting may impair drug absorption and lead to flare-ups. These women need careful urologic supervision.

A great deal of rest is required during pregnancy. Any illness or stress may bring on a crisis and necessitate changes in drug dosages. Families must understand that increasing drug dosages will not increase muscle strength and may precipitate a life threatening drug overdose. In general, however, drug dosages do not change during pregnancy. Many types of drugs are contraindicated in MG. These include many types of antibiotics, antiarrthythmics, local anesthetics such as procaine and xylocaine, some general anesthetics, morphine sulfate, meperidine, propranolol and other ß-blockers, magnesium sulfate and curare, all of which are commonly used in obstetrics. Demerol may be used for pain, and spinal or epidural anesthesia is preferred. The smooth muscle of the uterus is not affected by MG, however voluntary muscles may tire and necessitate a forceps delivery. Surgical delivery is hazardous for MG mothers because of surgical stress, anesthetic agents and postoperative complications related to respiratory complications.

Following birth, severe and sudden aggravation may occur. Drug dosages need careful monitoring and infections require aggressive treatment. Postpartum complications include sudden and devastating respiratory failure.

Breastfeeding is not absolutely contraindicated but anticholinesterase drugs as well as antibodies to acetylcholine are present in the milk.

Neonatal Myasthenia gravis (NMG): Maternal antiacetylcholine receptor antibodies (anti-AChR IgG) cross the placenta by passive transfer. Maternal titers correlate poorly with maternal disease and it is recommended that all MG mothers have titers done in pregnancy, on cord blood, and on their babies. There is, however, some immunologic protection of the baby during gestation. Babies of affected women may be somewhat small-for-dates as well.

Transient MG may appear in 12% of newborns of affected mothers. NMG symptoms noted in the first 12 to 24 hours of life include bulbar paralysis and respiratory failure, lethargy, muscle weakness, weak sucking, feeble cry and absent or weak Moro reflex; these are seen in 10% to 20% of these infants. Anticholinesterase drugs and respiratory support must be administered promptly. The natural resolution of NMG occurs within 10 days to 15 weeks, during which period titers gradually subside. Care should continue 3 to 6 months postpartum.

Seizure Disorders: Most epileptic syndromes are of unknown origin, and begin in childhood or adolescence. These women have a 1 in 30 risk of having children with epilepsy or seizures and genetic counseling may be desired. The most commonly associated fetal malformation is facial cleft; this can occur if either parent is epileptic.

About 50% of all women have no change in seizure activity in pregnancy, 20 to 25% have an increase, and a small number have fewer seizures. Those who have 1 or more seizures monthly are more likely to have seizure activity aggravated during pregnancy than those whose seizures occur less than once every three months. Those carrying male fetuses are twice as likely to have more seizures. Psychological stress, physical fatigue and sleep deprivation may contribute to a lower seizure threshold. The most significant seizures in pregnancy are those which cause generalized convulsions or tonic-clonic episodes because they pose a greater potential risk of fetal hypoxia; petit mal (absence) seizures, pose no particular increased risk during pregnancy.

Very rarely, seizures begin for the first time during pregnancy; even more rarely they are present only during pregnancy. Women having their first seizure during the postpartum period may be treated with drugs for two weeks; Dilantin is often given in such cases. Other causes of postpartum seizures may be eclampsia, arteriovenous malformation, meningioma, or cortical venous thrombosis.

Blood concentrations of anticonvulsant drugs are altered during pregnancy because of changes in how these drugs bind to protein; free (unbound) drug concentrations should be measured for greater accuracy. Seizure medications are all problematic for the fetus; those most commonly prescribed are reviewed below:

DRUG	MINOR ANOMALIES	MAJOR ANOMALIES & COMPLICATIONS	COMMENTS
Dilantin (phenytoinz; diphenylhydantoin)	Craniofacial & digital	Cleft lip & palate: delayed growth & cognitive development; poor vit. K metabolism	Also caused by genetic & environmental factors
Tegretol (carbamazepine)	Similar to above	Similar to above	---
Tridione (trimethadione & paramethadione)	Fetal trimethadione syndrome; craniofacial	Heart defects; delayed growth & psychomotor development; neural tube defects; poor vit. K metabolism	Contraindicated in pregnancy
Depakene or Depakote (Valporate)	Not described	No data	Contraindicated in pregnancy
Mysoline (primidone)	No data	Heart defects; delayed growth & development, retardation when used with other anticoagulants	Limited information
Phenobarbital	Facial & other minor defects	Poor vit. K metabolism	Limited information
Valium (diazepam)	No data	Facial clefts	Limited studies
Zarontin (ethosuximide)	Inadequate data	No data	No information
Clonazepam (clonopin)	Inadequate data	No data	No information

The risk that seizure activity poses to the pregnancy varies with the type of seizures and their cause, the woman's age, any electroencephalogram (EEG) abnormalities, and the length of seizure-free intervals. If possible, drug therapies should be gradually replaced with nutritional and herbal therapies over a 6 to 12 month period before conception to avoid fetal effects. A naturopath should oversee drug reduction and withdrawal. Seizure control should be maintained for at least 6 months prior to conception. When drugs are necessary during pregnancy, a single drug should be used whenever possible. Keep the following points in mind:

1. Plasma volume increases and dilutes serum drug levels
2. Plasma protein binding of some drugs may be reduced, thus changing the amount therapeutically available.
3. The liver may metabolize some drugs more efficiently.
4. In some instances renal clearance may increase.
5. Absorption of drugs from the bowel may be reduced in some cases.
6. Certain drugs which are used in pregnancy may have detrimental interaction with other drugs.
7. Folic acid reduces the level of phenytoin, although folate is needed in pregnancy, doses of 100 to 1000 mcg. are recommended in conjunction with phenytoin therapy.

Women with good seizure control are likely to have a good maternal and fetal outcome. Some doctors recommend termination of labor with surgery in the following situations: when there is a grand mal seizure during labor; in the presence of a neurologic deficit which may limit the mother's ability to cooperate in an emergency; poor seizure control in late pregnancy in spite of treatment; daily psychomotor or weekly grand mal seizures; a previous history of severe seizures during heavy physical or mental stress.

Medications must be continued during labor to prevent seizures that may be prompted if drugs are withdrawn suddenly. Phenytoin, Valium (used for control of an ongoing seizure but not to prevent seizures), and phenobarbital should be available in IV form. Postpartum, oral contraceptives have not been found to exacerbate epilepsy, although they may affect the metabolism of antiepileptic drugs.

Newborn: Babies are at risk for postpartum withdrawal from maternal barbiturate medications and can experience hyperexcitability, occasional seizures, tremulousness and impaired sucking. The use of drugs to ease withdrawal symptoms is not recommended in most cases, but phenobarbital is the best to use (2 to 3 mg/kg/day) if necessary. Vitamin K supplies may be also low in babies whose mothers have been taking barbiturates.

Breastfeeding is not contraindicated in women who have seizure disorders; however, significant amounts of phenobarbital can be transmitted in the milk, and changing medications is recommended.

Drugs interfering with vitamin K metabolism lead to bleeding during the first 24 hours of life in 50% of newborns at risk. Clotting factors should be checked (vitamin K dependent factors and prothrombin time) and 1 mg. of injectable vitamin K or another form of supplementation should be administered after birth. Continued supplementation may needed if clotting factors remain abnormal.

Spinal cord injuries: Trauma is the main cause of spinal cord injuries and partial or complete paralysis the result. Paraplegia is a partial or complete paralysis below the waist. Tetraplegia (quadriplegia) is partial or complete paralysis from the neck down. The level of spinal injury correlates with the amount of mobility a woman retains. Damage in the neck (C1 to C7) affects all four limbs. Injuries from C3 to C5 leave little upper body mobility and injuries from C5 to C7 leave limited hand use. Injuries to T1 through T12 have mobility impairment of the lower limbs and injuries from L1 to L5 affect muscles in the limbs and abdominal muscles. Bowel and bladder function are usually impaired as well. Fertility is not affected.

Be sure to check for anemia, decubital ulcers and infections before and during pregnancy, when pressure sores may be a continuing problem due to weight gain and circulatory changes. Pulmonary and renal function should be evaluated. Chronic urinary tract infections may be a problem and prophylaxis with nitrofurantoin is recommended.

Paraplegic women may require an indwelling urinary catheter from late pregnancy through birth. Deep venous thrombosis is a possible problem when mobility is compromised. Autonomic hyperreflexia is serious with spinal cord damage (called a lesion) above T5-6. Sudden reflex sympathetic discharge of nerve impulses below the level of the lesion causes abrupt systolic and diastolic hypertension, sweating, blotching of the skin, anxiety and often intense headaches. This may be induced by skin or visceral stimuli such as bladder distention with a blocked catheter or bowel distention due to constipation, infections, dilation of the anal sphincter during an exam, cervical dilation during labor and breastfeeding. Examining mother in a semi-sitting position will minimize the risk of stimulating autonomic hyperreflexia. Cerebral hypertension may lead to aphasia (loss of ability to speak or comprehend), hemiplegia (paralysis of one side of the body), convulsions, coma and death. Management includes elevation of the head, evaluation of bowel and bladder status and antihypertensive drugs.

Labor will be felt in women who have sustained damage below T11, T12, or L1. Women with lesions from T5-6 to T10 have painless labor but may be aware of uterine contractions. Lesions of the *cauda equina* cause relaxed perineal muscles. A pudendal block may be used to relax muscles in spasm if needed.

If the injury is at T6 or above, autonomic hyperreflexia is a frequent complication of labor causing the blood pressure to rise during each contraction, accompanied by a painful headache. Because of this possibility some recommend continuous blood pressure monitoring and EKG to evaluate the cardiac rhythm. Hypertensive medication with rapid onset, offset reactive drugs, continuous fetal

1134

monitoring and consultation with an anesthesiologist during the antepartum period may also be advisable. Women who have high cervical spine lesions will need ventilatory support available during labor.

Polyneuropathies: Polyneuropathy is the bilateral, symmetrical and simultaneous dysfunction of nerves due to an underlying disease or damage. The most common types are secondary to metabolic disease such as diabetes or malnutrition and progress slowly over several months or years. Tingling, numbness and burning pain are some of the symptoms seen. In developing countries polyneuropathies may be caused by thiamine deficiency.

In the United States **Guillian-Barre syndrome** may occasionally occur in pregnancy. This is an acute, rapidly progressing form of polyneuropathy characterized by muscular weakness and mild sensory loss in the extremities. It is usually triggered by an infection, surgery or a vaccination. If ventilatory assistance is needed the prognosis is grave; otherwise, milder cases can go to term. Newborns of affected mothers are not themselves affected.

Hearing impairment: Deafness includes all conditions which require a hearing aid. People may be born deaf, become deaf in childhood or adulthood; an ear, nose and throat specialist will know if the condition is genetic, if this is a concern. The most common types of deafness affecting women of childbearing age include hereditary otosclerosis (see chapter on Ear Problems and Hearing Impairment in the section on Problems That Can Occur At Any Time) or less commonly infection of the middle ear, meningitis, tumors, accidents, congenital effects of maternal German measles, or, very rarely, Méniére's disease, which affects fluid levels in the middle ear and may increase the likelihood of falling as pregnancy advances. However, may woman will experience fewer attacks during pregnancy. Other ear conditions are usually not affected. There are no contraindications to pregnancy in hearing impaired women. (Campion, 1991)

Visual impairment: Visual impairment ranges from needing glasses to total blindness. Partial loss of sight takes many forms and may mean difficulty seeing clearly, no central or peripheral vision, only tunnel vision, seeing as through cracked glass or only high color contrasts. Only 10% of the visually impaired are totally blind. Vision may gradually be reduced because of illness and some types respond to surgery. Only a few forms of visual impairment are genetic. Very few eye conditions are affected by pregnancy. If the impairment is secondary to a tumor, high blood pressure which occurs during pregnancy may present a problem. Edema in the hands may make touch less sensitive in latter pregnancy, but this will resolve after birth. Falling may occur more easily as the center of gravity changes with advancing pregnancy. Otherwise, pregnancy and parenting impose the practical problems faced by all visually impaired people. (Campion, 1991)

Reproductive Organ Disease

Endometriosis: Endometriosis is the growth of normal uterine endometrial tissue in areas outside the endometrium. It may extend to adjoining structures such as the uterine tubes and ovaries. Painful periods and deep pain with yoni penetration characterize this condition. Although it has been associated with infertility, most women with endometriosis are fertile. There is no evidence of increased risk for pregnancy-related complications from the disease itself other than ectopic pregnancy; however, surgery may leave the endometrium or other organs scarred. A scarred endometrium may increase the risk of abnormal placental attachment.

Reproductive cancers:

Cervix: Fifteen years ago, cervical cancer was the most common gynecological malignancy, it now ranks third in incidence and second in fatality rate for reproductive cancers. This is primarily due to early detection with PAP smears.

Cure rate are similar with radiation and surgery, the two modalities used by bio-technical practitioners. All studies to date show that the majority of cervical cancers are squamous and that untreated squamous dysplasia can lead to invasive malignancy. Dysplasia ranges from mild to severe to carcinoma *in situ*. The incidence of carcinoma *in situ* is increasing and becoming more prevalent in younger women.

Conization is one means of treating the mildest forms of microinvasive cervical cancer and carcinoma *in situ*. It involves cutting a cone shaped section from the cervical os. There are four important issues which arise for women who have had conization of the cervix as part of their therapy:

1. The risk of recurrent cervical dysplasia. Recurrences may complicate pregnancy, as it is more difficult to evaluate the cervix after previous therapy and during pregnancy. Previous therapy also increases the possibility of invasive malignancy concealed beneath mildly dysplastic cells. Procedures such as repeat conization used to distinguish this problem pose great risks during pregnancy.

2. The risk of iatrogenic postconization infertility. This is hard to quantify since associated venereal disease may also impair fertility, but a relationship may exist. Conization may promote the invasion of undetected organisms. The cervix has four defined functions in fertility: it provides the fertile mucous which allows the sperm to ascend into the uterus and tubes, it serves as the sphincter of the uterus to maintain pregnancy, the endocervical epithelium may serve as a holding place for sperm and provide some transformation process to

enhance fertilization, and it produces mucous which helps isolate the fetus from the flora of the yoni. If conization removes enough endocervical tissue to interfere with these processes, fertility may be impaired, but firm statistics about such risks are not available since conization techniques and the amount of tissue removed varies.

3. The risk of iatrogenic cervical looseness (incompetence) which may occur with conization, or as a result of a congenital cervical weakness such as intrauterine DES exposure. This may be difficult to distinguish from simple premature labor, but if the maternal diet is adequate and no contractions were perceived prior to the loss, looseness can be assumed. Premature birth may be as much as three times more common when a loose cervix exists.

4. Iatrogenic cervical stenosis. Scarring due to conization may compromise the cervical opening, interfering with cervical dilation or labor, making PAP smears difficult and theoretically impairing fertility (if the cervical opening is very tiny). Lines of normal cervical stress may be altered and can lead to severe tearing of the upper yoni or cervix. This can result in poor healing and subsequent cervical looseness. When the cervix is rigid from scarring, a careful exam of the upper vault of the yoni and cervix should be done postpartum to rule out lacerations.

Recurrent cervical dysplasia in pregnancy: There is no evidence that pregnancy increases the frequency of recurrent dysplasia. Those that have undergone therapy should delay pregnancy for at least 3 months (preferably 6) to allow for healing. PAP smears should be done every 3 months for the first 2 years after therapy.

The recurrence rate is influenced by the original therapy used. All therapies leave some tissue in which viruses are still present, which may lead to recurrent dysplasia. Conization, which removes the most tissue, has the lowest recurrence rate but has significant associated obstetric complications (see above). Cryocautery and carbon dioxide laser surgery have somewhat higher recurrence rates (still less than 12%) but have as few known obstetric consequences.

Dysplasia detected in pregnancy is managed as in the nonpregnant woman, but conization is avoided whenever possible and endocervical curettage is not performed. If biopsy finds no cancer cells, treatment should not be undertaken in pregnancy. Shallow conization, if used at all, should be undertaken as a diagnostic maneuver to discover invasive cells rather than as therapy. Cytotoxic agents and retinoic acid are both contraindicated in pregnancy.

Ovarian cancer: Most women who have ovarian cancer have no significant family history. Primary treatment is with surgery and usually includes hysterectomy. Scar tissue adhesions may be a problem in those who retain their uteri, which can sometimes be corrected. With no undue postsurgical complications, some women can conceive.

Radiotherapy for ovarian tumors will often leave a woman infertile. Women who have received chemotherapy may be told that there appears to be no lasting genetic damage to future fetuses, but there has not been sufficient time to draw conclusions about remote effects. Most studies describing the effect of chemotherapy on pregnant women have been derived from populations of women with unrecognized pregnancy at the onset of therapy. The embryo is relatively protected from the maternal circulation and therefore chemotherapy is felt to have little effect at that time. After implantation, chemotherapy may cause miscarriage during the first eight weeks.

The risk of reactivation of the cancer during pregnancy depends upon how thoroughly the situation was investigated. A second laparoscopy is sometimes performed after treatment. However, even though there are no known ovarian tumors which are specifically activated by the hormones of pregnancy, most such tumors are rich in sex steroid receptors and the possibility of reactivation is real.

Following women for tumor recurrence is hindered in pregnancy due to physical and hormonal changes. Teratogenic reports on various drugs are few with the exception of methotrexate therapy, which is strictly contraindicated in pregnancy. The newer the drug, the less information concerning its side effects is available, and all cancer drugs should be used cautiously.

Women who have had previous chemotherapy should know that some drugs (notably doxorubicin drugs such as Adriamycin and daunorubicin drugs such as Cerubidine) can cause cardiac problems in the recipient. A cardiac exam should take place prior to pregnancy or as early in pregnancy as possible. Cisplatin causes renal damage and renal function tests should be performed if it has been used. Bleomycin causes permanent lung damage. Alkylating agents may cause myelodysplasia and impaired bone marrow reserve. A CBC with platelets should be recommended during preconception counseling. Treatment with drugs such as vincristine or vinblastine may lead to significant neurologic impairment, including autonomic dysfunction with severe postural hypotension or constipation.

Cancer of the vulva: The expected incidence of vulval cancer during pregnancy is 1 in every 8000 pregnancies. Treatment is by vulvectomy, surgical removal of the affected tissues. There are no adverse fetal effects. A yoni delivery is possible in a woman who has undergone surgery. (Gleicher, 1985, p. 1104)

Cancer of the yoni: The most common symptom is abnormal bleeding from the yoni. DES daughters are most at risk. Surgical removal of the cancerous areas may necessitate surgical birth. (Gleicher, 1985, p. 1105)

Breast cancer: If breast cancer appears during pregnancy, diagnosis may be obscured by the normal breast changes which occur at that time. It does not seem that previously treated breast cancer is restimulated by the hormones of pregnancy.

Each case must be examined individually to determine the recurrence rate of the specific type of cancer involved. Some researchers have reported that pregnancy after treatment seems to increase survival rates, although intact fertility after chemotherapy may cause the favorable prognosis. The following recommendations have been suggested for women wishing to conceive:

1. Women with a history of disease at stage II or worse or patients with any metastases should probably not conceive.
2. Delay conception for 1 year after all treatment is discontinued.
3. It may be somewhat safer for those with estrogen-receptor positive tumors than receptor negative tumors to become pregnant.

Respiratory Disorders

Asthma: The most common pulmonary problem of young women is asthma, with symptoms of airway resistance such as painful breathing, wheezing and cough. Symptoms may vary and can be related to different sections of the airway. Emotional issues play a large role in the overall etiology of asthma and some therapists may be skilled at working with these issues. Acupuncture and homeopathic remedies can also be helpful. Stress reduction is an important consideration, as well as assessing possible allergies, environmental, climate and geographic factors which may be impacting the severity of symptoms. If Asthma is atopic (due to allergies) the child has a 1 in 10 chance of inheriting some allergic condition; if both parents are affected, the chance is 1 in 3. For non-atopic asthma, the risk for children is less clear (Campion, 1991)

About .4% to 1.3% of all pregnant women are asthmatic. Most have no change in symptoms, some have a remission and a few get worse. Women with severe symptoms before conception do less well when breathing is further compromised by the enlarging uterus. Those with attacks only at night or with exercise may actually have a cardiac condition, but they will usually have other signs of heart disease as well.

The most common form of asthma is an inherited immunologic disorder. A family history is typical. Inhaled antigens evoke a circulating antibody response. Upon re-exposure to the antigen by inhalation, an antigen-antibody complex forms and combines with receptors on the surface of lung cells. Women should avoid known triggers (i.e. things they are allergic to) during pregnancy.

Bronchospasm associated with systemic vasculitis, acute bronchitis, exercise, aspirin, or exposure to occupational agents may bring on an asthma attack. Such common agents as animal dander, fumes from plastics, formaldehyde, grains, isocyanates, metals, proteolytic enzymes in detergents, textiles, tobacco, fuel combustion exhausts, and western red cedar wood may precipitate an attack.

Medications should be reviewed before conception. The drugs for asthma cross the placenta but none have been associated with fetal defects, with the possible exception of steroids (the link to cleft lip is being questioned). If steroids are absolutely necessary, aerosol agents are better than oral drugs since there is less systemic absorption. However, fetal oxygenation is vital to the health of the baby and when this is jeopardized, the benefit of the drug outweighs the risk. Severe asthma is a life threatening problem for mother and fetus and needs to be taken seriously.

A *beta*-sympathomimetic inhaler is the first drug to try. The *beta*-2 agonist Terbutaline is relatively specific, and is considered the safest for pregnancy. Albuterol, a ß-1 and ß-2 agonist is in pregnancy category C; it may cause cardiac side effects such as rapid heart rate and irregularities of heart's rhythm, as well as tremors and anxiety, although such symptoms are more likely to develop with IV therapy than when inhaled. These drugs may cause elevated blood glucose levels in diabetics. Salbutamol has been widely used in pregnancy. Ephedrine also seems to be relatively safe, but epinephrine, sold over-the-counter as Primatine mist, is not recommended in pregnancy. Cromlyn may be used as an inhaler to prevent an attack, but is for prophylaxis only. Theophylline has been widely used but may cause nausea and tachyarrythmias in some, especially when given IV. Laboratory tests to determine a count of total blood eosinophils (TEC) may be useful in monitoring the effectiveness of therapy. In adequately treated asthmatics, the TEC is less that 500 mm^3.

No long term harm to the fetus or breastfeeding newborn has been noted with the drugs recommended above, although occasional side effects include jitteriness, tachycardia and arching of the back due to spasm.

Steroids should be used only if all other forms of therapy prove useless. Inhalers with beclomethasone may reduce or eliminate the need for oral prednisone, reducing the total amount of drug absorbed by the system. Side effects from long term use include an increase in monilial (yeast) infections of the upper respiratory and gastrointestinal tracts as well as osteoporosis. If a woman changes from oral to inhaler therapy, the oral medication should be slowly tapered off by gradually reducing the dosage by 1 mg or less daily if the dose has been less than 10 mg daily of prednisone. Maternal adrenal activity and secretion of urinary estriol will be suppressed if more than 30 mg. of prednisone are taken daily. The baby's pituitary adrenal axis does not seem to be impaired.

Asthma during labor: Asthma attacks in labor are unusual. A *beta*-sympathomimetic inhaler should be used if breathing becomes difficult. If steroids are needed to control asthma in labor, use hydrocortisone 100 mg. IM at 6 hour intervals to prevent hypothalami-pituitary adrenal axis suppression. The regular use of asthma drugs during pregnancy can inhibit normal uterine activity and may lead to start and stop contraction patterns during labor. Epidural anesthesia is preferred over general to minimize the risk of respiratory infection. Fetal and maternal mortality may be increased in very severe cases, but in general the outlook is good.

Cystic Fibrosis (CF): This is the most common lethal autosomal recessive genetic disorder. It occurs in 1 in every 2000 Caucasians, 1 in every 17,000 African Americans and rarely in Native Americans or Oriental peoples.

CF has multisystem involvement in which mucus secretions behave in an abnormal way. It results in obstructive lung disease, hepatic cirrhosis, intestinal obstruction, pancreatic exocrine insufficiency and secondary diabetes. Survival rates are better than ever due to prophylactic bronchial care, pancreatic enzymes and vitamins supplementation. A high protein, low fat diet is recommended.

Most affected girls live well into the reproductive years. In severe cases where chronic illness is characterized by repeated lung infections, obstructive lung diseases, intestinal malabsorption and poor nutrition, menstruation is often delayed to the age of 15 or later.

Preconception counseling should include advice regarding bringing the lungs to optimal functioning with postural drainage several times daily. All infections should be treated promptly. Good nutrition and normal weight prior to conception will help a woman carry the pregnancy. Medications should be reviewed and those containing iodine avoided due to undesirable fetal effects.

During pregnancy no additional measures are needed to treat CF. There is an increased risk for secondary diabetes in those with CF. CF screening is recommended for the baby. Breastfeeding is not contraindicated but it is wise to check sodium levels in the milk as CF causes excessive loss of sodium in sweat.

Keep CF in mind when checking the newborn from a family with a history of unusual pulmonary or gastrointestinal symptoms.

α_1-Antitrypsin Globulin Deficiency: This rare homozygotic syndrome should be suspected with a family history of obstructive emphysema, early onset of emphysematous chronic obstructive pulmonary disease, or bilateral radiographic evidence of basilar pulmonary emphysematous changes. It should also be considered in those with cirrhosis of the liver, moderate enlargement of the liver and mild abnormality of liver function.

The diagnosis is likely when α_1-globulin is absent on protein electrophoresis and is confirmed by measurement of low levels of serum α-antitrypsin. The normal serum concentration of α_1-antitrypsin is 212 ± 21 mg/dl. Deficiency results in chronic lung disease. Young women with the above problems should be screened for this disorder; if found, genetic counseling is recommended.

Women with active α_1-Antitrypsin Globulin Deficiency have similar problems as those with active chronic hepatitis, but little hard data is available at this time. This condition may not affect the successful outcome of pregnancy.

Bronchiectasis: Bronchiectasis is a dilation of a bronchial tube which secretes large amounts of pus. This condition may be congenital or acquired via infection. It may produce extreme weakness and necessitate postural drainage and physiotherapy. Other than the obvious respiratory impairment this represents, no specific information is available on its effect during pregnancy.

Extrinsic Restrictive Lung Disorders: These include pleural disease, kyphoscoliosis, pectus excavatum and ankylosing spondylitis. They can make pregnancy more difficult, although an occasional pregnant woman has such uncommon conditions in a form severe enough to cause pulmonary or cardiac insufficiency, the primary concerns during gestation.

Pulmonary Embolic Disease (PED): The risk of PED is increased for women who have previously experienced deep vein thrombosis and emboli outside of pregnancy, although the exact recurrence rate is unknown. There are varying opinions about what interventions are necessary. If testing is called for, a bilateral ascending venography may be performed. If this examination is normal, a baseline impedance plethysmography is indicated and no anticoagulants are prescribed. If the venogram shows extensive previous thrombosis, some recommend treating the woman prophylactically throughout gestation. If medication is deemed appropriate, subcutaneous heparin may be used prophylactically during pregnancy and continued for 6 weeks or more postpartum. However, most emboli occur within the month postpartum, and are most likely to appear during the first 3 days after birth.

Sarcoidosis: This is a worldwide systemic granulomatous disorder of unknown etiology which affects all ethnic groups. It usually involves the thoracic lymph nodes and, more rarely, the lungs. More than half of the patients have minimal pulmonary disease which does not appreciably affect pulmonary function (stage 1). Most feel sarcoidosis improves with pregnancy, but may worsen again postpartum.

Those with Stage 2 and 3 disease have more restrictive disease with lung tissue stiffness that occurs with or without obstructive features, for which steroids may be prescribed. Diagnosed women should have an extensive lung evaluation before conception to exclude every treatable cause. Corticosteroid or more recently methotrexate treatment may be indicated for women with the following conditions:

1) Extrathoracic, cerebral, and serious hepatic and renal involvement
2) Hypercalcemia
3) Persistent systemic symptoms including fever and any serious or functional organ involvement that is not spontaneously regressing
4) Eye and nervous system involvement

Sarcoidosis is predictably stable during pregnancy and sometimes symptoms improve or disappear entirely. Inactive or resolving disease usually requires no treatment. Active disease may improve during pregnancy but then worsen again 3 to 6 months postpartum in about one half of all affected women. Pregnancy is contraindicated for women who have the following risk factors:

*Vital lung capacity <1 liter (absolute limit is 700 ml.)
*Pulmonary hypertension (cor pulmonale is an absolute contra-indication)
*Painful breathing when at rest
*Symptoms requiring high dose of steroids (>15 mg. prednisone daily)

No special management is necessary for the average case in pregnancy. It is not transmitted to the fetus. Affected women may be very sensitive to Vitamin D and should take no extra supplements. (Gleicher, 1985, p. 977)

Skeletal and Joint Disorders

Amputation or missing limbs: There are no medical problems during pregnancy for women missing a limb. Those wearing a prothesis may experience poor fit due to weight gain and rashes around the cuff may be a problem. Center of balance problems may worsen as pregnancy advances.

Ankylosing Spondylitis: Ankylosing spondylitis is also known as **Marie-Strümpell Disease**. It is a chronic, progressive form of arthritis distinguished by the inflammation and eventual ankylosis of a number of joints, primarily involving the spine and adjacent structures. (Ankylosis refers to abnormal immobility and fixation of a joint due to pathological changes in the joint or the surrounding tissue.) It is much more common in young men than women, but recent data suggests this disease exists in a mild form that affects both sexes equally. It begins between ages 20 and 30 as insidious low back pain with marked morning back stiffness which improves with moderate physical activity during the day. It slowly moves upward to encompass the entire spine, leading to fusion of the sacroiliac joints and lumbar spine with obliteration of the normal lumbar lordosis (curve). As it progresses, the dorsal and cervical vertebrae bow forward, causing a stooped position. The inflammation involves areas of tendon insertion around the vertebrae and the joints. Calcification leads to bony ankylosis.

The course of the disease seem largely unaffected by pregnancy although patients have more back pain during the second and third trimesters. No fetal problems arise and mechanical complications of birth are few. Children of affected mothers have a 1 in 10 chance of having the condition.

Bone cancer: Bone cancer that develops during pregnancy is rare. Treatment is with surgery, and sometimes chemotherapy and radiation. Delay in the treatment of aggressive benign and slow-growing lesions increases maternal morbidity. Delay in treating high-grade malignancy increases maternal morbidity and mortality. Fetal risks depend upon the type of treatments as well as the gestational age. No information is available regarding pregnancy risk for women who have previously been diagnosed and treated for bone cancer. (Gleicher, 1985, pp. 1092-5)

Dwarfism: Disorders of bone and cartilage that are associated with short stature are referred to a skeletal dyscrasias or chondrodystrophies, achondroplasia is the most common. Diabetes, spinal compression and cardiorespiratory problems may complicate the picture. All of these conditions may be associated with pelvic deformities so severe that normal birth is impossible. Evaluation must be made on an individual basis. (Gleicher, 1985, p. 1031)

Fibrous dysplasia: In this disorder normal bone structure is replaced with fibroosseous connective tissue. In most cases only one bone is affected.

Deformities tend to occur on one side of the body only, with skin lesion appearing on the affected side. Pregnancy appears to stimulate activity in dysplastic tissues. (Gleicher, 1985 p. 1030)

Kyphoscoliosis: This disorder of the spine causes it to curve to the side with an accompanying anteroposterior hump. During pregnancy, perinatal mortality may be increased, possibly due to maternal hypoxia. There may be associated abnormalities of the bony pelvis which require surgical delivery.

Hyperostosis: Hyperostosis refers to an overgrowth of bone. Osteopetrosis and osteopoikilosis may complicate pregnancy and labor because of pelvic deformities or systemic complications. (Gleicher, 1985, p. 1030)

Bone disease: Failure of bone mineralization may be due to malnutrition (such as vitamin D deficiency) or malabsorption, liver disease, drugs (especially anticonvulsants which disturb vitamin D absorption), or renal insufficiency. Problems related to Vitamin D deficiency are particularly prevalent among Asian, Indian, and Pakistani women. **Rickets** during childhood may stunt bone growth and lead to a small pelvis, particularly in the anteroposterior diameter. Laboratory tests for serum 25-OHD concentration can help determine if a deficiency currently exists. If deficiency is discovered, begin with a bolus dose of 5000 IU daily until body stores are restored; a subsequent dose of 100 to 400 IU daily is sufficient. Asymptomatic or mild vitamin D deficiency can cause serious problems in the fetus, presumably due to subnormal levels of fetal calcium. (Gleicher, 1985, p. 1025)

Osteoporosis: This disorder occurs when the bones undergo gradual demineralization, leaving them fragile and easily damaged; it is very rare in women of childbearing age. **Necrosis of the femoral head** may occur with sudden onset of severe pain in the hip.

Some inherited metabolic disorders such as **Marfan's syndrome** and **osteogenesis imperfecta** cause poor mineralization of the bones.

Osteogenesis imperfecta: Also called **Lobstein disease**, manifestations of this genetic disorder range from mild bone fragility to severe fragility with multiple fractures and early death. Blue sclera are common in the more severe forms. The incidence of fractures does not increase during pregnancy but old breaks which resulted in deformities may result in cephalopelvic disproportion. Abnormal platelet function, dental problems and hypermetabolism are also concerning complicating factors. Ultrasound may be used to diagnosis some forms in the fetus. Pregnancy is not encouraged in women who have severe forms of this condition. (Gleicher, 1985)

Osteomalacia: This is the adult form of low-calcium rickets with absence of bone growth. The principal causes are Vitamin D deficiency, malabsorption or poor metabolism. It is more common in cultures where women are veiled or work in dark environments. In modern times it may be found in women from Pakistan, Northern India, Iran and Bedouin tribes. Bone deformities with easy fractures gradually develop with complaints of backache, muscular weakness and numb, prickly feelings in the arms and legs. Pregnancy and labor are not affected unless pelvic deformities have developed. Calcium lactate in a dose of 5 grams daily and Vitamin D in doses of 10,000 UI daily should be sufficient to treat mild to moderate conditions. In severe conditions, give 30,000 IU of Vitamin D daily; IV calcium may need to be given as well. (Gleicher, 1985, p. 1028-9)

Pseudoxanthoma elasticum: This disorder is characterized by degeneration of elastic tissue of the skin, eye and cardiovascular system. Skin changes usually begin after the age of 20 with areas becoming lax, overlapped and relatively inelastic with yellowish raised areas. Similar changes may occur in the mouth, rectum and yoni mucosae. Eye changes noted on ophthalmic exam include reddish-brown marks radiating from the optic disk. Heart problems include insufficiency, hypertension, premature calcification of the vessels, weakness or absence of pulse in the extremities. Nosebleeds, upper gastrointestinal tract hemorrhage and severe uterine bleeding may also occur. Out of 25 pregnancies in 8 affected women, severe episodes of gastrointestinal bleeding and heart problems have been noted. None had problems during labor or birth. (Gleicher, 1985, p. 310)

Rheumatoid arthritis: This chronic inflammatory disease involves joints symmetrically; it waxes and wanes in severity. About 20% of those affected have a complete remission, which usually occurs during the first year of illness. Three to four times more women are affected than men and onset is typically during the childbearing years. Fertility is normal and the risk that a child will contract the disease is unpredictable but very small. It is diagnosed by the presence of multiple chronically inflamed joints. Once a diagnosis is firmly established, most patients have IgM autoantibody to y-globulin (the rheumatoid factor) in their serum. Since this antibody rarely appears in other conditions, active arthritis with consistently negative tests for this antibody should cause a search for other conditions such as syphilis, lupus, psoraistic arthritis, or ankylosing spondylitis or a variant thereof.

Remission of rheumatoid arthritis frequently occurs during pregnancy and 74% experience this in the first trimester. Unfortunately the disease reappears in a more severe form postpartum, with peak reoccurrences 4 to 6 weeks after birth. A pregnancy protein termed PZP (pregnancy zone protein) or α_2.PAG (pregnancy-associated glycoprotein) achieves higher levels during pregnancy in those subjects who have remissions than in the 26% who do not. How these proteins relate to rheumatoid arthritis is not understood.

Juvenile rheumatoid arthritis (JRA) or Still's disease: This variant is similar to rheumatoid arthritis but appears in childhood and often causes severe polyarthritis. Total remission in adolescence is the rule. Rarely pregnancy may exacerbate the disease or onset may occur during pregnancy.

Aspirin is considered one of the best drugs to treat this disorder aspirin is considered one of the best but should be stopped prior to delivery, with a substitution of steroids such as prednisone, if necessary. Other, newer drugs have no established record regarding relative safety in pregnancy and should be carefully investigated regarding their possible effect on the fetus.

Arthritic syndromes and birth: The enlarging uterus may cause breathlessness, especially in those with spinal arthritis. Women should pace their days, allowing planning their activities to allow for rest. A physiotherapist can help women plan a program of exercise that addresses her specific physical condition. Those with chronic arthritis tend to have low hemoglobins, so watch for anemia in pregnancy. If separating the legs is difficult, exams should be done with the woman lying on her side. Birth poses no special problem unless the hips are deformed or the legs cannot be separated to allow for birth; the joints may cause mechanical problems making it difficult for the woman to assume certain positions. Those who have had a hip replacement will probably require a surgical birth. Jaw, neck, and other joint disease might complicate the administration of general anesthesia. Coping with pain, reduced mobility and function, tiredness and uncertainty regarding the course of the illness all produce anxiety and stress for those with arthritis. Drug types and doses should be assessed for breastfeeding safety. Breastfeeding will require creative positioning to minimize maternal discomfort. (Campion, 1991)

Scoliosis: Scoliosis is a curvature of the spine sideways in either an S or a C shape due to a weakness in the spinal column which buckles due to unstable rotational forces during the growth period, which stops at about age 25. It tends to be more severe in girls because they grow more rapidly. Surgery can be used to correct the curvature in some cases. A small minority of women who have severe scoliosis may have some breathing difficulty, but otherwise pregnancy poses no problems.

Spina bifida: This occurs when two or more vertebra fail to form properly, leaving a gap; this can be as minor as a small section of missing bone causing no impairment whatsoever to an opening through which spinal nerves are protruding which may lead to paralysis below the defect. With better surgical techniques, many women with spina bifida now reach childbearing age. Severe incontinence and/or poor kidney function may be good reasons to avoid pregnancy, as these pose a threat to maternal health, otherwise pregnancy is not contraindicated. Muscle spasms, pressure sores and kidney infections may occur more frequently during pregnancy. Pelvic deformities are the only reason a surgical birth might be necessary.

Skin Disorders

Dermatitis Herpetiformis: This subepidermal blistering dermatosis usually occurs during the late teens or early twenties. It appears on the extensor surfaces as groups of vesicles that are very pruritic. Direct immunofluorescence of normal skin demonstrating IgA deposition in the dermoepidermal area is diagnostic. In nonpregnant women the lesions respond to sulfapyridine and sulfones or prolonged use of a gluten-free diet. The use of sulfa drugs near term may cause kernicterus in the baby, so treatment with drugs is best delayed until breastfeeding is finished.

Psoriasis: Psoriasis produces well demarcated raised red plaques which may appear anywhere on the body. Areas of rubbing or trauma such as the scalp, knees, elbows, genitalia, and buttocks are most often affected. The cause is not known. Psoriasis improves in pregnancy in 50% of cases. Treatment during pregnancy should be limited to ultraviolet B light or topical agents. (Gleicher, 1985, p. 1148)

Atopic dermatitis: This is an intensely itchy skin disorder often found in conjunction with other allergies. The skin is dry, often scaly and often thickened and hardened. The folds of skin such as the back of the knees are often affected. It may remit during pregnancy. (Gleicher, 1985, p. 1148)

Erythema nosodum: These lesions appear as a rash consisting of tender red or purple nodules over the shins. They may complicate sarcoidosis and tuberculosis as well as other infections, drug therapy and inflammatory bowel disease. New lesions appear as others are resolving and each lasts a few days to a few weeks. The entire cycle may last several months, accompanied by fever and joint pain. If no other complicating factors are present, an isolated presentation of this condition does not adversely affect pregnancy. Symptoms may worsen with pregnancy and steroids are commonly used to control them. (Gleicher, 1985, p. 1149)

Ichthyoses: These disorders of cornification are characterized by scaling skin. They may be mild and relatively common in the form of autosomal dominant ichthyosis vulgaris, or severe, such as autosomal recessive lamellar ichthyosis. Some forms are lethal. Mild ichthyosis does not seem to impact pregnancy.

Sterol sulfatase deficiency is the biochemical defect in X-linked recessive ichthyosis. This disorder affects one in every 60,000 males. Placental sterol sulfatase deficiency was found in all the placentas of male offspring who developed ichthyosis. This placental abnormality has been recognized to be associated with low to absent maternal serum and urine estriols and often results in post-term pregnancies that fail to go into labor spontaneously. For more information contact: Ichthyosis First, Box 410453, San Francisco, CA 94141.

Pemphigus Erythematosus: This is a variant of pemphigus vulgaris which is frequently associated with other immunologic disease such as thymoma, myasthenia gravis, systemic lupus erythematosus and rheumatoid arthritis.

Pemphigus Vulgaris: This intraepidermal autoimmune blistering disease is clinically similar to herpes gestationes. It is associated with 14% fetal mortality rate; there is evidence of placental transmission. However, this death rate was associated with maternal and fetal immunodeficiency from high doses of corticosteroids and azathioprine along with overwhelming cytomegalovirus pulmonary infection. Live-born infants of affected mothers may have transient lesions lasting 1 to 2 weeks.

Porphyria: Porphyria cutanea tarda (PCT) and varigate porphyria (VP) often flare during pregnancy. They tend to flare in women taking oral contraceptives, so the hormonal influence of pregnancy acts in the similar fashion. This disease produces skin blisters. Treatment includes avoiding sunlight, phlebotomy and occasionally antimalarial drugs (which should be avoided during pregnancy).

Erythema multiforme: This disorder is a reaction to a vast number of antigens such as drugs, bacteria, parasites, etc. Itchy, red, lesions can occur anywhere on the baby, but are most often found on the palms and soles of the feet. Attacks can be more frequent in pregnancy. Drug therapy includes antihistamines and steroids.

Acrodermatitis enteropathica: This inherited defect of zinc absorption leads to diarrhea and dermatitis of the perineum, around the mouth and in inguinal areas. Treatment is with increased oral zinc supplementation. (Gleicher, 1985, p. 1149)

Fox-Fordyce disease and hidradenitis suppurativa: These inflammatory conditions of the apocrine glands both improve during pregnancy; however postpartum rebound can be severe. (Gleicher, 1985, p. 1146)

Rare Collagen Diseases:

Periarteritis nosoda (PAN): There are a few reports of women having this condition during pregnancy and the fulminant vasculitis (inflammation of blood vessels) seems uninfluenced; however few women survive gestation.

Polymyositis: This disorder of unknown origin is characterized by an inflammation of many muscles simultaneously, producing muscular weakness. The problem develops slowly and may appear at any age. Since this condition is rare and severe with a high mortality rate, information on its course in pregnancy scarce.

Skin cancers:

Basal cell carcinoma: These slow-growing tumors appear in light-exposed areas. They may present as a translucent papule with or without pigment, ulceration, or a raised border with a few overlying vessels, or a scaling papule or patch. Removal by a skilled surgeon is simple and cure rates are good, even during pregnancy. Other skin cancers, with the exception of melanoma, are found most often in older individuals. (Gleicher, 1985, p. 1069)

Melanoma: Skin cancer may appear during pregnancy. If it is confined to the epidermal layer, the survival rate for pregnant women who receive surgery is the same as for the nonpregnant. If cancer has penetrated further into the skin layers, the prognosis is worse for pregnant women. (Gleicher, 1985, p. 1149)

1150

White Blood Cell Disorders

Neutropenia: Noncancerous white cell disorders include neutropenia and agranulocytosis secondary to drugs or other environmental exposure. Neutropenia (low neutrophils) is also seen in a variety of systemic disorders. Agranulocytosis (lack of granulocyte production) is usually an acute event, generally drug induced. It is an ominous development and unless its cause is recognized and eliminated it can lead to overwhelming infection. Pregnancy outcomes depend on identification and treatment of the underlying cause; this is preferably done before conception.

Acute leukemia: This is a malignant disorder of blood cells characterized by accumulation of primitive cells that are not completely mature in the bone marrow and peripheral blood. There are six subtypes of this disease. Symptoms include bone and joint pain, palpitations, painful breathing, fever, and bleeding from mucus membranes or the gastrointestinal tract. White blood counts may rise to 100,000 blasts/mm combined with low platelets and anemia. Transfusions with blood products and antibiotics are used to maintain the blood during pregnancy; chemotherapeutic agents commonly used produce a variety of fetal problems such as prematurity, decreased blood counts, and certain defects. Childhood leukemia has the highest recovery rate. Girls with acute lymphoblastic leukemia (ALL) that were treated with chemotherapy and radiation usually develop normally and have healthy pregnancies with normal babies. Pregnancy does not appear to adversely affect the remission duration in leukemia or the effectiveness of therapy. The recurrence rate for acute leukemia appearing after age 10 is relatively high compared to leukemia treated in early childhood, with accompanying anemia, thrombocytopenic bleeding, infection and poor pregnancy outcome. (Gleicher, 1985, p. 1150-3)

Acute nonlymphoblastic leukemia (ANLL): This type of leukemia is more common in adults. Remission with drugs can be achieved, but is usually short. Some recommend bone marrow transplant after one remission. Although normal infants have been born even with chemotherapeutic drugs being used during pregnancy, the outlook for the mother is grim due to the disease process itself.

Chronic leukemia: Chronic lymphocytic leukemia (CLL) and chronic myelogenous leukemia (CML), also called chronic granulocytic leukemia (CGL), is rare in women of childbearing age. In men it can be aggressive and rapidly progressive. Little information is available regarding pregnancy, but conception is probably best avoided.

CML occurs most often in younger women. Although successful pregnancies have been reported, they are rare because treatment often causes ovarian failure. Some drugs (especially hydroxyurea) are also mutagenic and should be avoided in women contemplating pregnancy. Pregnancy should also be avoided if the prospective biological father is being treated with any such drugs. Pregnancy in early untreated cases may do well, since thrombocytopenia and complications due to infections are unusual and mild. Transfusion for anemia may be the only support needed. Spleen enlargement may cause pain in 75% of cases. Radiation to reduce this has not had obvious fetal effects. Survival after diagnosis averages 3.5 years. Pregnancy does not unfavorably influence the disease. Infants of untreated mothers seem to be normal.

Hodgkin's disease: This cancer is considered universally fatal without treatment. It presents with painless enlargement of a superficial lymph node of the neck, underarm or inguinal areas. Better outcomes occur with irradiation, chemotherapy or a combination of these two modalities. A number of successful pregnancies with normal deliveries have been reported in women who have been previously treated. Sterility in treated men has been reported and they may wish to store sperm before treatment. If a woman has uncontrolled disease or is still in therapy, pregnancy is a poor choice, as drugs are teratogenic. For women in remission or who are considered cured there is no evidence of relapse during pregnancy. (Gleicher, 1985 p. 1061)

Non-hodgkin's lymphoma: Tumors of the lymph nodes and lymphoid tissue are very rare among women in their childbearing years. However, when they occur, they tend to be poorly responsive to treatment, with a high relapse rate. Pregnancy is best avoided.

1152

References and further reading

(Material in this section is synopsized from de Swiet unless otherwise noted in the text)

Campion, Mukti Jain, The Baby Challenge, Tavistock/Routledge, New York, 1991.

de Swiet, Michael, Medical Disorders in Obstetric Practice, Blackwell Scientific Pub., Oxford, Eng., 1984.

Gabbe, Steven, et.al., ed., Obstetrics: Normal and Problem Pregnancies, 2nd ed., Churchill Livingstone, New York, 1991.

Gleicher, Norbert, Principles of Medical Therapy in Pregnancy, Plenum Medical Book Co., New York, NY, 1985.

Kolder, Veronika, OB, editing comments, May, 1995.

Pritchard, Jack, et.al., William's Obstetrics, 17th ed., Appleton-Century-Crofts, New York, 1985.

Stein's Infectious Disease, 4th ed., 1994.

Talbott, J., Gout, Grune & Stratton, New York NY, 1967, pp. 146-148

Washam, V., The One-Hander's Book: A Basic Guide to Daily Living, John Day Co., NY, 1973.

APPENDIX

Obtaining Products and Publications Mentioned in This Text

Arista Surgical Supply, 67 lexington Ave., New York, NY 10010-1898 (212) 679-3694/(800) 223-1984

Astroglide is manufactured by Biofilm, Inc., 3121 Scott St., Vista, CA 92083.

Around the Moon distributes The Lens, a 100 power magnifying lens used for checking salvia and amniotic fluid for ferning. P.O. Box 3325, Applegate, OR, 97530 800-797-FERN

Bectin & Dickenson (B & D) produce disposable syringes lubricated only with a tiny bit of silicone.

Books for Midwives Press, Downs Court, 29, The Downs, Altrincham, Cheshire, England, WA14 2QD, 061-929-0190, catalgogue of British textbooks, some of which are not published in North America.

Breast shells and pumps may be ordered from the following suppliers:
Ameda/Egnell, 765 Industrial Dr. Cary, IL 60013
Graham-Field, Inc., 400 Rabro Dr. East, Hauppauge, NY 11788
Medela, Inc., 4610 Prime Parkway, P.O. Box 660, McHenry, IL 60051
Netsy Co., 34 Sunrise Ave., Mill Valley, CA 94941 (shells only)
Pharmic, 1878 S. Redwood Rd., Salt Lake City, UT, 84104 (shells only)

Cascade HealthCare Products (equipment), **Birth and Life Bookstore** (<u>Imprints</u> catalogue of textbooks and books for parents) and **Moonflower Birthing Supply** (herbs, remedies and vitamins) 141 Commercial St. NE, Salem, OR 97301, (503) 371-4445/orders (800) 443-9942. Source of textbooks, equipment, herbs, homeopathic remedies and many *in vitro* lab kits.

Childbirth Graphics, P.O. Box 21207, Waco, TX 76702-1207, (800) 299-3366. A wide variety of teaching aides and related supplies for teaching about birth for educators of midwives as well as parents.

ICEA, P.O. Box 20048, Minneapolis, MN, 55420, (800) 624-4934, publishes <u>Bookmarks</u>, a catalogue of books on all aspects of childbirth.

Energique Inc., P.O. Box 121, Woodbine, IA, 51579/consult (712) 647-2890/order (800) 869-8078. A wide variety of unusual herbs, homeopathic combination remedies and ointments, Bach Flower remedies (Rescue Remedy and others) and nutritional supplements. Happy to work with midwives.

General Medical Supply is not a mail order company, but they will sell retail in small quantities. They have locations in 50 places across the country and are the largest hospital suppliers in the country. Check your Yellow Pages or the business to business Yellow Pages to find out if they have an office near you.

Henry Shein, Inc., 5 Harbor Park Dr., Port Washington, NY 10050, (800) 772-4346. Hyp-Rho-D brand Rh- immune globulin can be ordered with proper DEA ID. They also carry instruments and many other non drug items that do not require a DEA #. Shein makes its own name brand Uristix (protein & glucose and one with 9 tests in all) that are half the price of Ames (etc.) They come in bottles of 50.

Herbs and homeopathic remedies: See the chapter on Health Care Modalities in the Practice Makes Perfect section.

Loving Lift belly supporters, Moore Products, P.O. Box 647, Belmont, CA 94002-9854, (415) 592-8174/(800) 457-1567. Also **Baby Hugger**, by Trennaventions, RR 1, Box 253 D, Derry, PA, 15627, (412) 694-5283 and **Jeunique Natal Support** International, Inc., 19501 E. Walnut Dr., City of Industry, CA, 91748, (909) 598-8598.

NF formulas Inc., 9755 SW Commerce Circle, C-5, Wilsonville, OR 97070-9602 (503) 682-9755. High quality nutritional supplements, happy to work with midwives.

Rainbow Light Nutritional supplements, 207 McPherson St., Santa Cruz, CA 95060 (800) 635-1233.

Scientific Botanicals, P.O. Box 31131, Seattle, WA 98103 (206) 527-5521. Carry oil-based oral vitamin K (Quinone). They will not sell to unlicensed practitioners, so enlist a doctor or CNM if necessary.

Standard Process Labs., Inc., P.O. Box 652, Milwaukee, WI 53201. (800) 558-8740. Source for many fine nutritional supplements and Collinsonia root tablets. Glandular extracts, some herbs, etc., all very high quality and organic. Sold only through practitioners who they authorize to distribute (chiropractors and naturopaths). Will consider independent midwives on an individual basis. Ask about a service representative in your area.

Thorne Research, Seattle, WA, 98188; (800) 228-1966. Carries a variety of high quality supplements.

1156

Journals of interest to midwives:

BIRTH, Blackwell Science, Inc., 238 Main St., Cambridge, MA, 02142, (6170 876-7000 individual subscription one year $40.00

Capsules and Comments in Perinatal and Women's Nursing, Journal Circulation, Mosby, 11830 Westline Industrial Dr.,, P.O. Box 46908, St. Louis, MO 63146-9934. (800) 453-4351. More or less the US equivilant to MIDIRS, quarterly, individual subscription $39.95.

Midwifery Today, P.O. Box 2672, Eugene, OR 97402, (503) 344-7438. Individual subscription (US) $35.00 for one year (four issues), $65.00 for two years.

MIDIRS, 9 Elmdale Rd., Clifton, Bristol BS8 ISL, England, (0272) 251791. Subsription rate fsor UK student £27.00/individual £32.00/Europe individual £38.00/rest of world individual £42.00. This journal provides a variety of abstracts of articles of interest to midwives. Tends to include much of political interest to the UK, but provides a unique international perspective on many topics.

Midwifery, Sales Promotion Dept., Churchill-Livingston Journals, Robert Stevenson House, 1-3 Baxter's Place, Edinburgh, EH1 3AF, UK, individual (US) $93.00 one year, quarterly, members of ICM, $75.00 1 year.

Mothering, PO Box 532, Mt. Morris, IL, 61054, (800) 827-1061, individual subscription 1 year $18.95, four issues.

Journal of Nurse-Midwifery, Journal Fullfillment Dept., Elsevier Science Pub. Co., 655 Avenue of the Americas, New York, NY 10010. Individual subscription $55.00 yearly for 6 issues.

The Birth Gazette, 42 The Farm, Summertwon, TN, 38483 (615) 964-2519. One year, individual subsecription $30.00 (4 issues).

The Compleat Mother, P.O. Box 209, Minot, ND 58702, (701) 852-2822. One year $12.00 (4 issues)

Illustration References

Unless otherwise noted, the drawings in this book are original renditions by Rhonda Wheeler using the following texts as references.

Baldwin, Rahima, Special Delivery, Celestial Arts, Berkeley, CA, 1986.

Bates, Barbara, A Guide to Physical Examination, 5th ed., J.B. Lippincott, Philadelphia, 1991.

Bland, B, & Montgomery, T, Practical Obstetrics, F. A. Davis, Philadelphia, 1935.

Carola, R., Harley, J., & Noback, C., Human Anatomy and Physiology, McGraw-Hill, NY, 1990.

Davis, Elizabeth, Heart and Hands: A Midwife's Guide to Pregnancy and Birth, 2n ed., Celestial Arts, Berkeley, CA, 1987.

Ehrlich, A., Medical Terminology for Health Professionals, 2nd ed., Delmar Pub., 1993.

Fed. of Feminist Women's Health Centers, How to Stay Out of the Gynecologist's Office, Women to Women Pub., Los Angeles, CA 1981.

Gabbe, Steven, et. al. ed. Obstetrics: Normal and Problem Pregnancies, 2nd ed., Churchill Livingstone, New York, 1991.

Garrey, M., et.al., Obstetrics Illustrated, Churchill Livingstone, London, Eng., 1980.

op. cit., Gynecology Illustrated, Churchill Livingstone, London, Eng., 1978.

Gaskin, Ina May, Spiritual Midwifery, The Book Pub. Co., Summertown, TN, 1978.

Greenhill, J., Principles and Practice of Obstetrics, W. B. Saunders, Co., Philadelphia, PA, 1951.

Hegner B. & Caldwell, E., Nursing Assistant, 6th ed., Delmar Pub., Albany, NY 1992.

Hellman, L, et.al., William's Obstetrics, 14th ed., Appleton-Century-Crofts, New York, 1971.

Kapit, W. & Elson, L., Anatomy Coloring Book, 2nd ed., Harper Collins College Pub., NY 1993.

Kitzinger, S., The Complete Book of Pregnancy and Birth, Alfred Knopf, NY, 1989.

Lichtman, R., & Papera, S., Gynecology: Well-woman Care, Appleton & Lance, Norwalk CT, 1990.

Maye's Textbook of Obstetrics, 1953.

McLennan, C., Synopsis of Obstetrics, 8th ed., C.V. Mosby Co., St. Louis, MO 1970.

Moloy, H., Evaluation of the Pelvis in Obstetrics, 3rd ed., Plenum Medical Book Co., NY, 1975.

Moore, Keith, & T. Persaud, The Developing Human: Clinically Oriented Embryology, 5th ed., W. B. Saunders Co., Philadelphia, PA, 1993.

Myles, Margaret, Textbook for Midwives, Churchill Livingstone, New York, NY, 1981.

Olds, Sally, et.al., Obstetric Nursing, Addison-Wesley, Pub., Menlo Park, CA, 1980.

Oxhorn, Harry, Human Labor and Birth, 5th ed., Appleton-Century-Crofts, Norwalk, CT, 1986.

Samuels, Mike & Nancy, The Well Pregnancy Book, Summit Books, NY, 1986.

Solomon, E., & Philips, G., Understanding Human Anatomy and physiology, W.B. Saunders, Co., Phil., 1987.

Stoppard, Marian, Pregnancy and Birth Book, Ballantine Books, NY, 1985.

Thomas, C. ed., Tabor's Cyclopedic Medical Dictionary, F.A. Davis, Philadelphia, PA, 1985.

Tortora, Gerard & Anagnostakos, N., Principles of Anatomy and Physiology, 5th ed., Harper & Row Publishers, New York, NY 1987.

Varney, Helen, CNM, Nurse-Midwifery, 1st. ed., Blackwell Scientific Pub., Boston, MA 1980.

Whitley, Nancy, A Manual of Clinical Obstetrics, J.B. Lippincott Co., Philadelphia, PA 1985.

INDEX

Blood mole 720
Blood pressure
  assessment of, 420
  equipment, about, 344
  high, 1011
  interpretation of, 1010
  interpreting readings, 1010
  labile, about, 1012
  low, 1010
  low, dizziness and, 972
  midpregnancy findings, 830
Blood type and factor, explained 580
Blood vessels
  about, 142
  distended in healthy pregnancy, 829
Blood volume, contracted
  after fetal demise, 871
  and abnormal clotting, 138
Blood volume, expanded
  affect on blood pressure, 828
  and heart problems, 1016
  and postdatism/postmaturity, 877
  and varicose veins, 1057
  in normal pregnancy, 194
Bloody show
  as a sign of active labor, 822
Blue Cohosh 787
Blue-green algae as a protein source 220
Body frame size, assessment of 417
Bonine, for nausea 758
Borage oil
  to soften the cervix, 787, 788
Boron, (table) 208
Brachial plexus pain 1028
Bradley childbirth education 644
Bradycardia
  about, 987
  defined, 374
Brain
  about, 124
  tumors of, 1088
Braxton-Hicks contractions
  about the term, 11
  and postdatism, 878
Breastfeeding
  as a requirement for care, 552
  during pregnancy, 590
  in Western culture, 587
  prenatal concerns regarding, 587
  prenatal preparation for, 589
  previous surgery and, 587
  with burn scars, 589
Breasts

about, 177
augmented, to examine, 444
changes during pregnancy, 444, 668,
  670
disorders of, 182
fibrocystic changes of, 182
history of cancer, 1137
reduction or augmentation and
  breastfeeding, 587
support of, 590
to examine, 438
Breech birth
  clinical considerations for, 817
  discussing risks of, 812
Breech presentation
  chiropractic technique to turn, 809
  distinguishing from vertex via internal
    exam, 486
  tilt exercise to correct, 805
Brewer, Dr. Thomas
  and Gail, books by, 833
  toxemia hotline number, 833
Bromide (table) 292
Brompheniramine 283
Bronchiectasis 1141
Bronchitis 968
Bruising easily 1060
Budd-Chiari syndrome 1086
Bulb of the vestibule, about 164
Bulbocavernosus muscle
  anatomy of, 168
  attachment to sphincter, 170
  examination of, 479
Bulimia
  history of, 568
  weight gain and, 246
Cadmium poisoning 1036
Caffeine
  about, 272
  in food and drugs, (table) 272
Calcitonin, about 134
Calcium
  as clotting factor, 138
  dietary importance of (table), 208
  for hypertension, 1014
  leg cramps and, 955
  pregnancy needs for, 224
Calories
  adequate, spare protein for use, 218
  diet low in, 639
  metabolic demands for, 220
  protein and, 218
Cambodian cultural practices 598